hypertension, 12, 18, 47, 54, 74, 79, 128, 152, 153, 175, 190, 196, 204, 248, 251, 271, 272, 309–318
hypervigilant, 227
hypotension, 21, 43, 45, 47, 57, 74, 81, 116, 149, 153, 190, 359, 366
hypoxia, 20, 226, 272, 366
inattention, 13, 20, 80, 225, 227, 228, 249
incontinence, 2, 11, 17, 19, 20, 29, 33, 43, 68, 176–183
intoxication, 86, 87, 227, 264, 273, 402
ischemia, 74, 75, 79, 126, 127, 151, 247, 322, 325–327
jaundice, 10, 12, 410, 459, 567
joint, 5, 6, 49, 54, 149, 163–165, 277, 278, 283, 284, 286–289, 291
keratitis sicca, 131
kidney, 4, 7, 8, 42, 43, 77–79, 125
kyphosis, 13, 165, 306, 344, 571
labyrinthitis, 142, 148–152, 364
lacrimal, 131
lentigo senilis, 492
lethargy, 183, 190, 201, 228, 250, 424, 427, 429
lung, 7, 111, 171, 360, 396, 397, 399, 403
lymph nodes, 163, 410, 470, 471, 477, 483, 485, 508, 549, 550, 552, 553
memory, 13, 33, 49, 80, 83, 104, 208, 237, 244, 245
mental status, 1, 2, 13, 15, 17, 21, 24, 104, 108, 114, 156, 183, 214, 217, 225, 227–229, 241, 245, 256, 268, 272, 335, 337, 340, 364, 405, 424, 523, 527
mood, 19, 51, 56, 57, 61, 63, 89, 90, 97, 105, 209, 210, 212, 239, 246, 252, 268, 269
movement, 13, 15–16, 26, 100, 143–145, 152, 166, 167, 169, 258, 262, 286, 379, 394
murmur, cardiac, 345, 346
nail, finger, 16, 437, 502
nail, toes, 13, 327, 502
neuropathy, 25, 50, 51, 57, 130–131, 150–152, 168, 180, 250, 263, 326, 327, 329, 447, 449–451, 455, 456, 468, 470, 549, 574
nipple discharge, 442
nodules, 287, 288, 445, 459, 460, 504, 559
nose, 16, 132, 262, 466, 467, 475, 496, 509, 577
nystagmus, 148, 385, 388, 389
odor, 14, 116, 175, 183, 436, 437, 525
oliguria, 79, 420, 421, 428, 557
oropharynx, 405, 411, 476, 477, 485, 568
osteoporosis, 42, 47, 97, 113, 165, 170, 171, 193, 201, 272, 293–299
ovary, 438–440, 459, 536, 539
palate, 384, 411, 475, 476, 485, 486
papule, 436, 437, 483, 495, 498, 499, 502–504, 507, 509
paralysis, 264, 268, 364, 367, 372, 396, 397, 429, 513, 515
penis, 187, 201–203, 499, 505
perineum, 186, 433, 435, 573
periodontal, 7, 112, 301, 474, 479–481, 483, 485, 487, 488
pharynx, 476, 531, 568
posture, 4, 13, 16, 262, 385
prostate, 4, 76, 111, 118, 119, 165, 171, 176
pruritis, 434–438
pulse, 13, 26, 88, 90, 202, 310, 311, 322, 324–327, 336, 339, 344, 345, 348, 366, 382, 406, 424, 450, 458, 508
pupil, 6, 15, 122, 123
pustule, 499, 500, 509
rectocele, 181, 434, 438
rectum, 429, 438, 439, 543, 572–574
red eye, 131
retinopathy, 121, 122, 125–126, 130, 447, 449–450
rhinitis, 202, 270, 298
rib, 338, 411
scalp, 5, 131, 141, 466, 484, 491, 492, 496, 503, 504, 507
scoliosis, 14, 170, 306
sepsis, 46, 184–188, 227, 241, 244, 331, 420, 524, 525, 554, 556–557, 560
sinus, 42, 75, 79, 149, 218, 287, 335, 336, 338, 341, 344, 345
smell, 6, 110, 112, 114
somnolence, 45, 57, 118, 119, 228, 258, 262, 392, 411, 415
spasm, 57, 164, 166, 171, 179, 180, 203, 279, 281, 314, 379, 384, 570, 573
speech, 6, 14, 136, 141, 228
spine, 4, 149, 151, 162, 163, 166–170, 279, 281, 282, 288, 295–299, 304, 306, 399, 471, 551
swallowing, 7, 24, 34, 114, 118, 368, 370, 372, 479, 481–483, 488, 568, 576
tachycardia, 51, 57, 78–80, 87, 112, 118, 119, 187, 218, 270, 310, 313, 314, 335, 337
tachypnea, 187, 557
testes, 188
thrombophlebitis, 508
thyroid, 61, 78, 114, 151, 152, 156, 171, 200, 210, 213, 262, 268, 272, 298, 303, 348, 360, 385, 386, 448, 456–461
toe, 6, 14, 162, 164, 167, 168, 291, 321, 325–327, 450, 508
tongue, 6, 262, 380, 381, 411, 457, 458, 467, 476, 477, 483, 485–487
tremor, 13, 57, 85, 87, 88, 248, 250, 378–393
tympanometry, 139, 140
ulcer, 25, 54, 109, 111, 113, 118, 122, 131, 226, 317, 324, 325, 329–330, 332, 372, 450
urethra, 176, 181, 419, 438
urinary incontinence, 2, 10, 11, 17, 175–183
uterine prolapse, 434, 438
vagina, 181, 203, 433 438
varicose veins, 324
vertigo, 134, 142, 144, 145, 148–152, 499
vision, 6, 118, 119, 121–124
vulva, 433–438
wakefulness, 226, 255, 258, 264
weight gain, 13, 115, 118, 119, 441, 454, 457
weight loss, 14, 17, 23, 108–120, 182
wheezes, 400, 403
wrist, 16, 256, 258, 278, 386, 393, 457, 464
xerostomia, 111, 466, 467, 474, 478, 481–482

Office Care Geriatrics

D. S. BANGERA MD.

Office Care Geriatrics

EDITORS

THOMAS C. ROSENTHAL, MD

Professor and Chair
Department of Family Medicine
School of Medicine and Biomedical Sciences
University at Buffalo
Buffalo, New York

MARK E. WILLIAMS, MD

Ward K. Ensminger Distinguished Professor of Geriatric Medicine
Chief, Division of General Medicine and Geriatrics
University of Virginia School of Medicine
Charlottesville, Virginia

BRUCE J. NAUGHTON, MD

Associate Professor
Chief, Division of Geriatrics
School of Medicine and Biomedical Sciences
University at Buffalo
Buffalo, New York

Lippincott Williams & Wilkins
a Wolters Kluwer business
Philadelphia • Baltimore • New York • London
Buenos Aires • Hong Kong • Sydney • Tokyo

Acquisitions Editor: Sonya Seigafuse
Managing Editor: Nancy Winter
Developmental Editor: Lauren Aquino
Project Manager: Jennifer Harper
Senior Manufacturing Manager: Benjamin Rivera
Marketing Manager: Sharon Zinner/Adam Glazer
Design Coordinator: Teresa Mallon
Production Services: Laserwords Private Limited
Printer: Edwards Brothers

530 Walnut Street
Philadelphia, PA 19106 USA
LWW.com

Printed in the USA

Library of Congress Cataloging-in-Publication Data

Office care geriatrics / edited by Thomas Rosenthal, Mark Williams,
Bruce Naughton.
p, ; cm.
Includes bibliographical references and index.
ISBN 0-7817-6196-4
1. Geriatrics. 2. Primary care (Medicine) I. Rosenthal, Thomas.
II. Williams, Mark E. III. Naughton, Bruce.
[DNLM: 1. Geriatrics—methods. 2. Aging—physiology. 3. Health
Services for the Aged. WT 100 O32 2006]
RC952.7.O324 2006
618.97—dc22

2006011624

Care has been taken to confirm the accuracy of the information presented and to describe generally accepted practices. However, the authors, editors, and publisher are not responsible for errors or omissions or for any consequences from application of the information in this book and make no warranty, expressed or implied, with respect to the currency, completeness, or accuracy of the contents of the publication. Application of this information in a particular situation remains the professional responsibility of the practitioner.

The authors, editors, and publisher have exerted every effort to ensure that drug selection and dosage set forth in this text are in accordance with current recommendations and practice at the time of publication. However, in view of ongoing research, changes in government regulations, and the constant flow of information relating to drug therapy and drug reactions, the reader is urged to check the package insert for each drug for any change in indications and dosage and for added warnings and precautions. This is particularly important when the recommended agent is a new or infrequently employed drug.

Some drugs and medical devices presented in this publication have Food and Drug Administration (FDA) clearance for limited use in restricted research settings. It is the responsibility of the health care provider to ascertain the FDA status of each drug or device planned for use in their clinical practice.

To purchase additional copies of this book, call our customer service department at (800) 638-3030 or fax orders to (301) 223-2320. International customers should call (301) 223-2300.

Visit Lippincott Williams & Wilkins on the Internet: at LWW.com. Lippincott Williams & Wilkins customer service representatives are available from 8:30 am to 6 pm, EST.

10 9 8 7 6 5 4 3 2 1

This text is dedicated to all those physicians and providers who entered school intent on assisting as many patients as possible to live the healthiest life possible. May all our patients live long enough to know of our respect for elders.

Contents

Contributors List ix
Preface xiii
Acknowledgments xv
Color Insert

1 The Approach to the Elderly Patient 1
Mark E. Williams

Section I Caring for the Older Patient: Management Principles

2 Principles of Care for Older Persons 18
Mudanai Sabapathy and Bruce J. Naughton

3 Office-Based Caregiver Support 28
Jane Marie Thibault and James G. O'Brien

4 Rational Drug Therapy in the Elderly 40
Robert L. Dickman

5 Pain Control 48
Michael P. Temporal

6 Loss and Bereavement in the Elderly 59
Donald P. Bartlett, Marlon Russell Koenigsberg, and Jeffrey M. Moll

7 Management of the Surgical Patient 73
Peter Pompei

8 Substance Abuse 82
Robert Mallin

9 Elder Abuse: "It Shouldn't Hurt To Be Old" 95
Patricia A. Bomba

Section II Functional Consequences of Common Syndromes

10 Weight Loss in the Elderly Patient 108
Russell G. Robertson

11 Visual Impairment in the Elderly 121
Shariar Farzad, David Sarraf, and Anne L. Coleman

12 Hearing Difficulty 134
Roseanne C. Berger and Robert F. Burkard

13 Dizziness, Syncope, and Falls in the Elderly 147
Richard Brunader and Janet Leah Retke

14 Low Back Pain in the Elderly 162
Kim Edward LeBlanc

15 Urinary Disorders 175
Richard J. Ackermann

16 Sexual Function and the Older Adult 196
Fran E. Kaiser

17 Evaluation and Treatment of Depression 207
Robin R. Whitebird, Richard L. Heinrich, Patrick J. O'Connor, and Leif I. Solberg

18 Delirium 225
Sidney T. Bogardus, Jr.

19 Chronic Memory Impairment 236
Thomas C. Rosenthal

20 Sleep Disorders 254
Tarannum Alam and Cathy A. Alessi

21 Schizophrenia and Anxiety in Late Age 266
Kim S. Griswold

Section III Chronic Disease in the Older Patient

22 Musculoskeletal Problems in the Elderly 276
Kim Edward LeBlanc

23 Metabolic Bone Disease 293
Ailleen Heras-Herzig and Theresa A. Guise

24 Hypertension and Lipid Disorders 309
Vinod R. Patel and Thomas C. Rosenthal

25 Peripheral Arterial Disease 320
Gregory S. Cherr

26 Cardiac Disease 335
Tarek Helmy, Amar D. Patel, and Nanette K. Wenger

27 Heart Failure 354
Richard W. Pretorius

28 Cerebrovascular Disease and Stroke 363
William D. Smucker

29 Tremor 378
Lesley D. Wilkinson, Carol Stewart, and Nancy Tyre

30 **Pulmonary Disease in the Elderly 395**
Eleanor M. Summerhill

31 **Renal Function and Failure 414**
Robert D. Lindeman

32 **Gynecology and Breast Disease 432**
Barbara A. Majeroni

33 **Diabetes and Thyroid Disorders in the Elderly 445**
Sara E. Young, Richelle J. Koopman, and Arch G. Mainous III

34 **Immune and Inflammatory Disease in Older Adults 462**
David R. Thomas

35 **Oral Conditions 474**
Jude A. Fabiano

36 **Common Dermatologic Conditions in Aging 491**
Charles A. Cefalu and Lee Nesbitt

37 **Prevention and Treatment of Pressure Ulcers: An Evidence-Based Approach 511**
Robert E. Pieroni

38 **Neoplastic Disease 530**
Kenneth G. Schellhase

39 **Hematology 546**
Gerald L. Logue

40 **Common Infections in the Elderly 554**
William A. Woolery

41 **Common Gastrointestinal Disorders in the Elderly 563**
Kristen M. Robson and Anthony Lembo

Index 581

Contributors List

RICHARD J. ACKERMANN, MD Director of the Geriatrics Fellowship Program, Department of Family Medicine, Medical Center of Central Georgia; Professor, Department of Family Medicine, Mercer University School of Medicine; Family Health Center, Macon, Georgia

TARANNUM ALAM, MD Advanced Geriatric Fellow, Geriatric Research Education and Clinical Center, Veterans Administration Greater Los Angeles Healthcare System, Sepulveda, California; Multicampus Program in Geriatric Medicine and Gerontology, University of California, Los Angeles, California

CATHY A. ALESSI, MD Professor, Multicampus Program in Geriatric Medicine and Gerontology, University of California, Los Angeles, California; Associate Director, Clinical Programs, Geriatric Research Education and Clinical Center, Veterans Administration Greater Los Angeles Healthcare System, Sepulveda, California

DONALD P. BARTLETT, PhD Clinical Assistant Professor, Psychologist, Department of Family Medicine, State University of New York at Buffalo, Buffalo, New York

ROSEANNE C. BERGER, MD Associate Professor, Department of Clinical Family Medicine, University at Buffalo, Buffalo, New York; Attending Staff, Department of Family Medicine, Kaleida Health Care Center, Williamsville, New York

SIDNEY T. BOGARDUS JR., MD Associate Professor, Department of Internal Medicine, Yale University School of Medicine, New Haven, Connecticut

PATRICIA A. BOMBA, MD, FACP Clinical Assistant Professor, Department of Medicine, University of Rochester, Rochester, New York; Clinical Assistant Professor, Department of Medicine, State University of New York Upstate Medical University, Syracuse, New York; Vice President and Medical Director, Department of Geriatrics, Med America Insurance Company, Excellus BlueCross BlueShield, Rochester, New York

RICHARD BRUNADER, MD Associate Professor of Family Medicine, Department of Family and Community Medicine, University of California; Staff Physician, Department of Family Medicine, University of California Medical Center, Sacramento, California

ROBERT F. BURKARD, PhD Professor, Departments of Communicative Disorders and Sciences, and Otolaryngology, University at Buffalo, Buffalo, New York

CHARLES A. CEFALU, MD, MS Professor and Chief, Section of Geriatric Medicine, Department of Family Medicine, Louisiana State University Health Sciences Center; Medical Director, Geriatric Medicine, Department of Family Medicine, Medical Center of Louisiana, New Orleans, Louisiana

GREGORY S. CHERR, MD, RVT Assistant Professor, Department of Surgery, State University of New York at Buffalo; Attending Vascular Surgeon, Registered Vascular Technologist, Department of Surgery, Buffalo General Hospital, Buffalo, New York

ANNE L. COLEMAN, MD, PhD Professor of Ophthalmology and Epidemiology, Francis and Ray Stark Chair of Ophthalmology, Jules Stein Eye Institute, University of California, Los Angeles, California

ROBERT L. DICKMAN, MD Jaharis Family Chair of Family Medicine, Tufts University School of Medicine, Boston, Massachusetts

JUDE A. FABIANO, DDS Associate Professor, Department of Restorative Dentistry, School of Dental Medicine, University at Buffalo; Attending Staff, Department of Dentistry, Kaleida Health Care System, Buffalo, New York

SHARIAR FARZAD, MD Resident, Department of Ophthalmology, Jules Stein Eye Institute, University of California, Los Angeles, California

KIM S. GRISWOLD, MD Associate Professor, Departments of Family Medicine, Psychiatry and Social and Preventive Medicine, State University of New York at Buffalo; Attending in Family Medicine, Department of Family Medicine, Buffalo General Hospital, Buffalo, New York

THERESA A. GUISE, MD Professor of Internal Medicine, University of Virginia; Gerald D. Aurbach Professor in Endocrinology, Department of Internal Medicine, Charlottesville, Virginia

RICHARD L. HEINRICH, MD Associate Clinical Professor, Department of Psychiatry, University of Minnesota; Hospice Medical Director, Hospice of the Lakes, Geriatric Division, HealthPartners Medical Foundation, Minneapolis, Minnesota

TAREK HELMY, MD, FACC Assistant Professor, Department of Medicine, Division of Cardiology, Emory University School of Medicine; Director of the Cardiac Catheterization Laboratory at Grady Memorial Hospital, Atlanta, Georgia

AILLEEN HERAS-HERZIG, MD Assistant Professor of Research, Department of Internal Medicine, Osteoporosis and Metabolic Bone Disease Clinic, University of Virginia, Charlottesville, Virginia

FRAN E. KAISER, MD, AGSF, FGSA Chief Executive Officer, Kaiser and Associates; Adjunct Professor of Medicine, Saint Louis University, St. Louis, Missouri; Clinical Professor, Department of Medicine, University of Texas at Southwestern, Medical Center; Dallas, Texas

MARLON RUSSELL KOENIGSBERG, PhD Clinical Assistant Professor, Department of Family Medicine, State University of New York at Buffalo, Psychologist, Department of Family Medicine, Kaleida Health Care Center, Buffalo, New York

RICHELLE J. KOOPMAN, MD, MS Assistant Professor, Department of Family Medicine, Medical University of South Carolina, Charleston, South Carolina

KIM EDWARD LEBLANC, MD, PhD Marie Lahasky Professor and Chairman, Department of Family Medicine, Louisiana State University School of Medicine, New Orleans, Louisiana

ANTHONY LEMBO, MD Assistant Professor, Department of Medicine, Harvard Medical School; Director, Gastrointestinal Motility, Department of Medicine, Beth Israel Deaconesss Medical Center, Boston, Massachusetts

ROBERT D. LINDEMAN, MD Professor Emeritus, Department of Medicine, University of New Mexico School of Medicine, Albuquerque, New Mexico

GERALD L. LOGUE, MD Professor and Head, Division of Hematology, Department of Medicine, University at Buffalo, Erie County Medical Center, Buffalo, New York

ARCH G. MAINOUS III, PhD Professor and Director of Research, Department of Family Medicine, Medical University of South Carolina, Charleston, South Carolina

BARBARA A. MAJERONI, MD Associate Clinical Professor, Department of Family Medicine, State University of New York at Buffalo; Attending Physician, Department of Family Medicine, Erie County Medical Center, Buffalo, New York

ROBERT MALLIN, MD Associate Professor, Department of Family Medicine Psychiatry, Medical University of South Carolina; Medical Staff, Department of Family Medicine, Medical University of South Carolina Hospital, Charleston, South Carolina

JEFFREY M. MOLL, MD Clinical Assistant Instructor, Department of Psychiatry, State University of New York at Buffalo; Resident, Department of Psychiatry, Erie County Medical Center, Buffalo, New York

BRUCE J. NAUGHTON, MD Associate Professor and Head, Division of Geriatric Medicine, Department of Medicine, University at Buffalo School of Medicine, Buffalo, New York

LEE NESBITT, MD Chairman, Department of Dermatology, Louisiana State University School of Medicine, New Orleans, Louisiana

JAMES G. O'BRIEN, MD Smock Endowed Chair in Geriatrics, Department of Family and Geriatric Medicine, University of Louisville; Active Staff, Department of Family and Geriatrics, University of Louisville Hospital, Louisville, Kentucky

PATRICK J. O'CONNOR, MD, MPH Clinical Associate Professor, Department of Community and Family Medicine, University of Minnesota Medical School; Senior Clinical Investigator, HealthPartners Research Foundation, Minneapolis, Minnesota

AMAR D. PATEL, MD Fellow, Cardiovascular Diseases, Department of Medicine, Emory University School of Medicine, Atlanta, Georgia

VINOD R. PATEL, MD Clinical Assistant Professor, Department of Family Medicine, University at Buffalo, Buffalo, New York

ROBERT E. PIERONI, MD Professor Emeritus, Department of Internal Medicine and Family Medicine, University of Alabama School of Medicine, Program Tuscaloosa, Alabama; Attending Physician, Department of Internal Medicine, Druid City Hopital Regional Medical Center, University of Boulevard, Tuscaloosa, Alabama

PETER POMPEI, MD Associate Professor, Department of Internal Medicine, Stanford University School of Medicine; Associate Program Director, Department of Internal Medicine Residency at Stanford Hospital and Clinics, Stanford, California

RICHARD W. PRETORIUS MD, MPH Associate Professor, Department of Clinical Family Medicine, University at Buffalo, Buffalo, New York

JANET LEAH RETKE, PT, MAOM Supervising Physical Therapist, Department of Physical Medicine and Rehabilitation, University of California, Davis Medical Center, Sacramento, California

RUSSELL G. ROBERTSON, MD Associate Professor, Department of Family and Community Medicine, Medical College of Wisconsin, Milwaukee, Wisconsin

KRISTEN M. ROBSON, MD Clinical Assistant Professor, Department of Medicine, Tufts University School of Medicine, Boston, Massachusetts; Staff Physician, Department of Gastroenterology, Lahey Clinic, Burlington, Massachusetts

THOMAS C. ROSENTHAL, MD Professor and Chairman, Department of Family Medicine, School of Medicine and Biomedical Sciences, University at Buffalo, Buffalo, New York

MUDANAI SABAPATHY, MD Fellow in Geriatrics, State University of New York at Buffalo, Department of Geriatrics, Millard Filmore Gates Circle Hospital, Buffalo, NewYork

DAVID SARRAF, MD Assistant Clinical Professor, Department of Ophthalmology, Jules Stein Eye Institute, University of California School of Medicine; Greater Los Angeles VA Healthcare Center, King/Drew Medical Center, Los Angeles, California

KENNETH G. SCHELLHASE, MD, MPH Assistant Professor, Department of Family and Community Medicine and Health Policy Institute, Health Services Research, Medical College of Wisconsin, Milwaukee, Wisconsin; Active Staff, Department of Family and Emergency Medicine, Waukesha Memorial Hospital, Waukesha, Wisconsin

WILLIAM D. SMUCKER, MD, CMD Professor, Department of Family Medicine, Northeastern Ohio Universities College of Medicine, Rootstown, Ohio; Associate Director, Family Medicine Center of Akron, Department of Family Medicine, Summa Health System, Akron, Ohio

LEIF I. SOLBERG, MD Clinical Professor, Department of Family Medicine and Community Health, University of Minnesota Medical School; Director for Care Improvement Research, HealthPartners Research Foundation, Minneapolis, Minnesota

CAROL STEWART, MD, FAAFP Assistant Professor, Department of Family Medicine, David Geffen School of Medicine at University of California, Los Angeles; Residency Core Faculty, Les Kelley Family Health Center, Santa Monica, California

ELEANOR M. SUMMERHILL, MD, FACP, FCCP Assistant Professor, Division of Pulmonary and Critical Care, Department of Medicine, Brown Medical School, Providence Rhode Island; Director, Internal Medicine Residency Program, Memorial Hospital of Rhode Island, Pawtucket, Rhode Island

MICHAEL P. TEMPORAL Associate Professor, Department of Community and Family Medicine, Saint Louis University, St. Louis, Missouri; Associate Residency Director, Saint Louis University, Southern Illinois Health Care Foundation, Department of Family Medicine, St. Elizabeth's Hospital, Belleville, Illinois

JANE MARIE THIBAULT, MA, MSSW, PhD Associate Clinical Professor, Department of Family and Geriatric Medicine, School of Medicine, University of Louisville, Louisville, Kentucky

DAVID R. THOMAS, MD, FACP, AGSF, GSAF Professor, Department of Medicine, Division of Geriatric Medicine, Saint Louis University Health Sciences Center, St. Louis, Missouri

NANCY TYRE, MD Associate Physician Diplomat, Residency Faculty, Department of Family Medicine, University of California, Les Kelley Family Health Center, Santa Monica, California

NANETTE K. WENGER, MD Professor, Department of Medicine (Cardiology), Emory University School of Medicine; Chief of Cardiology, Department of Medicine (Cardiology), Grady Memorial Hospital, Atlanta, Georgia

ROBIN R. WHITEBIRD, PhD Community Faculty, School of Social Work, University of Minnesota; Research Associate, HealthPartners Research Foundation, Minneapolis, Minnesota

LESLEY D. WILKINSON, MD Associate Professor, University of California, Los Angeles, California

MARK E. WILLIAMS, MD Ward K. Ensminger Distinguished Professor of Geriatric Medicine, Department of Internal Medicine, University of Virginia School of Medicine, Charlottesville, Virginia

WILLIAM A. WOOLERY, DO, PhD, CMD, FACOFP Clinical Assistant Professor, Department of Family and Community Medicine, School of Medicine, Mercer University, Macon, Georgia

SARA E. YOUNG, MD Instructor, Department of Family Medicine, Medical University of South Carolina, Charleston, South Carolina

Preface

Developing a comprehensive care plan for a geriatric patient requires exceptional "perceptive knowledge," which is challenging to explain but is a skill set demonstrated by primary care clinicians every day. Consider the "hidden object" page of *Highlights for Children*, a magazine our children received, which had a picture page filled with hidden objects such as a ball, spoon, scissors, and so on. We know what the object of interest should look like, and we engage a process by which we move lines in and out of focus until the image of interest emerges. This combination of knowledge and perception skills is "perceptive knowledge." By analogy, the typical medical textbook reminds us that a clinical situation will have certain items or clinical clues. However, having a check list of clues is different from actually perceiving their presence or absence. The perceptive challenge for the clinician is: "What crucial hidden clues are present and will I find them given a limited amount of time?"

Several times each day, the primary care clinician seeks the key elements (the clues) in a patient's history or physical examination. These clues, often "hidden" to the patient, lead to the diagnosis and treatment. We have asked the authors contributing to this text to recognize the challenge in this work and to point out the "hidden pictures" obscured within the complex presentation of illness in older adults. We have then asked them to go one step further, to not simply point out the pictures but to enhance the clinician's skill at finding the hidden picture as he or she moves from patient to patient. We want the clinician to understand the "how" and the "why."

If we have been successful, the proficient primary care clinician will observe a patient to have a shuffling gait in the office hallway, incorporate the patient's complaint of declining libido in the examination room, and consider the diagnosis of Parkinson disease. This is in spite of four other good clinicians looking at the same specific complaints in isolation and missing the common thread. Arriving at the answers for each patient requires the experience, intellect, perceptive knowledge, and selective use of information sources by a seasoned clinician. This text strives to sharpen perceptive capacity while connecting it to accumulated knowledge. The chapters will affirm perceptions that fit (or do not fit) a diagnosis and lead the clinician to evidence-based treatment decisions.

In the elderly, not all interventions improve wellness, relieve suffering, or reduce mortality. Modern medicine provides several interventions for most clinical predicaments, but not all interventions are justifiable or can be delivered with a risk acceptable to the patient's circumstance, philosophy, life expectancy, or capacity to sustain the potential tribulations implicit in an intervention. The basis of geriatric medicine is to ensure that elderly people get the best care available, not necessarily the most care available. Today's clinician must balance an increasingly complex set of options, values, and realities.

The editors, all of them geriatric primary care clinicians, realize that most of us have only 90 seconds to use a clinical reference while in the midst of seeing patients. Therefore, each chapter offers a differential diagnosis list. We have included a special index for signs, symptoms, and anatomy to provide quick answers to the problems that patients present with. (Patients cough, they do not declare "pneumonia.") We believe that busy clinicians will also appreciate the depth of each chapter and leave the text open on their desk for more casual reading at the end of work hours. When used this way, the clinicians will acquire a broader understanding of the key issues relevant to the care of the elderly patient and feel more confident about the quality of their evidence-based management. In all cases, the clinicians can be assured of being led into the vast arena of geriatric care by experienced and knowledgeable geriatric clinicians.

We have included chapters that focus on issues of sleep, appetite, sexuality, body changes, stamina, physiology, and personality changes expected in healthy aging. The chapters on healthy aging provide a framework for understanding the challenges of aging and disease. Treatment recommendations include the standard medical tools augmented by modifications in activities, diet, and exercise that are important in reducing morbidity. Patient education recommendations and resources are also included where appropriate.

The authors of the chapters have focused on describing a clinically relevant "how-to" approach to diagnosis and treatment. This approach incorporates meta-analyses, published literature, and existing evidence-based reviews, such as the Cochrane Collaboration, to predict outcomes relevant to the patient's quality of life. The level of evidence for recommendations is rated according to the following scale: Level A (single high-quality or multiple randomized controlled trials or meta-analysis), level B (small randomized controlled trials, observation data, and cohort studies that have been consistent), and level C (consensus/expert opinion).[1] With patience and motivation each clinician will incorporate our text with his or her perceptive knowledge to address the needs of the geriatric patient because, in the long run, patients need care plans tailored to their own unique circumstances.

Thomas C. Rosenthal, MD
Mark E. Williams, MD
Bruce Naughton, MD

[1]Siwek J, Gourlay ML, Slawson DC, Shaughnessy AF. How to write an evidence-based clinical review article. *Am Fam Physician* 2002;65:251–258.

Acknowledgments

We wish to thank Andrew Danzo, a Medical Editor on staff at the University at Buffalo. He worked extensively with chapter authors to help achieve the meaning intended. We wish to thank Ethel Sharp, who did considerable work chasing down information, tracking submissions and communicating with all of us.

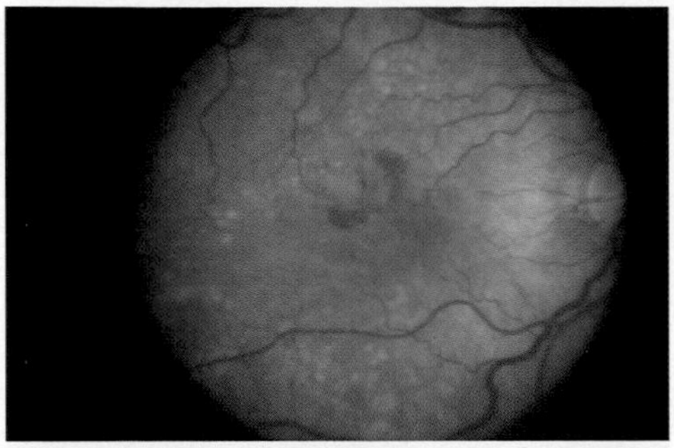

Figure 11.1 Acute wet form age-related macular degeneration with subretinal hemorrhage and scattered large drusen.

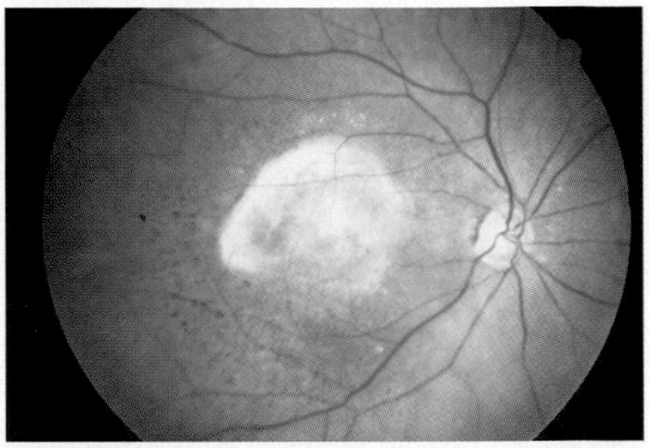

Figure 11.2 End-stage wet form age-related macular degeneration with inactive subretinal fibrosis (''disciform scar'').

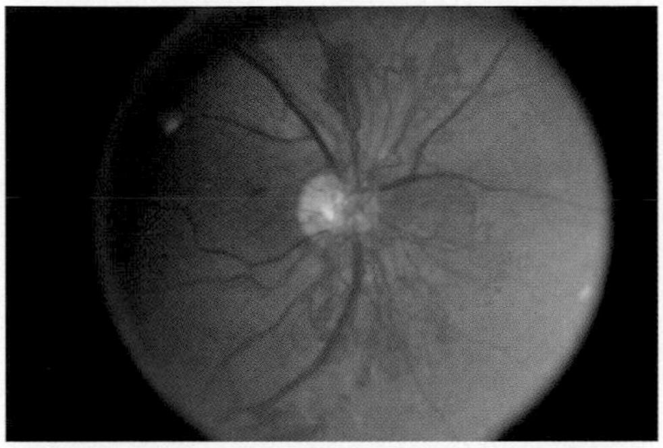

Figure 11.3 Florid neovascularization of the disc in a patient with proliferative diabetic retinopathy.

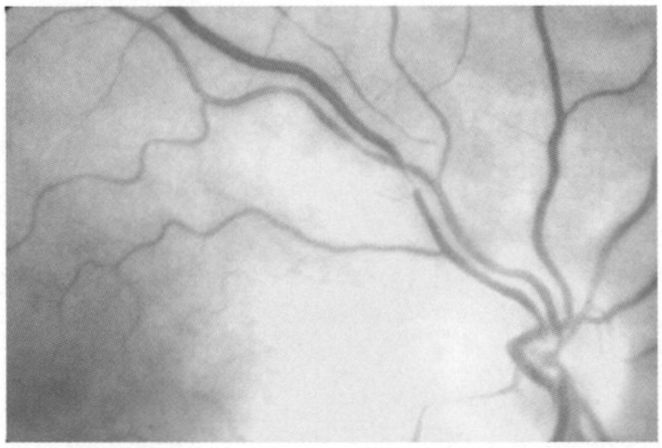

Figure 11.4 Hypertensive retinopathy with arterial narrowing and arteriovenous nicking.

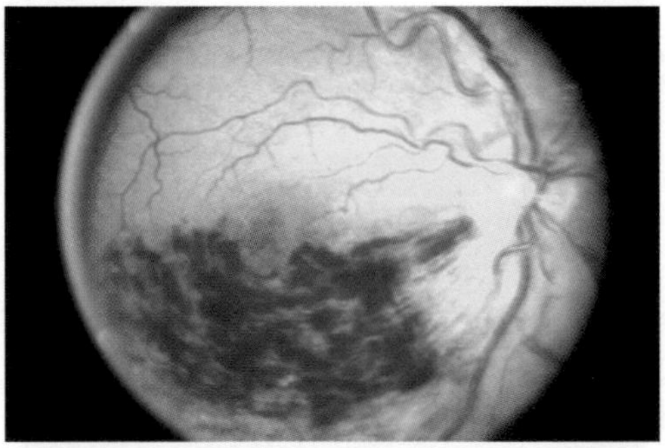

Figure 11.5 Inferotemporal branch retinal vein occlusion with sectoral flame-shaped hemorrhages.

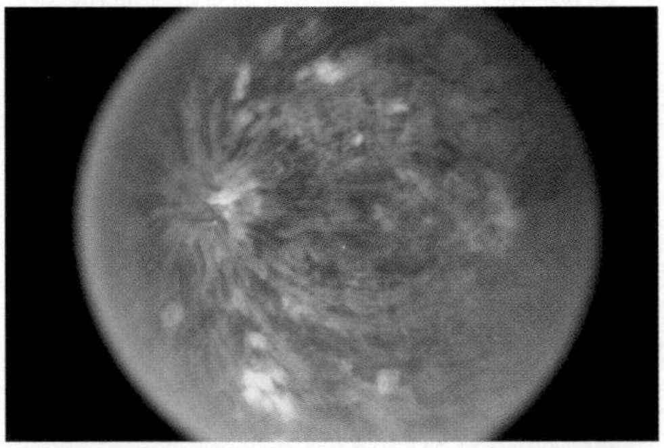

Figure 11.6 Diffuse intraretinal hemorrhages with scattered cotton wool spots in a patient with CRVO.

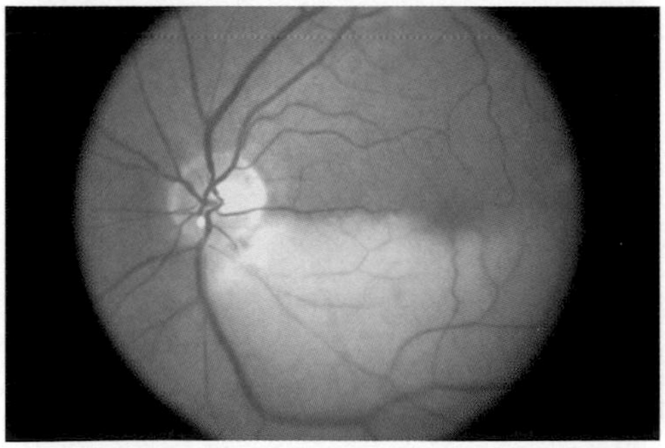

Figure 11.7 Inferotemporal branch retinal artery occlusion showing a proximal Hollenhorst plaque with sectoral retinal edema and pallor.

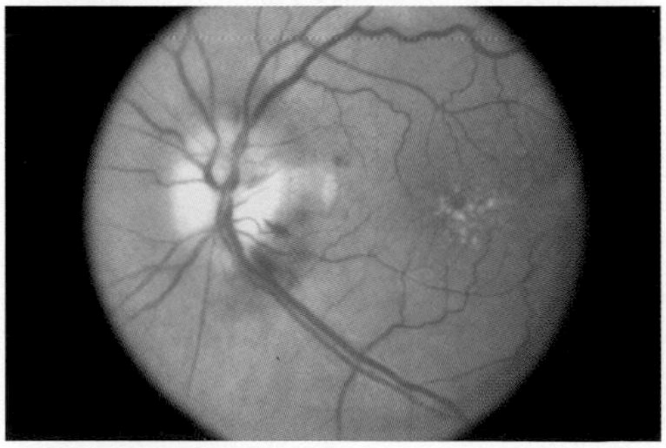

Figure 11.8 Nonarteritic anterior ischemic optic neuropathy with disc edema and peripapillary flame-shaped hemorrhages.

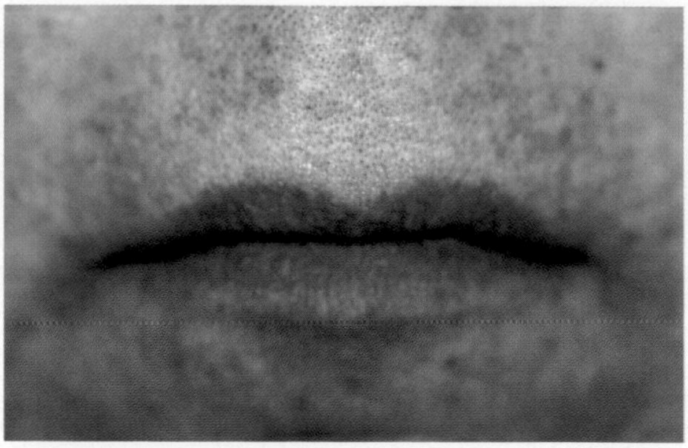

Figure 35.1 Normal appearance of lips.

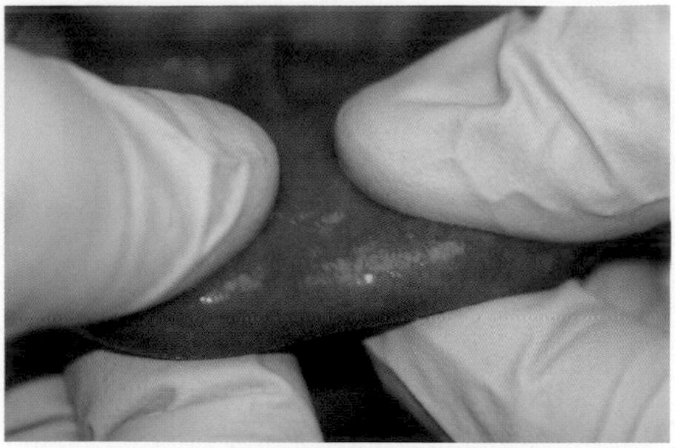

Figure 35.2 Bidigital palpation on lower lip.

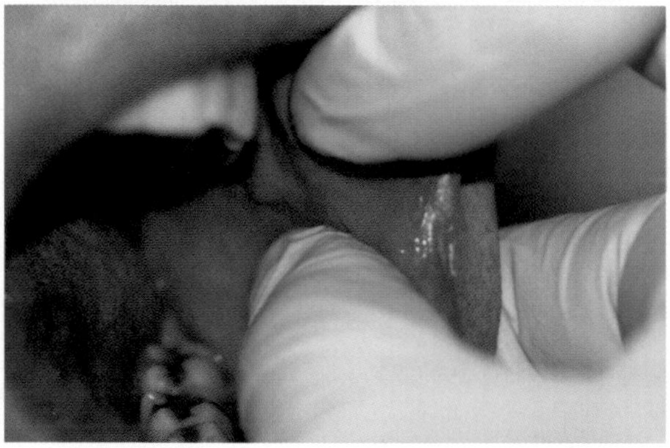

Figure 35.3 Bidigital palpation of buccal mucosa.

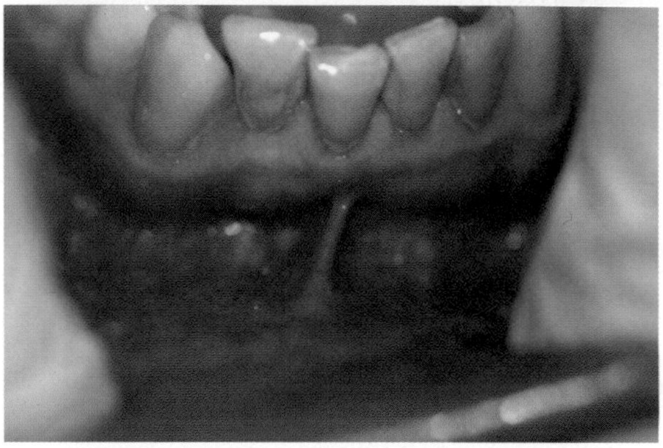

Figure 35.4 Visual examination of anterior buccal vestibule, mandibular arch.

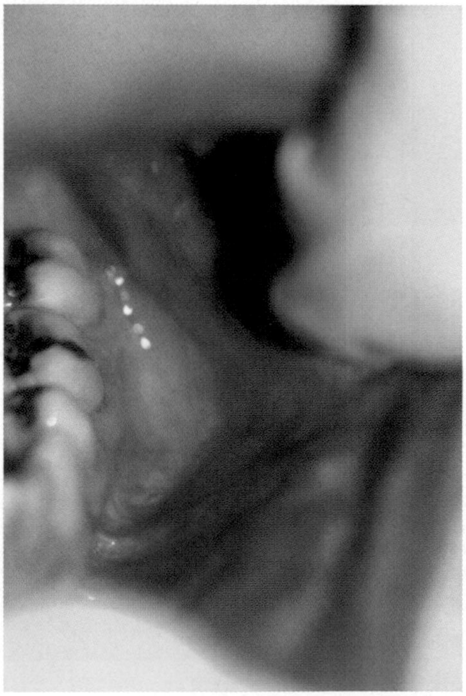

Figure 35.5 Visual examination of posterior buccal vestibule, mandibular arch.

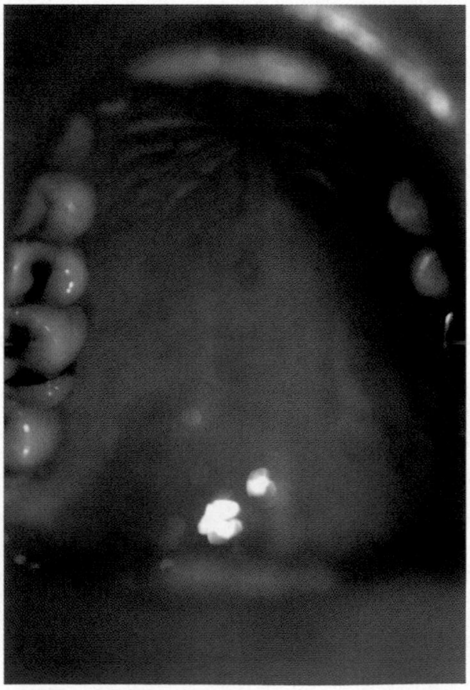

Figure 35.6 Visual examination of hard palate.

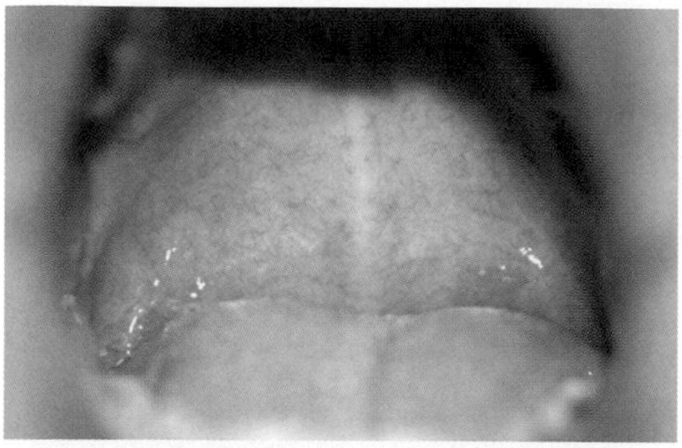

Figure 35.7 Visual examination of soft palate.

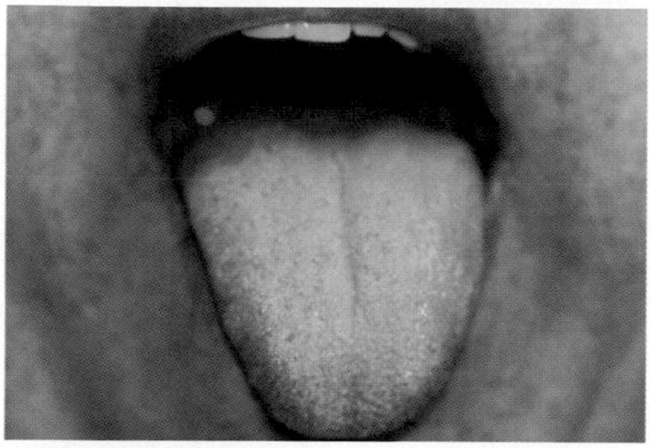

Figure 35.9 Visual examination of dorsal surface of tongue.

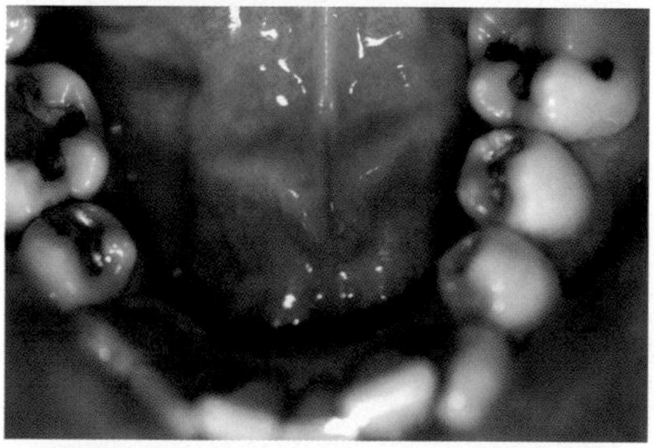

Figure 35.11 Visual examination of floor of the mouth, including Wharton ducts.

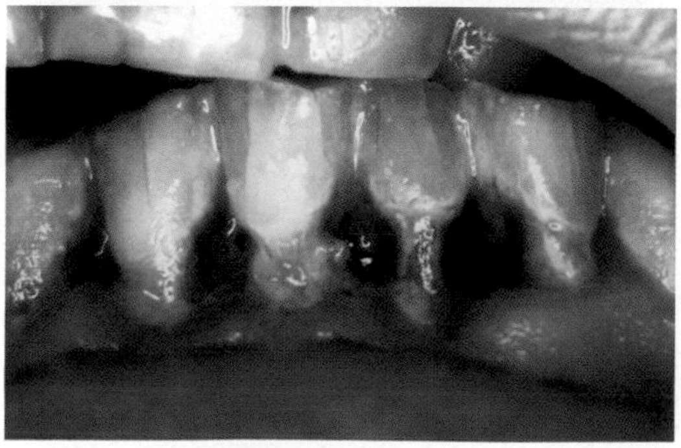

Figure 35.13 Root surface caries.

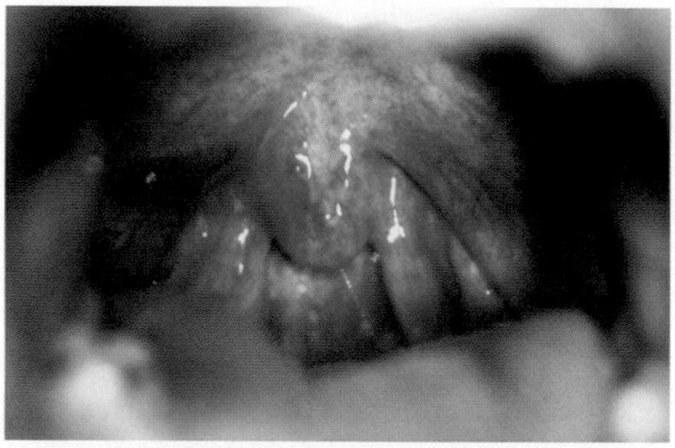

Figure 35.8 Visual examination of oropharynx.

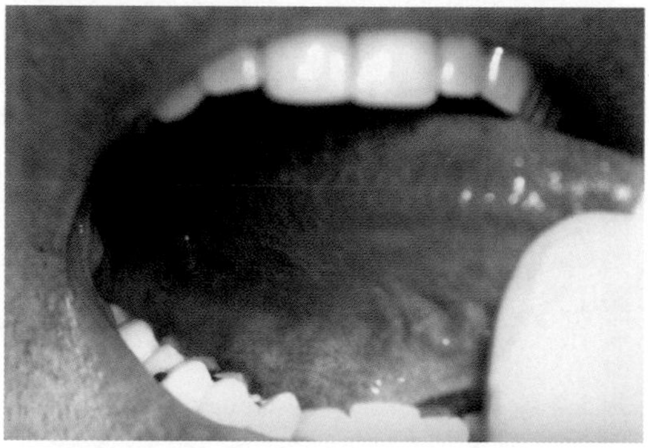

Figure 35.10 Visual examination of lateral surface of tongue, including lingual tonsil.

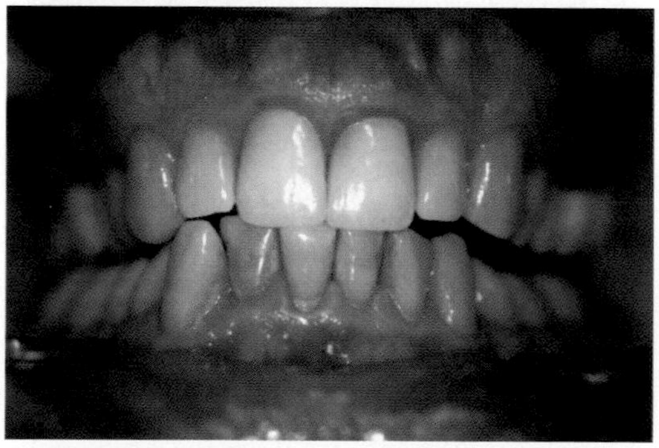

Figure 35.12 Visual examination of anterior gingival and teeth.

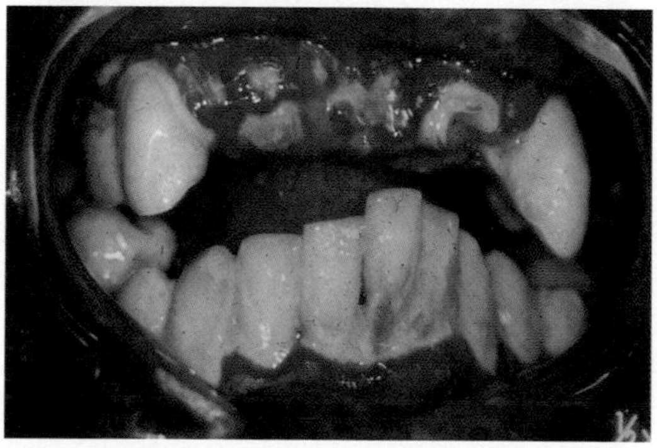

Figure 35.14 Severe periodontal disease.

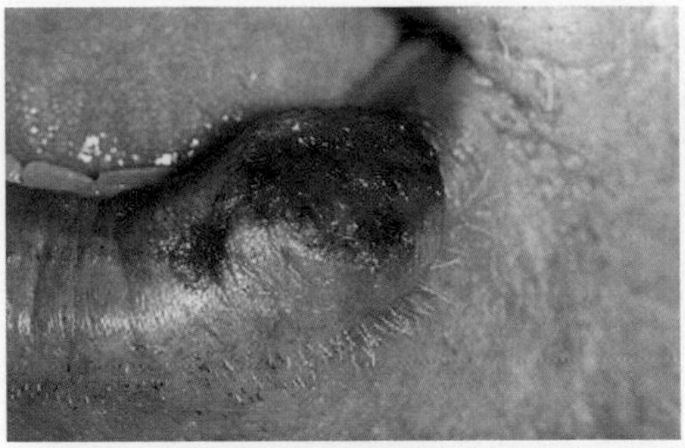

Figure 35.15 Advanced oral cancer of lower lip.

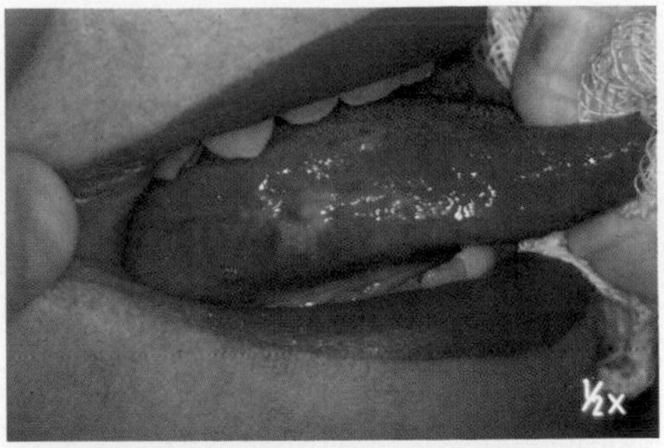

Figure 35.16 Oral cancer of lateral border of tongue. Note red and white areas of lesion.

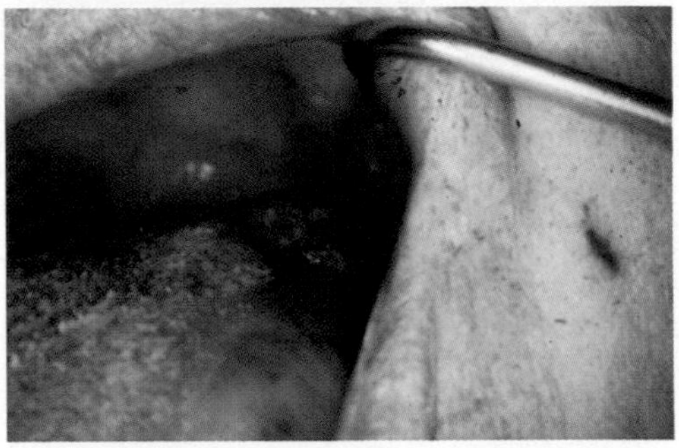

Figure 35.17 Oral cancer of posterior tongue/lingual tonsil.

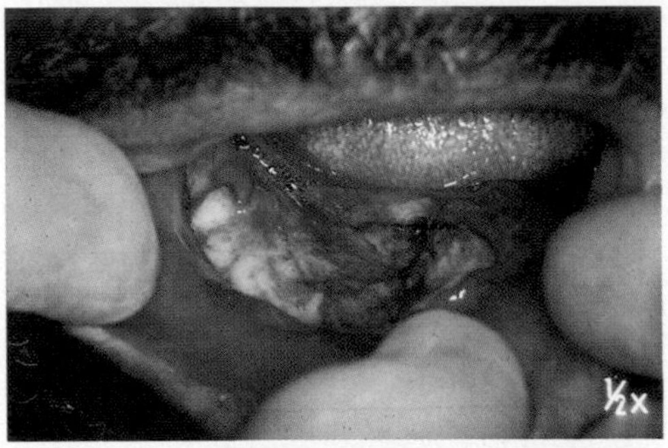

Figure 35.18 Advanced oral cancer of floor of the mouth.

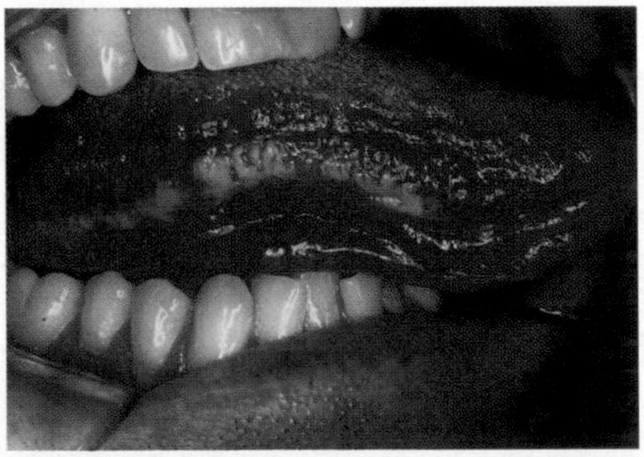

Figure 35.19 Candidiasis of lateral border of the tongue.

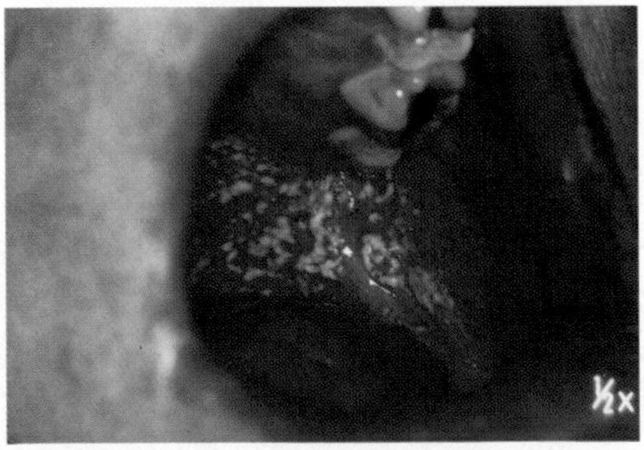

Figure 35.20 Candidiasis of soft palate.

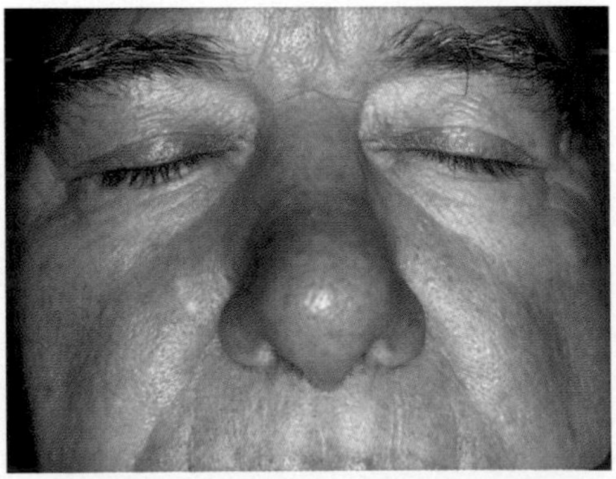

Figure 36.1 Lesions of sebaceous hyperplasia.

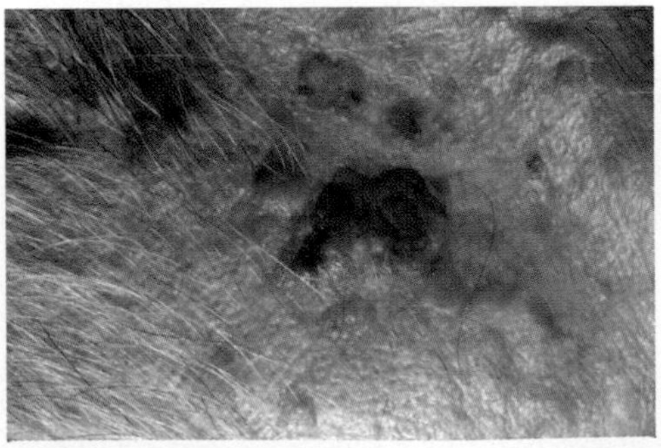

Figure 36.2 Lesions of seborrheic keratoses.

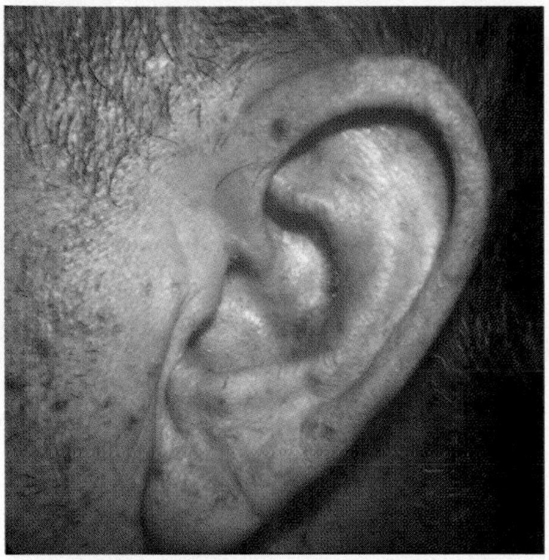

Figure 36.3 Appearance of the lesions of venous lakes, or benign venous angiomas, in the ear.

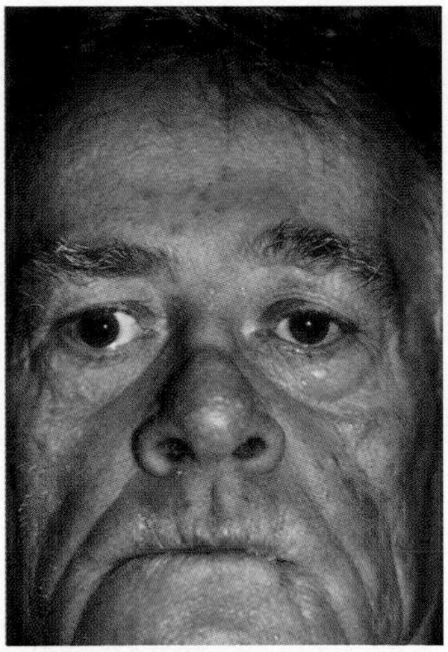

Figure 36.4 Seborrheic dermatitis—appearing as a greasy scaling and erythema of the scalp and skin areas.

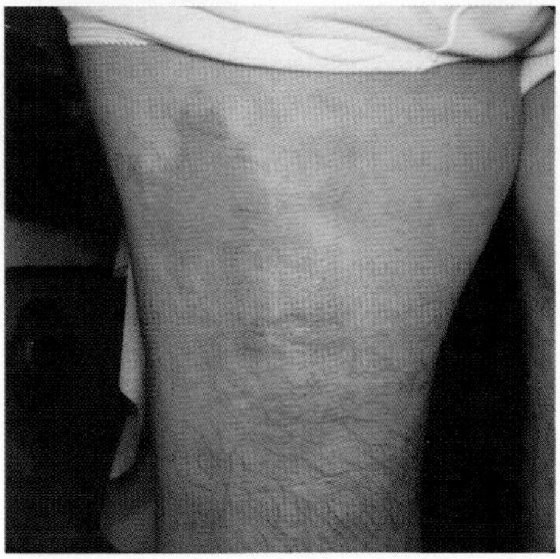

Figure 36.5 Allergic contact dermatitis, presenting as vesicles or bullae in the area in contact with an allergen.

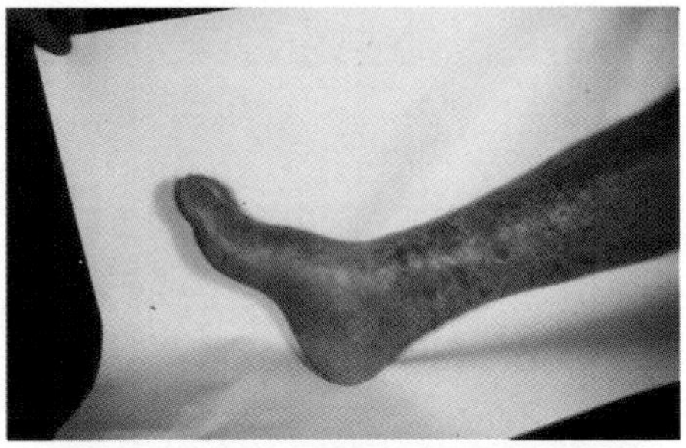

Figure 36.6 Stasis dermatitis, characterized by red, edematous areas of the skin.

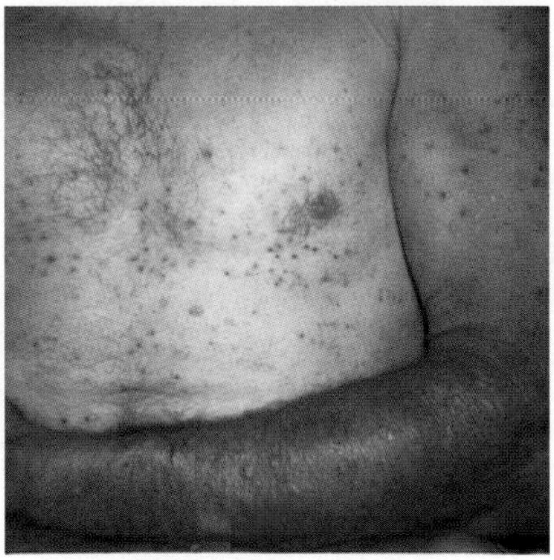

Figure 36.7 Neurodermatitis or lichen simplex chronicus.

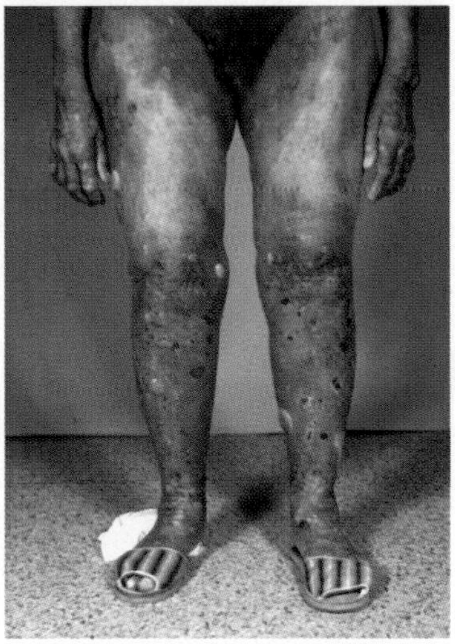

Figure 36.8 Bullous pemphigoid localized to the lower extremities.

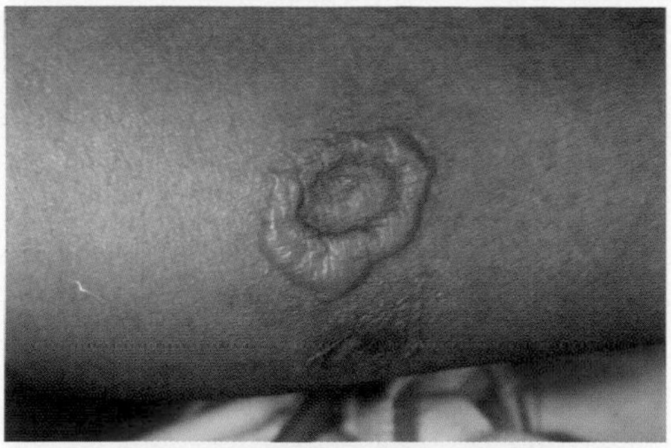

Figure 36.9 Erythema multiforme bullosum appearing as large hemorrhagic bullae on an erythematous base without scaling.

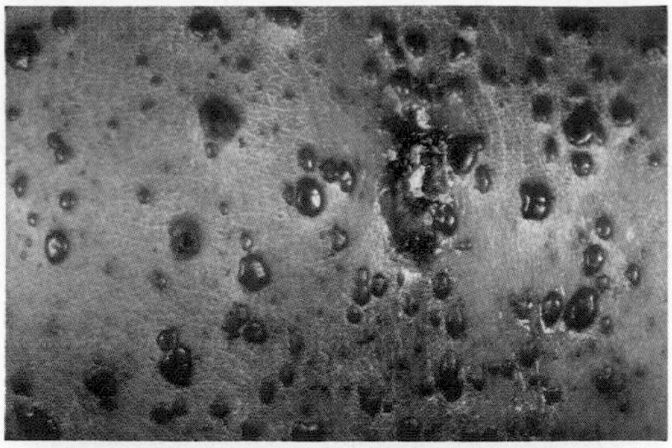

Figure 36.10 Herpes zoster (shingles), presenting as a grouped band of inflammatory vesicles and bullae following the pattern of a dermatome distribution.

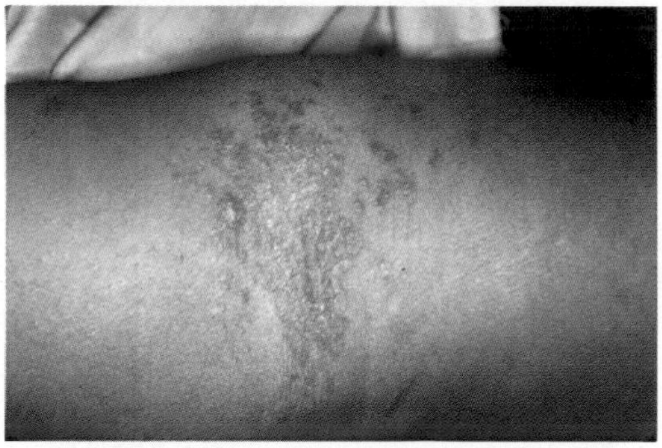

Figure 36.11 Candidiasis.

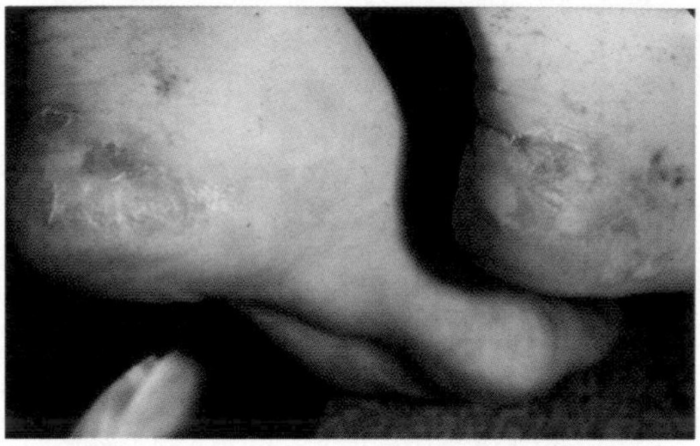

Figure 36.12 Tinea pedis, or athlete's foot.

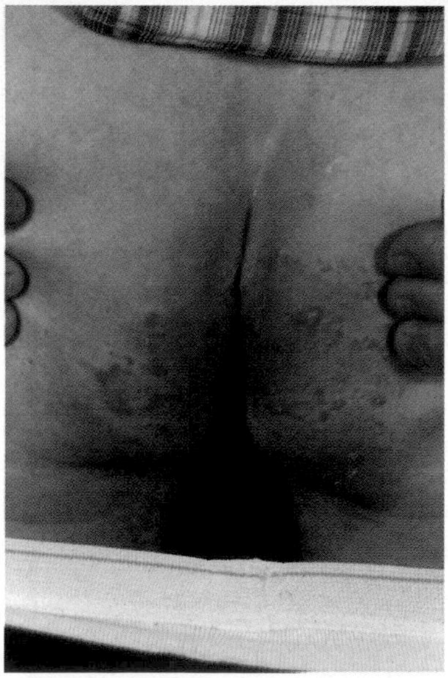

Figure 36.13 Tinea cruris, or jock itch or crotch itch, presenting as erythematous scaling dermatitis.

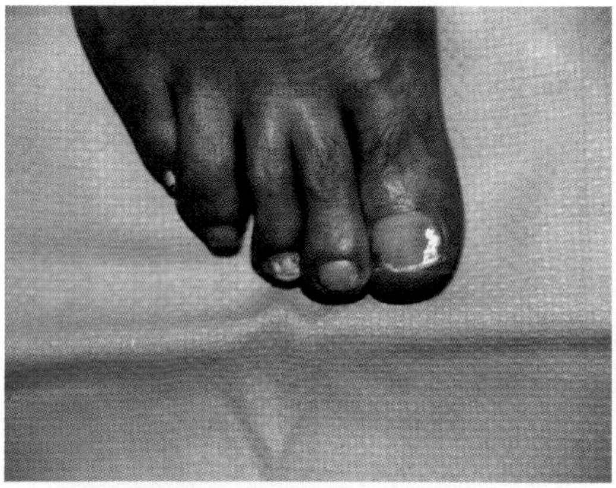

Figure 36.14 Onychomycosis of toenails.

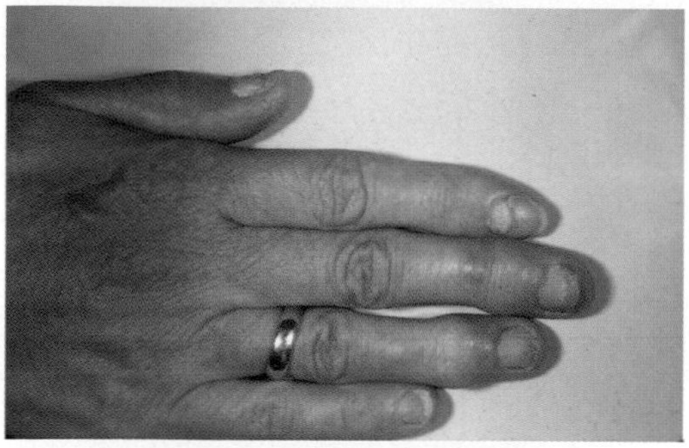

Figure 36.15 Onychomycosis of fingernails.

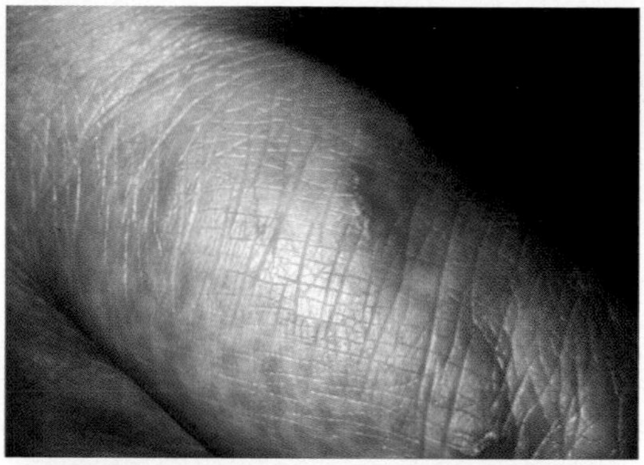

Figure 36.16 Scabies, characterized by linear burrows or crooked or raised lines.

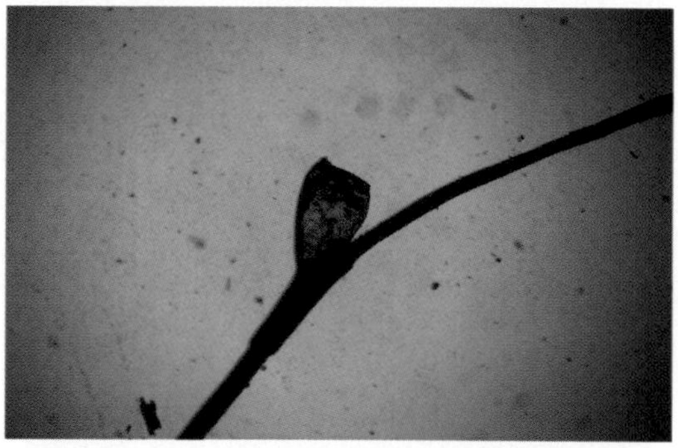

Figure 36.17 Pediculosis—presence of eggs on the hair shaft.

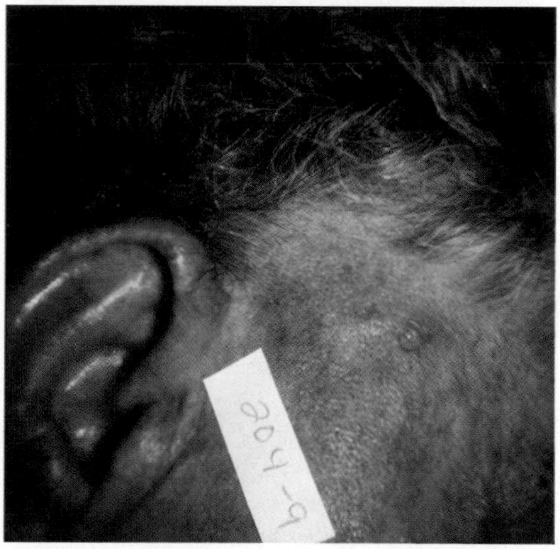

Figure 36.18 Lesions of actinic keratoses, or solar keratoses, appearing as a single pinhead-sized area of white scale or multiple flat, rough, or slightly elevated scaly macules or papules on a hyperemic base measuring 0.2 to 1.5 cm.

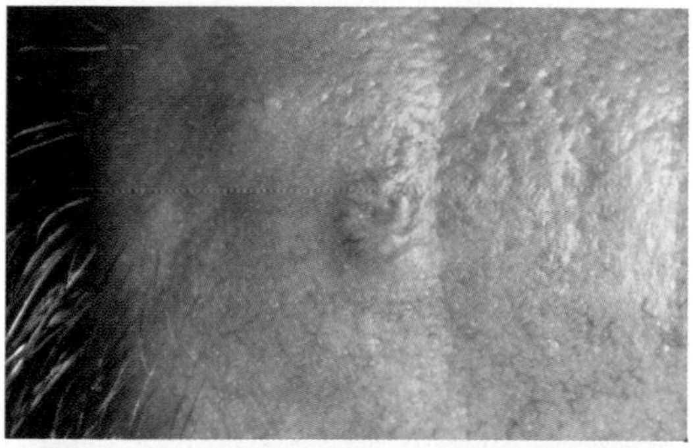

Figure 36.19 Basal cell carcinoma of the nodular type.

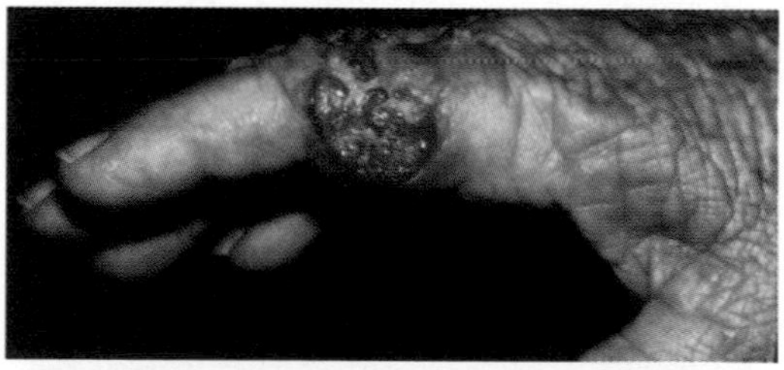

Figure 36.20 Squamous cell carcinoma—in the fingers.

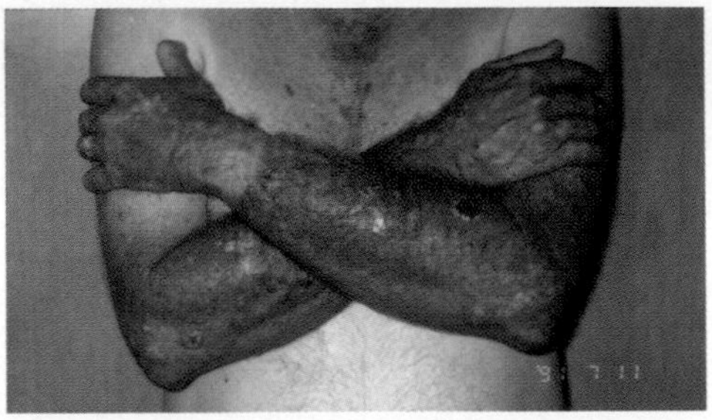

Figure 36.21 Squamous cell carcinoma—in the arms.

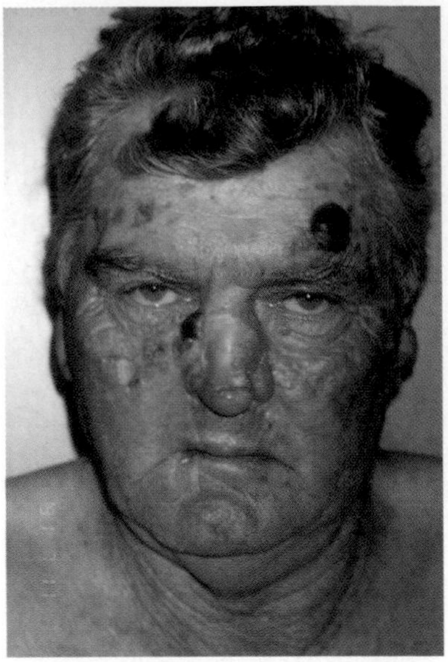

Figure 36.22 Squamous cell carcinoma—on the face.

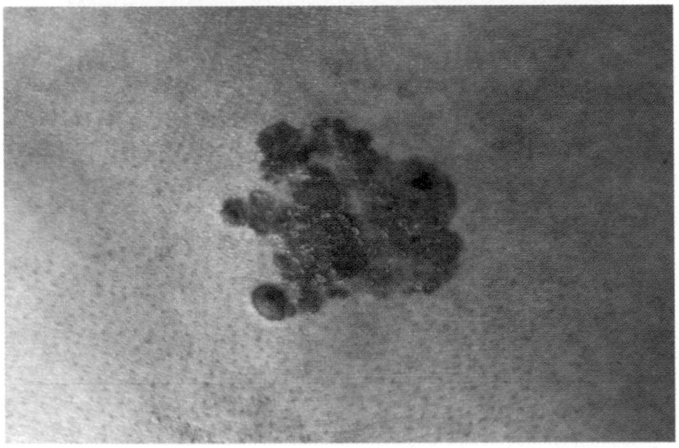

Figure 36.23 Bowen disease, characterized by a slow-growing patch of scaling skin with a sharp irregular border and areas of crusting.

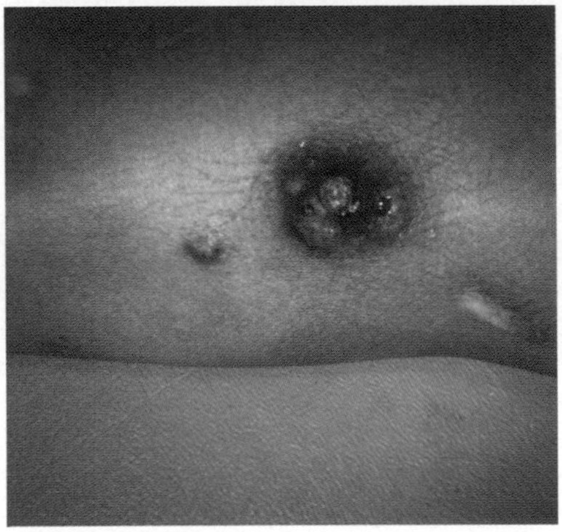

Figure 36.24 Dysplastic nevus.

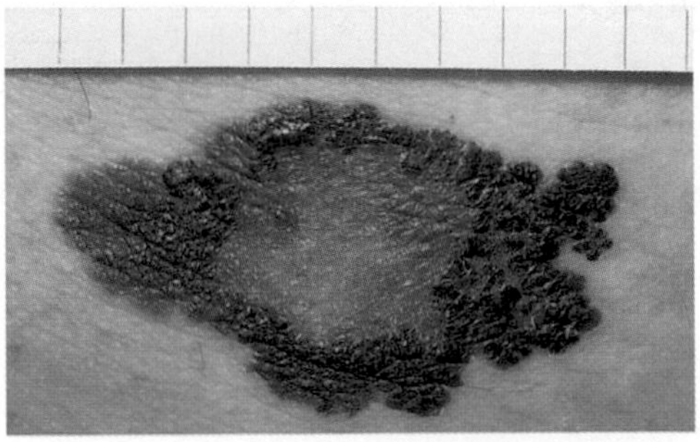

Figure 36.25 Melanoma—"A, B, C, D, E" (*a*symmetry, *b*order irregularity, *c*olor variegation, *d*iameter of the lesion, *e*levation) criteria for evaluation of pigmented lesions.

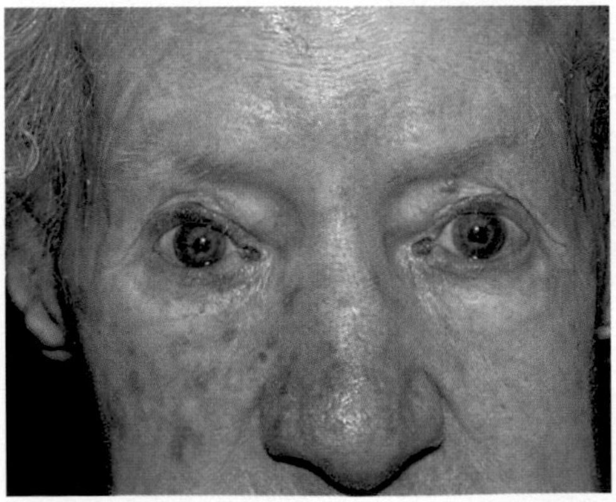

Figure 36.26 Rosacea, presenting in the central facial region and the nasal area.

1

The Approach to the Elderly Patient

Mark E. Williams

CLINICAL PEARLS 1

REVIEWING OUR PERCEPTIONS OF AGING 2

GENERAL PRINCIPLES TO IMPROVE CARE OF ELDERLY PEOPLE 2

The Psychology of the Examiner 2
Increasing Your Perceptive Capacity 3
Show Reverence for the Patient 3
Creating a Healing Atmosphere 3
Biological and Psychological Uniqueness Increases with Aging 4

CLINICALLY RELEVANT DIFFERENCES BETWEEN YOUNG AND OLD PEOPLE 4

How the Body Ages 4
Changes in Height 4
Body Composition 4
Skin and Connective Tissue 4
Musculoskeletal Changes 5
Changes in the Nervous System 5
Changes in the Special Senses 6
Changes in the Cardiovascular System 6
Changes in the Respiratory System 7
Changes in the Gastrointestinal System 7
Renal Function 8
Hematopoietic Tissues 8
The Implications of Age-Related Physiologic Changes 9

PRESENTATION OF ILLNESS IN OLDER PERSONS 10

CHANGES IN THE CLINICIAN'S PERSPECTIVE 10

THE IMPORTANCE OF FUNCTION 12

PERFORMING THE GERIATRIC ASSESSMENT 12

Appearance 12
Dress (Diagnostic Clues from Clothing) 13
Language 14
Behaviors 15

SUMMARY 16

CLINICAL PEARLS

- Chronologic age and biologic age are not the same.
- As we age we become more unique and differentiated, hence care must be individualized.
- Because old age is counterpoised against the certainty of death, preventive strategies focus on the quality of remaining life rather than on extending the quantity of life.
- The ability to live independently is a critical issue.
- Elderly people often present with symptoms that must be managed even when the underlying cause is not clear.
- A major barrier to a full observation is having things fall into familiar context (habit).
- The clinical interview (taking the history) is the "physical examination" of the intellect.
- Shoes tell the story of their owner.
- Linguistic analysis can assist in determining intellectual vitality, mental status, educational attainment, and emotional state.

The increasing biologic uniqueness of older persons as they age requires that their medical care be individualized.

The physician must be aware of his or her own attitudes and beliefs regarding aging and death and how these views influence the physician–patient relationship. As physicians, we must understand how elderly people behave when they are ill and know how to interpret a changing constellation of multiple disease possibilities and interrelationships. The physician requires knowledge, skills (especially in physical diagnosis), and the willingness and discipline to carefully evaluate each situation and to formulate a specifically tailored care plan. Because of the magnitude and complexity of medical, psychological, and social problems in older persons, an effective physician must cooperate with other members of the health care team. The accumulation and constant refinement of these skills reflect the maturity and scientific grounding of the physician.

Elderly persons require an approach and a clinical perspective that differs substantially from the medical evaluation of younger persons. The spectrum of symptoms is broader, the manifestations of distress are more subtle, and the implications for maintaining independence are more compelling. Improvement is sometimes less dramatic and slower to appear. The differential diagnosis is often different in older patients compared to younger patients, and chronic illnesses are more common. In addition, the presentation of disease is frequently nonspecific in elderly people. The most common presenting complaints are mental status changes, behavioral changes, urinary incontinence, gait disturbance or a fall, and weight loss. As a result of this, nonspecific presentation symptoms are difficult to interpret.

The benefits of rehabilitation need to be emphasized when developing an effective, comprehensive plan of care for functionally impaired older persons. Most medical interventions during old age derive their value from their influence on the person's maintenance of independent living. An older person's ability to manage daily activities cannot be determined confidently from the length of the problem list. The crucial issue is the elderly person's ability to function because the discomfort and disability produced by even incurable conditions may often be modified. A conventional disease-specific perspective may not lend itself to developing strategies that best serve the older patient.

REVIEWING OUR PERCEPTIONS OF AGING

The way we think about elderly people strongly influences the way we provide care to them. Because many of us have stereotypes about aging and elderly people, it is important for us to keep an open mind while we focus our current perceptions. The striking increase in average life expectancy during the 20th century rates as one of the major events of our time. We are in the midst of a social revolution, not in new ideology, but in our changing population pattern. For the first time in human history, infants in fortunate nations such as ours can expect to live well into their seventies and beyond. This demographic revolution increases pressure on resources because it also creates further social change and new opportunities for older persons. Such rapid changes have left most of us living with outdated, generally negative attitudes about aging and elderly people. Most of us still view old people as being physically decrepit or in rapid, inevitable decline. Mentally, they are viewed as forgetful or childish, with little ability to learn and adapt; socially and economically, they are often considered a burden. The same outmoded beliefs are embedded in many of our health care and social programs. With such stereotypes, where is the expectation and encouragement for their continuing capacity to enrich their own lives and to enrich society?

These deep-seated cultural stereotypes do not describe accurately the new wave of elderly persons or their potential contributions to society. Today's aging individuals are mostly far from decrepit. Less than 25% experience any disability and <5% are in nursing homes. Intellectually, they thrive when given new opportunities to learn and grow. Given suitable occupation, they work with zest and competence well beyond the traditional age of retirement. Many have an emotional maturity and the kind of wisdom that comes only with age. In short, chronologic age has virtually lost its meaning as a useful index of individual capacity.

To be sure, many old people have special needs for health care and other supports. But these cannot be provided knowledgeably without abandoning the old stereotypes, creating a broader public understanding of today's elderly population and its potential relationship to the rest of society. Such understanding will bring recognition of the many ways our later years can be more a culmination of life than a prelude to death.

GENERAL PRINCIPLES TO IMPROVE CARE OF ELDERLY PEOPLE

The fact that you are reading this chapter says a lot about your interest and commitment to improve your care for elderly people. It is important that you commit yourself to excellence. Mediocrity has no place in the care of elderly people. Your self-discipline is necessary to maintain focus and avoid distractions.

The Psychology of the Examiner

The psychology of the examiner is the first consideration. Careful geriatric clinicians must be able to focus their attention and awareness. The nature of the clinician's inner state should be one of complete attention to the patient's concerns and appreciating the special aspects of the moment. The examiner's overall intention is to help and to be of assistance to a person implicitly asking for relief from distress, for guidance, or for support. In addition, the clinician's technique reflects his or her grounding and maturity. You must be totally focused on the patient, with no thoughts or inner dialogue on any other matter. You are giving the other person your most priceless possession, your undivided attention.

Increasing Your Perceptive Capacity

The second principle is to work hard to increase your perceptive capacity. This is not as easy as it sounds. There are three types of knowledge: General, specialized, and perceptive. General knowledge is what is in the textbook or encyclopedia. Take "basketball" as an example. If we look "basketball" up in an encyclopedia we get a particular type of information: The history of the game, number of players on a team, basic rules, referees' signals, and a listing of championship teams in the past. Specialized knowledge is what an informed fan would know: Which teams had a good recruiting year, which team plays well against a particular opponent, whose star player has a nagging injury. This body of knowledge is not found in the encyclopedia. The third type of knowledge is perceptive knowledge: What is it like to be out on the basketball court with the ball in a game situation. This framework helps us appreciate that most health care education is either general or specialized knowledge: Lists, tables, flowcharts, algorithms, decision trees, or clinical pathways. This important information has its place in clinical care. But very little time is spent educating learners on how perceptions guide one on what *to do*.

One difficulty in sharing perceptive knowledge is that we have a limited perceptive vocabulary. It is cumbersome to describe perceptive insights without a descriptive vocabulary. Another factor limiting the sharing of perceptive knowledge is that there are few role models with the requisite experience who are also willing to communicate their techniques and expose their vulnerabilities to others. In geriatrics there has also been a lack of students with an interest in the perceptions gained through a caring relationship with an elderly patient.

Show Reverence for the Patient

Francis Ward Peabody said in a classic 1927 monograph in the Journal of the American Medical Association that the art of caring for the patient is to care for the patient. He also wrote, "The treatment of a disease may be entirely impersonal; the care of a patient must be completely personal." This succinct advice epitomizes the need for the craftsmanship of caring.

One of my sons collects sports cards. Although I cannot tell the valuable cards from the common ones, I can sort them accurately by watching how he handles them. The rare rookie card of a star athlete is handled with a sense of reverence. In fact, we infer value by observing how people touch objects they perceive to be valuable. There is a precious delicacy of the touch, with attention to each nuance in movement. The pottery bowl (or a rare book, for example) commands total concentration and an obvious appreciation for value. In the same way, it is easy to tell the student (or resident or attending physician) who is "caring for the patient" by how he or she takes the patient's hand to begin the physical examination. Again, there is a sense of conscious appreciation, respect, and reverence.

Creating a Healing Atmosphere

Conscientious information gathering requires awareness of the premise and dynamics of the clinical encounter and structuring the environment to facilitate communication. The attitudes of physicians and other health care personnel strongly influence the quality of information available from the history. The premise of the clinical relationship is the expectation of reducing morbidity and improving function and quality of life by whatever means possible. It is important to emphasize the premise, which is not necessarily to eliminate the cause of the distress (which may be impossible in many circumstances) but to help relieve the distress itself, because the presence of disease and the development of symptoms are not always closely related. This key insight frees health care providers from the frustration, anxiety, and sense of vulnerability that results from cure-oriented expectations.

Attention to a few specific environmental considerations can improve communication by facilitating sensory input to the older person and putting them at ease. Because some older people have visual impairments, techniques to improve nonverbal cues become useful. For example, to improve visual information, physicians should avoid having a strong light behind them (such as a window) because it puts the face in silhouette. Another useful technique is to reduce the distance between participants. As a rule of thumb, the optimal distance is that at which the interviewer begins to feel uncomfortably close. For individuals with hearing impairment, the volume of the voice must be raised without raising the pitch. Shouting, which raises the pitch, defeats the purpose because high-frequency sounds are characteristically affected more profoundly than lower-frequency sounds in the aging ear. Shouting can also produce significant discomfort because the failing ear may become more sensitive to loud sounds.

Environmental conditions can improve communication by relaxing and comforting the older person. Office equipment should be practical and comfortable. Plush furniture may be stylish and handsome but dysfunctional for persons with painful backs, hips, or knees. Older persons often prefer a simple straight-backed chair with armrests (for possible assistance in standing). Another important way to improve communication is to sit down. The importance of sitting is inversely proportional to the time available for the encounter: The less the time available, the greater the importance of sitting. In addition to providing a common level for eye contact, sitting helps neutralize the appearance of impatience and haste. The appearance of impatience inhibits communication by magnifying a hierarchic relationship (physician over patient) rather than establishing a partnership to solve problems. The professional may nonverbally communicate that he or she is more interested in the problem or disease than in the person who is experiencing the distress.

Biological and Psychological Uniqueness Increases with Aging

As we age, we become more unique and differentiated and less like one another. There is more biologic variability among octogenarians than neonates. Anyone who has attended a high school or college reunion can attest to the fact that some individuals age very slowly over a 10-year period while other individuals seem to have aged several decades. Because of this increasing biologic variability with aging, our approach must be individualized. A "one-size-fits-all" strategy will not fit an older person.

CLINICALLY RELEVANT DIFFERENCES BETWEEN YOUNG AND OLD PEOPLE

What is aging? Aging is a nearly ubiquitous biologic process characterized by progressive, predictable, inevitable evolution and maturation until death. Aging is not the accumulation of disease, although aging and disease are related in subtle and complex ways. A fundamental principle is that biologic age and chronologic age are not the same. Different individuals age at different rates, and aging occurs in different organ systems at different rates, influenced primarily by the individual's socioeconomic status and lifestyle choices. For example, smoking cigarettes seems to accelerate aging in the pulmonary and cardiovascular systems.

Normal aging in the absence of disease is a remarkably benign process. In physiologic terms, normal aging involves the steady erosion of organ system reserves and homeostatic controls. This erosion is evident only during periods of maximal exertion or stress. The limits of homeostatic maintenance eventually reach a critical point (usually in advanced age), such that relatively minimal insults cannot be overcome, resulting in the person's death over a relatively short time. Consequently, any morbidity apparent to the person is compressed into the last period of life. Deviations from this ideal represent the effects of superimposed disease.

Aging also causes important changes in body composition and in the structural elements of tissues. Between age 25 and 75, the lipid compartment expands from 14% to 30% of the total body weight, whereas the total body water (mainly extracellular water) and lean muscle mass decline. This change in body composition has important implications for nutritional planning, metabolic activity, and the use of drugs by older persons. For example, the lipid-soluble drugs such as diazepam remain in the bodies of older persons for a much longer time than they remain in younger persons. Aging changes have also been documented in connective tissue and the isomeric forms of structural proteins.

How the Body Ages

Difficulties in making health care decisions result when normal aging changes are not appreciated or are misinterpreted. Because of this, a knowledge of the anatomy of aging is fundamental to our care.

Changes in Height

All individuals lose height as they age but with great variability both in the age of onset and the rate of loss. On average, approximately 5 cm are lost by the age of 80. Changes in posture, changes in the growth of vertebrae, a forward bending of the spine, and compression of the disks between the vertebrae cause a loss in trunk length. Increased curvature of the hips and knees, along with decreased joint space in the trunk and extremities, contributes to a loss of structure. In the feet, joint changes and a flattening of the arches can also contribute to the loss of standing height.

Body Composition

Lean body mass is lost with age; this reduction is mainly a decrease in muscle mass, with some decrease in bone and viscera. Hormonal changes seem to influence these losses. The fall in the level of estrogen (and adrenal androgens) is proportionally much greater in women than that in the level of total androgen (adrenal plus testicular) in men. Other organs also show losses: The liver and kidneys, for example, lose approximately a third of their weight between age 30 and 90. The prostate differs; it doubles in weight between age 20 and 90.

Skin and Connective Tissue

Little change occurs with aging in the outer layer of the skin called the *stratum corneum*. The contact area between the dermis and the epidermis decreases, and the number of deeper basal cells and pigment-producing cells, called *melanocytes*, is reduced. With advancing age, the number of Langerhans cells, which come from the bone marrow and provide assistance to the immune system, is also modestly reduced. The reduction of these cells is striking in the skin that has been exposed to sunlight; this reduction is thought to contribute to the development of sun-related skin cancers.

The content of collagen, a basic chemical building block of skin, decreases with age, which results in less skin elasticity. The collagen fibers in younger skin exhibit an orderly arrangement similar to fibers in a rope. These fibers become coarser and random with aging, resembling a mass of unstirred spaghetti. Alterations in elastic tissue cause a loss of resiliency and produce wrinkles.

Hair changes play a prominent role in the perception of age. Hair graying results from a progressive loss of melanocytes from the hair bulbs. The loss of these pigment cells is more rapid in the hair than in the skin, possibly because of the rapid proliferation of cells during hair growth. The graying of hair in the axilla is thought to be one of the most reliable signs of aging. There is a decease in the number of hair follicles on the scalp. Changes in the growth rate of hair depend upon the site. The growth rate of scalp, pubic, and armpit hair declines; however, possibly because of hormonal changes, an increase in growth of facial hair is sometimes seen in elderly women. An increased growth of eyebrow, nostril, and ear hair occurs in elderly men.

Musculoskeletal Changes

A decrease in muscle weight relative to total body weight characterizes advanced age. Aging changes in the muscles include a decrease in muscle strength, endurance, size, and weight relative to total body weight. However, the late onset of these changes and their unpredictable rate of appearance suggest that they may not be due to aging but rather due to inactivity, nutritional deficiency, disease, or other long-standing conditions. Curiously, both the diaphragm and the heart, two muscles that work continuously, appear to be relatively unchanged by aging. Age-related chemical changes occur in the cartilage, the substance that provides the lubricating surface of most joints. Because cartilage contains no blood vessels, it depends upon the blood supply of the synovium (the tissue that produces joint fluid) for nutrients that pass through the joint fluid. The water content of cartilage decreases, and changes in the deeper structures such as the underlying bone may influence the cartilage and may reduce its ability to adapt to repetitive stress.

Bone loss is a universal aspect of aging that occurs at highly individual rates. Aging affects and reduces the bone cells that produce bone more severely than those cells that reabsorb bone. Although bone remodeling occurs throughout life, the balance between the amount of bone reabsorbed and the amount of bone formed is impaired with aging; the growth of bone slows and the bone begins to thin and become more porous. The internal latticework of bones loses its horizontal supports, which significantly compromises its strength.

The skull appears to thicken with age. All the skull dimensions increase, but greater increases are noted deep in the skull and in the frontal sinuses. Bone growth has also been demonstrated well into advanced age in the ribs, fingers, and femur. These changes in the hip may be important because growth in the mid portion of the bone results in a wider but weaker bone.

Conditioning, nutrition, vascular and neurologic abnormalities, and hormones influence the degeneration in the muscles and bones. Conditioning is the most significant influence because disuse or underuse produces marked declines in bone and muscle structures. Nutrition affects bone and mineral metabolism, and blood vessel and neurologic abnormalities accelerate muscle degeneration. In addition, a variety of hormones—growth hormone, estrogens, androgens, and many others—modify the musculoskeletal integrity.

Changes in the Nervous System

The brain's weight declines with age, but this decline appears to be in a few specific places rather than overall. Atrophy of the gray matter is usually moderate in healthy older people, as compared with a more extensive loss of cells in older people with dementia. From age 30 to 70, the blood flow to the brain decreases by 15% to 20%. With aging, there is a loss of neurons in the gray matter, cerebellum, and hippocampus that seems to be involved in some aspects of memory function. Less dramatic losses occur in deeper brain structures. For some nerves, the density of their interconnections seems to be reduced with aging. However, there is a slow and continued growth of the terminal dendritic connections between nerves, which suggests a possible repatterning of the nervous system.

Age-related changes in certain neurotransmitters occur in specific parts of the central nervous system. The catalyzing and synthesizing enzymes of acetylcholine, acetylcholinesterase and choline acetyltransferase decline significantly with age. These decreases are most prominent in the caudate nucleus. Changes in glutamic acid decarboxylase have also been reported. The decrements are significant and also seem to affect the caudate nucleus. A 40% loss of binding sites for dopamine agonists and antagonists occurs with age. Similar aging changes have been observed in cortical and pineal β-adrenergic receptors. Changes in membrane fluidity with age may impair receptor function. Binding sites for serotonin in the frontal cortex and hippocampus are reduced with age.

Aging changes in brain structure and biochemistry do not necessarily affect thinking and behavior. Basic language skills and sustained attention are not altered with aging, but some aspects of cognitive ability do seem to change, the earliest being the ability to retain large amounts of information over a long period. Naming tasks and abstraction are altered late in life. However, none of these changes develops uniformly or inevitably, and many older people continue to perform at levels that are comparable to, or even exceed, those of much younger people.

Changes in the Special Senses

Vision

With age, the tissues around the eyes atrophy and fat around the eye is lost; this may result in the upper lid drooping and the lower lid turning inward or outward. The decreased production of tears combined with atrophy around the eye increases the chances of eye infection. Changes in the cornea can also occur, although they are usually related to disease and not aging. The iris becomes more rigid, the pupil becomes smaller, and changes occur around the lens, predisposing the person to glaucoma. As newer lens fibers proliferate at the periphery, older fibers migrate to the center to form a denser central section. This process is like continually forming a ball of yarn. The lens progressively accumulates yellow substances, possibly from a chemical reaction involving sunlight and the amino acids in the lens. These substances reduce the amount of light and color entering the eye, and this yellow filtering causes the lens to become less transparent to the blue part of the color spectrum. To older eyes, blue appears greenish blue.

Changes in the retina have not been clearly identified, although blood vessel disease involving the retina is common. Changes in the blood supply to the retina and possibly the pigmented layer of the retina can cause macular degeneration, one of the most common causes of vision loss in older people.

The most common change in vision associated with aging is called *presbyopia*, a condition in which it becomes harder to focus on nearby objects. This is mainly due to decreased elasticity of the lens and atrophy of the ciliary muscle that controls the lens shape. Presbyopia affects men and women equally and begins in the early twenties, although it is usually not noticeable until 20 or 30 years later. Eyeglasses usually correct the problem. As individuals age, they adapt more slowly to abrupt changes from light to dark areas. So consistent is this correlation with age that a person's age may be predicted to within 3 years on the basis of this performance. These changes are not trivial—after 2 minutes of reduced illumination, young people's eyes are almost five times more sensitive than older people's eyes; after 40 minutes, there is a 240-fold difference.

Hearing

The external auditory canal atrophies, resulting in thin walls and decreased cerumen production. The tympanic membrane thickens and often appears dull and white. Ossicular joints can develop degenerative changes. Significant inner ear changes take place, such as loss of hair cells in the organ of Corti, loss of cochlear neurons (especially at the basal end), capillary thickening in stria vascularis, and degeneration of the spiral ligament. Whether aging in the absence of excessive noise exposure can produce these changes is unknown.

Hearing loss for pure tones, presbycusis, increases with age in both men and women. Higher frequencies are more affected than lower frequencies. Overall, the loss is slightly milder for women than for men. Decrements occur with aging not only in the absolute threshold of tones of varying frequency but also in the differential threshold—the point at which changes in pitch are detectable. Between age 25 and 55, pitch discrimination declines linearly; but after the age of 55 the decline is steeper, especially for very high and low frequencies. Pitch discrimination plays an important role in speech perception. Speech discrimination declines with age, even when pure tone hearing loss is taken into account. Speech intelligibility declines by $<5\%$ from age 6 to 59, but deteriorates rapidly thereafter, dropping by $>25\%$ from peak levels after age 80. With ambient noise or indistinct speech, older people hear even less.

Taste

The evidence regarding taste sensitivity is inconclusive and varies both among individuals and the substance tested. The tongue atrophies with age, which may result in diminished taste sensation; however, the number of taste buds remains unchanged, and the responsiveness of these taste buds appears to be unaltered.

Smell

The sense of smell declines rapidly after the age of 50 for both men and women, and the parts of the brain that are involved in smell degenerate significantly. By age 80, the detection of smell is almost 50% poorer than that at the peak capacity. Taste and smell work together to make the discrimination and enjoyment of food possible. As individuals age, they may have trouble recognizing a variety of blended foods by taste and smell.

Touch

In general, the response to painful stimuli diminishes with aging. Sensitivity of the cornea of the eye to light touch declines after the age of 50 (touch sensitivity to the nose begins to decline by age 15). Pressure touch thresholds on the index finger and the big toe decline more in men than in women.

Changes in the Cardiovascular System

With aging, the heart tends to show disease in the heart muscle, heart valves, and coronary arteries. It is unclear whether any age-related changes of the heart occur in the absence of disease. The cells responsible for producing heartbeats become infiltrated with connective tissue and fat. Similar but less dramatic changes occur in other parts of the heart's electric system. Poor blood supply does not seem to be an underlying cause. Age-related declines in cardiac contractility include a prolonged contraction time, decreased response to various medications that ordinarily stimulate the heart, and increased resistance to electric stimulation (normally these changes do not result in disease). The elastic properties of the heart muscle are altered.

Changes in the blood vessels also occur as individuals age. Irregularities in size and shape develop in the cells that line blood vessels, and the layers in the blood vessel wall become thickened with connective tissue. The large arteries increase in size and thickness. The extent of blood flow within various organs varies: In the kidney it may decrease by 50% and in the brain by 15% to 20%.

The cardiovascular system responds less efficiently to various stresses with age. The maximum heart rate changes in a linear fashion and may be estimated by subtracting the person's age from 220. The resting heart rate and the amount of blood pumped by the heart over time (cardiac output) do not change. The cardiac output with work may increase, although there is a decrease in the maximum heart rate. This increase in cardiac output occurs because the amount of blood pumped with each beat (stroke volume) increases to compensate for the decreased heart rate with age. Following stress, it takes longer for the heart rate and blood pressure to return to resting levels.

Whether blood pressure increases as an inevitable consequence of aging is unknown. Several studies have shown that aging is associated with an increase in blood pressure. Stiffness within the blood vessels is thought to be the reason for this increase; however, an age-associated increase in blood pressure is not found in individuals who live in isolated, less technologically developed societies or in people who grow old in a special environment such as a psychiatric institution.

Changes in the Respiratory System

The trachea and large airways increase in diameter as people age. Enlargement of the end units of the airway results in a decreased surface area of the lung. Decreased lung elasticity contributes to the increase in lung volumes and to the reduced amount of surface area. The decreased elasticity causes the chest to expand and the diaphragm to descend. The ends of the ribs calcify to the sternum, producing stiffening of the chest wall, which increases the workload of the respiratory muscles.

The consequences of these aging changes are an increased likelihood that pulmonary disease and progressive declines in measurements of lung function will be developed. From age 20 to 80, the vital capacity declines linearly. The functional residual capacity increases from approximately 20% of the total lung capacity at the age of 20 to 35% at the age of 60. The decrease in arterial partial pressure of oxygen (Po_2) (i.e., increased A–a O_2 gradient) is largely due to ventilation–perfusion (V/Q) mismatch. Elastic recoil of the lungs decreases with age, airways tend to collapse, and the closing volume increases steadily. The well-perfused, dependent parts of the lung show the most airway closure, thus causing V/Q mismatch. Carbon monoxide diffusion capacity decreases with age; the contribution of this change in gas exchange to the decreased arterial Po_2 is unknown.

Maximum oxygen consumption (Vo_2max) is a measure used to understand the overall cardiopulmonary function. Vo_2max declines progressively with age but is also substantially influenced by exercise, so that conditioned older persons may obtain values exceeding those of the much younger. Endurance training can increase the lung capacity of sedentary older persons.

Changes in the Gastrointestinal System

On the whole, the gastrointestinal tract shows less age-associated change in function than other systems. The lining of the gut maintains an extraordinary capacity for replacing itself. Age-related dental changes do not necessarily lead to the loss of teeth. Poor dental hygiene is a more important factor than age in this dental loss. Usually, the losses are caused by cavities or periodontal (gum) disease, both of which can be prevented by good care. With age, the location of cavities changes, and an increasing amount of root cavities and cavities around existing sites of previous dental work are seen. Tooth loss leads to changes in diet and can increase the likelihood of malnutrition. False teeth reduce taste sensation and do not completely restore normal chewing ability. Alterations in swallowing are more common in older people without teeth. As people age, they do not chew as efficiently as younger people and tend to swallow larger pieces of food. Swallowing in older people takes 50% to 100% longer, probably because of subtle changes in the swallowing mechanism.

Esophagus and Stomach

Changes in esophageal motility with normal aging have been labeled *presbyesophagus*. Although a high incidence of absent peristalsis after swallowing and frequent nonperistaltic repetitive contractions were initially reported as cardinal features of presbyesophagus, more recent studies in healthy older persons have demonstrated that the principal abnormality is decreased amplitude of esophageal contraction during peristalsis. All other measures of esophageal motility, including relaxation of the lower esophageal sphincter and onset, speed, and duration of contraction wave, do not differ on the basis of age. Moreover, the decreased amplitude of peristalsis does not appear to cause clinical symptoms. Therefore, esophageal motility disorders in older persons are due to diseases such as diabetes mellitus, central nervous system disorders, or neuropathies rather than aging.

With aging, the gastric mucosa and smooth muscles thin, and the gastric wall shows increased leukocytes and aggregation of lymphoid tissue. Gastric motility is normal. Whereas age-related atrophy of parietal cells occurs and acid secretion decreases, achlorhydria signifies disease.

The Small and Large Intestine

The small intestine shows a modest amount of atrophy of the lining. Changes in the large intestine include atrophy of the lining, changes within the muscle layer, and blood vessel abnormalities. Approximately 30% of people who are 60 years or older have diverticula in the lining of the large intestine. The likelihood of diverticuli increases with age. The condition results from increased pressure inside the intestine, which is caused by a disorder of intestinal muscle function. Weakness in the bowel wall near blood vessels is another contributing factor.

Direct measurements of the speed with which substances are transported through the small intestine have not shown any age-related changes when people are not eating. However, on eating, elderly people show reduced intestinal muscle contractions. Because the food transport in the large intestine slows down, constipation is common. Subtle changes occur in the coordination of large intestinal muscle contractions. The number of certain narcotic (opiate) receptors increases with aging, and this increase may lead to significant constipation when narcotics are ingested.

The intestine's ability to absorb foods, as well as drugs, generally does not change significantly. Changes can occur in the metabolism and absorption of some sugars, calcium, and iron. Highly fat-soluble compounds such as vitamin A appear to be absorbed faster as age increases. The activity of some enzymes such as lactase, which helps in the digestion of some sugars (particularly those found in dairy products), appears to decline, but the levels of other enzymes remain normal. The absorption of fat may change, but this may relate more to changes in the pancreas and the digestive enzymes it produces rather than the ability of the intestine to absorb fat.

Liver and Pancreas

The liver decreases in size with age. The shape of the liver adjusts to the contours of adjacent organs. Aged liver cells contain increased lipofuscin pigment. Reductions occur in the smooth endoplasmic reticulum, mitochondria, and Golgi membrane. The mean volume of hepatocytes increases. There is reduced regenerative ability, possibly because of reduced protein and ribonucleic acid (RNA) synthesis. The most common structural change in the pancreas is acinar atrophy. High incidence of intralobular and interlobular fibrosis has been reported.

The liver and pancreas maintain adequate function throughout life; age-related hepatic or pancreatic failure does not occur. The P-450 microsomal oxidase and nicotinamide adenine dinucleotide phosphate (NADPH)–cytochrome *c* reductase systems of the liver decline in efficiency with age. Bilirubin excretion changes very little. Trypsin secretion is moderately decreased, but other pancreatic enzymes and bicarbonate production appear to be unchanged.

Renal Function

Renal mass decreases by 25% to 30% with age. Cortical loss predominates. A subset of nephrons with long loops of Henle are reduced. These nephrons, with glomeruli located in the inner third of the cortex, play a key role in producing concentrated urine. The number of glomeruli decreases; sclerosis occurs in up to 30% of those remaining. Glomeruli also show loss of capillary loops, decreased epithelial cells, and increased mesangial cells. The filtering surface is reduced. The renal basement membrane changes, with increased hydroxylation of amino acids and increased content of sugars. Interstitial fibrosis occurs in the renal pyramid. Diverticular changes in the distal tubule increase with age. Renal vascular changes include afferent arteriole spiraling and decreased size of arcuate and interlobular arteries. Loss of cortical nephrons increases medullary blood flow.

Cross-sectional and longitudinal studies of large populations have shown a steady age-related decline in creatinine clearance. Linear declines of 1% per year from age 40 to 90 have been determined, with recent evidence suggesting a steeper fall at very advanced ages. In some older persons studied for as long as 18 years, absolutely no fall in creatinine clearance was observed—a few showed an increase. The fall in glomerular filtration rate (GFR) leads to reduced renal clearance of some drugs and reduced urinary acidification. The abilities to maximally dilute and maximally concentrate urine are reduced to a greater extent than is GFR. The renin–angiotensin–aldosterone axis is poorly responsive to volume depletion in older people. The ability of older persons to retain sodium maximally under conditions of plasma volume contraction is also reduced. The ability of the aging kidney to metabolize various hormones, such as insulin, parathormone, calcitonin, and glucagon, has not been adequately studied. Changes in the production of erythropoietin have not been documented.

Hematopoietic Tissues

The hematopoietic tissues, such as the gut mucosa, have remarkable regenerative capacities, perhaps accounting for their maintenance with age. The normal values for red cell number and size, hemoglobin concentration, and hematocrit are essentially unchanged. The average life span of red blood cells remains constant, although red cells in older people may be more fragile. Blood volume is usually well maintained. The amount of active bone marrow diminishes with age and marrow fat increases. The functional reserve for hematopoiesis—the ability to accelerate the production of red blood cells—is reduced in older people, but the response to hemorrhage, although impaired, remains adequate.

Anemia, although common, is not a normal physiologic consequence of aging. It always has a cause other than age, most commonly malnutrition, blood loss, or presence of a malignancy. White cell and platelet numbers are unchanged with age. The function of neutrophils and mononuclear cells may be affected by aging. Healthy older people do not show defects in macrophages. Infection or bleeding leads to a brisk outpouring of neutrophils and platelets. Production and consumption of complements are decreased during infection.

The Implications of Age-Related Physiologic Changes

What are the general implications of these age-related physiologic changes? First, advancing age results in increasing differentiation and biologic uniqueness. As a result of this increasing differentiation over time, algorithmic approaches, clinical pathways, rigid guidelines, and other strategies of diagnostic investigation and resource allocation are likely to be less than optimal if they are based solely on age criteria. Health providers, clinical investigators, and health policy makers must recognize that this increasing variability assumes greater relevance with age.

The second implication of growing older is that biologic systems minimally affected by age are often profoundly influenced by socioeconomic status and lifestyle circumstances, such as cigarette smoking, physical activity, nutritional intake, and economic advantage. Although the precise mechanisms by which socioeconomic status and lifestyle factors induce physiologic changes are unknown, some exposures seem to accelerate physiologic aging. The potential interactions of environmental and physiologic conditions are shown in Figure 1.1. The upper curve represents the maximal potential performance for a given system, such as the musculoskeletal system or cardiovascular system. Ideally, this curve is almost horizontal, with minimal decrements in maximal performance over time. The position and slope of this curve may be affected by various environmental factors. For example, cigarette smoking in youth may reduce the optimal respiratory potential in later years. The lower curve represents the rate of atrophy when the system is at rest (never stressed). The system always functions at some point between the two curves. Because the curves diverge over time, three inferences are apparent. First, age-related physiologic changes are generally of a lesser magnitude than environmental and conditioning factors. Second, self-maintenance becomes more important as people age. In other words, the possibility of significant decline increases as a person ages. Finally, unless a person is in near optimal condition, advancing age suggests a greater chance for improvement. As a result, the prevalent pessimism about aging cannot be supported by the available evidence.

The third consequence of aging physiology is the prospect of living with diminishing resources with which to meet increasingly complicated environmental demands. The decline in functional reserve is often compounded by losses of social status, income, family support (e.g., death of a spouse), and self-esteem. Disease processes may reduce physical and mental capabilities. These changes in capacity may appear magnified by rapidly changing social expectations. For example, knowledge of computer systems and multiple communication platforms is becoming an increasingly important social skill. Computer literacy is a virtual prerequisite for many employment opportunities, regardless of the level of previous contributions. The complexity of changing social expectations may be especially problematic for persons who have developed a self-reliant lifestyle and self-image. In addition, some older persons may be victims of changes in the physical environment. Some neighborhoods, fashionable decades ago, may have deteriorated into high-crime areas.

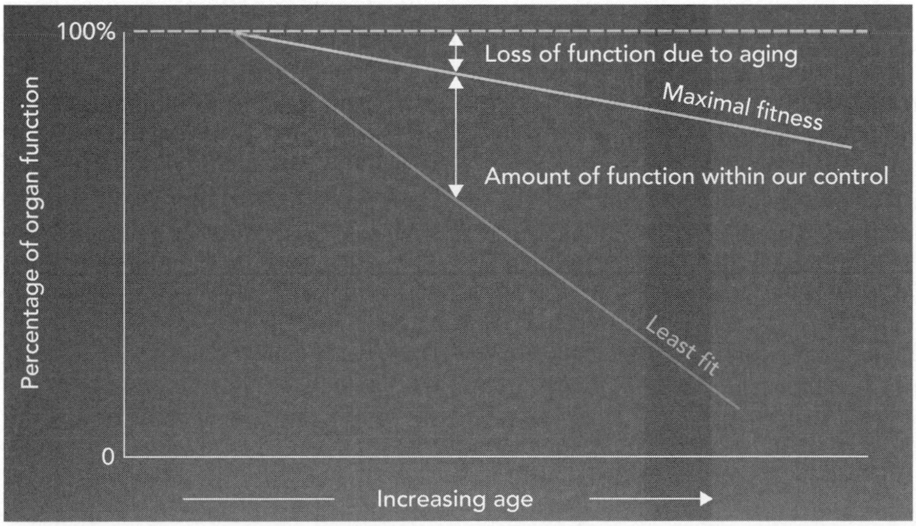

Figure 1.1 The effects of age on organ function.

PRESENTATION OF ILLNESS IN OLDER PERSONS

Three issues influence the presentation of disease in an older person: The underreporting of illness, changes in the patterns of illness, and altered responses to illness. A common myth is that older persons are hypochondriacal and frequently burden the health care system with trivial complaints. In fact, older people may underreport significant symptoms of illness. The reasons for underutilization of health care services by older persons may result from personal attitudes and social isolation. One prevalent attitude is ageism: The belief that all old people are the same and that they are falling apart. The manifestations of disease may be dismissed as age-related changes, leading people to say, "What do you expect at my age?" A second factor contributing to the underreporting of illness by older persons is the perception of an unresponsive system of care. This apparent unresponsiveness may take several forms, such as inconvenient office locations, inadequate parking facilities, abbreviated encounters with physicians, and apparently disinterested or discourteous health personnel. In the emergency room, older people are asked about their financial coverage before their chief complaint.

Depression is another factor limiting the desire in some older persons for interaction with the health care system. This condition reduces the desire for improvement—"What do I have to gain?" Depression is a significant geriatric illness because it is both prevalent and treatable. Denial, another reason suggested for the underreporting of illness by older persons, may result from fear of economic, social, or functional consequences. Economic fears may be justified because of the high cost of clinical encounters, especially for persons who have saved their resources without planning for unstable and unprecedented economic trends. A final relevant psychological factor is the isolation often experienced by many older persons. Isolation reduces opportunities for receiving reactions to personal appearance, state of health, ideas, or attitudes.

The second issue influencing the presentation of illness in some older persons is an altered pattern or distribution of illness. Some conditions such as hip fracture, Parkinson disease, or polymyalgia rheumatica are virtually confined to the later stages of life. In addition, some disease processes are more prevalent in old age. Examples of conditions with an increased prevalence in older persons include cardiovascular disorders, malignancy, malnutrition, myxedema, and tuberculosis. Because of these altered patterns of illness, the physician must understand the epidemiologic implications in the interpretation of various signs and symptoms. For example, jaundice, a sign often suggesting viral hepatitis in young people, usually results from gallbladder disease or malignancy in older persons.

The accumulation of multiple chronic disorders is another special feature of illness presentation in older persons. Four of every five older persons have at least one chronic illness. Symptoms of one condition may either exacerbate or mask symptoms of another, frequently complicating the clinical evaluation. For example, symptomatic arthritis may mask the expression of severe cardiovascular disease if a person, by limiting physical activity, does not stress the heart.

The third issue influencing presentation of disease is the altered response of older persons to illness, yet another dimension of geriatric health behaviors. A person's perception of illness may be modified by attitudinal factors, social factors, and changes in the sensory organs. Manifestations of clinically important disease may be attenuated in older persons, particularly in those who are frail and disabled. For example, angina pectoris may be absent or less dramatic in older persons with ischemic cardiac disease. A final factor relevant to the geriatric encounter is that symptoms in one organ system may reflect abnormalities in another. An acutely ill older person frequently presents with confusion, anorexia, urinary incontinence, unsteady gait (or the effects of a fall), or combinations of these symptoms and other symptoms. For example, an older person with a urinary tract infection may present with confusion and disorientation. Because of this nonspecific presentation of illness, the physician must exercise meticulous attention to expeditiously evaluate acute changes in an older person's health status.

CHANGES IN THE CLINICIAN'S PERSPECTIVE

How critical is it for the physician to determine the precise nature of the underlying disease when helping an elderly person cope with illness? Certainly, the quest to define the disease causing a person's distress is important when the disease is reversible, remediable, or both. Almost by definition, this search is not a dominant issue in the management of many chronic conditions, such as heart failure or chronic arthritides. Nonetheless, the clinical algorithm that mandates the initial "ruling out" of the remediable disease permeates clinical teaching and practice. Since the 17th century, the first principle of medical practice has been the mandate to define the one disease that underlies a patient's distress. Treatment directed at this underlying disease represents the most direct and effective way to alleviate symptoms. Despite the overwhelming success of this disease–illness paradigm, its limitations cannot be disregarded: Some features of illness (the manifestations or symptoms of distress) are independent of disease (the anatomic or physiologic derangement). Many diseases do not necessarily produce illness, and the quality of the illness may not be predictable from knowledge of the disease. For example, knowing the extent of disease in a patient with rheumatoid arthritis does not allow one to predict confidently the patient's capacity to work.

The search for reversible disease, although important, is a secondary issue in the management of chronic illness and may even be detrimental if the physician–patient relationship is predicated on uncovering reversible disease.

Three arguments that favor the precise determination of the underlying disease are particularly compelling: (i) Identifying the reversible or remediable disease is obviously rewarding, (ii) clinical uncertainty is thereby reduced, and (iii) accurate prognosis through an understanding of the condition's natural history should be useful. But do these arguments pertain to chronic illness in an elderly person?

The discovery of reversible disease in chronically ill elderly patients remains an important medical responsibility. However, this search for remediable disease should not be the only focus of the clinical encounter. If it is the focus, what is the basis of the doctor–patient relationship when all reversible diseases have been excluded? Contrary to the situation in acute illness, in which the expeditious discovery of remediable disease is an imperative, the search for reversible disease in chronically ill people can be pursued in a more leisurely manner. Most experienced physicians readily define and treat remediable conditions in their elderly patients. Often, iatrogenic problems (especially drug toxicities and unnecessary procedures) are identified as the reversible processes.

A disease-specific focus, however, de-emphasizes the dominant issue in the management of chronic illness, which is the maximization of the patient's productivity, creativity, well-being, and happiness. This goal of improving patient function and satisfaction to the utmost is usually achieved without curing the underlying disease.

The need to reduce clinical uncertainty, to leave no stone unturned, is another rationale for defining disease in the setting of chronic illness. A common argument is that a patient may be spared unnecessary diagnostic procedures once the underlying condition is totally defined. The decision about how far to proceed with the diagnostic evaluation is ultimately a joint contract between the patient and the physician. The benefit of a diagnostic procedure derives from the likelihood that it will yield meaningful information. In chronic illness in elderly people, the information meaningful for the definition of disease is elusive. Diagnostic tests are an exercise reflecting more the need to allay clinicians' anxiety than the need to resolve clinical uncertainty, and they are often counterproductive. If it is justifiable to make illness the primary concern of both participants, many diagnostic and screening tests become irrelevant.

The third argument for defining disease in chronically ill people is to allow accurate prognosis. Because prognosis generally involves estimating the remaining life span, its value is maximal in diseases that markedly influence longevity. For such diseases, prognostic estimates facilitate therapeutic decisions. For example, treatment regimens that are especially toxic or risky are usually reserved for circumstances in which longevity is immediately threatened. Small reductions in life expectancy are a less important concern in the management of chronic diseases and become nearly irrelevant for many elderly people. Even for some less chronic problems, many patients seem to prefer improved quality of life to extended life span.

Another factor that limits the utility and accuracy of prognostic estimates in geriatric patients relates to the constancy of the human life span. If the age at which patients have their first infirmity continues to increase, then the overall period of infirmity must decrease, assuming that life span remains constant. In view of this compressed morbidity, delaying the onset of progression of chronic illness becomes as important as curing the underlying chronic disease. Furthermore, most of the disability experienced by elderly people results from diseases (such as atherosclerosis, diabetes mellitus, osteoarthritis, or chronic obstructive pulmonary disease) that represent exaggerations of normal age-related physiologic decline, thereby raising them above a clinical threshold. Because the problem is one of rate, not of decline, a "cure" would require defining the determinants of the threshold. For example, what specific factors determine the clinical threshold above which a physician should prescribe medications for elderly patients with glucose intolerance? Does the maintenance of a euglycemic state or a normal hemoglobin A_{Ic} level with medications constitute a cure? Defining these threshold determinants and their relation to the quality of illness is a matter of some urgency. Otherwise, "prognosis" will continue to predict the number of chronic diseases at death—hardly an overriding patient concern. Even such a limited prognostic inference is confounded because elderly people manifest such wide biologic variability.

Understanding the difference between illness and disease is part of the treatment of elderly people, with function rather than disease as the focus. The effective physician appreciates that an increase in diagnostic capability does not substitute for care. And diagnostic efficiency does not necessarily improve the patient's quality of life or life expectancy. In fact, functioning can often be improved without knowledge of what disease the patient has, but knowledge of the illness can provide the necessary information. For example, treatment of urinary incontinence due to detrusor instability focuses on reduction of bladder contractions, increase of bladder capacity, and improvement of confidence and self-esteem. Treatment does not depend on knowing whether the bladder instability is due to brain trauma, cerebrovascular accidents, dementia caused by Alzheimer disease, or any other irreversible process. Knowledge of the illness, rather than the underlying disease, allows the physician to help the patient to a greater degree. When the patient is treated in this way, both physician and patient avoid the disappointment and frustration of not being able to define or cure the primary disease that underlies the illness of urinary incontinence.

When a diagnosis does need to be made, it can usually be done more effectively in the elderly patient by reversing the usual order of the diagnostic thought process. In younger patients, there are four basic parts to the diagnostic formulation: The first is etiology, which may range from bacteria to poverty; the second is anatomy (i.e., what would be seen if the patient's body were dissected today); the third is pathophysiology; and the fourth is the functioning of the patient. In elderly people, the key points remain the same, but the order of importance—the order in which these factors need to be considered—tends to be reversed. Functioning is the first step to consider.

THE IMPORTANCE OF FUNCTION

The ability to continue living independently is a critical issue for all elderly persons. Loss of this ability is a serious illness, which, in the United States, often leads to institutionalization. In some instances, the loss of independence is a manifestation of overt organ system dysfunction (such as severe heart failure), but this is an exception. Why should an elderly person with reasonably well-preserved visceral, mental, and musculoskeletal function be afflicted with the illness of loss of independence?

Manual dexterity, extensively validated in numerous studies, appears to be intimately and principally associated with the ability to live independently. Manual function is quantified by timing the performance of simple tasks (such as writing a sentence, opening a door, or stacking checkers). In one study, the least sensitive of the manual tasks surpassed any other traditional measure studied in terms of sensitivity, including a battery of standard assessments and findings on physical examination, in predicting disability. The quantification of manual inefficiency in elderly patients provides important information for making clinical decisions that relate to the probability that the patient will lose independence. This reference holds in spite of the enormous differences in other characteristics seen in groups of elderly people.

An important implication of these observations is that measurements of illness, when they are properly quantitated, are superior to strictly disease-oriented indices in defining certain health needs. Because of the ubiquity of chronic diseases and the lack of objective physiologic markers of aging, most geriatric assessments use measurements of disability (or illness). Even in the studies just described, no difference in pathoanatomic state (disease) could be discerned in the functioning of the rheumatologic, neurologic, ophthalmologic, or other organ systems. We do not know how to account for the difference in manual ability; yet, as a vital sign of functioning, the measurement reflects the risk of the loss of independence, and an impairment in hand function may even be responsible for this loss.

PERFORMING THE GERIATRIC ASSESSMENT

The assessment of the elderly person begins the moment the clinician sees the patient and continues until the clinical encounter is complete. We reveal ourselves to others through the choices that we make in our appearance, dress, language, and behaviors. Human choices are not random, so appreciating the nature of this self-expression can be very useful. Each of us is cultivating a "look." It is not a random event in the way we wear our hair, the fit of our clothing, what we choose to show off about ourselves, and the things we wish to hide. Incongruities in this self-presentation are important diagnostic clues and require further inquiry. The appreciation and identification of these incongruities is crucial to diagnosing dementing illnesses. In this regard, the clinical interview becomes the "physical examination" of the intellect. This section reviews a basic framework of the fundamental observations within each of the categories of appearance, dress, language, and behavior.

Appearance

The initial appreciation of a patient derives from an impression of his or her body in overview, as well as specific features of the individual's uniqueness. These identifying characteristics form the observational basis of a person's individuality and provide essential clues to the person's inner and outer state. A fundamental question is whether the patient looks acutely ill, chronically ill, or generally well. Does the apparent age (how old the patient looks) match the chronologic age (how many birthdays has the patient celebrated)? The apparent age may reflect overall health and well-being more accurately than the chronologic age. Some nonagenarians look decades younger than their years and their life expectancy seems to correlate with their apparent age. One *caveat* is that surgery or severe illness may cause such a young-appearing person to seem to age many years over just a few weeks.

An observant clinician notes the patient's body size, shape, and proportions. For example, is the patient overweight or are there signs of weight loss such as temporal wasting or, if more severe, loss of the buccal fat pad? Increases in abdominal fat may suggest a metabolic syndrome, with increased risk of diabetes mellitus and premature vascular disease. Skin findings may be obvious over the face, arms, legs, or other areas of exposed skin. Is there the pallor of anemia, the bronze tone of jaundice, the lemon yellow tint of pernicious anemia, the hyperpigmentation of Addison disease, the ruddy complexion of hypertension or alcoholism, or the ecchymosed arm of a recent fall or possible abuse?

Some diseases create specific appearances that in some circumstances allow the likely diagnosis to be made on sight. Reviewing the classic artwork of Dr. Frank Netter for conditions such as parkinsonism, myxedema, depression, acromegaly, and chronic lung disease can refresh your memory and sharpen your skills. Do not be in a rush to make a spot diagnosis. Our intent is to be accurate in appreciating the truth in the light of the moment—the reality of the patient's predicament.

Look carefully at the patient's overall habitus and posture. The hunched forward position of kyphosis reflects previous anterior vertebral compression fractures. The presence of assistive devices such as wheelchairs, canes, or walkers provides obvious clues of ambulation difficulty. Musculoskeletal deformities such as amputations, the arthritic changes of rheumatoid arthritis, the unilateral contractures of cerebrovascular disease, or the frontal bossing of Paget disease may be immediately visible.

Notice the presence of adventitious movements. Restlessness is a worrisome sign in a bedfast or nursing home patient and suggests delirium until proven otherwise. Virtually any medical condition is a potential cause of delirium, but the common factors to consider are drug toxicity, infection, metabolic disorder, or acute cardiac, pulmonary, or neurologic event. Alcohol or drug withdrawal is an underappreciated cause. Often, individuals in withdrawal will have damp feet. In addition to restlessness, any stereotypic limb movements such as tremor, chorea, or athetosis provide clues to the person's neurologic or behavioral status. Head bobbing from side to side suggests tricuspid insufficiency, whereas forward and backward bobbing (de Musset sign) reflects a wide pulse pressure, usually from aortic insufficiency. Occasionally, elderly people with severe behavioral problems or psychiatric illness will quietly rock back and forth in their chair.

The presence of makeup in an older woman generally implies well-being (or recent improvement if the patient has been ill). Care in the application implies functionally adequate vision and reasonable upper extremity motor coordination. Overapplication may reflect vanity and a strong desire to look much younger. Heavy eyebrow pencil may be an attempt to hide eyebrow hair loss perhaps due to hypothyroidism, systemic lupus erythematosus, syphilis, or heavy metal toxicity. The time of the last hairdo implies the last time an older woman felt reasonably well. Check the hair length to see how far the hair has grown (approximately 1.25 cm every 6 weeks). Perfume suggests well-being or is used for camouflage. If the patient is wearing nail polish, the distance from the cuticle to the line of polish gives the approximate date of application because nails grow approximately 0.1 mm per day. Picked at nail polish reflects nervousness and agitation. Toenail polish suggests unusual flexibility or a friendly helper.

Dress (Diagnostic Clues from Clothing)

Observing the older person's choice of clothing helps in appreciating his or her socioeconomic status, personality, culture, interests, and state of health. However, the interpretation must be circumspect: The clothing may have come from a second-hand store. Nonetheless, a disciplined observer can tell the affluent person who is trying to look less conspicuous by dressing down from the garments of a less economically advantaged elderly person. Incongruities should also be noted: An expensive but frayed suit could signify change in fortune.

Pay attention to the style and fit of the clothing. Check the belt for the amount and rate of weight gain or loss. A rule of thumb is approximately 7 kg per belt loop. The thickest dark black mark reflects the usual belt hole and fainter marks suggest more recent changes. Cerebral dominance can sometimes be inferred from the differential wear on the shirt cuffs, with the more worn, shiny texture indicating the dominant side. Bulges in shirt or pants pockets may give clues to the patient's personal mythology. Although it is not usually practical or appropriate to ask, it would be fascinating and quite revealing to observe what people choose to keep with them in their pockets, wallets, or purses. (What specific items do you keep with you? What is the personal significance of each item?) The person who shows up in the clinic wearing pajamas or a nightgown probably has a major chronic illness. If they also have a suitcase with them, they have been hospitalized in the past and are expecting to be hospitalized today.

Notice the patient's choice of clothing material and color. What basic statements are they making? Are they drawing attention to themselves or trying to blend in? Is the clothing trendy, flashy, tasteful, conservative, or practical? What economic status does the clothing reflect? What is being hidden and what is being revealed? The person who is totally covered up may have photosensitivity. Neck coverings such as a scarf or turtleneck outfit could be hiding a thyroidectomy or tracheostomy scar. What does the person feel comfortable in showing off about himself or herself? An elderly woman wearing a sweater on a hot summer day might have the cold intolerance or hypothyroidism, whereas an elderly man feeling comfortable wearing only a short sleeve cotton shirt to the clinic in the winter suggests an increased risk of hypothermia. Uniforms provide immediate inferences to the person's occupation and their value to the individual. Hobbies or special interests, such as fishing or Masonic membership, may be reflected on a necktie or tie tack. The elderly man wearing a Phi Beta Kappa tie is trying to tell you something.

Burns on clothing can reflect impaired mental status, inattention, or drug effect. A rosette of small round burns under the neck on the anterior chest (rosette sign) produced from cigarette ash falling onto the chest suggests a smoker with coexistent drug or alcohol abuse. Some occupations and hobbies requiring welding or soldering can increase the risk of burns on clothing.

The degree of fastidiousness is also important because people pay less attention to self-care when they are ill. Stains on clothing can be a clue to hobbies or occupation (e.g., painting or plastering) or poor hygiene (e.g., dirt, food, or body fluids). The absence of sweat in the presence of fever suggests anhidrosis. A fishy odor of sweat can be a sign of schizophrenia, uremia, zinc oxide, or excess fish oil supplementation. Sweat (or urine) that smells like violets raises the question of possible turpentine ingestion.

Stains on underclothing reflect general hygiene and state of health. Orange or red staining of undergarments suggests rifampin (could this person have tuberculosis?). The color of stool stains may be a clue to ingestion or illness, such as the light tan (acholic) color in liver disease. Darker than normal stool color suggests gastrointestinal bleeding (maroon, purplish black, or tarry) and ingestion of iron (greenish black), charcoal (coal black), and bismuth (dark gray black). Mineral oil ingestion produces an oily stain on undergarments because the anal sphincter cannot completely contain oil (although it can differentiate and contain solid, liquid, and gas).

Urine stains can come in a variety of colors, each with its own differential. Red urine can be a sign of hematuria, porphyria, phenolphthalein or aniline dyes, and ingestion of beets (this is called *beeturia* and is a sign of iron-deficiency anemia; the red beet pigment is transported across the gut wall by the iron transport system and is filtered by the kidneys). Dark brown urine suggests hemoglobinuria, myoglobinuria, methemoglobinuria, bilirubinuria, or ingestion of phenol, cresol, or phenhydrazine. Urine that turns black is a clue to alkaptonuria, while orange urine suggests that the patient is taking rifampin, senna, or pyridium. Bluish green urine is sometimes seen in *Pseudomonas* infection or on ingestion of methylene blue.

Shoes tell the story of their owner. Notice the coordination of the shoes with the rest of the clothing. The type of shoe is informative: Casual, work, walking, dressy, athletic, and so on. Are the shoes well cared for or is there a pattern of neglect?

If the patient is only wearing one shoe or if one shoe has an open toe consider gout, trauma, arthritis, or bunions. Shoes with no laces or laces that are undone imply significant edema, inflamed feet, or limited dexterity. The patterns of shoe wear also provide important information. Excess wear on the toe relative to the heel suggests foot drop. Differential wear on one side is seen in hemiparesis, leg length discrepancy, and scoliosis.

Ornaments are quite interesting reflections of our personality and interests. The amount and quality of jewelry reflects the taste and economic status of the owner. Rings can provide clues to education, age (calculate from class ring graduation year), clubs, organizations, and marital status (obviously not infallible). The absence of a ring heralded by a light-toned shiny band of skin at the base of a finger may suggest depression or suicide. A tight-fitting ring implies edema, whereas a loose, wrapped ring reflects weight loss. A black stain under a gold colored ring or necklace is a soft sign of diabetes mellitus.

Tie tacks, necklaces, earrings, pins, medallions, and key chains may indicate hobbies, clubs, education, profession, and religious beliefs. A person wearing a copper bracelet has arthritis and believes in talisman. Some people wear their Social Security Number on their jewelry. The first digit of the Social Security Number indicates the region of the United States from which the card was applied (first three digits indicate the state).

Language

Appearance and dress form the basis of our initial impressions of the patient and their general state of health. After this stage of static observations, a dynamic communication occurs between the physician and patient. Language is a major part of this interaction.

The first part of the language assessment is called *paralanguage*, which deals with the rate and delivery of speech. In essence, paralanguage addresses the manner of speech. How do the patients say what they say? The aphasia classification of fluency is based on paralanguage. The strength of a person's voice is a useful marker of overall "vitality." This concept can be especially helpful in assessing a familiar patient over the telephone. Illness seems to compromise the patient's voice projection, providing a clue to a change in his or her status. Paralanguage also addresses the speech rate, pitch, volume, degree of articulation, and quality of the delivery. For example, anxious individuals may speak at a rapid rate at a higher than normal pitch. Soft speech may be a clue to parkinsonism. Another aspect of paralanguage concerns pauses and pause intervals. The pause interval is the time from the end of your utterance to the beginning of the person's response. Normally, this interval varies on the basis of the content. Strong emotionally charged content tends to shorten the pause interval. Unfamiliar content lengthens the interval. If you were asked, "Give me a one-sentence summary of the second law of thermodynamics," there might be a pause. The importance of appreciating pause intervals is that if the pauses are always short we might consider hyperthyroidism, autonomic overactivity, or anxiety. Excessive pause intervals might signify depression, parkinsonism, medication effect, or myxedema.

Another component of language assessment is a general linguistic analysis. This is an analysis of the content of the communication. In other words, does the language make sense? The key question is "Are the thoughts complete?" Can the person communicate a coherent flow of concepts or ideas? Some individuals show digressions from the main theme of the conversation, digressing from the digressions, and never returning to the main point. We all know people who communicate this way, so a deviation from their normal communication pattern is more revealing than a stable communication pattern. Incomplete thoughts reflect more significant communication difficulty. Does the patient show awareness of the implications of answers (insight), anticipation of an answer, or evidence of abstract thinking? These would tend to show higher cortical function. Humor does not always indicate higher function unless it is spontaneous to the moment. Some very demented elderly people can relate extremely humorous stories from a well-practiced repertoire.

The linguistic analysis can become even more specialized. The person's choice of words may be a marker of intellectual vitality. The descriptive richness is revealed in colorful verbs and adjectives. The use of personal pronouns may mirror the emotional distance. For example, the use of the word "my" often indicates emotional closeness ("my doctor asked me to see you today"). The complexity of syntax also reflects overall education and mental capacity.

Specific content issues include evidence or examples of dysfunction, rate of progression, and the nature of adaptations. While evaluating mental status, it is useful to see whether the person can take a "mental walk" and use his or her imagination to provide spatial information. For example, "Mrs. Smith, if you met me at the front door of your house and you invited me inside, tell me what we would see." People with dementia have difficulty using their imagination and find this task extremely challenging. Context specificity refers to the concept that the boundaries of the answer are contained in the question. People with dementia may easily answer a question but not within the appropriate boundary. For example, "What specific plants did you plant in your garden?" "I planted annuals and perennials" is a few categories of abstraction removed from the intent of the question.

Behaviors

Observing behaviors is easy, but interpreting them is difficult. It is extremely easy to overly extrapolate behavioral observations. Nonetheless, some emotions are clearly revealed in gestures. Context is critical in interpreting behaviors. The overall harmony and congruence of the observations are the keys to understanding the meaning of a behavior. Contradictions (apparent incongruities) are very revealing. For example, a nervous laugh reflects both amusement and extreme discomfort.

The core of our emotional life is conveyed on the 25 square inches of the human face. Nothing is as well known as the subtle nuances of facial expression that ripple across the countenance like waves on the ocean. In fact, the change in expression reflecting an altered mood is very slight. Most details of facial expression primarily consist of eye and mouth expressions.

The Use of the Eyes

According to the mythologist Joseph Campbell, the 12th-century troubadours of Europe said "the eyes are the messengers of the heart—they search for what the heart seeks to possess." Eye movement sends a variety of emotion. For example, eyes that are downcast with the face turned away shows low self-esteem. Gaze aversion occurs if the topic makes one feel uncomfortable or guilty. If medical students are asked a question they think they should be able to answer but cannot, their eyes immediately look toward their feet. In grief, the brow is furrowed and the eyes are clenched. The eyes of depression sometimes view the world through partially closed lids: The eyebrows are always involved, often slightly raised and bent into an inverted "V." Raised eyebrows suggest disbelief, and the jaw muscles may tighten. A sideways glance reflects suspicion, uncertainty, or rejection. Frowns are easily recognized as signs of displeasure or confusion.

Normally, there is eye contact during 30% to 60% of a conversation. Limited eye contact implies that the person is hiding something, perhaps a sense of low self-esteem. Eye contact increases if one feels defensive, aggressive, or hostile. Excessive eye contact (over 60%) implies that the person is interested in the other person more than the subject of the conversation (the extremes are lovers and fighters).

Abstract thinkers seem to have more eye contact than concrete thinkers. Perhaps they have a better ability to integrate information and are less distracted by eye contact. Eye contact with a slight one-sided smile means that the person is weighing your actions.

If the lower eyelid rises, it shows plainly that the person is not sure they believe what you are telling them. If the lower lid, in addition to being raised, is brought in toward the nose, it indicates frank disbelief. If your message is not registering, the upper lid will be lowered and the eyeball will be slightly raised to meet it. If the upper lid completely covers the iris to the pupil of the eye, the patient's mind is sluggish. If the upper lid covers the top half of the pupil, it indicates the patient is indifferent. When the pupil is exposed by the upper lid coming down only to the top edge of pupil, the patient is interested and attentive. If the upper lid covers half the width of the top arc of the iris, the mind is very attentive—if the upper lid touches the edge of the iris, it is a positive indication that the mind is very attentive, but feelings have been aroused. Proptosis suggests hyperthyroidism. More specific eye observations are covered elsewhere.

The Mouth and Smile

The mouth also clearly transmits the inner state of the person. In sadness or depression, the mouth is often stretched and the lip margins may be thinned. The mouth tends to show anger by being tightly compressed. An open mouth with clenched teeth and tightly drawn eyes suggests significant pain.

Interpreting smiles is a useful skill to cultivate. The simple smile is open and relaxed, with the mouth pulled up toward the ear and the eyes slightly closed with a tight lower lid. False smiles tend to be less relaxed with eyes that are open and the corners of the mouth moved lateral rather than up toward the ear. This smile is polite but has no depth or sense of sincerity.

Arm and Hand Movements

Arm and hand movements are another core element of behavior. Gestures are hand signals that send visual signs of openness, doubt, frustration, inner conflict, and self-esteem. For example, a clinched fist shows determination or aggression. A broad scissors movement (resembling a basketball referee's call of "no basket") suggests "no way." Finger pointing is assertive. Palm movements also convey useful information. A hard karate chop onto an open palm suggests a desire to cut through a problem. Holding both palms up is often a sign that implores for agreement, whereas having both palms down is a restraining gesture for people to remain cool headed. Palms facing directly ahead as if stopping traffic are front-repelling and signify protest. Palms with the back facing ahead are embracing, and reflect a comfort seeker. Sidewise palms (like a hand shake) while talking suggest a desire for negotiation.

Open hands signal sincerity, openness, and pride as does unbuttoning the coat. Arms crossed on chest can be a sign of defensiveness or simply a posture of comfort. One useful clue is to check the hands to see if they are relaxed or fistlike? Standing with hands on hips implies readiness or dedication.

Placing the hand to the cheek with the forefinger pointing reflects the patient's critical evaluation. Chin stroking is a sign of consideration or that the patient is making a judgment. Pinching the bridge of the nose (usually with closed eyes) indicates great concern and thought over the decision. Nose twitching is a sign of doubt or negation (beware—sometimes a nose itches, but you can tell the difference). The hand covering the mouth suggests astonishment, self-doubt, or deceit.

There are several gestures that reflect signs of frustration. For example, arms spread while hands grip the edge of the table is a posture demanding attention. Sitting with the hand on the occiput with the head bowed down is another reflection of inner frustration. As mentioned in the preceding text, a fist is a clue to determination, extreme emphasis, or anger. Tugging at the ear reflects a desire to interrupt.

Signs of inner conflict include perspiration that may indicate nervousness, infection or a withdrawal syndrome, or hand pinching and fidgeting. These fidgeting gestures imply a need for reassurance. Finger gestures such as thumb sucking, nail biting, or picking at the cuticle or nail polish convey anxieties, inner conflicts, and apprehensions. Tightly clenched hands show an intense inner tension, as does hand wringing. A pointed finger says, "look there" and is often used to reprimand, admonish, discipline, or to drive home a point. Gripping the wrists suggests needing self-control; they reflect putting on the brakes.

Signs of low self-esteem include placing the palm to the back of the neck; this is a defensive, bending posture. On the other hand, steepling the fingers as if in prayer reflects confidence and self-control. The hand height when steepling if high can show a proud, smug demeanor.

Sitting and Standing Postures

Sitting on the edge of the chair implies readiness and a person who is action oriented. The patient who sits leaning back with crossed legs and making a kicking movement reflects an inner boredom and impatience. A patient (or more commonly a family member) sitting with their leg over the arm of the chair signals indifference and an uncooperative attitude. A family member sitting with the chair back to their chest is a sign of dominance or aggression. Leaning back with hands supporting the head signals a sense of superiority, whereas fidgeting implies nervousness. The patient who sits tugging at his or her pants suggests that decision-making is in process. Sitting with locked ankles signals inner tension and significant stress. On the other hand, sitting with the hands at the back of the neck, leaning back, with a straight posture and the shins out suggests authority and self-confidence.

Standing postures are also very revealing to the observant physician. The pace, stride length, and posture signal the emotions and overall vitality. Frail individuals tend to walk slower and without the usual rhythmic cadence of a healthy person's gait. A rapid walk with free hand swing means that the person is goal oriented and used to pursuing objectives. Walking with one's hands always in their pockets suggests a person who is secretive, critical, and enjoys playing the role of a devil's advocate. The elderly person who scuffles with his or her head down signals dejection. Individuals who walk with their hands on their hips denote sudden bursts of energy. These individuals are sprinters rather than long-distance runners. Walking with one's hands behind the back with head bowed and at a slow pace shows that one is preoccupied. Persons who walk with their chin raised, arm swing exaggerated, and legs stiff reflect self-satisfaction and pomposity.

Finally, there are some miscellaneous behaviors that can be seen frequently in the clinical setting. The head tilted to the side is often an attempt at persuasion. Moving close to speak confidentially can be an aggressive gesture that is used to dominate or direct. Short breaths can signify respiratory distress or general frustration. "Tsk, tsk" implies frustration or disgust, whereas rapid jerky movements reflect nervousness. "Whew" suggests relief, and frequent throat clearing reflects nervousness. Jingling money in pockets may show preoccupations.

SUMMARY

The approach to the medical evaluation of elderly persons requires a perspective different from that needed for younger persons. The spectrum of complaints is different, the manifestations of distress more subtle, the implications for function more important, and improvements sometimes less dramatic and slower to appear. The differential diagnosis of various problems is often different. Presentations are frequently nonspecific (i.e., mental status changes, behavioral changes, urinary incontinence, gait disturbance, or weight loss). The crucial issue is the elderly person's ability to function. Understanding the difference between illness and disease is a prerequisite to the care of patients affected by incurable disorders. Educated palliation in the absence of substantive information about this discrepancy is the art of medicine. Because elderly patients often present with several chronic diseases, many of which are irreversible, cure-oriented physicians are especially vulnerable to frequent disappointments. More importantly, although many chronic conditions are incurable, the discomfort or disability they produce may be substantially modified. If this concept is not realized and addressed, elderly patients with irreversible chronic diseases may receive less than optimal care from physicians seeking cures. The degree to which we, as physicians, can assist chronically ill people reflects our understanding of human discomfort and our sensitivity to personal distress. If we maintain a purely disease-specific focus, we may have difficulty thinking about strategies to best serve the patient. Defining pathologic entities may be less complicated than intervening in the illness of the patient, but the latter constitutes healing.

SELECTED READING

Fitzgerald F. The bedside Sherlock Holmes. *West J Med.* 1982;137:169–175.

Jones TV, Williams ME. Rethinking the approach to evaluating mental functioning of older adults: The value of careful observations. *J Am Geriatr Soc.* 1988;36:1128–1134.

Williams ME. Clinical implications of aging physiology. *Am J Med.* 1984;76:1049–1053.

Williams ME. Geriatric assessment. *Ann Intern Med.* 1986;104:720–721.

Williams ME. *The American Geriatrics Society's complete guide to aging & health.* New York, NY: Harmony Books; 1995:494.

Williams ME. Clinical evaluation of the elderly patient. In: Hazzard WR, Bierman EL, Blass JP, et al. eds. *Principles of geriatric medicine and gerontology,* 4th ed. New York, NY: MacGraw-Hill; 1999

Williams ME. Sherlock Holmes at the bedside: The case of the missing patient. *J Am Geriatr Soc.* 2003;51:1813.

Principles of Care for Older Persons

2

Mudanai Sabapathy *Bruce J. Naughton*

CLINICAL PEARLS 18

ORGANIZATION OF CARE 19
Ambulatory Care 19
Care in the Hospital 19
Care in the Long-term Care Facility 19

TRANSITIONS IN CARE 20

COMMON COMPLICATIONS 20
Delirium 20
Medication Management 20
Infections 22
Pneumonia 24
Constipation 25
Pressure Ulcers 25

FUNCTIONAL DECLINE AND REHABILITATION 25

PALLIATIVE CARE AND END OF LIFE CARE 26

CLINICAL PEARLS

- Chronic disease management and prevention of functional impairment are major goals of elder care across delivery sites.
- Interdisciplinary comprehensive assessment and long-term interdisciplinary management improve outcomes.
- Implement systems to improve safety across sites of care.
- Recognize delirium as a major adverse event in an acute illness.
- Reduce adverse drug events and polypharmacy.
- Avoid treatment of asymptomatic bacteriuria.
- Treat pneumonia at home and in the nursing home when possible.
- Anticipate functional decline during acute illness.
- Establish indications for palliative care early and review the indications following a significant change in clinical condition.
- Learn to recognize symptoms of dying.

CASE: PART ONE

An 85-year-old woman is transferred from a nursing home to the emergency department (ED) with drowsiness and increased confusion. The patient has a history of stroke, hypertension, angina, type 2 diabetes mellitus, and osteoarthritis. She is on multiple medications. She normally ambulates with a two-wheeled walker and is dependent in several activities of daily living (ADLs). She was at her baseline the day prior to the ED visit but was found to be lethargic and incontinent of urine on the morning of admission. She was not able to ambulate and refused her breakfast.

Chronic diseases and functional impairment are major challenges in the care of the older patient. Patients aged 75 years and older are different from the young, both in terms of physiology and the frequent presence of multiple comorbidities. Among older patients, acute illness is often an acute exacerbation of one or more underlying chronic conditions. Stabilization, relief of symptoms, preservation and/or restoration of function, and prevention of recurrences are the primary aims of treatment in the older adult, regardless of whether care is provided at home, in the hospital, or at the nursing home.

In general, for patients older than 75 years with cognitive and/or functional impairment and for patients with multiple chronic illnesses, the principles of management of acute illness and chronic conditions are similar. Care is directed toward preventing exacerbations, maintaining function, and providing good pain control while avoiding adverse drug effects, infections, and injury.

Evaluation of symptoms in older adults involves the recognition that different illnesses may present with similar symptoms. For example, the episode of delirium described in the above clinical vignette has many potential etiologies, including infection, cardiovascular events, adverse drug effects, constipation, and dehydration. Evaluation should begin with an understanding of the patient's baseline functional status, a detailed history, and a thorough physical examination. Particular attention should be paid to the patient's medication list and medications that may be bought over the counter. Older individuals often take several vitamin and herbal supplements, and side effects from such medications should be considered when evaluating the patient's symptoms.

Programs or efforts that begin with a detailed assessment of the older patient's medical, functional, cognitive, and social status and address acute and chronic issues concurrently have been shown to improve outcomes.[1–4] Outcome measures must include the patient's values and goals. For example, older patients by themselves or through a health care proxy may choose to forego artificial nutrition and hydration or other forms of treatment when faced with a heavy burden of chronic illness and advancing age.

ORGANIZATION OF CARE

Ambulatory Care

A primary care approach combining an initial interdisciplinary, comprehensive assessment with long-term interdisciplinary outpatient management has been shown to improve outcomes for targeted older adults.[5] The assessment involves physical, psychosocial, and environmental factors that impact on the well-being and function of older individuals. The use of an organized approach employing objective measurements helps target key areas of functional status. Evaluation areas include ADLs, cognition, mood, social supports, gait and falls, nutrition, sensory impairments, incontinence, polypharmacy, elder abuse, pressure sores, pain, and advance directives.[6]

A primary care clinician who organizes and coordinates outpatient care that meets the complex needs of functionally impaired older adults may achieve outcomes similar to those of an interdisciplinary team. In these cases, the care plan inevitably includes services delivered by an *ad hoc* multidisciplinary team. Geriatric assessment centers have been developed to implement preorganized interdisciplinary teams and enhance traditional primary care management.

Care in the Hospital

Hospital programs have embraced the patient-centered care model. These models include intensive review of medical care with a view to minimizing the adverse effects of procedures and medications. They have established protocols for prevention of disability and for early rehabilitation. Hospital programs implement discharge planning early in the admission to develop a continuum of care plan. Taken together, these interventions reduce the incidence of delirium, lower the frequency of discharge to institutions for long-term care, and reduce health care costs.[1,2,4] Some programs use geographically defined units with specialized personnel. Others have enhanced the training of existing hospital personnel who serve patients meeting the criteria throughout the hospital.

In some facilities, a practitioner can order geriatric hospital services for at-risk older adults during hospitalization as a holistic service. Alternatively, the practitioner may act more independently, applying the principles of careful medication management and medical procedure review to minimize adverse outcomes, and ordering specialty services such as physical therapy as needed. Either pattern may reduce functional loss and the length of hospital stay if implemented with input from social workers and rehabilitation services.

Care in the Long-term Care Facility

Long-term care residents are usually dependent in three or more ADLs and have one or more sources of disability, such as Alzheimer disease, multi-infarct dementia, stroke, chronic heart disease, chronic obstructive pulmonary disease (COPD), and osteoarthritis. Care is multidisciplinary, involving the collaboration of physicians, nurses, nursing aides, physical therapists, speech therapists, occupational therapists, and social workers.

The federal Medicare program requires a physician to see the nursing home resident at least once every 30 days for the first 90 days after admission and at least once every 60 days thereafter. Physician visits may be alternated with visits by a nurse practitioner. Because the physician may see the patient infrequently, a Minimum Data Set (MDS) has been developed to help the nursing staff recognize and evaluate common clinical syndromes that occur in nursing home residents. Certain answers on the MDS trigger the use of resident assessment protocols (RAPs) to facilitate nursing staff-to-physician communication about clinical issues.[7]

Many nursing homes do not have daily attendance by a physician and depend upon telephone contact with a physician. As a result, physician orders are frequently given over the telephone. Many facilities use nurse-driven guidelines or protocols for common acute illnesses such as pneumonia. This standardization reduces medication error and the need to hospitalize patients for management of many acute illness episodes. Regular presence of a nurse practitioner or a physician assistant provides support to the nursing staff and families while promoting management of acute illnesses in the nursing home.

TRANSITIONS IN CARE

CASE: PART TWO

While in the emergency room the patient developed fever. Urinalysis was positive for nitrite and leukocyte esterase, and microscopic evaluation revealed many bacteria and white cells. Chest x-ray was negative and a complete blood count showed significant leukocytosis. After urine and blood cultures were obtained, the patient received one dose of IV ceftriaxone. Shortly after the administration of ceftriaxone, the patient developed a maculopapular rash on the chest and back.

Exchange of information between care settings is vital for patient safety and to prevent complications arising from poor coordination of clinical services. This interface is called *transitional care*. Transitional care is a set of actions designed to ensure the coordination and continuity of health care as patients are transferred between different care settings. In the absence of coordination, care must be provided without full knowledge of the problems addressed, services provided, medications prescribed, or preferences expressed by the patient in the previous setting.[8] Poorly executed care transitions result in medication errors[9] and failure to address the primary purpose of a transfer. In the above case, the nursing home was aware of the allergy to ceftriaxone, but failure to convey the information led to an avoidable hospital admission.

Concise information on diagnosis, allergies, and medication management is vital for safe and efficient transition of care. Transitional care may be improved by keeping the patient and caregiver informed and using advanced practice nurses.[10] Care pathways and protocols, integration of acute and long-term care,[11] identification of patients at risk for complications and poor outcomes,[8] and electronic medical records can improve transitional care.

COMMON COMPLICATIONS

Delirium

Delirium is the most common complication of acute hospitalization among older adults. Delirium is a marker for increased morbidity, mortality, and functional decline as well as prolonged hospital stays and increased costs. Approximately 50% of older adults who experience delirium during hospitalization are already delirious upon presentation to the ED. Therefore efforts to prevent delirium depend on whether the patient is at home, in a nursing home, or in the hospital.

Age and preexisting cognitive impairment are two important and easily identified risk factors for delirium. Other risk factors include poor premorbid functional status, visual and hearing impairment, and Parkinson disease. Features of delirium include acute onset, fluctuating course, inattention, plus disorganized thinking and/or altered level of consciousness.[12] Inattention, a hallmark of delirium, can be assessed by asking the patient to say the days of the week backwards.

Acute illnesses associated with fever, such as pneumonia or urinary tract infections (UTIs), and conditions that cause hypoxia, such as COPD or congestive heart failure, are major precipitants of delirium.[13] Other preventable precipitants include medications, particularly polypharmacy, pain, urinary retention, fecal impaction, and dehydration. Benzodiazepines, narcotics and anticholinergic medications including tricyclic antidepressants, medications for urinary incontinence, and antihistamines are commonly associated with delirium.

Delirium in the Hospital

A comprehensive and systematic approach to preventing delirium has been shown to reduce the rate of the incidence and prevalence of delirium.[14] (see Table 2.1) Delirium prevention programs are associated with an overall improvement in ADLs, immobility, dehydration, and cognitive status.[14] For patients aged 65 years and older admitted to an orthopaedic surgery service with hip fracture, a routine geriatric consultation focused on discontinuation of medications known to precipitate delirium, early mobilization, and removal of Foley catheters significantly reduced postoperative delirium. Another trial focused on avoiding the use of benzodiazepines and anticholinergic medications also found a significant reduction in the hospital rate of delirium.[15]

Delirium Outside the Hospital

These principles may also be applied in the home and at a skilled nursing facility. Particular emphasis on avoiding medications known to precipitate delirium reduces the incidence of delirium. The need for hospitalization and length of stay may also be reduced if medications associated with delirium are promptly stopped or significantly reduced should delirium occur (see Table 2.2).

Medication Management

Adverse Drug Events at Home

Older adults are at increased risk for, and experience a disproportionate amount of, adverse drug events. Sound medication management is a fundamental tenet of good geriatric medicine practice. In all settings, medication lists should be reviewed at each contact with an eye toward

TABLE 2.1
DELIRIUM/BEHAVIOR ASSESSMENT AND INTERVENTION

Part I: RN's initial screen	Part II: Intervention (Interdisciplinary)
Mental status evaluation ■ Cognitive impairment ■ Delirium Review assessment with physician Precipitating factors: ■ Pain ■ Fecal impaction ■ Acute medical illness: • Dehydration (BUN/creatinine ratio >18) • Urinary tract infection • Pneumonia • Stroke • Fracture • Postoperative state • Foley catheter • Restraints Environmental stimuli (noise, sleep disruption, disruptive roommate): ■ Avoid benzodiazepines ■ Avoid anticholinergics ■ Simplify pain regimen (minimize p.r.n) ■ Consider synergistic agents (such as neuroleptics or antidepressants that supplement behavior treatment) Review with physician evidences of psychosis: ■ Hallucinations ("I see those children") ■ Delusions ("This is a nice hotel") ■ Paranoia ("That medicine is poison")	Implement Behavior Measurement Scale For delirious patients or individuals with reports of behavior disturbances: Record all categories of behavior that occur during each shift for first 24 h postadmission 1. Treat underlying medical factors 2. Treat precipitating factors: • Remove precipitating medications • Immobility 3. Provide family support 4. Use nonpharmacological intervention for: • Physically nonaggressive behavior • Episodes triggered with ADL care

RN, registered nurse; BUN, blood urea nitrogen; ADL, activities of daily living.
From Naughton BJ, Saltzman S, Ramadan F, et al. A multifactorial intervention to reduce prevalence of delirium and shorten hospital length of stay. *J Am Geriatr Soc.* 2005;53(1):18–23.

limiting medications to those that have specific indications and are essential to address immediate acute and underlying chronic conditions. Medication dosage should be adjusted to the individual's conditions, remembering that failure to adjust for age-associated changes in renal function is a common source of error. See Table 2.3 for commonly used medications to be avoided in older adults with specific diagnoses. Pharmacists can provide valuable support in making dosage adjustments.

Cardiovascular medications including antihypertensives, central nervous system (CNS) medications, antibiotics, diuretics, and nonopioid medications are commonly implicated.[16,17] Preventable events include inappropriate choice of drugs, drug interactions, or drug allergy.[18] Patients suffer needlessly from adverse effects of medications if they do not, or cannot, report symptoms or when physicians ignore the patient's complaints about symptoms. Strategies include developing educational materials for patients, using translation services, and increasing patients' access to outpatient pharmacists to discuss medications and side effects. Home health care agencies should collect data on all the medications used, prescription and nonprescription.[19]

Adverse Drug Events in the Hospital

Hospitalization often results in the addition of medications to combat a growing list of comorbidities. In fact, some studies that have controlled for comorbidities, age, and multiple medications have found comorbidity to be a stronger predictor of adverse events than age.[20] For example, an adult with preexisting cognitive impairment and parkinsonism is at a much higher risk for developing delirium when a psychotropic medication is administered, than is a patient of similar age without those comorbidities.

Allergic reactions with itching, nausea, and vomiting are the most frequent events associated with antibiotics.[21] The next most common adverse events are hepatic and renal toxicity followed by cardiovascular effects expressed as bradycardia, hypotension, and arrhythmia. CNS effects,

TABLE 2.2
MEDICATIONS ASSOCIATED WITH DELIRIUM

Prescription Drugs	Over-the-Counter Medications and Complementary/Alternative Medications
■ Central-acting agents: a. Sedative hypnotics (benzodiazepines) b. Anticonvulsants (barbiturates) c. Antiparkinsonian agents (benztropine, trihexyphenidyl) ■ Analgesics: a. Narcotics (meperidine) b. Nonsteroidal anti-inflammatory drugs ■ Antihistamines (hydroxyzine) ■ Gastrointestinal agents: a. Antispasmodics b. H_2 blockers ■ Antinauseants: a. Scopolamine b. Dimenhydrinate ■ Antibiotics: a. Fluoroquinolones ■ Psychotropic medications: a. Tricyclic antidepressants b. Lithium ■ Cardiac medications: a. Antiarrhythmics b. Digitalis c. Antihypertensives (β-blockers, methyldopa) 1. Miscellaneous: a. Skeletal muscle relaxants b. Steroids	■ Antihistamines (diphenhydramine, chlorpheniramine) ■ Antinauseants (dimenhydrinate, scopolamine) ■ Liquid medications containing alcohol ■ Mandrake ■ Henbane ■ Jimson weed ■ *Atropa belladonna* extract

From Alagiakrishnan K, Wiens CA. An approach to drug-induced delirium in the elderly. *Postgrad Med J.* 2004; 80(945):388–93.

usually sedation and confusion, account for another 10% of adverse events.[21]

Dosing errors (overdosing and underdosing) account for nearly 60% of prescribing errors.[22] Prescribing medications in spite of a known allergy accounts for another 16% of errors.[22] The factor most commonly associated with medication error is failure to account for a pathophysiologic state (heart failure or renal insufficiency) or condition (advanced age) that requires dosage adjustment.[23]

Adverse Drug Events in the Nursing Home

Nursing home residents typically suffer from multiple medical problems. They undergo long-term drug treatment, with weakening physiologic reserve. Aging-related pharmacokinetic and pharmacodynamic changes increase the risk of adverse drug reactions. Nursing home patients commonly receive long-term medications associated with adverse effects, including narcotics, antihistamines with strong anticholinergic effects, sedatives/hypnotics, gastrointestinal/antispasmodic agents, antidepressants, platelet inhibitors, and iron supplements.[24] The medication list should be regularly reviewed by the physician and pharmacist to minimize errors, particularly whenever there is a change in the functional status.

The transition of care from the nursing home to the hospital and back is a particularly vulnerable time. Changes to medications should be highlighted and explicit reasons for starting new medications or discontinuing existing medications should be provided.

Infections

Urinary Tract Infections

UTI is the most frequent bacterial infection in residents of long-term care facilities. Ninety percent of uncomplicated UTIs are caused by uropathogenic strains of *Escherichia coli*. Enterobacteriaceae, such as *Klebsiella, Enterobacter*, and *Proteus; Pseudomonas*; gram-positive bacteria, such as *Staphylococcus saprophyticus* and *Enterococcus* also cause UTIs. *Staphylococcus aureus* in the urine may indicate hematogenous seeding and an occult systemic infection. Candiduria may indicate the presence of immunosuppression,

TABLE 2.3

COMMONLY USED MEDICATIONS TO BE AVOIDED IN OLDER ADULTS WITH SPECIFIC DIAGNOSES

Diagnosis	Avoid
Anorexia/weight loss	Fluoxetine Digoxin >0.125 mg/d
Benign prostate hyperplasia Overflow incontinence	Oxybutynin (Ditropan) Tolterodine (Detrol) Decongestants (pseudoephedrine) Anticholinergic drugs (hydroxyzine, TCAs)
Congestive heart failure	NSAIDs TCAs Pioglitazone and rosiglitazone Metformin
Cognitive impairment	Anticholinergic drugs (diphenhydramine [Benadryl], oxybutynin [Ditropan]) Muscle relaxants Benzodiazepines
Chronic renal failure	Enoxaparin Fondaparinux Propoxyphene ACE inhibitors NSAIDs COX-2 inhibitors Potassium supplements Spironolactone Metformin Chlorpropamide
Essential hypertension (first-line treatment)	Verapamil α-Blockers Clonidine Verapamil/diltiazem combined with β-Blockers
Falls	Diuretics administered at bedtime Benzodiazepines TCAs Conventional antipsychotic drugs Muscle relaxants
Hiatal hernia Reflux disease Iron deficiency anemia Receiving warfarin	Alendronate and risedronate NSAIDs Iron ($FeSO_4$) >325 mg/d NSAIDs COX-2 inhibitors Aspirin

TCAs, tricyclic antidepressants; NSAIDs, nonsteroidal anti-inflammatory drugs; ACE, angiotensin-converting enzyme; COX-2, cyclooxygenase-2.
Adapted from Ramadan F, Masoodi N. Commonly used medications to avoid in adults with specific diagnoses. *Pharmacol Geriatr Ser.*

obstruction, or neutropenia. Symptomatic infection is a frequent cause of morbidity and hospital transfer. External drainage systems in men with incontinence double the frequency of UTI.

However, there is a high prevalence of asymptomatic bacteriuria in long-term care facilities, ranging between 15% to 30% among men and 25% to 50% among women. Asymptomatic bacteriuria is associated with chronic illnesses, impaired bladder function, and incontinence interventions. The greater the functional impairment, including dementia, the more likely the patient is to have asymptomatic bacteriuria. Those with chronic indwelling catheters are always bacteriuric.

As a result, UTI is significantly overdiagnosed and overtreated in this population. Many older individuals have urine cultures positive for bacteria at any time and there is substantial diagnostic difficulty in differentiating symptomatic from asymptomatic infection in the elderly.

Clinical deterioration without localizing findings and nonspecific symptoms such as anorexia, malaise, fatigue, or weakness are frequently misinterpreted as UTI in the presence of a culture positive for infection.[25] The resulting use of antimicrobials contributes to the high prevalence of resistance in nursing homes.

One exception to a policy of withholding antibiotics for asymptomatic infections is the *Proteus* species. Patients with *Proteus* bacteria should be treated because of the organisms' propensity to induce formation of urinary stones.[26] Otherwise, antimicrobial treatment of asymptomatic bacteriuria does not decrease symptomatic infection or improve survival. Antibiotics are associated with increased adverse effects, emergence of resistant organisms, and increased cost.

Pneumonia

Pneumonia at Home

Community-acquired pneumonia is the fifth leading cause of death in people older than 65 years in the United States. *Streptococcus pneumoniae* is the most frequent cause followed by *Haemophilus influenzae*. Pneumonia due to gram-negative bacilli occurs in patients with debility, prior use of antibiotics, decreased activity, diabetes, alcoholism, and incontinence. Older adults are also at greater risk of infection with group B streptococci, *Moraxella catarrhalis*, and *Legionella* species, although the incidence is low.[27] Elderly patients may present with nonspecific symptoms. They have a lower frequency of pleuritic chest pain, in addition to absence of fever, less pronounced rales, and altered mental status. All adults older than 65 years should receive polyvalent pneumococcal vaccine.[28]

Pneumonia in the Hospital

Hospital-acquired pneumonia remains a major cause of mortality and morbidity in older adults. Risk factors include severe acute or chronic illnesses, malnutrition, prolonged hospitalization, cigarette smoking, alcoholism, and COPD. Also, treatments with cytotoxics and corticosteroids, antacids and histamine type 2 blockers, nasogastric tubes, mechanical ventilation, and sedation alter host defenses.[29]

Hospital-acquired pneumonia in the first 4 days of hospitalization is often due to community-acquired pathogens such as *S. pneumoniae* or *H. influenzae*. In contrast, hospital-acquired pneumonia after 5 days is more often caused by aerobic gram-negative bacilli or methicillin-resistant *Staphylococcus aureus* (MRSA). Prior broad-spectrum antibiotic use is a risk factor for colonization or infection with *P. aeruginosa*, *Acinetobacter*, MRSA, and other resistant bacteria.[27] Empiric treatment of late-onset hospital-acquired pneumonia should include antipseudomonal agents until *P. aeruginosa* is excluded as the causative agent.

Pneumonia in the Nursing Home

Pneumonia is a leading cause of morbidity, hospitalization, and mortality among the elderly living in nursing homes. Silent aspiration, poor functional status, nasogastric feeding, swallowing difficulties, confusion, the presence of obstructive lung disease, tracheostomy, and advancing age are risk factors. *S. pneumoniae* remains the predominant cause followed by *H. influenzae* and *M. catarrhalis*.[28,29] Nursing home residents with pneumonia can be treated successfully in the nursing home (Evidence Level A).[30,31] Guidelines have been formulated to assist the provider in selecting oral or parenteral antibiotics for the treatment of nursing home–acquired pneumonia.[32]

Hospitalization has only a marginal effect on immediate survival, even when residents are severely ill. It has no effect on immediate or 2-month mortality among those less severely ill, but hospitalization is associated with a substantial decline in the functional status. The presence of nurse practitioners or physician assistants in the skilled nursing facility has been associated with prompt treatment and a reduced need for hospitalization.[32]

Clostridium difficile Diarrhea

Clostridium difficile is the most commonly diagnosed cause of infectious hospital-acquired diarrhea. Nursing home patients are at particularly high risk of colonization with *C. difficile* because of frequent antibiotic administration, frequent hospitalizations and nosocomial exposure, and age.[33] Nursing home residents with diarrhea should therefore be tested for *C. difficile* toxin in the stools, particularly after antibiotics or hospitalization.

The spectrum of disease caused by *C. difficile* ranges from asymptomatic colonization to severe pseudomembranous colitis and occasional bowel perforation and death. The term *Clostridium difficile*–associated diarrhea (CDAD) is used to describe symptomatic manifestations of the disease. Most of these patients have been exposed to antimicrobials that reduce normal colon bacteria and "colonization resistance" of the large intestine. As a result, *C. difficile* becomes dominant. Whether colonization progresses to disease is determined by age, comorbidities, and other factors that are as yet unknown.

The ability of *C. difficile* to form spores that are resistant to many disinfectants allows it to remain viable in the environment for long periods. The incidence of CDAD has increased dramatically with the use of third-generation cephalosporins and other broad-spectrum antibiotics. CDAD prolongs hospital stays and increases health care costs.[34] The incidence of CDAD is reduced by careful selection of specific antibiotics, hand washing by health care workers, and room and instrument cleaning.

Recurrent CDAD may be experienced by patients both at home or in the nursing home. Prompt recognition and treatment can prevent rehospitalization. It is recognized by the presence of recurrent diarrhea with leukocytosis and is more common after community-acquired *C. difficile* infection or in the presence of chronic renal failure. Approaches to prolonged treatment (6 weeks) include the use of pulsed doses of vancomycin (125 mg every other day to keep *C. difficile* in the spore state yet with minimal effects on normal fecal flora), the administration of anion-exchange resins to absorb *C. difficile* toxin (such as 4 g of cholestyramine three times daily), or the use of agents to antagonize *C. difficile* (such as *Saccharomyces boulardii* or *Lactobacillus* strain GG) (Evidence Level B).[35]

Constipation

Constipation is common among older adults. Defecatory problems not only cause discomfort and anxiety but also are major contributors to delirium, urinary retention, intestinal obstruction, and sigmoid volvulus. Constipation may cause fever and leukocytosis, and increase the risk of perforation of the colon secondary to ischemic necrosis.

Periodic objective assessment for constipation in adults should be incorporated into routine nursing and medical care. This is particularly important in patients unable to report symptoms because of cognitive or communication difficulties, older adults on medications such as anticholinergic drugs, opiates, and calcium and iron supplements, and those with impaired mobility.

Pressure Ulcers

Pressure ulcers are among the most common adverse events to occur among hospital and nursing home patients. The prevalence of pressure ulcers among hospitalized patients varies from 3% to 11%, the highest rates among medical and surgical intensive care unit (ICU) patients. The incidence of pressure ulcer development among nursing home residents increases with the length of stay in a facility. More than 20% of residents develop a pressure ulcer after 2 years in a nursing home.

Typically, deep pressure ulcers begin as superficial stage II lesions, which deteriorate over weeks. However, some of the most severe pressure ulcers occur as a result of pressure-related deep tissue damage causing subcutaneous necrosis under normal-appearing skin. The latter are seen over the heels and sacrum and are evident 12 to 24 hours after a precipitating event. The extent of necrosis may not be apparent until 2 to 3 weeks after transfer from the hospital to the nursing home, when an ulcer that had appeared to be stage II suddenly becomes a stage III or IV ulcer.[36]

Intrinsic risk factors leading to pressure ulcers include age >75 years, age-related skin changes, limited mobility, neuropathy (diabetes and spinal cord injury), dementia, or coma. Bowel or bladder incontinence provides a source of moisture and bacterial contamination that promotes skin breakdown. Poor nutritional status compounds the problem because patients are unable to meet the increased metabolic demands of wound healing.

Pressure is the most important extrinsic factor. Patients who are seated or bedridden for extended periods are prone to the development of pressure-induced skin damage. Friction and shearing forces occur as a patient is repositioned in bed or transferred from the bed to a wheelchair. Patients elevated at an angle of 30 degrees or more are particularly susceptible to shearing force damage.[37]

Therefore, interventions to prevent pressure injury include mobilization, repositioning, and the use of pressure management devices. Even in the critical care setting, mobility should be encouraged through range of motion exercises, physical therapy for strengthening and transfers, and occupational therapy interventions to prevent loss of mobility and function.

Interventions to reduce shear damage include moisturizing the skin to decrease the surface tension; using draw sheets, lift sheets, or transfer aids to assist in moving patients; and maintaining the head of the bed at below 30 degrees–Fowler position. The latter can be difficult in patients with respiratory impairment or who are at risk for aspiration. These patients would be considered at greater risk for shearing force damage and should have their sacrococcygeal area monitored more closely for skin breakdown.[38]

FUNCTIONAL DECLINE AND REHABILITATION

Sarcopenia, the loss of muscle mass with age, results in diminished strength and contributes to falls, injury, and loss of independence. Deconditioning, particularly common after an acute illness, superimposed on sarcopenia further decreases functional capacity. A multidisciplinary assessment should be done following an acute illness for risk of falls, mobility and balance, independence with ADLs and instrumental ADLs, and cognitive function. This evaluation determines the rehabilitation plan, including where care is best provided.

Hospital-at-home models have been developed as a means of providing acute hospital-level care in the home. These models may reduce the incidence of adverse events associated with acute illness among older adults, including functional decline.[39]

However, rehabilitation to functional status is one of the more common unmet needs among community-dwelling older adults. A ready transition to rehabilitation services shortens the disability period and the length of hospital stay. Rehabilitation may be provided at home, at a skilled nursing facility, or at the hospital. Social resources and the intensity of service required determine the site for rehabilitation care. The rehabilitation care should include an evaluation of the patient's functional needs, medication review and adjustment, home safety assessment, and discharge planning tailored to persistent functional impairment.

PALLIATIVE CARE AND END OF LIFE CARE

> **CASE: PART THREE**
>
> The patient was switched to levofloxacin. The infection responded to treatment with resolution of leukocytosis and fever. A repeat urinalysis was negative for infection. However, the patient developed delirium and had poor oral intake. The patient's premorbid condition included advanced dementia. She had issued advance directives indicating that she would want palliative care instead of life-prolonging treatment once the diagnosis of advanced dementia was established. Palliative care was initiated after discussion with the health care proxy, and she died peacefully 7 days after admission.

Palliative care should begin at home or in the nursing home and be thought out before the patient is transferred to the hospital. If transferred to an emergency room or hospital, advance directives should receive respectful priority. Failure to recognize the appropriateness of palliative care and to communicate the indication for palliative care to the family is a major barrier in providing care for patients at the end of life.

Palliative care aims to relieve the suffering and improve the quality of life of patients with advanced illnesses. Palliative care skills include communication with patients and family members; management of pain or other symptoms; psychosocial, spiritual, and bereavement support; and coordination of an array of medical and social services. Palliative care can and should be offered simultaneously with other medical treatments.[40]

Physicians should be alert to the signs of impending death. As patients get near to death they become increasingly weary, weak, and sleepy. They become less interested in getting out of bed or receiving visitors and disinterested in things happening around them, occasionally with features of agitated anguish. Few of these features will be new ones. However, what should suggest to the clinician that the terminal phase is starting is that most of the above become evident at the same time.[41]

Signs of impending death include audible retained respiratory secretions (death rattle), respirations with mandibular movement (jaw movement increases with breathing), cyanosis of extremities, and no radial pulse.[42] Pain management should continue, if indicated, and the family should be informed of the natural process being expressed.

REFERENCES

1. Applegate WB, Miller ST, Graney MJ, et al. A randomized, controlled trial of a geriatric assessment unit in a community rehabilitation hospital. *N Engl J Med.* 1990;322(22):1572–1578.
2. Reuben DM, Borok GM, Wolde-Tsadik G, et al. A randomized trial of comprehensive geriatric assessment in the care of hospitalized patients. *N Engl J Med.* 1995;332(20):1345–1350.
3. Naughton BJ, Saltzman S, Priore R, et al. Using admission characteristics to predict return to the community from a post-acute geriatric evaluation and management unit. *J Am Geriatr Soc.* 1999;47:1100–1104.
4. Landefeld CS, Palmer RM, Kresevic DM, et al. A randomized trial of care in a hospital medical unit especially designed to improve the functional outcomes of acutely ill older patients. *N Engl J Med.* 1995;332(20):1338–1344.
5. Burns R, Nichols LO, Martindale-Adams J, et al. Interdisciplinary geriatric primary care evaluation and management: Two-year outcomes. *J Am Geriatr Soc.* 2000;48(1):8–13.
6. Devons CAJ. Comprehensive geriatric assessment: Making the most of the years. *Curr Opin Clin Nutr Metab Care.* 2002;5:19–24.
7. Elon RD. Omnibus budget reconciliation act of 1987 and its implications for the medical director. *Clin Geriatr Med.* 1995;11(3):419–432.
8. Coleman EA. Falling through the cracks: Challenges and opportunities for improving transitional care for persons with continuous complex care needs. *J Am Geriatr Soc.* 2003;51(4):549–555.
9. Boockvar K, Fishman E, Kyriacou CK, et al. Adverse events due to discontinuations in drug use and dose changes in patients transferred between acute and long-term care facilities. *Arch Intern Med.* 2004;164(5):545–550.
10. Naylor M, Brooten D, Campbell R, et al. Comprehensive discharge planning and home followup of hospitalized elders: A randomized clinical trial. *JAMA.* 1999;281:613–620.
11. Eng C, Pedulla J, Eleazer G. Program for All-inclusive Care for the Elderly (PACE): An innovative model of integrative geriatric care and financing. *J Am Geriatr Soc.* 1997;45:223–232.
12. Inouye SK, van Dyck CH, Alessi CA, et al. Clarifying confusion: The confusion assessment method, a new method for detection of delirium. *Ann Intern Med.* 1990;113:941–948.
13. Rummans TA, Evans JM, Krahn LE, et al. Delirium in elderly patients: Evaluation and management. *Mayo Clin Proc.* 1995;70(10):989–998.
14. Inouye SK. A practical program for preventing delirium in hospitalized elderly patients. *Cleve Clin J Med.* 2004;71(11):890–896.
15. Naughton BJ, Saltzman S, Ramadan F, et al. A multifactorial intervention to reduce prevalence of delirium and shorten hospital length of stay. *J Am Geriatr Soc.* 2005;53(1):18–23.
16. Hanlon JT, Schmader KE, Koronkowski MJ, et al. Adverse drug events in high risk older outpatients. *J Am Geriatr Soc.* 1997;45(8):945–948.
17. Gurwitz JH, Field TS, Harrold LR, et al. Incidence and preventability of adverse drug events among older patients in the ambulatory setting. *JAMA.* 2003;289(9):1107–1116.
18. Meredith S, Feldman PH, Frey D, et al. Possible medication errors in home healthcare patients. *J Am Geriatr Soc.* 2001;49(6): 719–724.
19. Lau DT, Kasper JD, Potter DE, et al. Hospitalization and death associated with potentially inappropriate medication prescriptions among elderly nursing home residents. *Arch Intern Med.* 2005;165(1):68–74.
20. Bates DW, Miller EB, Cullen DJ, et al. Patient risk factors for adverse drug events in hospitalized patients. *Arch Intern Med.* 1999;159(21):2553–2560.
21. Kanjanarat P, Winterstein AG, Johns TE, et al. Nature of preventable adverse drug events in hospitals: A literature review. *Am J Health Syst Pharm.* 2003;60(17):1750–1759.
22. Lapointe NM, Jollis JG, Medication errors in hospitalized cardiovascular patients. *Arch Intern Med.* 2003;163(12):1461–1466.
23. Lesar TS, Briceland L, Stein DS, et al. Factors related to errors in medication prescribing. *JAMA.* 1997;277(4):312–317.
24. McMurdo ME, Gillespie ND. Urinary tract infection in old age: Over-diagnosed and over-treated. *Age Ageing.* 2000;29(4): 297–298, UI: 10985436
25. Nicolle LE. Urinary tract infection in geriatric and institutionalized patients. [Review] [19 refs]. *Curr Opin Urol.* 2002;12(1):51–55, UI: 11753134
26. Mandell GL, Bennett JE, Dolin R, et al. *Principles and practice of infectious diseases,* 6th ed. Vol. I, Elsevier Science; 2005:832,835–836.
27. Lynch JP III. Hospital-acquired pneumonia: Risk factors, microbiology and treatment. *Chest.* 2001;119(2):373s–384s.
28. Loeb M. Pneumonia in the Elderly. *Curr Opin Infect Dis.* 2004; 17(2):127–130.

29. Schwartz DB. Hospital acquired pneumonia—evolving knowledge. *Curr Opin Pulm Med.* 2004;10(suppl 1):S9–S13.
30. Mylotte JM, Naughton B, Saludades C, et al. Validation and application of the pneumonia prognosis index to nursing home residents with pneumonia. *J Am Geriatr Soc.* 1998;46(12):1538–1544.
31. Naughton BJ, Mylotte JM, Ramadan F, et al. Antibiotic use, hospital admissions, and mortality before and after implementing guidelines for nursing home-acquired pneumonia. *J Am Geriatr Soc.* 2001;49(8):1020–1024.
32. Naughton BJ, Mylotte JM. Treatment guideline for nursing home-acquired pneumonia based on community practice. *J Am Geriatr Soc.* 2000;48(1):82–88.
33. Thomas DR, Bennett RG, Laughon BE, et al. Postantibiotic colonization with clostridium difficile in nursing home patients. *J Am Geriatr Soc.* 1990;38(4):415–420.
34. Wilcox MH, Cunnliffe JG, Trundle C, et al. Financial burden of hospital acquired clostridium difficile infection. *J Hosp Infect.* 1996;34:23–30.
35. Bartlett JG. Clinical practice. Antibiotic-associated diarrhea. *N Engl J Med.* 2002;346(5):334–339.
36. Bennett RG, O'Sullivan J, DeVito EM, et al. The increasing medical malpractice risk related to pressure ulcers in the United States. *J Am Geriatr Soc.* 2000;48(1):73–81.
37. Cannon BC, Cannon JP. Management of pressure ulcers. *Am J Health Syst Pharm.* 2004;61(18):1895–1905; quiz 1906–7.
38. Arnold MC. Pressure ulcer prevention and management: The current evidence for care. *AACN Clin Issues.* 2003;14(4):411–428.
39. Leff B, Burton L, Guido S, et al. Home hospital program: A pilot study. *J Am Geriatr Soc.* 1999;47(6):697–702.
40. Morrison RS, Meier DE. Clinical practice. Palliative care. *N Engl J Med.* 2004;350(25):2582–2590.
41. Furst CJ, Doyle D. The terminal phase. *Oxford textbook of palliative medicine*, 3rd ed. Oxford University Press; 2003:1119–1133.
42. Morita T, Ichiki T, Tsunoda J, et al. A prospective study on the dying process in terminally ill cancer patients. *Am J Hosp Palliat Care.* 1998;15:217–222.

Office-Based Caregiver Support

3

Jane Marie Thibault ***James G. O'Brien***

- CLINICAL PEARLS 28
- INTRODUCTION: WHY SHOULD PHYSICIANS BE CONCERNED ABOUT CAREGIVERS? 29
- DEMOGRAPHICS OF CAREGIVING: WHO ARE CAREGIVERS? WHAT ARE THEIR CHARACTERISTICS? 30
- STYLES OF CAREGIVING 30
- EFFECTS OF CAREGIVING: WHAT HAPPENS TO HEALTH? 30
- CAREGIVING RESEARCH: WHAT DOES IT INDICATE? 31
- INTERVENTION: HOW CAN THE CAREGIVER'S BURDEN BE REDUCED? 31
- WHAT IS THE PHYSICIAN'S ROLE? 32
- ANGER 36
- WHAT RESOURCES ARE AVAILABLE TO THE PHYSICIAN? 36
- SUMMARY 38

CLINICAL PEARLS

- All patients should be asked, "Do you have caregiving responsibilities for someone who is chronically ill or disabled?"
- Persons who accompany patients to an office visit should be asked, "What caregiving services do you provide for my patient?"
- To help caregivers realize the effects of caregiving on their health, invite them to complete a "Caregiver Self-assessment Questionnaire."
- Have readily available in your office local, state, and national resources related to aging and caring for older adults.
- Encourage caregivers to join a caregiver support group.
- Develop a professional referral network of local geriatric social workers and counselors, the Alzheimer's Association, and the local Agency on Aging.
- Enable caregivers to realize that they are an essential part of your patient's health care team.

Fading Memory

My friend sits in the corner.
In reverie, he is reminiscing with his past
Trying to find his way through a vast
Wasteland with few remaining markers.

It is hard watching the lights of cognition
go out, one by one, breaking our connection.
He is leaving me, his mind slipping away from
our reality, back toward the security of the womb.

While the threads, holding him within my world,
Gradually unravel, is his mind truly blank?
Or is he slowly entering the Elysian Fields with
A new existence that he cannot share with me?

John I. Coe
The Pharos/Summer, 2004[1]

INTRODUCTION: WHY SHOULD PHYSICIANS BE CONCERNED ABOUT CAREGIVERS?

The health care delivery system is increasingly dependent on family and other volunteer caregivers to provide a variety of services to ill and frail elders (see Table 3.1). Although they are trained to assume responsibility for individual patients,[2] physicians are discovering that they are increasingly called upon to interact with caregivers of older adults in two significant ways. First, physicians who care for older adults, especially frail elders, often find themselves actively involved in communicating with, supporting, and instructing their patients' caregivers, recognizing and supervising them as a significant (yet often unacknowledged) part of the health care team. Second, primary care clinicians frequently treat midlife and older adult patients who have assumed responsibilities for the care of ill elders and are subjected to the documented stresses of the caregiving situation.

Whether the person is the physician's patient or the relative of the patient, the physician has a vested interest in helping the caregiver stay physically and emotionally healthy throughout the period for which he or she has caregiving duties.

The "vested interest" lies in the fact that caregivers play a significant role in the medical care of ill elders, especially those with dementia.[3] Because of caregivers' proximity to their patients, often living in the same home, physicians depend on them to observe and report patients' change over time—for diagnostic, treatment, and management purposes. Caregivers are increasingly required to implement, oversee, supervise, and assist with medical interventions such as administering medication, including injections; providing wound care; monitoring blood sugar levels; arranging transportation for medical visits; and providing personal care, all of which are not covered by medical insurance.

Providing daily care for another, in addition to working outside the home and/or managing his or her own life, involves a great deal of extra, time-consuming work, which can create a "dual life" for the caregiver. This dual life, which is often very stressful, can have negative effects on the caregiver's physical and emotional health. Inevitably, when a caregiver's health declines and the ability to care for the patient fails, the latter will be negatively affected. Ham et al. state, "The good caregiver can be the therapeutic tool to maintain optimal function despite (patient) disability. The challenge is to ensure that the caregiver is operating optimally and that the more dependent phase of the patient's illness can be postponed for as long as possible."[4]

In an attempt to meet the challenge of caring for the caregiver, the American Psychiatric Association, the American Association for Geriatric Psychiatry, The American Geriatrics Society, and the American Medical Association (AMA), have developed guidelines and recommendations for working with caregivers, especially for those caring for persons with dementia.[5] These guidelines are sorely needed because the older population's need for care is rising steadily. Statistics indicate that as the population of people aged 65 and older expands, the prevalence of functional disability and the need for help in the performance of activities of daily living also increases.[6] Most of the help required is provided by informal caregivers—family members, friends, and neighbors who offer primarily voluntary services to frail and chronically ill older adults living in the community. Their numbers are significant and growing. As long ago as 1988, a Duke University survey of 602 randomly selected family practice patients aged 40 years and older found that 25% (153) of the patients had caregiving responsibilities for noninstitutionalized relatives.[7]

In contrast with the responsibility for provision of normal child care, which decreases over time and is generally planned and expected, the combination of

TABLE 3.1

CHARACTERISTICS OF THOSE PROVIDING INFORMAL CARE FOR OLDER ADULTS (NATIONAL CENTER FOR CAREGIVING, 2004)

Characteristic	Percentage (%) Unless Noted
Average age	46 y
Female gender	75
Ethnicity	
Asian American	32
African American	29
Hispanic American	27
Whites	24
Caregiver's relationship	
Daughter	26.6
Other female relative	17.5
Son	14.7
Wife	13.4
Husband	10.0
Other male relative	8.6
Other female nonrelative	5.7
Other male nonrelative	1.8
Care for	
Parents	38
Spouses	11
Nonrelative	15–24
Employed full- or part-time	66
Duration of assistance	
1–4 y	Most
>5 y	20
Average time spent caring for a person aged 65+ y	20 h per wk
Caregivers spending >40 h per wk in caregiving role	20
Persons with dementia cared for at home by family members	67–75
Workers in United States with elder care responsibilities	25

increasing dependency of the ill elder and caregiving situations may last over many years, and are unplanned and at times unexpected. As a result, caregiving to elders can engender greater stress and spark stress-related disorders. Behavioral problems and incontinence of the patient; the strenuous physical labor involved in bathing, ambulating, dressing, and feeding; increased housework; sleep deprivation; the need to defer personal goals; financial difficulties; and family conflicts about care are just a few of the most common stressors experienced by care providers. Additionally, anticipation of increasing burden as the patient's frailty increases is a negative factor. Because caregiving affects both physical and mental health, investigators recommend that "providers should routinely ask about caregiving responsibilities when taking a middle-aged or older individual's medical history."[7]

Frequently those offering help are elderly themselves—women and men who have needs of their own, which they often neglect.

Schulz and Beach, coinvestigators of the Caregiver Health Effects Study, have found that "family caregivers perform an important service for society and their relatives... at considerable cost to themselves.... Some caregivers are at increased risk for serious illness. ... Caregivers who report strain associated with caregiving are more likely to die than noncaregiving controls."[8] Informal caregivers often experience and describe their own health as being poorer than that of their noncaregiving peers.[9] Almost all the studies on caregivers' mental health indicate that they experience a higher level of depressive symptoms than persons not involved in care.

DEMOGRAPHICS OF CAREGIVING: WHO ARE CAREGIVERS? WHAT ARE THEIR CHARACTERISTICS?

Long-term care may be defined as the provision of services that are required over an extended period, usually lasting for the remainder of a person's life. Until the middle of the 20th century, most long-term care services were provided by family members. With the enactment of the Medicare and Medicaid programs in the mid-1960s, the expanded funding for health care needs of older adults enabled the development of a variety of institutional modes of care. The current continuum of long-term care comprises informal and formal home-based services; adult day care; assisted living facilities; personal, intermediate, and skilled nursing home care; and hospice care. Because of the availability of such a variety of formal services, there may be an impression that most older adults are cared for either in institutional settings or in their own homes by professional aides or health care providers.

This is not the case. Informal caregivers continue to provide an enormous proportion of caregiving services, especially for patients in the early and middle stages of chronic illness. According to the statistics compiled by the Family Caregiver Alliance of the National Center for Caregiving (2004),[10] there are approximately 1.6 million persons living in 17,000 nursing homes in the United States. In the community, however, there are approximately 52 million informal and family caregivers providing services to individuals aged 20 and older who are ill or disabled.

When caregiving responsibilities are sequential, duties may continue for many years, especially for women. For example, after providing years of service to her ill father, a daughter may then have to care for her mother as she becomes frail, after which she may care for her in-laws and then her ill husband.

STYLES OF CAREGIVING

Caregivers may be characterized by the quality of their association with the person(s) for whom they are providing care. The fact that a person is designated a caregiver by the patient does not mean that she or he is providing good or even adequate care. Unfortunately, although they are in the minority, poor or even abusive caregivers exist. On a continuum of quality of involvement, caregivers may be classified as follows:

1. Fully engaged caregivers in partnership with the patient and health care team
2. Adequate caregivers
3. Providers of minimal care
4. Noncooperative caregivers
5. Neglectful caregivers
6. Overinvolved caregivers
7. Abusive caregivers
8. Seriously ill or heavily burdened caregivers (who are, themselves, a focus of concern).

It is essential that the physicians consider the baseline quality of service that a caregiver can reasonably provide. They must also keep in mind that the capacity to provide care can fluctuate with the person's biopsychosocial and employment situations and demands.

EFFECTS OF CAREGIVING: WHAT HAPPENS TO HEALTH?

Persons who provide services to older adults may experience both satisfaction and burden in their efforts to give care. Much of the early research focused on the concept of burden, which refers to "the physical, psychological or emotional, social, and financial problems that can be experienced by family members caring for impaired older adults."[11] The gathering evidence, in addition to the knowledge of prominent national figures who have succumbed to Alzheimer disease, such as President Reagan and actor

Kirk Douglas, have made the negative effects of caregiving so widely known that a survey of >1,000 adults sponsored by the Alzheimer's Association in October 2004, revealed that "Americans are as afraid of becoming an Alzheimer caregiver as they are of getting the disease itself."[12] The results of this survey led to the proposal of S. 2533/H.R. 4595 to the 108th Congress. Known as the *Ronald Reagan Alzheimer's Breakthrough Act of 2004*, this act will provide assistance and tax relief to caregivers if passed.[13]

CAREGIVING RESEARCH: WHAT DOES IT INDICATE?

The significance of caregiver burden, the measurement of its correlates, and the development of interventions to ameliorate burden have been subjects of gerontological research for more than a quarter of a century. As early as 1979, labeling spouses of disabled elderly men as *hidden patients*, Fengler and Goodrich warned that the process of caregiving placed the caregiver at risk for impairment of physical, emotional, and social well-being.[14]

Evidence strongly suggests that caregiver burden has dramatic negative effects on various aspects of health and that older caregivers are more negatively affected than younger ones.[15] The previously mentioned Caregiver Health Effects Study investigated the impact of caregiving on elderly spouses. Results showed that caregiver participants who experienced strain had mortality risks that were 63% higher than those not experiencing strain or in noncaregiving control group situations. Although some of the caregiver situations included recipients with dementing disorders, dementia caregiving was not the primary focus in this study. Results of other studies indicate that caring for persons with dementing diseases causes even more strain on the caregiver. The most common symptoms of caregiver strain include anxiety, depression, greater use of psychotropic medication, and a negative self-rating of physical health.[4]

A longitudinal study of 86 caregivers and 95 comparison participants found that persons caring for patients with a high degree of behavioral disturbance and/or for those who were admitted to long-term care facilities experienced greater deterioration in their emotional and physical health status than control participants did.[16] A Swedish study designed to investigate the consequences of living with a demented person found that spouses, not children, suffered from the highest levels of stress.[17]

A 13-month study comparing 69 spousal caregivers of demented elders with a matched, noncaregiving sample found that caregivers showed decline on three different measures of cellular immunity. Clinically, the caregivers reported increased instances of upper respiratory infections. The caregivers with the lowest levels of social support and those who were most disturbed by behavioral disturbances suffered the most negative effects in immune function.[18]

In general, disruptive problem behaviors have been found to cause more caregiver stress than either cognitive or functional impairment. A study of the total impact of specific problem behaviors of demented elders on caregiving found that the reactions of caregivers to disruptive behaviors were correlated with the caregivers' deterioration of physical and mental health and loss of financial resources.[19] However, the specific manner in which caregivers react to or cope with these behaviors may differ, causing them to experience greater or lesser stress. Some caregivers appear to adapt over time, whereas others succumb to the stress.[9]

INTERVENTION: HOW CAN THE CAREGIVER'S BURDEN BE REDUCED?

Research indicates that effective interventions for the relief from burden include (i) assessment of levels of both burden and satisfaction, (ii) provision of information to the caregiver, and (iii) skills training. The key to developing effective interventions is knowing what causes a particular caregiver's feelings of burden. In a classic study of the correlates of feelings of burden, Zarit et al. found that frequent visits from other family members to the ill elder eased the caregiver's feelings of burden, even in situations of extensive cognitive impairment, behavior problems, functional disabilities, and long duration of illness (Evidence Level A).[20] Gottlieb and Wolfe critically reviewed 17 empirical studies that connected the coping styles of caregivers of persons with dementia to caregiver health and morale.[21] Seven studies found that poor mental health in caregivers was related to the use of "wishfulness and fantasy" as their primary coping mechanism.

Two types of coping styles were associated with positive mental health—"acceptance coping" and "practical problem solving." In "acceptance coping," caregivers resign themselves to the reality of the situation and waste no energy wishing that the reality were other than it is. This allows them to focus their energy on the person and on caregiving tasks. "Practical problem solving," which is also called *instrumental coping response* involves the ability to accomplish daily caregiving and self-care tasks with competence and even creativity. Acceptance coping, which was defined as a positive emotion-focused strategy, was associated with positive mental health in three studies. Practical problem solving or instrumental coping responses were found in four studies (Evidence Level B).

These simple approaches are well within the supportive and instructional domain of the physician. One of the best ways a physician can help a caregiver is to refer the caregiver to the Alzheimer's Association or a similar support group. Most groups are both educational and supportive. Observing others in a similar situation and sharing caregiving strategies enable the caregiver to relinquish unrealistic fantasies and hopes for cure and feel less emotionally isolated. Some Alzheimer's Associations provide mock "prescription" pads with their telephone numbers and meeting schedules to physicians so that they may write a formal prescription to attend a support group meeting. Also, treating the caregiver as part of the patient's health care "team" can afford opportunities for the physician to encourage creative responses to difficult caregiving situations (Evidence Level C).

A recent study of the effects of the caregiving environment on survival time of the care recipient included quality of caregiver, health and presence of depression, spousal relationship, and caregiver coping styles as environmental variables. The only correlation found was that between specific caregiver coping styles and survival time of the care recipient with Alzheimer disease.[22] Caregiver wishfulness–intrapsychic coping (i.e., anticipating a miracle, daydreaming, fantasizing, and attempting to change their feelings about their situation) and instrumental and acceptance coping (i.e., engaging in specific, behavior-based problem-solving techniques and realistic acceptance of the caregiving situation) were the predominant styles. When compared with the previously mentioned caregiver variables, wishfulness–intrapsychic coping was associated with shorter care-recipient survival time. Instrumental and acceptance coping had no effect on survival time.

In light of the above findings, McClendon et al.[22] suggest that interventions should promote the reduction of wishfulness–intrapsychic approaches to coping because these behaviors may be detrimental to care recipients. Kitwood summarizes the recommendations more simply by stating that the effective and satisfied caregiver is able to "be with the care receiver in his or her world, rather than doing things to or for the care receiver."[23] Wishfulness coping pulls the caregiver away from the recipient emotionally. The caregiver who copes with the stress of the situation by engaging in escapist fantasy or wishful thinking refuses to allow herself or himself to enter the "world" of the person with dementia, reducing the former's psychological availability to the recipient. Emotional distancing may result in caregiving that is unresponsive to the recipient's physical, emotional, and social needs and that depersonalizes the recipient—a situation that may result in "excess disability,"[24] early placement in a nursing home, and/or ultimately decreased survival time.

One example of a promising intervention that includes most of the recommendations discussed in the preceding text is a "psychoeducative group program" provided for caregivers of demented persons living at home in Canada.[25] This program, which is composed of fifteen 2-hour weekly sessions, was designed to improve the caregivers' ability to cope with stress by teaching cognitive self-appraisal and new coping strategies. Caregivers were taught to assess the stressful situation and determine the cause of stress. When a specific behavior was problematic, they were taught behavioral interventions to decrease the problem. When the stressor was caused by the caregivers' interpretation of the problem, they were taught such emotion-focused strategies as reframing—looking at the situation from a different perspective or reinterpreting the situation. They were also encouraged and taught how to seek greater levels of social support. Results showed a 14% decrease in stressful reactions to negative care-recipient behaviors, as compared to a 5% decrease in the control group who participated in a general caregiver support group. In addition, the frequency of behavior problems also decreased. The investigators did not focus specifically on the eradication of escapist–wishful thinking coping strategies, but an increase in their sense of competence may have served to reduce such nonproductive behavior in caregivers (Evidence Level B).

Caregivers often fail to take advantage of educational and support groups because of lack of time, transportation, respite, discomfort in group settings, and a general hesitancy to leave the patient with another person. Responding to these impediments and recognizing the increase in the number of adults who use the Internet for health information, an increasing number of attempts are being made to provide on-line support and education for dementia caregivers.

WHAT IS THE PHYSICIAN'S ROLE?

The AMA promotes a "physician–caregiver–patient partnership approach" to elder care.[3] In this model, physicians provide information, referral, and support to caregivers; they also monitor the functioning of caregivers to promote their physical and emotional health.

An essential factor in the implementation of this model is the caregiver's attitude toward the patient's physician. The ability of the caregiver to carry out his or her responsibilities and provide optimal care over time is highly dependent on the caregiver's belief and trust that the physician (who has often been chosen by the patient and may not be the first choice of the caregiver) is providing the best possible care for the older patient. Without this basic trust, the caregiver–physician relationship can become hostile and ultimately detrimental to the patient. According to focus group responses to an informal, unpublished assessment, by Thibault in 2004, of caregivers who are themselves gerontologic practitioners and in correspondence with the principles of quality geriatric care espoused by Ham et al.[4] caregivers appear to value physicians who demonstrate the following characteristics:

1. Respectful, caring attitude toward the patient
2. Respectful attitude toward the caregiver, recognizing that he or she can provide reliable information and has a right to ask questions
3. Willingness to communicate clearly and promptly across practice settings, especially during times of transition from one setting to another, (e.g., from home to hospital)
4. Accessibility of office space and appointment hours

5. Geriatrics knowledge base and expertise
6. Willingness to educate the caregiver personally or through reading material or recommended community resources
7. Willingness, when necessary, to refer the patient to and confer with other providers—both medical and nonmedical
8. Willingness to offer encouragement and support
9. Sensitivity to financial burden

These characteristics correspond closely to the elements of high-quality geriatric care discussed in the introductory chapter of this book: Recognition of biologic and psychological uniqueness, which requires an individualized approach to care; physician's awareness of his or her own personal views about aging and death; the ability to focus fully on the patient; enhanced specialized and perceptive capacity; reverence for the patient; creation of a healing atmosphere; and emphasis on function through "the maximization of the patient's productivity, creativity, well-being, and happiness."[26]

In their discussion of family stresses, Ham et al. cite the following as the most significant sources of strain when caring for a dependent elder: Disturbed nights with diminished and interrupted sleep, aggressive or abusive patient behavior, urinary and fecal incontinence, need for help with basic activities of daily living, and ingratitude on the part of the patient.[4] Caregiver characteristics that correlate with increased stress include frailty, poor health, alcohol dependency, emotional instability, and other caregiving responsibilities (e.g., caring for grandchildren, a disabled spouse, or more than one elder). Financial burden is also a source of stress. Having found that increased use of formal services, including nursing home placement, leads to increasing burden, Brown et al. suggest that burden should be evaluated routinely as part of geriatric assessment.[27]

The following case demonstrates a typical patient situation, a variety of caregiver expectations, correlation of feelings of burden, and a need for sensitive and specific physician responses.

CASE: PART ONE

One month ago, Mrs. R., aged 69, and Mr. R., aged 74, relocated from a city 900 miles away to be closer to their only child, Ms. J., aged 38, a recently divorced executive and mother of two sons, aged 10 and 12. Ms. J. has been your patient for 10 years.

Five years before their relocation, Mr. R. was diagnosed with Parkinson disease. Mrs. R. reports that since the move, he has experienced increased immobility and difficulty communicating, declining short-term memory, and frequent episodes of irritability. Mrs. R. was diagnosed with type 2 diabetes 2 years ago, gives herself insulin injections, and successfully manages her disease, although she did not find the time to visit her physician before her relocation. She also suffers from arthritic knees and hands and states that she is often in considerable pain. Mrs. R. was the primary caregiver for her mother, who lived in the couple's home for 15 years and died 6 months ago at the age of 101 and had suffered from a vascular dementia for 16 years.

The couple lives in a new one-story patio home a mile from their daughter's house and two blocks from your office. They did not bring past medical records with them.

The couple has not yet made any new friends. Mrs. R. states that they have been too busy to join a church or any other social group. She also reveals that the couple is responsible for after-school child care of their grandsons, which would interfere with socialization.

Mrs. R. states that she has chosen you to be their physician for the following reasons: (i) Your office is located close to their home and (ii) her daughter has recommended you because she thinks you are a kind, caring, and capable primary care physician. Although you are not trained in geriatrics, as was their former physician, Mrs. R. states that she believes you will be able to provide the couple with excellent care.

Ms. J., who has been silent and holding back tears, states wearily that she is worried about her parents and that the move has not gone as smoothly as she had expected. She shakes her head when you ask her to explain what she means. As the family leaves your office, Ms. J. looks back at you and forms the following words silently, "I need to talk with you—I'll call."

How should you proceed, recognizing that you are now caring for two generations of this family, each with his or her individual needs? Of course, procuring past medical records and conducting your own physical, cognitive, and functional assessment are the basic tasks. In the domain of perception, one of the first questions that must be answered is, "How does each person relate to the other in terms of decision making and physical and emotional caregiving and receiving?" Another is, "What are the goals of care for Mr. R. as a patient, Mrs. R. as both a patient and her husband's caregiver, and Ms. J. as a patient and caregiver of both her parents and children?"

Answers to the following questions will guide your care of this extended family over time:

1. How emotionally intact is this family—how healthy are their long-term family dynamics?
2. How involved is Ms. J. in her parents' lives? How involved do Mr. and Mrs. R. want her to be in their health maintenance and care?
3. What is Mrs. R.'s perceived level of burden and what is her caregiver coping style? What is their daughter's?
4. Does each have long-term care insurance?
5. What is their level of emotional and physical independence?
6. Does Mrs. R. have any cognitive deficits? Is she still grieving the loss of her mother? Is she experiencing

stress related to the long period of care she provided her mother?

7. Who made the decision to relocate and how difficult has the move been? How much is the couple grieving the loss of friends, social roles, familiar activities and surroundings, and so on? What are all the reasons for their relocation at this particular time?
8. What are Mr. and Mrs. R.'s end-of-life care preferences?
9. What are the issues of privacy and confidentiality that need to be addressed? If Mrs. R. can give permission for you to talk with Ms. J. about their care, there is no problem. What can be done if she does not grant that permission?

During the course of the following 6 months you perceive that the person providing the lion's share of caregiving is Mrs. R., who is responsible for offering emotional and/or physical care for the following persons:

1. Mr. R., whose cognition and function are deteriorating quickly
2. Two grandsons, aged 10 and 12, for whom she provides after-school care 5 days per week from 3:30 to 7:00 PM, including supervision of outdoor play, homework, and provision of dinner; she also baby-sits for them when Ms. J. is traveling for work at least one weekend per month
3. Daughter Ms. J., who has a very high-stress, demanding job and is in emotional turmoil and grief because of an unwanted divorce and her parents' problems.

CASE: PART TWO—9 MONTHS LATER

Mrs. R. has been hospitalized, because of a mild stroke, which has left her with a moderate level of right-sided weakness. She has begun physical therapy and you would like her to be admitted to an inpatient rehabilitation unit for 2 weeks of more intensive therapy. She has been under considerable stress, and you believe that the respite from caregiving is necessary to her recovery. Also, there is some doubt that she would care for herself at home and would force herself back into the caregiver role if allowed to return home so soon, even with the intervention of home health care. You discuss the plan with the family, but all three adamantly refuse to anything but a home health care solution. Ms. J., who insinuates that if you had returned her call earlier, her mother might have been spared the effects of the stroke, states that she will take advantage of the Family Leave Act and stay at home for 2 weeks to care for her parents. You disapprove of this arrangement, realizing that Ms. J., whose blood pressure has been too high and unresponsive to medication, is placing herself under increased stress. However, the family will not consider any other alternative and you must balance your own knowledge of optimal care with the needs of the family. You order physical and occupational therapy and the services of a home health aide to help bathe both Mr. and Mrs. R.

Ms. J.'s health is also of concern. She scores in the mildly depressed range on the Beck Depression Scale but refuses to consider taking an antidepressant. You advise her to join a caregiver support group offered by the Alzheimer's Association and to engage in private family counseling for help with her marital dissolution grief and the behavioral problems she is now experiencing with both boys. You are aware of Ms. J.'s ill-concealed hostility toward you. You openly acknowledge and discuss the anger and you reinterpret it for her. Although any realistic fault should be admitted, you gently point out that much of her anger, directed solely at the physician, may, to a large degree, have its basis in her anger toward her father for being ill, her sons for their negative behavior, her husband for leaving her, and her mother's inability to care for her and her sons.

CASE: PART THREE—18 MONTHS LATER

Mr. R.'s health has declined dramatically and he is dying. When Mrs. R. returned home from the rehabilitation unit after her stroke, she found that her husband's Parkinson disease had worsened to such an extent that she needed home health aides to help her care for him. As the disease progressed, even 18 hours of home health aide per day was not adequate for his needs, necessitating Mr. R.'s relocation to a nursing home.

Problems become focused on end-of-life care after Mr. R. has lived in the facility for 4 months. He continues to decline, and at this time he is having increasing difficulty breathing. He has experienced one incident of aspiration pneumonia because of difficulty swallowing and now can no longer eat. You tell Mrs. R. and Ms. J. that he is dying and inform both of the need for decisions to be made about his end-of-life care. You have living wills for both Mr. and Mrs. R.; Mr. R.'s was made by his wife because he was not capable of understanding the concept when he entered your practice. Mrs. R. understands her husband's nearness to death and does not want him to be intubated or placed on a ventilator. She states that she does not want him to suffer any longer and that she is willing to "let him go."

Ms. J., on the other hand, wants "everything done" for her father. She believes that he still has some quality of life and does not want to die. She also states that her religion considers not placing him on a ventilator equivalent to euthanasia. She pulls you aside and informs you that her father's retirement benefits—a generous pension and excellent health and long-term care insurance that includes her mother—will end when he dies; it does not include an extension for Mrs. R. The couple's funds have been spent on Mr. R.'s home health and nursing home care; without the pension, Mrs. R. will have few resources—just the patio home and $900 of her own monthly Social Security payment (Mr. R. worked for the state and does not get Social Security). Ms. J. pleads with you to keep her father alive for as long as possible, for her mother's well-being. You sense her panic and increasing anger when you tell her that her mother, who has durable power of attorney for Mr. R., has the right to make the decision.

How are you?

Caregivers are often so concerned with caring for their relative's needs that they lose sight of their own well-being. Please take just a moment to answer the following questions. Once you have answered the questions, turn the page to do a self-evaluation. During the last week, I have . . .

1. Had trouble keeping my mind on what I was doing	Yes	No
2. Felt that I couldn't leave my relative alone	Yes	No
3. Had difficulty making decisions	Yes	No
4. Felt completely overwhelmed	Yes	No
5. Felt useful and needed	Yes	No
6. Felt lonely	Yes	No
7. Been upset that my relative has changed so much from his/her former self	Yes	No
8. Felt a loss of privacy and/or personal time	Yes	No
9. Been edgy or irritable	Yes	No
10. Had sleep disturbed because of caring for my relative	Yes	No
11. Had a crying spell	Yes	No
12. Felt strained between work and caring for my relative	Yes	No
13. Had back pain	Yes	No
14. Felt ill (headaches, stomach problems or common cold)	Yes	No
15. Been satisfied with the support my family has given me	Yes	No
16. Found my relative's living situation to be inconvenient or a barrier to care	Yes	No
17. On a scale of 1 to 10, with 1 being "not stressful" and 10 being "extremely stressful," please rate your current level of stress		
18. On a scale of 1 to 10, with 1 being "very healthy" to 10 being "very ill," please rate your current health compared to what it was this time last year		

Comments: (Please feel free to comment or provide feedback.)

Self-evaluation:

To determine the score:

1. Reverse score questions 5 and 15. (For example, a "No" response should be counted as a "Yes" and a "Yes" response should be counted as a "No".)
2. Total the number of "Yes" responses.

To interpret the score:

Chances are you are experiencing a high degree of distress:

- If you answered "Yes" to either or both questions 4 and 11; or
- If your total "Yes" score equals 10 or more; or
- If your score on question 17 is 6 or higher; or
- If your score on question 18 is 6 or higher.

Next Steps – Caregiver

- Consider seeing a doctor for a checkup for yourself.
- Consider having some relief from caregiving. (Discuss with the doctor or a social worker the resources available in your community.)
- Consider joining a support group.

Figure 3.1 Caregiver Self-assessment Questionnaire. *(continued)*

Next Steps – Physician

Any "Yes" responses to the questions on the Caregiver Self-assessment Questionnaire suggest that:

- The caregiver needs further assessment to determine the need for counseling/intervention.
- The caregiver might benefit from a medical checkup or referral to their personal physician. (Suggest they take the questionnaire to show.)
- The caregiver might benefit from joining a support group.
- The caregiver should be encouraged to arrange some relief from caregiving.
- The physician should consider a referral to social services.

Figure 3.1 *(continued)*

The secondary caregiver is Ms. J., who finds herself responsible for providing emotional and/or physical care for the following persons:

1. Her mother, with whom she has an emotional dependency and about whom she feels very protective and anxious
2. Her father, with whom she has not had a warm and nurturing relationship during the course of her life; she perceives her father as very judgmental and demanding of her mother, herself, and her sons
3. Her sons, aged 10 and 12, both of whom are having difficulty understanding why their father no longer lives with them; the older boy has begun misbehaving in school.

It is at this point that many physicians feel frustrated because of the paucity of options for active care. Frustration can lead to emotional abandonment of the family and an unhappy death for all concerned. What can you do to ease the end-of-life conflicts facing these two caregivers?

1. You can facilitate a mother–daughter discussion about Ms. J.'s concerns about her mother's financial well-being and ask the hospital social worker to meet with the two to discuss eligibility for services and programs after Mr. R.'s death.
2. You may also recommend the involvement of hospice for the availability of the chaplaincy and social work services, as well as help with the payment of medications.
3. You can help the family, empathizing with them in their pain, and discuss why intubation and feeding tubes may be in the best interests of the patient at this time. You tell Ms. J. and Mrs. R. that you believe that comfort care, the goal of which is to keep Mr. R. comfortable and free of pain, is most appropriate at this time.
4. Since Mr. R.'s condition deteriorated unusually rapidly, you can discuss the possibility of an autopsy to better determine the cause of death in the future.
5. Following the death of Mr. R., acknowledging him in some public way, either by visitation at the funeral home or by a sympathy card to both Mrs. R. and her daughter, is likely to be very much appreciated.
6. Shortly after the funeral, you can schedule an appointment to see Mrs. R. in your office to determine how she is handling her bereavement. Refer to a bereavement-counseling program (often offered by hospice) if she is having trouble with depressed mood or any of the vegetative signs of depression. Recommend the same to Ms. J.

ANGER

Caregivers frequently direct frustration and anger toward the physician. Experiencing a caregiver's anger can be unpleasant and cause the physician to adopt withdrawal or defensive behaviors. Sometimes the physician is at fault. Often, however, as in the case with Ms. J., the hostility is the result of pent-up frustration at the situation itself. The following are steps the physician can take to diffuse a caregiver's anger:

1. Acknowledge and address the fact that the caregiver is angry, even when only nonverbal behavior demonstrates the anger
2. Work with the caregiver (and patient, when appropriate) to identify the underlying cause of the negative feelings
3. Recognize that unaddressed anger will interfere with the quality of care
4. Express concern for the caregiver's burden
5. Suggest a counselor or support group if the anger is not caused by physician behavior and is a result of general frustration
6. If all of the above strategies fail to improve the situation and the unresolvable anger is interfering with the quality of patient care, withdraw from the case, giving at least 30 days' notice to both patient and caregiver.

WHAT RESOURCES ARE AVAILABLE TO THE PHYSICIAN?

A. Caregiver Assessment:

Physicians can identify persons who are providing care for others by making the following inquiries:

1. Ask patients of all ages, "Do you have the responsibility for caring for someone with a chronic illness or disability?"

Provide the following information to the caregiver to facilitate efficient office visits:

1. Inform the caregiver that you consider him/her a part of the patient's health care team, in partnership with you (and any other providers in your office).

2. Give both the patient and caregiver a copy of "Talking with Your Doctor: A Guide for Older People," provided by the National Institute on Aging. Order from: 1-800-222-2225

3. Develop guidelines for the use of your services, so that patients and caregivers know what to expect in terms of accessibility. Create a one-page handout titled "How to make the best use of an office visit"

   Physician Name:________________________________

   Office Number:________________________________

   Office Hours:________________________________

   Email address:________________________________

   a. Prior to the visit discuss the upcoming visit with the patient. Make a list of both of your concerns and questions and bring two copies, one that I can place in the chart and one on which you can take notes. Write your concerns in order of importance.

   b. Make sure the patient is wearing hearing aids and glasses. Ask me to speak more loudly or slowly, if necessary.

   c. You are welcome to audio tape-record the visit.

   d. Bring all medications with you, including over-the-counter medications, herbs, nutraceuticals, and medications prescribed by other physicians.

   e. Keep a notebook with all of the patient's medical information.

   f. Call ahead to see whether I am more than 45 minutes behind schedule.

   g. If you have questions between visits, I can be reached at the following times __________. Allow ________time for response.

      If you use e-mail, I prefer to use that instead of a telephone call.

      If I am unavailable, please call____________________.

4. Determine who the primary caregiver is, (the family spokesperson/contact in issues and decisions relating to the patient, who may or may not have a durable power of attorney).

5. Encourage the patient to appoint a durable power of attorney and health care surrogate.

6. Encourage the patient to make a living will and discuss this with both the patient and caregiver.

7. Explain who will attend the patient if he/she is hospitalized.

8. Develop a list of local agencies serving elders, home health agencies, assisted-living facilities, nursing homes, and geriatric case managers.

Figure 3.2 Caregiver guide to office visits.

2. Ask older adult patients, "Do you have someone on whom you depend regularly for care of any kind?"
3. Ask persons who regularly accompany an older patient to office visits, "What are your caregiving responsibilities?" Once caregivers have been identified, their name, telephone number(s), and address should be recorded in the patient's chart.
4. The AMA has created and recommends the use of an instrument titled "The Caregiver Self-assessment Questionnaire" (see Fig. 3.1) to help physicians identify caregivers at risk of deteriorating health.[28] The following process is suggested:

After identifying a caregiver, they should then be asked to respond to "The Caregiver Self-assessment Questionnaire." (This could be completed in the waiting room prior to the visit.) Phrase this request in the following way: "Caregiving responsibilities can have an effect on the caregiver's health, and I am as concerned about your well-being as that of my patient, because he/she is dependent on you. In order to help you, would you please fill out this questionnaire? With the information you give me, I may be able to provide you with suggestions to help you."

B. Caregiver Education:

Have copies of The 36-Hour Day (Mace ML, Rabins PV. Baltimore, MD: Johns Hopkins Press; 1999)[29] to lend to caregivers. This is now a "classic" family oriented guide to practical aspects of caring for persons with dementia. It provides information on the various stages of dementia and the patients' concomitant behaviors, and it also suggests ways in which caregivers can attend to their own needs (see Fig. 3.2). The physician's office may also keep a supply of brochures and information from local agencies, such as the Area Agency on Aging and the Alzheimer's Association, in the waiting room. Please see section on "Suggested Readings and Resources" at the end of this chapter for further information and services.

SUMMARY

In their analysis of the relationship of family caregivers and the health care system, based on the United Hospital Fund's Families and Health Care Project begun in 1996, the editors Carol Levine and Thomas Murray assert that "As the population ages and the health care system focuses on cost containment, family caregivers have become the frontline providers of most long-term and chronic care."[2]

One result of the growing phenomenon of caregiving is that the culture of the caregiver can often clash with the culture of traditional medicine, wherein the physician has the primary responsibility for decision making about chronic and terminal care. What is becoming apparent is that the "best practice" is one in which all players—including the patient, when possible—are considered part of the health team. In the team approach to elder care, each participant has a distinctive part to play, and the roles can frequently overlap. To provide optimal care, all players of the team must listen carefully and empathically to one another, recognizing material, social, emotional, and spiritual needs.[26] By acknowledging her or his membership as part of this team and by promoting a safe and compassionate milieu for both patient and caregiver, the physician caring for older adults may experience new and gratifying opportunities to grow both professionally and personally.

REFERENCES

1. Coe J. Fading memory. *The Pharos.* 2004; Summer.
2. Levine C, Murray T. *The cultures of caregiving: Conflict and common ground among families, health professionals, and policy makers.* Baltimore, MD: Johns Hopkins University Press; 2004.
3. Schulz RS, Martire LM. Family caregiving of persons with dementia: Prevalence health effects and support strategies. *Am J Geriatr Psychiat.* 2004;12:240–249.
4. Ham RJ, Sloane PD, Warshaw GA. *Primary care geriatrics*, 4th ed. St. Louis: Mosby; 2000.
5. American Medical Association. http://inova.org/inovapublic.srt/caregivers/caregivereng.pdf, 2004.
6. Administration on Aging. *A profile of older Americans: Disability and activity limitations.* 2003, www.aoa/gov/2003.
7. Andolsek KM, Clapp-Channing NE, Gehlbach SH. Caregivers and elderly relatives: The prevalence of caregiving in a family practice. *Arch Intern Med.* 1988;148:2177–2180.
8. Schulz R, Beach SR. Caregiving as a risk factor for mortality: The caregiver health effects study. *N Engl J Med.* 1999;282(23):2215–2219.
9. Dunkin JJ, Anderson-Hanley C. Dementia caregiver burden: A review of the literature and guidelines for assessment and intervention. *Am Acada Neuro.* 1998;51(1):S53–S60.
10. Family Caregiver Alliance. *Selected caregiver statistics.* 2004.
11. George LK, Gwyther LP. Caregiver well-being: A multidimensional examination of family caregivers of demented adults. *The Gerontologist.* 1986;26(3):253–255.
12. www.als.org.Media/newsreleases/2004/100404_caregiver.aswp, 2004.
13. http://olpa.od.nih.gov/legislation/108/pendinglegislation/reaganalzheimer.asp, 2004
14. Fengler AP, Goodrich N. Wives of elderly disabled men: The hidden patients. *The Gerontol.* 1979;19:175–183.
15. Clipp EC, George LK. Dementia and cancer: A comparison of spouse caregivers. *The Gerontol.* 1986;33(4):534–541.
16. Baumgarten M, Hanley JA, Infante-Rivard C. Health of family members caring for elderly persons with dementia. *Ann Intern Med.* 1994;120:126–132.
17. Graftström M, Fratiglioni L, Sandman PO. Health and social consequences for relatives of demented and non-demented elderly. A population-based study. *J Clin Epidemiol.* 1992;45(8): 861–870.
18. Kiecolt-Glaser JK, Dura JR, Speicher CE. Spousal caregivers of dementia victims: Longitudinal changes in immunity and health. *Psychosom Med.* 1991;53:345–362.
19. Robinson K, Adkisson P, Weinrich S. Problem behaviour, caregiver reactions, and impact among caregivers of persons with Alzheimer's disease. *J Adv Nursing.* 2001;36(4):573–582.
20. Zarit SH, Reever KE, Bach-Peterson J. Relatives of the impaired elderly: Correlates of feelings of burden. *J Geront.* 1980;20:649.
21. Gottlieb BH, Wolfe J. Coping with family caregiving to persons with dementia: A critical review. *Aging Ment Health.* 2002;6:325–342.
22. McClendon MJ, Smyth KA, Neundorjer MM. Survival of persons with Alzheimer's disease: Caregiver coping matters. *The Gerontol.* 2004;44(4):508–519.
23. Kitwood T. *Dementia reconsidered: The person comes first.* Philadelphia, PA: Open University Press; 1997.

24. Sabat SR. Excess disability and malignant social psychology: A case study of Alzheimer's disease. *J Com Appl Soc Psych.* 1994;4: 157–166.
25. Hébert R, Lévesque L, Vézina J, et al. Efficacy of a psychoeducative group program for caregivers of demented persons living at home: A randomized controlled trial. *J Geront Soc Sci.* 2003;58B:S58–S76.
26. Williams ME. *The approach to the elderly patient.*
27. Brown LJ, Potter JF, Foster BG. Caregiver burden should be evaluated during geriatric assessment. *J Am Geriatr Soc.* 1990;38: 455–460.
28. http://inova.org/inovapublic.srt/caregivers/caregivereng.pdf, 2004.
29. Mace ML, Rabins PV. *The 36-hour day.* Baltimore, MD: Johns Hopkins Press; 1999.

SUGGESTED READINGS AND RESOURCES

Eldercare Locator
A national directory of community services
(800)-677-1116
www.aoa.gov/naic/elderloc.html

Guide to the Family and Medical Leave Act
National Partnership for Women and Families
http://www.dol.gov/asp/programs/guide/fmle.htm

Family Caregiver Alliance
(415)-434-3388
www.caregiver.org

National Alliance for Caregiving
(301)-718-8444
www.caregiving.org

National Family Caregivers Association
(800)-896-3650
http://www.nfcacares.org/

Tips for Caregivers of People With Alzheimer Disease
National Institute on Aging
http://www.alzheimers.org/pubbs/careguide.htm

Can We Talk? Families Discuss Older Parents' Ability to Live Independently
AARP
http://research.aarp.org/il/ind_liv.pdf

Eldercare at Home
AGS Foundation for Health in Aging
http://www.healthinaging.org/public_education/eldercare/contents.php

Explaining Medicare to Caregivers
Center for Medicare Education
http://futureofaging.org/publications/data/V3N10.pdf

Rational Drug Therapy in the Elderly

4

Robert L. Dickman

- CLINICAL PEARLS 40
- PHARMACOLOGIC CONSIDERATIONS 41
- POLYPHARMACY 42
- ADVERSE DRUG REACTIONS 42
- SPECIFIC PROBLEM DRUGS IN THE ELDERLY 43
- CLINICAL STRATEGIES 46
- CONCLUSION 47

CLINICAL PEARLS

- Continuously review your patient's medications with an eye to stopping or reducing as many as possible.
- Explore nonpharmacologic treatment for problems.
- Simplify the regimen.
- Start low, go slow.
- Always consider over-the-counter and alternative medication while assessing your patient's drug regimen.
- Do not attribute all symptoms, such as fatigue and memory loss, to old age before considering that they may represent an adverse drug reaction.
- Always balance long-term benefits against short-term problems when considering a specific pharmacologic agent.
- Be aware of underuse of pharmacologic agents in the elderly.
- Be mindful of prescription costs when selecting a drug regimen.

There is perhaps nothing that better characterizes a "geriatric" approach to patient care than the appropriate management of pharmacologic agents in this age-group. Indeed, most primary care clinicians find themselves continually reevaluating older patients' medication lists, seeking to reduce dosages or eliminate medications altogether. It is the purpose of this chapter to acquaint the primary care physician with the basic pharmacodynamics and pharmacokinetics in the elderly to engender a rational approach to drug treatment in this age-group. In addition, we discuss the concepts of, and the reasons for, polypharmacy and adverse drug reactions. We also review a number of "problematic" medications commonly used by primary care clinicians in the outpatient setting that pose particular problems in this age-group.

Currently, people older than 65 constitute approximately 14% of the US population, but they use approximately 30% to 40% of all prescription and over-the-counter medications. Given our large "baby boomer" population, it is estimated that by the year 2035 a full 20% of the population will be older than 65, and the percentage of medication use will rise proportionally.[1] Further, the fastest growing segment of our population is the over-85 age-group, whose use of medication is proportionally greater than that of other seniors. The average person older than 65 uses 4.5 prescription medications daily, whereas the average institutionalized patient uses 7 prescription medications daily. Put in economic terms, the annual prescription drug expenditure per senior was $559 in 1992 and $1,205 in 2000, and the average prescription cost increased by 49% during this period. This economic burden does not even begin to take into account the cost of adverse drug treatment, including hospitalization. It is estimated that 28% of all hospital admissions for this age-group are for drug-related problems and that 70% of those are for adverse drug reactions.[2] Given the sizable and growing prevalence of polypharmacy, it behooves all primary care clinicians who care for older persons to approach this aspect of care rationally and cautiously.

PHARMACOLOGIC CONSIDERATIONS

Pharmacokinetics is the aspect of pharmacology that considers all the factors that contribute to the amount of drug presented to a receptor site. These include absorption, distribution, metabolism, and excretion. There are a number of important pharmacokinetic changes in older persons that indicate prescribing habits in this age-group.

Despite a small increase in achlorhydria and a decrease in gastric motility and gastrointestinal (GI) blood flow in elderly persons, drug absorption from the GI tract is not affected in any significant way. There is little data available on the absorption of transdermal, transbuccal, or transbronchial medications and, in elderly patients, no reason to assume any significant changes in absorption from these routes.

Only a very small reduction in serum albumin level is found as age advances, and therefore, the binding of drugs to carrier proteins is usually not affected.[3] In patients who are hypoalbuminemic for any reason (e.g., malnutrition), the amount of unbound bioactive drug may be greater, and therefore, a similar measure of total drug concentration (bound and unbound) might have a greater pharmacologic effect.

The plasma concentration of any medication will be affected by the total volume in which it is distributed. Because total body water decreases in the elderly, hydrophilic drugs such as warfarin, for dosages similar to those for younger people, will have higher plasma concentration when given to older people. Conversely, fat-soluble drugs such as benzodiazepines can accumulate in older people because of an increase in body fat, and therefore, these medications will have a much longer half-life in elderly patients.

Hepatic metabolism in the elderly and its effect on pharmacokinetics is not well understood. Drugs are metabolized in the liver in two phases. Phase I (oxidation and reduction) may be impaired in this group of patients, but phase II (conjugation) appears to be unaltered.[3] Further, hepatic blood flow and liver size are reduced, which influences

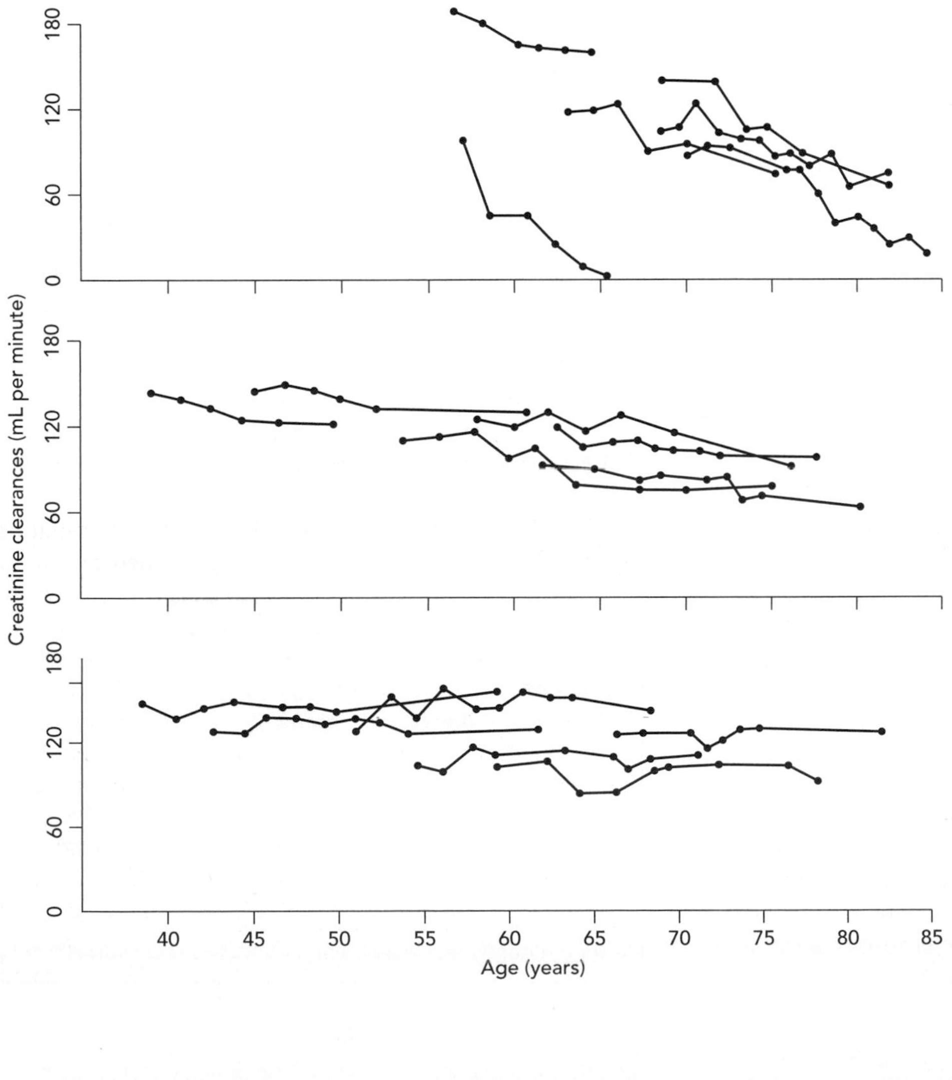

Figure 4.1 Age changes in creatinine clearance of male subjects studied serially in the Baltimore Longitudinal Study of Aging.
(Reprinted from Masoro EJ. Physiology of aging. In: Tallis R, Fillit H, Brocklehurst JC, eds. Brocklehurst's Textbook of Geriatric Medicine, 5th ed. London: Churchill Livingstone, 1998:88, with permission).

"first-pass" effects of a number of medications. Therefore, drugs that depend on this hepatic flow, such as isosorbide and lidocaine, should be started at lower dosages.

Changes in renal physiology in the elderly have by far the most profound effect on pharmacokinetics in this age-group. It is commonly thought that renal function declines by approximately 10% per decade after the age of 50 in "normal" elderly. These data, however, were based on older cross-sectional studies. Longitudinal studies of "normal aging" suggest that as many as 30% of octogenarians have preserved renal function (see Fig. 4.1).[4] It is important, therefore, to have some knowledge of he patients' renal function over time to accurately gauge the effect of renal function on drug use. Furthermore, because the total protein content may be decreased and muscle mass also diminished in this age-group, both the serum blood urea nitrogen (BUN) and creatinine levels may be lower than that indicated by the actual creatinine clearance. Although a specific formula may be employed to calculate creatinine clearance in the elderly, its use in the ambulatory setting is not practical. Suffice it to say that potentially nephrotoxic drugs (e.g., aminoglycosides) and those primarily excreted by the kidney (e.g., digoxin) should be used with extreme caution in this age-group.

Pharmacodynamic changes in the elderly are more difficult to quantify. Pharmacodynamics considers the effect of drugs on receptors. In many cases, similar serum levels of medications can have profoundly different effects in older versus younger patients. This was demonstrated in the classic study by Greenblatt et al.,[5] which showed a more pronounced effect of a long-acting benzodiazepine in older versus younger patients with the same serum level of the drug. On the other hand, β-adrenergic receptor site sensitivity is reduced in the elderly, so more isoproterenol may be necessary to increase the heart rate in the elderly. Similarly, the depressive side effects of β-blockade in this population will also be reduced. In summary, both the pharmacokinetic and pharmacodynamic changes seen in the elderly must be kept in mind when prescribing for patients of this age-group. Particular consideration should always be given to changes in renal function and altered receptor sensitivity.

POLYPHARMACY

When considering special topics that characterize the care of the elderly, polypharmacy is usually at the top of the list. Every time a new geriatric patient is seen in the office, he or she is requested to bring all of his or her medication. These must include over-the-counter and herbal medicines and can sometimes require a shopping bag to transport! There are a variety of reasons for the multiple medications that many older patients use. First of all, such people have many complaints and diseases. Because more people are living into the eighties and nineties, there is simply more time for problems to develop. Conditions such as degenerative joint disease, osteoporosis, and atrial fibrillation are classic examples of problems, the prevalence of which increases with age.

Second, we have many more medications available for use today than we did 20 years ago. Angiotensin-converting enzyme (ACE) inhibitors, angiotensin-receptor blockers (ARB), cholinesterase inhibitors, osteoporosis medications, and the newer nonsteroidal anti-inflammatory drugs (NSAIDs) are but a few that come to mind. Third, older patients often visit several doctors and communication between them is poor. Often, each physician will treat the particular organ dysfunction for which he or she is responsible with little regard for the other medications the patient may be taking.

Finally, there is yet another reason for polypharmacy in this population: Drug marketing and promotion. It is estimated that the pharmaceutical industry spends on average about $10,000 per doctor for marketing and promoting its products. Physicians are constantly being bombarded with new agents or new formulations of old agents, all of which are reputed to be superior and worthy of prescribing. Evaluating these "presentations," particularly when they are accompanied by lavish dinners, or for that matter even simple office supplies, is particularly difficult. Similarly, patients themselves are witness to countless media advertisements, many of which seem to at least suggest that the products will make them young again. Therefore, direct consumer advertising helps promote the polypharmacy we all see every day in our offices.

ADVERSE DRUG REACTIONS

CASE ONE

Mr. C. is an 89-year-old man brought to the office by his daughter because of inability to care for himself. He was found by a social worker in his out-of-state home to be very confused, with severe weight loss and rotting food in the refrigerator. On arrival at the office, he is emaciated and disoriented. He has a past history of congestive heart failure and anxiety. His medications include digoxin (Lanoxin) 0.25 mg q.d., diazepam 5 mg b.i.d., furosemide 20 mg q.d., and potassium chloride (K-Tabs) 10 mEq q.d.

On physical examination his blood pressure is 100/50 and his pulse is 60. His heart shows a 2/6 systolic ejection murmur. His chest is clear and he has no edema. He scores 15 out of 30 on the Mini-Mental State Examination. There are no lateralizing neurologic signs. His laboratory data are remarkably normal but for a digoxin level of 3.5 μg/mL. His electrocardiogram shows sinus bradycardia with first-degree atrioventricular block. He is admitted to the hospital and given IV fluids; digoxin is withheld and diazepam is tapered. After 4 days, he "wakes up" and wonders what his daughter has done by taking away his house. He spends the next year traveling independently, visiting his children and grandchildren.

This actual case is a dramatic example of the degree to which adverse drug reactions and inappropriate prescribing can affect the quality of patients' lives. On the other hand, countless cases of adverse drug reactions occur every day with less life-threatening events than this case, but which can be equally devastating. Adverse drug reactions occur much more frequently in older patients; some studies repeat a rate as high as 17% in this age-group.[6] These can be characterized in a variety of ways. This case illustrates two of them. First, inappropriate prescribing of medications known to adversely affect the elderly is perhaps the most potentially devastating. Mr. C. received a long-acting benzodiazepine, which is rarely a drug of choice in the elderly (this will be discussed later in this chapter). Second, prescribing too large a dose of a particular medication can lead to a toxic reaction such as the one we saw in the case. In this example, digoxin (Lanoxin) (whose use in nontachycardic congestive heart failure could be questioned in the first place) at such high doses could (and almost always does) lead to toxicity. Furthermore, when monitoring the effects of digoxin (Lanoxin), drug levels alone will not be sufficient and clinical judgment is paramount.

Another kind of adverse drug reaction results from a normally expected side effect, which, when placed in the context of the geriatric patient with polypharmacy, can be catastrophic. The best examples of this are agents (psychoactive and antihypertensive agents) that can cause some postural hypotension. In the context of an unstable, frail elderly patient with some autonomic dysfunction, a postural blood pressure drop can lead to a fall or a hip fracture. NSAIDs, which may adversely affect renal function, could be the final blow in an octogenarian whose glomerular filtration rate is already significantly decreased.

It is also important to keep in mind that drugs that can be expected to cause "nuisance" side effects in younger people can be extremely troublesome when they occur in the elderly. The best example of this is the anticholinergic effect seen with a variety of medications, including antihistamines, antiparkinson medications, and those drugs used to treat urge incontinence. Rather than a slightly dry mouth and a bit of constipation, a frail elderly man with benign prostatic hypertrophy can develop acute urinary retention or fecal impaction when using these drugs. Difficulty in controlling prothrombin times, particularly elevated ones, can be catastrophic in a frail elderly patient who falls and develops intracerebral bleeding as a result of this elevation.

Finally, a large variety of adverse drug reactions can result directly from drug–drug interactions. Given the problem of polypharmacy in this age-group, it is not hard to see how this can occur. These interactions can occur through a variety of mechanisms. First, certain medications when used together will each be treating a drug effect, not a disease. Proton pump inhibitors (as a result of NSAID use), positive inotropic agents (following calcium channel blockers), and anticholinergic and cholinergic bladder stimulators are but a few examples of this phenomenon.

Other examples of drug interactions are those in which two separate drugs, when used together, compete for the same binding sites. Examples include erythromycin and cimetidine, warfarin and allopurinol, or ciprofloxacin and phenytoin with benzodiazepines. Similarly, drugs that are simultaneously excreted by the kidneys, such as digoxin and amiodarone, can lead to toxicity of one or the other. Finally, additive effects of multiple agents can produce a whole host of adverse reactions. For example, thiazide-induced hypokalemia can precipitate digitalis toxicity. An NSAID, when used concurrently with ACE inhibitors, can induce worsening renal function in this particular age-group.

SPECIFIC PROBLEM DRUGS IN THE ELDERLY

Although there is no medication—over-the-counter, prescription, or alternative—that cannot have serious adverse consequences when given to older persons, there remain a number of "problematic" drugs that should be avoided or given very cautiously in this population. In 1991, Beers et al. published a classic article in which explicit criteria were given for determining inappropriate medication use in nursing homes.[7] This article was updated in 1997 in an effort to make it more applicable to the general geriatric population, as well as to review new medications that had recently come to the market.[8] Table 4.1 lists those prescribing concerns and the medications to which they could be applied.

There are a few *caveats* for the primary care physician when reviewing these problem medications. First, it is important to understand that this table was generated by a panel of six experts; others might legitimately disagree with some of their choices. Second, none of these drugs is absolutely contraindicated in elderly people. Finally, the list is by no means exhaustive.

There are a number of medications or classes of medications that deserve special mention and should be avoided at almost all costs. Long-acting benzodiazepines should generally not be used in older people. As we saw in our case example, diazepam in particular is a potentially dangerous drug in this age-group. Its prolonged half-life and altered pharmacodynamics allow it to cause profound sedation, confusion, and even delirium when given in "normal" doses to the elderly. Flurazepam (Dalmane), a long-acting benzodiazepine used as a hypnotic, can produce excessive sedation and increase the incidence of falls and fractures. Even short-acting benzodiazepines should be used cautiously in this age-group, particularly for the "treatment" of delirium in hospitalized and nursing home patients. Many clinicians have seen delirium secondary to lorazepam treated with more lorazepam!

TABLE 4.1
FINAL PRESCRIBING CRITERIA CONSIDERING DIAGNOSIS

Summary of Prescribing Concern	Applicable Medications	High Severity
Propoxyphene should generally be avoided in the elderly. It offers few analgesic advantages over acetaminophen, yet has the side effects of other narcotic drugs	Propoxyphene and combination products	No
Of all the available nonsteroidal anti-inflammatory drugs, indomethacin produces the most central nervous system side effects and should therefore be avoided in the elderly	Indomethacin (Indocin, Indocin SR)	No
Phenylbutazone may produce serious hematologic side effects and should not be used in elderly patients	Phenylbutazone (Butazolidin)	No
Pentazocine is a narcotic analgesic that causes more central nervous system side effects, including confusion and hallucinations, more commonly than other narcotic drugs; additionally, it is a mixed agonist and antagonist; for both reasons, its use should generally be avoided in the elderly	Pentazocine (Talwin)	Yes
Trimethobenzamide is one of the least effective antiemetic drugs, yet it can cause extrapyramidal side effects; when possible, it should be avoided in the elderly	Trimethobenzamide (Tigan)	No
Most muscle relaxants and antispasmodic drugs are poorly tolerated by the elderly and lead to anticholinergic side effects, sedation, and weakness; additionally, their effectiveness at doses tolerated by the elderly is questionable; whenever possible, they should not be used by the elderly	Methocarbamol (Robaxin), carisoprodol (Soma), oxybutynin (Ditropan), chlorzoxazone (Paraflex), metaxalone (Skelaxin), and cyclobenzaprine (Flexeril)	No
Benzodiazepine hypnotics with extremely long half-life (often days) in the elderly produce prolonged sedation and increase the incidence of falls and fractures. Medium- or short-acting benzodiazepines are preferable	Flurazepam (Dalmane)	Yes
Because of its strong anticholinergic and sedating properties, amitriptyline is rarely the antidepressant of choice in the elderly	Amitriptyline (Elavil), chlordiazepoxide–amitriptyline (Limbitrol), and perphenazine–amitriptyline (Triavil)	Yes
Because of its strong anticholinergic and sedating properties, doxepin is rarely the antidepressant of choice in the elderly	Doxepin (Sinequan)	Yes
Meprobamate is a highly addictive and sedating anxiolytic and should be avoided in elderly patients; those using meprobamate for prolonged periods may be addicted and use of the drug may need to be withdrawn slowly	Meprobamate (Miltown, Equanil)	Yes, if recently started
Because of increased sensitivity to benzodiazepines in the elderly, smaller doses may be effective and safer. Total daily doses should rarely exceed the suggested maximum dose	Lorazepam (Ativan), 3 mg; oxazepam (Serax), 60 mg; alprazolam (Xanax), 2 mg; temazepam (Restoril), 15 mg; zolpidem (Ambien), 5 mg; triazolam (Halcion), 0.25 mg	No
The long half-life of chlordiazepam in the elderly (often several days) produces prolonged sedation and increases the risk of falls and fractures; short- and intermediate-acting benzodiazepines are preferred if a benzodiazepine is required	Chlordiazepoxide (Librium), chlordiazepoxide–amitriptyline (Limbitrol), clidinium–chlordiazepoxide (Librax), and diazepam (Valium)	Yes
Of all antiarrhythmic drugs, disopyramide is the most potent negative inotrope and may therefore induce heart failure in the elderly; it is also strongly anticholinergic; when appropriate, other antiarrhythmic drugs should be used	Disopyramide (Norpace, Norpace CR)	Yes
Because of decreased renal clearance of digoxin, doses in the elderly should rarely exceed 0.125 mg daily, except when treating atrial arrhythmias	Digoxin (Lanoxin)	Yes, if recently started
Dipyridamole frequently causes orthostatic hypotension in the elderly; it has been proved beneficial only in patients with artificial heart valves; whenever possible, its use in the elderly should be avoided	Dipyridamole (Persantine)	No
Methyldopa may cause bradycardia and exacerbate depression in the elderly; alternative treatments for hypertension are generally preferred	Methyldopa (Aldomet), methyldopa–hydrochlorothiazide (Aldoril)	Yes, if recently started

(continued)

TABLE 4.1
(continued)

Reserpine imposes unnecessary risk in the elderly because it induces depression, impotence, sedation, and orthostatic hypotension; safer alternatives exist	Reserpine (Serpasil); reserpine–hydrochlorothiazide (Hydropres)	No
Chlorpropamide has a prolonged half-life in the elderly and can cause prolonged and serious hypoglycemia; additionally, it is the only oral hypoglycemic agent that causes SIADH; it should be avoided in the elderly	Chlorpropamide (Diabinese)	Yes
Gastrointestinal antispasmodic drugs are highly anticholinergic and generally produce substantial toxic effects in the elderly; additionally, their effectiveness at doses tolerated by the elderly is questionable; all these drugs are best avoided in the elderly, especially for long-term use	Dicyclomine (Bentyl), hyoscyamine (Levsin, Levsinex), propantheline (Pro-Banthine), belladonna alkaloids (Donnatal and others), and clidinium–chlordiazepoxide (Librax)	Yes
All nonprescription and many prescription antihistamines have potent anticholinergic properties; many cough and cold preparations are available without antihistamines and are safer substitutes in the elderly	Examples include single and combination preparations containing chlorpheniramine (Chlor-Trimeton), diphenhydramine (Benadryl), hydroxyzine (Vistaril, Atarax), cyproheptadine (Periactin), promethazine–dexchlorpheniramine (Polaramine)	No

SIADH, syndrome of inappropriate antidiuretic hormone secretion.
Reprinted from Beers MH: Explicit criteria for determining potentially inappropriate medication use by the elderly: An update. *Arch Intern Med.* 1997;157:200–300. Copyright 1997, American Medical Association, with permission.

The use of narcotic analgesics in the frail elderly is always a delicate balance. Constipation, somnolence, and occasionally, confusion should be expected and balanced against the particular pain syndrome one wishes to ameliorate. Pentazocine (Talwin) and meperidine (Demerol) are particularly poor choices in the elderly. They have many side effects and appear to be less effective for this age-group. Unfortunately, chronic pain syndromes can make the "golden years" anything and may require aggressive management in a multidisciplinary fashion. Pain medications, when used, should be in the smallest dose, with an anticipatory treatment of constipation. Local treatments (e.g., lidocaine [Lidoderm] patch and injections) along with physical therapy can lessen the need for systemic analgesics.

Although the use of tricyclic antidepressants in treating depression has generally been supplanted by selective serotonin reuptake inhibitors (SSRIs) and newer compounds, they will occasionally be prescribed for older people. In a study by Willcox et al., which evaluated inappropriate prescribing for community-dwelling elders, at least 500,000 patients were found to be on amitriptyline.[9] The anticholinergic effects of these medications are particularly bothersome in older people, who often complain of severe dry mouth and constipation when taking them. In addition, they are notorious for causing postural hypotension and may aggravate dementia. If in the rare occasion a tricyclic is indicated, always start with the lowest possible dose to achieve the therapeutic benefit. For patients on these medications, consider a "drug holiday" (by tapering and substituting an SSRI for a tricyclic whenever possible). In an occasional patient, amitriptyline in low doses can sometimes be an effective hypnotic agent and is often used in the management of chronic pain syndromes.

Chlorpropamide, a sulfonylurea used to treat diabetes, is essentially contraindicated in the frail elderly. It is notorious for producing prolonged hypoglycemia, which can masquerade as worsening dementia in this age-group and can, in rare instances, produce the syndrome of inappropriate antidiuretic hormone secretion and subsequent hyponatremia, which may present as an acute delirium as well. Dipyridamole (Persantine) should not be used in elderly patients. It often causes postural hypotension, which, as was discussed in the preceding text, can precipitate falls with particularly catastrophic consequences.

In view of the current controversies surrounding the use of cyclooxygenase-2 (COX-2) NSAIDs, it behooves the family physician to use these drugs extremely cautiously in the elderly. Although only rofecoxib has been removed from the shelves, physicians should prescribe the other COX-2 inhibitors only as a last resort, if at all. Even when using a traditional NSAID, occult GI bleeding often without pain is a common side effect that occurs more frequently in the elderly. Worsening renal failure and edema occur less commonly but can be very worrisome. It is remarkable how many elderly patients, when treated aggressively with physical therapy and acetaminophen (Tylenol), can achieve relief from their arthritic complaints and avoid the use of NSAIDs altogether.

There are a large number of other problematic medications for older people. Muscle relaxants such as cyclobenzaprine (Flexeril); older medications such as meprobamate, methyldopa, and reserpine; and GI antispasmodics such as chlordiazepoxide/clidinium (Librax) are but a few examples of the large number of medications which should be avoided in older people. The antihistamine diphenhydramine (Benadryl) deserves particular mention. It is commonly used by seniors as an over-the-counter hypnotic agent, often in combination with acetaminophen. Prolonged sedation, confusion, and anticholinergic symptoms are common side effects caused by this drug in the elderly.

CLINICAL STRATEGIES

There is little doubt that stopping or reducing medications will often do more good for older patients than starting new ones. Often patients have been placed on medications for acute problems and are left on them indefinitely. Psychotropic medications and antidepressants are particularly good examples of this problem. In many patients, the medications used to treat acute delirium or a depressive episode are given even long after the event is over. It is much better to prove a patient needs a medicine, than to keep him on it if he doesn't.

The use of physical therapy for musculoskeletal complaints is very effective and much less toxic than the use of chronic NSAIDs. Referring a patient to a senior community center can help in case of depression and even allow for the avoidance of antidepressant medications. Relaxation techniques are very effective in controlling anxiety and can take the place of anxiolytics. Lifestyle modification can help patients with high blood pressure and elevated cholesterol levels and obviate the need for antihypertensives and statins.

Medications that require an every 4- or 6-hour dosing should be avoided in the frail elderly. Even with prepared weeklong pill containers, older patients can have trouble with twice-a-day dosing. Patients will often forget to take their medications, and before adding another to achieve the desired effect, physicians should pay close attention to the compliance issue. Other factors that contribute to poor compliance include living alone, lack of support system, numerous physical impairments such as degenerative joint disease and generalized weakness, and cognitive, visual, and hearing deficits. I have seen a number of hospitalized patients who, when given what they were supposed to be taking at home, became profoundly hypotensive and even obtunded on the medical floor.

When you do decide to introduce a new medication in the elderly patient, always begin at the lowest possible dose and gradually advance it, depending on both its therapeutic effect and potential side effects. This is particularly true for psychoactive medications but is also applicable for antihypertensive medications, analgesics, and almost all other prescriptions used in the treatment of older persons. On the other hand, it is also important to achieve therapeutic levels when choosing a drug measurement for your patient. Keeping patients on subtherapeutic levels of some drugs (e.g., antidepressants) risks side effects and drug interactions without the benefit of the medication's therapeutic effect.

Over-the-counter antihistamines, decongestants, and NSAIDs are frequently utilized by patients, and their usage is never reported unless the patient is asked. Megavitamins and a large variety of herbal supplements are often present in the medicine cabinets of seniors. Physicians know of many of the potential adverse reactions associated with antihistamines, decongestants, and nonsteroidals but have much to learn about the herbal preparations. A necessary first step, however, requires our awareness of their use.

As is the case with presentations of diseases in older people, adverse drug reactions may present in atypical ways. Just as delirium, or for that matter dementia, may represent the first manifestation of sepsis or congestive heart failure, it can also be the only indication of an adverse drug reaction. Every time a physician evaluates the complaints of a frail elderly person, drug toxicity should be the first consideration. Careful withdrawal of medicines rarely has catastrophic effects, whereas the reflexive maintenance of a pharmacologic regimen often does. Once again, always remember: It is better to prove that a patient needs a medicine than to keep him or her on it when not required.

CASE TWO

An 85-year-old mildly demented man living in an assisted-living facility with his wife has been diagnosed with stage III congestive heart failure. Because of elevated serum low-density lipoprotein and triglyceride levels, the patient is placed on 40 mg of atorvastatin (Lipitor) and 600 mg of gemfibrozil to control these problems. Within 3 weeks, he develops significant muscle cramps and is hospitalized with rhabdomyolysis.

Although this reaction is not common, it is an example of overzealous and unrealistic prescribing. There is little evidence that decreasing cholesterol or triglyceride levels in individuals older than 85 will prolong life. It will certainly have no effect (except perhaps an adverse one) on the quality of life as well. Other examples of aggressive treatment in octogenarians include management of systolic hypertension and "tight" glucose control in patients with diabetes in this age range.

CASE THREE

A 92-year-old man with persistent systolic hypertension is seen in the office. The patient is totally asymptomatic but suffers from severe degenerative joint disease and an unstable gait. He has a loud aortic stenosis murmur. A decision is made to begin amlodipine (Norvasc) 5 mg q.d., which has little effect on his blood pressure. The dose is then increased to 10 mg a day, and a diuretic is added. There is minimal change in the patient's systolic pressure while sitting but he develops postural hypotension, with two or three brief syncopal events in the last month. He also claims that he has not felt "quite right" since starting the medications. After stopping amlodipine (Norvasc) and the diuretic, his blood pressure remained at approximately 170/80 but he felt completely well.

Although the data on systolic hypertension in the elderly clearly favors treatment, it should not be the only factor considered when making treatment choices for the very old. Further, most studies do not include patients in their late eighties or nineties. Most patients in this age-group prefer feeling well in the short-term rather than enduring discomfort for some "potential" long-term benefit. This should not be misconstrued to imply that we never treat these people preventatively. Treatment should be instituted if the systolic blood pressure can be reasonably controlled with no ill effects.

This chapter clearly has as its major take-home message the need to treat elderly patients with as few medications as possible and in the lowest possible dose. On the other hand, underuse of medications in this population can be problematic as well. Osteoporosis may be one example. There are countless frail, stooped-over elderly women who have never even been told of osteoporosis by their physician, much less evaluated and treated for it. Other examples would include the lack of aggressive pain management, the underdiagnosis and treatment of depression, and lack of stroke prevention. Ascribing all symptoms to "degenerative" disease, or old age for that matter, will potentially miss treatable disease. Elderly onset rheumatoid arthritis, diastolic heart failure, and ataxia secondary to normal pressure hydrocephalus are but a few examples of conditions that should be diagnosed and treated in the elderly.

Given the extraordinary financial burden that prescription drugs have on our patients, their insurance companies, and our society in general, it behooves us all to be mindful of drug costs when choosing therapeutic agents. The cost of first-line antihypertensives (e.g., β-blockers and diuretics) is a fraction of that of "newer" medications. Acetaminophen (Tylenol) or generic ibuprofen is cheap when compared to COX-2 NSAIDs. Amoxicillin or trimethoprim–sulfamethoxazole as an initial treatment for bronchitis or sinusitis is generally effective and costs approximately 10% of that of the newer fluoroquinolones such as levofloxacin. Regardless of your patient's prescription drug program, cost-effective prescribing should be a part of everyday practice.

CONCLUSION

In conclusion, a rational and cautious approach to pharmacotherapy in the senior population is perhaps the most important aspect of good geriatric health care. Knowledge of geriatric pharmacology and the prompt recognition of adverse drug reactions will allow the primary care physician to approach geriatric prescribing cautiously and confidently. Always thinking about ways to "streamline" the medical regimen will never harm and will sometimes help the overall health of the clinician's senior patients. Many geriatricians have helped patients more by stopping medications than by starting them. Given the large number of geriatric patients who will be seeking care in the next 10 years, every primary care clinicians should be well prepared to care for them. Rational drug therapy is the cornerstone of good geriatric health care.

REFERENCES

1. Lombardi TP and Kennicut JD. *Promotion of a safe medication environment: Focus on the elderly and residents of long-term care facilities Medscape Pharmacists.* 2001;2. www.medscape.com.
2. Chutka DS, Takahashi PY, Hoel RW, et al. Inappropriate medications for elderly patients. *Mayo Clin Proc.* 2004;(79):122–139.
3. Avorn J. and Gurwitz JH. Principles of pharmacology. In: Cassell CK, Cohen HJ, Larsen EG, eds. et al. *Geriatric medicine*, New York, NY: Springer-Verlag; 1997:50–75.
4. Beers MH. Explicit criteria for determining potentially inappropriate medication use by the elderly: An update. *Arch Intern Med.* 1997;157:200–300.
5. Greenblatt DJ, Sellers EM, Shader RI, et al. Drug therapy: Drug disposition in old age. *N Engl J Med.* 1982;306:1081–1088.
6. Classen DC, Pestotnik SL, Evans RS, et al. Adverse drug events in hospitalized patients: Excess length of stay, extra costs, and attributable mortality. *JAMA.* 1992;277:301–306.
7. Beers MH, Ouslander JG, Fingold SF, et al. Inappropriate medication prescribing in skilled-nursing facilities. *Ann Intern Med.* 1992;117:684–689.
8. Beers MH, Ouslander JG, Rollinger I, et al. Explicit criteria for determining inappropriate medication use in nursing home residents. *Arch Intern Med.* 1991;151:1825–1832.
9. Willcox SM, Himmelstein DU, Woolhandler S, et al. Inappropriate drug prescribing for the community-dwelling elderly. *JAMA.* 2004;272:292–296.

Pain Control

5

Michael P. Temporal

CLINICAL PEARLS 48

THE MECHANISM OF PAIN 49

PAIN CLASSIFICATION 49

EVALUATION OF PAIN 50
Evaluation of Pain in the Cognitively Impaired 51

GOALS OF PAIN MANAGEMENT 51
Nonpharmacologic Pain Therapies 52
Pharmacologic Management 53
Surgical Intervention 57

CONCLUSION 57

ACKNOWLEDGMENT 57

CLINICAL PEARLS

- Pain is not a normal part of aging.
- Even in the cognitively impaired, any complaint of pain must be taken as real.
- A patient's report of pain is the most reliable gauge of effectiveness of therapy.
- Many older adults are reluctant to report pain, but as the "fifth vital sign," pain should be assessed at every encounter.
- Older persons will often not use the specific word "pain" but readily describe symptoms of burning, ache, soreness, and stiffness or hurting.
- The goal of chronic pain management is improved function and quality of life; the elimination of pain is usually not possible.
- Pain scales can help track the effectiveness of management strategies over time and can be adapted to cognitive or sensory impairments.
- The biopsychosocial context is important in understanding and managing painful conditions for both the patient and the provider.
- Routine rather than as-needed dosing of medications for persistent pain results in better pain control.
- A multidisciplinary approach using multiple modalities in addition to medications is usually needed to manage persistent pain.
- Nociceptive pain is treated stepwise, progressing from nonopiate analgesics and nonsteroidal anti-inflammatory drugs (NSAIDs) to opiate analgesics.
- Neuropathic pain frequently responds to antidepressants, anticonvulsants, and topical agents, but conventional agents are also needed.
- Combination analgesic/narcotic medications are limited to the total daily dose of the nonnarcotic agent. All sources of prescribed and over-the-counter analgesics, especially acetaminophen, aspirin, and ibuprofen, must be considered.
- When dosing analgesic medications, avoid the maximum recommended dose for long periods; titrate to the lowest effective dose by being cognizant of drug–drug, hepatic, and renal adjustments.
- When prescribing prolonged use of an NSAID, consider the use of concomitant proton pump inhibitors or misoprostol to decrease the risk of gastric irritation.
- When prescribing narcotic analgesics, anticipate constipation and nausea and institute prophylactic therapy as indicated.

Pain is an unpleasant sensory and emotional experience associated with actual or potential tissue damage. Management of pain is probably the most frequent reason for seeking health care. From one quarter to one half of the community-dwelling older population suffers important pain problems. At least as many, if not more, older adults have pain problems in the nursing home. Nearly 85% of older adults are affected by painful conditions and diseases associated with pain, including osteoarthritis, rheumatoid arthritis, cancer, herpes zoster, temporal arteritis, polymyalgia rheumatica, and atherosclerotic disease. Other common conditions include low back disorders, gout, and headache. The incidence of persistent pain increases with age, affecting 34% of those aged 75 to 79 and 50% of those older than 95.

The physical effects of pain can result in loss of mobility, deconditioning, and restriction in function. This can lead to complicating painful conditions including falls, pressure sores, and incontinence. Pain can be a symptom of underlying inflammation or infection and contributes to delirium and worsening cognitive impairment.

The effects of pain are not just physical but also include emotional and psychosocial responses. Depression, fatigue, alteration of sleep or appetite, and social withdrawal are common responses to painful conditions. The perception of pain and response can be culturally mediated and altered by previous painful experiences or associated events.

Although pain in the elderly is generally accepted as common, the inadequate treatment of pain, unfortunately, is also common. In nursing homes, up to one fourth of those who report daily noncancer pain have no analgesic medications on order. Effective pain evaluation depends on understanding the underlying process contributing to pain, concomitant disease states, and the careful assessment of pain, including severity, associated symptoms, and its effect on function and quality of life. Management will often be multidisciplinary and include pharmacologic and nonpharmacologic approaches. The goal of pain management is not the elimination of pain but the restoration or improvement of function.

THE MECHANISM OF PAIN

Pain is a complex, subjective and unpleasant sensation derived from sensory stimuli and modified by memory, expectations, and emotions. The experience of pain involves transduction of noxious stimuli in sensory nerves to electric impulses. These impulses are then transmitted along thick, myelinated A-delta fibers and thin unmyelinated C-fibers to the dorsal horn of the spinal cord, thalamus, and cerebral cortex, areas responsible for the perception and discrimination of painful sensations. Modulation of pain, both inhibitory and excitatory, occurs along the peripheral nervous system and central nervous system (CNS) to respond and adapt to the stimulus. One component of this adaptive phenomenon is neuroplasticity. This is the capacity of neurons to change function, chemical profile, or structure, thereby altering their pain sensory function, and is an important feature of persistent pain.

Older people generally feel less acute pain in response to a specific injury compared to younger adults. This may be due to deterioration of the peripheral C-fibers. This does not mean that older people do not feel pain. Indeed, older persons are more likely to develop persistent pain because of an increased capacity for temporal summation and sensitization of nerves in the spinal cord. Following a painful stimulus, older persons will maintain a hyperexcitable state longer than younger persons; therefore repeated, separate stimuli will result in more pain. The function of endogenous opioids tends to decline in the elderly as well, reducing the natural capacity for pain relief.

PAIN CLASSIFICATION

Pain can be classified broadly as nociceptive or neuropathic (see Table 5.1), and as acute or persistent. Inflammatory pain and functional pain can have predominant nociceptive or neuropathic components.

> **CASE ONE**
>
> An 80-year-old woman presents with stiffness and ache in her knees following an outing with her family. She has had arthritis and used doses of over-the-counter analgesics as needed, but she experienced incomplete relief. She is hesitant to tell you about the pain because she does not want "strong medication" but describes the pain as severe (7/10) and says that it is making her afraid to leave home.

Nociceptive pain results from the activation of pain receptors by noxious stimuli. It may have a somatic or visceral component, which can help differentiate the location of the activated receptors. Somatic pain originates from deep tissue injury or cutaneous injury, is often easily localized, and is described as dull, achy, or gnawing. Conditions include fractures and muscle pulls. Deep somatic pain can be less easily localized. Visceral nociceptive pain results from injury to an organ, organ system, or supporting tissue (e.g., pleura or peritoneum). It is also described as diffuse, dull, achy, or gnawing. It is poorly localized and radiates from its location. Examples include bowel obstruction and tumor infiltration. In community-dwelling elderly, the prevalent types of pain are joint, leg, and back pain. Pain in joints, an old fracture site, and malignancy are more prevalent in nursing home elderly. Generally, nociceptive pain responds to analgesic medications.

> **CASE TWO**
>
> A 75-year-old man with long-standing diabetes describes a sensation in his legs throughout the day that makes walking and sitting uncomfortable. He feels a burning sensation in his feet that is especially pronounced at night, and mere contact with the bedsheet causes intense discomfort. Aspirin and acetaminophen have not helped the condition at all. His hemoglobin A_{IC} level has been maintained at 7%.

Neuropathic pain results from damage to peripheral or secondary afferent neurons or damage at higher levels of the CNS, resulting in abnormal signal generation (ectopic

TABLE 5.1
DIFFERENTIAL DIAGNOSIS OF NEUROMUSCULAR PAIN (729.1)

Nociceptive Pain	Neuropathic Pain
Inflammatory pain Bursitis (727.0), osteoarthritis (715.09), rheumatoid arthritis (714.0), pleurisy (511.0), gout (274.9), pseudogout (712.29), tumor infiltration	**Nerve compression** Raduculitis (729.2), inflammatory demyelinating polyradiculoneuropathy (357.89)
Infection Peritonitis (567.9), infectious arthropathy (711.9x), dental caries (521.09), osteomyelitis (730.2x)	**Infection** Trigeminal neuralgia (350.1), postherpetic neuralgia (053.19), HIV sensory neuropathy (042)
Trauma Fracture, osteoporosis (733.00)	**Trauma** Entrapment neuropathy (355.9), compressive myelopathy from spinal stenosis (724.00)
Pressure Cervical (721.0) and lumbar (721.3) spondylosis, pressure sore (707.0), bowel obstruction (560.9)	**Metabolic disorder** Painful diabetic neuropathy (250.6x), nutritional deficiency-related neuropathy (357.4)
Musculoskeletal disorder Myofascial syndromes (729.1), strain (843.9), leg cramps (729.82), low back pain (724.2), disc disease (722.9)	**Surgery** Phantom limb pain (353.6), postmastectomy pain (611.71)
Nonspecific Migraine headache (346.9x), tension headache (784.0)	**Irradiation** Postradiation plexopathy (990)
	Neurotoxin Chemotherapy-induced polyneuropathy (357.6), alcoholic polyneuropathy (357.5)
	Psychological Somatization (306.9)

HIV, human immunodeficiency virus.

or spontaneous), propagation, or perception. It is often due to neural damage from surgery, radiation, and side effects of medications or disease processes (e.g., tumor infiltration, compression, and stroke). Common causes of neuropathic pain in the elderly include postherpetic neuralgia, diabetic neuropathy, and radiculopathy. The description of neuropathic pain commonly includes burning, tingling, or stabbing. Other common descriptions may include hot or cold sensation, raw or itchy skin, and dull aching pain. Medications are aimed at interfering with signal propagation.

Often, pain cannot be distinctly classified as nociceptive or neuropathic. Back pain, headache, and vascular pain may have features of both. Most persistent pain has both nociceptive and neuropathic symptoms.

Acute pain is generally associated with tissue damage, and the pathology is generally readily apparent. It is limited in duration and is not usually associated with long-term effects on the patient's quality of life or with progressive disease. After a relatively limited healing period, which ranges from hours to days, the pain receptors involved return to a normal resting stimulus threshold. Examples include tissue injury from trauma or surgery. Treatment includes common analgesic medications.

Chronic or persistent pain exists after an acute process should have resolved or may be associated with no specific injury. Typically, pain lasting for >3 months is considered persistent. The American Geriatrics Society Panel on Persistent Pain in Older Persons prefers the term *persistent* to *chronic* to help reduce the negative images associated with the latter term, such as treatment failure, malingering or long-standing psychiatric problems, or drug-seeking behavior. Persistent pain can be categorized as malignant or nonmalignant. Malignant persistent pain usually has a pathology and is indicative of a life-limiting disease such as cancer, end-stage organ dysfunction, or human immunodeficiency virus (HIV) infection. It may have both nociceptive and neuropathic elements and therefore responds to opioid, nonopioid, and adjuvant agents. Persistent pain may be present for months to years or can be sporadic. Often, there is no detectable pathology because the injured area in question is physically remote from the original area of stimulation.

EVALUATION OF PAIN

Many misconceptions lead to elderly persons underreporting pain to health care providers (see Table 5.2). Consequently, significant pain complaints may be missed if not routinely asked about at each medical encounter. Older persons will often not use the specific word "pain" but will readily describe the discomfort, hurt, or ache that they have. The assessment of pain must include the type, severity, onset, location, and duration of pain and previous therapies.

Developing a common language to assess the patient's pain is important in the initial evaluation and measurement of the success of various interventions. The severity of pain may vary over the course of the day, so asking about both the current intensity of pain and the worst pain over the last 24 hours is helpful. Rating the intensity of pain as mild, moderate, or severe is important, but using a numeric

TABLE 5.2
BARRIERS LEADING TO UNDERREPORTING OF PAIN

Pain considered normal part of aging
Expectation that doctor/nurse knows when pain occurs
Fear that pain may indicate progression of disease
Fear of needing additional lab test and expense
Belief that there are no (or no adequate) treatments available
Concern of use of strong opioid medications

scale (0 to 10 or 0 to 100 with "0" being no pain and "10 or 100" the worst pain in the patient's life) may give a better range of pain assessment. Another instrument, the Functional Pain Scale rating, incorporates both severity and interference with daily activities. Zero relates to no pain or interference with daily activities; "1" relates to tolerable pain not interfering with activities; "2" to tolerable pain that interferes with some activities; "3" to intolerable pain but being able to use the phone, watch television, or read; "4" to intolerable pain and not being able to do the same activities that are possible with a rating of "3"; and "5" to intolerable pain and inability to communicate verbally.

Also, it is helpful for the patient to describe the quality of the pain (i.e., sharp, burning, or dull), duration (i.e., transient, intermittent, or persistent), and to identify the location and direction of radiation of pain (i.e., superficial or deep, localized or diffuse). Pain questionnaires such as the McGill Pain Inventory help prompt the patient to describe pain and are useful tools for monitoring improvement. The patient should be asked about aggravating and relieving factors. The present pain management regimen and previous treatments and their responses should be evaluated because they can significantly impact treatment options.

Although specific causes of pain should always be sought, many times pain in the elderly will not have a clear onset or single etiology. Some specific pain syndromes, such as trigeminal neuralgia, herpes zoster neuralgia, or temporal arteritis, present with classic features. However, many examples exist of atypical presentation of illness that in younger persons is typically painful (e.g., infection and myocardial infarction). Pain can also be secondary to a concomitant disease. Painful neuropathy from diabetes, peripheral vascular disease, and stroke should be considered. Pain therapy will be most successful in these situations by modifying the underlying disease, and pain may respond to more than just medication. Glucose control is the cornerstone in managing diabetic complications.

The objective signs of acute pain may include pallor, sweating, tachycardia, and facial grimacing. The patient who presents with persistent pain will likely not have these symptoms, and objective findings on examination can be a challenge. Unsuspected causes of pain can include dental or oral pathology, nocturnal leg cramp, and poststroke contractures. Physical examination should include careful evaluation of the location of pain and identification of common referral patterns. Palpation for trigger points and inflammation, and maneuvers to reproduce pain should be sought. The range of motion, as well as a complete neurologic examination, should be documented. The scope of the workup will depend on the patient's prognosis, goal of care, and advance directives.

Laboratory testing options include hemoglobin level and hematocrit, fasting glucose level, and chemistry profile for liver and renal function. Evaluation of uric acid for gout pain and alkaline phosphatase for Paget disease or other bone involvement may be warranted. Radiologic examination should depend on suspected underlying processes (i.e., spine films for compression fracture or computed tomography scan/magnetic resonance imaging for spinal stenosis).

Finally, it is important to have a sense of the impact that pain has on the person's life. Physical function and limitation need to be identified. Social supports and coping strategies must be assessed. Some patients may rely on their network of family and friends or find support through their spiritual life and religious or other civic organizations. In geriatric patients small improvements in physical function can have dramatic improvements in well-being. Improving independence through mobility and completion of activities of daily living or returning to enjoyable activities with improved extremity function can result from improved pain control.

The emotional and psychosocial impact of pain is important to acknowledge. If anxiety or depression are significant contributors or responses to the painful experience, coping strategies need to be prescribed. The inability to sleep because of pain can have a profound effect on daily activity; the success of pain control may simply be the ability to get a few hours of restful sleep. The response to pain may be fear, anxiety, anger, and loneliness.

Undermanaged pain can lead to depression, and depressed mood can make the perception of pain worse. However, patients may be diagnosed with a mood or thought disorder and treated with a psychotropic medication when the actual problem is unrecognized and untreated pain. The use of mild analgesics may reduce the use of psychotropic drugs.

Evaluation of Pain in the Cognitively Impaired

An estimated 45% to 80% of nursing home patients have some chronic pain. There is no reason to assume that those with cognitive impairment are any less able to feel pain. Self-report should not be used as a sole means of pain assessment. Although the patients may be unable to speak of their pain, decreased appetite, increased irritability, poor sleep, and agitated behaviors may be symptoms of pain. Other nonspecific signs may include grimacing, teeth grinding, sighing, groaning, breathing heavily, or resistance to care. Assessments by family or caregivers will certainly help in evaluating the effectiveness of pain management strategies. The family should be asked about how the older person has manifested pain or discomfort in the past. The use of a visual scale of happy to tearful faces can be used to help speech-impaired persons to rate their pain. Simple, directed yes–no questions are also helpful.

GOALS OF PAIN MANAGEMENT

Effective pain management is multidisciplinary and includes pharmacologic and nonpharmacologic options (see Table 5.3). The complete elimination of pain is not a

TABLE 5.3
PAIN MANAGEMENT STRATEGIES

Nonpharmacologic Measures ⟷	Analgesic Medications ⟷	Adjuvant Medications
Rehabilitation	Acetaminophen	
Psychological maneuvers	Aspirin	Anticonvulsants
Anesthesiology	Nonacetyl salicylates	Topical agents
Surgical intervention	NSAIDs	SSRI
Nerve stimulation	COX-2 inhibitors	SNRI
Complementary medicine	Weak opioids	TCA
Lifestyle interventions	Potent opioids	Antispasmodics
Education	Steroids	

NSAID, nonsteroidal anti-inflammatory drug; COX-2, cyclooxygenase-2; SSRI, selective serotonin reuptake inhibitor; SNRI, serotonin–norepinephrine reuptake inhibitor; TCA, tricyclic antidepressant.

necessary goal of treatment. Improved function and the ability to cope with painful stimuli may be more reasonable. Identifying the specific goals that the patient may have for pain treatment will help in developing a rational plan. Understanding what the patient can or will do to participate in pain management is crucial when considering nonpharmacologic strategies. An inability to cooperate with an extensive physical therapy regimen does not mean that the patient cannot benefit from restorative care services. Clarification of perceptions of pain management is equally important to decrease the chance of rejecting a helpful therapy because of unwarranted fear of addiction or "being drugged up." Identifying specific functional goals such as activities, abilities, or socialization make for more measurable success.

Families and patients (as well as care staff) need ongoing education and reinforcement of the knowledge that pain is not a normal part of aging. Inadequate pain management is often the result of inadequate recognition and inquiry. Some patients will not report pain because they do not want to bother anyone or they assume that there is no treatment. They may refuse or restrict treatment because of feared side effects.

Nonpharmacologic Pain Therapies

Physical therapies and exercise have the advantage of improving strength, flexibility, and endurance. As learned interventions, they allow the individual and caregivers a sense of control in symptom management. This works best in the cognitively intact and motivated patient, but some element of physical therapies can be instituted in all cases of pain. A simple exercise program can be developed for any individual, tailored to his or her abilities and preferences and titrated incrementally to its success. Hot or cold therapies may help decrease local inflammation or improve circulation to a painful area. Simple products such as a hot water bottle or ice cubes can be employed. Precautions are necessary so that prolonged contact does not cause damage to the local tissue and surrounding structures. Concomitant use of a skin vasodilating agent such as analgesic balm, methyl salicylate cream, or capsaicin should be avoided.

While randomized trials have not demonstrated its utility in chronic low back pain, transcutaneous electrical nerve stimulation (TENS) continues to be used for mild to moderate pain in older individuals. It works through counterstimulation of the pain-transmitting nerves. Careful assessment for the optimal placement and electrical setting for patient comfort and effectiveness is important in the long-term success of this modality. Other muscle stimulation techniques that physical therapy can provide include massage and ultrasound heat treatments. Orthotic devices can be helpful in improving body alignment and stability. They can also be helpful in decreasing the risk or managing the consequences of contracture.

Occupational therapy can be used to help improve the endurance and effectiveness of self-care activities and identify compensatory strategies for improved function. The focus is on completion of everyday activities of self-care to promote independence. Adaptive equipment is an important rehabilitative tool for the impairment that the pain causes. Alteration of the home environment can help minimize hazards.

Psychological maneuvers can be a helpful intervention for pain management. The cognitive behavioral therapies are helpful when the patient has sufficient cognition to understand the source of pain, its effects, and coping strategies (Evidence Level B). As a coping strategy, cognitive behavioral therapy may help the person accept some level of pain and change self-defeating thought patterns in response to pain.

The goal of relaxation techniques is to control the focus of attention, shifting it away from the painful stimuli. Self-directed repetitive focus on a word, sound, phrase, or prayer allows the person to direct attention to a different focus and develop a passive distraction from the unwanted stimulus. Even in the cognitively impaired, gentle tones of voice and redirected conversation can help decrease the focus from pain to more favorable experiences. Likewise, progressive relaxation or breathing techniques can provide a sense of control over one's body, taking control away from the painful stimulus.

Complementary or alternative therapies will commonly be employed by a patient or his or her family. Some therapies may be culturally embedded as a learned response to pain and suffering. Although few of these therapies have evidence of efficacy, the clinician must be reasonably assured that the proposed therapy will not be harmful or costly to the patient. The use of acupuncture, homeopathic, chiropractic, and spiritual healing may have a beneficial effect on the patient and should not be discounted.

Mixing of the various available techniques can help augment the success of any single therapy. This in turn can decrease the amount of medication used for pain control. Making a variety of interventions available to the patient can give them a sense of control to utilize specific techniques for specific circumstances.

Pharmacologic Management

Aging affects the metabolism, distribution, and excretion of nutrients and drugs. Liver function may be impaired, and competing enzyme systems may slow the metabolism of drugs. Serum albumin level decreases, allowing more free drug to circulate. Renal function and clearance may also be impaired, resulting in accumulation of drugs and making the elderly more sensitive to doses of medication or to be at higher risk for side effects. An assessment of current renal function is essential when initiating pain medications. In general, the starting doses of medication should be 25% to 50% of the dose prescribed for younger patients and titrated more slowly to allow time to determine steady state effect and hopefully minimize side effects (Evidence Level C). Routine dosing of medication is recommended rather than prescription on an as-needed basis. Often, by the time the patient takes the medicine on an as-needed basis, the pain is more severe and requires higher doses for pain relief. Scheduled dosing may also decrease the anxiety associated with anticipating the next dose of medication and will certainly improve the administration of necessary drugs in the long-term care setting (Evidence Level A).

Nonopioid Pain Medications

Among the nonopioid analgesics, acetaminophen is for mild to moderate pain (see Table 5.4). It is inexpensive and available in liquid, pill, and suppository formulations. Although not an anti-inflammatory drug, its action is through *N*-methyl-D-aspartate (NMDA) receptors and substance P. In regular scheduled dosages of 2 to 4 g per day, it provides excellent pain relief for musculoskeletal disorders. Lower total doses should be used in people of smaller frame or in those who have experienced poor nutrition or weight loss. The American Geriatrics Society recommends a 50% to 75% dose reduction in the setting of liver or renal disease or excessive alcohol consumption. Combination medications that have acetaminophen should be considered in the total daily dose taken. Toxic drug–drug interactions include rifampin, phenytoin, carbamazepine, barbiturates, and warfarin.

Nonsteroidal anti-inflammatory drugs (NSAIDs) are indicated mainly for short-term use in inflammatory arthritic conditions and acute rheumatic disorders. They can also be helpful in combination with opioids for treating bone pain from cancer. NSAIDs vary greatly in their potency, analgesic and anti-inflammatory effect, and side effects. Patients may respond better to one class of

TABLE 5.4
NONOPIOID ANALGESICS IN THE ELDERLY

Generic Name	Brand Name	Initial PO Dose (mg)	Total mg/24 h
Acetaminophen	Tylenol	650 q6h	4,000 (2–3 g in case of liver disease)
Aspirin	Bayer, Ecotrin	325–650 q6h	4,000
Celecoxib	Celebrex	100 q24h	400
Choline magnesium trisalicylate	Trilisate	500 q12h	3,000
Diclofenac potassium	Cataflam	50 q8h	150
Diclofenac sodium	Voltaren	50 q8h	150
Diflunisal	Dolobid	250 q12h	1,000
Etodolac	Lodine	200 q8h	1,200
Fenoprofen	Nalfon	200 q6h	3,200
Flurbiprofen	Ansaid	50 q12h	300
Ibuprofen	Advil, Motrin	200 q6h	3,200
Ketoprofen	Orudis	25 q8h	300
Nabumetone	Relafen	500 q24h	2,000
Naproxen	Naprosyn, Aleve	220 q12h	1,500
Salsalate	Disalcid	500 q12h	3,000
Sulindac	Clinoril	150 q12h	400
Tramadol	Ultram	25 q6h	300
Valdecoxib	Bextra	10 q24h	10
Corticosteroid	Prednisone	5 q.d.	60

Most nonspecific NSAIDs should be used cautiously in the elderly and are contraindicated in the setting of advanced renal disease. Close monitoring is expected.

NSAIDs over another, but using multiple NSAIDs only increases the risk for toxicity.

Aspirin is the prototypic anti-inflammatory agent. It is a potent anti-inflammatory agent because of the inhibition of prostaglandin, and it irreversibly binds to platelets. However, it must be given every 4 to 6 hours and even in usual doses can cause gastric irritation and bleeding. High doses or regular use can cause tinnitus or nephrotoxicity. As an alternative, nonacetylated salicylates have the advantage of potentially fewer gastrointestinal (GI) side effects and are not nephrotoxic in standard doses. Agents include choline magnesium trisalicylate (Trilisate) and salsalate (Disalcid). All are available as generic oral preparations, making them an attractive cost-effective option (Evidence Level B). Although they are not as potent prostaglandin inhibitors as other NSAIDs, they can be very effective pain relievers. They should be avoided in patients sensitive to aspirin. They can be dosed every 8 to 12 hours.

There are numerous NSAIDs available in both parenteral and oral preparation. These agents act by nonselective inhibition of cyclooxygenase-1 (COX-1) and COX-2, accounting both for their effects and side effects. Pain relief often occurs at doses lower than the anti-inflammatory dose, and some agents are indicated only for short-term use (<5 to 10 days). Ibuprofen and naproxen (Naprosyn) are very effective in providing anti-inflammatory and analgesic effect. Chronic use of NSAIDs must be considered in light of the well-known toxicities, and close monitoring in the older patient is essential. GI effects can range from mild nausea or dyspepsia to severe bleeding. The upper GI damage associated with nonselective NSAIDs may be lessened by the concomitant use of misoprostol or proton pump inhibitors (Evidence Level A). The use of H_2 receptor antagonists has not been proved to prevent gastric ulcers or gastroduodenal ulcer complications associated with the use of nonselective NSAIDs.

Nephrotoxic effects can include proteinuria, renal insufficiency, peripheral edema, and hypertension. Sulindac is the only nonspecific NSAID with reported fewer renal side effects. With reversible platelet inhibition, NSAIDs can increase bleeding, and prothrombin time must be monitored when administered with warfarin. NSAIDs can also precipitate congestive heart failure (CHF), hyperkalemia, and CNS dysfunction.

Selective COX-2 inhibitors are an acceptable alternative for patients who have inadequate relief with acetaminophen for symptomatic osteoarthritis and mild to moderate pain. Recent concerns about the association of COX-2 inhibitors and cardiac disease warrant careful discussion with patients or their surrogates, and the lowest effective dosing regimen should be utilized. COX-2 inhibitors tend to have less GI prostaglandin inhibition and are associated with less GI toxicity, but ulceration and bleeding have been reported. Like other NSAIDs, the COX-2 inhibitors can increase blood pressure and cause edema through sodium retention; they can also cause renal insufficiency. Caution is advised if the patient has hypertension, is on an angiotensin-converting enzyme inhibitor, or has heart failure because the addition of COX-2 can lead to CHF exacerbation.

Celecoxib (Celebrex) 200 mg per day has been effective for both osteoarthritis and rheumatoid arthritis. Current recommendations of celecoxib are 400 mg on day 1 for acute pain, and then 200 mg b.i.d. p.r.n. With dosages ranging from 100 to 400 mg per day for osteoarthritis and 200 to 800 mg per day for rheumatoid arthritis, celecoxib has been as effective as naproxen 1,000 mg per day or diclofenac 150 mg per day for the management of pain. Valdecoxib (Bextra) starting at 12.5 mg per day up to 25 mg per day has also been comparable to naproxen 1,000 mg per day. Rofecoxib (Vioxx) has been removed from the market.

Topical Agents

Topical agents (see Table 5.5), including capsaicin, methyl salicylate, trolamine salicylate, and camphor preparations, are as effective as either monotherapy or adjunctive therapy for localized pain in joints and muscles, but they are not practical for diffuse pain. Capsaicin works by depleting the applied area of substance P and preventing further formation over time, so that pain signals are less readily transmitted (Evidence Level C). Topical salicylates have limited efficacy but may have a beneficial effect through local irritation overriding pain signals or the generation of local heat. Also, if applied in excess to a large area of skin or to broken skin or mucous membranes, systemic salicylate side effects and enhanced anticoagulant effect can occur. Thorough hand washing by patients or others who apply capsaicin is necessary to avoid transference or inadvertent contact with mucous membranes, which can result in burning and stinging. Available in both a standard (0.025%) and high-potency (0.075%) preparation, capsaicin may be helpful in postherpetic neuralgia but must be applied several times a day. Initial tolerance can be improved with concurrent use of topical lidocaine.

Anesthetic gels including ketamine, lidocaine, or compounded products for transcutaneous absorption can be considered, especially in a patient unable to take oral medication. Long used in the palliative care setting,

TABLE 5.5
TOPICAL AGENTS

Agent	Brand Name
Lidocaine 5% patch	Lidoderm
Camphor/phenol	Campho-Phenique, Sarna
Methyl salicylate/menthol	Ben Gay
Trolamine salicylate	Aspercream
Capsaicin 0.025%	Capsin
Capsaicin 0.075%	Zostrix HP

TABLE 5.6
OPIOID ANALGESICS IN THE ELDERLY

Medication	Forms	Initial	Interval (h)	Equipotent Dose to 30 mg PO Morphine
Codeine	Tylenol no. 2–no. 4	15–60 mg	6–8	200 mg
Oxycodone	Percocet, Percodan, Tylox	5 mg	6–12	20 mg
Oxycodone SR	OxyContin	10 mg	12	20 mg
Hydrocodone	Vicodin, Lortab	5 mg	6	30 mg
Morphine	Roxanol, MSIR	10 mg	4–6	30 mg PO/10 mg IV
Morphine SR	MS Contin	30 mg	12	30 mg PO/10 mg IV
Morphine ER	Kadian	20 mg	24	30 mg PO/10 mg IV
Hydromorphone	Dilaudid	2 mg	4–6	7.5 mg PO/1.5 mg IV
Methadone	Dolophine	5 mg	8	
Fentanyl patch	Duragesic	25 μg/72 h	200 μg/72 h	

compounded agents can include opioid medications for adjunctive pain relief.

Opioid Pain Medications

Opioid medications (see Table 5.6) are probably the original pharmaceuticals. They can be administered orally, intramuscularly, or intravenously, and some are also available in transdermal formulations. Various products are immediate-release, sustained-release, and controlled-release (compounded with both immediate- and delayed-release formulations). Commonly, the oral opioids are combined with acetaminophen, aspirin, or ibuprofen, which can have the advantage of lowering the total dose needed of either medication. However, this also has the effect of providing a ceiling that limits the total dose that can be administered.

A common concern of both patients and providers is potential overuse or addiction to narcotic pain medications. It is important to understand the distinction between physical dependence, analgesic tolerance, and addiction. Physical dependence refers to the acquired physiologic adaptation of the continued need for medication. Tolerance refers to the need for higher doses to attain the same effect. This phenomenon is common to many medications and requires gradual dose reduction when changing the medication or taking the person off it. Addiction refers to the pathologic behavior of impaired control or compulsive use of the drug despite harm. The risk of addiction in older patients is mostly associated with a previous history of substance abuse. In regularly scheduled doses of narcotic pain medication, older persons tend not to escalate their requirements.

Tramadol is a unique agent with pain relief comparable to the opioids. Tramadol is primarily a centrally acting analgesic with effects through norepinephrine and serotonin inhibition, blocking pain transmission in the spinal cord, and secondarily a blocker of CNS μ-opioid receptors. It has a low potential for abuse. Starting at 25 to 50 mg, tramadol has rapid absorption, peaks in 2 hours, and has a half-life of 6 hours. It is also available in a fixed dose 37.5 mg combination with acetaminophen, 325 mg. Although not likely to be abused or lead to respiratory depression, it can cause significant nausea, drowsiness, sweating, and constipation. Tramadol should be avoided or used cautiously in combination with tricyclic antidepressants (TCAs), selective serotonin reuptake inhibitors (SSRIs), and monoamine oxidase inhibitors (MAOIs) because of the risk of causing seizures.

Codeine, hydrocodone, and oxycodone are considered lower-potency opioids when given in combination with aspirin and acetaminophen. Originally available as immediate-release, short-acting agents, sustained-release formulations have been developed. Propoxyphene is a commonly used agent, but is probably no more effective than the acetaminophen it is combined with, and is associated with the accumulation of metabolites and CNS toxicity in chronic use. Propoxyphene should be avoided for chronic use in the elderly.

Morphine is the standard preparation to which all opioid medications are compared. Available as immediate-release liquid, tablet, rectal, IV, and IM administration, it can be convenient for initial drug titration and management of breakthrough pain. Long-acting preparations in a number of unique extended-release products are available, but patients need to be warned that biting or chewing the vehicle can result in immediate release of the drug with toxic effects. An extended-release morphine (Kadian) has encapsulated medication that can be sprinkled from the capsule and mixed with food or given through feeding tube.

In many patients with persistent pain, it is worthwhile to switch to an alternate agent when tolerance has developed rather than continue dose escalation of the same medication. When changing between opioids, the new agent may be started at one half to two thirds of the equivalent analgesic dose and then titrated to response. If the quality or character of the pain has changed, however, an evaluation for a new source of pain may be indicated.

When prescribing opioid medications, it is important to have a bowel regimen in place to anticipate constipation as a side effect. This should include physical activity when possible and increased fiber or stool softeners (docusate sodium) to maintain liquid in the stool. Lactulose, a nonabsorbed sugar, will also help maintain liquid stool and can be titrated to effect. An alternative osmotic laxative is polyethylene glycol (MiraLax), which some find easier to drink and is not sweet in flavor. Despite all this, a stimulant laxative such as senna concentrate (Senokot) is needed to stimulate the bowel musculature. Magnesium laxatives should be avoided in renal impairment.

An interesting area of study is the use of dextromethorphan to potentiate the action of opioid analgesics. Dextromethorphan directly antagonizes the NMDA receptors, which then blocks the central sensitization and development of opioid tolerance.

Methadone, although commonly prescribed for opioid addiction, can also be written for analgesia. It is an agonist at the μ-opioid receptor that has greater efficacy than morphine with repeated doses. Although a single dose of 15 mg oral morphine has an analgesic equivalency of 10 mg oral methadone, with repeated dosing relatively smaller amounts of methadone are needed. Methadone is a synthetic compound and may be used in patients with morphine allergy. It has a long half-life, so initial response may be slower and duration of effect may also be prolonged. The College of Physicians and Surgeons of Ontario recommends starting dosages in the frail elderly to be as low as 2.5 mg orally once per day, with incremental dose changes every 5 to 7 days and close monitoring for systemic toxicity (Evidence Level C).

Adjuvant Medications

Other medications are important in the management of neuropathic pain (see Table 5.7). Multiple randomized control trials have demonstrated the efficacy of TCAs, gabapentin, opioid analgesics, tramadol, and lidocaine 5% patch for neuropathic pain.

Antidepressants have a dual role of treating mood disorders and independently addressing pain symptoms. TCAs work through various degrees of inhibition of norepinephrine and serotonin receptors. SSRIs are effective and have a more favorable side effect profile than older agents. Atypical antidepressants include norepinephrine and dopamine reuptake inhibitors (NDRIs), serotonin–norepinephrine reuptake inhibitors (SNRIs), and serotonin-2 antagonist reuptake inhibitors (SARIs). These agents may have analgesic qualities as well. The analgesic effect is independent of the antidepressant effect.

TCAs have analgesic properties in low doses, but the analgesic effect increases with higher doses and over

TABLE 5.7
ADJUVANT MEDICATIONS

Medication	Brand Name	Initial Dose	Interval (h)	Not to Exceed in Young Adults/24 h
		Anticonvulsants		
Carbamazepine	Tegretol	100 mg	8–12	—
Clonazepam	Klonopin	0.5 mg	6–8	—
Gabapentin	Neurontin	100 mg	8–24	3,600 mg
Phenytoin	Dilantin	100 mg	12–24	10–20 μg/mL serum level
		Antidepressants		
Doxepin	Sinequan	25 mg	8–24	300 mg
Duloxetine	Cymbalta	30 mg	24	60 mg
Fluoxetine	Prozac	10 mg	24	60 mg
Imipramine	Tofranil	25 mg	12–24	150 mg
Nortriptyline	Pamelor	10 mg	24	75 mg
Paroxetine	Paxil	10 mg	24	40 mg
Sertraline	Zoloft	25 mg	24	200 mg
Venlafaxine	Effexor	25 mg	8–24	200 mg
		Muscle Relaxants		
Baclofen	Lioresal	5 mg	8–12	80 mg
Carisoprodol	Soma	350 mg	8–24	1,400 mg
Tizanidine	Zanaflex	2 mg	12–24	36 mg

time. Dosing should begin with the lowest available strength, given at bedtime and then titrated over weeks and increased to maximum efficacy as dose-related side effects allow. The tertiary amines, imipramine, amitriptyline, clomipramine, and doxepin, were originally studied but may have intolerable side effects in the elderly. The quaternary amines tend to cause less central activity and hypotension and may be better tolerated in older persons. These include desipramine, nortriptyline, protriptyline, and amoxapine. All tricyclics should be used with caution in patients with cardiac disease, glaucoma, urinary retention, and autonomic insufficiency.

Serotonin reuptake inhibitors were introduced as novel antidepressants and have been found useful in a variety of conditions including panic disorder, generalized anxiety, chronic fatigue, premenstrual syndrome, and chronic pain. Their role in pain management is likely related to depression and anxiety that are somatically mediated (Evidence Level B). Common side effects include headache, stimulation or sedation, cardiac effects (e.g., bradycardia or tachycardia), GI effects (e.g., change in appetite, nausea, vomiting, or diarrhea), sedation, lowered seizure threshold, tremor, or tinnitus.

The SNRIs include venlafaxine and duloxetine. Early studies of venlafaxine demonstrated pain relief. Duloxetine, which is a balanced SNRI, works centrally through sodium channels and is the first U.S. Food and Drug Administration (FDA)-approved treatment for the management of painful diabetic peripheral neuropathy (Evidence Level A). The recommended dosage is 60 mg once daily, but 30 mg capsules are also available.

The anticonvulsants can have a significant role in the management of neuropathic pain. They work by stabilizing neuronal membranes and altering sodium, calcium, and potassium channels, and they may affect other neurotransmitters in modulating pain. Phenytoin was first noted to have properties in pain relief, and it was originally started at 100 mg three times a day and titrated to patient response. Serum levels must be monitored, and side effects are common. Folate supplementation is necessary to decrease the risk of drug-induced peripheral neuropathy and megaloblastic anemia (Evidence Level B). Carbamazepine has FDA approval for trigeminal neuralgia pain. Available in both short- and extended-release preparations, dosing begins at 100 mg at bedtime and is titrated to effect. It has significant side effects, including a black-box warning for aplastic anemia and agranulocytosis, so baseline complete blood count should be obtained (Evidence Level A).

Gabapentin has been studied in patients with postherpetic neuralgia, painful diabetic neuropathy, mixed neuropathic syndromes, phantom limb pain, Guillain-Barré syndrome, and acute and chronic spinal cord injury pain, and it is an effective agent in the elderly. Dosing begins at 100 to 300 mg at bedtime and is titrated up to three times a day to total doses of 3,600 mg. Its absorption is not affected by food. It is generally well tolerated and has notably fewer cognitive side effects than other anticonvulsants. Side effects include somnolence, dizziness, and less frequently, GI symptoms and peripheral edema (Evidence Level A).

Local anesthetics have been tried for pain relief, as well as for their effect on membrane stabilization and flux of sodium channels. The topical lidocaine 5% patch is indicated for postherpetic neuralgia. It can be cut to fit the area of pain. It is safe and easily tolerated but should be dosed such that no more than three patches are applied for 12 hours to the affected area, with at least a 12-hour off period between applications to avoid systemic absorption and possible interaction with class I antiarrhythmics. Local skin irritation has been reported.

Finally, antispasmodics may be indicated for the spasticity associated with chronic conditions, as well as for augmentation of other analgesic agents. Used alone, they are not effective pain treatments. All antispasmodic agents can cause significant sedation. Tizanidine (Zanaflex) has been found to help muscle spasm, as well as persistent pain symptoms. It should begin with low doses at bedtime and slowly titrated daily or b.i.d. (Evidence Level B).

Surgical Intervention

Referral to anesthesiologists and pain management centers is appropriate for patients with complex persistent pain. Spinal injections of opioids and implantable pain delivery devices or electrical stimulation devices may be considered. Local or trigger point injections may temporarily improve participation and effectiveness of rehabilitation (Evidence Level C).

CONCLUSION

The clinician has many opportunities to help manage older people's complaints of pain. Through careful evaluation, the underlying and contributing factors can be defined and a variety of pharmacologic and nonpharmacologic treatments employed. The severity and effectiveness of response can be followed even in the cognitively impaired. Restoration of function, and improvement in sleep, mood, and daily activities are the most important results of effective pain management.

ACKNOWLEDGMENT

The author appreciates the assistance of Erin Frankford, Pharm.D. in preparing the accompanying tables.

SELECTED READING

American Geriatrics Society Panel on Persistent Pain in Older Persons. The management of persistent pain in older persons. *J Am Geriatr Soc*. 2002:50:S205–S224.

American Pain Society. *Principles of analgesic use in the treatment of acute pain and cancer pain*, 5th ed. Glenview, Ill: American Pain Society: 2003:16.

Ballantyne J, ed. *The Massachusetts General Hospital handbook of pain management*, 2nd ed. Philadelphia, PA: Lippincott Williams & Wilkins; 2002.

Ballantyne J, Mao J. Opioid therapy for chronic pain. *N Engl J Med.* 2003;349(20):1943.

College of Physicians and Surgeons of Ontario. *Evidence-based recommendations for medical management of chronic non-malignant pain.* 2000.

Galer BS, Gammaitoni AR. More than 7 years of consistent neuropathic pain relief in geriatric patients. *Arch Intern Med.* 2003;163:628.

Gloth FM. Pain management in older adults: Prevention and treatment. *J Am Geriatr Soc.* 2001;49:188–199.

Gloth FM III, Scheve AA, Stober CV, et al. The functional pain scale: Reliability, validity, and responsiveness in an elderly population. *J Am Med Dir Assoc.* 2001;2(3):110–114.

McCarberg BH, Dachs R. *Managing pain: Dispelling the myths*. American Academy of Family Physicians, Leawood, KS; 2003.

Melzack R. The McGill Pain Questionaire (MPQ). *Pain.* 1975;1: 277–299.

Melzack R. The short form McGill Pain Questionnaire. *Pain.* 1987; 30:191–197.

Raphael J, Leo RJ, Singh A. Pain management in the elderly: Use of psychopharmacologic agents. *Ann Long Term Care: Clin Care Aging.* 2002;10:37–45.

Rudy T, ed. *Persistent pain in older adults: An interdisciplinary guide for treatment*. New York, NY: Springer Publishing Company; 2002.

Schnitzer TJ. Managing chronic pain with tramadol in elderly patients. *Clin Geriatr*. 1999;7:35–45.

Scudds RJ, Robertson McD. Empirical evidence of the association between the presence of musculoskeletal pain and physical disability in community-dwelling senior citizens. *J Pain.* 1998;75:229–235.

Temporal, M. Chronic Pain. In: Mengel MB, ed. *Family medicine: Ambulatory care and prevention*. McGraw Hill, New York, NY; 2005.

6

Loss and Bereavement in the Elderly

Donald P. Bartlett *Marlon Russell Koenigsberg* *Jeffrey M. Moll*

CLINICAL PEARLS 59

INTRODUCTION 59
Terminology 60

NORMAL GRIEF 60
Differential Diagnosis of Normal Grief and Depression 61

COMPLICATED GRIEF 61

BEREAVEMENT CARE 62
Gradually Shift to Palliative Care 62
Establish a Bereavement Register 64
Identify Patients at High Risk 64
Assess and Assist Anticipatory Grieving 64
Counsel the Dying Patient 66
Provide Support to the Family while the Patient is Dying 66
Attend the Funeral and Write a Letter of Condolence 67
Assist in the Grieving Process 68
Monitor for Poor Bereavement Outcome 70
Treat Complicated Grief and Depression 70

CONCLUSIONS 71

CLINICAL PEARLS

- Normal grief does not unfold in a series of predictable stages. It is a set of common reactions (e.g., shock, denial, and sadness) that vary in intensity and gradually diminish over time.
- Complicated grief is a syndrome characterized by delayed or incomplete adaptation to loss.
- Symptoms of complicated grief or major depressive disorder lasting beyond 6 months, or suicidal thinking at any time, indicates a need for mental health evaluation and treatment.
- Gradually shifting to palliative care enables consideration of anticipatory grief issues for both patients and families.
- A bereavement register enables tracking of patients and families for proactive case management to overcome isolation in elderly bereaved.
- Writing a letter of condolence can be a simple yet powerful act that comforts the family and provides a bridge to bereavement care.
- Grief is universal, yet the experience is always idiosyncratic.
- Help the bereaved by listening well, gently probing for more, and accepting their experience.

INTRODUCTION

The prevalence of bereavement increases with age, making it a significant challenge for older adults whose health and adaptive capacities may already be compromised.[1] Family physicians and general internists often provide care for multiple generations of a family over long periods, developing a rapport that is valuable at times of loss. They are in a unique position to identify the bereaved, track the course of their experiences, screen for complications, and provide support throughout the process.

Bereavement is a significant health risk for many patients.[1,2] Within 5 years of the death of a spouse, mortality from ischemic heart disease increases between 20% and 35%.[2] Grief reactions are also associated with high-risk health behaviors, development of high blood pressure,[2] and increased use of alcohol and tobacco.[1] Unresolved grief is related to an increase in the incidence of anxiety and depressive disorders, which in turn negatively affect the course of many chronic diseases.[2] There is also a related increased risk of suicide attempts in the bereaved.[1] These health risks increase the burden on an already overtaxed health care system and on individual providers. After the loss of a spouse, there is an increased rate of clinic visits by widowed persons.[1] Furthermore, studies of bereavement in the elderly have found that normal grief symptoms can persist up to 4 years after the death of a spouse.[2]

This chapter briefly reviews guidelines for the identification and management of bereavement in the primary care office. Although the focus is on helping spouses and families through the grieving process, we also address the challenge of assisting dying patients with managing their own anticipatory grief.

Terminology

Interpretation of guidelines and relevant research requires consistent terminology. The terms *loss, bereavement, mourning*, and *grief* are often used interchangeably, with some confusion. We present the following definitions as common ground for discussions on the assessment and treatment of grief reactions.[3–5]

Loss: The permanent separation from and deprivation of something or someone of value and attachment. The loss may be physical (tangible) or psychosocial (symbolic). Some examples of loss include death of a loved one, loss of a beloved object (e.g., house burning down), loss of functioning or independence (e.g., decreased mobility or amputation), or a significant change in one's life (e.g., entry into a nursing home).

Bereavement: The period after a loss during which mourning occurs and grief is experienced.

Mourning: The culturally defined process by which people adapt to loss. "Mourning refers to the social expression of grief . . . and it includes rituals and behaviors that are specific to each culture and religion"[6] (page 130). For example, in Navajo culture the public rituals of mourning occur for only 4 days.[4]

Normal Grief: The unique personal response to separation and loss. The grief response includes psychological, behavioral, social, and physical reactions including shock, disbelief, overwhelming sadness, anxiety, poor sleep and eating patterns, fatigue, headache, and social withdrawal. Types of grief[4,6] include:

- *Anticipatory Grief:* A grief reaction that occurs in anticipation of an impending loss. This includes anger, guilt, anxiety, irritability, sadness, feelings of loss, and/or a decreased ability to perform usual tasks.[4]
- *Acute Grief:* Grief occurring at the time of death or in the first few days/weeks after death. It may include denial, intense crying spells, panic attacks, derealization (a sense of unreality), emotional numbness, and a variety of somatic symptoms that can seem exaggerated or frightening to family and friends.
- *Chronic Phase of Normal Grief:* Refers to intense grief that subsides during the first year and may then return as temporary waves or pangs of grief at certain times, such as the anniversary of the spouse's death, birthdays, or specific reminders. This exacerbation of grief is episodic, and grief reactions diminish in frequency and intensity with time.[6]

Complicated Grief: A syndrome characterized by delayed or incomplete adaptation to loss.[1] Complicated grief occurs when symptoms do not resolve over time and/or increase in intensity.

NORMAL GRIEF

Misdiagnosis of grief reactions often occurs because intense symptoms of grief are seen as indicators of depression or dementia. Accurate differential diagnosis requires a clear model of normal grief and algorithms to distinguish normal grief from complicated grief and depression.

Initially, normal grief was described as occurring in stages.[7] The classic Kubler-Ross stages included denial, anger, bargaining, depression, and acceptance. Bowlby theory of attachment[7] postulated the following series of stages: Shock and numbness, yearning and searching (i.e., separation anxiety and denial of the reality of the loss), disorganization (i.e., depression, despair, or difficulty planning for the future), and reorganization and positive readjustment. Research now indicates that grief does not unfold in so orderly a manner[1] but often comes in unpredictable waves, with some stages or reactions being more prominent than others.[8] Practitioners who are preoccupied with a rigid stage model often misdiagnose normal grief as complicated grief or depression. Unfortunately, patients who are aware of the stage model often feel they are not grieving "the right way" if their reactions vary. A clinically useful way to view normal grief is as a set of common reactions that vary in intensity but diminish over time. The commonly observed reactions[1,4,7] are as follows:

Sadness: Overwhelming sadness is of course the central feature of grief. Surviving family and friends may be unable to talk about the deceased without crying. Initially, some weepiness may be constantly present. In normal grief, the frequency and intensity of crying gradually diminishes.

Shock: Symptoms of shock include disorientation, emotional numbness, cognitive slowing, and fluctuating dissociation. This is more common in acute grief immediately following death but may recur after an intense trigger (e.g., autopsy results). Persistence beyond 6 months is an indication of complicated grief.[1]

Denial: Some patients may refuse to talk about their relative's death, may resist bequeathing the deceased's possessions, or may leave intact previous plans involving the deceased. Others may avoid objects or situations related to the deceased or may avoid talking about them altogether. These behaviors can be an initial adaptive reaction to protect the self from pain of loss and fear of the future. However, normal grieving eventually entails a gradual acceptance of the loss and a growing accommodation to new roles and situational demands.

Separation Distress: Episodic intense yearning for the deceased and thoughts about the deceased are characteristics of separation distress. However, after 6 months most bereaved patients exhibit less frequent and less intense symptoms of separation distress.[1]

Anger: Anger is a common reaction to stress. Hostility may be directed toward the deceased, health care providers, family, and others. When present, this largely resolves within 6 months.

Guilt: Commonly, surviving family members experience pangs of guilt that they did not do enough for the deceased. They may feel that they should have been more alert to signs of deterioration or acted more assertively to seek emergency medical care. Temporary expressions of guilt are normal and gradually subside over time.

Acceptance and Adaptation: Normal grief is characterized by the episodic expression of the symptoms described in the preceding text, which gradually diminish over time and show marked improvement by 6 months. Some reactions may last 2 years or more but the overall course is one of less intense grief and increasing functional ability. The adapting patient shows increasing self-confidence, trust in others, acceptance of the loss, expressed belief that life is still meaningful, and a willingness to accept new life roles.[1]

Differential Diagnosis of Normal Grief and Depression

A patient's history of a recent major loss may predispose the physician to not consider medical comorbidities that may be contributing to the patient's current depressive symptoms. It is important to rule out the existence of undiagnosed medical conditions that may present with depressive symptoms. This workup should include a thorough medical history and physical examination, review of prescribed and over-the-counter medications for side effects and polypharmacy, screening for substance abuse or herbal treatments that may impact mood, Mini-Mental State Examination, thyroid panel, complete blood count, basic chemistry panel, vitamin B_{12} and folate levels, and serum drug levels (if the patient is taking medications such as theophylline or digitalis). Toxicology screen and an electrocardiogram may also be indicated. A more complete discussion and table of medical differential diagnosis of depressive symptoms in the elderly are given in Table 17.5.

Having ruled out medical comorbidities, the clinical challenge is to distinguish normal grief from clinical depression. The presentation of normal grief and depression usually begin to diverge between 3 and 6 months after the loss. Periyakoil and Hallenbeck[9] outline the following differential indicators for normal grief and depression:

Temporal Variation: Grief diminishes over time and is experienced in waves triggered by memories or cues that remind the person of his or her deceased partner. Depression is often defined by a persistent sadness or dysphoria that can become chronic without treatment.

Negative Self-image: Grieving patients present a relatively normal self-image. Depressed patients often show a pervasive sense of worthlessness.

Anhedonia: The ability to experience pleasure and enjoy special moments with family is still present in patients who are grieving. Depressed patients often show an inability to experience pleasure.

Hopelessness: Whereas depressed patients often present with a marked sense of hopelessness, the grieving patient shows a capacity to think about and anticipate the future.

Response to Support: Patients who are grieving may withdraw temporarily, but at other times they will seek or appreciate social support to help them through the grieving process. Depressed individuals are more likely to persistently withdraw from social contact and derive little solace from it.

Preoccupation with Death: Grieving patients may show some occasional preoccupation with death and may express a desire to be with the deceased. However, these patients do not experience the persistent and active suicidal ideation or intent that can be present in clinical depression.

COMPLICATED GRIEF

Some bereaved patients seem to "get stuck." For these patients the more intense symptoms of normal grief (e.g., denial, sadness, and numbness) do not diminish over time. Prigerson and Jacob's extensive research on bereavement reactions has identified complicated grief as a syndrome distinct from normal grief and depression.[1] The diagnostic criteria for complicated grief[1] are given in Table 6.1.

Complicated grief produces greater functional impairment than normal grief[1] but is not as severe as depression. Complicated grief is also associated with adverse health outcomes if untreated (including high blood pressure, ulcerative colitis, suicidal ideation, cancer, and cardiac events).[1] The careful differential diagnosis of complicated grief and depression is important because treatment of

TABLE 6.1
PROPOSED DIAGNOSTIC CRITERIA FOR COMPLICATED GRIEF

Person must meet all four criteria

Criterion A

Person has experienced the death of a significant other and response involves three of the four following symptoms, experienced at least daily or to a marked degree:

- Intrusive thoughts about the deceased
- Yearning for the deceased
- Searching for the deceased
- Excessive loneliness since the death

Criterion B

In response to the death, four of the eight following symptoms experienced at least daily or to a marked degree:

- Purposelessness or feelings of futility about the future
- Subjective sense of numbness, detachment, or absence of emotional responsiveness
- Difficulty acknowledging the death (e.g., disbelief)
- Feeling that life is empty or meaningless
- Feeling that part of oneself has died
- Shattered worldview (e.g., lost sense of security, trust, or control)
- Assumption of symptoms or harmful behaviors of, or related to, the deceased person
- Excessive irritability, bitterness, or anger related to the death

Criterion C

The disturbance (symptoms listed in the preceding text) endures for at least 6 months

Criterion D

The disturbance causes clinically significant impairment in social, occupational, or other important areas of functioning

Reprinted with permission, Prigerson HG, Jacobs SC. Perspectives on care at the close of life. Caring for bereaved patients: "All the doctors just suddenly go". *JAMA.* 2001;286(11):1369–1376.

complicated grief differs from that of depression (discussed in the subsequent text).[1]

Complicated grief, normal grief, and depression share some core symptoms (e.g., sadness, guilt, and appetite and sleep disturbance). In fact, during the first few weeks or months, normal grief and/or complicated grief may be indistinguishable from depression.[9] One should begin careful monitoring for complicated grief and/or depression by approximately 6 months.[1] Compared to normal grief, the distinguishing feature of complicated grief is a preoccupation with the deceased that does not diminish over time (see Table 6.2). This may include intrusive thoughts about the deceased, yearning and searching for the deceased, or assuming certain behaviors or mannerisms of the deceased. Complicated grief does not include the persistent vegetative signs that characterize major depression.

The presence of suicidal ideation should prompt an immediate psychiatric referral at any point in the course.

BEREAVEMENT CARE

Presented in the subsequent text are guidelines for bereavement care.[3,8,10] To enhance clinical relevance, the guidelines are presented in an approximate sequence of care as patients are followed from anticipatory grief to acute grief, and through bereavement to resolution.

Gradually Shift to Palliative Care

Introduce palliative care concepts and interventions long before exhausting curative care regimens. This gradual introduction of a second focus on reducing suffering and improving quality of life is responsive to patient and family needs throughout the course of illness and avoids an abrupt, stressful shift at a later date.[11,12]

Patients vary in their receptiveness to medical information and decision making. Check how much the patient wants to know (e.g., "Some of my patients like to know the full details about their condition, they read up on it and ask many questions; some of my patients do not want much detail, they just want to know about the treatment plan. What about you?"). Check who else should be included in education and decision making (e.g., "Is there anyone else who should be involved in these discussions?"). Recheck these points from time to time—over the course of a terminal illness, patients often vary in their desire for information and comfort in including family members in the discussions.

TABLE 6.2
DIFFERENTIAL DIAGNOSIS[a]

	Normal Grief	Complicated Grief	Depression
Overview	The grief response includes psychological, behavioral, social, and physical reactions that may come in waves of sadness, shock, disbelief, anxiety, anger, guilt, irritability, and feelings of loss Gradually, unevenly, these diminish with time The capacity to think about and anticipate the future gradually returns	What begins as normal grief fails to resolve Grief symptoms plateau or worsen with time Denial may persist—there is continued difficulty acknowledging the death The bereaved may continue to feel purposeless; their future seems futile They may continue to feel numb, detached, and emotionally unresponsive They may be very irritable, bitter, or angry about the death	In major depression, intense sadness is persistent rather than fluctuating, as in normal grief Depression is also characterized by persistent vegetative signs that are not as prominent as those in complicated grief
Temporal	Intense symptoms of acute grief begin to subside after a few weeks and gradually (but unevenly) diminish over a year or two By 6 mo, there is marked improvement Temporary intense waves of grief may be triggered by special days or other reminders The overall course is one of less intense grief and improved functioning	Bereaved patients "get stuck" The intense symptoms of normal grief do not diminish over time; functioning fails to improve Sometimes symptoms and functioning actually worsen over time	Depressive symptoms are more continuous and persistent Symptoms such as negative mood and social withdrawal are present most days
Social	Patients who are grieving may withdraw temporarily, but at other times they will seek or appreciate social support to help them through the grieving process The ability to enjoy everyday pleasures and special moments with family gradually returns Certain pleasures may be accompanied by guilt (i.e., "I should not be enjoying myself—my husband died"), but this decreases with time	Individuals continue to be preoccupied and have difficulty with extended socialization and enjoyment of everyday activities Pervasive feelings of loneliness and isolation are present.	Depressed individuals are more likely to persistently withdraw from social contact and derive little solace from it Well-meaning attempts to break one's routine with some pleasurable activity may be met with apathy or aggravation and are rarely helpful in lifting the spirits Depressed patients often show an inability to experience pleasure (anhedonia)
Cognitive	There is an initial preoccupation with the death, including images and thoughts of what could have or should have been done, but this lessens with time Recollection of pleasant memories gradually returns The ability to discuss the deceased without overwhelming emotion gradually improves	Preoccupation with the deceased persists unabated, with yearning, searching, and intrusive thoughts about the deceased A shattered view of self and environment continues, including the feeling that life is empty or meaningless and that part of oneself has died, or a lost sense of security, trust, or control	Depressed patients often show a pervasive sense of worthlessness and/or hopelessness, which is often associated with persistent and active suicidal ideation or intent The risk of suicide is highest in the depressed elderly
Functional impairment	Individuals may initially show decreased ability to perform usual tasks. In the very old, slowed reaction times and decreased ability to adjust to new situations complicate this, as does frailty or cognitive impairment The adapting patient shows increasing self-confidence, trust in others, acceptance of the loss, expressed belief that life is still meaningful, and a willingness to accept new life roles	Complicated grief produces greater functional impairment than normal grief, but does not rise to the severity of depression	Depression includes clinically significant impairment in social, occupational, or other important areas of functioning

[a]Differential diagnosis of medical conditions is covered in Table 17.5.
Portions adapted from Prigerson HG, Jacobs SC. Perspectives on care at the close of life. Caring for bereaved patients: "All the doctors just suddenly go". *JAMA*. 2001;286(11):1369–1376, and Periyakoil VS, Hallenbeck J. Identifying and managing preparatory grief and depression at the end of life. *Am Fam Physician*. 2002;65(5):883–890.

Establish a Bereavement Register

A bereavement register enables tracking of patients who are receiving palliative care or approaching the end of life and identifying families currently in bereavement.[2] If the practice already maintains a death register, this can be expanded to create a bereavement register for spouses and family members of recently deceased patients.[13] Many grieving geriatric patients, especially those with little family and social support, tend to suffer in silence until worsening emotional or health problems bring them to the physician's office. The bereavement register can be a prompt for assertive bereavement care and result in proactively reaching out to bereaved patients.[2]

Identify Patients at High Risk

Patients on the bereavement register should be screened for salient risk factors. Davidson presents an assessment tool[3,14] incorporating the following indicators that can be useful in systematically assessing risk. The factors cited in the subsequent text can be assessed through a clinical interview or chart review and by drawing on staff knowledge of the patient and family:

1. Deaths that are unexpected, untimely, or in some way shocking
2. Relationships with the deceased that were ambivalent or dependent (i.e., clinging)
3. Poor family coping (i.e., high conflict, low cohesiveness, or poor expressiveness)
4. Lack of social support
5. Personal vulnerability of the bereaved (i.e., poor self-esteem or low trust in others)
6. Previous history of psychiatric illness, psychotropic medications, or intolerance to stress
7. Use of alcohol or illicit drugs to assist in coping
8. Concurrent losses, crises, or stressors, especially change of residence
9. Prolonged caregiving with significant emotional strain
10. Bereaved individual's belief that death was preventable
11. Not viewing the body of the deceased

Older caregivers of dying patients are at particular risk for complicated grief reactions. Most older persons die of disabling conditions that require support from family for an extended period of time.[15] Family caregivers assume the burdens of time, logistic management, physical tasks, financial costs, and emotional burdens, as well as mental and physical health risks.[16] An elderly spouse may not have the personal resources to assume all these burdens. The amount of emotional strain the caregivers experience profoundly impacts their anticipatory and acute grief. Caregivers who report being under the most strain are most likely to be depressed, neglect their own health, and have increased mortality. Once their caregiving burden is lifted by the death of their spouse, they begin to take better care of themselves, but their depressive symptoms tend to linger. Caregivers who report little strain show a pattern more similar to normal grief, but with more depressive and weight loss symptoms after the death.[15]

Older caregivers should be carefully monitored during physician visits. If necessary, the caregiver should be seen alone briefly during patient visits to the office. The needs of caregivers vary, and plans should be individually tailored. There is good evidence that "listening well" is important. Caregivers whose physicians listened to their needs and opinions about the patient's illness were significantly less likely to be depressed and to report that caregiving compromised their personal lives.[17]

Recommend to the caregiver (with the patient present) to seek and regularly spend time away from the caregiver role. Explain that this has been shown to be better for both the caregiver and the patient. Encourage discussion on this issue.[10,16,18] Other specific practical suggestions to reduce the burdens and obtain help and support may be found in the article by Rabow et al.[16]; see also the section "Suggested Readings and Resources" and Chapter 3.

Assess and Assist Anticipatory Grieving

Some research suggests that assistance with anticipatory grieving helps spouses accept and adapt to the loss sooner.[19] Families can be provided with information about end-of-life services available from local self-help groups, hospices, and other social and mental health agencies, as well as national resources for caregiving and support (see the section "Suggested Readings and Resources"). Emphasize that such resources offer useful help and practical ideas for all families going through this phase, not just for people who are struggling.[10] Providers can also assess anticipatory grief and begin to enable the grieving process by employing some of the communication techniques suggested for dying patients, as given in Table 6.3.

The physician and clinic staff can assist the family with practical issues.[10] This might include providing information and support for decision making; discussing goals of care and advance-care planning; determining wishes, preferences, hopes, and fears; providing emotional and social support; and referring to specific services to meet identified social needs (e.g., access to care and help in home, school, work, transportation, rehabilitation, medications, counseling, equipment, and community resources).[10]

With increasing age comes increasing familiarity with death and loss. Typically, older people have already experienced the death of other people close to them. Multiple losses close in time often have a compounding effect. For the older spouse of a dying patient, many of life's other roles have diminished (e.g., parent or provider), so the loss of the patient may represent the loss of his or her last major role. This can have a profound effect on self-image, which is worth discussing at an opportune time.

Clinic staff should also begin to anticipate adapting interventions to the family's culture and religious beliefs. Clements[22] provides a set of culturally sensitive questions

TABLE 6.3
COMMON CONCERNS OF DYING PATIENTS

Concerns	Sample Explorative Questions
Health and Health Care	
■ Physical symptoms (e.g., pain, nausea, and loss of mobility) ■ Mental awareness ■ Treatment/care ■ Involvement in medical decisions ■ Treatment as a "whole person"	What has been most difficult about this illness for you? What are you most worried about? What matters the most to you now? How do you want me, as your doctor, to help you in this situation? What are the barriers to feeling secure and in reasonable control as you go through this illness?
Behavioral and Emotional Concerns	
■ Behavioral reaction (e.g., not coping, not being "strong," losing control, or losing one's mind) ■ Loss of autonomy	What has been the emotional impact on you? What are your concerns about your illness? Can you tell me about a time you feel you coped well with a difficult situation in your life?
Existential/Religious Concerns	
■ Achieving a sense of completion, meaning of illness, life's accomplishments, legacy ■ Coming to peace with God ■ Death (fear of the afterlife, fear of the unknown)	How have you made sense over why this is happening to you? Are your religious beliefs important to you in this illness? What role have these beliefs taken in facing difficult issues in the past? Do you find yourself thinking back over your life? What do you still want to accomplish? What do you want your children and grandchildren to remember about you? How might you be able to continue to be a presence in their lives after you are gone?
Social Concerns	
■ Family and friends (i.e., being a burden while dying, impact of death on them, and abandonment) ■ Helping others	Who are the most important people in your life now? Who do you depend on? Who do you confide in about your illness and reactions? What has been the impact of this on your spouse? What are your concerns about your family? Are there important relationships that need healing or strengthening? Do the important people in your life know what they mean to you? Are there ways you can help your family now to prepare for and deal with your death?
Practical Concerns	
■ Financial/practical worries ■ Preparing for death ■ Having funeral arrangements planned	What are the practical concerns you have been thinking about? Have you discussed your preferences for funeral arrangements with someone? Have you shared your advice about future financial or other practical issues with your family or others?

Adapted from Buckman R. *How to break bad news.* Baltimore, MD: Johns Hopkins University Press; 1992;[20] Periyakoil VS, Hallenbeck J. Identifying and managing preparatory grief and depression at the end of life. *Am Fam Physician.* 2002;65(5):883–890; Steinhauser KE, et al. Factors considered important at the end of life by patients, family, physicians, and other care providers. *JAMA.* 2000;284(19):2476–2482;[21] Lo B, Quill T, Tulsky J. Discussing palliative care with patients. ACP-ASIM end-of-life care consensus panel. American college of physicians-American society of internal medicine. *Ann Intern Med.* 1999; 130(9):744–749.

that communicate respect for the family's unique heritage and give the family some autonomy in structuring bereavement care:

- What are the family's cultural traditions and rituals for coping with dying, the deceased's body, and honoring the deceased?
- What are the family's beliefs about what happens after death?
- What does the family feel to be a normal expression of grief and acceptance of the loss?
- What does the family consider to be the roles for each member in coping with the death?
- Are certain types of death less acceptable (e.g., suicide) or are certain types of death especially difficult to handle for the family's culture (e.g., the death of an infant or child)?

Counsel the Dying Patient

Dying older patients, in addition to anticipating their own loss of life, often struggle to cope with many other losses: Decreased autonomy; loss of physical abilities, simple pleasures, activities, home, future celebrations they will miss; and anticipated (or actual) loss of family and friends. They grieve over these compounding losses in individual, personal ways that encompass the spectrum of human functioning. In addition to the reactions of normal grief described in the preceding text, they may be dealing with a variety of worries, as well as spiritual and existential issues. It is important for the primary physician to inquire about these issues and demonstrate sensitivity and receptivity to the difficult content.

With dying patients and their families, it is particularly important to not emphasize stages of grief. The risk is that the patient who dies without "completing the stages" may leave the family feeling like they have failed. Discussing common grief reactions (see preceding text) is more helpful.

Take the lead and ask about and address common anticipatory grief issues. Even if the patient does not initiate such discussions, ask about common concerns (Table 6.3). Asking about such issues indicates your receptiveness to discussing them. Patients who are initially reluctant to address them will often note this and bring it up another day.[9]

Individualize the plan and patient education. In follow-up visits, expect to repeat patient education and revisit earlier decisions. Explain common elements of grief reactions and provide patient education materials. Goals of increased survival, comfort, cognitive function, and physical function often compete. Individually tailor the plan to meet the patient's stated preferences about treatment options and priorities of care. Emphasize and respect the patient's autonomy. Assist the patient in achieving a sense of control in preparing for death—this may include discussing options in health care, finances, funeral arrangements, and legal issues and documenting preferences. Other useful interventions may focus on patient/family education about the dying process, visiting a hospice, consulting with legal/financial experts, and so on.

Anticipate the management of common end-of-life problems. Regularly reassess and adjust plans for management of pain and symptoms (e.g., dyspnea, constipation, anorexia, and nausea). Facilitate psychosocial support and the development of a plan for the time of death. Encourage the patient to make use of supportive family and friends, giving receptive people specific helpful tasks.

Help an avoidant patient face realities. However, there is little evidence that an approach of "breaking through the denial" is effective. It is better to focus on including the patient in decision making.

1. *Empathize:* "This must be very difficult for you to discuss. . . . "
2. *Emphasize autonomy:* "I want to help you have some control over important decisions regarding . . . " (e.g., medical treatment in various circumstances, family financial decisions, or child custody arrangements)
3. *Expand focus:* From medical concerns to personal and family tasks that could humanize the final phase of life (e.g., saying good-bye or connecting with family members)
4. *Present this as a chance to address final issues:* "I am concerned that if we only focus on your immediate medical needs, we will miss the chance to plan together for. . . . "

If the patient requests the physician to hasten death, it may be a result of significant physical factors that can be ameliorated. If persistent, this is suggestive of clinical depression. In the absence of such factors, this provides an opportunity to ask about fears, concerns, and preferences for end-of-life care.

Deal with the practicalities of end-of-life issues. Address ethical and legal issues of health proxy, confidentiality and family involvement, surrogate decision making, and advanced care planning. Address insurance and financial issues pertinent to the patient's situation and prognosis.

Provide Support to the Family while the Patient is Dying

Communication: While the patient is dying, careful active listening is more important than talking. Touch base with each person present and ask if they have questions or concerns. Talk openly about the dying process and observed clinical changes—it will inform the family and help make it acceptable to ask questions.[3] Encourage open discussion of issues presented in the previous section on "Counsel the Dying Patient."[4,10]

Contact: For patients dying at home, speak regularly with their family. Make clear that you are available for them when needed.[10,16,18] Consider home visits. In institutional settings, spend time in the room with the dying patient and family. Touch base frequently when you cannot be there. When doctors stay away from the room out of respect for the family's privacy, the family may worry that the doctor is not available or is avoiding the dying patient.[3]

Educating Family/Friends: "The person who is dying cannot be cured, but can be helped through the experience with acceptance, touch, listening, and support."[23]

Check the family members' understanding of the condition, treatment, prognosis, and patient's wishes. Help them talk about physical and emotional changes they have noticed in the patient. Remind the family members that the dying person may still hear them, and encourage family members to talk to the dying patient and reminisce about good times in the past and happy memories. Inquire about pictures and mementos in the room to facilitate orientation to family and reminiscing.[3]

Prepare family and friends present for common physical changes in the body during the final stage of life by explaining these changes in normal, nonalarming terms.[3,23] Explain that: "Most people with a fatal illness become increasingly frail in their final weeks and eventually die peacefully. The physical systems that maintain life often slow down before they stop. This creates physical changes you might notice that are a normal, natural part of the process. If you are comfortable providing some hands-on care, there are some simple things you can do to help keep them comfortable." If family/friends present are interested, suggest hands-on care options, such as those in Table 6.4.[23] Tailor the specific items and suggestions to suit the patient's condition and setting. Respect family's/friends' comfort in providing or not providing such care.

Attend the Funeral and Write a Letter of Condolence

The decision to attend the funeral depends on the relationship between the physician and the patient and his or her family. Attending a funeral or memorial service may assist the family in the grieving process and make it easier for them to consult the doctor about grief issues in the months ahead.

Similarly, a letter of condolence from the deceased's physician can be meaningful to a grieving family and can serve as an implicit invitation to continue to consult the physician throughout the bereavement period. However, many doctors avoid writing this letter and minimize its importance. Common explanations include being too busy, not knowing the patient well enough, not having seen the patient recently, and diffusion of responsibility among clinic staff. In addition, writing the letter may force doctors into the uncomfortable position of facing their own sense of loss and failure.[24] However, failure to write a letter can alienate a bereaved family and reinforce a view of the medical world as cold and uncaring.

Bedell et al.[24] offer helpful suggestions for writing a meaningful letter. She recommends beginning with a simple and direct expression of sorrow (e.g., "I want to offer my condolences on your profound loss") while avoiding patronizing clichés (e.g., "it was meant to be" or "I know how you feel"). Including personal references to the deceased's work, family, or interests indicates to the family that you knew the deceased as more than just a patient. One can also comment on the deceased's nobility and courage in coping with his or her illness. It can be appropriate to express appreciation for the opportunity to assist in the patient's care.

Bedell provides the following summary:

> "In a medical world shaped by technologic advances in the care of patients, we must maintain our humanity in our interactions with patients and their families, particularly when we share with them some of the most profound moments of life and death. After a patient dies, when we all

TABLE 6.4
NORMAL PHYSICAL CHANGES IN FINAL STAGES OF LIFE

Physical Changes	Explanation	Hands-on Care Options
Cooling of skin, changes in color	Circulation is decreasing	Keep person comfortable with sheet or light blanket
Sleeping more	Metabolic changes may make the person more difficult to arouse	Individuals may still be able to hear; continue to sit and talk quietly, reminisce
Decreased appetite and thirst	Decreased need	Do not force food/drink; ice chips, small cups or syringe of thin juices, and wet swabs help keep mouth and lips comfortable
Incontinence of bladder and/or bowel	Relaxation of muscles	Pad bed, clean and turn patient when needed, and use ventilation and air fresheners
Disorientation	Circulation to brain is decreasing, metabolic changes may contribute	Identify self by name regularly when talking
Restlessness	Circulation to brain is decreasing, metabolic changes may contribute	Try talking quietly, soothing music, touch, light massage to calm the patient
Gurgling sounds from throat	Normal result of decreased fluid intake and decreased coughing	Tilt head to the side to allow secretions to drain and wet swab lips and mouth
Change in breathing	Decreased control of breathing may cause irregular pattern, with rapid shallow breathing broken by lengthening pauses	Can try elevating head and upper body slightly, or turning person to side

Adapted from Long MC. Death and dying and recognizing approaching death. *Clin Geriatr Med.* 1996;12(2):359–368.

feel helpless, the best care we can provide is our expression of concern and sympathy in a letter of condolence."[24] (Bedell SE, Cadenhead K, Graboys TB. The doctor's letter of condolence. *N Engl J Med.* 2001;344(15):1162–1164)

Assist in the Grieving Process

Proactive Case Management: Grieving spouses may withdraw from family and friends and avoid contact with clinics and doctors. The very old are more likely to experience social isolation and mobility impairment. Isolation increases the risk of complicated grief, depression, and anxiety disorders. Consequently, it is important to assertively monitor grieving patients to assess physical and psychiatric status, overall functional level, and issues of home safety. The primary care clinician may also need to draw on existing social supports or facilitate use of community social resources.

Hegge and Fischer provide recommendations for the functional assessment of grieving spouses in Table 6.5.[19] This assessment can be accomplished during an office examination or as part of a home visit. Many factors affect the functional aspect of grief, so individual responses should be assessed rather than assumed. For example, Hegge and Fischer[19] provide evidence that the expression of grief varies with a widow's age. Senior widows (aged 60 to 74) are often faced with the task of learning new life skills and establishing a new identity distinct from their spouses'. They may fear becoming too dependent on their children and may look to friends for their primary support after the acute grief period. Social withdrawal is a risk of complicated grief and depression. Senior widows should be encouraged to reconnect with social networks and community activities. For this age-group, obtaining a pet can be therapeutic and can help fill the void at home.

On the other hand, elderly widows (as defined by Hegge—aged 75 and older) are more often facing issues related to their own physical decline and mortality. These patients and their families may be struggling with possible placement in a higher level of care. Psychologically, an elderly widow may be preoccupied with thoughts of her own death. These widows, whose support systems have been reduced by disability and death, are more likely to depend heavily on their children throughout the bereavement period. Older widows may need closer surveillance for nutritional deficits, confusion, disorientation, and accident proneness. Despite these challenges, elderly widows can move more swiftly through the grieving process if they have been in longer-term caretaking roles and have had more opportunity for anticipatory grieving.[19] (No similar definitive studies for widowers were identified. However, there is considerable consensus in the literature that men and women share an age-related vulnerability to complicated grief resulting from progressive physical decline, social isolation, and cognitive slowing.)

TABLE 6.5
FUNCTIONAL ASSESSMENT

Individual grief reactions

- Current components of grief reactions
- Use of effective coping strategies (e.g., keeping busy, relying on familiar routines, visits with others, reflecting on memories, prayer, or meditation)
- Use of ineffective coping strategies (e.g., social isolation, self-blame, excessive sleep, or overreliance on alcohol and/or medications)

Physical functioning

- Nutrition
- Sleeping patterns
- Accident-prone tendencies

Psychological functioning

- Depressive symptoms
- Anxiety symptoms
- Confusion, disorientation (assess carefully to avoid a false label of dementia)
- Preoccupation with one's own death

Social functioning (monitor availability and quality of support, as well as overdependence on support systems)

- Family support systems
- Friend, neighbor, and clergy support systems
- Need for grief support group

Self-care

- Activities of daily living, instrumental activities of daily living
- Taking care of physical health needs
- Ability to competently manage own affairs and make decisions about practical matters
- Need for assistance with finances, legal issues, and home management

Portions adapted from Hegge M, Fischer C. Grief responses of senior and elderly widows. Practice implications. *J Gerontol Nurs.* 2000;26(2):35–43.

Communication Techniques: Cognitive abilities of healthy older persons show a slow decline with age in several areas. These include learning and recall of new information, ability to generate problem-solving strategies in new situations, nonverbal creative thinking, flexible reasoning, and speed of information processing. Behaviorally, older persons have difficulty with word finding, verbal fluency, complex visual–spatial tasks (e.g., performance is poorer and slower), and overall reaction time. The normal grieving older adult, having decreased cognitive ability to cope with novel situations, may appear more confused or demented than a younger grieving person. In the primary care office, health care professionals may need to provide additional structure and time for these interviews. For example, if open-ended questions fail to yield information about important areas of functioning, the primary doctor should take the initiative in asking about specific common concerns.

Recommended core communication strategies are shown in Table 6.6.

Encouraging Adaptive Activities: In addition to facilitating grieving, the provider can encourage a number of adaptive activities that support adjustment to a new phase of life:

- Review previous successful coping strategies to determine whether they are relevant to the current loss.[19]
- Simple writing tasks (e.g., instructing patients to write about their experiences and emotions during the bereavement period) have been shown to improve health and psychiatric status and even immune function.[1]
- Encourage prayer and/or meditation.[19]
- Social contact and support has been shown to buffer stress and prevent depression.[1]
- Provide health education (including nutrition counseling, accident prevention).
- Develop an active daily routine, learning new life skills (e.g., financial management, computer skills).

Pharmacotherapy: There is little support for pharmacologic interventions as a "treatment" for normal grief. Most experts discourage the ongoing use of medications because they may interfere with the normal grief process.[9,25,26] Convincing research data are lacking. Pharmacologic treatment of complicated grief and depression are discussed in the subsequent text (see section "Treat Complicated Grief and Depression").

Primary physicians are often asked to provide some medication to acutely grieving adults to help them sleep, but there is little research to guide pharmacotherapy of grief-related insomnia in the elderly. Benzodiazepines are discouraged in the ambulatory elderly even for very short-term use because of increased risk of residual sedation, cognitive changes, falls, hip fractures, and poor sleep architecture.[27] Trazodone has been used off-label for insomnia, but because there is little evidence that trazodone improves sleep in nondepressed people[28] and that it has more significant side effects (including orthostatic hypotension, cardiac arrhythmias, dry mouth, and priapism) than alternatives,[27,28] it is not recommended for management of acute grief in the elderly. Although all hypnotics carry risks in the ambulatory elderly, the nonbenzodiazepine hypnotics that work as more selective benzodiazepine-receptor antagonists (SBRAs), including zaleplon, zolpidem, and eszopiclone, appear to be more promising, on the basis of the limited available research. The onset and duration of action is relatively short, leading to less residual sedation, cognitive changes, falls, or disturbance of sleep architecture than benzodiazepines.[27] Common side effects, including drowsiness, dizziness, and headache, are dose dependent.[29] In adults, the SBRAs are all effective in improving sleep latency, but the improvement of total sleep time is related to the dose and, possibly, the drug half-life.[29] For all these drugs, the recommended dose for people older than 65 is approximately half the adult dose because these drugs tend to have higher peak levels and longer half-lives in older people. Although good studies that directly compare these newer hypnotics in the

TABLE 6.6
COMMUNICATING WITH OLDER BEREAVED PATIENTS

A. Effective strategies
- Use the deceased's name
- Acknowledge the death ("I am sorry Betty is gone")
- Talk about the deceased and memories ("What are you remembering about Julio today?")
- Answer questions about his/her death ("Do you have questions about Bill's illness or treatment?")
- Talk about grief feelings ("How has Doris' death affected you?")
- Label and normalize expressed feelings ("You are very angry at him for leaving you with these financial problems. It has been very rough on you handling this on top of everything else. Some of my patients have also felt kind of guilty about being angry at the dead, but it is very normal. Do you feel like that too?")
- Educate about normal grief (i.e., common reactions, "waves" and triggers, and variability)
- Allow for individual variation. Some patients want to talk, some just want quiet company, and some want to be alone. Some want to keep busy, whereas others want to hide under the covers. Some people cry profusely; others appear stoic. Most people vary over time. Explain that family members will vary in their grief response (e.g., just because someone does not cry or wants to keep busy does not mean they do not care). Explaining this to patients also makes it clear that you, as physician, are accepting such variations

B. Harmful strategies to avoid
- Avoid being casual or aloof (brief comments such as "Call me" or "How are you?" with nothing further)
- Avoid telling patient what to think, feel, or believe ("Do not feel guilty," "You should be glad it went quickly," "They are happy now," or "It is God's will")
- Avoid disallowing patient's feelings ("Be strong" or "You should be getting over this by now")

Portions adapted from Prigerson HG, Jacobs SC. Perspectives on care at the close of life. Caring for bereaved patients: "All the doctors just suddenly go". *JAMA.* 2001;286(11):1369–1376. and Periyakoil VS, Hallenbeck J. Identifying and managing preparatory grief and depression at the end of life. *Am Fam Physician.* 2002;65(5):883–890.

elderly are lacking, it would be reasonable to hypothesize that the SBRAs with longer half-lives might show greater improvement in total sleep, as well as greater side effects of increased residual sedation, falls, and hip fractures, than shorter-acting SBRAs. The respective mean half-lives in adults are approximately 1 hour for zaleplon, 2.6 hours for zolpidem, and 6 hours for eszopiclone,[30] with some studies finding approximately 50% longer half-lives in the elderly. In view of the paucity of pertinent research, a short course (seven to ten pills, p.r.n.) of the shorter-acting SBRA hypnotics (zaleplon or zolpidem) is preferred but should be prescribed cautiously, using the recommended geriatric dose with precautions against residual sedation and fall. Any sedating drug is probably a poor choice in an elderly ambulatory patient who is already at risk for falls (e.g., mobility impaired).

Monitor for Poor Bereavement Outcome

Assess the bereaved families' risk for poor bereavement outcome (e.g., complicated grief and/or depression) and link to appropriate services as needed.

Good Bereavement Outcome: Grief becomes less intense over time. Most preloss activities are resumed and new activities are added. Grief can be cued by anniversary dates, songs, and other memories, but this is temporary and normal functioning and quality of life is reestablished.[1,3]

Poor Bereavement Outcome: Grief lasts for 6 months to 2 years with little or no decrease in its intensity, inability to resume preloss life activities, and inability to enjoy pleasant events and experiences.[1,3]

Treat Complicated Grief and Depression

Major depressive disorder during bereavement should be treated by following the guidelines for its treatment in the elderly. Specifically, selective serotonin reuptake inhibitors, cognitive therapy, and interpersonal therapy have been shown to be effective and well tolerated[31] (for more information, see Chapter 17).

There is a growing body of literature indicating that complicated grief does not respond as well as depression to many current treatments for depression. There is some weak evidence to support the use of paroxetine. Tricyclic antidepressants have not been found to be effective, and their use in the elderly is generally discouraged.[1] Because the diagnostic criteria for complicated grief have been developed recently and are not currently included in the *Diagnostic and Statistical Manual of Mental Disorders*, randomized controlled trials of treatments specific to complicated grief are largely forthcoming.

Several behavioral psychotherapy treatments have shown positive results in helping complicated grief patients resolve lingering bereavement issues and adapt to a new life: Traumatic grief treatment, cognitive-behavior therapy for complicated grief, and family-focused grief therapy. Referral to mental health professionals proficient in these approaches should be considered.

Traumatic grief treatment is an exposure-based treatment derived from empirically supported posttraumatic stress disorder treatment.[32] First through imaginal exposure, then through *in vivo* exposure, patients are repeatedly exposed to the most distressing elements of their traumatic experience (in this case, the death of a loved one) until habituation occurs and overall emotional reactivity diminishes. During this process the therapist also corrects distorted cognitive schemas (e.g., "I could have done more") that have repeatedly triggered and maintained a complicated grief response. Initial studies have indicated that traumatic grief treatment reduces emotional intensity, increases positive memories of the deceased, improves overall functional level, increases the breadth of social activities, and reduces comorbid anxiety and depression.[33]

Various forms of cognitive-behavior therapy for complicated grief have recently been favorably reviewed.[34–36] These therapies are focused on helping patients to cognitively reconstruct the meaning of their world in a way that facilitates emotional catharsis and behavioral adaptation. Therapeutic processes focus on both loss-oriented coping (e.g., looking at photographs, crying about the loss, and understanding one's attachment to the deceased) and restoration-oriented coping (e.g., learning the new skills necessary to adapt to a new life). The patients are helped to integrate the loss into their present life and develop a new social identity.

Family-focused grief therapy[37] is another promising development for bereaved individuals and their families. This therapy is based on the empiric finding that the psychosocial health of bereaved individuals is strongly correlated with the level of family functioning. The therapeutic focus is on family communication, cohesiveness, conflict resolution, and facilitation of shared grief. Initial studies demonstrate that family-focused grief therapy can minimize the psychiatric comorbidity often associated with complicated grief.

Bereaved patients can benefit from these developing therapies if referrals for behavioral assessment and treatment of complicated grief are made to palliative care organizations and/or to therapists with specialty training in grief therapies.

The presence of symptoms of complicated grief or major depressive disorder after 6 months or the presence of suicidal thinking indicate a need for psychiatric evaluation and treatment.[1] However, many bereaved elderly patients may refuse a psychiatric referral and prefer to be seen by their primary care clinician.

As with depressed patients, elderly patients being treated for complicated grief should be closely monitored until symptoms have significantly diminished. Arrange for the patient to be seen by their primary care clinician, a mental health professional, or the combination every 1 to 2 weeks.

During each follow-up visit, evaluate complicated grief symptoms, functioning, treatment adherence, motivation, side effects, suicidal ideation, and lethality. Reflect any progress and reassure when possible. Consider treatment modifications, including the addition of counseling.

CONCLUSIONS

Bereavement care for geriatric patients will continue to put increasing demands on primary care clinicians. Elderly patients who are grieving not only need direct assistance with bereavement but also present with accelerated complications of chronic disease if grief is unresolved.

This chapter presents a best practices model for bereavement care in primary medicine. Although there are no randomized controlled trials of geriatric bereavement care, the existing palliative care guidelines[10] provide an excellent resource for those interested in a comprehensive review.

REFERENCES

1. Prigerson HG, Jacobs SC. Perspectives on care at the close of life. Caring for bereaved patients: "All the doctors just suddenly go". *JAMA*. 2001;286(11):1369–1376.
2. Lemkau JP, et al. A questionnaire survey of family practice physicians' perceptions of bereavement care. *Arch Fam Med*. 2000;9(9):822–829.
3. Davidson KM. Evidence-based protocol. Family bereavement support before and after the death of a nursing home resident. *J Gerontol Nurs*. 2003;29(1):10–18.
4. Casarett D, Kutner JS, Abrahm J. Life after death: A practical approach to grief and bereavement. *Ann Intern Med*. 2001;134(3): 208–215.
5. Rando TA. *Grief, dying, and death: Clinical interventions for caregivers*. Illinois, IL: Research Press Company; 1984.
6. Brindley P, Emery B, Pereira J. Grief and bereavement. In: Ratnaike R, ed. *Practical guide to geriatric medicine*. New York, NY: McGraw-Hill; 2002.
7. Penson RT, Green KM, Chabner BA, et al. When does the responsibility of our care end: Bereavement. *Oncologist*. 2002;7(3): 251–258.
8. Osterweiss M, Solomon F, Green M, eds. *Bereavement: Reactions, consequences, and care*. Washington, DC: National Academy Press; 1984.
9. Periyakoil VS, Hallenbeck J. Identifying and managing preparatory grief and depression at the end of life. *Am Fam Physician*. 2002; 65(5):883–890.
10. National Consensus Project for Quality Palliative Care. Clinical practice guidelines for quality palliative care, executive summary. *J Palliat Med*. 2004;7(5):611–627.
11. Lo B, Quill T, Tulsky J. Discussing palliative care with patients. ACP-ASIM end-of-life care consensus panel. American college of physicians-American society of internal medicine. *Ann Intern Med*. 1999;130(9):744–749.
12. Alexander CS, Back A. *Integrating palliative care into the continuum of HIV care: An agenda for change*. Promoting Excellence in End-of-Life Care; Robert Wood Johnson Foundation. April 2004. Available from: http://www.promotingexcellence.org/hiv/hiv_report/index.html. Accessed November 30, 2004.
13. Charlton R, Sheahan K, Smith G, et al. Spousal bereavement–implications for health. *Fam Pract*. 2001;18(6):614–618.
14. Kissane DW, McKenzie DP, Bloch S. Family coping and bereavement outcome. *Palliat Med*. 1997;11(3):191–201.
15. Schulz R, Beach SR, Lind B, et al. Involvement in caregiving and adjustment to death of a spouse: Findings from the caregiver health effects study. *JAMA*. 2001;285(24):3123–3129.
16. Rabow MW, Hauser JM, Adams J. Supporting family caregivers at the end of life: "They don't know what they don't know". *JAMA*. 2004;291(4):483–491.
17. Block SD. Perspectives on care at the close of life. Psychological considerations, growth, and transcendence at the end of life: The art of the possible. *JAMA*. 2001;285(22):2898–2905.
18. Kasuya RT, Polgar-Bailey P, Takeuchi R. Caregiver burden and burnout. A guide for primary care physicians. *Postgrad Med*. 2000; 108(7):119–123.
19. Hegge M, Fischer C. Grief responses of senior and elderly widows. Practice implications. *J Gerontol Nurs*. 2000;26(2):35–43.
20. Buckman R. *How to break bad news*. Baltimore, MD: Johns Hopkins University Press; 1992.
21. Steinhauser KE, Christakis NA, Clipp EC, McNeilly M, et al. Factors considered important at the end of life by patients, family, physicians, and other care providers. *JAMA*. 2000;284(19): 2476–2482.
22. Clements PT, Vigil GJ, Manno MS, et al. Cultural perspectives of death, grief, and bereavement. *J Psychosoc Nurs Ment Health Serv*. 2003;41(7):18–26.
23. Long MC. Death and dying and recognizing approaching death. *Clin Geriatr Med*. 1996;12(2):359–368.
24. Bedell SE, Cadenhead K, Graboys TB. The doctor's letter of condolence. *N Engl J Med*. 2001;344(15):1162–1164.
25. Ratnaike R, ed. *Practical guide to geriatric medicine*. New York, NY: McGraw-Hill; 2002
26. Barker L, Burton J, Zieve P, eds. *Principles of ambulatory medicine*, 4th ed. Philadelphia, PA: Williams & Wilkins; 1995.
27. Scott M, Stigleman S, Cravens D. Clinical inquiries. What is the best hypnotic for use in the elderly? *J Fam Pract*. 2003;52(12): 976–978.
28. James SP, Mendelson WB. The use of trazodone as a hypnotic: A critical review. *J Clin Psychiatry*. 2004;65(6):752–755.
29. Walsh JK. Pharmacologic management of insomnia. *J Clin Psychiatry*. 2004;65(suppl 16):41–45.
30. Lexi-Comp Online. *Lexi-Comp, Inc*. Available from: http://www.crlonline.com. Accessed May 1, 2005.
31. Nathan PE, Gorman JM. *A guide to treatments that work*, 2nd ed. New York, NY: Oxford University Press; 2002.
32. Harkness KL, Shear MK, Frank E, et al. Traumatic grief treatment: Case histories of 4 patients. *J Clin Psychiatry*. 2002;63(12): 1113–1120.
33. Shear MK, Frank E, Foa E, et al. Traumatic grief treatment: A pilot study. *Am J Psychiatry*. 2001;158(9):1506–1508.
34. Neimeyer RA. Reauthoring life narratives: Grief therapy as meaning reconstruction. *Isr J Psychiatry Relat Sci*. 2001;38(3–4): 171–183.
35. Neimeyer RA, ed. *Meaning reconstruction and the experience of loss*. Washington, DC: American Psychological Association; 2001.
36. Neimeyer RA, Prigerson HG, Davies B. Mourning and meaning. *Am Behav Sci*. 2002;46(2):235–251.
37. Matthews LT, Marwit SJ. Complicated grief and the trend toward cognitive-behavioral therapy. *Death Stud*. 2004;28(9): 849–863.

SUGGESTED READINGS AND RESOURCES

American Academy of Family Physicians
www.familydoctor.org
Under the heading "Cancer" there are patient education handouts about caregivers, end-of-life issues, palliative care, and grieving

American Association of Retired Persons (AARP)
www.aarp.org/life/endoflife
Extensive information on estate planning, wills, other legal matters, hospice, palliative care, funeral planning, and links to other web resources for patients and professionals

Center to Advance Palliative Care
www.capcmssm.org
Palliative care resources for health care professionals and organizations

End-of-Life Palliative Education Resource Center
http://www.eperc.mcw.edu/
Resource materials for health care professionals and health educators

Hospice Foundation of America
http://www.hospicefoundation.org/
Information on hospices; extensive list of links, resources, and organizations; includes section for caregivers

National Library of Medicine (US)—Medline Plus
www.nlm.nih.gov/medlineplus/bereavement.html
Collection of links to high-quality patient resources on grief and bereavement. Some are also available in Spanish

Promoting Excellence in End-of-Life Care
www.promotingexcellence.org
End-of-life and palliative care resources for clinicians and researchers

Red Cross
http://www.redcross.org/services/hss/care/family.html
Family Caregiving series of classes offered at local Red Cross Chapter

Caregiver Resource Directory of Beth Israel Hospital (New York City)
http://www.netofcare.org/
Information and resources for caregivers

The American Gerontological Society Online Caregiver Guide
http://www.healthinaging.org/public_education/eldercare/
A comprehensive online book for caregivers of elderly

The National Family Caregivers Association (NFCA) and the National Alliance for Caregiving (NAC)
http://www.familycaregiving101.org/
Information and resources for caregivers

US Administration on Aging, National Family Caregiver Support Program
http://www.aoa.gov/prof/aoaprog/caregiver/carefam/carefam.asp
Information and resources for caregivers

Management of the Surgical Patient

7

Peter Pompei

CLINICAL PEARLS 73

PREOPERATIVE ASSESSMENT AND MANAGEMENT 74
Cardiovascular System 74
Respiratory System 76
Kidney and Metabolism 77
Neuropsychiatric Concerns 78

POSTOPERATIVE MANAGEMENT OF SPECIFIC MEDICAL PROBLEMS 79
Cardiovascular Problems 79
Pulmonary and Thromboembolic Problems 79
Kidney Failure 79
Fluid and Nutrition Management 80
Delirium and Postoperative Cognitive Decline 80

CLINICAL PEARLS

- Operative therapy can be an effective management option for many health problems affecting older persons.
- Surgery can be done with few complications in older patients.
- Risk indices that help stratify patients and practice guidelines to optimize management have been developed for cardiac, pulmonary, and neuropsychiatric problems.
- Consider discontinuing angiotensin-converting enzyme (ACE) inhibitors before surgery.
- Most medications can be taken with small sips of water on the morning of surgery.
- β-Blockers have been shown to decrease the risk of cardiovascular events during surgery.
- Effective prophylactic measures exist for patients who are at risk for bacterial endocarditis, thromboembolism, and delirium.
- Respiratory complications can be reduced by using incentive spirometry and early mobility after surgery.
- Generally give two thirds of the usual dose of insulin for a morning procedure and one half for an afternoon procedure. Hold oral hypoglycemics.
- Restore a euthyroid state before elective procedures.
- Pain or a distended bladder may raise blood pressure postoperatively.
- Ten percent to 30% of older patients suffer postoperative cognitive decline that lasts for months or may be permanent.
- Effective chronic disease management through comprehensive preoperative assessment and attentive perioperative care can minimize complications of surgical interventions.

Use of health care services by older persons is high and disproportionate to the number of persons aged 65 years and older in the population. This holds true for the special case of operative interventions as well. Currently, it is estimated that of all adults operated on each year, one third are in the 65 years and above age-group. Among persons who reach the age of 65, at least half will undergo surgery in the remaining years of their lives. Advances in technology that address the diseases afflicting older persons are partly responsible for these utilization patterns. Common surgeries that older persons undergo include cataract extraction and intraocular lens implantation, revascularization procedures, joint replacements, cholecystectomy, and bowel resections.

Another reason for the increased number of surgical procedures among older persons is the recent significant decline in operative risk. Over the last 50 years, operative mortality among patients aged 80 years and older has decreased from approximately 10% to below 3%. This change has been ascribed to advances in anesthesiology and newer surgical techniques, including safer anesthetic agents and limited-access approaches such as laparoscopic procedures. Because the complication rates for urgent and emergent procedures remain high for older persons—three to ten times greater than for younger persons—planned procedures with sufficient time to optimize the management of a patient's health status are always preferred. Operative risk has consistently been found to be related to the burden of comorbidity rather than to the age of the patient. Consistent findings are that, even among patients aged 75 years and older, those with few comorbid conditions have a low risk of complications, and this risk is directly related to the number and severity of coexisting illnesses. Although the functional reserve of any organ may decline with advancing age, it is the presence of disease processes, chronic and acute, that significantly compromise homeostatic mechanisms.

The generalist physicians caring for the older person during the perioperative period have several responsibilities. First, they are frequently called on by surgical colleagues to identify and modify risk factors that may predispose the patient to specific complications. Second, to reduce the risk of complications, they must optimally manage all the acute and chronic medical problems of the patient throughout the perioperative period. Third, whenever possible, generalist physicians should initiate and maintain appropriate preventive strategies to reduce the risk of selected complications. Finally, they should understand, as fully as possible, the wishes and advance directives of the patient in case of a serious complication. A discussion about personal values and wishes, preferences for future interventions, and the surrogate decision makers to be involved when necessary can be critical in ensuring a comprehensive patient-centered treatment plan.

PREOPERATIVE ASSESSMENT AND MANAGEMENT

Evaluating a patient's risk for select complications and intervening to modify these risks are important functions of the preoperative assessment. The most common complications involve the respiratory, cardiac, and neuropsychiatric systems, so these require special attention. Ensuring the optimal management of concurrent medical problems and instituting preventive measures to reduce the risk of morbidity and mortality from a surgical procedure are other important functions of a preoperative assessment. Most of the evidence-based approaches for assessing and managing patients before surgery are organ or system based.

Cardiovascular System

Hypertension is one of the most commonly encountered chronic diseases affecting the cardiovascular system. Perioperative complications from hypertension including stroke and myocardial infarction are associated with both excessive elevations and wide fluctuations of blood pressure. Patients with well-controlled hypertension should be maintained on their antihypertensive regimen as much as possible throughout the perioperative period. For elective procedures, the morning doses of the patients' medications should be taken with a sip of water before the induction of anesthesia. The one exception to this recommendation relates to angiotensin-converting enzyme (ACE) inhibitors, which may interact with anesthetic agents to cause severe hypotension; some recommend that this class of medication be withheld on the morning of surgery.[1] According to the Joint National Committee on Prevention, Detection, Evaluation, and Treatment of High Blood Pressure, when the preoperative diastolic blood pressure exceeds 110 mm Hg, surgery should be delayed.[2] The blood pressure should be reduced gradually with medications over several weeks, although this decision must be made in conjunction with a full understanding of the potential benefits and urgency of the proposed operative intervention. Hypertension is often a marker for vascular diseases that are associated with adverse surgical outcomes. It is reasonable to assess older patients with hypertension with a detailed history and physical examination to uncover coronary disease, congestive heart failure, and cerebrovascular disease and obtain an electrocardiogram, looking for changes of ischemia or left ventricular hypertrophy. Because hypertension can lead to chronic kidney disease, it is useful to measure the serum creatinine level and estimate the glomerular filtration rate.

Cardiac complications of noncardiac surgery are among the most serious, and a number of risk indices have been developed over the years. As the ability to reliably predict the patients who are at risk for cardiac complications improved, practice guidelines were developed to identify and manage this risk. The stepwise algorithm advocated by the American College of Cardiology (ACC) and the American Heart Association (AHA) is updated regularly to incorporate the latest evidence from clinical trials.[3] According to this guideline, the clinician should consider three major factors in sequence: Clinical predictors of risk, the functional capacity of the patient, and the risks specific to the planned surgery. As shown in Table 7.1, clinical predictors are grouped as minor, intermediate, or major. It is notable that advanced age is categorized as a minor clinical predictor, acknowledging that the increased operative risk to older persons is attributable to accumulated medical problems and not age alone. Patients with intermediate or minor clinical predictors of risk are next assessed for functional capacity, as defined in Table 7.2. Those with minor or no clinical predictors who also have moderate or excellent functional capacity can proceed to the operating room. For patients who

TABLE 7.1
CLINICAL PREDICTORS OF INCREASED PERIOPERATIVE CARDIAC RISK FOR NONCARDIAC SURGERY

Minor Predictors	Intermediate Predictors	Major Predictors
Advanced age	Mild angina pectoris	Unstable coronary syndromes
Abnormal ECG	Prior myocardial infarction	Significant dysrhythmias
Rhythm other than sinus	Compensated or prior heart failure	Decompensated heart failure
Low functional capacity	Diabetes mellitus	Severe valvular disease
History of stroke	Renal insufficiency	
Uncontrolled hypertension		

ECG, electrocardiogram.
From Eagle KA, Berger PB, Calkins H, et al. *ACC/AHA guideline update for perioperative cardiovascular evaluation for noncardiac surgery: A report of the American College of Cardiology/American Heart Association Task Force on Practice Guidelines (Committee to update the 1996 Guidelines on perioperative cardiovascular evaluation for noncardiac surgery).* American College of Cardiology; 2002. Available at: http://www.acc.org/clinical/guidelines/perio/dirIndex.htm used with permission.

have either minor clinical predictors and poor functional capacity or intermediate clinical predictors and moderate or excellent functional capacity, the degree of risk associated with the planned surgery is considered. If the surgical risk is low or intermediate, as listed in Table 7.3, the patients can proceed to the operating room. Delaying the noncardiac surgery for additional testing and management is recommended for the following three groups of patients: (i) Those who are undergoing a high-risk surgery who have poor functional capacity, (ii) those undergoing a high-risk procedure who have intermediate clinical predictors, (iii) those who have major clinical predictors, irrespective of their functional capacity or the surgical risk. As with all practice guidelines, the algorithm is intended to assist physicians in meeting the needs of most patients in most circumstances; individual treatment plans are best made jointly by the treating physician and the patient.

Accumulating evidence supports the use of β-blocker therapy perioperatively to reduce the risks of cardiac complications in noncardiac surgery.[4] Despite variations in drug administration (i.e., oral vs. parenteral; initiating the drug either weeks before or immediately before the surgery; discontinuing the drug immediately, at 48 hours, at hospital discharge, at 7 days, or at 30 days; or titrating the dose to different heart rates), β-blockers have been found to significantly decrease postoperative cardiac ischemia, myocardial infarction, and death. The number of patients who would need to be treated in order to achieve benefit is fewer than ten. The success of empiric β-blocker therapy in reducing cardiac risk may obviate the need for preoperative noninvasive testing in some patients.

Valvular heart disease can predispose surgical patients to congestive heart failure, myocardial ischemia, and endocarditis. Severe aortic stenosis, one of the major clinical

TABLE 7.2
EXAMPLES OF ACTIVITIES THAT HELP STRATIFY PATIENTS ACCORDING TO FUNCTIONAL CAPACITY

Poor Functional Capacity (Maximal Energy Expenditure $\leq$4 METs)	Moderate/Excellent Functional Capacity (Maximal Energy Expenditure >4 METs)
■ Eating, dressing, using the toilet	■ Climbing a flight of stairs or walking up a hill
■ Walking indoors around the house	■ Running a short distance
■ Walking a block or two on ground level	■ Scrubbing floors or moving furniture
■ Doing light housework—dusting, washing dishes	■ Playing golf, bowling, dancing
	■ Swimming, singles tennis, skiing

METs, metabolic equivalents.
From Eagle KA, Berger PB, Calkins H, et al. *ACC/AHA guideline update for perioperative cardiovascular evaluation for noncardiac surgery: A report of the American College of Cardiology/American Heart Association Task Force on Practice Guidelines (Committee to update the 1996 Guidelines on perioperative cardiovascular evaluation for noncardiac surgery).* American College of Cardiology; 2002. Available at: http://www.acc.org/clinical/guidelines/perio/dirIndex.htm used with permission.

TABLE 7.3

RISKS OF CARDIAC COMPLICATIONS ASSOCIATED WITH SPECIFIC NONCARDIAC SURGERIES

High Risk (>5%)	Intermediate Risk (<5%)	Low Risk (<1%)
■ Emergent major surgeries ■ Aortic and other major vascular surgery ■ Peripheral vascular surgery ■ Prolonged procedures with large fluid shifts and/or blood loss	■ Carotid endarterectomy ■ Head and neck surgery ■ Intraperitoneal and intrathoracic surgery ■ Orthopaedic surgery ■ Prostate surgery	■ Endoscopic procedures ■ Superficial procedures ■ Cataract surgery ■ Breast surgery

From Eagle KA, Berger PB, Calkins H, et al. *ACC/AHA guideline update for perioperative cardiovascular evaluation for noncardiac surgery: A report of the American College of Cardiology/American Heart Association Task Force on Practice Guidelines (Committee to update the 1996 Guidelines on perioperative cardiovascular evaluation for noncardiac surgery).* American College of Cardiology; 2002. Available at: http://www.acc.org/clinical/guidelines/perio/dirIndex.htm used with permission.

predictors in the ACC/AHA practice guideline reviewed in the preceding text, can be asymptomatic and difficult to distinguish from the more benign aortic sclerosis common in older persons. If the systolic murmur is heard with the stethoscope placed over the right clavicle, the chances of moderate or severe aortic stenosis are increased. Patients with this finding should be examined for the following clinical findings: (i) Reduced carotid artery volume, (ii) delayed carotid artery upstroke, (iii) reduced intensity of the second heart sound, and (iv) maximum intensity of the murmur over the second right intercostal space. If three of these four findings are present, the risk of significant aortic stenosis is sufficient to warrant confirmation by an echocardiogram.[5]

Certain valvular abnormalities and other cardiac conditions increase the risk of endocarditis for some operative interventions. According to the AHA, patients in the high-risk category for endocarditis are those with prosthetic heart valves, complex cyanotic congenital heart disease, surgically constructed systemic–pulmonary shunts or conduits, or a previous history of endocarditis. Patients in the moderate-risk category are those with other congenital cardiac malformations, acquired valve dysfunction, hypertrophic cardiomyopathy, and mitral valve prolapse with regurgitation and/or thickened valve leaflets. Prophylaxis is not recommended for patients with the following conditions: Previous coronary artery bypass grafts, cardiac pacemakers, and a history of rheumatic fever without valve dysfunction. It is recommended that both high- and moderate-risk patients undergoing procedures that involve the respiratory tract (e.g., tonsillectomy, surgeries involving the respiratory mucosa, and rigid bronchoscopy) and the genitourinary tract (e.g., prostate surgery, cystoscopy, and urethral dilation) be given endocarditis prophylaxis. High-risk patients undergoing gastrointestinal tract surgery (e.g., sclerotherapy for esophageal varices, esophageal dilation, biliary tract surgery and endoscopy, and surgery involving intestinal mucosa) also require prophylaxis; for patients in the moderate-risk category, prophylaxis is considered optional. The recommended antibiotic regimens[6] according to procedure and patient-risk category are shown in Table 7.4.

Respiratory System

Pulmonary complications occur even more commonly than cardiovascular problems among older surgical patients. There are important age-related changes in the respiratory system, such as a decline in alveolar elasticity and an increase in chest wall stiffness, that predispose patients to atelectasis and diminished expiratory flow rates. Many surgical procedures involve a general anesthetic and confine the patient in a supine position for several hours. These factors, especially when combined with an abdominal incision, contribute to a reduced functional residual capacity and increased airway resistance. The patient- and surgery-related effects on the respiratory system contribute to hypoventilation, small airway closure, secretion retention, and attendant hypoxemia and pulmonary infections. Multifactorial risk indices have been developed and validated to improve our ability to identify those patients at highest risk for respiratory complications. Factors that are consistently related to an increased risk of postoperative pulmonary complications include type of incision (abdominal or thoracic), advanced age, functional status, impaired cognitive function, and recent smoking. Other factors that are not consistent between studies include body mass index of ≥ 27 kg per m^2; recent weight loss (>10% in the last 6 months); a history of cancer, angina, cerebrovascular disease, or renal insufficiency; an incision length ≥ 30 cm; and an American Society of Anesthesiologist (ASA) class ≥ 3.[7,8] Because many of these factors are not modifiable, there is still considerable work to be done to develop a practice guideline that can help physicians reduce the rate of

TABLE 7.4
PROPHYLACTIC ANTIBIOTIC REGIMENS FOR PATIENTS AT RISK FOR BACTERIAL ENDOCARDITIS

Dental, Oral, Respiratory Tract, or Esophageal Procedures	
Standard Regimen	
Amoxicillin	2 g orally 1 h before procedure
Amoxicillin/Penicillin-Allergic Patients	
Clindamycin	600 mg orally 1 h before procedure
or	
Cephalexin or cefadroxil	2 g orally 1 h before procedure
or	
Azithromycin or clarithromycin	500 mg orally 1 h before procedure
Patients Unable to Take Oral Medications	
Ampicillin	2 g intravenously or intramuscularly within 30 min before procedure
Penicillin-Allergic Patients Unable to Take Oral Medications	
Clindamycin	600 mg intravenously within 30 min before procedure
or	
Cefazolin	1 g intravenously or intramuscularly within 30 min before procedure
Genitourinary and Gastrointestinal (excluding esophageal) Procedures	
High-risk Patients	
Ampicillin and gentamicin	IV or IM administration of ampicillin 2 g, plus gentamicin 1.5 mg/kg (not to exceed 120 mg), 30 min before the procedure; followed by ampicillin 1 g IM/IV or amoxicillin 1 g, orally 6 h after initial dose
High-risk Patients Allergic to Ampicillin/Amoxicillin	
Vancomycin and gentamicin	Intravenous administration of vancomycin 1 g, over 1–2 h plus gentamicin 1.5 mg/kg IM/IV (not to exceed 120 mg); complete injection/infusion within 30 min of starting procedure
Moderate-risk Patients[a]	
Amoxicillin or ampicillin	Amoxicillin 2 g orally 1 h before procedure, or ampicillin 3 g IM/IV within 30 min of starting procedure
Moderate-risk Patients Allergic to Ampicillin/Amoxicillin	
Vancomycin	1 g IV over 1–2 h; complete infusion within 30 min of starting procedure

[a]Patients with prosthetic heart valves and those with a previous history of endocarditis are considered to be in the high-risk category and should not be considered for this regimen.
IV, intravenous; IM, intramuscular.
Adapted from Dajani AS, Taubert KA, Wilson W, et al. Prevention of bacterial endocarditis: Recommendations of the American Heart Association. *JAMA.* 1997;277:1796 used with permission.

pulmonary complications. In the meantime, physicians can play an important role by encouraging patients in the preoperative period to practice coughing and deep breathing exercises, master the use of the incentive spirometer, and work toward early mobility after the surgery.

Kidney and Metabolism

Because of their role in drug metabolism and fluid and electrolyte balance, it is important to assess kidney and metabolic functions preoperatively so that these can be optimally managed throughout the perioperative period. The reduced number of glomeruli and fall in kidney blood flow with advancing age contribute to a decline in creatinine clearance. Because muscle mass also decreases with age, the serum creatinine level may remain normal and cannot be used in isolation to estimate kidney function. Although several formulae have been proposed to estimate creatinine clearance in older persons, the following two methods have gained wide acceptance:

1. Cockcroft-Gault:[9]

$$C_{Cr}(\text{mL per minute}) = \frac{[140 - \text{age (y)} \times \text{weight (kg)}]}{[72 \times S_{Cr}\ (\text{mg per dL})]}$$

where C_{Cr} is creatinine clearance and S_{Cr} is serum creatinine
(This formula is for men; the estimate is adjusted for women by multiplying the result by 0.85.)

2. Abbreviated equation of the Modification of Diet in Renal Disease study group:[10]

$$\text{Estimated glomerular filtration rate (mL/minute/}\\ 1.73\ \text{m}^2) = 186 \times (S_{\text{Cr}})^{-1.154} \times (\text{age})^{-0.203}$$

(The estimate is adjusted for women by multiplying the result by 0.742 and for African-Americans by multiplying the result by 1.210.)

Both calculations have been endorsed as useful methods for estimating glomerular filtration rate in adults by the National Kidney Foundation.[11] It is acknowledged that these estimates, based on commonly available clinical information, are sufficiently accurate to allow the clinician to make appropriate dose adjustments for the medications metabolized by the kidneys.

A considerable number of older surgical patients have type 2 diabetes, a condition that increases the risk of infectious and cardiovascular complications. Managing blood glucose level during the perioperative period is complicated by several factors. The tissue damage and stress associated with surgery stimulates the release of insulin counter-regulatory hormones—epinephrine, glucagon, cortisol, and growth hormone. These, in turn, act by promoting gluconeogenesis or by blunting insulin release or insulin action. In addition, insulin clearance can be compromised and nutritional intake is likely to be highly variable around the time of a surgery.

Management strategies have been developed to optimize blood sugar control perioperatively.[12] For patients with diet-controlled diabetes, no special interventions are recommended before the procedure. Blood sugar levels are monitored perioperatively, and hyperglycemia is treated with short-acting insulin. Patients receiving oral hypoglycemic agents should withhold the medication on the day of surgery, and hyperglycemia can be corrected with short-acting insulin until the oral agent can be resumed. For patients receiving once-daily insulin injections, dosing on the morning of the surgery will depend on the timing of the surgery: Two thirds of the dose for a morning procedure and one half of the dose for an afternoon procedure. An intravenous infusion of glucose is recommended at a rate of 5 g of glucose per hour. If multiple insulin injections are used to manage a patient's diabetes, one half to one third of the morning dose is administered preoperatively with an intravenous infusion of glucose. The greatest risk of serious complications is from hypoglycemia, so the goal for diabetes control perioperatively is for blood sugar levels to range between 150 and 200 mg per dL.

Thyroid diseases, although less common than diabetes, can be associated with significant complications if unrecognized and untreated. As many as 10% of older hospitalized patients, in whom nonspecific and atypical manifestations are common, may have hypothyroidism. Untreated hypothyroidism can impair drug metabolism and cause central nervous system depression and respiratory insufficiency. Rapid correction of hypothyroidism is possible in cases of trauma or other emergency surgeries: Intravenous administration of 300 to 500 μg of L-thyroxine can improve the metabolic rate within 6 hours. Corticosteroids are commonly administered simultaneously to avoid depletion of adrenal reserves associated with the improved metabolic rate. Hyperthyroidism occurs in $<1\%$ of hospitalized older patients. Fever, tachycardia, and congestive heart failure are the most common complications of untreated disease. Older patients may become hyperthyroid after being exposed to nonionic contrast radiography. It is important to restore a euthyroid state before elective procedures. When faced with an urgent surgery, treatment with 1,000 mg of propylthiouracil by mouth and a β-blocker to manage catecholamine surges is an option. Steroids are often given simultaneously both to avoid cortisol depletion and to lower serum thyroxine and thyroid-stimulating hormone levels.

Older persons are at high risk for nutritional deficits and many consume alcohol on a regular basis. Poor nutrition is a well-established risk factor for pneumonia, poor wound healing, and many other postoperative complications. It is difficult to measure nutritional status, and the strongest predictor of adverse outcomes such as prolonged hospitalization, frequent readmissions, and increased mortality is serum albumin.[13] Therefore, in addition to a careful history and physical examination to assess for malnutrition, a serum albumin level determination can be helpful in assessing risk. Optimizing preoperative nutritional status is recommended; parenteral nutritional supplements have not consistently shown benefit. Regular alcohol use can predispose older patients to disastrous complications of alcohol withdrawal syndrome postoperatively. All patients should be systematically screened for alcohol use, and preoperative prophylactic benzodiazepines can be considered for individuals at high risk for developing an alcohol withdrawal syndrome.[14]

Neuropsychiatric Concerns

Cognitive and affective disorders are common among older patients and contribute to complications and poor outcomes after surgery. These conditions are also notoriously under-recognized, so a preoperative, systematic evaluation of every patient is important. Delirium is the most common postoperative neuropsychiatric complication, and preoperative and intraoperative factors have been identified as risk factors. In a study of older persons undergoing noncardiac surgery, the following factors were found to increase the risk of delirium: Age $\geq$70 years; cognitive impairment; limited physical function; a history of alcohol abuse; abnormal serum sodium, potassium, or glucose level; intrathoracic surgery; and abdominal aneurysm surgery. Two percent of patients with no risk factors developed delirium compared to 10% with two risk factors and 50% with three or more.[15] Prior knowledge of these risk factors allows for more vigilant management strategies. A targeted medical intervention for older patients admitted with hip fractures successfully reduced the incidence of delirium from 50% to 32%. The intervention focused on oxygenation, fluids and electrolytes, pain management, unnecessary medications, bowel and bladder function, nutrition, early mobilization, prevention and management of postoperative medical complications, and orientation cues.[16]

POSTOPERATIVE MANAGEMENT OF SPECIFIC MEDICAL PROBLEMS

The intraoperative management of patients is the purview of our colleagues in anesthesiology. It is useful to review the record of the operative course, noting vital signs, volume of medication administration, duration of anesthesia, and any comments about what transpired in the operating and recovery rooms. This will assist the physicians in managing the medical conditions commonly encountered in older persons who undergo surgery. The physicians must also remain mindful of the important goal of restoring the patient to an optimal level of functioning. Early mobilization and resumption of self-care activities will help reduce the risk of thromboembolism, improve respiratory mechanics, minimize cardiovascular deconditioning, and reduce muscle loss.

Cardiovascular Problems

When notified of an elevated blood pressure postoperatively, it is important to consider noncardiovascular causes such as pain or a distended bladder. Volume status and whether any usual antihypertensive medications were mistakenly omitted are other causes to consider. The correction of any of these conditions is straightforward. If the elevated blood pressure is related to essential hypertension, several medications are available for parenteral administration: β-Blockers, calcium channel blockers, ACE inhibitors, and drugs that block both α- and β-receptors. Parenteral vasodilators such as hydralazine are generally avoided because diastolic filling can be seriously compromised by these medications if the patient has a hypertrophic cardiomyopathy secondary to chronic hypertension.

Cardiac rhythm disturbances occur commonly and can precipitate myocardial ischemia and heart failure. Older persons are at increased risk for developing postoperative supraventricular tachycardias, especially if there is a history of supraventricular dysrhythmias, asthma, heart failure, premature atrial complexes on a preoperative electrocardiogram, or if the patient has had a vascular, abdominal, or thoracic procedure.[17] When a supraventricular tachycardia occurs, it is important to attempt to restore sinus rhythm with infusions of adenosine, a β-blocker, or a calcium channel blocker. If the rhythm is that of atrial fibrillation, conversion to sinus rhythm can be attempted with electrical cardioversion or amiodarone. Alternatively, rate control using β-blockers or calcium channel blockers may alleviate symptoms. Spontaneous reversion to sinus rhythm often occurs within 6 weeks of the surgery. If atrial fibrillation persists for >24 to 48 hours, it is important to consider anticoagulation therapy to reduce the risk of stroke.

Heart failure can be precipitated postoperatively by excessive fluid administration, cardiac ischemia, or a new rhythm disturbance. It can be extremely challenging to ensure optimal ventricular filling pressures on the basis of the clinical assessment of volume status in older persons by physical examination and standard laboratory parameters alone. Although some have argued for the use of pulmonary artery catheters in high-risk patients, studies have not shown a mortality benefit for this intervention.[18]

Pulmonary and Thromboembolic Problems

Early mobilization, deep breathing exercises, and incentive spirometry are key factors in reducing the risk of atelectasis and pneumonia postoperatively. In addition to these problems, venous thrombosis and pulmonary embolism are common and serious complications experienced by older surgical patients. Because both conditions can be associated with significant morbidity even with effective treatment, prophylaxis has become an important strategy. Recommended prophylactic regimens differ on the basis of the type of surgery.[19] For patients older than 60 undergoing general surgery, the current recommendations include postoperative treatment with low-dose unfractionated heparin, low-molecular-weight heparin, or intermittent pneumatic compression devises. Older patients having elective hip or knee replacement surgeries or hip fracture surgery can be effectively managed with low-molecular-weight heparin or adjusted-dose warfarin (international normalized ratio target 2.5, range 2 to 3). Low-molecular-weight heparins are cleared by the kidneys and dose adjustment may be required for patients with an estimated creatinine clearance below 30 mL per minute. The duration of prophylactic treatment has been debated, but recent evidence suggests that patients treated for 4 to 6 weeks after a hip or knee replacement have fewer episodes of venous thromboembolism, with an acceptably low risk of major bleeding complications.[20]

Kidney Failure

Postoperative kidney failure is a serious complication associated with a high mortality. Preoperative impaired kidney function, seen commonly among older patients, is an important risk factor for this complication. The kidneys are vulnerable to even transient reductions in cardiac output and to the toxic effects of anesthetic agents and other medications. Early signs of acute renal failure can include oliguria, isosthenuria, and an increase in serum creatinine. When impaired renal blood flow is responsible for acute kidney failure, the urine sodium level will typically be <40 mEq per L and the urine-to-plasma creatinine ratio will be >10. Treatment is directed at optimizing intravascular volume and cardiac output. In contrast, when acute tubular necrosis is the mechanism of kidney failure, granular or epithelial cell casts are often present in the urine sediment, the urine sodium level will be >40 mEq per L, and the urine-to-plasma creatinine ratio will be <10. Identifying and eliminating nephrotoxic medications while meticulously maintaining a euvolemic state are the key principles to effectively manage this syndrome. Dialysis is rarely required but may be necessary if the patient develops pulmonary edema, hyperkalemia, metabolic acidosis, or encephalopathy. Finally, obstructive nephropathy is an important cause of acute kidney failure, especially in older men. Bed rest, preexisting prostatic hypertrophy, and medications with anticholinergic properties conspire to precipitate acute urinary retention and kidney failure. This condition is readily reversed by placing a urinary bladder catheter, and ongoing management requires attentive monitoring of fluid and electrolyte derangements during the anticipated brisk postobstructive diuresis.

Fluid and Nutrition Management

It is important to consider the expected changes in body composition and fluid regulation that complicate managing older persons during the perioperative period. With aging, irrespective of body weight, there is a relative increase in body fat with a reciprocal decrease in muscle, total body water, and intracellular water. Maintaining adequate hydration in older persons can be impaired by a reduced sensation of thirst and an impaired ability of the kidneys to concentrate the urine and conserve water. The normal mechanisms for maintaining volume homeostasis are further compromised during the perioperative period because of the hormonal responses to the trauma of tissue damage. The stress-related release of antidiuretic hormone will promote fluid retention, a fact to be taken into account when administering postoperative intravenous fluids to avoid iatrogenic volume overload. Although no formula can guarantee the optimal fluid, electrolyte, and calorie administration for an individual patient, the following guideline has been recommended as a useful starting point.[21] To approximate intracellular volume for persons aged 65 to 85 years and weighing 40 to 80 kg, use 25% to 30% of body weight (in kg) for men and 20% to 25% for women. **Estimates of the daily metabolic requirements of older patients in the basal state per liter of intracellular volume are as follows:**

Water	100 mL
Energy	100 kcal
Protein	3 g
Sodium	3 mmol
Potassium	2 mmol

For example, an 80-year-old woman who weighs 55 kg has an estimated intracellular volume of 11 L. To maintain water balance in a basal state, the infusion rate for intravenous fluids would be between 45 and 55 mL per hour. It is reassuring to know that this estimate of daily volume requirements is comparable to the recommendation of many nutritionists: 30 mL/kg body weight/day. Regular, systematic monitoring of volume status is necessary to accommodate changing conditions and the individual patient response to the fluid and electrolyte administration.

Adequate nutrition is essential in the perioperative period, when wound healing increases the need for energy in the form of calories. Hospital nutritionists can be helpful in calculating caloric needs and in documenting caloric intake. A wide variety of nutritional supplements have been developed to achieve the energy goals of hospitalized older persons with a variety of comorbid conditions. There is limited empiric evidence to guide us on optimal routes of administration; however, enteral supplements are preferred for patients with a functioning gastrointestinal tract, and parenteral supplements are limited to those patients in whom enteral feeding is not possible.

Delirium and Postoperative Cognitive Decline

Brain dysfunction is a common complication of older surgical patients, and the two most common syndromes are delirium and postoperative cognitive decline. Delirium has been recognized since antiquity as a transient disorder characterized by abrupt onset, confusion, inattention, and altered consciousness. When older surgical patients are systematically observed for this condition, it has been shown to affect 10% to 50% of them. The syndrome is certainly underreported and probably significantly under-recognized as well. For patients and their families, delirium can be a frightening experience, and it has consistently been shown to be associated with increased morbidity and mortality. The most common risk factors have been described earlier in this chapter, and the most common precipitating events have been found to be metabolic derangements, drugs, infections, and cardiorespiratory disorders. Of intraoperative factors that might be expected to be precipitants, anesthetic agent, hypotension, bradycardia, and tachycardia have not been shown to be associated with delirium. On the other hand, intraoperative blood loss is linked to delirium; even after taking the preoperative risk factors into account, patients with a postoperative hematocrit <30% had an increased risk (odds ratio = 1.7; 95% CI, 1.1 to 2.7) of delirium.[15] Prevention is the best strategy for managing the problem of delirium in older surgical patients, but when this fails, treatment involves identifying and correcting the precipitating factor and providing supportive care. Only when there is a risk that the patient will cause harm to himself or herself or others should drug therapy be considered. Low doses of the traditional or atypical antipsychotic medications can effectively suppress violent and aggressive behaviors but should be used sparingly.

Postoperative cognitive decline is another syndrome of cognitive dysfunction that is characterized by acquired abnormalities in learning and memory. It was first described after cardiac surgery but has more recently been observed after a variety of noncardiac surgical procedures, including those done under regional anesthesia. As many as 10% to 30% of older patients may suffer cognitive decline of varying severity that lasts for months and may be permanent. No etiology has been established for this condition; specifically, studies have documented no relationship to intraoperative hypotension, hypoxemia, or the type of anesthesia.[22] Given our limited understanding of this syndrome, effective preventive or treatment strategies are unknown. The prevalence and significance of postoperative cognitive dysfunction among older persons is sufficient to support the recommendation for a careful preoperative assessment of cognition. A quantitative measure of cognition will serve as a useful baseline and facilitate early detection of subtle postoperative abnormalities.

REFERENCES

1. Fleisher LA. Preoperative evaluation of the patient with hypertension. *JAMA.* 2002;287(16):2043–2046.
2. Chobanian AV, Bakris GL, Black HR, et al. The seventh report of the Joint National Committee on Prevention, Detection, Evaluation, and Treatment of High Blood Pressure: The JNC 7 report. *JAMA.* 2003;289:2560–2571.
3. Eagle KA, Berger PB, Calkins H, et al. *ACC/AHA guideline update for perioperative cardiovascular evaluation for noncardiac surgery: A report of the American College of Cardiology/American Heart Association Task Force on Practice Guidelines (Committee to update the 1996 Guidelines on perioperative cardiovascular evaluation for noncardiac surgery).* American College of Cardiology; 2002. Available at: http://www.acc.org/clinical/guidelines/perio/dirIndex.htm.
4. Auerbach AS, Goldman L. β-blockers and reduction of cardiac events in noncardiac surgery: Scientific review. *JAMA.* 2002;287: 1435–1444.
5. Etchells E, Glenns V, Shadowitz S, et al. A bedside clinical prediction rule for detecting moderate of severe aortic stenosis. *J Gen Intern Med.* 1998;13:699–704.
6. Dajani AS, Taubert KA, Wilson W, et al. Prevention of bacterial endocarditis: Recommendations of the American Heart Association. *JAMA.* 1997;277:1794–1801.
7. Brooks-Brunn JA. Validation of a predictive model for postoperative pulmonary complications. *Heart Lung.* 1998;27:151–158.
8. Arozullah AM, Khuri SF, Henderson WG, et al. For the National Veterans Administration Surgical Quality Improvement Program. Development and validation of a multifactorial risk index for predicting postoperative pneumonia after major noncardiac surgery. *Ann Intern Med.* 2001;135:847–857.
9. Cockroft DW, Gault MH. Prediction of creatinine clearance from serum creatinine. *Nephron.* 1976;16:31–41.
10. Levey AS, Boach JP, Lewis JB, et al. An more accurate method to estimate glomerular filtration rate from serum creatinine: A new prediction equation, Modification of Diet in Renal Disease Study Group. *Ann Intern Med.* 1999;130(6):461–470.
11. National Kidney Foundation Kidney Disease Outcome Quality Initiative Advisory Board. Part 5. Evaluation of laboratory measurement for clinical assessment of kidney disease. *Am J Kidney Dis.* 2002;39(2, Suppl 1):S76–S110.
12. Jacober SJ, Sowers JR. An update on perioperative management of diabetes. *Arch Intern Med.* 1999;159(20):2405–2411.
13. Gibbs J, Cull W, Henderson WG, et al. Preoperative serum albumin level as a predictor of operative mortality and morbidity: Results from the National VA surgical risk study. *Arch Surg.* 1999;134: 36–42.
14. Spies CD, Rommelspacher H. Alcohol withdrawal in the surgical patients: Prevention and treatment. *Anesth Analg.* 1999;88(4): 946–954.
15. Marcantonio ER, Goldman L, Orav EJ, et al. The association of intraoperative factors with the development of postoperative delirium. *Am J Med.* 1998;105:380–384.
16. Marcantonio ER, Flacker JM, Wright RJ, et al. Reducing delirium after hip fracture: A randomized trial. *J Am Geriatr Soc.* 2001;49: 516–522.
17. Polanczyk CA, Goldman L, Marcantonio ER, et al. Supraventricular arrhythmia in patients having noncardiac surgery: Clinical correlates and effect on length of stay. *Ann Intern Med.* 1998;129: 279–285.
18. Sandham JD, Hull RD, Brant RF, et al. Pulmonary artery catheters do not reduce mortality among high-risk surgical patients. *N Engl J Med.* 2003;348:5–14.
19. Geerts WH, Heit JA, Clagett PG, et al. Prevention of venous thromboembolism (Sixth ACCP consensus conference on antithrombotic therapy). *Chest.* 2001;119:132S–175S.
20. Eikelboom JW, Quinlan DJ, Douketis JD. Extended-duration prophylaxis against venous thromboembolism after total hip or knee replacement: A meta-analysis of the randomized trials. *Lancet.* 2001;358:9–15.
21. Miller RD. Anesthesia for the elderly. In: Miller RD, ed. *Anesthesia.* New York, NY: Churchill Livingstone; 1986:1801–1818.
22. Moller JT, Cluitmans P, Rasmussen LS, et al. Long-term postoperative cognitive dysfunction in the elderly ISPOCD1 study. *Lancet.* 1998;351:857–861.

Substance Abuse

8

Robert Mallin

CLINICAL PEARLS 82

EPIDEMIOLOGY OF SUBSTANCE USE DISORDERS IN THE OLDER PATIENT 83
Alcohol and Aging 83
Alcohol Use Disorders in the Older Patient 83
Other Drug Abuse in the Elderly 83
Tobacco Use and Older Adults 84

PRACTICAL MANAGEMENT OF SUBSTANCE USE DISORDERS IN OLDER PATIENTS 85
Screening and Assessment 85
Diagnosis of Substance Abuse versus Substance Dependence 85
Intervention 86
Acute Intoxication or Withdrawal Potential 87

BIOMEDICAL CONDITIONS AND COMPLICATIONS 89

EMOTIONAL/BEHAVIORAL CONDITIONS AND COMPLICATIONS 89

READINESS TO CHANGE (RESISTANCE TO TREATMENT) 90

RELAPSE RISK 90
Program Level 0.5—Early Intervention 90
Program Level I—Outpatient Treatment 90
Program Level II—Intensive Outpatient Treatment/Partial Hospitalization 90
Program Level III—Residential/Inpatient Treatment 90
Program Level IV—Medically Managed Intensive Inpatient Treatment 90

TREATMENT 90
Primary Care of the Patient in Recovery 91
Abstinence 91
Meeting Attendance 91
Sponsor Contact 92
Emotional Symptoms 92
Physical Health 92
Exercise 92
Leisure Activities 92
Compulsive Behavior 92
Legal Issues 92
Family and Relationship Issues 92
Spiritual Support 92

COMMON MEDICAL PROBLEMS IN RECOVERY 92
Sleep Disorders 92
Pain 93
Anxiety Disorders 93
Depression 93
Over-the-Counter and Prescription Medication Use 93

CLINICAL PEARLS

- Substance use disorders are common in the elderly and present less straightforwardly than they do in younger patients.
- Look for alcohol abuse and prescription drug abuse in the older patient. Illegal drug use and opioid abuse are very uncommon.
- Social isolation and loss of spouse, family member, close friends, and physical health are important risk factors for substance abuse in the older patient.
- Moderate alcohol intake (60 mL per day for men and 30 mL per day for women) may be too much for the older patient.
- Once the patient has crossed into substance dependence, efforts at modification of use are more difficult and abstinence appears necessary.
- For the older patient with a substance dependence disorder, abstinence from addictive substances is the most appropriate recommendation.

EPIDEMIOLOGY OF SUBSTANCE USE DISORDERS IN THE OLDER PATIENT

Alcohol and prescription drug misuse affect up to 17% of those aged 60 years and older, an invisible epidemic because of the difficulty of diagnosis, the shame associated with the illness, and ageism.[1] Comorbid chronic illness, medication use, physiologic changes, and social issues associated with aging combine to put the older patient at increased risk for a substance use disorder. In addition, these factors contribute to a greater impact of substance use disorders on older adults compared to the young. Substance abuse may increase the older patient's risk of social decline, injury, and illness.[2]

Older adults tend to favor alcohol and prescription drugs. Illicit drug use is rare among individuals older than 60, with the exception of those with antecedent substance use. In the community, alcohol abuse occurs in 2% to 10% of the older population. In the population of older patients treated in primary care clinics, excessive alcohol use may be prevalent in as high as 12% of women and 15% of men.[3] In the emergency room, the prevalence of alcohol dependence is 15%.[4] For Medicare beneficiaries, alcohol-related hospitalizations account for 1.1% of admissions, approximating the prevalence of myocardial infarction. From 2% to 3% of older patients in the community receive prescriptions for opioids, and these medications rarely cause problems. Benzodiazepines comprise 17% to 23% of drugs prescribed for older patients and are far more problematic in causing sedation, ataxia, memory problems, and delirium.[5] Among drinkers, 15% report nightly use of sedatives,[6] and benzodiazepines are associated with an increased risk of falls.[7]

Alcohol and Aging

There is no evidence that *moderate* alcohol consumption causes cognitive impairment in older individuals. However, older patients experience higher blood alcohol levels (BALs), given the same amount of alcohol consumed, than do their younger counterparts because of declining hepatic metabolism and renal excretion[8] (see Table 8.1). Unfortunately, alcohol abuse or dependence can have a profound effect on multiple areas of the older patient's health (see Table 8.2).

TABLE 8.1
AGE-RELATED CHANGES THAT AFFECT ALCOHOL METABOLISM

Decreased production of alcohol dehydrogenase
Increase in percentage of body fat
Decrease in lean body mass
Decrease in total body water

Because of the interaction of comorbid states and alcohol consumption, most authorities recommend a downward adjustment of moderate alcohol intake in the older patient (Evidence Level C). The recommendations for the general population are to avoid more than two drinks daily for men and no more than one daily for women. Men are cautioned not to drink more than four drinks in any given day, and women not to exceed three on any given day.[9] For patients older than 65, it is recommended that they do not consume more than one drink daily and less than three on any given day.[10] Comorbid states, medications, and social considerations should result in lower recommendations.

Alcohol Use Disorders in the Older Patient

Because of the significant impact that excessive alcohol intake has on the older patient, emphasis has been placed on problem drinking rather than the traditional considerations of alcohol dependence. Reliance on rigorous *Diagnostic and Statistical Manual of Mental Disorders, Fourth Edition* (*DSM-IV*) criteria for alcohol dependence would underestimate the problem among the elderly. It has been suggested that the terms *alcohol abuse* and *alcohol dependence* be abandoned for the older patient and replaced with the concepts of *at-risk* and *problem drinkers*. The "at-risk" drinker is defined as an older patient drinking more than recommended (greater than one drink daily) and whose pattern of use, although not yet causing problems, can bring about negative consequences for the drinker or those around him or her. The "problem drinker" is already experiencing these problems as the result of excessive alcohol use.[11]

Elderly drinkers are often further classified as those with early versus late onset of drinking. Early onset drinkers are described as having problematic drinking that began before the age of 40. These patients are often long-standing alcoholics who have continued their abusive drinking patterns as they age. They often have psychiatric disorders in addition to their substance use disorders. Late-onset drinkers in contrast do not display problematic drinking until after the age of 50. Often, they begin heavy alcohol intake after the loss of a loved one, or as the result of poor adjustment to retirement or other losses. They tend to be healthier than the early onset drinkers and tend to respond better to treatment. It is thought that about one third of problematic older drinkers are of this late-onset variety.[12] Risk factors for late-onset drinkers can be found in Table 8.3.

Other Drug Abuse in the Elderly

Abuse of prescribed substances is more often a concern among older patients because illicit drug use is uncommon. Opioids are not commonly prescribed for older adults and do not frequently lead to addiction. Tolerance to opioids

TABLE 8.2
DIFFERENTIAL DIAGNOSIS INTERNATIONAL CLASSIFICATION OF DISEASES, NINTH REVISION(ICD-9) CODES

Alcohol abuse	305.0
Alcohol dependence	303.0
Alcohol withdrawal	291.81
Alcohol withdrawal delirium	291.0
Alcohol-induced persisting amnestic disorder (Korsakoff psychosis, Wernicke-Korsakoff)	291.1
Alcohol-induced persisting dementia	291.2
Opioid dependence	304.0
Sedative, hypnotic, or anxiolytic dependence	304.1
Tobacco use disorder	305.1
Comorbid States Worsened by Alcohol Dependence and ICD-9 Code	
Dementia	
Alcohol-related	291.2
Wernicke-Korsakoff	291.1
Alzheimer	331.0
Immune system disorders	279.3
Liver disease (cirrhosis, hepatoma, hepatitis, alcoholic fatty liver)	571.2
Gastrointestinal bleeding (varices, gastritis, peptic ulcer)	535.5
Osteoporosis	733.0
Malnutrition	263.9
Stroke	436.0
Cardiovascular disease (hypertension, cardiac dysrhythmias, myocardial infarction, cardiomyopathy)	414.0
Psychiatric disorders (depression, anxiety)	311.0

decreases with age, as do the frequency and severity of side effects. This is thought to be secondary to increased receptor sensitivity.[13]

Benzodiazepines are often encountered as a problem in the elderly and may be overused. In some communities, 25% of the older than 65 population takes tranquilizer or hypnotic medications at any given time.[14] Whereas younger adults may not experience physiologic dependence until after 6 months or more of regular use, older patients may become dependent in as little as 3 months.[15] The adverse effects of chronic benzodiazepine use are outlined in Table 8.4.

Tobacco Use and Older Adults

Smoking declines with age. The prevalence of smoking in the United States is 23.4%, but after the age of 65 this decreases to 15% in men and 11% in women. Because tobacco abuse causes >400,000 deaths in the United States annually and >4 million older Americans smoke, the burden on the health of older patients is greater for tobacco abuse than any other abused substance. There is significant comorbidity between tobacco use and alcohol abuse. From 60% to 70% of male alcohol users smoke, and the prevalence of smoking among alcoholics is >80%.[1] The

TABLE 8.3
RISK FACTORS FOR LATE-ONSET PROBLEMATIC DRINKING

- Gender (men have greater risk than women)
- Family history of alcohol abuse
- Diagnosis of substance use disorder earlier in life
- Loss of spouse
- Losses (e.g., retirement, impairment of senses, decreased mobility, or declining health)
- Psychiatric disorders
- Other substance use (e.g., benzodiazepines, illicit drugs, or tobacco)
- Psychoactive prescription drugs

TABLE 8.4
ADVERSE EFFECTS OF CHRONIC BENZODIAZEPINE USE IN ELDERLY PATIENTS

- Diminished psychomotor performance
- Loss of coordination
- Diminished reaction time
- Daytime drowsiness
- Ataxia
- Falls
- Labile emotional state
- Confusion
- Rage
- Amnesia

decrease in risk begins almost immediately after smoking cessation, and older smokers are more likely to quit than younger patients.

PRACTICAL MANAGEMENT OF SUBSTANCE USE DISORDERS IN OLDER PATIENTS

Methods for identifying substance use disorders include screening and assessment, intervention, detoxification, treatment, and aftercare. Although these methods are similar for all ages, special considerations and expertise are required when applied to the older patient.

Screening and Assessment

Social isolation, ageism, retirement, and chronic illness reduce the likelihood that the older patient's substance abuse will be noticed by others. However, almost 90% of adults older than 65 see a physician on a regular basis. These visits provide an opportunity for health care providers to play a central role in the identification of substance use disorders in this population.

The use of common screening tools such as the CAGE (cutting down, annoyed, guilty, and eye-opener) (see Table 8.5) and Michigan Alcoholism Screening Test (MAST) can identify patients with alcohol problems at relatively high sensitivity. In the older patient, removing the *C* question, "Have you ever felt the need to cut back on your drinking?," appears to strengthen the CAGE specificity without significantly reducing its sensitivity.[16] The MAST has been modified to the Short Michigan Alcoholism Screening Test—Geriatric Version (SMAST—G) (see Table 8.6).[17]

Apart from screening tests, laboratory markers (see Table 8.7) may identify patients who require further evaluation. Biochemical markers such as γ-glutamyl transferase, mean corpuscular volume, and carbohydrate-deficient transferrin have low sensitivity and specificity but are useful when used with other screening tools.[18]

TABLE 8.5
CAGE (CUTTING DOWN, ANNOYED, GUILTY, AND EYE-OPENER) QUESTIONS

Have felt that you should *cut down* on your drinking?
Have people *annoyed* you by criticizing your drinking?
Have you ever felt bad or *guilty* about your drinking?
Have you ever had a drink first thing in the morning (*eye-opener*) to steady your nerves or get over a hangover?

Score: One to two "yes" responses should require further evaluation

Ewing JA. Detecting alcoholism. The CAGE questionnaire. *JAMA*. 1984;252(14):1906.

TABLE 8.6
SHORT MICHIGAN ALCOHOLISM SCREENING TEST—GERIATRIC VERSION

1. When talking with others, do you ever underestimate how much you actually drank?
2. After a few drinks, have you sometimes not eaten or have had to skip a meal because you did not feel hungry?
3. Does having a few drinks decrease your shakiness or tremors?
4. Does alcohol sometimes make it hard for you to remember parts of the day or night?
5. Do you usually take a drink to relax or calm your nerves?
6. Do you drink to take your mind off your problems?
7. Have you ever increased your drinking after experiencing a loss in your life
8. Has a doctor or nurse ever said he or she was worried or concerned about your drinking?
9. Have you ever made rules to help you manage your drinking?
10. When you feel lonely, does a drink help?

Score: Two or more "yes" responses indicate an alcohol problem

Diagnosis of Substance Abuse versus Substance Dependence

A positive screen requires the clinician to differentiate between substance dependence and physical dependence. The term *substance dependence* is synonymous with addiction; however, the term *physical dependence* is not. Physical dependence refers to a physiologic state of adaptation of specific receptors in the brain such that when a drug is taken for a period of time and subsequently stopped, a predictable withdrawal syndrome is experienced. This phenomenon may occur in or out of the context of addiction. Substance dependence or addiction is a pattern of drug use that is most simply described as a loss of control over the use of a substance such that the person with this disease will use drugs despite the continued occurrence

TABLE 8.7
RED FLAGS THAT SHOULD SIGNAL CONCERN ABOUT POSSIBLE SUBSTANCE ABUSE IN OLDER PATIENTS

1. Episodes of delirium
2. Worsening dementia
3. Recent exacerbation of chronic illness
4. Increasing isolation
5. Weight loss and decreased appetite
6. Persistent pain without clear cause
7. Sleep disturbance
8. Depression
9. Impaired self-care
10. Anxiety
11. Intermittent tremor
12. Irritability and difficulty managing anger
13. Violence
14. Driving problems

TABLE 8.8
DIAGNOSTIC AND STATISTICAL MANUAL OF MENTAL DISORDERS, FOURTH EDITION (DSM-IV) CRITERIA FOR SUBSTANCE DEPENDENCE

A maladaptive pattern of substance use, leading to clinically significant impairment or distress, as manifested by three (or more) of the following occurring at any time in the same 12-mo period:

1. Tolerance, as defined by either of the following:
   a. A need for markedly increased amounts of the substance to achieve intoxication or the desired effect
   b. Markedly diminished effect with continued use of the same amount of the substance
2. Withdrawal, as manifested by either of the following:
   a. The characteristic withdrawal syndrome for the substance
   b. The same (or closely related) substance taken to relieve or avoid withdrawal symptoms
3. The substance is often taken in larger amounts or over a longer period than was intended
4. There is a persistent desire or unsuccessful effort to cut down or control substance use
5. A great deal of time is spent in activities necessary to obtain the substance, use the substance, or recover from its effects
6. Important social, occupational, or recreational activities are given up or reduced because of substance use
7. The substance use is continued despite knowledge of having a persistent or recurrent physical or psychological problem that is likely to have been caused or exacerbated by the substance

Modified from American Psychiatric Association. *Diagnostic and statistical manual of mental disorders IV.* Washington, DC: American Psychiatric Press; 1994:181.

of important negative consequences of the drug use. The essential difference between substance abuse and dependence is that the person with substance abuse retains some control over its use and can modify that use in response to negative consequences. The person with substance dependence appears to be unable to exercise control over his or her drug use despite these negative consequences. From a practical point of view, the difference may be seen as one of number and severity of consequences. The more severe and numerous the consequences in the face of continued drug use, the more likely the patient will meet the criteria for substance dependence (see Table 8.8).

The patient who is engaged in substance abuse may benefit from a reduction in the amount and frequency of drug use, and in the face of consequences they may modify the use. Once the patient has crossed into the area of substance dependence, however, efforts at modification of use are more difficult, and abstinence appears to be the only way to effect a recovery from the compulsive use of addictive substances.

Intervention

Intervention tactics vary widely and may be as informal as a statement about the patient's behavior and drinking or may be as formal and complex as a facilitated meeting between the patient and loved ones to convince him or her to enter a residential treatment program. For at-risk drinkers, brief interventions may be effective, resulting in significant reduction in alcohol consumption and the consequences that follow.[19]

Feedback on at-risk drinking behavior may be the simplest form of intervention. For a patients who appears to be drinking more than the recommended amount and are having a few alcohol-related problems, a statement from their physician (such as, "Mr. Smith, I am concerned that you are drinking too much and that it is having a negative impact on your health.") may be sufficient to help the patients modify their behavior. Brief interventions are most effective when they are nonconfrontational and supportive in nature. They may be used to effect change in a variety of behaviors and may include some of the characteristics listed in Table 8.9. The use of motivational interviewing techniques may enhance and improve outcomes.[1]

For patients with substance dependence that is complicated by significant denial, a more formal approach to intervention is appropriate. This involves a formal meeting between the patients and persons important in their life. It is typically facilitated by an experienced addiction specialist. Typically, during these interventions, persons concerned about the patient describe their observations of and experiences with his or her substance use. These are often dramatic and powerful experiences that break through the patient's system of denial. They are effective in approximately 80% of cases.[20]

When considering further treatment for patients with substance dependence, the use of the American Society of Addiction Medicine Patient Placement Criteria (see Table 8.10) provides both a framework for assessment and a means of referring patients to appropriate levels of service.[21] Using the assessment dimensions as a guide, the physician can evaluate the patient with a substance use disorder.

TABLE 8.9
CONTENTS OF BRIEF INTERVENTIONS FOR OLDER AT-RISK DRINKERS

Questions that address what the patient already knows about alcohol consumption and the risks associated with drinking
Questions to uncover the reason why the at-risk drinker is consuming more than the recommended amount of alcohol
Education about the specific problems that appear to be affecting the at-risk drinker
Education about potential problems associated with increased alcohol consumption
Education about drinking patterns for patients in the age-group of the older at-risk drinkers
Strategies for the goal of cutting down on quantity and frequency of alcohol consumption
Strategies for managing roadblocks to the reduction of alcohol use
Written contract on goals and strategies

TABLE 8.10
AMERICAN SOCIETY OF ADDICTION MEDICINE PATIENT PLACEMENT CRITERIA

Assessment Dimensions

1. Acute intoxication and/or withdrawal potential
2. Biomedical conditions and complications
3. Emotional/behavioral conditions and complications
4. Treatment acceptance/resistance
5. Relapse potential
6. Recovery potential

Levels of Care

1. Level 0.5 Early intervention
2. Level I Outpatient treatment
3. Level II Intensive outpatient/partial hospitalization
4. Level III Medically monitored intensive inpatient treatment
5. Level IV Medically managed intensive inpatient treatment

Acute Intoxication or Withdrawal Potential

Acute intoxication or withdrawal potential is a dimension of assessment that determines the need for medical management to prevent life-threatening complications of withdrawal. Alcohol and other sedative–hypnotic drugs have a predictable course of withdrawal when physically dependent patients cease the use of these drugs (see Table 8.11). Table 8.12 presents some of the characteristics that increase the risk of alcohol withdrawal in patients. Older patients often have more severe withdrawal than their younger counterparts and may respond adversely to medications used to treat withdrawal symptoms. Whereas younger patients with mild withdrawal may be treated as outpatients, older patients are best treated for sedative–hypnotic withdrawal as inpatients (Evidence Level C).[22]

Benzodiazepines remain the drugs of choice for alcohol withdrawal (Evidence Level B), but when treating older patients the clinician may be faced with increased symptoms of alcohol withdrawal associated with increased intolerance to the side effects of benzodiazepines, making the treatment a difficult balancing act. Lorazepam appears to be the safest empiric choice among the various benzodiazepines for treating alcohol withdrawal in the elderly[23] (Evidence Level C). In an older population that is taking more medications, caution is required to avoid interactions.

The use of withdrawal scales such as the Clinical Institute Withdrawal Assessment (CIWA) (see Table 8.13) may help reduce the doses needed to accomplish symptom control in this population.

Other withdrawal syndromes that are common in the older patient involve barbiturates and benzodiazepines, both of which may present in the same manner as alcohol withdrawal and have the same treatment. Anticonvulsants such as gabapentin and carbamazepine have been found to be cross-tolerant with alcohol and have been used with success in sedative–hypnotic withdrawal in younger patients (Evidence Level A). There have been no clinical trials to date with older patients, but it is reasonable to assume that these medications would be effective in this group (Evidence Level C).

Opioid addiction is uncommon in the older patient group, but physiologic dependence for patients on long-term opioid therapy is not unusual. Opioid dependence may present with diarrhea, abdominal cramping, nausea, diaphoresis, piloerection, and mydriasis. Although not life threatening, unlike sedative–hypnotic withdrawal, it is most uncomfortable. Symptoms may be controlled with low-dose opioids or buprenorphine. Clonidine is used extensively in younger populations, but older patients

TABLE 8.11
SIGNS AND SYMPTOMS OF ALCOHOL WITHDRAWAL

Development of a combination of the following several hours after cessation of a prolonged period of heavy drinking

1. Autonomic hyperactivity: Diaphoresis, tachycardia, elevated BP
2. Tremor
3. Insomnia
4. Nausea or vomiting
5. Transient visual, tactile, and auditory hallucinations or illusions
6. Psychomotor agitation
7. Anxiety
8. Generalized seizure activity

BP, blood pressure.

TABLE 8.12
RISK FACTORS ASSOCIATED WITH SIGNIFICANT ALCOHOL WITHDRAWAL

1. Age >40 y
2. Male gender
3. Daily consumption of more than 750 mL of liquor
4. Drinking around the clock to maintain steady blood levels of alcohol
5. Excessive drinking for over 10 y
6. Development of tremulousness and anxiety within 6–8 h of cessation
7. History of seizures, hallucinations, delusions with alcohol withdrawal
8. Presence of an acute medical problem, such as pneumonia
9. Alcohol level ≥250 mg/dL on admission

Score

0–2 factors: Low risk for severe withdrawal
3–7 factors: Moderate risk
7–9 factors: High risk

Modified from Fleming MF. Pharmacologic management of nicotine, alcohol and other drug dependence. In: Fleming MF, Barry KL, eds. *Addictive Disorders*. St. Louis: Mosby–Year Book; 1992:49.

TABLE 8.13

CLINICAL INSTITUTE WITHDRAWAL ASSESSMENT (CIWA) WITHDRAWAL ASSESSMENT SCALE

Patient__________ Date______ Time_____ BP___/___
Age___ Race/Sex__ Drugs of choice (Primary)____ Other__

1. Autonomic Hyperactivity

Pulse rate	min
0	<80
1	81–100
2	101–110
3	111–120
4	121–130
5	131–140
6	141–150
7	>150

Sweating (observation)

0 No sweating
1 Barely perceptible sweating, palms moist
2
3
4 Beads of sweat obvious on forehead
5
6
7 Drenching sweats

2. Hand tremor: Arms extended and fingers spread apart

Observation

0 No tremor
1 Not visible
2
3
4 Moderate with patients arms extended
5
6
7 Severe, even with arms not extended

3. Anxiety: Ask, "Do you feel nervous or anxious?"

Observation

0 No anxiety, at ease
1 Mildly anxious
2
3
4 Moderately anxious
5
6
7 Severe equivalent to panic

4. Transient tactile auditory or visual disturbances: Ask, "Have you any itching, pins and needles sensations, or any burning or numbness, or do you feel bugs crawling on or under your skin? Are you aware of sounds around you and are they harsh? Are you hearing things that you know are not there? Does the light appear too bright? Does it hurt your eyes? Are you seeing anything that is disturbing to you?"

Observation

0 Not present
1 Present but minimal
2
3 Moderate
4 Frequent
5
6
7 Hallucinations almost continuous

(*continued*)

TABLE 8.13
(continued)

5. Agitation:

Observation

0	No tremor
1	Somewhat more than normal activity
2	
3	
4	Moderately fidgety and restless
5	
6	
7	Paces back and forth during most of the interview, or constantly thrashes about

6. Nausea or vomiting: Ask, "Do you feel sick to your stomach or have you vomited?" Include recorded vomiting since last observation

Observation

0	Not present
1	Very mild
2	
3	
4	Moderate
5	
6	
7	Severe

7. Headache: Ask, "Does your head feel full? Does it feel like there is a band around your head? Do not rate for lightheadedness; otherwise rate severity.

Observation

0	Not present
1	Very mild
2	
3	
4	Moderate
5	
6	
7	Severe

Modified from Shaw JM, Kolesar GS, Seller EM, et al. Development of optimal treatment tactics for alcohol withdrawal. *J Clin Psychopharmacol.* 1981;1:383–387.

often do not tolerate the hypotensive effects of this drug (Evidence Level C).

Nicotine withdrawal may become a problem for the older smoker who has been hospitalized for another problem and cannot get out of the hospital to smoke. Symptoms include irritability, difficulty concentrating, anxiety, and nausea and may contribute to other symptoms of delirium that may be from other causes. Although not studied specifically in the elderly, nicotine replacement therapies are often used in older patients with good results (Evidence Level C).

BIOMEDICAL CONDITIONS AND COMPLICATIONS

As age increases, there are significant increases in length of stay and frequency of discharge to an extended care facility following treatment for substance abuse[23] (Evidence Level B). Chronic illnesses such as hypertension, diabetes, and coronary artery disease and multiple medications complicate detoxification and treatment. Recovery programs often require a high degree of medical management for a wide variety of medical conditions.

EMOTIONAL/BEHAVIORAL CONDITIONS AND COMPLICATIONS

Suicide rates increase with age. Substance use disorders are the most common comorbid condition, after depression, associated with suicide.[24] Consequently, some patients may need to be hospitalized in a unit that can manage suicidal patients. The difference between a substance-induced mood disorder and major depression may be difficult to discern. It is easier when the patient improves with abstinence, but the decision to begin treatment for depression is difficult. Weighed against potential side effects, most experts begin antidepressive medication early in the belief that it can only help the patient with mood disturbance (Evidence Level C). Comorbid psychiatric conditions including dementia and delirium are worsened by abused substances and by medications used in withdrawal. Often, addressing the etiology of cognitive impairment must wait until months after the detoxification process, but then, improvement may continue for up to 2 years.

READINESS TO CHANGE (RESISTANCE TO TREATMENT)

Acceptance of the diagnosis of a substance dependency problem is difficult for most patients, but it may especially be so in the elderly, who may have accentuated feelings of shame about addiction. If the patient is resistant, the question of leverage comes up. Often, leverage for older patients is different from their younger counterparts. For the younger patient, the influence of job responsibilities and pressures often drive him or her to treatment. In the older patient, retirement and financial security may reduce this pressure and family pressure is often necessary. For example, a family may decide that Grandma cannot baby-sit the grandchildren until she gets treatment for her drinking problem.

RELAPSE RISK

Risk of return to substance use affects the clinician's decisions about the level of treatment. For patients with little impulse control and little insight into their problem, relapse risk may be great. Compliance with other medical regimens may provide insight to relapse potential. Patients who have a history of noncompliance have more difficulty than those who have successfully managed their medication regimens.

What type of support is available to the patients? Do they have family and friends who are available to support their recovery? Are they isolated and living alone? Are they in an environment that can support their functional abilities? Often, older patients spend more time in residential treatment programs because they do not have significant support at home. Once the dimensions have been determined, consideration can be given to the appropriate level of service. The greater the severity of dimensions, the greater the intensity of the program that may be necessary.

Program Level 0.5—Early Intervention

Program level 0.5 is the level of care that refers to the patient who may be drinking more than the recommended quantity but has not yet reached the level of a patient who meets the criteria for substance dependence. Treatment at this level consists of advice about appropriate levels of drinking using motivational interviewing techniques.

Program Level I—Outpatient Treatment

Program level I is intended for patients who have a diagnosis of substance dependence or abuse and need organized outpatient treatment. These patients are not at risk for significant withdrawal, have no or manageable comorbid conditions, and have a good support network. Generally, these services address issues such as knowledge deficits about addiction and treatment, cognitive behavioral therapies, motivational interviewing, and introduction to Alcoholics Anonymous (AA) or other appropriate 12-step recovery programs.

Program Level II—Intensive Outpatient Treatment/Partial Hospitalization

Services in program level II provide an intense experience in alcohol and drug treatment on the outpatient level. Usually meeting for several hours three or more times weekly, the focus is on comprehensive biopsychosocial assessments, with individualized treatment plans and specific treatment goals that are developed with the help of the patient. Patients who have some resistance to treatment and may have a risk of relapse may do better in this setting than in Level I programs.

Program Level III—Residential/Inpatient Treatment

Twenty-four hour live-in programs are recommended for patients at high risk of relapse, who may have failed lower-intensity treatment programs, and who need more care than can be managed in the lower-intensity programs.

Program Level IV—Medically Managed Intensive Inpatient Treatment

Program level IV treatment has physician management and may be ideal for the patient with significant comorbid states or who has a high risk of withdrawal that will require medical management. Typically, 24-hour medical, psychiatric, and nursing care are available in these settings.

TREATMENT

Although reduced alcohol intake is a reasonable goal for the patient who is drinking more than the recommended quantity of or abusing alcohol, abstinence is the only reasonable recommendation for the patient who is addicted. There is good evidence to suggest that there is a direct relationship between intensity and length of substance abuse treatment and success in abstinence[25] (Evidence Level B). The goals of addiction treatment are given in Table 8.14. Treatment programs that focus on older patients should

TABLE 8.14
GOALS OF TREATMENT

Resolving knowledge deficits about the disease of addiction
Identifying defenses
Overcoming denial
Improving skills in handling affective material
Orientating to Alcoholics Anonymous (or other 12-step programs)
Encouraging family services

have specific characteristics. There should be staff who are experienced and interested in working with older patients, and there should be adequate connections with services for older patients. Group activities should be age-specific, supportive, and less confrontational than groups created for younger patients. There focus of problem solving should be around issues such as depression, loneliness, and loss[26] (Evidence Level C).

Flexibility may be especially important in treatment programs that focus on older patients. Treatment may have to be interrupted for medical or psychiatric treatment. Most treatment programs introduce patients to 12-step recovery programs such as AA. Fellowships are essential to the success of AA and rely on identification with members, so it is important that they are age appropriate. Patients who attend aftercare programs after initial substance use treatment are more likely to maintain abstinence than those who do not (Evidence Level B). Involvement in AA has been shown to be a predictor of long-term abstinence (Evidence Level B).

Primary Care of the Patient in Recovery

Although treatment centers encourage patients to speak to their physicians about their recovery many are reluctant to do so. The lack of familiarity that many primary care doctors have with recovery reinforces that reluctance. Older patients seem to have more concern about the shame associated with their diagnosis. In the long view, however, it is likely that the primary care clinician will have more contact than other health care professionals with the patient in recovery and, consequently, would benefit from an understanding of the principles of recovery.

The most important factor in working with these patients may be a nonjudgmental, supportive relationship. The physician should convey concern, respect, and empathy by using open-ended questions and active listening. Affirmation of the patient's success will build the therapeutic relationship more effectively than giving advice.

Often, if the patient has undergone addiction treatment, an aftercare contract has been completed. These contracts are generally negotiated in treatment and spell out the tasks needed to prevent relapse. They frequently address issues such as frequency of attendance at 12-step recovery meetings, attendance in aftercare therapy groups, an agreement to begin and maintain a relationship with a sponsor, and drug screening. Generally, they also include an agreement about who is to be informed of the patient's progress and the need to name a primary care clinician who can cooperate with this process.

In a routine primary care visit, it is not reasonable to cover each of these points. But it should be possible to cover one or two in each visit, thereby covering the entire list over time.

Abstinence

The cornerstone of recovery from addiction is abstinence. Strictly interpreted, abstinence implies that the patient is consuming no mood-altering substances except under the direction of a physician. It is the recovering person's responsibility to be sure that the physician who may be prescribing a mood-altering substance knows that the patient is in recovery and has some understanding of the disease of addiction and recovery. This concern should include over-the-counter medications and dietary supplements, which may have the potential to result in relapse.

The patient should be cautioned to avoid medications that may affect mood or contain alcohol, or those for which the effect may be unknown. The willingness with which patients turn the decisions about medication to negotiations with their physicians can be a good indicator of the sustainability of their recovery. Maintaining abstinence, as well as preventing relapse, is the primary daily task of a patient in recovery. The primary care clinician can help by monitoring the process. A straightforward question such as "Have you had any mood-altering substances, either prescribed or otherwise, since our last visit?" is appropriate.

Some aftercare contracts call for random urine drug screens. For some patients this is a critical tool. The primary care clinician should negotiate an agreement with the patient that allows the physician to ask for a drug screen, should the question arise.

Meeting Attendance

The usual recommendation is that the patient attends at least 90 meetings in the first 90 days of recovery (Evidence Level C). The patient's sponsor should be involved in the negotiation to step down the frequency after the first 90 days. An elderly patient's health and ability to travel should play a role in these decisions.

Involvement in the fellowship of meetings has been shown to be important and should be assessed. Are the patients forming new relationships in the meetings? Are they getting involved in the setting up or breaking down process of the meeting? Are they doing service work, such as making coffee, helping other recovering persons, chairing meetings?

Some patients have difficulty connecting in 12-step recovery groups. They may complain of religious issues associated with many recovery groups. These are often spiritual in nature but most are not religious. Encourage the patient to try different groups to find one that is acceptable. Often, contacting someone in AA who has a similar occupation or background can increase the patient's comfort.

Sponsor Contact

Serious involvement in a 12-step recovery program requires a sponsor. Patients are encouraged to find someone of the same sex who has qualities they respect to ask to sponsor them. Often sponsorships begin as temporary relationships but evolve into permanent relationships. Frequent contact with one's sponsor is encouraged but is negotiated between the sponsor and the patient. Although some sponsors prefer to remain anonymous with regard to a patient's primary care clinician, many are willing to work closely with the doctor to maximize the patient's chances to avoid relapse. A vague or hesitant answer to the question "What step are you and your sponsor working on?" is a red flag that should prompt further inquiry.

Emotional Symptoms

Patients in early recovery often deal with newly emerged or rediscovered emotions. Fear, anger, guilt, and depression are all emotional traps that can lead to relapse if not handled constructively. Individual or group psychotherapy can be intense, particularly for patients with comorbid psychiatric diagnoses. Twelve-step recovery programs use the acronym HALT to remind patients in early recovery to avoid getting too Hungry, Angry, Lonely, or Tired, lest they relapse.

Physical Health

Patients with addiction often neglect their physical health and their health surveillance may be delayed. Patients in successful recovery are likely to be vigilant about medication compliance and keeping appointments and will demonstrate appropriate concern about their physical health. Ignoring their health may be a sign of relapse.

Exercise

Patients in active addiction seldom maintain an adequate exercise program. On the other hand, patients in recovery may become compulsive about exercise as a replacement for their drug use. Exercise is to be encouraged. In reasonable amounts, it improves overall health and replaces the time formerly spent drinking or using drugs. It can be a cornerstone of a patient's recovery.

Leisure Activities

Drinking and drug use consume the patients' time. In recovery, they may discover that they have forgotten how to have fun while sober. Encouraging patients to engage in social activities through their 12-step recovery group is one way to promote healthy leisure activity. Patients should be cautioned about leisure activities around people who are using or abusing alcohol or other drugs early in recovery. The temptation of access to drugs or alcohol can overwhelm a weak moment.

Compulsive Behavior

The transfer of compulsive behavior from drugs to other behaviors is common during early recovery. Compulsive eating, purging, exercise, work, gambling, and sex should be addressed as a continuum of the addictive personality. They often lead to relapse.

Legal Issues

Legal consequences complicate many recovery experiences. The patient should seek professional assistance from attorneys knowledgeable about the consequences of addictions.

Family and Relationship Issues

Addictions impact and often destroy relationships. Recovery is not an automatic cure and conflict is inevitable. Virtually all families should enter family therapy and consider joining partnership programs such as Al-Anon.

Spiritual Support

Understanding that the heart of the 12-step recovery program is spiritual, the physician should encourage the patient to continue to pursue spiritual growth. Recognition that this is not the same as pursuit of religion may be important to some patients.

COMMON MEDICAL PROBLEMS IN RECOVERY

As many as 20% of primary care office visits have some form of substance abuse associated with them. The number of patients who are in recovery from addictive disorders is unknown. Physicians are often faced with problematic medical complaints from patients who are in various stages of recovery.

Sleep Disorders

Insomnia is common, especially early in recovery, and may be a symptom of withdrawal, especially from opiates or sedative–hypnotics. Reassurance that a normal sleep pattern will return is often the only intervention necessary. Unfortunately, this can be a slow process and may take months to resolve. Sleep hygiene education is often useful. Avoiding hypnotics, especially benzodiazepines, barbiturates, and zolpidem, is appropriate. Tricyclic antidepressants are probably safe but are also best avoided unless depression is present.

Pain

The appropriate treatment of pain is an important part of caring for the individual in recovery. Inadequate treatment of pain has proved to be as risk laden as overprescribing in terms of relapse. Pain tolerance in recovering addicts may be reduced, and tolerance to analgesics may be increased, even after recovery. Offering acetaminophen and nonsteroidal anti-inflammatory agents is appropriate. If these are ineffective, short-term use of narcotic analgesics is appropriate. They should be dose adjusted to relieve pain and followed by a detox plan if necessary. The recovering addict may become physically dependent quicker than other patients.

Safe use of these agents may be improved by engaging the sponsor or spouse to provide accountability, monitoring adherence to the prescribed dosing schedule, and paying attention to other areas of recovery.

Long-term opiate use has been shown to be safe for the treatment of chronic benign pain in nonaddicted individuals. No similar evidence exists for those in recovery. Therefore, avoidance of controlled substances in patients recovering from addiction is good policy. Referral to a pain management specialist who understands addiction is an alternative.

Anxiety Disorders

Anxiety is common in early recovery and often a symptom of withdrawal. Avoidance of controlled substances (including clonazepam) is important. Behavioral approaches, buspirone, β-blockers, and selective serotonin reuptake inhibitors may be helpful and safe.

Depression

Depressive symptoms may have been present before abuse and, during recovery, may be induced by substance withdrawal. The latter condition will resolve with abstinence. Comorbid depression negatively affects recovery and should be treated. Antidepressants appear to be safe in recovery, but psychotherapy is equally effective.

Over-the-Counter and Prescription Medication Use

Any mood-altering substance has the potential to contribute to relapse. Patients need to know this and be encouraged to ask for the physician's guidance before using any medication. Self-prescribing should be discouraged. It is advisable to have an agreement with the patient that you will be apprised of any medications or supplements he or she is taking. Some addictive substances are currently not controlled. The physician should be aware of all components of medications prescribed. Headache preparations may contain butabarbital or butorphanol. Even tramadol, although not controlled, has been associated with relapse.

REFERENCES

1. Blow FC. Special issues in treatment: Older adults. In: Graham AW, Schultz TK, Mayo-Smith MF, eds. *Principles of addiction medicine*, 3rd ed. Chevy Chase, MD: American Society of Addiction Medicine; 2003:581–607.
2. Gambert SR, Katsoyannis KK. Alcohol-related medical disorders of older heavy drinkers. In: Beresford TP, Gomberg E, eds. *Alcohol and aging*. New York, NY: Oxford University Press; 1995:70–81.
3. National Institute on Alcohol Abuse and Alcoholism (NIAAA). *The physician's guide to helping patients with alcohol problems*. Rockville, MD: National Institutes of Health; 1995.
4. Reid MC, Anderson PA. Geriatric substance abuse. *Med Clin North Am*. 1997;81:999–1016.
5. D'Archangelo E. Substance abuse in later life. *Can Fam Physician*. 1993;39:1986–1993.
6. Adams WL. Potential for adverse drug-alcohol interactions among retirement community residents. *J Am Geriatr Soc*. 1995;43:1021.
7. Sheahan SL, Coons SJ, Robins CA. et al. Psychoactive medication, alcohol use and falls among older adults. *J Behav Med*. 1995; 18:127.
8. Adams W. Alcohol and substance abuse. In: Duthie EH, Katz PR, eds. *Practice of geriatrics*. Philadelphia, PA: WB Saunders; 1998:307–316.
9. Gunzerath L, Faden V, Zakhari S, et al. National Institute on Alcohol Abuse and Alcoholism report on moderate drinking. *Alcoholism: Clin Exper Res*. 2004;28:829–847.
10. Sattar SP, Petty F, Burke WJ. Diagnosis and treatment of alcohol dependence in older alcoholics. *Clin Geriatr Med*. 2003;19: 743–761.
11. Blow FC, ed. *Substance abuse among older adults (Treatment Improvement Protocol No. 26)*. Rockville, MD: Center for Substance Abuse Treatment; 1998.
12. Atkinson RM, Turner JA, Kofoed LL, et al. Early vs late onset alcoholism in older persons: Preliminary findings. *Alcohol Clin Exp Res*. 1985;9:513–515.
13. Solomon K, Manepallli J, Ireland GA, et al. Alcoholism and prescription drug abuse in the elderly. *J Am Geriatr Soc*. 1993;41: 57–69.
14. Kirby M, Denihan A, Bruce I, et al. Benzodiazepine use among the elderly in the community. *Int J Geriatr Psychiatry*. 1999;14: 280–284.
15. Petrovic M, Pevernagie D, Mariman A, et al. Fast withdrawal from benzodiazepines in geriatric inpatients: A randomized double-blind, placebo-controlled trial. *Eur J Clin Pharmacol*. 2002;57: 759–764.
16. Hinkin CH, Castellon SA, Dickson-Furhrman E, et al. Screening for drug and alcohol abuse among older adults using a modified version of the CAGE. *Am J Addict*. 2001;10:319–319.
17. Blow FC, Gillespe BW, Barry KL, et al. Brief screening for alcohol populations in elderly populations using the Short Michigan Alcohol Screening Test- Geriatric Version (SMAST-G). *Alcohol Clin Exp Res*. 1998;22:31A.
18. Sattar SP, Petty F, Burke WJ. Diagnosis and treatment of alcohol dependence in older adults. *Clin Geriatr Med*. 2003;19(4):763–776.
19. Blow FC, Barry KL. Older patients with at-risk and problem drinking patterns: New developments in brief interventions. *J Geriatr Psychiatry Neurol*. 2000;13(3):115–123.
20. Johnson V. *I'll quit tomorrow*. New York, NY: Harper& Row; 1980.
21. Mee-Lee D, Shulman MA. ASAM placement criteria and matching patients to treatment. In: Graham AW, Schultz TK, Mayo-Smith MF, eds. *Principles of addiction medicine*, 3rd ed. Chevy Chase, MD: American Society of Addiction Medicine; 2003:453–465.
22. Brower KJ, Mudd S, Blow FC, et al. Severity and treatment of alcohol withdrawal in elderly versus younger patients. *Alcohol Clin Exp Res*. 1994;18(1):196–201.
23. Peppers MP. Benzodiazepines for alcohol withdrawal in the elderly and patients with liver disease. *Pharmacotherapy*. 1996;16(1): 49–57.

24. Kraemer KL, Mayo-Smith MF, Calkins DR. Impact of age on the severity, course, and complications of alcohol withdrawal. *Arch Intern Med.* 1997;157(19):2234–2241.
25. Finney JW, Moos EH. Effects of setting, duration and amount on treatment outcomes. In: Graham AW, Schultz TK, Mayo-Smith MF, eds. *Principles of addiction medicine,* 3rd ed. Chevy Chase, MD: American Society of Addiction Medicine; 2003:443–451.
26. Schonfield L, Dupree LW. Treatment approaches for older problem drinkers. *Int J Addict.* 1995;30:1819–1842.

9

Elder Abuse: "It Shouldn't Hurt To Be Old"*

Patricia A. Bomba

CLINICAL PEARLS 96

DEFINITIONS 96

PUBLIC HEALTH ISSUES 96
Incidence and Prevalence 96
Mortality Rates 97
Elder Abuse as a Geriatric Syndrome 97

WHEN TO SUSPECT ELDER ABUSE AND NEGLECT 98
Vulnerability 98
Risk Factors 98
"Red Flags" 99
Family Situations 99
Caregiver Issues 99
Cultural Issues 99

TYPES OF ABUSE 99
Physical Abuse 99
Psychological Abuse 100
Sexual Abuse 100
Domestic Violence of Late Life 100

TYPES OF NEGLECT 100
Abandonment 100
Self-Neglect 101

FINANCIAL EXPLOITATION 101

SCREENING FOR ABUSE 101
National Clinical Guidelines Recommendation Statement 101
Academic Geriatric Experts Recommendation 102
Practical Clinician Tool 102

CLINICAL ASSESSMENT 102
Setting 102
History 102
Physical Examination 102
Assessing Mental Capacity 104
Capacity versus Competence 105
Laboratory 105

MANAGEMENT 105
Principles 105
Recommendation 106
Reporting 106

DOCUMENTATION 106

SUMMARY 106

*MedAmerica is a leading long-term care insurer committed to raising awareness of elder abuse. "It Shouldn't Hurt To Be Old" is the title of an awareness campaign developed by Lifespan to publicize the hidden problem of elder abuse. Lifespan began an Elder Abuse Prevention service in 1987. MedAmerica is a partner in Lifespan's Elder Abuse Consortium.

CLINICAL PEARLS

- Elder abuse is a hidden public health issue.
- Elder abuse results in increased mortality rates and unnecessary suffering, injury pain, decreased quality of life, and loss or violation of human rights.
- Elder abuse is under-recognized, underreported, and underprosecuted.
- Financial exploitation is common and often associated with other types of abuse.
- Neglect is the most prevalent form of elder abuse.
- Any vulnerable older adult is at risk of mistreatment.
- Perpetrators are family members in most cases.
- Self-report cannot be relied upon to identify cases.
- Self-report may be compromised by cognitive impairment, fear, family situations, caregiver, and cultural issues.
- Elder abuse may be missed by failure to consider the diagnosis.
- The ethical challenge is to balance our professional duty to protect the safety of the vulnerable elder with the elder's right to self-determination.
- Reporting elder abuse to protective services is mandatory in most but not all states.

Elder abuse (also known as *elder mistreatment*) refers to intentional actions by a caregiver or other person who stands in a trusting relationship to the elder, which cause harm (whether or not harm was intended) or create a serious risk of harm to a vulnerable elder. The concept also includes failure by a caregiver to satisfy the elder's basic needs or protect the elder from harm. Elder abuse is a growing problem in every community and among all social strata and is under-recognized, underreported, and underprosecuted. It is an independent risk factor of increased mortality rates in older adults.[1] Elder abuse includes acts of commission and omission and involves medical, psychological, social, legal, ethical, financial, and environmental concerns.

Health care professionals are in a pivotal position to identify and intervene on behalf of their victimized patients. To do so, all health care professionals must maintain a high index of suspicion for elder abuse, neglect, and financial exploitation in all health care settings. This implies a commitment to screenings of all elders and an understanding of how to perform more detailed diagnostic assessments when needed. All members of the health care team, especially physicians, nurses, and social workers, must know when to refer patients for additional assessment and when and how to use community resources effectively. The ethical challenge for the physicians is to balance their professional duty to protect the safety of vulnerable elders with the elder's right to self-determination.

DEFINITIONS

Elder abuse is an all-inclusive term representing all types of mistreatment or abusive behavior toward older adults. These may be acts of commission or omission, or neglect. They may be intentional or unintentional. Whether a behavior can be labeled as abusive, neglectful, or exploitive depends on its frequency, duration, intensity, severity, consequences, and cultural context. In discussions with older adults, the term *elder mistreatment* may be preferred. It is also recognized that victims of domestic violence grow old.

Definitions and legal terminology vary from state to state. Experts recognize elder abuse as the willful infliction of injury, unreasonable confinement, intimidation, or cruel punishment with resulting physical harm, anguish, or mental illness. As defined by the National Center on Elder Abuse,[2] physical abuse is the use of physical force that results in injury, physical pain, or impairment. Sexual abuse is defined as nonconsensual sexual contact of any kind with an elderly person. Psychological abuse is defined as the infliction of anguish, pain, or distress through verbal or nonverbal acts. Neglect, the most prevalent form of elder abuse, is defined as the refusal or failure to fulfill any part of a person's obligations or duties to an elder, including the provision of goods or services, which are necessary to avoid physical harm, mental anguish, or mental illness. Abandonment is defined as the desertion of an elderly person by an individual who has assumed responsibility for providing care for an elder or by a person who has physical custody of an elder. Financial exploitation is the illegal or improper use of an elder's funds, properties, or assets. It is the fastest growing form and is frequently linked with other types of abuse.

PUBLIC HEALTH ISSUES

Incidence and Prevalence

In the preceding decade, five community surveys showed that 5% of older adults report experiencing instances of domestic elder abuse, neglect, and financial exploitation. The lack of consistency in terminology used among the 50 states and variation in reporting standards contribute to inadequate incidence and prevalence data. To obtain more valid incidence data, the Congress mandated a national study in 1996. A "sentinel" approach was employed, similar to previous federally sponsored child abuse surveys. This methodology assumes that reported cases present only the proverbial "tip of the iceberg" and that many more cases in the community are never reported. Through a random sampling process, 20 counties were selected to serve as the sample sites. In each county, information on the cases was obtained from the local Adult Protective Services agency and a specifically trained group of individuals, or the sentinels, who were drawn from agencies that normally serve older people, such as hospitals, clinics, law enforcement agencies, senior citizens programs, and banking institutions. The results of the National Elder Abuse Incidence Study[3] estimated that nearly a half a million persons aged

60 and older living in domestic settings were abused, neglected, or exploited in the United States in 1996. Of this total, only 70,942 cases were reported and substantiated by Adult Protective Services. The remainder were not reported but were identified by the "sentinels." In other words, for every case reported to the Adult Protective Services, it is assumed that there were five cases that were not reported. Further projecting the estimates—recognizing those that were never reported nor recognized—it was estimated that there were between 820,000 and 1.86 million abused older people in the country.

As a point of comparison, the 1996 US Cancer Statistics for older adults reveals 133,000 cases of colon cancer per year, 66,000 cases of cervical cancer per year, and 185,000 cases of breast cancer per year. The incidence of elder abuse and neglect cases increased by 128% between 1986 and 1996. The National Center for the Prevention of Elder Abuse estimates a 60% increase since 1996.[4] The most frequently cited prevalence figure is 32 seniors per 1,000.

Mortality Rates

Elder abuse results in increased mortality rates.[1] Dr. Mark Lachs evaluated data from the New England Established Population for Epidemiological Studies of the Elderly, which followed an annual health survey of 2,812 community-dwelling adults aged 65 or older. He compared these data against reports of elder abuse and neglect made to the local Adult Protective Service over a 9-year period. The survival rates of the nonabused and abused were tracked. By the 13th year following the initiation of the study, 40% of the nonabused group was still alive, compared to 17% of those seen for self-neglect. Only 9% of those seen for elder mistreatment were still living. No other significant factors predictive of mortality were found, including age, gender, income, functional status, cognitive status, diagnosis, and social support.

Elder Abuse as a Geriatric Syndrome

Over the last two decades, studies have documented physicians' failure to diagnose a variety of common conditions in elderly people in the course of "usual and customary care." Examples include dementia, depression, and general functional decline. Geriatricians have conceptualized these entities as "geriatric syndromes," or common clinical problems that rarely have a single, underlying, pathophysiologic process, which is typically sought in the pure medical model. More often, there are several contributing factors that shape the clinical presentation. Typically, environmental factors play a prominent role. Interventions are multiple and directed at specific pathology, as well as contributing environmental factors. Elder abuse has many of the characteristics of a geriatric syndrome.

Framing elder abuse as a geriatric syndrome provides a conceptual starting point from which the physician and health care professional can begin to address mistreatment, from screening to management. Definitive diagnosis and management requires a comprehensive evaluation of all potentially contributing factors. The relative contribution of comorbid medical conditions, environmental factors, and social influences must be determined before rational interventions are developed.

From the perspective of physicians, Dr. Mark Lachs identified three major causes generic to the problem of family violence: Clinical and academic discomfort, time and reimbursement constraints, and perceived impotence.[5] Many physicians feel uncomfortable inquiring about domestic violence and may feel clinically incompetent because they lack formal training. Family violence does not fit neatly within the traditional medical paradigm of symptoms, diagnosis, and treatment. Personal identification with patients may preclude the proper evaluation of family violence.

From an academic perspective, additional research focused on elder abuse and neglect is urgently needed. Time and reimbursement constraints hinder evaluation of elder abuse, which is a time-consuming process. A complete assessment may not be practical, particularly if discovery occurs in the midst of a routine evaluation. Scheduling a longer follow-up visit or referral is essential. Awareness of available community resources provides professionals with an important timesaving advantage.

Unfortunately, many physicians perceive that they are unable to make a difference. Some express the belief that it was the duty of the victims to separate from an abusive environment and that they doubted that counseling would achieve a positive outcome. Some physicians express unsatisfactory outcomes with previous patients, which created skepticism that they could serve any useful role. This attitude views the problem as a social issue and, therefore, places it outside their professional boundaries. Signs and symptoms of elder abuse may be dismissed as inevitable aspects of aging or ascribed to comorbid diseases (see Table 9.1).

Fractures can be attributed to osteoporosis. Direct reports of abuse may be dismissed as manifestations of dementia, delirium, delusion, or confusion, or even side

TABLE 9.1
SIGNS AND SYMPTOMS OF ELDER ABUSE VERSUS ASPECTS OF AGING OR COMORBID DISEASE

Abuse	Normal Aging
Lacerations	Skin tears
Multiple bruises	Coagulopathy on excess warfarin (Coumadin)
Multiple fractures	Osteoporosis
Depressed mood	Depression
Reports abuse	Dementia
Confusion, head trauma	Alcoholism, metastatic illness

effects of polypharmacy. Depression and pain may be underreported by the patient and therefore unrecognized and untreated by the physician. Because chronic pain can lead to depression, social isolation, and neglect, early identification is critical.

Failure to thrive is often blamed on general frailty, when in fact it can be the result of the deliberate withholding of food or medicines by a care provider. Unless clinicians consider elder abuse in the differential diagnosis of these presentations, these "false-negatives" will continue.

WHEN TO SUSPECT ELDER ABUSE AND NEGLECT

CASE ONE

Mrs. S., who is 75 years old and suffers from moderate dementia, is accompanied to her doctor's visit by her husband of 50 years. Mrs. S. has been a patient for only about 1 year, and the reason for the change of physicians is never broached. Mr. S. explains that her dementia causes her to give inaccurate answers to most health questions. Often during the examination, when he speaks for Mrs. S., she gets "weepy" and this causes him to tell her to stop crying and answer the questions asked of her.

Although the doctor has suggested assistance at home, Mr. S. "forgets" to follow up or refuses nursing visits at home when a nurse arrives. Mr. S. feels he can take care of his wife alone and that she is "fooling" the doctor about her memory loss.

Relevant issues:

- Why did they leave their previous doctor?
- Have they had multiple doctors over the last few years (i.e., "doctor hopping")?
- Do the medical professionals allow Mr. S. to speak for his wife? Do they believe that because she is demented, nothing she says is accurate? Why is she never alone?
- Why does she get "weepy" when her husband intervenes? Is there a pattern?
- Are Mr. S.'s opinion about his wife's dementia and his resistance to outside services "red flags" for possible abuse or neglect?

Vulnerability

Although there is no single explanation for elder abuse and neglect, one central element is vulnerability—any condition that allows another person to take advantage of the victim. It is not the same as being cognitively impaired, although cognitive impairment can certainly lead to vulnerability. There are multiple ways in which a person can be vulnerable, including being seriously medically ill, physically or emotionally dependent, lonely, depressed, or grieving. Fear, early life experiences, substance use, and personality traits also contribute to vulnerability.

Risk Factors

The National Elder Abuse Incidence Study[3] published in 1998 found that the median age of the victims was 76.5 years and that elders aged 80 years and older were abused two to three times more often than younger people. Half of the abused individuals were physically dependent on others. Women were abused more often than men, even after accounting for their proportion in the aging population. The perpetrators were family members (often with a history of substance abuse) in 90% of the cases. The remaining 10% were caregivers, companions, "scam artists," and others. The study found that the most frequent reporters of elder abuse to Adult Protective Services were family members; hospitals were responsible for 17.3% of such reports, whereas physicians, nurses, and clinics in the community reported only approximately 8% to 10% of cases. Individuals having more contact with "social systems," such as Medicaid clients, were more frequently reported as victims (see Table 9.2A, B).

High-risk factors for abuse include poor health, cognitive and functional impairment in the elder, substance abuse or mental illness on the part of the elder or abuser, dependence of the abuser on the victim, shared living arrangements, social isolation, external factors causing stress, and a history of domestic violence. A number of recent studies have demonstrated that medical disease plays a greater role in abuse than previously recognized.[6] Independent risk factors for elder mistreatment include dementia, depression, and malnutrition. Other common associated clinical diagnoses include alcohol abuse, psychosis, and executive dysfunction. A recent study examined the prevalence and 3-year incidence of abuse among postmenopausal women and found that they were exposed to abuse at similar rates

TABLE 9.2
RISK FACTORS FOR VICTIMS AND PERPETRATORS

A. Victim Risk Factors
Poor health
Cognitive or functional impairment
Substance abuse or mental health illness in the elder
Substance abuse or mental health illness in the abuser
Dependence of the elder on the abuser
Shared living arrangements
Social isolation
External factors causing stress
History of domestic violence

B. Perpetrator Risk Factors
Psychiatric disorders
Dependence of abuser on victim
External stressors
Caregiver burnout
Lack of experience/education
Substance abuse or mental health illness in the abuser

TABLE 9.3
MOST COMMON DIAGNOSES ASSOCIATED WITH ELDER ABUSE

Dementia and other cognitive disorders
Depression
Alcohol and substance abuse
Mental health disorders, including psychosis
Executive dysfunction
Malnutrition, dehydration, and starvation
Pressure sores
Falls and fractures

to younger women. The study concluded that abuse poses a serious threat to their health (see Table 9.3).[7]

"Red Flags"

Elder mistreatment must be considered whenever:

1. there are unreasonable delays in seeking medical attention between the injury or illness and the clinical assessment;
2. the history from the victim and the perpetrator significantly differs or when explanations are implausible or vague;
3. lab test or x-ray results are suggestive of abuse or inconsistent with the history and physical examination;
4. there are frequent emergency room visits for exacerbation of chronic disease despite a comprehensive plan for medical care and adequate resources, particularly if different facilities are used;
5. patients practice "doctor hopping" (frequent changes in clinicians); or
6. a functionally impaired or cognitively impaired patient presents for follow-up without a caregiver.

Family Situations

Excess family stress can trigger elder abuse. Discord in the family, a history and pattern of violent interactions within the family, social isolation or the stresses on one or more family members who care for the older adult, and lack of knowledge or caregiving skills can all contribute to elder mistreatment. The financial burdens of health care for an aging parent or living in overcrowded quarters can trigger elder abuse. These situations can be especially difficult when the adult child has no financial resources other than those of the aging parent.

Social isolation can also signal that a family may be in trouble and at risk for abuse. The isolation can be a strategy for keeping abuse a secret or may be a result of the stress of caring for a dependent older family member. Isolation cuts off family members from outside help and support and also makes it harder for outsiders to see and intervene in volatile or abusive situations.

Caregiver Issues

Caregiver stress is a significant risk factor for abuse but does not cause or is not a cause of elder abuse. Caregivers frequently experience intense frustration and anger. This can lead to a range of abusive behaviors when they are thrust into a demanding daily routine without appropriate training and information about how to balance the needs of the older person with their own. The risk of elder abuse is even greater when an older person is seriously ill or physically or cognitively impaired. In such stressful situations, caregivers often feel trapped or hopeless and are unaware of available resources and assistance.

In addition to stress, other factors that can lead to abuse in a frail older person include mental or emotional illness, addiction to alcohol or other drugs, job loss or other personal crises, financial dependency on the older person, and a tendency to use violence to solve problems. Sometimes, the older adult may be physically abusive to the caregiver, especially when the older person has psychiatric illness or cognitive impairment.

The problem may be compounded by a caregiver's perception of duty to his or her parent. This feeling can cause the caregiver to think that the older person deserves and wants only his or her care and that respite or residential care is a betrayal of the older person's trust.

Dependency is another contributing factor in elder abuse. When the caregiver is financially dependent on an impaired older person, there may be financial exploitation. When the reverse is true, the caregiver may experience resentment that leads to abusive behavior.

Cultural Issues

Certain societal attitudes make it easier for abuse to continue without detection or intervention. A familiar example is society's belief that what goes on in the home is a private "family matter." Shame and embarrassment often make it difficult for older persons to reveal abuse. There is also variation across diverse cultural and ethnic communities of what is considered "abuse." Research demonstrates that reports of abuse in some ethnic groups are four times higher than in others.[8]

Religious or ethical belief systems sometimes allow for mistreatment of family members, especially women. Those who participate in these behaviors do not consider them abusive. In some cultures, women's basic rights are not honored, and older women in these cultures may not realize they are being abused.

TYPES OF ABUSE

Physical Abuse

Bruises, welts, cuts, wounds, and cigarette, rope, and burn marks easily raise suspicion, particularly if they are present

TABLE 9.4
WHEN TO SUSPECT PHYSICAL OR PSYCHOLOGICAL ABUSE

A. When to Suspect Physical Abuse

Bruises, welts, cuts, wounds
Cigarette, rope, or burn marks
Blood on the person or clothing
Injuries, including fractures and sprains
Painful body movements, unrelated to illness

B. When to Suspect Psychological Abuse

Sense of resignation or hopelessness
Passive, helpless, withdrawn behavior
Fearful, tearful, anxious, clinging behavior
Self-blame for life situation or caregiver behavior

at multiple sites, are bilateral or shaped like objects (such as a belt or fingers). Injuries including fractures, strains, and dislocations, particularly those involving the upper body or untreated injuries in various stages of healing must signal concern to the health care professional. Painful body movements unrelated to illness, and a change in demeanor or activity level should also raise suspicion (see Table 9.4A).

Psychological Abuse

Psychological abuse results from verbal assaults, insults, threats, intimidation, humiliation, or harassment. It can also result from intentionally isolating or ignoring an elder person, failing to provide companionship, making unannounced changes in routine, or failing to provide important information. One should suspect this type of abuse when an older person exhibits a sense of resignation or hopelessness, as well as passive, helpless, withdrawn behavior, or when the patient appears fearful, tearful, anxious, or clinging (Table 9.4B).

Sexual Abuse

Discussing sexual issues openly is difficult for many elderly women because they were raised in a time when the topic was taboo. Becoming a victim of sexual abuse represents the worst form of lost dignity, and sexual abuse is a criminal act. Victims may feel profound shame or embarrassment that family, friends, or the community will discover the abuse and that they will be shunned. Blood on the person or torn, stained, or bloody underclothing may be a manifestation of sexual abuse. Other potential manifestations include bruises around the breasts, genitals, or inner thighs; unexplained venereal disease or genital infections; vaginal bleeding or unexplained anal bleeding; and difficulty in walking or sitting without evidence of musculoskeletal disease.

Domestic Violence of Late Life

Intergenerational and marital violence can persist into old age and become factors in elder abuse. In some instances, elder abuse is simply a continuation of abuse that has been occurring in the family over decades. If a woman has been abused during a 50-year marriage, she is not likely to report abuse when she is very old and in poor health.

Sometimes, a woman who has been abused for years may turn her rage on her husband when his health fails. If there has been a history of violence in the family, an adult child may "turn the tables" on the abusing parent by withholding nourishment or overmedicating the parent.

TYPES OF NEGLECT

CASE TWO

Mr. J. is a 68-year-old widower with a long history of alcohol abuse who has lived alone for almost 10 years. He had worked as an upper-level manager in a major company for 30 years and took an early retirement. He was released from the hospital following a recent stroke. The only relative to agree to live with him is a daughter who has a history of "issues" with her father. His daughter obtains his power of attorney before he is discharged. All believe that this will allow bills to be paid for utilities, food, aide service, and so on, and will limit the amount spent on alcohol.

After three office visits are cancelled and rescheduled, Mr. J. is seen by his physician. He is unshaven, has very poor hygiene, and is wearing old, soiled clothes. When asked about the aide service, he explains it stopped when Medicare quit paying. He also relates that his daughter told him there is not enough money coming in each month for more help and that the additional cost of a new minivan to help transport him allows little money for anything else.

Relevant issues:

- Despite a high probability that the household income is more than adequate to meet existing needs, why is Mr. J. in such poor shape?
- Is a new minivan the best way to transport Mr. J. or is it for other uses? Who owns it?
- Despite obvious need, why is there no aide service in the home—what can the doctor do to "push" the issue?

Abandonment

Not honoring the wishes of an older adult who lacks capacity is a form of abandonment. Family and friends may fail to recognize the lack of capacity and ignore, neglect, or abandon the patient. Lack of capacity may lead one to live in squalor; a change in the quality of the living situation can be a clue to incapacitation.

TABLE 9.5
WHEN TO SUSPECT NEGLECT

Pressure sores
Unclean appearance
Inadequate food or meal preparation
Underweight, frail, dehydrated appearance
Inappropriate use of medications
Inadequate utilities
Unsafe or unclean environment
Neglected household finances

Self-Neglect

Neglect is the most prevalent form of elder abuse. Self-neglect is failure to live safely in one's own environment. Because of the implied value judgments in evaluating living circumstances, it is difficult to assess this as a form of elder mistreatment. Some elders may not recognize how detrimental their actions are and how vulnerable the living setting is. Elders living in the community who experience clinically significant psychiatric or depressive symptoms and/or cognitive impairment are at risk for the development of self-neglect and may be candidates for interventions.[9]

Self-neglect occurs when adults are not willing or able to perform essential self-care tasks such as obtaining food, clothing, adequate shelter, adequate medical care, goods, and services necessary to maintain personal hygiene and general safety, and managing financial affairs. Poor overall self-care, such as poor personal hygiene, is a major indication of self-neglect. Inadequate food or meal preparation may result in weight loss, malnutrition, or pressure sores. Manifestations of self-neglect also include unattended or untreated health problems or failure to provide necessary prosthetic devices, dentures, glasses, hearing aids, or durable medical equipment. Inadequate utilities (e.g., improper wiring, no heat, and no running water) suggest hazardous or unsafe living conditions. Unsanitary living conditions (e.g., dirt, fleas, and lice on the person; soiled bedding; fecal/urine smell; and inadequate clothing) can represent a public health hazard. Neglected household finances can add to the problem (see Table 9.5).

FINANCIAL EXPLOITATION

Financial exploitation is the fastest growing form of abuse and is frequently linked with other types of abuse. With this type of mistreatment, a trusted individual (new or old) takes advantage of the vulnerability of an older adult, either by design or by accident. Typically, three elements are present in financial abuse: a vulnerable older adult, a trusted individual who takes advantage of the vulnerability of the older adult, and control over the older person that results in a change in assets. Manifestation of control includes intimidation, threats, coercion, abuse, persuasion, or isolation. Safeguards include an independent evaluation of the older adult before any change of assets, a fair exchange of assets, and written legal agreements between the parties.

Seniors are susceptible to overpayment for goods and services or unnecessary services from con artists who prey on vulnerable people. Financial exploitation must be considered if there is an abrupt or unexplained change in power of attorney, wills, or other legal or financial documents. It must be suspected if an elder's signature is found on unusual financial transactions or for titles to the elder's possessions. Missing checks or money or credit card bills from clothing or electronic equipment suppliers are all potential signs of financial abuse. An unexplained decrease in the elder's bank account should raise a red flag. Missing belongings, particularly the unexplained disappearance of valuable possessions, obviously raise concerns (see Table 9.6).

TABLE 9.6
WHEN TO SUSPECT FINANCIAL EXPLOITATION

Overpayment for goods and services
Unexplained change in POA, wills, and legal documents
Missing checks or money
Unexplained decrease in bank account
Missing belongings

POA, power of attorney.

SCREENING FOR ABUSE

Health care professionals must be aware of elder mistreatment and consider the possibility of abuse in any patient with unusual clinical findings or in vulnerable circumstances. Presently, there is no standardized approach to screening (see Table 9.7).

National Clinical Guidelines Recommendation Statement

The U.S. Preventive Services Task Force (USPSTF) found insufficient evidence to recommend for or against routine screening of older adults or their caregivers for elder abuse.[10,11] The USPSTF found no existing studies that determine the accuracy of screening tools for identifying violence among older adults in the general population and no studies that examined the effectiveness of interventions in older adults. Lack of such evidence requires an "I" rating (insufficient evidence to recommend for or against) for elder abuse screening. The evidence for the effectiveness of case-finding tools was not reviewed. The recommendation statement advised all clinicians to be alert to the physical and behavioral signs and symptoms associated with abuse and neglect. Patients in whom abuse is suspected should receive proper documentation, treatment, and referral to appropriate resources, as well as suitable follow-up.

TABLE 9.7
WHEN TO SUSPECT ELDER MISTREATMENT

Delays between injury or illness and assessment
History from victim and perpetrator differs
Implausible or vague explanations
Frequent ED visits for illness despite plan of care and adequate resources
Functionally impaired patient presents without caregiver
Cognitively impaired patient presents without caregiver
Lab or x-ray results inconsistent with history
"Doctor hopping"

ED, emergency department.

The American College of Obstetricians and Gynecologists and American Medical Association recommend that physicians routinely ask elderly patients direct, specific questions about abuse.[12]

Academic Geriatric Experts Recommendation

A recent review of elder abuse screening and assessment instruments concluded that there is much to be done to achieve consensus on what constitutes appropriate screenings.[13] Asking routine screening questions as part of a geriatric assessment does more than simply screen for elder mistreatment; it provides a signal to the elder that it is a safe topic to explore with the health care professional.

Practical Clinician Tool

A high index of suspicion leads to early recognition and intervention. For clinicians in busy practices, a simple one-page tool (see Figs. 9.1 and 9.2) provides the principles of assessment and management, best practice guidelines, and screening questions. The intent of the tool is to raise awareness and maintain a high index of suspicion for elder abuse, neglect, and financial exploitation.

Screening and assessment instruments have been developed to assist health care professionals in identifying elder abuse. The Hwalek-Sengstock Elder Abuse Screening Test is a 15-item instrument that measures physical abuse, vulnerability, and potentially abusive situations.[14] Scofield et al. modified this as a 6-item brief, rapid screening instrument[15] consisting of the following:

1. Are you afraid of anyone in your family?
2. Has anyone close to you tried to hurt or harm you recently?
3. Has anyone close to you called you names, put you down, or made you feel bad recently?
4. Does someone in your family make you stay in bed or tell you that you are sick when you know you are not?
5. Has anyone forced you to do things you did not want to do?
6. Has anyone taken things that belong to you without your approval?

CLINICAL ASSESSMENT

Framing elder abuse as a geriatric syndrome affirms the need for a multidimensional assessment, including an assessment of mental capacity, because elder mistreatment encompasses a broad range of behaviors, events, and circumstances. Coupled with an assessment and investigation by the Adult Protective Services, an interdisciplinary care plan can be developed that includes appropriate interventions.[16]

Setting

A quiet relaxing environment helps put the person at ease. It is important to gain and maintain trust with the patient by empathic listening and asking nonthreatening questions. It is a red flag if a potential victim is not allowed to speak privately. After speaking with an elderly person about alleged abuse, never attempt to compare versions with the alleged abuser. Doing so may endanger the victim and tip off the alleged abuser to the reason for your inquiry. In these discussions, assume that the victim's statements are true and make it clear to them that abusive behavior is wrong and it is not the victim's fault. Victims need to be assured that they are not alone and that help is available. If self-neglect is a consideration, a home assessment is essential if it can be arranged.

History

Historical items of interest include comorbid medical and surgical conditions and review of the patient's cognitive and functional status. Because depression and anxiety are often related to elder abuse, screening for these conditions is often productive. Undertake a thorough review of all medications, including over-the-counter medicines, herbs, and supplements, and review adherence to the medication regimen. When assessing for alcohol and substance abuse, it is critical to understand the patient's perception of the problem. Be attentive to vague references to sexual advances and to any past history of neglect, abuse, or domestic violence and examine the older person's perception of the action and the cultural context in which the action occurred.

A complete psychosocial history helps define the social context. It is important to recognize any long-standing relationship problems between the victim and the possible perpetrator. Try to define the level of caregiving required and the amount of social support already in place. Inquire about financial resources and how they are managed.

Physical Examination

After conducting a clinical history, an appropriate focused physical examination is required, keeping in mind the various signs of elder mistreatment described earlier. The

MEDAmerica INSURANCE COMPANY
An Excellus Company
Home Office: Pitsburg, PA

Principles of Assessment and Management of Elder Abuse
Developed by Patricia A. Bomba, M.D., F.A.C.P., MedAmerica Medical Director

Assessment

Maintain an index of suspicion for elder abuse, neglect and financial exploitation.

History: *Assess*
- Comorbid medical and surgical conditions
- Cognitive status: Mentally retarded, developmentally disabled, Alzheimers disease and related memory disorders
- Functional status: ADLs and performance status
- Trajectory of decline in status
- Medication history and compliance
- Alcohol and substance use
- Vague references to sexual advances
- Past neglect, abuse, or domestic violence

Psychosocial History: *Assess*
- Depression, anxiety, PTSD, suicide risk
- Longstanding relationship problems between victim and perpetrator
- Quality of life
- Caregiving and social support
- Financial resources
- Patient's, family's, and caregiver's cultural and spiritual beliefs

Assessment:
- Order and evaluate appropriate diagnostic labs and x-rays

Diagnostic Terms:
Elder Abuse—all-inclusive term for all forms of elder mistreatment
Abuse—act of commission
Neglect—act of omission
Mistreatment—term preferred by seniors

Types of Elder Abuse:
- Physical
- Sexual
- Psychological
- Financial exploitation
- Self-neglect
- Abandonment
- Domestic violence of late life

Results of Elder Abuse:
- Unnecessary suffering, injury, pain, decreased quality of life, loss or violation of human rights
- Increased mortality rates

Lachs, M. 1998, JAMA 280(5):428-32

Suspect Elder Abuse, Neglect, Financial Exploitation

General:
- Delays between injury or illness and assessment
- History from victim and perpetrator differs
- Implausible or vague explanations
- Frequent ED visits for illness despite plan of care and adequate resources
- Functionally impaired patient presents without caregiver
- Cognitively impaired patient presents without caregiver
- Lab or x-ray results inconsistent with history
- "Doctor hopping"

Physical Abuse:
- Bruises, welts, cuts, wounds, cigarette/rope burn marks
- Blood on person, clothes
- Injuries: Fractures, sprains
- Painful body movements, unrelated to illness
- Pressure sores

Psychological Abuse:
- Sense of resignation or hopelessness
- Passive, helpless, withdrawn behavior
- Fearful, tearful, anxious, clinging
- Self-blame for life situation or caregiver behavior

Neglect:
- Unclean appearance
- Inadequate food or meal preparation
- Underweight, frail, dehydrated
- Inappropriate use of medications
- Inadequate utilities
- Unsafe or unclean environment
- Neglected household finances

Financial Exploitation:
- Overpayment for goods, services
- Unexplained change in POA, wills, legal documents
- Missing checks, money
- Unexplained decrease in bank account
- Missing belongings

Modified Ohio EA & DVLL Screening Tool, NEAN 13(2) 2001:35

Management and Monitoring

Assess for safety: Is there immediate danger?

Yes → Immediate referral

No ↓

Does the patient accept intervention?

Yes →
- Implement a safety plan
- Provide emergency information
- Educate the patient
- Develop goals of care
- Alleviate causes of abuse
- Refer patient and family for services
- Arrange follow-up

No ↓

Does the patient have the capacity to refuse treatment?

Yes →
- Implement a safety plan
- Provide emergency information
- Educate the patient
- Develop goals of care
- "Gentle persuasion"
- Arrange follow-up

No →
- Refer to APS
  - Financial Management
  - Guardianship
  - Court proceedings
- Refer to geriatric consultation team
- Arrange follow-up

Modified AMA Diagnostic and Treatment Guidelines on Elder Abuse and Neglect, 1992

Figure 9.1 Front page of Elder Abuse "Tool". ADLs, activities of daily living; PTSD, posttraumatic stress disorder; ED, emergency department; POA, power of attorney; APS, adult protective services (Copyright 2002 Patricia Bomba, M.D., F.A.C.P./MedAmerica—All Rights Reserved—www.MedAmericaLTC.com).

MEDAmerica INSURANCE COMPANY

Principles of Assessment and Management of Elder Abuse
Developed by Patricia A. Bomba, M.D., F.A.C.P., MedAmerica Medical Director

As health care professionals, our challenge is to balance:
1. Duty to protect the safety of the vulnerable elder
2. Elder's right to self-determination

VALUES

- Treat elders with honesty, compassion, respect
- Goals of care should focus on improving quality of life and reducing suffering

PRINCIPLES: Rights of Older Adults

- Right to be safe
- Retain civil and constitutional rights, unless restricted by courts
- Can make decisions that do not conform to social norms if no harm to others
- Have decision-making capacity unless courts decide otherwise
- May accept or refuse services

BEST PRACTICE GUIDELINES

- First, **DO NO HARM**
- Interest of the senior is the priority
- Avoid imposing your personal values
- Respect diversity
- Involve the senior in the plan of care
- Establish short-term and long-term goals
- Recognize the senior's right to make choices
- Use family and informal support
- Recommend community-based services before institutional-based services, whenever possible
- In the absence of known wishes, act in the best interest and use substituted judgment

Adapted and modified from A National Association of Adult Protective Services Administrators (NAAPSA) consensus statement.

SCREENING QUESTIONS

- Are you afraid of anyone in your family?
- Has anyone close to you tried to hurt or harm you recently?
- Has anyone close to you called you names or put you down or made you feel bad recently?
- Does someone in your family make you stay in bed or tell you you're sick when you know you aren't?
- Has anyone forced you to do things you didn't want to do?
- Has anyone taken things that belong to you without your OK?

Modified 15-item H-S/EAST screening tool by Australian Women's Health Survey (Scofield, 1999)

Figure 9.2 Back page of Elder Abuse "Tool". (Copyright 2002 Patricia Bomba, M.D., F.A.C.P./ MedAmerica—All Rights Reserved—www.MedAmericaLTC.com).

examination may also provide an opportunity for further confidential discussion because caregivers can be politely asked to leave the examining room. A mental status examination is useful to determine whether a person suffers from cognitive deficits sufficient to impair the person's judgment.

Assessing Mental Capacity

Mental capacity relates to a cluster of mental skills people use in everyday life to perceive and react to the risks in the environment. These skills include memory, logic, ability to calculate, and the "flexibility" to turn attention from one task to another. Generally, decision-making capacity refers to the ability to:

- understand and process information;
- make reality-based decisions about one's lifestyle and deportment that are in character with one's beliefs and values over time;
- communicate these decisions;
- carry out the activities of daily living; or

- direct others to carry out personal wishes to meet the essential needs for food, clothing, shelter, and medical care.

Different capacities are required for different tasks, such as marrying or divorcing, agreeing to a medical procedure or test, agreeing to a new living situation, executing a will, or making a donation. A finding that the patient lacks capacity to make a health care decision does not imply a lack of capacity for any other purpose. Similarly, a patient's lack of capacity to make a financial decision does not imply a lack of capacity to make health care decisions. Capacity assessment should include a detailed history from the patient, as well as collateral history from family and caregivers; physical examination that includes screens for cognition; function, and mood; and tests to exclude reversible conditions. Pertinent questions would include:

- Is the patient able to make and express choices in relation to this particular medical intervention?
- Is the patient able to provide reasons for his or her choices?
- Do the patient's reasons have some basis in fact and reality?
- Is the patient able to understand and appreciate the potentially harmful consequences of his or her chosen course of action?

Failure to recognize lack of capacity can lead to increased disability, complications of disease states, loss of independence, and death.

Capacity versus Competence

The physician must also assess the patient's ability to provide informed consent. For legal and proper consent, the person consenting must have sufficient mental capacity and be able to understand the implications and ramifications of his or her actions. Moreover, an individual who is stronger or more powerful should not coerce the older person. The stronger individual may attempt techniques to isolate the weaker person, promote dependency, or induce fear or distrust.

Undue influence and mental capacity are distinct. The key issue is whether the individual can act freely. Although diminished capacity may contribute to a person's vulnerability to undue influence, cognitive assessment cannot reliably identify undue influence. Only the courts decide undue influence and competence.

In summary, capacity depends on one's ability to understand the act or transaction, the consequences of taking or not taking action, and the consequences of making or not making the transaction; to weigh choices; make a decision; and commit to the decision.

Laboratory

There are no specific laboratory tests to order; however, monitoring drug levels, ordering appropriate diagnostic testing, and considering diagnostic x-rays in the settings of trauma are sometimes indicated.

Examples of useful laboratory findings in identifying specific conditions are included in Table 9.8.

TABLE 9.8
EXAMPLES OF LABORATORY FINDINGS FOR IDENTIFYING SPECIFIC CONDITIONS

Laboratory Findings	Specific Condition
BUN/creatinine level	Dehydration
Glucose level	Diabetes
PT/PTT/platelets	Coagulopathy
Liver function test	Alcohol abuse
Thyroid function test	Hypothyroidism, hyperthyroidism
Albumin level	Nutritional assessment
Fractures	Consider bone survey
Urinalysis	Source for fever

BUN, blood urea nitrogen; PT, prothrombin time; PTT, partial thromboplastin time.

MANAGEMENT

As noted earlier, the management challenge for health care professionals is to balance the duty to protect the vulnerable elder with the elder's right to self-determination. To do so requires a commitment to basic values, including treating elders with honesty, compassion, and respect, and recognition of the fact that goals of care should focus on improving quality of life and reducing suffering (see Table 9.9).

Principles

The National Association of Adult Protective Services Administrators (NAAPSA) consensus statement[17] outlines the basic principles and best practice guidelines that are meaningful for all health care practitioners and other professionals concerned with elder abuse. For this reason, a modified version was adapted for inclusion on the single-page Principles of Assessment and Management of Elder Abuse Tool (Figs. 9.1 and 9.2).

TABLE 9.9
INTERVENTIONS

Document well in medical records
Report to Adult Protective Services
Engage law enforcement
Refer to geriatric medicine teams
Enhance social supports
Provide numbers for women's shelters
Work with district attorneys to provide testimony

Recommendation

There are three essential questions to consider when one suspects elder mistreatment:

1. Is the patient safe?
2. Does the patient accept intervention?
3. Does the patient have the capacity to refuse treatment?

If there is imminent danger, then immediate action and referral for appropriate intervention is necessary. If the patient is presently safe, there is time to develop trust with him or her and the caregiver. If the patient accepts intervention, the health care professional must implement a safety plan, provide emergency information, educate the patient that abuse is wrong, develop goals of care, alleviate the cause of abuse, refer the patient and family for appropriate services, and, importantly, arrange follow-up. In the event the patient refuses intervention and has capacity, the same series of steps should be followed, with follow-up appointments assuming greater importance. A follow-up phone call from the physician or nurse often provides helpful contact in these situations. If the patient refuses intervention and lacks decisional capacity, the clinician should refer the patient to Adult Protective Services, including arrangements for financial management, guardianship, and advocacy for possible court proceedings. Close follow-up of these high-risk cases is critical to a successful outcome. In complex cases, referral to a geriatric consultation team for comprehensive assessment may be helpful, if such consultation is available.

Reporting

Reporting elder abuse to protective services is mandatory in most but not all states. As of 2005, New York, Delaware, Wisconsin, Colorado, New Jersey, and South Dakota did not have such services. In 42 states, failure to report elder abuse is a punishable offense. Self-neglect is not reportable in 15 states. Section 164.512 of the Health Insurance Portability and Accountability Act (HIPAA) outlines uses and disclosures where consent is *not* required. Victims of abuse, neglect, or domestic violence are excluded. This exception allows legal disclosure to other professionals involved in care and treatment, protection, and legal matters concerning a patient. Using their professional judgment, the covered entities are encouraged to cooperate with disclosure requests from the court, law enforcement, lawyers in legal proceedings, Adult Protective Services, and other "health care providers" to facilitate information exchange when needed to serve or protect patients.

DOCUMENTATION

Patients should receive proper documentation of the incident, symptoms, and physical findings. Photographs should be taken as indicated. The size of the injuries should be measured and recorded. Appropriate body maps should be included in office notes. These notes may become a critical component of future legal proceedings on behalf of the victim. Physicians must be prepared to engage law enforcement and work with district attorneys to provide testimony. Well-documented medical records are often sufficient and preclude the need for testifying in court.

SUMMARY

Elder abuse is a growing but hidden problem in our society. Health care professionals can—and must do better. We must heighten the awareness of this problem in our everyday practice setting, acknowledge its existence, and expand our comfort level while questioning our patients. More durable solutions for this major public health issue must take place on the medical, psychological, social, and legal levels, and care must be carefully coordinated among multiple systems. For health care professionals, the cases are demanding and often frustrating; and for older adults, the solutions are difficult and frequently unacceptable. For the present, part of the solution lies in framing elder abuse as a geriatric syndrome, utilizing an interdisciplinary approach to integrate community resources, developing an evidence base through rigorous research, and increasing professional and community awareness of this hidden epidemic.

REFERENCES

1. Lachs MS, Williams CS, O'Brien S, et al. The mortality of elder abuse. *J Am Med Assoc*. 1998;280:428–432.
2. Available at www.elderabusecenter.org/basic/index.html. Accessed July 2004.
3. National Center on Elder Abuse. *National elder abuse incidence study: Final report*. Washington, DC: American Public Health Services Association; 1998. Available at: http://www.elderabuse center. org. Accessed September 2004.
4. National Committee for the Prevention of Elder Abuse. 2003. Available at: http://www.preventelderabuse.org. Accessed September 2004.
5. Lachs MS. Preaching to the unconverted: Educating physicians about elder abuse. *J Elder Abuse Neglect*. 1995;7:1–12.
6. Dyer CB, Pavlik VN, Murphy KP, et al. The high prevalence of depression and dementia in elder abuse or neglect. *J Am Geriatr Soc*. 2000;48:205–208.
7. Mouton CP, Rodabough RJ, Ravi SL, et al. "Prevalence and 3-year incidence of abuse among postmenopausal women. *Am J Public Health*. 2004;94:605–612.
8. Lachs MS, Williams C, O'Brien S, et al. Older adults. An 11-year longitudinal study of adult protective service use. *Arch Intern Med*. 1996;156:449–453.
9. Lachs MS, Williams C, O'Brien S, et al. Risk factors for reported elder abuse and neglect: A nine-year observational cohort study. *Gerontologist*. 1997;37:469–474.
10. Nelson HD, Nygren P, Mclnerney Y, Klein J. Screening for family and intimate partner violence: Recommendation statement. *Ann Intern Med*. 2004;140:382–386.
11. Nelson HD, Nygren P, Mclnerney Y, Klein J. Screening women and elderly adults for family and intimate partner violence: A review of the evidence for the U.S. preventive services task force. *Ann Intern Med*. 2004;140:382–386,387–404.

12. American Medical Association Council on Scientific Affairs. *Diagnostic and treatment guidelines on elder abuse and neglect.* Chicago, IL: American Medical Association; 1992.
13. Fulmer T, Guadagno L, Dyer C, et al. Progress in elder abuse screening and assessment instruments. *J Am Geriatr Soc.* 2004;52:297–304.
14. Hwalek M, Sengstok M. Assessing the probability of abuse of the elderly: Towards the development of a clinical screening instrument. *J Appl Gerontol.* 1986;5:153–173.
15. Scofield M, Reynolds R, Mishra G, et al. *Vulnerability to abuse, powerlessness and psychological stress among older women.* Callagan, NSW : University of Newcastle, Women's Health Australia Study; 1999.
16. Dyer C, Gleason M, Murphy K, et al. Treating elder neglect: Collaboration between a geriatrics assessment team and adult protective services. *South Med J.* 1999;92:242–244.
17. A National Association of Adult Protective Services Administrators (NAAPSA) Consensus Statement. Available at http://www.elderabusecenter.org/pdf/publication/ethics.pdf. Accessed November 2004.

SUGGESTED READINGS AND RESOURCES

National Center on Elder Abuse
1201 15th Street, N.W., Suite 350
Washington, DC 20005-2842
(202) 898–2586
(202) 898–2583 (fax)
ncea@nasua.org
www.elderabusecenter.org

Clearinghouse on Abuse and Neglect of the Elderly (CANE)
University of Delaware
Department of Consumer Studies
Alison Hall West, Room 211
Newark, DE 19716
(302) 831–3525
CANE-UD@udel.edu
http://www.elderabusecenter.org/default.cfm?p=cane.cfm

National Committee for the Prevention of Elder Abuse
1612 K Street, N.W.
Washington, DC 20006
(202) 682–4140
(202) 223–2099 (fax)
ncpea@verizon.net
http://www.preventelderabuse.org

The American Bar Association Commission on Law and Aging
Commission on Law and Aging
American Bar Association
740 15th Street, N.W.
Washington, DC 20005-1022
(202) 662–8690
(202) 662–8698 (fax)
abaaging@abanet.org
www.abanet.org/aging

Eldercare Search
(Featuring a search by city, zip, county for General Info, Long-term Care Ombudsman, Elder Abuse Prevention, Health Insurance Counseling, Prescription Assistance, and Legal Assistance)
1-800-677-1116 (toll-free, Monday through Friday, 9:00 AM to 8:00 PM [ET])
http://www.eldercare.gov/Eldercare/Public/Home.asp

National Association of State Units on Aging
1225 I Street, N.W., Suite 725
Washington, DC 20005
(202) 898–2578
NCEA@nasua.org
http://www.nasua.org/

National Center for Victims of Crime
2000 M Street, N.W., Suite 480
Washington, DC 20036
(202) 467–8700
(202) 467–8701 (fax)
webmaster@ncvc.org
http://www.ncvc.org/ncvc/main.aspx?dbName=DocumentViewer&DocumentID=32350

International Network for the Prevention of Elder Abuse
http://www.inpea.net/

National Elder Abuse Incidence Study
http://www.aoa.gov/eldfam/elder_rights/elder_abuse/ABuseReport_Full.pdf

US Senate Hearing on Elder Abuse-2003
http://frwebgate.access.gpo.gov/cgibin/getdoc.cgi?dbname=108_senate_hearings&docid=f:93251.pdf

Monroe County, NY Elder Abuse Site
http://www.elderrespect.org/

American Psychological Association–Elder Abuse and Neglect
http://www.apa.org/pi/aging/elderabuse.html

MedAmerica Insurance Company
(To obtain laminated copies of the Practical Clinician's Tool, CD, and other provider materials)
www.MedAmericaLTC.com

Weight Loss in the Elderly Patient

10

Russell G. Robertson

CLINICAL PEARLS 108

LEXICON 109

WEIGHT CHANGES IN THE HEALTHY AGING ADULT 110

CAUSES OF WEIGHT LOSS 110
Gastrointestinal Causes of Weight Loss 111
Psychiatric 112
Inflammatory, Infectious, and Chronic Diseases 112
Neurologic 112
Medications 112
Other Causes 112

PHYSIOLOGY OF WEIGHT LOSS 112
Metabolism 113
Biochemical Changes 113
Hormonal Changes 113
Osteoporosis 113

ASSESSMENT 113

WEIGHT REDUCTION 115

MANAGEMENT 115
Nutritional Interventions 115
Tube Feeding 116
Environmental Factors 118
Physical Activity 118
Medications and Weight Loss 118

CONCLUSION 119

ACKNOWLEDGMENT 120

CLINICAL PEARLS

- Among healthy people, total body weight tends to peak in the sixth decade of life.
- Involuntary weight loss is not a normal part of aging and usually represents some underlying disease process.
- Clinically important weight loss is defined as the loss of 10 pounds (4.5 kg) or >5% of the body weight over 6 to 12 months and is associated with a doubling of mortality over 4 to 5 years.
- Individuals who lost >10% of their body weight between the age of 70 and 75 had significantly higher mortality risk during the following 5 years.
- Weight maintenance is associated with a decreased incidence of death.
- Thirty-six percent of deaths in an at-risk population could have been avoided if early nutritional intervention to prevent weight loss had been initiated.
- Resting energy expenditure (REE) becomes the greatest part of energy expenditure because of a decline in physical activity and may represent 60% to 75% of the total daily energy requirements of healthy elderly subjects.
- Reduced physical activity, decreased REE, and lower lean body mass reduce energy demand by up to 1,200 kcal per day in men and 800 kcal in women between the age of 20 and 80.
- Depression is a common cause of weight loss.
- There is a correlation between weight loss and deterioration of mental status, as measured by the Mini-Mental State Examination and the Geriatric Depression Scale.
- A trial of antidepressants should be considered for patients with weight loss and possible depression.

- The use of just three medications reduces an individual's ability to taste and may lead to anorexia.
- The first line of treatment for weight loss is to supplement with high-density, high-protein formulas that supply 240 to 360 calories and 10 to 14 g of protein per 240-mL can.
- The relaxation of dietary restrictions instituted for an underlying disease may be considered if they are a barrier to meeting energy needs.
- The most promising intervention to increase muscle mass and strength in older persons is progressive resistance training.

Detecting the existence of weight loss in the elderly is unlike many other diagnostic challenges because it requires the ability to see what is no longer there. It is like looking at two photos that at first glance appear similar until it becomes apparent that select and often obscure items in one are absent from the other. The failure to make this clinically essential assessment has profound implications. This is because weight loss is a common problem in older adults and has been associated with adverse outcomes, such as decreased functional status, institutionalization, and increased mortality.[1] Clinicians must understand that weight loss is not a normal part of aging and usually represents some underlying disease process, especially when it is an unexplained clinical finding in apparently healthy individuals.[2,3] That weight loss may be one of the first clinical markers of Alzheimer disease underscores the importance of paying attention to what may be an easily overlooked data point.[4] Weight loss remains independently associated with mortality even after adjustment for baseline health status.[5]

One study found that individuals who lost >10% of their body weight between the age of 70 and 75 had a significantly higher mortality risk during the following 5 years compared to those who lost <5%.[6] Low body weight and weight loss are powerful predictors of morbidity including higher rates of infection, increased risk of decubitus ulcers, and poor response to medical therapy.[7,8] This involutional process leads to and is a consequence of energy dysregulation, results in the atrophy of muscle, and accelerates the loss of independence.[3]

The fact that the average 75-year-old person has three chronic medical conditions and is on five prescription medications poses real challenges to the clinician caring for the aged. The sometimes evocative and occasionally urgent medical needs of the elderly have the potential to obscure what may be subtle changes that should trigger aggressive weight management.[1,9]

Body weight is determined by a complex interaction of calorie intake, absorption, and utilization.[7] The challenge of weight loss is multifaceted, with different clinical and metabolic effects depending on specific underlying triggers.

Low body weight in elders may reflect either their usual weight or a weight loss. Therefore, the most precise nutritional marker is measured weight loss over time because optimal weight in old age is a matter of considerable debate.[10] A number of population studies have shown a U-shaped relationship of body mass index (BMI) with mortality and have indicated some surprisingly high body weights associated with the lowest mortality.[10]

Among healthy people, total body weight tends to peak in the sixth decade of life. Once weight has peaked, there is relative stability, with longitudinal studies demonstrating a weight loss of 1 to 2 kg per decade thereafter.[7] In healthy elderly, there is an increase in fat tissue that balances a loss in skeletal muscle until very old age, when loss of both fat and skeletal muscle occurs.[11]

Clinically important weight loss can be defined as the loss of 10 pounds (4.5 kg) or >5% of the body weight over a period of 6 to 12 months. This amount of weight loss is associated with a doubling of mortality over 4 to 5 years.[12] Weight loss of >10% represents protein-energy malnutrition and impaired physiologic function including impaired cell-mediated and humoral immunity.[7] The challenge for physicians is that some patients may be undisturbed by their weight loss, or may even welcome it, and may mistakenly attribute the loss to their attempts to lose weight.[7]

LEXICON

There are a few key terms that have distinct definitions in weight management.

Cachexia: Weight loss may be a key feature, but cachexia more accurately represents the clinical consequences of chronic inflammation from a variety of causes. When weight loss due to cachexia occurs, it stems from the loss of fat-free mass, with muscle wasting as a key element. Cachexia is a kind of metabolic meltdown that often results in accelerated weight loss, loss of function, and a resistance to remediation. Cachexia may be associated with little or no weight loss in its early stages.

Sarcopenia: Sarcopenia specifically refers to decreased or diminished reserves of muscle and lean body mass.

Wasting: Wasting is the gradual loss of strength or substance. It is an unintentional loss of body weight (5% to 10%; BMI <28) coupled with a functional impairment in apparently healthy individuals, with loss in both the fat and fat-free compartments.

Failure to Thrive: Failure to thrive is weight loss, decreased appetite, poor nutrition, and inactivity, often accompanied by dehydration, depressive symptoms, and impaired immune function.

BMI: BMI is the ratio of weight in kg to the square of height in meters. Normal BMI for the elderly is 20 to 30.

Body Cell Mass: Body cell mass is the fat-free portion of cells within muscle, viscera, and the immune system.

Bodily Energy Requirements:

1. Resting energy expenditure (REE) is the energy required to maintain body temperature and

essential physiologic processes. This represents 60% to 75% of the total daily energy expenditures of healthy adults.
2. Diet-induced thermogenesis is the energy required to digest and process ingested food. It represents 10% to 15% of total daily body energy expenditure.
3. Energy of physical activity represents 10% to 30% of total body energy expenditure.

WEIGHT CHANGES IN THE HEALTHY AGING ADULT

The process of normal aging has inherent mechanisms that result in; changes in fat and muscle distribution, changes in taste and smell, and alterations in gastric and intestinal motility, all of which can affect appetite. These processes in combination with age-related changes in activity will ultimately result in incremental weight loss independent of any disease state. Among aging healthy people, total body weight peaks in the sixth decade of life.[7] This is the norm in developed nations where adult weight, which increases during middle age, generally remains stable in the healthy elderly until the ninth decade and then gradually falls.[11] Once an individual's weight has peaked, there is relative stability in total weight in the healthy elderly.[7]

However, lean body mass (fat-free mass) begins to decline at a rate of 0.3 kg per year in the third decade, and at age 60 in men and 65 in women the rate increases to a 0.5% annual decline in lean body mass.[13,14] These weight changes are largely attributed to a decline in physical activity. In the healthy elderly, an increase in fat tissue balances a loss in skeletal muscle mass until very old age, when the loss of both fat and skeletal muscle loss occurs.[11] Because fat-free mass declines as much as 40% between the age of 30 and 70, at any given body weight or BMI, older persons will be considerably fatter than their younger counterparts.[1]

There are also changes occurring at a cellular level, which reflect changes in cellular composition and associated intrinsic physiologic processes. Body cell mass is the fat-free portion of cells within the muscle, viscera, and immune system. Body cell mass declines steadily with age in healthy, successfully aging people. This mass is important because it directly predicts strength, and therefore functional status, and is the major determinant of energy needs.[15]

There are physiologic mediators of weight loss in healthy individuals that may also be mediators in the presence of disease and debilitation. Some loss of lean body mass is due to age-related declines in anabolic hormones (e.g., growth hormone, dehydro-3-epiandrosterone, and sex hormones), the adverse effects of accumulated free radicals, increased cytokines (interleukin-6 [IL-6] and tumor necrosis factor-α [TNF-α]), and the effects of intermittent acute illness and reduced activity levels.[1] These changes are interrelated with age-related loss of smell and taste and intestinal motility disorders such as constipation, gastroparesis, and dyspepsia.[16] Collectively, there seems to be a steady transformative process that leads to some degree of sarcopenia, even in successfully aging adults, and is universal. It is difficult to know whether the sarcopenia seen in the elderly is due to decreased physical activity or whether it leads to decreased physical activity.[15]

Therefore, it becomes apparent that normal weight changes in the elderly are the result of interrelated mechanisms that may originate at the level of intracellular processes reflected in cell composition and that may then impact digestive physiology, which leads to changes in compartmentalization of fat and muscle mass. These phenomena contribute to a decline in appetite, leading to a decline in the ingestion of nutrients needed to sustain physical activity that is required to delay or forestall loss of muscle mass, weakness, and sarcopenia—apoptosis at work.

CAUSES OF WEIGHT LOSS

The previous section details weight changes that are incremental and are consistent with the process of healthy aging. There is also a physiologic weight loss that is due to a gradually decreased intake of food throughout life. Between the age of 20 and 80, the mean energy intake is reduced by up to 1,200 kcal per day in men and 800 kcal in women. This is believed to be the result of decreased hunger, reflecting reduced physical activity, decreased REE, and loss of lean body mass, all producing lower demand in calories and food intake.[2] This is the physiologic weight loss (below the threshold of 5% annual weight loss) seen as a consequence of aging.

We will now examine the causes of weight loss that are nonphysiologic and exceed the 5% threshold. This is what may be considered protein-energy malnutrition, which is highly prevalent among the elderly and which, in addition to leading to an underweight condition, is an important cause of age-related declines in muscle mass.[17] Protein-energy malnutrition is often due to multiple factors. A circuitous relationship often exists among the causes that makes the isolation of a pivotal event or process and the subsequent development of a clinical approach to treatment challenging and, to a degree, frustrating. This unintentional or involuntary weight loss is associated with self-rated poor health, chronic disability, cancer, respiratory diseases, diabetes, and cardiovascular events such as heart attack and stroke.[18]

The term *nutritional frailty* is used to describe a dramatic decline in appetite and drastic decline in food intake. There can be a precipitous drop in body weight over a period of weeks and months that is recognized as a hallmark of terminal and unremediable decline.[2] When it is due to an illness, the prognosis is grave. However, when no definitive cause can be identified, patients may be amenable to treatment and have a better prognosis.[7]

Weight is mediated primarily by one's appetite. So long as an individual has adequate access to sources of food

TABLE 10.1
CLINICAL CAUSES OF WEIGHT LOSS

Malignant Neoplasms	Gastrointestinal Diseases	Psychiatric Disorders	Neurologic Disorders	Chronic Diseases, Infections, Inflammation	Medication Effects	Others
Gastrointestinal (153.9/159)	Peptic ulcer disease (533.90)	Depression (311)	Stroke (V17.1)	Pulmonary tuberculosis (11.9)	Anorexia (783.0)	Poverty
Hepatobiliary (155.56)	Inflammatory bowel disease (555.9)	Bereavement (V62.82)	Quadriplegia (344.0)	Mycotic diseases (V75.4)	Nausea (787.02)	Isolation
Hematologic (208.9)	Dysmotility syndromes (564.1)	Paranoia (297.1)	Multiple sclerosis (340)	Parasitic Infection (134)	Vomiting (787.03)	Alcoholism (303.0)
Lung (162.9)	Chronic pancreatitis (577.1)		Functional disabilities	Subacute bacterial endocarditis (421.0)	Diarrhea (787.91)	
Breast (174.9)	Colonic disorders (562.1)		Visual impairment (368.10)	HIV (042)	Dysgeusia (781.1)	
Genitourinary (188.0)	Constipation (564.0)		Alzheimer disease (290.0)	Cardiovascular disease (429.2)		
Ovarian (183)	Atrophic gastritis (535.2)			Pulmonary disease (519.9)		
Prostate (185)	Oral problems (528.9/529.9)			Renal failure (585)		
	Dysphagia (787.2)			Diabetes (250.0)		
				Hyperthyroidism (242.9)		
				Hypothyroidism (244.9)		

Adapted from references 7, 10, 14, 18, 20.

with sufficient caloric content and has the ability to eat independently or with assistance, intake and consequently one's weight is directly related to appetite. The mechanisms that maintain a healthy appetite are not completely understood.[19] Seemingly simple disruptions in physiologic processes that physicians may deem of little consequence in younger populations can have profound effects in the elderly. Peptic ulcer disease or gastroesophageal reflux disease may lead to loss of appetite.[19] A decrease in relaxation of the fundus of the stomach can result in early antral filling, causing early satiation.[13] Low-fat and sodium-restricted diets do not taste as good and are associated with weight loss, low albumin level, and orthostasis in nursing home patients.[14] Some patients with a history of anorexia nervosa relapse later in life and develop what is called *anorexia tardive*.[14] Causes of involuntary weight loss are listed in Table 10.1.

One of the most ominous causes of unintentional weight loss is cancer. In one series of patients, malignancies were the cause of weight loss in one third of all patients. The most common cancers were gastrointestinal, hepatobiliary, hematologic, lung, breast, genitourinary, ovarian, and prostate.[7]

Gastrointestinal Causes of Weight Loss

In two large studies evaluating causes of weight loss, gastrointestinal causes ranked second in one and first in the other. Peptic ulcer disease, inflammatory bowel disease, dysmotility syndromes, chronic pancreatitis, celiac disease, constipation, atrophic gastritis, and oral problems are some of the potential etiologies that can precipitate weight loss.[13] Malabsorption in the elderly presents with nonspecific weight loss and may be associated with diarrhea. The most common causes of malabsorption are bacterial overgrowth, pancreatic exocrine deficiency, and sprue.[14]

Oral problems deserve special attention. Several oral problems are associated with involuntary weight loss, including halitosis, poor oral hygiene, xerostomia, inability to chew, reduced masticatory force, nonocclusion, temporomandibular joint syndrome, inflammation, lesions, and oral pain.[5,12] Edentulousness is a strong predictor of weight loss and is associated with lower intake of calories, protein, and micronutrients such as calcium, and vitamins A, C, and E.[5] Periodontal disease, defined as a form of chronic inflammation in which periodontal pockets with at least 6 mm probing depth are present, was equal to edentulousness as a predictor of weight loss.[12] This disease is associated with an increase in systemic inflammatory mediators, including TNF-α, C-reactive protein, and IL-6, which play a large role in the physiology of weight loss.[12]

Psychiatric

An individual's emotional health plays a critical role in nutritional status. Depression may lead to apathy and an inability to care for self that includes inattention to nutritional needs.[7,14] Anxiety has been associated with several functional gastrointestinal disorders, including rumination and nonulcer dyspepsia, that are also known to contribute to weight loss through increased energy expenditure and loss of appetite.[7] Bereavement can cause significant weight loss in the elderly and is noticeably more pronounced in men.[14] More intense forms of mental disease such as paranoid disorders may lead to the development of paranoid delusions about foods and cause weight loss.[14]

Inflammatory, Infectious, and Chronic Diseases

Infection through tuberculosis (TB), fungal disease, parasites, subacute bacterial endocarditis, and human immunodeficiency virus (HIV) are occasional causes of unintentional weight loss.[7] Cardiovascular and pulmonary diseases cause unintentional weight loss through increased metabolic demand and decreased appetite and caloric intake.[7] Renal disease, as manifested by uremia, produces nausea, anorexia, and vomiting and diminishes appetite.[7] Connective tissue diseases may increase metabolic demand and disrupt nutritional balance.[7] Diabetes, hyperthyroidism, and hypothyroidism are the most common endocrine problems that cause weight loss. Hyperthyroidism occurs in up to 9% of elderly patients and can manifest as weight loss, apathy, and tachycardia.[14]

Neurologic

Neurologic injuries such as stroke, quadriplegia, and multiple sclerosis may lead to visceral and autonomic dysfunction that can impair caloric intake. Dysphagia from these neurologic insults is a common mechanism.[7] Functional disability compromising activities of daily living (ADLs) and instrumental activities of daily living (IADLs) is a common cause of undernutrition in older adults and may be the most overlooked.[13,21,22] Visual impairment from ophthalmic or central nervous system (CNS) disorders such as tremor can limit the ability of people to prepare and eat meals.[14]

The relationship between weight loss and Alzheimer disease deserves special consideration. Weight loss alone may be one of the earliest manifestations of Alzheimer dementia.[6,19] Approximately 50% of patients with dementia have protein-energy malnutrition, which in later stages is exacerbated by development of pseudobulbar dysphagia.[16] Diminished taste and smell combine with the hyperactivity of some patients with Alzheimer disease (i.e., pacing, agitation, and aggression) to cause an imbalance between intake and utilization.[11,14,19] Agnosia can develop, which makes it difficult to recognize edible objects and use utensils.[16]

Medications

The role of medications as both a primary and contributing cause of involuntary weight loss cannot be overlooked. According to one study, 12% of older adults take at least ten prescriptions and over-the-counter medications, with half taking at least five or more.[23] Medications can cause anorexia, nausea, vomiting, gastrointestinal distress, diarrhea, dry mouth, or changes in taste, and they can alter the intake, absorption, and utilization of nutrients.[14,19] Psychotropic medications and selective serotonin reuptake inhibitors (SSRIs) have been associated with weight loss.[19] In one cohort of community-living older adults, a linear relationship was found between the number of medications used and weight loss, suggesting that the medications were an independent cause of weight loss and additive to the disease processes for which they were prescribed.[23]

Other Causes

Poverty, living alone, and emotional isolation are associated with inadequate food intake. Not only may the elderly lack the motivation to prepare a meal but they may also have to choose between the purchase of food or medications.[13] Alcoholism, which is frequently overlooked in the elderly, can be a significant cause of weight loss and malnutrition.[14] Institutionalization appears to be a separate risk factor. From 30% to 50% of nursing home patients have inadequate food intake with malnutrition, and 21% of hospitalized patients consume <50% of required calories.[24]

PHYSIOLOGY OF WEIGHT LOSS

A basic understanding of what is transpiring at the cellular level is useful in conceptualizing weight loss. To better characterize this, remember that weight—or body mass—can be considered as composed of several compartments: Water and solid mass, lean tissue, fat tissue, and minerals (mostly bone).[19] Body cell mass describes the fat-free portion of cells within the muscle, viscera, and immune system. Several characteristics common to the elderly include a decreasing margin of homeostatic reserve and an increased likelihood of experiencing assaults to homeostatic balance.[2]

Metabolism

Basal metabolism in the elderly is distinctly different from that in younger people because most of the energy is spent while at rest. In the elderly, particularly those who are underweight, REE represents the greatest part of energy expenditure, constituting 60% to 75% of the total daily energy requirements.[17] The act of feeding itself has a thermic effect, defined as the increase in energy expenditure associated with food ingestion. It includes the energy costs of food absorption, metabolism, and storage and represents another 10% of total daily energy expenditure.[17] In sedentary elderly, as much as 85% of all energy expenditure involves almost no physical activity.[24] Fat-free mass is the principal determinant of REE and its effect depends on both its quantity and metabolic activity, which may be modulated by overall health and physical activity.[17] This feedback places the primarily sedentary elderly at risk for diseases that further contribute to cachexia, such as chronic urinary tract infections, decubitus ulcers, and malignancies. These diseases elevate resting metabolic rates that accelerate loss of body cell mass.[15]

Biochemical Changes

Anorexia, cachexia, chronic disease, and geriatric wasting lead to elevated levels of cytokines such as TNF, IL-6, and soluble IL-2 receptor.[24] The release of cytokines during chronic disease may be an important indication of frailty through induction of lipolysis, muscle protein breakdown, and nitrogen loss.[2] Sarcopenia is further induced by loss of α-motor neurons in the spinal column, loss of endogenous growth hormone production, inadequate protein intake, dysregulation of catabolic cytokines, loss of estrogen and androgen production, and reduced physical activity.[15]

Hormonal Changes

Aging is associated with marked decreases in insulin-like growth factors and insulin-like growth factor–binding proteins that may lead to decreased anabolic activity and contribute to increased catabolism and wasting.[25] It has been well documented that growth hormone secretion declines with age. This begins in the fourth decade of life and shows an incremental decrease with each decade thereafter. At age 70 to 80, approximately 50% of all subjects have no significant level of serum immunoreactive growth hormone at any time of the day. The decline in growth hormone secretion is a part of the etiology of the alterations in the insulin-like growth factors and insulin-like growth factor–binding proteins that are associated with aging.[25] These changes contribute to the decreases in lean body mass, increased adiposity, and impaired immune function that occur with aging and may also be a result of protoinflammatory cytokines such as TNF and IL-1β.[25] Appetite is the final common pathway through which these neurohumoral mechanisms act, including the newly discovered neurohormones leptin and the orexigen.[19]

Circulating cytokine levels have been found to be associated with higher mortality and functional disability in community-dwelling elderly.[24] Depression can be accompanied by dysfunction in the hypothalamic-pituitary axis that is characterized by higher circulating cytokine levels as well.[24]

Osteoporosis

A direct relationship exists between involuntary weight loss, osteoporosis, related fractures, and malnutrition.[26] There is evidence that protein depletion increases bone loss in elderly individuals and that the malnutrition associated with weight loss has a negative association with bone mineral density.[26] Because most energy expenditure in the elderly occurs while at rest, the resultant decline in mechanical load alters bone remodeling, leading to bone loss.[27] Hip fractures are associated with a decrease in calcium and protein intake and linked to decreases in levels of glucocorticoids and growth hormone and a disturbance in leptin levels.[27]

Of all the components of body cell mass, muscle cell mass declines the most with aging. This is due to a reduction in the number and size of type II muscle cells.[15] Decline in muscle mass and muscle action on bones contributes to the loss of bone mineral mass.[26] It is then no surprise that older, postmenopausal women who experience weight loss have increased rates of hipbone loss and a twofold greater risk of hip fracture. This is irrespective of current weight or intent to lose weight and is only partially reversed by exercise. As a result, any weight change should trigger an evaluation of bone density in women older than 60 years.[27]

ASSESSMENT

Once unintentional weight loss is suspected, a careful and stepwise evaluation ought to ensue that begins with a history and physical examination.[28] First and foremost, an effort to document weight loss through serial measurements is essential.[13] If there is uncertainty, the patient's weight should be evaluated weekly to look for trends and provide an objective measure for treatment.[19]

According to Bales and Ritchie,[2] the Council for Nutrition's Clinical Strategies in Long-Term Care recommends a workup for weight loss when any of the following four indicators are present: Involuntary weight loss of 5% in 30 days, weight loss of 10% in 180 days, a BMI of <21, or the patient leaving at least a quarter of his or her food uneaten for two thirds of meals over 1 week. These standards may be applicable to the outpatient setting and serve as a firm index against which one could verify the presence of significant weight loss.

Change in the fit of clothing is another index to be considered when assessing weight loss if reliable serial weights are unavailable.[14] More detailed indices of weight loss such as anthropometric measurements can be employed but are usually not necessary for most clinicians and may not be as useful as once thought.[14,16,17] Simple measurement of the BMI remains an easily obtainable and routinely available parameter of weight loss, with a BMI <20 to 21 indicative of an underweight condition.[17]

History and physical findings that are especially pertinent include evidence of changes in appetite, smell, or taste and the presence of abdominal pain, nausea, vomiting, diarrhea, constipation, and dysphagia. An initial panel of tests should include a complete blood count, sedimentation rate, urinalysis, comprehensive metabolic panel, thyroid-stimulating hormone (TSH) level, fecal occult blood testing, TB skin testing, and HIV testing if appropriate.[13,14,16,17,29] There is substantial evidence for performing a dental evaluation as a part of the initial evaluation[5,29] (Evidence Level C).

Because gastrointestinal causes are predominant, endoscopic evaluation of the upper and lower gastrointestinal tract, abdominal ultrasonography, and tests to exclude malabsorption are recommended as second-tier investigations.[20,28] In one series, diagnostic yields were the highest for fecal occult blood testing, sigmoidoscopy, thyroid function testing, upper endoscopy, and upper gastrointestinal series, whereas computed tomography scanning was not found to be useful.[29] Although prealbumin, albumin, and cholesterol levels and lymphocyte counts may help establish a diagnosis of malnutrition, they do not contribute to finding the etiology of unintended weight loss.[29] If investigations fail to reveal a clear cause, further age-related cancer screening would be advised, with emphasis on the gastrointestinal tract.[7]

Data on how the individual is functioning on a day-to-day basis is equally important. Measurements of the patient's autonomy and activity can be done with scales of ADLs and IADLs, which play an important role in determining REE.[7,17,21,22] Because of the correlation between weight loss and mental status changes, the Mini-Mental State Examination and the Geriatric Depression Scale can be useful.[29,30] When assessing the nutritional status of elderly patients, a well-validated and simple screening test is the Mini Nutritional Assessment (MNA).[18,31] The validity of the MNA was found to be substantial and significantly related to perceived weight loss over 1 year.[6]

Attention should be paid to social and functional problems, the availability of foods, the use of nutritional supplements, and daily caloric intake.[29] Elderly persons with weight loss should be observed while eating to assess their ability to manage utensils, to determine the amount of food eaten, denote the presence of chewing problems, assess difficulty in swallowing, identify visual difficulties, and assess whether they perceive the food as appetizing.[13] A medication review is necessary to look for polypharmacy, which is known to interfere with taste and cause anorexia. SSRIs can be anorectic; sedatives and narcotics may interfere with cognition and the ability to eat.[29] For nursing home patients, the resident assessment instrument, contained within the minimum data set required by Medicare, has been found to be a good predictor of changes in BMI and an early predictor of weight loss[32] (see Table 10.2).

TABLE 10.2
ASSESSMENT AND TESTING FOR WEIGHT LOSS

Historical assessment	5% weight loss in 30 d
	10% weight loss in 180 d
	BMI <21
	25% of food left uneaten over 7 d
	Change in fit of clothing
	Change in appetite, smell, or taste
	Abdominal pain, nausea, vomiting, diarrhea, constipation, dysphagia
	Medication review
Functional assessment	Activities of daily living
	Instrumental activities of daily living
	Mini-Mental State Examination
	Geriatric Depression Scale
	Mini Nutritional Assessment
	Resident assessment instrument from the minimum data set
	Observation of eating
Laboratory assessment	CBC, ESR, UA, CMP, TSH, fecal occult blood testing, TB skin test, and HIV if indicated
Procedural assessment	Dental evaluation
	Upper and lower endoscopy (if indicated)

BMI, body mass index; CBC, complete blood (cell) count; ESR, erythrocyte sedimentation rate; UA, urinalysis; CMP, cytidine 5′ -phosphate; TSH, thyroid-stimulating hormone; TB, tuberculosis; HIV, human immunodeficiency virus.
Adapted from references 2, 5, 7, 13, 14, 16, 17, 19–22, 28–30.

WEIGHT REDUCTION

A brief discussion of voluntary weight loss is warranted. Although we are in the midst of a national obesity epidemic, caution should be exercised when considering weight reduction measures in the elderly. Unlike younger people, the prognostic significance of excess weight in the elderly is controversial. Mild to moderate excess weight has not been associated with an increase in cardiovascular disease and all-cause mortality in elderly people.[27]

Although modest weight loss may be beneficial in overweight and healthy older individuals, even intentional weight loss has been associated with an increased risk of death in a frail elderly population after controlling for compromised health and functional status.[10] A study in elderly people with diabetes demonstrated that weight loss, whether voluntary or involuntary, predicted an increased risk of dying independent of baseline weight, preexisting illness, smoking, depression, or physical inactivity—even in overweight individuals.[33]

Adoption of current clinical guidelines for the treatment of excess weight and obesity in the elderly needs further evaluation.[27]

MANAGEMENT

Management of weight loss needs to begin with a discussion with the patient and family to establish expectations. Although it seems obvious that providing more food/energy should increase consumption and therefore body weight, in practice this goal is difficult to achieve because many of the factors causing nutritional frailty are not related to food access and supply.[2] Although efforts to improve nutritional status are often warranted, appropriate care provided late in the course of a disease may be palliative.[1]

Once it becomes apparent that the person is at risk for the consequences of weight loss and that treatment is appropriate, most therapeutic plans will include several simultaneous interventions. The first step is the identification and treatment of any specific underlying disease or other causative contributing conditions.[1] This might include addressing known chronic diseases and ensuring that their treatment has been optimized. Figure 10.1 provides an overview to the management of weight loss.[29]

Nutritional Interventions

It is extremely important, regardless of the cause, to begin early nutritional supplementation to achieve the best outcome.[29] One study revealed that 36% of deaths in an at-risk population could have been avoided or delayed if early nutritional intervention to prevent weight loss had been initiated.[10] Urgent reversal of weight loss through nutritional supplementation also reduces both fall risks and hip fractures.[13] Feeding requires a team approach. Educating caregivers on the nuances of feeding can have real benefits manifested as weight gain, particularly in patients with Alzheimer dementia.[6,30]

Total daily caloric requirements for the ambulatory elderly range from 30 to 35 kcal per kg; requirements are 40 kcal per kg for the malnourished and those with moderate illnesses.[14] The MNA identifies people at risk for malnutrition who do not yet have weight loss or low albumin levels. An MNA (see Fig. 10.2) score between 17 and 23.5 is much more amenable to successful intervention than a low score <17.[31] The following steps are recommended to get the most out of the MNA:

1. Calculate the patient's BMI
2. Assess risk factors for malnutrition such as isolation, nursing home placement, use of more than three medications, or the presence of pressure sores
3. Answer the MNA diet questions
4. Complete the sections on the subjective assessment of nutrition and general health.

A score on the MNA of over 24 is considered good. For these patients, attention should be directed at maintaining current nutritional health. A score <17 is indicative of protein-calorie undernutrition. It indicates a need for a comprehensive nutritional assessment and a survey of underlying diseases.[31] There is a large body of evidence demonstrating that oral supplementation results in mortality reductions and improved nutritional status.[34] Therefore, in most cases, the first line of treatment is to supplement orally with a high-density, high-protein formula in combination with positive environmental conditions.[6] The usual formula supplies 240 to 360 calories and 10 to 14 g of protein (20% or greater) per 240 mL can.[7,19]

Other measures include monitoring the consistency of food, learning patient preferences, determining favorite mealtimes, selecting preferred dietary supplements, and assessing the ability to self-feed and susceptibility to distractions.[19] As these characteristics become known, feedings can be modified according to the desires of the individual. Frequent small servings of food are preferred to larger servings that may be overwhelming and cause symptoms.[29] If supplemental snacks are used, they should be provided between meals so as not to decrease intake at mealtime.[7] Liquid supplements are preferable to solid supplements because of faster emptying times.[29] In a study of nursing home residents over a 2-month period, oral supplementation was associated with increased body weight and nutritional status in most malnourished patients, as well as in those at risk for malnutrition. In addition, the supplements chosen were convenient and well accepted.[2]

Patients who do not respond to oral supplementation may benefit from the relaxation of dietary restrictions instituted for an underlying disease.[7] Removing dietary limitations, even in diabetes, while continuing to monitor blood sugar levels, is sometimes necessary and acceptable.[29] Adding flavor enhancers that amplify the intensity of food

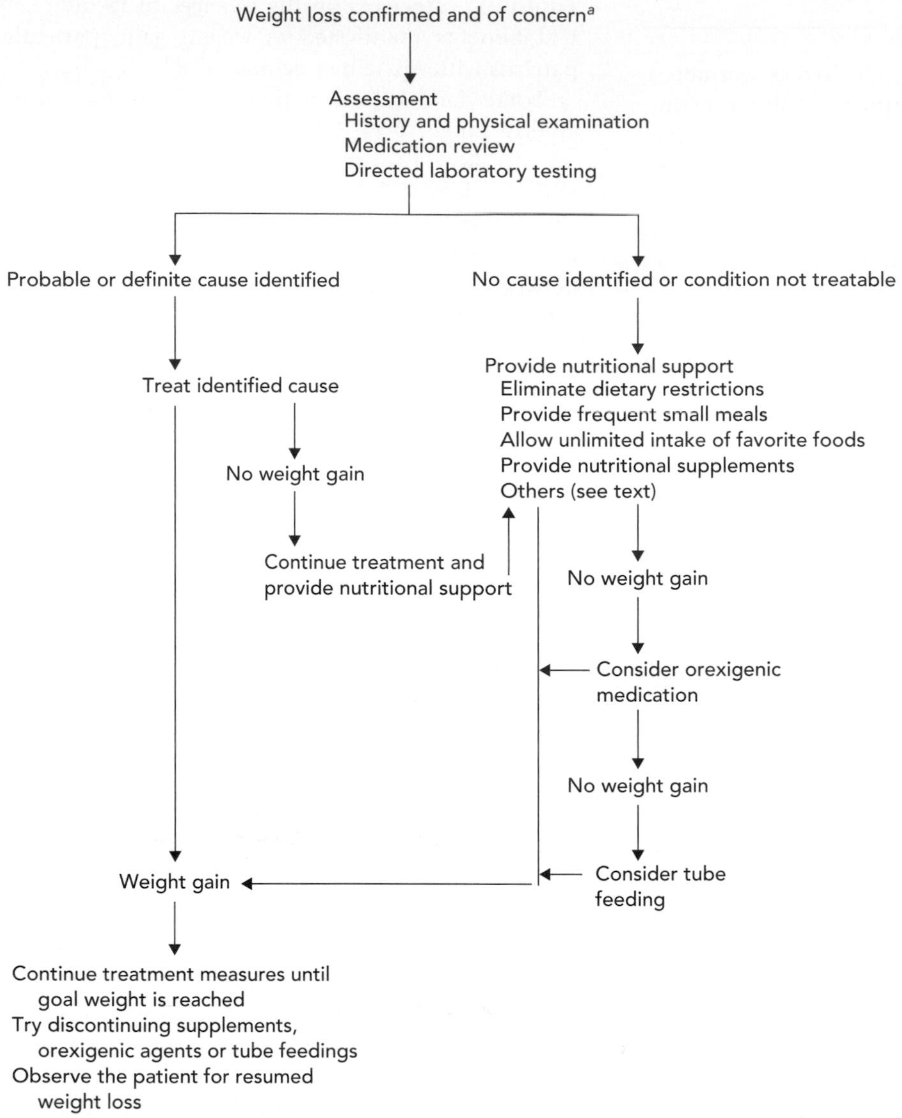

[a]Weight loss of concern is generally defined in several ways: (i) Loss of 5% to 10% of body weight in the previous 1 to 12 months or (ii) loss of 2.25 kg (5 lb) in the previous 3 months. Nursing home guidelines require evaluation if there is a 10% loss in the previous 6 months, a 5% loss in the previous month or a 2% loss in the previous week.

Figure 10.1 An approach to the management of the elderly patient with weight loss. (Huffman GB. Evaluating and treating unintentional weight loss in the elderly. *Am Fam Physician.* 2002;65(4):640–651).

odor in patients with hyposmia can be useful.[14,29] The addition of flavorings such as roast beef, ham, natural bacon, and cheese show short-term benefits.[2] Limited evidence suggests a potential benefit of creatine, especially when combined with exercise.[2] ω-3 Fatty acids in supplemental form alter cyclo-oxygenase and lipo-oxygenase activity and inhibit cytokine production. They too have been shown to be helpful.[2]

Tube Feeding

Tube feeding (either temporary or permanent) should be considered only for those patients unable to ingest sufficient calories orally.[7] Family members should understand that feeding tubes have risks and benefits. They are not a panacea because there is evidence showing that elderly demented persons given adequate calories in this manner may not gain weight.[19,29,35] Tube feedings neither prevent aspiration nor reduce suffering and may actually prolong suffering in patients with terminal diseases.[36,37] A unique complication of tube feeding in older adults is postprandial hypotension. The release of a vasodilator peptide from the gut after a bolus feeding may cause syncope and falls.[13] If tube feedings are to be considered, percutaneous endoscopic gastrostomy is the most successful methodology[2] (Evidence Level B).

Tube feeding formulas vary according to a patient's specific needs, and numerous brand names are available. Simple blenderized foods may be appropriate for patients

Last name:____________ First name:____________ Middle initial:_____Sex:_____Date:________

Age:__________ Weight (kg):__________Height (cm):__________

Complete the form by writing the points in the boxes. Add the points in the boxes, and compare the total assessment to the malnutrition indicator score.[a]

Anthropometric assessment **Points**

1. Body mass index (weight in kg ÷ [height in m]^2):
- a. <19 = 0 points
- b. 19 to <21 = 1 point
- c. 21 to <23 = 2 points
- d. >23 = 3 points

☐

2. Midarm circumference:
- a. <21 cm = 0 points
- b. 21 to ≤22 cm = 0.5 point
- c. >22 cm = 1 point

☐

3. Calf circumference:
- a. <31 cm = 0 points
- b. ≥31 cm = 1 point

☐

4. Weight loss during past 3 months:
- a. >3 kg = 0 points
- b. Does not know = 1 point
- c. 1 to 3 kg = 2 points
- d. No weight loss = 3 points

☐

General assessment

5. Lives independently (not in a nursing home or hospital):
- a. No = 0 points
- b. Yes = 1 point

☐

6. Takes more than three prescription drugs per day:
- a. Yes = 0 points
- b. No = 1 point

☐

7. Has suffered psychological stress or acute disease in the past 3 months:
- a. Yes = 0 points
- b. No = 1 point

☐

8. Mobility:
- a. Bed-bound or chair-bound = 0 points
- b. Able to get out of bed or chair, but does not go out = 1 point
- c. Goes out = 2 points

☐

9. Neuropsychologic problems:
- a. Severe dementia or depression = 0 points
- b. Mild dementia = 1 point
- c. No psychological problems = 2 points

☐

10. Pressure sores or skin ulcers:
- a. Yes = 0 points
- b. No = 1 point

☐

Dietary assessment

11. How many full meals does the patient eat daily?
- a. One meal = 0 points
- b. Two meals = 1 point
- c. Three meals = 2 points

☐

Points

12. Selected consumption markers for protein intake:
- a. At least one serving of dairy products (milk, cheese, yogurt) per day: ☐Yes ☐No
- b. Two or more servings of legumes or eggs per week: ☐Yes ☐No
- c. Meat, fish, or poultry every day: ☐Yes ☐No

0 or 1 yes answers = 0 points
2 yes answers = 0.5 point
3 yes answers = 1 point

☐

13. Consumes two or more servings of fruits or vegetables per day:
- a. No = 0 points
- b. Yes = 1 point

☐

14. Decline in food intake over the past 3 months because of loss of appetite, digestive problems, or chewing or swallowing difficulties:
- a. Severe loss of appetite = 0 points
- b. Moderate loss of appetite = 1 point
- c. No loss of appetite = 2 points

☐

15. Cups of fluid (e.g., water, juice, coffee, tea, milk) consumed per day (1 cup = 8 oz):
- a. <3 cups = 0 points
- b. 3 to 5 cups = 0.5 point
- c. >5 cups = 1 point

☐

16. Mode of feeding:
- a. Needs assistance to eat = 0 points
- b. Self-fed with some difficulty = 1 point
- c. Self-fed with no problems = 2 points

☐

Self-assessment

17. Does the patient think that he or she has nutritional problems?
- a. Major malnutrition = 0 points
- b. Moderate malnutrition or does not know = 1 point
- c. No nutritional problem = 2 points

☐

18. How does the patient view his or her health status compared with the health status of other people of the same age?
- a. Not as good = 0 points
- b. Does not know = 0.5 point
- c. As good = 1 point
- d. Better = 2 points

☐

Assessment total (maximum of 30 points): ☐[a]

[a]Malnutrition indicator score: ≥24 points = well nourished; 17 to 23.5 points = at risk for malnutrition; <17 points = malnourished.

Figure 10.2 Mini Nutritional Assessment. (Adapted with permission from Guigoz Y, Vellas B, Garry PJ. Assessing the nutritional status of the elderly: The Mini Nutritional Assessment as part of the geriatric evaluation. *Nutr Rev.* 1996;54:S59–S65).

with otherwise intact gastrointestinal tracts. Over the counter nutritional supplements may be easier to use. There are also formulations for patients with lactose intolerance. Patients with hypertonic or hypotonic states or with a need for greater protein supplementation may benefit from formulations specifically developed for these conditions.

Environmental Factors

Improvements in the environment can have a positive effect on feeding behaviors.[2] Increases in intake can be facilitated through providing companionship at mealtimes, optimizing preparation for taste and presentation, administering medications with meals to minimize adverse effects, avoiding gas-forming foods and beverages, managing bowel movements to avoid constipation and diarrhea, increasing physical activity to stimulate appetite and improve one's sense of well-being, and promoting oral health.[7] Easily distractible people should be somewhat isolated during mealtimes. Those who cannot self-feed require feeding assistance from staff or other caregivers.[19] The contributions of dietitians for specific nutritional guidance, speech therapists for treating dysphagia and related swallowing disorders, and social services personnel cannot be overestimated.[14,29]

Physical Activity

Physical therapy and activity should be encouraged to promote appetite and food intake.[29] The most promising intervention for increased muscle mass and strength in older persons is progressive resistance training, with a number of studies showing improved muscle mass, strength, balance, and endurance in older adults.[2] Strength training and protein-calorie supplementation were more likely to increase calories consumed than protein-calorie supplementation alone.[2] Habitual physical activity is more effective in the prevention of overweight than it is in the promotion of weight loss.[34] Even among frail older people, a physically active lifestyle can minimize the weight loss that often accompanies chronic disease, thereby maintaining some degree of health and function toward the end of one's lifespan.[34]

Medications and Weight Loss

Medications can cause nausea or vomiting, anorexia, dysgeusia, and dysphagia, and as a consequence, they need to be reviewed and, where indicated, discontinued.[14] Antihistamines, captopril, allopurinol, carbamazepine, levodopa, and digoxin have potentially adverse effects.[13] A review of all psychoactive medications should be undertaken because their potential to provoke weight loss may exceed their value in treating depression or other psychiatric disorders.[14]

Medications available to treat weight loss fall into two categories: Those that have U.S. Food and Drug Administration (FDA) approval for the treatment of conditions that may contribute to weight loss and those that are orexigenic and facilitate weight gain (see Table 10.3). The former category includes medications to treat conditions such as depression, peptic ulcer disease, gastroesophageal reflux disease, and constipation. Antidepressants, histamine

TABLE 10.3
OREXIGENIC MEDICATIONS

Medication	Dose	Side Effects
Mirtazapine	15 mg at h.s.	Orthostatic hypotension, worsening depression, hypomania, mania
Cyproheptadine	2 mg q.i.d.	Blurry vision, dry mouth, urinary retention, constipation, tachycardia, delirium
Megestrol acetate	200–400 mg b.i.d. (maximum 800 mg/d)	Adrenal insufficiency diabetes, deep vein thrombosis
Dronabinol	2.5 mg b.i.d. (maximum 10 mg/d)	Somnolence, dizziness, euphoria
Growth hormone	20 μg/kg three times a wk	Edema, carpal tunnel syndrome, diabetes, gynecomastia
Testosterone	100 mg injection/wk	Liver toxicity, gastrointestinal symptoms, contraindicated in men with prostate cancer and in women
Methylphenidate	2.5 mg b.i.d. (maximum 10 mg/d)	Arrhythmias, insomnia, nervousness

Adapted from Moriguti JC, Uemura Moriguti EK, Ferriolli E, et al. Involuntary weight loss in elderly individuals: Assessment and treatment. *Sao Paulo Med J.* 2001;119(2):72–77; Gazewood JD, Mehr DR. Diagnosis and management of weight loss in the elderly. *J Fam Pract.* 1998;47(1):19–25; Golden AG, Daiello LA, Silverman MA, et al. University of Miami division of clinical pharmacology therapeutic rounds: Medications used to treat anorexia in the frail elderly. *Am J Ther.* 2003;10(4):292–298.

blockers, proton pump inhibitors, metoclopramide, and medications used for the prevention of constipation are approved for the uses for which they are intended and have a risk profile that is well understood. On the other hand, and with the possible exception of mirtazapine, the orexigenic drugs have not been extensively studied in the elderly, have risk benefit profiles that require careful consideration, may have life-threatening side effects, and may not have been approved for use as an appetite stimulant by the FDA.[7,29]

Weight loss and depression are often intertwined.[24] Elevated circulating levels of cytokines have been observed in depressed individuals. ILs and TNFs are inhibited in individuals treated with tricyclic antidepressants.[24] The SSRIs and tricyclics have been extensively studied with regard to their effect on weight. SSRIs have been associated with initial weight loss (Evidence Level B). The benefits of tricyclics (Evidence Level B) may be offset by their anticholinergic side effects. Mirtazapine, an antidepressant with both noradrenergic and serotonergic properties, has been associated with increased appetite and weight gain and less nausea than the SSRIs (Evidence Level A).[16]

Given the known benefits, a trial of antidepressants should be considered for patients with weight loss and depression. Mirtazapine and traditional tricyclic antidepressants, if deemed safe, may be used. SSRIs should be avoided.[13,29]

Use of any of the following medications should be undertaken with care and only after a discussion with the patient and/or family member because they have not been widely studied in the elderly and are not FDA approved for the purpose of stimulating appetite.

Progestational agents such as megestrol acetate have been shown to stimulate appetite, produce weight gain, and decrease cytokine levels in patients with cancer wasting and acquired immunodeficiency syndrome (Evidence Level C).[2] In one study of patients with geriatric wasting, 12 weeks of treatment with megestrol improved appetite and induced weight gain. Megestrol also increased levels of prealbumin, albumin, and fat-free mass.[24] Another study in the frail elderly noted no weight gain but did demonstrate an increase in appetite and improvement in depressive symptoms.[16] Dosing ranges from 80 to 800 mg per day.[16,19,29] Megestrol should be discontinued if no effect on appetite is seen by 8 weeks.[1] Side effects include adrenal insufficiency, diabetes, and deep vein thrombosis.[16]

Dronabinol is a synthetic cannabinoid that has been shown to decrease nausea, improve appetite, and result in weight gain in patients with HIV. In a study of patients with Alzheimer disease, body weight increased but CNS side effects included somnolence, dizziness, euphoria, paranoid reactions, and "feeling high." The starting dose is 2.5 mg twice a day (before lunch and supper). Most patients respond with a maximum daily dose of 10 mg twice per day (Evidence Level C).[16,29]

Growth hormone and testosterone have been evaluated as orexigenic agents. Several short-term studies involving treatment with growth hormone in doses of 20 μg per kg subcutaneously three times per week resulted in body weight increases (Evidence Level B). Risks for chronic use include carpal tunnel syndrome, edema, arthralgias, gynecomastia, and diabetes, with one study showing increased mortality.[16] Because serum testosterone levels decrease in aging and systemic illnesses, supplementation has been attempted. Increases in lean muscle mass through protein synthesis and exercise performance have been shown to occur with doses equivalent to 100 mg of testosterone in weekly injections. Its use is contraindicated in carcinoma of the prostate, is controversial in women, and is associated with liver toxicity and gastrointestinal symptoms.[16] Testosterone needs more study before being recommended for the treatment of malnutrition and cachexia.[1]

Cyproheptadine is the oldest orexigenic medication. It is an antihistamine and a serotonin agonist. It has been studied largely in pediatric patients. The presence of anticholinergic side effects, which may cause blurry vision, dry mouth, urinary retention, constipation, tachycardia, and delirium in older adults, call into question its utility.[16,29] Methylphenidate is not recommended for long-term use but can be administered beginning at 2.5 mg per day up to 5 mg twice daily so long as heart rate is below 100 beats per minute.[19] Antipsychotic medications such as risperidone, olanzapine, and quetiapine should be used primarily to treat the behavioral consequences of psychosis and dementia and not as orexigenic agents despite evidence that weight gain may occur when they are prescribed.[16] Other medications that are being studied include the use of pentoxifylline, thalidomide, and melatonin.

Certain macronutrients that may promote anabolism, such as glutamine, arginine, and ω-3 fatty acids through the inhibition of proinflammatory cytokines with decreased levels of TNFs, are also receiving attention.[1,2]

CONCLUSION

The management of weight loss in the elderly is surprisingly complex, challenging, and often frustrating. Success requires that the clinician consider the whole person to resist the distraction of focusing on the management of chronic diseases at the expense of overall well-being. This concept of wholeness includes the physical, social, and emotional environment in which the individual lives. There is very good evidence that early nutritional supplementation reduces the potential for morbidity and mortality. The powerful and almost overarching role of depression cannot be overlooked in both the assessment and treatment of weight loss.

Because the treatment approaches range from the nearly innocuous to the relatively aggressive, it is the role of the clinician to inform the patient and family members of risks and benefits throughout any treatment program. In addition to the problems associated with weight loss, an understanding of the dynamics that lead to this condition generates a compelling argument for promoting wellness, as manifested through healthy levels of physical activity and societal engagement for all but the most compromised individuals. The adverse effects of a sedentary and intellectually unengaged existence clearly erode the essential and necessary life force of aging persons, increasing their vulnerability to disease and debilitation that may ultimately manifest weight loss.

ACKNOWLEDGMENT

I would like to acknowledge the assistance of Ms. Veronica Ruleford in the preparation of this text.

REFERENCES

1. Wallace JI, Schwartz RS. Epidemiology of weight loss in humans with special reference to wasting in the elderly. *Int J Cardiol.* 2002;85:15–21.
2. Bales CW, Ritchie CS. Sarcopenia, weight loss, and nutritional frailty in the elderly. *Annu Rev Nutr.* 2002;22:309–323.
3. Poehlman ET. Working group session report: Wasting in geriatrics and special consideration in design of trials involving the elderly subjects. *J Nutr.* 1999;129(1):308S–310S.
4. Guyonnet S, Nourhashemi F, Ousset PJ, et al. Factors associated with weight loss in Alzheimer's disease. *J Nutr Health Aging.* 1998;2(2):107–109.
5. Ritchie CS, Joshipura K, Silliman RA, et al. Oral health problems and significant weight loss among community-dwelling older adults. *J Gerontol Sci Med Sci.* 2000;55A(7):M366–M371.
6. Holm B, Soderhamn O. Factors associated with nutritional status in a group of people in an early stage of dementia. *Clin Nutr.* 2003;22(4):385–389.
7. Bouras EP, Lange SM, Scolapio JS. Rational approach to patients with unintentional weight loss. *Mayo Clin Proc.* 2001;76:923–929.
8. Poehlman ET, Dvorak RV. Energy expenditure, energy intake, and weight loss in Alzheimer disease. *Am J Clin Nutr.* 2000;71(2):650S–655S.
9. Centers for Disease and Control and the Merck Institute of Aging and Health.The state of aging and health in America. 2004; www.cdc.gov/aging.
10. Payette H, Coulombe C, Boutier V, et al. Weight loss and mortality among free-living frail ELDERS: A prospective study. *J Gerontol Sci Med Sci.* 1999;54A(9):M440–M445.
11. Wang PN, Yang CL, Lin KN, et al. A Controlled Study. Weight loss, nutritional status and physical activity in patients with Alzheimer's disease.. *J Neurol.* 2004;251:314–320.
12. Weyant RJ, Newman AB, Kritchevsky SB, et al. Periodontal disease and weight loss in older adults. *J Am Geriatr Soc.* 2004;52:547–553.
13. Moriguti JC, Uemura Moriguti EK, Ferriolli E, et al. Involuntary weight loss in elderly individuals: Assessment and treatment. *Sao Paulo Med J.* 2001;119(2):72–77.
14. Gazewood JD, Mehr DR. Diagnosis and management of weight loss in the elderly. *J Fam Pract.* 1998;47(1):19–25.
15. Roubenoff R. The pathophysiology of wasting in the elderly. *J Nutr.* 1999;129(1):256S–259S.
16. Golden AG, Daiello LA, Silverman MA, et al. University of Miami division of clinical pharmacology therapeutic rounds: Medications used to treat anorexia in the frail elderly. *Am J Ther.* 2003;10(4):292–298.
17. Sergi G, Coin A, Bussolott M, et al. Influence of fat-free mass and functional status on resting energy expenditure in underweight elders. *J Gerontol Sci Med Sci.* 2002;57A(5):M302–M307.
18. Wannamethee SG, Shaper AG, Whincup PH, et al. Characteristics of older men who lose weight intentionally or unintentionally. *Am J Epidemiol.* 2000;151(7):667–675.
19. Wang SY. Weight loss and metabolic changes in dementia. *J Nutr Health Aging.* 2002;6(3):201–205.
20. Hernandez JL, Riancho JA, Matorras P, et al. Clinical evaluation for cancer in patients with involuntary weight loss without specific symptoms. *Am J Med.* 2003;114:631–637.
21. Katz S, Ford AB, Moskowitz RW, et al. Studies of Illness in the Aged. The index of ADL: A standardized measure of biological and psychological function. *JAMA.* 1963;185:914–919.
22. Lawton MP, Brody EM. Assessment of older people: Self-maintaining and instrumental activities of daily living. *Gerontologist.* 1969;9:179–186.
23. Agostini JV, Han L, Tinetti ME. The relationship between number of medications and weight loss or impaired balance in older adults. *J Am Geriatr Soc.* 2004;52:1719–1723.
24. Yeh S, Wu SY, Levine DM, et al. Quality of life and stimulation of weight gain after treatment with megestrol acetate: Correlation between cytokine levels and nutritional status, appetite in geriatric patients with wasting syndrome. *J Nutr Health Aging.* 2000;4(4):246–251.
25. Gelato MC, Frost RA. IGFBP-3 functional and structural implications in aging and wasting syndromes. *Endocrine.* 1997;7(1):81–85.
26. Coin A, Sergi G, Beninca P, et al. Bone mineral density and body composition in underweight and normal elderly subjects. *Osteoporos Int.* 2000;11:1043–1050.
27. Ensrud KE, Ewing SK, Stone KL, et al. The Study of Osteoporotic Fractures Research Group. Intentional and unintentional weight loss increase bone loss and hip fracture risk in older women. *J Am Geriatr Soc.* 2003;51:1740–1747.
28. Lankisch PG, Gerzmann M, Gerzmann JF, et al. Unintentional weight loss: diagnosis and prognosis. The first prospective follow-up study from a secondary referral centre. *J Intern Med.* 2001;249:41–46.
29. Huffman GB. Evaluating and treating unintentional weight loss in the elderly. *Am Fam Physician.* 2002;65(4):640–651.
30. Riviere S, Gillette-Guyonnet S, Voisin T, et al. A nutritional education program could prevent weight loss and slow cognitive decline in Alzheimer's disease. *J Nutr Health Aging.* 2001;5(4):295–299.
31. Vellas B, Guigoz Y, Garry P, et al. The Mini Nutritional Assessment (MNA) and its use in grading the nutritional state of elderly patients. *Nutrition.* 1999;15(2):116–122.
32. Corbett CF, Crogan NL, Short RA. Using the minimum data set to predict weight loss in nursing home residents. *Appl Nurs Res.* 2002;15(4):249–253.
33. Wedick NM, Barrett-Connor E, Knoke JD, et al. The relationship between weight loss and all-cause mortality in older men and women with and without diabetes mellitus: The Rancho Bernardo Study. *J Am Geriatr Soc.* 2002;50:1810–1815.
34. Dziura J, Mendes de Leon C, Kasl S, et al. The Yale Health and Aging Study 1982–1994. Can physical activity attenuate aging-related weight loss in older people? *Am J Epidemiol.* 2004;159(8):759–767.
35. Potter JM. Oral supplements in the elderly. *Curr Opin Clin Nutr Metab Care.* 2001;4:21–28.
36. Winter SM. Terminal nutrition: framing the debate for the withdrawal of nutritional support ins terminally Ill patients. *Am J Med.* 2000;109(9):723–726.
37. Gillick MR. Rethinking the role of tube feeding in patients with advanced dementia. *N Engl J Med.* 2000;342(3):206–210.

Visual Impairment in the Elderly

11

Shariar Farzad David Sarraf Anne L. Coleman

- CLINICAL PEARLS 121
- REFRACTIVE ERROR AND CATARACT 122
- AGE-RELATED MACULAR DEGENERATION 123
- DIABETIC RETINOPATHY 125
- RETINAL VENOUS OCCLUSIVE DISEASE 126
- RETINAL ARTERIAL OCCLUSIVE DISEASE 128
- GLAUCOMA 129
- ANTERIOR ISCHEMIC OPTIC NEUROPATHY 130
- RED EYE 131
- EYELID PROBLEMS 131
- HERPES ZOSTER 131
- LOW-VISION REHABILITATION 132
- ACKNOWLEDGMENT 132

CLINICAL PEARLS

- Visual impairment affects 20% to 30% of persons aged 75 and older.
- Cataracts and refractive error are common; both are correctable, and correction improves quality of life.
- The dry form of age-related macular degeneration is common and antioxidant multivitamins may slow progression.
- The wet form of macular degeneration is the most common cause of blindness in the elderly and may respond to laser surgery or antiangiogenesis inhibitors.
- Glaucoma is the most common cause of blindness in the elderly African American population.
- Screening for glaucoma should take place every 1 to 2 years after age 50.
- Elevated intraocular pressure is not an absolute diagnostic criteria for glaucoma.
- Therapies aim to reduce intraocular pressure, protecting the optic disc and preserving visual fields.

Visual impairment, defined as visual acuity <20/40, increases exponentially with age, such that 20% to 30% of the population at age 75 years is affected (see Table 11.1 for a summary of the conditions that cause vision loss in the elderly). Blindness (visual acuity of 20/200 or worse) affects 2% of the population aged 75 years and older. Those aged 65 and older make up 12% of the US population, but they constitute 50% of the blind population. Cataract, age-related macular degeneration (ARMD), diabetic retinopathy, and glaucoma are the most common causes of blindness.

Among all office visits by older persons, 14% are to ophthalmologists, one of the highest rates among all specialty visits. Falls and car crashes, both associated with impaired vision, consume considerable medical resources. Impaired vision is linked to deterioration in the quality of life and in the activities of daily living of older persons.

The American Academy of Ophthalmology recommends a comprehensive eye examination every 1 to 2 years for

TABLE 11.1
SUMMARY OF CONDITIONS THAT CAUSE VISION LOSS IN THE ELDERLY (ICD-9 CODES)

Acute Painless	Acute Painful	Subacute and Chronic
Wet form ARMD (CNV) (362.52)	Primary angle closure glaucoma (365.20)	Nuclear sclerotic cataracts (366.19)
Vitreous hemorrhage (as in proliferative diabetic retinopathy) (362.02)	Secondary angle closure glaucoma (365.20) (e.g., neovascular glaucoma)	Cortical cataracts (366.19)
Central retinal vein occlusion (362.35)	Iritis (364.3)	Posterior subcapsular cataracts (366.19)
Branch retinal vein occlusion (362.35)	Iridocyclitis (364.3)	Atrophic ARMD (362.51)
Central retinal artery occlusion (444.9)	Corneal ulcer (370.0)	Diabetic macular edema (362.01)
Branch retinal artery occlusion (444.9)	Arteritic ischemic optic neuropathy (446.5) (e.g., temporal arteritis)	Diabetic macular ischemia (362.01)
Nonarteritic anterior ischemic optic neuropathy (362.51)	Herpes zoster keratitis (053.2)	Primary open-angle glaucoma (365.11)
Retinal detachment (361.00)	Herpes zoster uveitis (053.2)	Normal tension glaucoma (365.12)

ARMD, age-related macular degeneration; CNV, choroidal neovascularization.

persons aged 65 and older. The U.S. Preventive Services Task Force recommends annual vision testing. One third of all new cases of blindness can be avoided with effective use of available ophthalmologic services.

REFRACTIVE ERROR AND CATARACT

The two leading causes of visual impairment worldwide are refractive error and cataract, for which eyeglasses and surgical cataract extraction, respectively, are mainstays of treatment. Despite the considerable successes of these therapeutic options, many people do not receive adequate treatment for these problems.

Refractive error may be categorized as emmetropia (neutral refraction), ametropia, or presbyopia. Three forms of ametropia exist: Myopia (nearsightedness), hyperopia (farsightedness), and astigmatism (distorted vision).

Typically, older patients demonstrate increasing hyperopia, unless a cataract is present, which can induce a myopic shift. Although contact lens and laser refractive surgery are available for myopic and hyperopic refractive errors, these alternative forms of treatment have traditionally been used by younger persons.

After the age of approximately 40, emmetropic persons begin to develop progressive presbyopia, impaired ability to focus on near objects that is caused by gradual hardening of the lens and decreased muscular effectiveness of the ciliary body. Reading glasses or bifocal eyeglasses may be prescribed.

Monovision with laser *in situ* keratomileusis (LASIK) is currently an option for presbyopic or pre-presbyopic patients seeking refractive surgery. This procedure corrects one eye for reading while the fellow eye is corrected for distance. Implantation of an anterior chamber multifocal intraocular lens after cataract surgery is another option for the correction of presbyopia. Finally, a new form of surgery under investigation uses an expansion of the sclera in the ciliary body region adjacent to the equator of the lens, which allows the ciliary body greater ability to change the anterior curvature of the lens as an accommodation to delay the onset of presbyopia.

Cataracts (vision reducing lens opacities) occur in 20% of persons aged 65 years and 50% aged 75 years and older. Cataracts may be associated with increased glare, decreased contrast sensitivity, and decreased visual acuity. Several risk factors have been reported: Decreased vitamin intake, light (ultraviolet B) exposure, smoking, alcohol use, long-term corticosteroid use, and diabetes mellitus. The most important risk factor is increased age.[1] Different types of cataracts present with distinct effects on visual acuity. The three main types of age-related cataracts are nuclear, cortical, and posterior subcapsular cataracts.[2] Often, patients have more than one type of cataract.

Nuclear cataracts appear as yellowing and sclerosis of the lens nucleus, best distinguished on slit lamp examination. In a primary care setting, the direct ophthalmoscope can be used from an arm's length distance to judge for dimming of the red reflex caused by a central opacity in the lens. Nuclear cataracts are usually bilateral but exhibit varying degrees of asymmetry. They are slowly progressive and tend to cause greater impairment of distance vision than of near vision. Patients can present with a myopic shift in their refraction, permitting previously presbyopic individuals to read without reading glasses ("second sight"). Progressive yellowing of the lens causes decreased contrast sensitivity manifested by poor penetration of visible light onto the retina.

It is important to note that no degree of cataract will cause a Marcus Gunn pupil. Patients who present with more insidious onset of vision loss and a relative afferent pupillary defect warrant a more thorough ophthalmic examination to assess the health of the optic nerve and retina.

Cortical cataracts present early with formation of vacuoles and water clefts in the anterior and posterior lens cortex. These vacuoles can best be seen with a slit lamp on retroillumination or by using a direct ophthalmoscope to obtain a red reflex from an arm's length distance. As cortical changes progress, white wedge-shaped opacities, known as *cortical spokes*, can be seen at the lens periphery, projecting to the center of the lens. On retroillumination using a direct ophthalmoscope, the cortical spokes appear as shadows obscuring the red reflex. In more advanced cases, the peripheral cortical opacities can coalesce to involve the entire lens cortex, giving the lens a diffuse white and opaque appearance. Cortical cataracts are usually bilateral but tend to be more asymmetric than nuclear cataracts. They have greater variability in their rate of progression, and their effect on visual acuity depends on the location of the cortical opacity. Glare is commonly associated with cortical cataracts, as manifested by decreased vision when staring at a light source such as a car headlight. Less commonly, cortical cataracts can be the source of monocular diplopia.

Posterior subcapsular cataracts first present with a subtle sheen in the posterior cortical layers visible only by slit lamp examination. More advanced stages exhibit granular and plaque-like opacities on the posterior subcapsular cortex, which are best seen with retroillumination using a slit lamp or a direct ophthalmoscope. This type of cataract is more often seen in younger patients than in those with advanced nuclear or cortical cataracts. In addition to its age-related etiologies, it can also be associated with systemic or topical corticosteroid use, history of ocular inflammation, trauma, or exposure to ionizing radiation. Patients with posterior subcapsular cataracts often complain of glare and poor vision in bright settings. This is secondary to constriction of the pupil, which narrows the visual axis to that provided by the central cataractous lens.

When evaluating a patient with cataracts, a physician should objectively measure visual acuity. Distance vision using a Snellen chart as well as near vision using a reading card should both be checked. In a patient with cataracts, pinhole distance visual acuity is often better than that obtained with best refractive correction. In cases of posterior subcapsular and cortical cataracts, distance vision should be checked with the application of a light source directed at the patient's eyes to measure visual impairment caused by glare. The next step is correlation of the degree of media opacity with the degree of visual impairment.

In addition to careful examination of the macula and the optic nerve, a careful history detailing the time course of vision loss and the patient's baseline visual function is important. The main objective of this step is determining that the patient's eye is healthy enough to expect improved visual function after cataract surgery. Finally, consideration must be given to the patient's overall health and ability to undergo surgery, in addition to his/her ability to participate in postoperative care.

Cataract extraction is one of the most successful surgeries in medicine (90% of patients achieve vision of 20/40 or better). Approximately 1.5 million cataract procedures are performed each year in the United States alone. In inner cities and underdeveloped countries such as India, the demand for surgery has surpassed available resources.

Cataract extraction is safe and can be completed in <15 minutes under local or topical anesthesia. The surgery involves the sonographic breakdown and aspiration of the lens (phacoemulsification) through a 3 to 4 mm limbal (corneoscleral junction) incision. An artificial implant (intraocular lens) is placed in the capsular bag that is the only remnant of the native lens retained. A secondary laser procedure (capsulotomy) may be necessary to ablate subsequent capsular opacification that develops in 15% of patients. Typically, patients will require spectacles only for reading postoperatively, although the U.S. Food and Drug Administration (FDA) has recently approved the use of multifocal lens implants that may negate the use of glasses altogether.

AGE-RELATED MACULAR DEGENERATION

ARMD is the most common cause of blindness in older persons throughout the developed world. Approximately 1 in 27 Americans (10 million people) have reduced vision due to ARMD. Increased age is the most important risk factor, although a genetic predisposition also contributes. Other risk factors include smoking and hypertension. Fair-skinned persons are at greater risk of developing this disease than those who are black, in whom pigment may serve as a protective element.

Severe vision loss or central visual blindness is typically caused by the wet form of ARMD, defined by the presence of a choroidal neovascular membrane (CNVM). Less commonly, geographic atrophy of the retinal pigment epithelium (RPE) within the macular region noted in the late stage of the dry form of ARMD may explain the severe vision loss. The natural history of CNVM is progressive subfoveal growth with leakage, bleeding, and eventual fibrotic scarring, leading to central blindness.

The most common form of ARMD is the dry type characterized by drusen, which appear clinically as dull yellow deposits located in the submacular compartment deep to the retinal vessels (see Fig. 11.1). Drusen are classified by their number, size, and confluence. The presence of CNVM in the fellow eye and numerous, large confluent drusen represent the greatest risk for progression to the wet form of ARMD. Associated with the presence of drusen, RPE mottling or atrophy is a hallmark of the dry form of ARMD. Clinically, mottling of the RPE appears as a focal or geographic area of pigment clumping and depigmentation in the retina. Geographic atrophy is denoted by a large central and circumscribed area of RPE atrophy that exposes the underlying choroidal vessels. This type of atrophy represents the late stage of ARMD and can cause central blindness although CNVM is absent and the macula is dry.

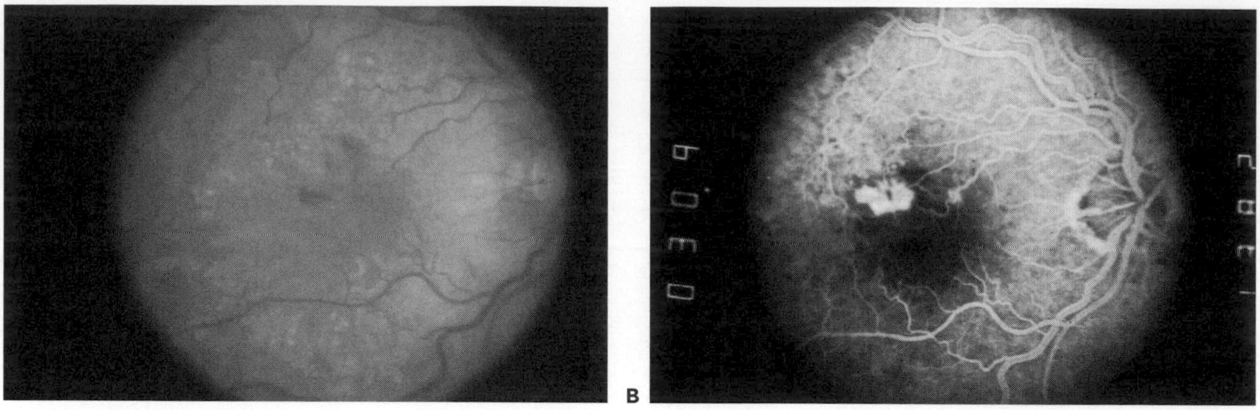

A B

Figure 11.1 **A:** Acute wet form age-related macular degeneration with subretinal hemorrhage and scattered large drusen. **B:** Fluorescein angiogram exhibiting a choroidal neovascular membrane corresponding to the previously noted area of intraretinal hemorrhage. (See color insert.)

It is important to identify the clinical markers for CNVM, which include subretinal heme, subretinal fluid, and the presence of a gray green membrane or pigment ring. On examination, subretinal heme can be differentiated from intraretinal heme by its deeper location with regard to the retinal vessels (Fig. 11.1). The end stage of the wet form of ARMD shows cicatrization or fibrotic proliferation known as a *disciform scar*, which clinically appears as an elevated white lesion in the macula (see Fig. 11.2).

In a primary care setting, patients older than age 50 with no prior diagnosis of ARMD who present with clinical markers of dry form ARMD should be referred to an ophthalmologist for routine monitoring on the basis of the stage of the disease. Early dry form ARMD warrants annual funduscopic examination, while the later stages of dry form ARMD require biannual examination.

The Age-Related Eye Disease Study (AREDS) found that the risk for the development of CNVM could be reduced by 25% when patients with high-risk drusen (numerous and large) are treated with high-dose multivitamin supplementation.[3] A combination multivitamin supplement containing β-carotene 25,000 IU, vitamin E 400 IU, vitamin C 500 mg, and zinc 80 mg is available as an over-the-counter preparation (Bausch and Lomb, Ocuvite PreserVision). This vitamin therapy, however, is contraindicated in smokers because of the increased risk of lung cancer due to the high-dose β-carotene component. Patients with the dry form of ARMD should be provided with an Amsler grid, a good home-monitoring tool, to regularly test for metamorphopsia (Evidence Level C). Those who develop sudden distortion or vision loss, signaling the development of CNVM, require urgent ophthalmological evaluation.

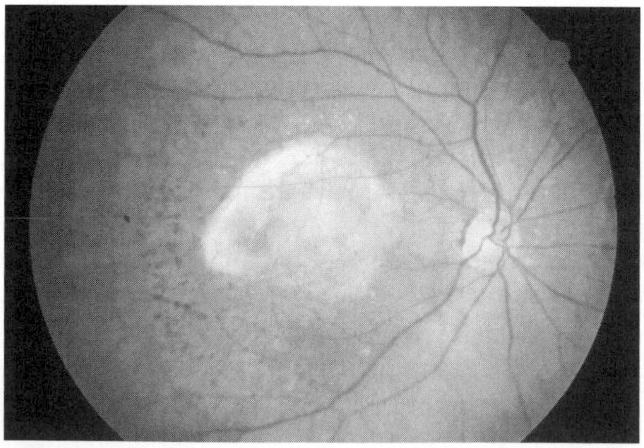

Figure 11.2 End-stage wet form age-related macular degeneration with inactive subretinal fibrosis ("disciform scar"). (See color insert.)

Laser therapy for CNVM has been beneficial, but only in circumstances when membranes are well defined (i.e., the margins of the lesion are clearly delineated on fluorescein angiography) and are extra- or juxtafoveal. The benefits of this therapy are limited, as 50% to 75% of lesions recur after laser therapy. Photodynamic therapy using porphyrin-derived dyes has been shown to be useful in those patients with subfoveal CNVM in whom conventional laser therapy will destroy the fovea. According to the Treatment of ARMD with Photodynamic therapy (TAP) study, 43% of patients receiving photodynamic therapy sustained moderate visual loss ($>$15 letters from baseline) after 1 year of follow-up versus 57% of patients not receiving the photoactivated dye laser treatment. Moreover, 16% of those receiving photoactivated dye laser treatment sustained an improvement in visual acuity while 7% showed improvement in the placebo group. These benefits continued after 2 years of follow-up but required as many as five sessions of photodynamic therapy.[4] Subfoveal membranes that were predominantly classical appeared to have the greatest response to photodynamic therapy, although a later study has shown marginal benefit for the treatment of small, purely occult subfoveal CNVM as well. Overall, the benefits of photodynamic therapy are not overwhelming, but photodynamic therapy is a relatively safe option for delaying vision loss in the wet form of ARMD.

Intravitreal injections of inhibitors to vascular endothelial growth factor (VEGF) have been validated as an adjuvant therapy for the wet form of ARMD (Evidence Level B). FDA approval has recently been obtained for the treatment of wet form ARMD with serial intravitreal injections of pegaptanib sodium (Macugen), an aptamer which blocks the 125 isoform of VEGF. The FDA approval was based on findings from two pivotal phase 2/3 randomized multicenter double-masked clinical trials involving approximately 1,200 patients with all subtypes of neovascular ARMD.[5] Results showed that among patients receiving 0.3 mg of Macugen, 70% lost less than three lines of vision compared with 55% of patients receiving control treatment ($p < 0.0001$), a 27% increased chance of stabilization after the first year. Macugen also helped limit progression to legal blindness by 50% compared to controls. Two-year clinical data from the studies demonstrated a continued treatment benefit with Macugen.

Other VEGF inhibitor therapies include the intravitreal injection of ranibizumab (Lucentis), an antibody fragment that inhibits all isoforms of VEGF, and its intravenous counterpart bevacizumab (Avastin), each of which is presently being investigated by the FDA and holds great promise for the treatment of wet form ARMD.

Another treatment modality for subfoveal CNV currently under investigation, anecortave acetate, targets proteases required for vascular endothelial cell migration. Anecortave acetate, an angiostatic steroid, is administered as a posterior juxtascleral depot application at 6-month intervals. Recent 12-month clinical outcomes have shown the drug to be efficacious in maintaining vision, preventing severe vision loss, and inhibiting subfoveal CNV lesion growth.[6]

Unfortunately, laser therapies and intraocular injections do not exist for the atrophic form of ARMD. RPE and photoreceptor transplantation with or without stem cells have been extensively investigated *in vitro* and in animal models but have not reached the clinical realm.

Numerous genetic conditions resulting in premature macular degeneration exist, for which the mutated sequence has been cloned and the protein product isolated. Mutations in ABCA4 (adenosine triphosphate [ATP]-binding cassette protein of the retina), a photoreceptor protein involved in molecular transport and exchange, leads to the development of Stargardt disease, in which macular drusenoid flecks and atrophy associated with central visual loss develop by the second or third decade of life. Stargardt macular dystrophy has been found to have perhaps some association with the dry or atrophic form of ARMD. Certain populations of patients with ARMD have been found to have an increased incidence of the heterozygous form of this mutation, but the data have been conflicting. Sorsby fundus dystrophy is associated with many of the features of ARMD. Visual loss, however, typically develops before the age of 50. The affected gene has been sequenced and the mutated protein, involved in extracellular remodeling, is TIMP-3 (tissue-inhibitor of metalloprotease-3). However, genetic studies have yet to uncover an association of this mutation with ARMD.

Most recently, much excitement has been generated by published studies from three separate centers that have uncovered as high as a 50% association of the high-risk forms of ARMD with a mutation in the complement factor *H* gene. In individuals homozygous for the risk allele, the likelihood of ARMD was found to be increased by a factor of 7.4. The complement factor *H* gene is located on chromosome 1 in a region that has been repeatedly linked to ARMD in family based studies,[7] and the protein is known to be a regulator of complement activation and may implicate inflammation in the progression of ARMD.

DIABETIC RETINOPATHY

Duration of disease and control of blood sugar represent the most important variables in the development and progression of diabetic retinopathy. After 10 years, 70% of those with type 2 diabetes demonstrate some form of retinopathy, and nearly 10% show proliferative disease. Diet control, exercise, proper glucose management with frequent daily glucose testing, and the use of oral hypoglycemics or insulin, or both, are crucial in maintaining glycosylated hemoglobin levels lower than 7%. The Diabetic Control and Complications Trial demonstrated that tight blood sugar control in patients with type 1 diabetes resulted in a long-lasting decrease in the rate of development and progression of diabetic retinopathy.[8] The UK Prospective Diabetes Study validated these results in the older population with type 2 diabetes. Tight blood-pressure control (140/80) with either β-blockers or angiotensin-converting enzyme inhibitors was also found to be an important factor in decreasing microvascular complications, such as the need for retinal laser therapy. Other systemic risk factors, including kidney function and serum cholesterol, may also influence the course of diabetic retinopathy and should be optimized. Angiotensin-converting enzyme inhibitors have been found to decrease progressive nephropathy in patients with diabetes and may have similar benefits to the retina.[9–12]

Nonproliferative diabetic retinopathy (NPDR) is characterized by retinal microvascular changes in the absence of neovascularization. Clinical findings upon funduscopic examination include microaneurysms, dot-blot intraretinal hemorrhages, retinal hard exudates with or without retinal edema, and nerve fiber layer infarcts (cotton wool spots). The Preferred Practice Patterns Committee of the American Academy of Ophthalmology in 1998 recommended the following timetable for ophthalmologic screening examination of patients with diabetes[13] (Evidence Level C):

1. Annually for no retinopathy or rare microaneurysms
2. Every 9 months for mild NPDR
3. Every 6 months for moderate NPDR

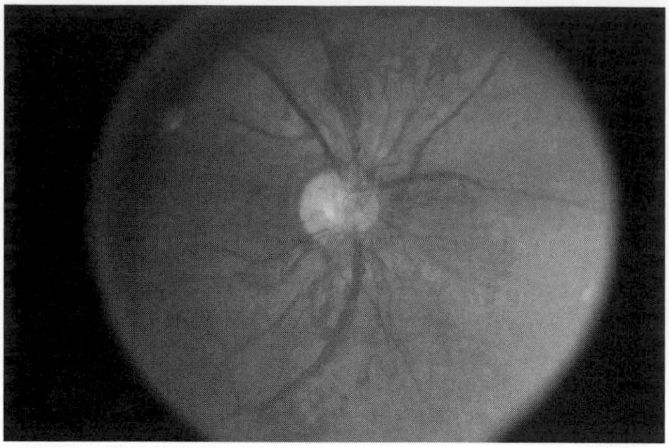

Figure 11.3 Florid neovascularization of the disc in a patient with proliferative diabetic retinopathy. (See color insert.)

Progressive ischemia as evidenced by increasing intraretinal hemorrhages, venous caliber changes such as beading or intraretinal microvascular abnormalities, and capillary nonperfusion on fluorescein angiography characterize the preproliferative stage of diabetic retinopathy. Patients with preproliferative diabetic retinopathy are at a 15% to 45% risk of progression to the proliferative stage.

The *sine qua non* feature of the proliferative stage is the presence of retinal or optic disc neovascularization (see Fig. 11.3). Proliferative diabetic retinopathy (PDR) can be complicated by vitreous hemorrhage or retinal detachment. Any patient with diabetes who has floaters and vision loss needs urgent referral to rule out vitreous hemorrhage, which is the most common cause of blindness.

There are two major indications for laser therapy in the setting of diabetic retinopathy: Diabetic macular edema and neovascularization. Clinically significant macular edema (CSME) refers to diabetic macular edema involving or threatening the fovea. Focal macular laser has been found to prevent vision loss in patients with diabetes (type 1 or 2) with CSME (Evidence Level A). The Early Treatment Diabetic Retinopathy Study showed about a 50% decline in the incidence of moderate vision loss (a drop of three or more lines on Snellen visual acuity) in patients with CSME treated with focal macular laser.[14] Patients with CSME should undergo fluorescein angiography to guide laser treatment and exclude macular ischemia as an alternative cause of vision loss. Recently, intravitreal triamcinolone acetonide (Kenalog) injection has become a popular adjuvant modality for the treatment of diabetic macular edema resistant to focal macular laser therapy. A multicenter prospective study is under way to assess focal macular laser and intravitreal triamcinolone acetonide (Kenalog) therapy head to head.

Panretinal photocoagulation (PRP) has been found to decrease the risk of severe vision loss in patients with diabetes with preproliferative or PDR. The Diabetic Retinopathy Study demonstrated an 11% incidence of severe vision loss in patients with high-risk PDR treated with PRP, but a 26% incidence in those who did not receive laser therapy during a 2-year follow-up.[15] Patients with low-risk PDR (i.e., less extensive neovascularization *not* associated with vitreous hemorrhage) and those with preproliferative retinopathy also benefited with PRP, although the margin of benefit was smaller. Nonclearing vitreous hemorrhage or tractional macular detachment may be addressed surgically by pars plana vitrectomy, membrane peeling, and endolaser. The beneficial effects of laser therapy have been attributed to the reduction of growth factors such as VEGF. Future adjuvant therapy for diabetic macular edema and PDR may include intraocular injections of inhibitors to VEGF (e.g., Macugen or Lucentis) that may decrease vasopermeability and the drive for vasogenesis.

RETINAL VENOUS OCCLUSIVE DISEASE

Branch retinal vein occlusions (BRVOs) and central retinal vein occlusions (CRVOs) typically affect individuals with arterial sclerosis, causing venous compression. More than 90% of patients are older than 50, with a mean age of onset in the sixties. The Eye Disease Case-Control Study identified the following major risk factors for the development of BRVO and CRVO:[16,17]

1. Hypertension
2. Diabetes mellitus (not a major independent risk factor in BRVO)
3. Cardiovascular disease
4. Open-angle glaucoma

Clinically, BRVO occur in the superotemporal retinal quadrant in more than 60% of cases. Visual field defects occur on the basis of the location of the vascular occlusion. Venous occlusion almost always occurs at the site of an arteriovenous crossing where the vessels share a common adventitial sheath, often preceded by arteriovenous nicking (see Fig. 11.4). Funduscopic examination findings include venous tortuosity and engorgement distal to the point of occlusion associated with sectoral intraretinal flame-shaped and dot-blot hemorrhages, cotton wool spots, and retinal edema distributed along the vascular arcade and retinal quadrant affected by the venous occlusion (see Fig. 11.5). In cases of hemiretinal vein occlusion (HRVO), a variant of BRVO, these findings are identified in the superior or inferior hemispheric retina. More chronic changes associated with BRVO and HRVO include collateralization and/or neovascularization. Chronic macular edema may be noted by the presence of hard lipid exudates, epiretinal membranes, and/or subretinal pigmentary changes or fibrosis. Permanent vision loss may be attributable to macular ischemia and/or macular edema; however, 50% to 60% of patients maintain a Snellen visual acuity of 20/40 or better.

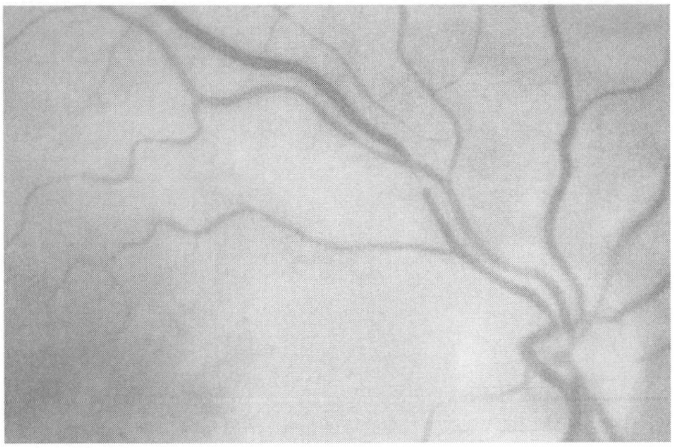

Figure 11.4 Hypertensive retinopathy with arterial narrowing and arteriovenous nicking. (See color insert.)

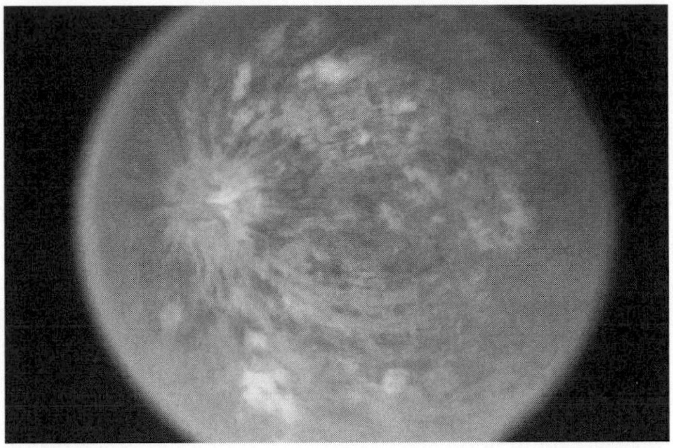

Figure 11.6 Diffuse intraretinal hemorrhages with scattered cotton wool spots in a patient with CRVO. (See color insert.)

Patients with BRVO should undergo a detailed ophthalmic examination by an ophthalmologist upon presentation followed by a repeat dilated fundus examination in 3 months (Evidence Level C). Fluorescein angiography can be of great value in detecting retinal ischemia and macular edema. Patients with retinal ischemia affecting a contiguous area greater than 5 disc diameters are at greatest risk for the development of retinal neovascularization, occurring in 40% of these cases. Elevated finer neovascular vessels must be differentiated from flat larger caliber collateral vessels that can also be present in case of ischemia. A clinical clue as to the presence of retinal neovascularization is nearby preretinal heme, which is often boat-shaped in nature. Iris neovascularization is rare and occurs in only 1% of cases.

Retinal photocoagulation therapy is indicated in special cases of BRVO. The Branch Vein Occlusion Study Group established the criteria for focal macular laser in BRVO as persistent macular edema with vision loss to <20/40 for >3 months. In these cases, treated eyes showed a near twofold increase in the rate of visual gain by two Snellen lines and a statistically significant increase in the number of eyes maintaining 20/40 or better vision.[18] Scattered laser therapy (quadrantic PRP) to the ischemic retinal quadrant was recommended in the presence of neovascularization to reduce the risk of vitreous hemorrhage and tractional retinal detachments.[19]

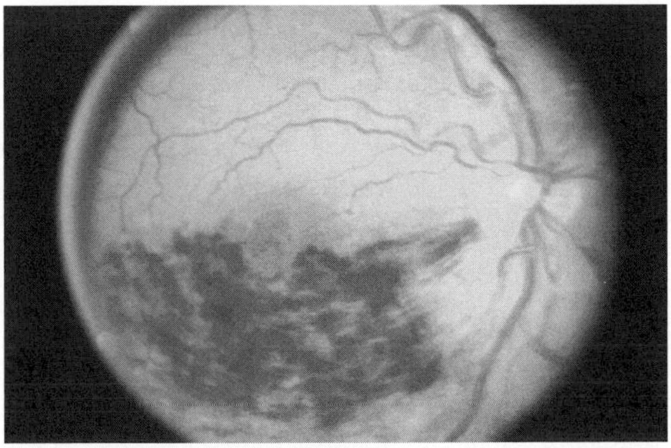

Figure 11.5 Inferotemporal branch retinal vein occlusion with sectoral flame-shaped hemorrhages. (See color insert.)

CRVO has a poorer prognosis and is associated with a more severe vision loss secondary to a more diffuse presentation of retinal edema, hemorrhages, and underlying ischemia. Optic nerve head edema with venous tortuosity and engorgement is seen throughout the retina (see Fig. 11.6). CRVO is subdivided into two categories on the basis of the degree of retinal ischemia present on fluorescein angiography. The ischemic subtype is classified by a contiguous area of retinal ischemia 10 or more disc diameters in size and is associated with a larger degree of retinal hemorrhages and more severe venous tortuosity.[20] The presence of a relative afferent pupillary defect can serve as a convenient clinical tool in classifying a case of CRVO as the ischemic subtype. Retinal neovascularization is rare; however, iris neovascularization is seen in approximately 60% of cases with ischemic CRVO. Iris neovascularization typically occurs within 3 to 6 months of the onset of CRVO.

The role of retinal photocoagulation in CRVO is limited to the presence of iris neovascularization. The Central Vein Study Group found no role in prophylactic PRP in CRVO. Similarly, focal macular laser for macular edema was also found to be of no benefit.[21] In cases of persistent macular edema with a relatively intact macular capillary network, periodic intravitreal triamcinolone injections may play a role in decreasing the degree of macular edema, and thereby restoring vision. Patients with CRVO must be evaluated by an ophthalmologist upon onset of symptoms, followed by monthly dilated funduscopic examinations and gonioscopy for 6 months. Early detection of iris and angle neovascularization is key to initiate PRP therapy to prevent the onset of neovascular glaucoma.[22]

RETINAL ARTERIAL OCCLUSIVE DISEASE

Retinal arterial occlusive disease is an important cause of acute painless vision loss in the elderly patient. The degree of visual deficit directly correlates to the area of retinal ischemia caused by the vascular occlusion. Central retinal artery occlusion often presents with severe vision loss (more than 2/3 of cases with ≤20/400 visual acuity), with the exception of cases in which a cilioretinal artery is present (15% to 30% of cases) maintaining vascular flow to the macula.[23] On the other hand, branch retinal artery occlusion may go undetected in cases involving the nasal or peripheral retina. Branch retinal artery occlusion involving the macula may be associated with sudden onset of vision loss, often as an altitudinal visual field defect.

Branch retinal artery occlusion results from an embolic or thrombotic event. The three main types of emboli include cholesterol emboli (Hollenhorst plaques) resulting from carotid artery stenosis, calcific emboli from cardiac valvular disease, and platelet fibrin emboli secondary to underlying large vessel arteriosclerosis. The most common source of retinal vascular emboli in patients older than 50 is the carotid artery (the heart for those under the age of 50). Other rare causes of emboli and underlying systemic diseases associated with branch retinal artery occlusion include the following:

1. Fat emboli from bone fractures
2. Infectious emboli from endocarditis
3. Emboli associated with cardiac myxoma
4. Talc emboli (associated with chronic intravenous drug use)
5. Systemic hypertension
6. Sickle cell disease
7. Hypercoagulation disorders (i.e., oral contraceptives, antiphospholipid syndrome, factor V Leiden deficiency)
8. Connective tissue disorders such as lupus erythematosus or giant cell arteritis
9. Inflammatory or infectious etiologies such as syphilis or toxoplasmosis

Clinically, branch retinal occlusion presents with sectoral retinal pallor and edema along the distribution of the occluded retinal artery (see Fig. 11.7). These changes occur as a result of retinal tissue infarction, which has been shown to occur 90 to 270 minutes after the onset of ischemia in animal studies. Careful funduscopic examination often reveals segmental flow in the involved artery along with attenuation of the vessel. Cotton wool spots indicative of focal retinal infarction may also be present. In cases associated with carotid artery disease, a Hollenhorst plaque may be visible as an intra-arterial refractile, yellow or white deposit, often at the site of a vessel bifurcation (Fig. 11.7). The peripheral retinal vasculature should always be examined to aid the diagnosis, as Hollenhorst plaques may cause transient posterior pole ischemia and later be dislodged into the smaller peripheral retinal arterioles. Over time,

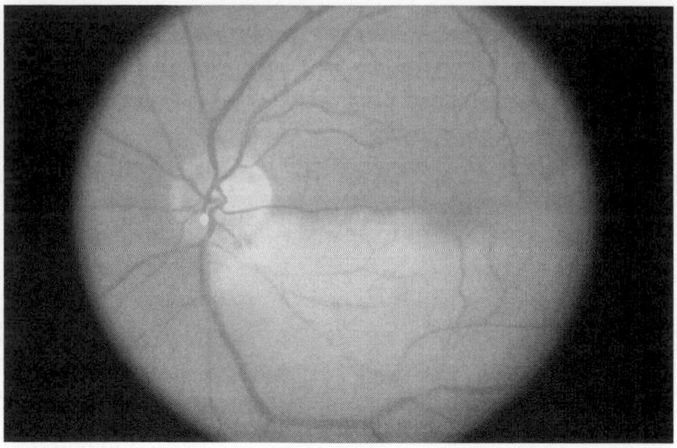

Figure 11.7 Inferotemporal branch retinal artery occlusion showing a proximal Hollenhorst plaque with sectoral retinal edema and pallor. (See color insert.)

recanalization of the occluded retinal artery occurs and flow is reestablished. Often, besides the remaining visual defect, the only visible sign of previous vascular occlusion is attenuation and sclerosis of the affected artery.[24]

As yet, no ocular therapy of proven value is available for branch retinal artery occlusion. In the presence of a Hollenhorst plaque where the patient presents to the office within minutes or a few hours of onset of vision loss, ocular massage and anterior chamber paracentesis may aid in restoring flow and preventing retinal infarction by dislodging the embolus into the peripheral retina. More importantly, patients should undergo systemic workup to treat any underlying disorders.

Central retinal artery occlusion presents with clinical findings similar to those seen in branch retinal artery occlusion in that the retina appears pale and edematous secondary to acute ischemia and infarction of the retinal nerve fiber layer. These changes span the entire retina, with the exception of macular sparing, which occurs when a cilioretinal artery is present. In the acute state, a cherry red spot may also be present in the macula, representing the intact choroidal vasculature beneath the foveola. Clinically, these changes may be subtle, depending on the time course in relation to the onset of ischemia. Detection of retinal pallor may be difficult and may necessitate comparison with the fellow eye. As in the case of branch retinal artery occlusion, flow through the central retinal artery is reestablished with time as the vessel recanalizes.

Treatment modalities for patients who present with acute onset of vision loss from central retinal artery occlusion include ocular massage, anterior chamber paracentesis, oral acetazolamide, and hyperbaric oxygen inhalation therapy.[25] However, none of these measures have been proved to be of therapeutic value in large-scale prospective trials. Causes of central retinal artery occlusion include emboli (cardiac or carotid), thrombosis, giant cell arteritis (1% to 2% of cases), collagen vascular diseases, hypercoagulation disorders, and trauma. Appropriate systemic workup and treatment of the underlying disorder may be the most important management step. Iris neovascularization (rubeosis) occurs in approximately 20% of cases (usually within 4 to 6 weeks of onset) and for this reason, a repeat ophthalmic examination is indicated 1 month after presentation of central retinal artery occlusion. PRP is necessary for cases in which rubeosis is present to prevent the onset of neovascular glaucoma.

GLAUCOMA

Glaucoma is the second most common cause of blindness worldwide, and in the United States it is the most common cause of blindness in black Americans. It affects >2.25 million Americans aged 40 years or older and results in >3 million office visits each year. The financial burden is considerable because of the prevalence and chronicity of this disease and the debilitation that results. Federal costs are reported to reach as high as $1 billion for glaucoma-related Medicare and Medicaid payments and disability.[26]

The definition of glaucoma, now defined as characteristic optic nerve head damage and visual field loss, has undergone a considerable evolution. Elevated intraocular pressure (IOP) is no longer considered an absolute criterion, although it is a very important risk factor. There are many different types of glaucoma, of which primary open-angle glaucoma (POAG) is the most common. Adults older than 50 should have screening for glaucoma every 1 to 2 years. Older adults with a family history positive for glaucoma, African American lineage, or other risk factors may need more frequent screening.

POAG is a chronic disease most commonly affecting older patients. Aqueous humor may access the filtration site, but the network is "clogged," resulting in impaired passage out of the angle. Slow aqueous drainage leads to chronically elevated IOPs causing insidious and painless vision loss. This is in contrast to acute angle-closure glaucoma, in which the aqueous outflow is suddenly blocked, IOP rises precipitously, and the patient presents with considerable redness and pain with acute vision loss. Pain may be so severe as to cause headache, nausea, and vomiting. Emergent ophthalmologic referral is required to reverse the angle closure and reduce the IOP through the use of aqueous suppressants including β-blocker and α_2-agonist eyedrops and oral acetazolamide (Diamox), miotics, and laser iridotomy. Conversely, the IOP rise in POAG is slow and much less severe. Patients with POAG are asymptomatic and may suffer substantial paracentral field loss and optic disc cupping (i.e., cup-to-disc ratio >0.5) before consulting an ophthalmologist, underscoring the importance of regular ophthalmologic screening in the older adult.[26]

Development of POAG is most likely multifactorial and polygenic. Initial pedigrees were found to demonstrate linkage to the 1q locus. Subsequent investigations have more precisely defined the *GLC1A* gene that encodes for myocilin, the trabecular meshwork–induced glucocorticoid response protein. Several other chromosomal loci, including those mapped to chromosomes 2, 3, 7, and 10, have also been found to be associated with the development of glaucoma.[27]

Management of POAG may be approached by the ophthalmologist in a stepwise manner. A variety of IOP-lowering medications, both local and systemic, exist (see Table 11.2 for side effects of selected eyedrops for glaucoma). Mechanisms of action include decreased aqueous production or increased aqueous outflow. Various eyedrop formulations are available; latanoprost (Xalatan) and more recently bimatoprost (Lumigan), prostaglandin analogs that increase uveal–scleral outflow, and brimonidine (Alphagan), an α_2-adrenergic agonist that decreases aqueous production, are two relatively new and effective drugs to reduce IOP (Evidence level A).

TABLE 11.2
SIDE EFFECTS OF SELECTED EYE DROPS FOR GLAUCOMA

Class	Side Effects
Aqueous Suppressants	
β-Blockers (e.g., timolol)	Bradycardia, dyspnea, asthma, heart failure exacerbations
α-Agonists (e.g., brimonidine)	Allergic conjunctivitis
Carbonic anhydrase inhibitors (e.g., dorzolamide)	Blurriness
Aqueous Outflow Facilitators	
Prostaglandins (e.g., latanoprost)	Pain, redness, increased eyelashes, iris pigmentation, cystoid macular edema
Miotics (e.g., pilocarpine)	Brow arch, blurriness, nyctalopia
Epinephrine (e.g., dipivefrin)	Palpitations, angina, cystoid macular edema

In the face of visual field progression despite maximal medications or intolerance to medications, argon laser trabeculoplasty (application of laser energy to the trabecular meshwork) can be effective in lowering IOP in approximately 50% of patients for 3 to 5 years. Intraocular surgery involves the creation of a fistula or filtration site to allow an alternative route of aqueous egress (trabeculectomy). Adjunctive antimetabolite use with 5-fluorouracil or mitomycin C has increased the success of this procedure in those patients at high risk of failure because of fibrosis and scarring of the filtration site.

Alternative surgeries for glaucoma include drainage devices or aqueous shunts. Drainage devices, which are made of a foreign material such as plastic, shunt fluid from the anterior chamber to the subconjunctival space. Ciliary body destructive procedures with cryotherapy or laser (cyclocryoablation or cyclophotocoagulation) may be used in patients with a poor visual prognosis.

Currently, studies are under way to better understand the pathophysiology of normal tension glaucoma (NTG). The most recent collaborative NTG study showed that the level of pressure influences the course of NTG, as evidenced by a slower rate of incident visual field loss in cases with 30% or more lowering of IOP. The disease course is highly variable, but often slow enough that half of the patients have no progression in 5 years. Possible risk factors for faster progression currently under study include female gender, history of migraine headaches, and the presence of disc hemorrhages. Some patients may experience greater benefit from lowering of IOP than others, but further research is needed to be able to identify those who are most likely to benefit.[28]

A question that has perplexed ophthalmologists for years has been whether to treat patients with ocular hypertension defined by an elevated IOP in the presence of an open angle and a normal optic nerve. Recently, the Ocular Hypertension Treatment Study found that at 60 months, the cumulative probability of developing POAG was 4.4% in the medically treated group and 9.5% in the observation group. There was little evidence of increased systemic or ocular risk associated with ocular hypotensive medication. Therefore, it was concluded that topical ocular hypotensive medication was effective in delaying or preventing the onset of POAG in individuals with elevated IOP. However, this does not imply that all patients with borderline or elevated IOP should receive medication. Clinicians should still use their better judgment in initiating pharmacologic treatment in those individuals at higher risk for developing glaucoma.[29]

ANTERIOR ISCHEMIC OPTIC NEUROPATHY

Anterior ischemic optic neuropathy (AION) is the most common form of acute optic neuropathy in patients older than 50. AION presents as an acute painless monocular vision loss always accompanied by a visual field defect. The most common form of visual field loss is altitudinal (superior or inferior). In unilateral cases, a relative afferent pupillary defect is present, indicating the asymmetry in optic nerve function. AION is classified into two categories: The nonarteritic form (nonarteritic anterior ischemic optic neuropathy [NAION]), which is caused by microvascular occlusion of the blood supply to the optic nerve attributed to atherosclerotic vascular disease, and the arteritic form (arteritic form of anterior ischemic optic neuropathy [AAION]), which occurs as a result of occlusive inflammatory disease in the setting of giant cell (temporal) arteritis.[30]

NAION is the more common of the two forms of AION and accounts for more than 90% of all cases. It affects a younger age-group, with a mean age of presentation of 60. The degree of vision loss is usually less severe than that seen in AAION, with 60% of patients maintaining a Snellen visual acuity of 20/200 or better. Risk factors for NAION include diabetes, hypertension, smoking, hyperlipidemia, history of migraines, vasculitis, and structural crowding of the disc (small cup-to-disc ratio).

Clinically, vision loss is accompanied by optic nerve head edema. The disc edema may present as diffuse or segmental, with associated pallor or hyperemia. However, pallor is less common and is more often associated with AAION. Disc hemorrhages along with cotton wool spots around the ischemic disc are easy clinical tools for detecting disc edema (see Fig. 11.8). A less subtle but accurate measure of edema is the blurring of vessels as they course over the disc margin. The contralateral eye must also be examined to detect any possible underlying risk factors such as an anatomically crowded disc or preexisting hypertensive or diabetic retinopathy.

Previous modes of treatment used for NAION have included hyperbaric oxygen therapy and optic nerve sheath decompression, neither of which has been shown to be beneficial.[31,32] There is no clear role for aspirin therapy in prophylaxis for fellow eye involvement.[33] Studies looking

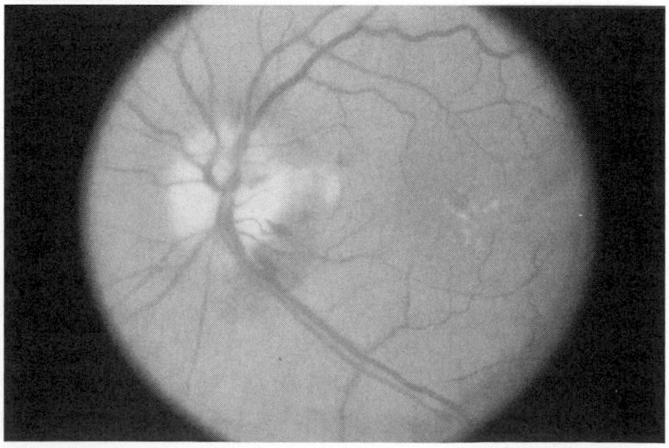

Figure 11.8 Nonarteritic anterior ischemic optic neuropathy with disc edema and peripapillary flame-shaped hemorrhages. (See color insert.)

at the role of neuroprotective agents as well as levodopa therapy are under way.[34] If left untreated, patients with NAION generally remain stable, with a very low rate of recurrence in the same eye, and approximately 40% of patients show three or more Snellen lines of visual recovery.

The AAION tends to occur in more elderly patients, with a mean age of presentation of 70 and a female preponderance of 2:1. More than 80% of patients report systemic symptoms of giant cell arteritis, which may include fever, weight loss, myalgias, jaw claudication, ear pain, temporal artery tenderness, scalp tenderness, and headaches. Clinically, AAION typically presents with a more pale presentation of disc edema than that seen in NAION, lacking the presence of hyperemic disc vessels and disc hemorrhages. Anatomical crowding of the disc is not a risk factor and its presence favors the diagnosis of NAION. Vision loss is often more severe, with patients usually presenting with a Snellen visual acuity <20/200.[35]

An elevated Westergren erythrocyte sedimentation rate in more than 84% of cases and a temporal artery biopsy positive for AION are diagnostic. However, a biopsy negative for AION is not exclusive and is seen in up to 9% of cases. Contralateral temporal artery biopsies should be considered in cases negative for AION with a strong clinical suspicion.[36] Immediate systemic corticosteroid treatment is crucial to avoid vision loss in the other eye. Patients rarely show any improvement in visual acuity in the affected eye. Consultation with a rheumatologist should be considered. The dosage of steroids may be tapered over the course of 1 year or longer, while monitoring for reduction of inflammatory markers and other systemic signs of active disease.

RED EYE

Red eye in elderly patients may be classified by cause: Benign or malignant. Malignant causes are typically associated with significant pain and vision loss, and they include corneal ulceration identified by the presence of a white corneal infiltrate. Emergent corneal scraping by an ophthalmologist to exclude an infection and the need for fortified antibiotic treatment is indicated. The presence of a corneal abrasion in the absence of an infiltrate or ulcer is prognostically much more favorable, but it is also associated with painful vision loss. It may be diagnosed with fluorescein staining and treated with antibiotic ointments with or without patching. First time presentation of anterior or posterior uveitis is relatively unusual in the older adult population. Suspicion should be aroused by the symptom of photophobia with vision loss; urgent ophthalmologic referral is required. Treatment may include corticosteroid eyedrop therapy, which can be complicated by cataract and increased IOP, and which is best prescribed by an ophthalmologist. Systemic investigations to exclude autoimmune diseases, systemic infections, and occult malignancies may be necessary.

Benign causes of red eye are typically painless and unassociated with vision loss and include blepharitis or dandruff of the eyelashes. Treatment includes lid hygiene, topical antibiotics, and gentle scrubbing with nontearing baby shampoo twice daily. Less commonly, viral conjunctivitis associated with mucous discharge and matting of the eyelids, especially in the morning, may be noted and treated supportively with warm compresses and education to limit spread of the infection to the other eye or to contacts.

Allergic conjunctivitis may affect older adults and is characterized by an itchy red eye and conjunctival infection and chemosis (swelling) upon examination. Patients are advised to avoid known precipitants such as pet dander or topical eyedrop medications. Management of allergic conjunctivitis includes systemic antihistamines, topical antihistamines or decongestants, and ophthalmic corticosteroids. Patients should be cautioned about side effects of topical ophthalmics. Ophthalmic corticosteroids should be prescribed by an ophthalmologist. Indications include inflammatory conditions of the eye and risks include secondary ocular infections, cataract formation, glaucoma, and corneal thinning.

Tears serve several important functions, including corneal lubrication, debris clearance, and immune protection. With age, tear production decreases, and older patients are prone to develop dry-eye syndrome or keratitis sicca, characterized by redness, foreign body sensation, and reflex tearing. Management includes tear replacement with artificial tears during the day and an ointment at bedtime. Temporary and permanent punctal plugs may be employed to retard tear egress through the nasolacrimal drainage system in more severe cases. Keratitis sicca may be associated with autoimmune disease; conditions such as Sjögren syndrome should be excluded.

EYELID PROBLEMS

Lid abnormalities are a common problem in older persons. Because of the gradual loss of elasticity and tensile strength that develops with age, secondary degenerative changes may take place. Blepharochalasis (drooping of the brow) and blepharoptosis (drooping of the eyelid) may cause cosmetic deformity and, if severe, may impair vision. Lid ectropion or entropion, eversion and inversion of the lid margins, respectively, can disrupt the ocular surface and cause discomfort for the patient. Various surgical procedures are available to address these problems.

HERPES ZOSTER

Herpes zoster ophthalmicus, or shingles, is a painful reactivation of varicella-zoster virus that not uncommonly affects older persons. Dermatomal distribution of weeping vesicles affecting the ophthalmic division of the trigeminal nerve is the classic presentation. Ocular involvement may be signaled by lesions on the tip of the nose (Hutchinson sign) and may include pseudodendritic keratopathy or uveitis. Suspicion of ocular involvement warrants a careful examination by an ophthalmologist. Oral acyclovir may shorten the course of disease and topical antivirals (e.g., trifluridine [Viroptic]) may be useful for corneal complications. More serious but far less common ocular findings may include anterior and posterior scleritis, optic neuritis, or even acute retinal necrosis, which requires more aggressive therapy, including intravenous acyclovir with or without intravitreal antiviral therapy to prevent blindness. Postherpetic neuralgia may be quite debilitating; various local ointments (e.g., capsaicin, lidocaine) or systemic medications (e.g., corticosteroids, tricyclic antidepressants) may be helpful.

LOW-VISION REHABILITATION

Despite considerable advancements in the medical treatment of ocular conditions, many patients, especially those with the wet form of ARMD, may ultimately sustain permanent visual loss. Visual training and the provision of visual aids are essential services available to the patient with low vision (visual acuity <20/60). Patients with low vision may develop useful adaptive skills with proper instruction. Eccentric viewing by ARMD patients with central macular pathology uses the principle of off-center fixation. The patient can benefit from formal training to find and use the most effective eccentric viewing points. Instruction in scanning and tracking, and other skills may help the patient integrate his or her visual environment. Various low-vision aids are available to improve one's ability to see both near and far. The finer detail required for reading is the most common indication for visual aids. Improved lighting is a simple modification that can enhance visualization of print. Selection of reading material using bold, enlarged fonts, and accentuated black-on-white contrast may also be helpful. Magnification is also commonly employed. Various devices such as high-plus spectacles, handheld magnifiers, stand magnifiers, and closed-circuit television can also enhance reading. Distance magnification may be achieved with the use of telescopic devices that can be handheld for spot viewing or spectacle mounted for continuous viewing. Talking devices, which are computers used to create voice synthesis such as those used at stoplights, or Braille may be especially helpful for those who have lost vision altogether.

ACKNOWLEDGMENT

This chapter was partly supported by research to prevent blindness grant number OP31 (Dr. Sarraf).

This chapter was modified from a chapter written by the same authors for the American Geriatrics Society's Geriatrics Review Syllabus.

REFERENCES

1. West SK, Valmadrid CT. Epidemiology of risk factors of age-related cataract. *Surv Ophthalmol.* 1995;39:323–334.
2. Kuszak JR, Deutsch TA, Brown HG. Anatomy of aged and senile cataractous lenses. In: Albert DM, Jakobiec FA, eds. *Principles and practice of ophthalmology.* Philadelphia, PA: Saunders; 1994:564–575.
3. Age-Related Eye Disease Study Group. A randomized, placebo-controlled, clinical trial of high-dose supplementation with vitamins C and E, beta carotene, and zinc for age-related macular degeneration and vision loss: AREDS report no. 8. *Arch Ophthalmol.* 2001;119(10):1417–1436.
4. Treatment of Age-Related Macular Degeneration with Photodynamic Therapy (TAP) Study Group. Photodynamic therapy of subfoveal choroidal neovascularization in age-related macular degeneration with verteporfin: Two-year results of 2 randomized clinical trials—TAP report 2. *Arch Ophthalmol.* 2001;119: 198–207.
5. Gragoudas ES, Adamis AP, Cunningham ET Jr, et al. Pegaptanib for neovascular age-related macular degeneration. *N Engl J Med.* 2004; 351(27):2805–2816.
6. D'Amico DJ, Goldberg MF, Hudson H, et al. Anecortave acetate as monotherapy for treatment of subfoveal neovascularization in age-related macular degeneration. *Ophthalmology.* 2003;110(12):2372–2383.
7. Klein RJ, Zeiss C, Chew EY, et al. Complement factor H polymorphism in age-related macular degeneration. *Science.* 2005;308(5720):385–389.
8. Diabetic Control and Complications Trial Research Group. The effect of intensive diabetic treatment on the progression of diabetic retinopathy in insulin-dependent diabetes mellitus. *Arch Ophthalmol.* 1995;113:36–51.
9. U.K. Prospective Diabetes Study Group. Efficacy of atenolol and captopril in reducing risk of macrovascular and microvascular complications in type 2 diabetes: UKPDS 39. *BMJ.* 1998;317(7160):713–720.
10. U.K. Prospective Diabetes Study Group. Intensive blood glucose control with sulfonylureas or insulin compared with conventional treatment and risk of complications in patients with type 2 diabetes (UKPDS 33). *Lancet.* 1998;352(9131):837–853.
11. Jain A, Sarraf D, Fong D. Preventing diabetic retinopathy through the control of systemic risk factors. *Curr Opin Ophthalmol.* 2003;14(6):389–394.
12. Ferris FL, Davis MD, Aiello LM III. Treatment of diabetic retinopathy. *N Engl J Med.* 1999;341(9):667–678.
13. Preferred Practice Patterns Committee, Retina Panel. *Diabetic retinopathy.* San Francisco, CA: American Academy of Ophthalmology; 1998.
14. Early Treatment Diabetic Retinopathy Study Research Group. Early photocoagulation for diabetic retinopathy. ETDRS report 9. *Ophthalmology.* 1991;98:766–785.
15. Diabetic Retinopathy Study Research Group. Photocoagulation treatment of proliferative diabetic retinopathy: Clinical application of Diabetic Retinopathy Study (DRS) findings: DRS report 8. *Ophthalmology.* 1981;88:583–600.
16. The Eye Disease Case-Control Study Group. Risk factors for branch retinal vein occlusion. *Am J Ophthalmol.* 1993;116:286–296.
17. The Eye Disease Case-Control Study Group. Risk factors for central retinal vein occlusion. *Arch Ophthalmol.* 1996;114:545–554.
18. Branch Vein Occlusion Study Group. Argon laser photocoagulation for macular edema in branch vein occlusion. *Am J Ophthalmol.* 1984;98:271–282.
19. Branch Vein Occlusion Study Group. Argon laser scatter photocoagulation for prevention of neovascularization and vitreous hemorrhage in branch vein occlusion: A randomized clinical trial. *Arch Ophthalmol.* 1986;104:34–41.
20. Central Vein Study Group; The Central Vein Occlusion Study. Baseline and early natural history report. *Arch Ophthalmol.* 1993;111:1087–1095.
21. The Central Vein Occlusion Study Group; The Central Vein Occlusion Study Group M Report. Evaluation of grid pattern photocoagulation for macular edema in central vein occlusion. *Ophthalmology.* 1995;102:1425–1433.

22. The Central Vein Occlusion Study Group; The Central Vein Occlusion Study Group N report. A randomized clinical trial of early panretinal photocoagulation for ischemic central vein occlusion. *Ophthalmology.* 1995;102:1434–1444.
23. Brown GC, Magargal LE. Central retinal artery obstruction and visual acuity. *Ophthalmology.* 1982;89:14–19.
24. Arruga J, Sanders MD. Ophthalmologic findings in 70 patients with evidence of retinal embolism. *Ophthalmology.* 1982;89:1336–1347.
25. Atebara NH, Brown GC, Cater J. Efficacy of anterior chamber paracentesis and carbogen in treating acute nonarteritic central retinal artery occlusion. *Ophthalmology.* 1995;102:2029–2034.
26. Tielsch JM. The epidemiology and control of open-angle glaucoma: A population-based perspective. *Annu Rev Public Health.* 1996;17:121–136.
27. Alward WL. The genetics of open-angle glaucoma: The story of GLC1A and myocilin. *Eye.* 2000;14(Pt3B):429–436.
28. Anderson DR. Collaborative Normal Tension Glaucoma Study. *Curr Opin Ophthalmol.* 2003;14(2):86–90.
29. Kass MA, Heuer DK, Johnson CA, et al. The Ocular Hypertension Treatment Study: A randomized trial determines that topical ocular hypotensive medication delays or prevents the onset of primary open-angle glaucoma. *Arch Ophthalmol.* 2002;120(6):701–713.
30. Arnold AC. Ischemic optic neuropathies. *Ophthalmol Clin North Am.* 2001;14:83–98.
31. Arnold AC, Hepler RS, Leiber M, et al. Hyperbaric oxygen therapy for nonarteritic anterior ischemic optic neuropathy. *Am J Ophthalmol.* 1996;122:535–541.
32. Ischemic Optic Neuropathy Decompression Trial Research Group. Optic nerve decompression surgery for Nonarteritic Anterior Ischemic Optic Neuropathy (NAION) is not effective and may be harmful. *JAMA.* 1995;273:625–632.
33. Beck RW, Hayreh SS, Podhajsky PA, et al. Spirin therapy in nonarteritic anterior ischemic optic neuropathy. *Am J Ophthalmol.* 1997;123:212–217.
34. Johnson LN, Guy ME, Krohel GB, et al. Levodopa may improve vision loss in recent onset, nonarteritic anterior ischemic optic neuropathy. *Ophthalmology.* 2000;107:521–526.
35. Aiello PD, Trautmann JC, McPhee TJ, et al. Visual prognosis in giant cell arteritis. *Ophthalmology.* 1993;100:550–555.
36. Boyev LR, Miller NR, Green WR. Efficacy of unilateral versus bilateral temporal artery biopsies for the diagnosis of giant cell arteritis. *Am J Ophthalmol.* 1999;128:211–215.

Hearing Difficulty

12

Roseanne C. Berger   *Robert F. Burkard*

CLINICAL PEARLS 134

HEARING AND AGING 135

DIFFERENTIAL DIAGNOSIS 136

PRESBYCUSIS 136
Screening 138
Physical Examination 139
Management 142

TINNITUS 143
Workup 143
Physical Examination 143
Laboratory and Imaging 143
Management 144

DIZZINESS AND BALANCE 144
History 144
Diagnostic Testing 144
Management 145

MÉNIÈRE DISEASE 145
Differential Diagnosis 145
Workup/Keys to Diagnosis 145
Laboratory/Imaging 145
Management 145

CONCLUSION 145

CLINICAL PEARLS

- "Loud talkers" typically suffer from sensorineural hearing loss, whereas "soft talkers" have conductive hearing loss.
- Functional hearing deficits can be identified in the examination room by creating background noise while looking away from the patient and asking a few simple questions.
- Patients complaining that people always yell may have a narrow range between audible and uncomfortably loud sound.
- Consider magnetic resonance imaging (MRI) with contrast when a patient presents with rapidly progressing unilateral sensorineural hearing loss or hearing loss associated with vertigo because these symptoms may be due to a vestibular schwannoma.
- High-resolution computed tomography scan effectively visualizes some conditions of the middle ear causing conductive hearing loss such as cholesteatoma or otosclerosis.
- Hearing aids make speech louder but not clearer.
- Aural/hearing rehabilitation programs minimize the effects of hearing impairment for patients using or refusing hearing aids.

Ninety percent of patients older than 80 years cope with difficulty in hearing conversations, instructions, or sounds that enrich, orient, or protect them. Hearing loss is in fact the third most common chronic condition of aging, following arthritis and hypertension.[1] The condition is more than a minor inconvenience. It contributes to impaired cognitive function, significant social and emotional handicap, and loss of independence.

This chapter reviews the etiology of hearing loss resulting from environmental insults and physiologic changes in the ear in response to aging (i.e., presbycusis or impaired audition in aging). Practical techniques for detecting hearing loss in the clinician's office and interpreting common diagnostic tests typically performed by audiologists are presented in conjunction with strategies for treatment, rehabilitation, and selection of assistive devices from the array of options on the market. Also included is a discussion of tinnitus, a frustrating hearing condition for both patients and their clinicians and its companion, vertigo.

HEARING AND AGING

A common prop in caricatures of frail, feisty, wrinkled, stooped old folks is a ram's horn strategically held next to the ear to capture sound. The image reflects behaviors that are symptomatic of impaired audition: Turning up the volume on the television or radio, speaking loudly, misinterpreting words, or disengaging from group discussions. However, hearing decline begins in the fourth decade. The extent and causes of hearing loss vary considerably across individuals; however, large cohort studies in Framingham, Wisconsin, Baltimore, Venice, Gothenburg (Germany), Denmark, and the United Kingdom consistently document the prevalence of the problem. Overall prevalence of hearing loss in a cohort of 3,753 persons aged between 48 and 92 years in the Beaver Dam, Wisconsin, study was estimated to be 45.9%.[2] Hearing declines at the rate of 0.5 to 0.7 dB per year for high-pitched sounds (i.e., frequencies of 2 to 4 kHz). This rate of decline quadruples in the seventh decade, particularly among men. Although this may vindicate those accused of "wife deafness," the gender gap virtually disappears by the ninth decade. According to Schuknecht,[3] there are multiple patterns, and therefore multiple underlying structural patterns, of age-related hearing loss, including sensory, neural, strial, and cochlear-conductive forms of presbycusis.

Human hearing translates vibrations into identifiable sounds ranging from the subtle drip of a leaky faucet to the startling clap of nearby thunder. The brain uses the difference in timing and level of signals arriving from a pair of ears to reliably locate the source of sound. Mechanical sound waves are captured by the saucer-shaped outer ear and travel through the auditory canal to the flexible eardrum (tympanic membrane [TM]) (see Fig. 12.1). The resulting vibration is transmitted to the first of three linked bones or ossicles in the middle ear: The malleus, incus, and stapes. The stapes, resembling a saddle, inserts into the oval window of the inner ear's cochlea. Because this membrane is much smaller than the eardrum and because the ossicles multiply incoming forces by their combined mechanical advantage, the pressure exerted on the cochlea is approximately 20 times stronger than that on the TM.[4] The cochlea, bearing a striking resemblance to the shell of the chambered nautilus, is filled with fluid. Specialized hair cells in the inner ear (cochlea), organ of Corti, pick up the transmitted cadence, opening up ion channels when the hairs (stereocilia) bend and leading to an intracellular depolarization. This completes the conversion of mechanical energy to electrical energy and leads to the release of neurotransmitters. The auditory branch of the eighth cranial nerve projects onto the cochlear nuclei, through the auditory brainstem to the medial geniculate body of the metathalamus, and, finally, to the primary auditory cortex of the temporal lobe. The cochlea also intercepts vibrations directly from surrounding bone, which serves as the basis for bone-conduction thresholds used audiometrically.

With age, alterations in the peripheral receptive organ contribute to presbycusis. Elasticity diminishes in the cartilage of the outer ear. Reduced numbers of active sebaceous glands produce drier and less viscous cerumen that is prone to obstruct the external auditory canal. Mechanical transmission of sound is affected by decreased elasticity, thinning of the TM, and calcification of the

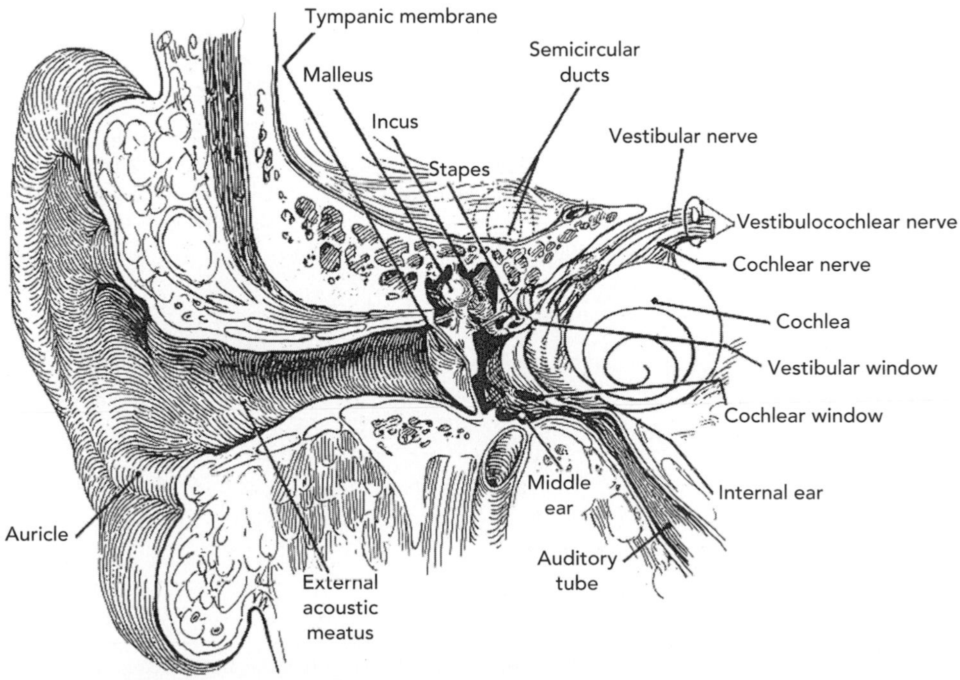

Figure 12.1 Anatomy of the ear. (Reprinted from *Stedman's medical dictionary*, 23rd ed, 1976:436 with permission of Lippincott, Williams & Wilkins.)

joints between the middle ear ossicles. The inner ear's organ of Corti, however, is most susceptible to age-related changes. The stria vascularis may atrophy. This network of endolymph-secreting capillaries generates a resting potential (called the *endolymphatic potential*) that sensitizes the hair cells in the cochlea.[5] Hair cell loss, most severe in the basal or high-frequency region of the cochlea, is responsible for the decline in pure-tone hearing in conjunction with loss of ganglion cells and reduction in fibers in the cochlear nerve. Hearing is also contingent on timely and accurate interpretation of information from the environment. Processing information in the temporal lobe may be affected by reduction in neuron number, size, or dendritic arborization.

DIFFERENTIAL DIAGNOSIS

Hearing deficits are categorized as conductive, sensorineural, or retrocochlear. A conductive hearing loss locates the problem to the middle or external ear. A sensorineural loss stems from inner ear structures (primarily the stria vascularis and cochlear hair cells). A retrocochlear loss involves portions of the auditory system that involve the eighth cranial nerve or central auditory nervous system. Once localized, the differential diagnosis includes age-related structural changes (i.e., impacted cerumen, tympanosclerosis, cochlear hair cell loss), infections, tumors, trauma, noise or other toxic exposures, genetic traits and congenital malformations. Tinnitus, often associated with hearing loss, is a troubling condition caused by the perception of sounds without an external source. Table 12.1 lists some conditions that are associated with hearing difficulty.

PRESBYCUSIS

CASE ONE

Mrs. B. is an active 84-year-old retired mathematician. She lives alone in a condominium within five miles of her daughter's family. Her routine includes attending daily aerobics workouts, playing bridge, reading, and watching televised news and dramas. The television volume is noticeably louder over the past several years and she is somewhat irritated because, in her opinion, her son-in-law does not speak distinctly. Her voice, on the other hand, is inappropriately loud for libraries or theater. Mrs. B. consents to an audiologic evaluation. Her audiometric results (see Fig. 12.2A) show that she has a bilateral, sensorineural hearing loss. She has a relatively mild hearing loss in the lower frequencies that increases to a moderate-to-severe hearing loss in the higher frequencies. Her tympanograms peak near ambient pressure (Fig. 12.2B), demonstrating normal middle ear function and confirming the audiometric results of a sensorineural hearing loss. When speech is loud enough, and in the absence of background noise, she has very good speech discrimination scores in each ear (100% in the right ear and 96% in the left ear).

This woman would be a good candidate for a hearing aid because her hearing loss in the lower frequencies is sufficient to make it difficult to hear speech at

TABLE 12.1
PARTIAL LIST OF CONDITIONS THAT CAUSE HEARING LOSS (ICD-9 CODES)

Conductive (389.0)	Sensorineural (389.1)	Retrocochlear (ICD-9)	Others
Bullous myringitis (384.01)	Autoimmune disease (279.4)	Neurofibromatosis type 2 (237.72)	Examination of ears and hearing (V72.1)
Cerumen impaction (380.4)	Ménière disease (386.00)	Meningioma (225.2)	Unspecified deafness (389.9)
Cholesteatoma (385.30)	Noise exposure (388.12)	Transient ischemic deafness (388.02)	Conversion disorder (300.11)
Glomus jugulare (227.6)	Medications (995.2)	Schwannoma (225.1)	
Ossicular disruption (385.2)	■ Aminoglycoside		
Otitis media (384.1)	■ Loop diuretics		
Otosclerosis (387.9)	■ Antineoplastic agents		
Serous otitis media (381.4)	■ Salicylates		
Tympanosclerosis (385.0)	Radiation exposure (V15.3)		
TM perforation (384.2)	Childhood infections		
	■ Mumps (072.8)		
	■ Measles (055.7)		
	■ Rubella (056)		
	■ Meningitis (047.9)		
	Syphilitic acoustic neuritis (094.86)		
	Sudden hearing loss (388.2)		
	Injury to acoustic nerve (951.5)		
	Multiple sclerosis (340)		
	Perilymphatic fistula (386.40)		

TM, tympanic membrane.

3 Frequency speech average
(500, 1000, 2000 Hz)

Mode	Right	Left
AC	38 dB	33 dB
BC	38 dB	35 dB

Speech Audiometry

Live SRT Disc CID W22 Tape

Test	Right	Left	BIN
SRT	40 dB	35 dB	dB
MASK	@ dB	@ dB	@ dB
DISC. SCORE	100%	96%	%
LEVEL	@ 80 dB	@ 75 dB	@ dB
MASK	@ dB	@ dB	

Audiogram Code

	AIR		BONE	
Ear	Un-masked	Masked	Un-masked	Masked
R	○ — ○	△ — △	<---<	[---[
L	X — X	□ — □	>--->	]---]

White ______ N.B ______ Noise

A Reliability : good ☑ fair ☐ poor ☐

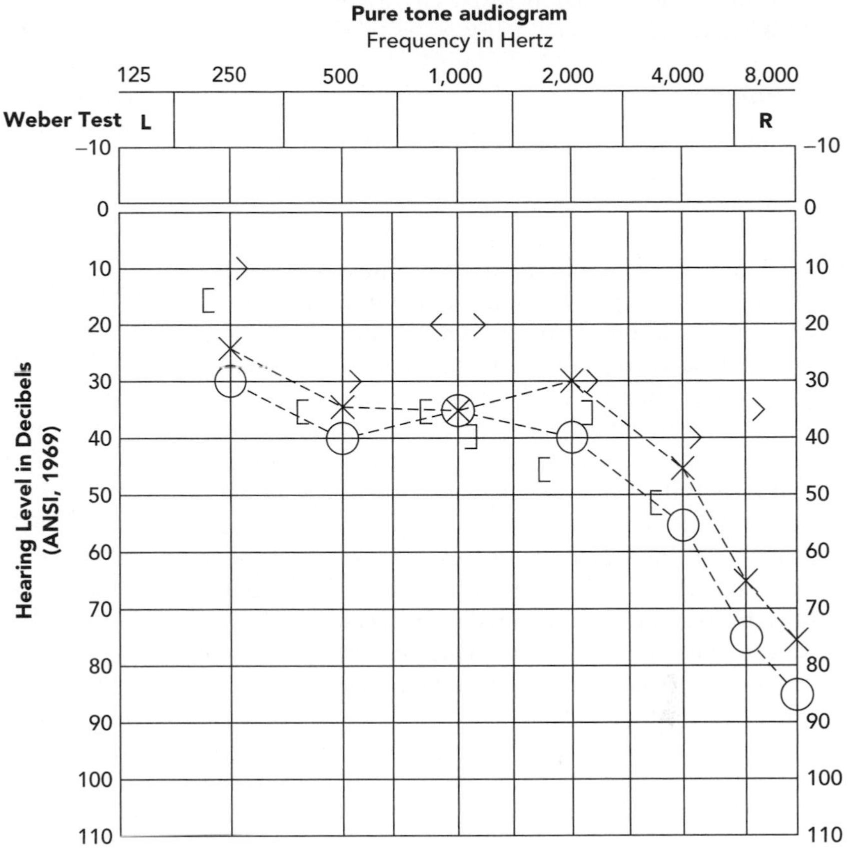

Masking Levels in Decibels		R	L	R	L	R	L	R	L	R	L	R	L
	Ac												
	Bc		55		65	65	65	65	60		75		

B

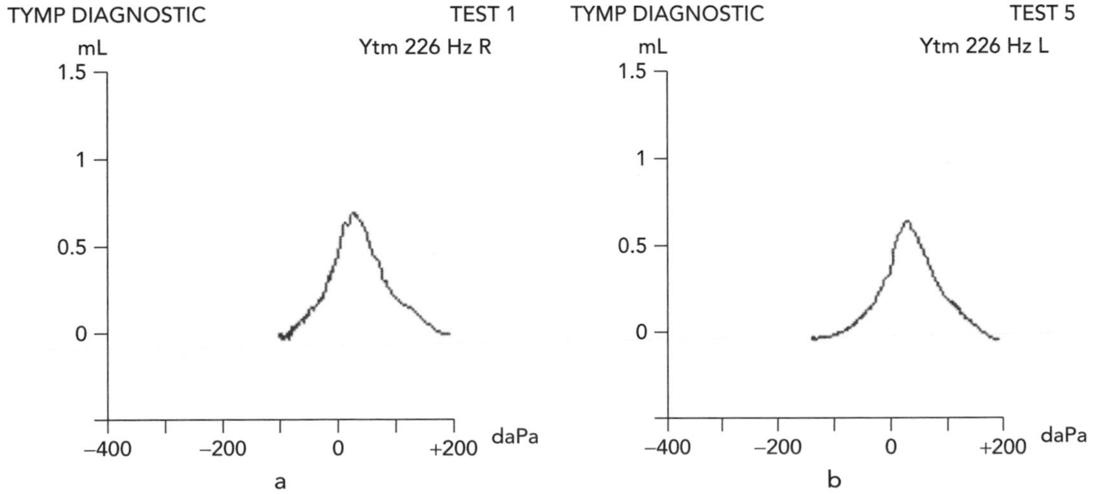

Figure 12.2 Audiometric results **(A)** tympanograms **(B)** of an 84-year-old woman with presbycusis.

conversational levels and her speech discrimination in quiet is excellent.

Screening

It has been reported that approximately 20% of physicians routinely screen their older patients for hearing loss.[6] Do not assume that the patient who easily converses face-to-face in a quiet examination room is free of significant hearing impairment. A more accurate picture is obtained by asking about hearing in the context of common situations. "Do you have difficulty hearing phone conversations?" "Is it difficult to hear when you are in a restaurant?" "Do you need to turn up the volume on the radio and television or does your family comment on your preferred listening volume?" Although patients are frequently accompanied by a spouse or child, resist the temptation to direct questions to them in lieu of the patient with an obvious hearing loss. Speaking directly to the patient promotes self-esteem, conveys respect, and demonstrates effective techniques for communicating with hearing-impaired listeners (e.g., maintain good eye contact, speak slowly without exaggerated lip movements or facial expressions, and rephrase rather than repeat misunderstood statements).[7]

The Hearing Handicap Inventory for the Elderly (HHIE), developed by Ventry and Weinstein (1982), identifies individuals with sufficient handicap to warrant professional follow-up. Research demonstrated adequate sensitivity and specificity for a self-administered ten-question version that can be completed in the office waiting room.[8,9] More recently, data from the 1971 to 1975 National Health and Nutrition Examination Survey (NHANES) and two established criteria for defining hearing loss (Ventry and Weinstein Scale and the High-Frequency Pure-Tone Average [PTA] Scale) were the basis for a seven-item questionnaire incorporating sociodemographic characteristics, as well as specific hearing loss questions (see Fig. 12.3). Scoring 3 of a possible 8 points is considered positive (sensitivity 80.1%; specificity 80.1%; odds ratio of 16.2 with 95% confidence interval).[10]

The medical, family, and social history are aimed at identifying causes of hearing difficulty. Past or present use of aminoglycoside antibiotics, quinine derivatives, loop diuretics such as furosemide or ethacrynic acid, and salicylates may suggest otoxicity contributing to hearing loss. A past history of chronic otitis media or mastoiditis may be accompanied by hearing loss. Although a commonly held belief is that hypothyroidism, diabetes, or multiple sclerosis is linked as well, the incidence among patients with these conditions does not appear different than that of the general population. Vocational, recreational, or situational sound exposure should be ascertained. The loud explosions of war, for example,

Clinical Scale to Detect Hearing Loss

Question	Points
1) Age:_____ ➢ 70 y.o. = 1 point	____
2) Sex: Male____ Female____ ➢ Male = 1 point	____
3) Highest grade attended ➢ < or = grade 12 = 1 point	____
4) Have you ever had deafness or trouble hearing in one or both ears? Yes_____, go to Question no. 5 No _____, go to Question no. 6 ➢ (no points assigned)	0
5) Did you ever see a doctor for hearing loss? Yes_____ No_____ ➢ Yes = 2 points	____
6) Without a hearing aid, can you usually hear and understand what a person says without seeing his face if that person whispers to you from across the room? Yes_____ No_____ ➢ No = 1 point	____
7) Without a hearing aid, can you usually hear and understand what a person says without seeing his face if that person talks in a normal voice to you from across the room? Yes_____ No_____ ➢ No = 2 points	____
3 or more points indicate positive score — TOTAL	_____

Figure 12.3 The seven-item screening questionnaire to detect hearing loss.

subjected many World War II veterans, now elderly, to noise and sound pressures capable of inducing acoustic trauma. Family history of hearing loss is commonly associated with age-related hearing loss.

Physical Examination

The clinical examination begins with listening to the patient's speaking voice. A monotonous tone or inappropriate volume may suggest hearing loss.[5] Loud talkers may have a sensorineural problem, whereas soft talkers more often have a conductive problem. Create background noise and negate lipreading by turning on a radio and turning away from the patient while asking a few questions. These maneuvers are effective in demonstrating hearing deficits that may not be reflected in an audiogram obtained under soundproofed laboratory conditions.

Inspection of the auditory canal for obstructing cerumen is essential. Removal of the material is a prerequisite for completing the examination and is often therapeutic. Low-pressure irrigation with warm water is the preferred technique. Application of hydrogen peroxide or products such as trolamine polypeptide oleate (Cerumenex) or carbamide peroxide (Debrox) for 3 days facilitates the procedure.

Middle ear landmarks may appear more pronounced when viewed through the more translucent TM of an elderly patient. White patches indicative of healed perforations, dullness from fibrosis, or redness visible behind the TM, with or without perforation (i.e., cholesteatoma), are among chronic findings that often herald hearing difficulty (see Table 12.2). These findings may interfere with the transmission of sound waves, causing a conductive hearing loss (see in the subsequent text).

TABLE 12.2
EXAMINATION FINDINGS ASSOCIATED WITH CHRONIC HEARING DIFFICULTY

Diagnosis	Description
Cholesteatoma	Redness visible behind TM with or without perforation Overgrowth of keratinizing squamous epithelium Cholesterol
Serous otitis media (secretory otitis)	Yellow TM Bulging with decreased bony landmarks and mobility indicates fluid in middle ear Retracted with no mobility or mobility on negative pressure indicates middle ear vacuum Air fluid level or bubbles possible
Large perforation	Interruption of TM Absent mobility
Healed perforation	Opaque white patch

TM, tympanic membrane.

Simple tests and maneuvers aid diagnosis in the examination room. Although individually subjective, collectively they accurately localize hearing loss and distinguish between conductive and sensorineural causes:

Whispered Voice:
The examiner places a finger in one ear canal and gently moves it to mask hearing, simultaneously testing hearing in the other ear by whispering one- and two-syllable words while standing 30 to 60 cm away. The patients should correctly repeat at least 50% of the softly whispered words.

Ticking Watch:
Mask hearing in one ear while moving a nonelectric watch toward the test ear and record the distance where the tick becomes audible. Compare results to those in normal patients.

Tuning Fork Tests:

Weber:
Place a vibrating tuning fork (usually a 128 or 256 Hz frequency) on the midline of the patient's head and ask where sound is best heard. Midline is the normal response. Sound lateralizes to the ear with poorer hearing in a conductive hearing loss or to the better ear if the etiology is sensorineural.

Rinne:
While monitoring time in seconds, ask the patient to indicate when he or she no longer hears sound from a vibrating tuning fork placed against the mastoid bone. While continuing to track time, place the tuning fork 1 to 1.25 cm away from the auditory canal and again ask the patient to indicate when sound disappears. Air-conducted sound is audible twice as long as bone-conducted sound in normal ears. Air-conducted hearing periods that are greater than one and less than two times as long as bone conduction suggest a sensorineural deficit. Bone-conduction times that are equal or greater than air-conduction time indicate conductive hearing loss.

Schwabach Test:
Examiners with normal hearing compare their perception of sound from a vibrating tuning fork placed on their mastoid bone with that of their hearing-impaired patient. The examiner will hear the vibration for a longer period than the patient with sensorineural hearing loss and for a relatively shorter period than the patient with conductive hearing loss.

Handheld Tympanometry/Audiometry:
Handheld or small desktop devices can generate tympanograms (see Test "Tympanometry") or assess hearing within a limited range for screening purposes. A handheld audiometer may generate multiple tone frequencies at one or more sound levels. Both tests require tightly sealing the

device into the ear canal for accuracy, and do not replace more thorough diagnostic testing.

Tympanometry:
Tympanograms measure the flow of sound energy passing from the outer to the middle ear with changes in ambient pressure. Acoustic impedance, the opposition to energy flow, or its inverse, acoustic admittance, is plotted against ear canal pressure. Figure 12.4 shows several tympanogram shapes. In a normal ear (Fig. 12.4A), the peak of the tympanogram is near ambient pressure. Disorders such as otitis media can cause the tympanogram to peak at negative pressure (Fig. 12.4B). Otitis media with effusion flattens the tympanogram (no peak—Fig. 12.4C). Shallow tracings are recorded with conditions such as otosclerosis (Fig. 12.4D), whereas larger peaks are generated with ossicular disruption or healed TM perforations (Fig. 12.4E). We can use acoustic impedance to measure the acoustic reflex, a contraction of the stapedius muscles in response to a loud sound. It presumes neurologic integrity of the eighth nerve and therefore can be used for determining the location of lesions (e.g., an eighth-nerve tumor).

Pure-Tone Audiogram:
The pure-tone audiogram is essential for accurate diagnosis and treatment planning for patients with hearing difficulty. Refer to an audiologist for a hearing test, unless you suspect an active pathology of the ear, and then to an otolaryngologist. The hearing test identifies the magnitude, as well as the configuration, of the hearing loss. Figure 12.2A shows the audiogram of the 84-year-old woman discussed previously. The x-axis is frequency in kHz and is plotted on a logarithmic scale, from 125 to 8,000 Hz. Frequency (in Hz, cycles per second of vibration, or kHz, thousands of cycles per second of vibration) is a physical representation of pitch: Low-frequency sounds are low in pitch, whereas

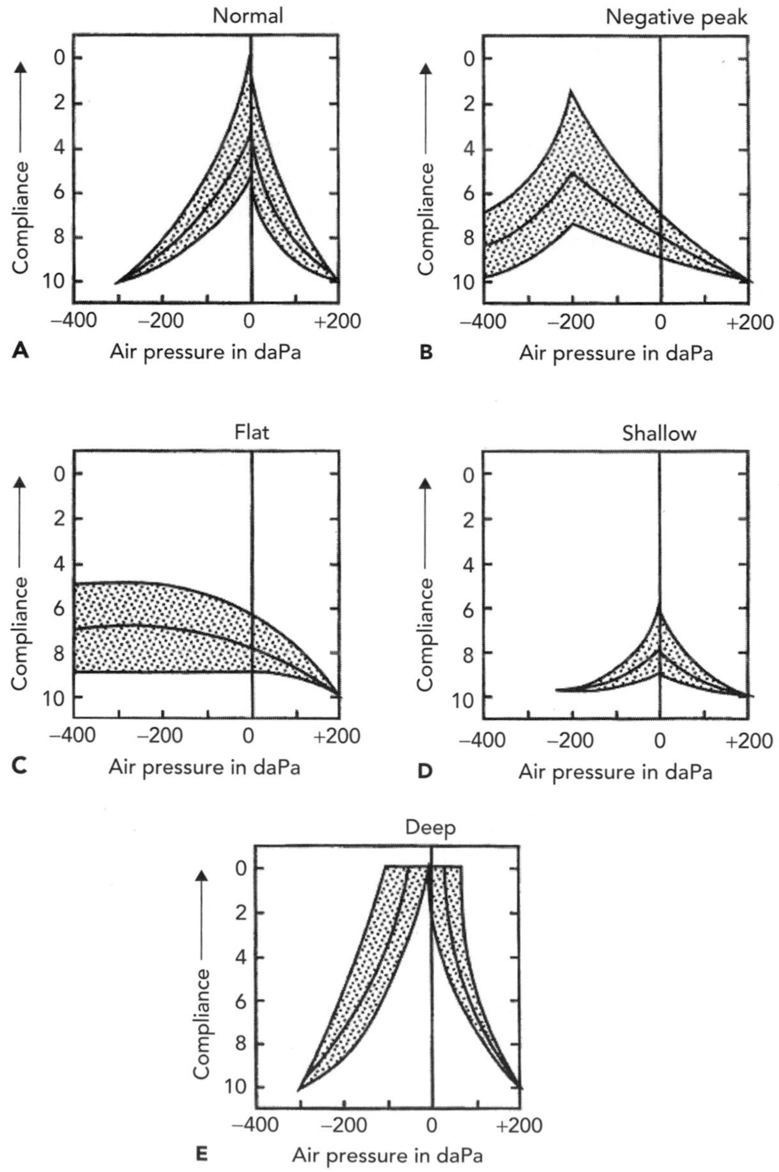

Figure 12.4 Tympanogram shapes—in a normal ear **(A)**, in case of disorders such as eustachian tube dysfunction **(B)**, in the presence of otitis media with effusion **(C)**, in conditions such as otosclerosis **(D)**, and in case of ossicular disruption or healed tympanic membrane perforations **(E)**. (Reprinted from F. Bess, Humes L. *Audiology the fundamentals*, 2nd ed. 1995, with permission of Lippincott Williams & Wilkins.)

TABLE 12.3
INTERPRETING AUDIOGRAM RESULTS FOR HEARING LOSS

Tone in Decibels (dB HL)	Degree of Hearing Loss
0–25	Normal hearing
25–40	Mild hearing loss
40–55	Moderate hearing loss
55–70	Moderately severe loss
70–90	Severe hearing loss
>90	Profound loss (legally deaf)

high-frequency sounds are high in pitch. In the cochlea, high-pitch sounds are encoded in the basal turn of the cochlea, whereas low-pitch sounds are represented in the apex. Altering the frequency (pitch) of the pure tone changes the region of the cochlea that is stimulated. The y-axis represents sound level in decibel (dB) hearing level (HL). The range 0 to 25 dB HL is normal. The greater the hearing loss, the greater the dB HL value (see Table 12.3).

It is important to understand that the dB scale is logarithmic and that someone with a threshold of 100 dB HL requires 100,000 times more sound pressure to hear that sound than does someone with a threshold of 0 dB HL. The value 0 dB HL represents the average hearing threshold of a large group of otologically and audiologically healthy subjects. Conversational speech is often at a level of roughly 50 dB HL, whereas speech presented at 90 to 100 dB HL is uncomfortably loud and speech at levels of 120 dB HL or more is painful.

The arithmetic mean of the audible or threshold tone in decibels at 500, 1,000, and 2,000 Hz is called the *PTA*. Symbols denote the test ear and signal type. "O," often printed in red, is the right ear air-conduction symbol. "X," often printed in blue, is the left ear air-conduction symbol. The symbols "<" and ">" are the unmasked right and left ear bone-conduction symbols, respectively, obtained by placing a vibrator on the skull, which bypasses the outer and middle ear systems.

Some patients complain that family and friends are always yelling at them. These are the individuals who may have a very narrow range of usable hearing, or dynamic range. The point where sound becomes uncomfortable may be the same as that for people with normal hearing (e.g., 90 dB HL), but the difference between this uncomfortable level and their hearing threshold (e.g., 80 dB HL) is very small. This can be a challenge for both the speaker and the hearing-impaired listener because most of the time speech will either be inaudible or uncomfortable for the hearing-impaired listener.

Modern hearing aids incorporate special algorithms (called *compression*) in an attempt to help the hearing-impaired individual with a reduced dynamic range. Many patients with sensorineural hearing loss have loudness recruitment. For example, a person with normal hearing might hear a tone at 0 dB HL, and his or her threshold of discomfort might be 100 dB HL. This is the person's usable range of hearing, or dynamic range, and in this example the dynamic range is 100 dB. A hearing-impaired person might have a threshold of 80 dB HL and still have a threshold of discomfort of 100 dB HL, and therefore he or she has a very limited dynamic range of 20 dB. Compression is a technique that provides a lot of amplification to soft sounds and much less amplification for loud sounds. This permits more effective amplification for those with a limited dynamic range.

Speech Recognition:
Spoken words challenge elders with an intermingled assortment of frequencies of varying levels. Therefore, the speech recognition threshold (SRT) is often performed to complement pure-tone audiometry. The SRT is determined by presenting two-syllable words, with equal stress on each syllable (called *spondees*), at decreasing levels to each ear until only 50% are correctly recognized. The SRT should agree with the PTA. Speech recognition is then tested at a louder and more comfortable or "suprathreshold" level. This is often called *speech discrimination testing*. For one popular test of speech discrimination, 50 single syllable words are presented, and the patient repeats the words heard. A patient with normal hearing will repeat nearly 100% of the words correctly. The percentage of correct words is often reduced in accordance with the degree of hearing difficulty, but the correlation between these two variables in not strong.

Special Tests for Populations with Testing Challenges:
Profound cognitive or motor impairments do not preclude hearing assessment in elders. The normal inner ear actually produces sounds ("cochlear echoes") in response to sounds introduced into the ear canal. A probe microphone placed in the ear canal can detect these cochlear echoes, called *otoacoustic emissions* (*OAEs*), which are thought to be generated by the outer hair cells of the inner ear. Scalp electrodes can be used to measure brain activity in response to brief sounds. Although many such responses can be recorded (and are collectively referred to as *auditory evoked potentials*), the response most commonly used clinically (both for threshold estimation and site-of-lesion testing) is the auditory brainstem response (ABR). Lesions of the eighth cranial nerve, pons, or midbrain can be identified by certain changes in the ABR pattern. In the elderly patient unwilling or unable to respond behaviorally, the ABR can be used to determine hearing impairment. For example, a patient suspected of exaggerating his or her hearing loss (perhaps to claim workers' compensation for work-related, noise-induced hearing loss) might warrant using an electrophysiologic estimation of hearing threshold.

Nuclear Magnetic Resonance Imaging:
When is magnetic resonance imaging (MRI) reasonably indicated? The response to this actively debated question must consider history, presenting symptoms, audiologic findings, patient's age, and cost. The patient with clear neurologic signs (e.g., unilateral facial paresis), unilateral or asymmetric hearing loss, or sudden hearing loss with persistent vertigo requires an MRI with gadolinium enhancement. Gadolinium is well tolerated, contains no iodine, and does not present a problem with renal excretion.

The image will identify space-occupying lesions such as slow-growing benign vestibular schwannomas (sometimes incorrectly called *acoustic neuromas*), glomus jugulare tumors, meningiomas, or pontine gliomas, as well as demyelinating diseases such as multiple sclerosis or leukodystrophies. Visualizing a vascular growth (e.g., a vascular tumor such as a glomus jugulare) through the TM also demands imaging. Imaging is less urgent for conditions known to be slowly progressing in the presence of stable hearing loss and no focal neurologic findings. A history consistent with the hearing loss is also reassuring (e.g., a history of occupational noise exposure). Persistent vertigo without a viral prodrome (suggesting labyrinthitis) warrants further investigation and, possibly, imaging. Similarly, persistent vague complaints of unsteadiness, as opposed to lightheadedness, warrant investigation for a tumor compressing the eighth nerve.

Management

Medical

Conductive Hearing Loss
Diagnosis dictates treatment. Referral to an otolaryngologist is appropriate for cases of conductive hearing loss that require or may benefit from surgical intervention. Chronic TM perforation, cholesteatoma, ossicular disruption, and otosclerosis fall into this category.

Sensorineural Hearing Loss
Sudden, often unilateral, hearing loss requires immediate referral for prompt treatment with steroids and/or antiviral medications either systemically or directly into the middle ear. Eighth-nerve tumors can also present with sudden hearing loss. In such cases, the consultant may order imaging studies.

Rehabilitation

In most elderly patients with hearing loss, the goal is assessing and minimizing hearing handicap. Hearing handicap scales in combination with the audiogram are useful in the diagnostic and rehabilitation process.[11] However, the rehabilitation prescription is contingent on the individual's lifestyle and communication needs. Family and friends may contribute valuable information to the assessment.

Hearing Aids

Hearing aids and other amplification devices are much maligned for their inability to screen out background noise, difficulty in manipulating the settings, stigma, and cost. With proper fitting, training, and support, however, these devices often produce gratifying results. Modern digital devices continuously sample the environment and adjust amplification as required. The circuits also offer noise suppression or filtering features for noisy environments. Costs for advanced digital technology are in the $2,500 range for one device. Hearing aids range in size from those that are totally contained in the ear canal to those that fit snugly behind the ear. More severe hearing losses often require larger devices. Smaller hearing aids, although more discreet, require considerable manual dexterity to adjust, install, or remove from the ear.

Hearing aids do not correct all changes in hearing that result from sensorineural hearing loss. Changes in sound processing, for example, persist and the hearing aid may only distort some sounds and make others too loud or not loud enough. Hearing function may also suffer if patients cannot afford two aids. Binaural information is important for locating the direction of a sound and therefore protects elders. Furthermore, two aids assist in listening to signals when there is a lot of background noise. The nuances of selecting, fitting, and, in the case of digital technology, programming devices is complex. Therefore, it is advisable for the primary care clinician to refer patients to clinical audiologists, professionals well grounded in administering and interpreting hearing tests, as well as designing appropriate interventions.

Cochlear Implants

Cochlear implants are an option for elderly patients with severe to profound hearing loss. Typically, this is due to sensorineural hearing loss, although in some cases those with mixed hearing loss (a conductive and sensorineural hearing loss) are candidates for this device. The implant bypasses the cochlea and electrically stimulates the auditory nerve fibers of the inner ear. An external processor converts acoustical energy (sound) into electrical current. An electrode array is surgically implanted into the inner ear, delivering current to the appropriate region of the cochlea in accordance with the sound's frequency. This sophisticated device produces excellent results in many patients, but it remains a costly alternative that is not always reimbursed by insurers.

Assistive Listening Devices

Theaters, houses of worship, and other public gathering spots often install assistive listening devices for their audiences. The systems translate microphone sounds into electromagnetic fields (or in some cases, FM radio frequencies or infrared signals) that are received by individuals who have telephone coils in their hearing aids or who borrow special receivers. Extraneous background noise is therefore less troublesome to the listener. This tends to increase the level of the signal relative to that of the noise and makes it easier to understand the signal. It should be noted that personal assistive listening devices can also be purchased. It is, for example, possible for individuals to have their hearing aids fit with FM devices that receive input from an external microphone. When the microphone is held close to the lips of a speaker in a noisy environment, this greatly enhances the ability of the hearing-impaired listener to follow the conversation.

Aural rehabilitation

Aural rehabilitation is an important adjunct to amplification. It minimizes the effects of hearing impairment, while maximizing the benefits of amplification. Patients learn to use visual cues (e.g., lipreading), select appropriate settings for hearing aids, and manipulate their listening environment to minimize communication difficulties. Without counseling, daily hearing aid utilization declines for new users. Even minimal amounts of counseling can significantly decrease the most commonly reported difficulties of the elderly: Listening in the presence of background noise, dexterity concerns, and the belief that hearing loss is not significant enough to warrant a hearing aid.[11] Self-help groups contribute to rehabilitation. Self Help for Hard of Hearing people is a national organization for the hearing impaired, with many local chapters. Contact information can be found in the section "Suggested Readings and Resources."

TINNITUS

Tinnitus, the perception of sound without an external source, can be a frustrating condition for patients and treating physicians. When chronic, the ringing, buzzing, hissing, roaring, or other sounds cause patients to become desperate and depressed. The primary care clinician must manage these and other comorbidities, educate patients about behaviors that exacerbate tinnitus, and refer when appropriate.

The prevalence of tinnitus increases with age and is more common in men. One theory is that tinnitus arises from environmental or degenerative damage to the auditory system, creating an imbalance between central auditory excitation and inhibition. This theory is supported by positron emission tomography (PET) and functional MRI studies.[12] Tinnitus can be categorized as objective (audible by the clinician as well as the patient) and subjective. Although objective tinnitus represents $<1\%$ of all cases, it includes conditions that may be correctable. Vascular fistulas, shunts, carotid stenosis, vascular compression on the auditory nerve, palatal myoclonus, or stapedial muscle spasticity are possible etiologies.

Workup

The history provides clues to the etiology and potential interventions. As with hearing loss, noise exposure, prior ear infections, or use of ototoxic medications (e.g., salicylates, nonsteroidal anti-inflammatory drugs, aminoglycoside antibiotics, loop diuretics, and chemotherapeutic agents including platinum-based antineoplastic agents and vincristine) are important. Arteriosclerosis, hypertension, and diabetes mellitus have systemic effects on vascular and neurologic function that contribute to both hearing loss and tinnitus. The quality and timing of the sound is significant. Pulsatile tinnitus in synchrony with the cardiac cycle suggests turbulent blood flow in stenotic vessels, vascular malformations, or anemia. A clicking rhythmic sound may suggest myoclonus of the palatal, tensor tympani, or stapedius muscles. Anxiety, depression, living alone, and unemployment exacerbate the perceived severity of tinnitus, as does excessive alcohol intake and insomnia.

The tinnitus history sometimes seems improbable. It is important to be alert for stories that are likely or unlikely to be linked to tinnitus. Hearing voices or music is a hallmark of auditory hallucinations and justifies psychiatric referral. On the other hand, sensorimotor acts (e.g., pushing on a tooth, jaw movement, and cervical thrust) commonly modify tinnitus. One particularly noteworthy form, gaze-evoked tinnitus, is associated with resection of a vestibular schwannoma.[13] In some respects it might be considered an auditory equivalent of phantom limb pain because it is heard in the deaf ear in response to eye movements. Cacace et al.[14] reported several case studies of what they termed *cutaneous-evoked tinnitus* following eighth-nerve resection, where tinnitus was elicited by touching the back of a hand or by finger manipulations. A recent case study[15] reported a woman who had gaze-evoked and cutaneous-evoked tinnitus. The latter was triggered by genital stimulation. It is imperative to listen to patient complaints about tinnitus because some very unusual forms exist.

Physical Examination

In addition to a thorough examination of the ear and assessing the function of the fifth, seventh, and eighth cranial nerves, auscultation of the heart and carotids and postauricular region may be rewarding. Vestibular function should also be assessed.

Laboratory and Imaging

Testing is dictated in part by clinical findings but may include tests for conditions leading to high-output cardiac states (anemia/hyperthyroidism). Doppler flow studies or echocardiograms contribute to diagnosing pulsatile tinnitus that is audible on examination. Although tinnitus can occur in patients with normal hearing, audiologic testing can also indicate the need for MRI with gadolinium enhancement. Unilateral high-frequency hearing loss combined with poor speech discrimination suggests the possibility of a vestibular schwannoma, whereas evidence of cochlear damage rarely requires imaging.[16]

Management

Refer patients with suspected objective tinnitus or vestibular schwannoma to an otolaryngologist, neuro-otologist, or neurosurgeon. The need for treatment of vascular stenosis must consider the critical nature of the lesion as measured on angiogram and the effect on the patient's life.

Detailed psychophysical studies have demonstrated that patients perceive pitch, loudness, and complexity of their tinnitus differently. Tinnitus retraining therapy (TRT) aimed at habituating patients to the tinnitus sounds rather than obliterating them claim improvement in 75% of patients. The multidisciplinary approach employs counseling and broadband noise generators. Hypnosis, biofeedback, and relaxation therapy have not been impressive.[16]

A variety of drugs have been used in attempts to treat tinnitus but none have been approved by the U.S. Food and Drug Administration for this purpose. To date, there is little or no evidence that they lead to significant improvements beyond placebo. *Ginkgo biloba* appeared very promising in several randomized clinical trials but firm conclusions were thwarted by variations in dose and formulation.[16]

Masking tinnitus by amplifying environmental noise with a hearing aid provides benefit in some patients. For those with hearing loss, the device can serve two purposes: Amplification and tinnitus masking. Masking devices alone can be used to mask tinnitus when a hearing aid is not needed, and combination devices (tinnitus masker and hearing aid) have been found to provide benefit in some tinnitus sufferers.

The American Tinnitus Association (ATA) is an excellent source of information for physicians and patients and can locate local tinnitus support groups (see section "Suggested Readings and Resources").

DIZZINESS AND BALANCE

The vestibular system shares an end organ with the auditory system—the membranous labyrinth—which includes the three semicircular canals, the utricle, saccule, and cochlea. Some drugs (e.g., the aminoglycosides) are both ototoxic and vestibulotoxic, and a number of disorders affect both the auditory and vestibular systems (e.g., vestibular schwannomas and Ménière disease).

History

The history should distinguish between true vertigo and a more vague sense of lightheadedness or imbalance because the causes differ. True vertigo (the sensation of the patient or the room spinning) often indicates a lesion of the peripheral vestibular system, whereas sensations of imbalance or lightheadedness may emanate from the peripheral vestibular system, the central nervous system, or systemic problems such as low blood pressure. Furthermore, postural instabilities leading to complaints of a sense of unsteadiness may reflect sensory problems (e.g., of the visual, somatosensory, and/or vestibular systems), central deficits, or problems of motor output (e.g., of the antigravity muscles of the legs). Similarly, reports of visual problems during head movement could be the result of a deficit anywhere in the reflex loop involved in the vestibular–ocular pathway (i.e., vestibular end organ; eighth nerve; vestibular nuclei; medial longitudinal fasciculus; cranial nerve nuclei and nerves III, IV, and VI; the extraocular muscles; and/or the visual system). The complex nature of the vestibulo-ocular and postural control systems makes the identification of the underlying cause of dizziness and balance disorders difficult. It is not unusual for patients to go from their primary care clinician to a variety of specialists (e.g., cardiologist, otolaryngologist, neurologist) with no conclusive diagnosis.

Dizziness is prevalent in the elderly,[17] as are balance problems.[18] Falls in the elderly often lead to hip fractures, and falls are the leading cause of accidental death in the elderly, leading to billions of dollars of health care costs annually in the United States.[19] Dizziness is subjective, and a questionnaire is often the best way of qualifying the dizziness problems. More details concerning the diagnosis and management of dizziness can be found in Chapter 13.

Diagnostic Testing

A number of tests are available to investigate vestibular and balance function. Tests of vestibular function often evaluate eye movements. In order to keep eyes focused on a target of interest, the head moves in one direction while eyes must move in the opposite direction. It is the vestibular system that senses the head movement and causes these reflexive eye movements (called the *vestibulo-ocular reflex*). The recording of eye movements can be done using electrodes (called *electronystagmography* [*ENG*]) or video goggles (called *video nystagmography*). Eye movements are monitored under a variety of conditions, including when the patient is at rest, is put into various positions, is following a moving pattern of lights, and when he or she is spun around in a rotary chair, and when warm or cool water or air is introduced into the ear canal.[20] Dynamic posturography is useful for quantifying balancing abilities under conditions where sensory input from the various sensory modalities contributing to balance (i.e., vestibular, visual, somatosensory) is manipulated. This allows identification of the relative contributions of these senses to balance function. This test battery also allows evaluation of motor abilities during balance. Other tests in this battery evaluate reflexive responses to the movements of the platform the patient is standing on.[20] Although dynamic posturography is generally not useful for site-of-lesion testing, it provides useful information about functional balance abilities, can determine whether postural instability arises from sensory versus motor function, and may be useful for generating a balance rehabilitation program.

Management

In the absence of a medically treatable cause, a vestibular rehabilitation program, typically provided by a physical therapist, may help alleviate dizziness.[21] As in tinnitus, support groups for those with dizziness or balance problems can be helpful. The Vestibular Disorders Association (VEDA) (see section "Suggested Readings and Resources" for contact information) can provide information about dizziness and balance disorders and has information about local chapters.

MÉNIÈRE DISEASE

Ménière disease is a debilitating disorder whose classical signs include hearing loss, tinnitus, and dizziness. The vestibular and auditory systems share common end organs. Conditions affecting the membranous labyrinth, composed of three semicircular canals—the utricle, saccule, and the cochlea—may therefore affect balance, as well as hearing. Ototoxic medications, for example, are often vestibulotoxic.

Differential Diagnosis

Ménière disease, also known as *endolymphatic hydrops*, is thought to be the result of abnormally high fluid pressure within the cochlea. The symptoms include (classically) a fluctuating, low-frequency hearing loss; episodic vertigo; roaring tinnitus; and a feeling of fullness in the ear. Its prevalence is approximately 1% in the United States.

Vestibular schwannomas must be considered in cases involving unilateral hearing loss without tinnitus, and often the symptoms of vestibular schwannoma are similar to those of Ménière disease.

In elderly patients, particularly those with known vascular disease, vertebrobasilar transient ischemic attacks or stroke must be considered along with cerebellar hemorrhage. Hearing loss may not accompany these conditions but, because of its ubiquitous nature, may be present in the elderly patient.

Workup/Keys to Diagnosis

The classical symptoms of Ménière disease are fluctuating low-frequency hearing loss, a feeling of fullness in the ear(s), episodic vertigo (the room or the patient is spinning), and a roaring tinnitus. In truth, often only a subset of these symptoms is present and patients may describe tinnitus differently. The hearing loss may not fluctuate and can involve the high frequencies. The symptoms may occur as self-limited episodes that increase in frequency for several years and then stabilize or decrease.

The etiology of vertigo is typically in the peripheral vestibular system. In the absence of vertigo, the cause of imbalance or lightheadedness is more difficult to localize. It may reflect a problem in the vestibular or central nervous system or systemic problems such as hypotension.

Laboratory/Imaging

All patients with vestibular complaints should have an audiogram. The battery of audiologic testing for patients with Ménière disease also includes a vestibular workup, including the recording of eye movements (called *ENG*) during postural manipulations, visual pursuit tasks, calorics, and rotary chair. ENG results will help elucidate the need for head and neck MRI. When the onset of symptoms is acute in the elderly population, an MRI should be obtained to evaluate the possibility of stroke or posterior fossa bleed.

Management

Meclizine, antiemetics, diuretics, and low-sodium diets are used to control the symptoms of Ménière disease. Benzodiazepines may be tried if first-line medications fail. Otolaryngologists will consider surgical intervention for resistant cases. Endolymphatic shunts, transtympanic injections of gentamicin, labyrinthectomy, or vestibular neurectomy are treatment options. Each of these surgical treatment modalities can provide relief from at least some of the symptoms of Ménière disease. However, no one treatment is effective for all (or even most) patients with Ménière disease.

CONCLUSION

Although hearing difficulty is common and often tolerated by elderly patients, it has consequences that often go unrecognized by physicians. Interventions may enhance quality of life, as well as offer enhanced safety and independence. The underlying conditions are often benign, but the astute clinician needs to consider the possibility of more ominous causes, such as eighth-nerve tumors, vascular tumors, stroke, or sudden hearing loss that require rapid intervention. Managing hearing loss is best done by a team approach with audiologists, physicians specializing in hearing disorders, and primary care providers.

REFERENCES

1. Weinstein, BE. Hearing loss in the elderly: A new look at an old problem. In: Katz J, ed. *Handbook of clinical audiology*, 5th ed. Philadelphia, PA: Lippincott Williams & Wilkins; 2002:597–604.
2. Divenyi P, Simon H. Hearing in aging: Issues old and young. In: *Current opinion in otolaryngology & head and neck surgery*, Vol. 7(5). Philadelphia, PA: Lippincott Williams & Wilkins; 1999.

3. Schuknecht HF. *The pathology of the ear*. Cambridge, MA: Harvard University Press; 1974.
4. Suplee C. *Everyday science explained*. Washington, DC: National Geographic Society; 1996.
5. Seidel H, Ball J, Dains, J et al. eds. *Mosby's guide to physical examination*. St. Louis, MO: CV Mosby Company; 1987.
6. Jerger J, Chmiel R, Wilson N, et al. Hearing impairment in older adults: New concepts. *J Am Geriatr Soc*. 1995;43:928–935.
7. Cassel CK, Walsh JR. *Geriatric medicine volume I medical, psychiatric and pharmacological topics*. New York, NY: Springer-Verlag; 1984.
8. Weinstein B. Validity of a screening protocol for identifying people with hearing problems. *Am Soc Hear Assoc*. 1986;28:41–45.
9. Jupiter T, DiStasio D. An evaluation of the HHIE-S as a screening tool for the elderly homebound population. *J Acad Rehab Audiol*. 1998;31:11–21.
10. Reuben D, Walsh K, Moore A. et al. Hearing loss in community-dwelling older persons: National prevalence data and identification using simple questions. *J Am Geriatr Soc*. 1998;46:1008–1011.
11. Sims D, Burkard R, Rehabilitation for presbycusis In: Hof P, Mobs C, eds. *Functional neurobiology of aging*. New York, NY: Academic Press; 2001:635–645.
12. Folmer R, Martin WH, Shi Y. Tinnitus: Questions to reveal the cause, answers to provide relief. *J Fam Pract*. 2004;53:532–540.
13. Wall M, Rosenberg M, Richardson D. Gaze evoked tinnitus. *Neurology*. 1987;37:1034–1036.
14. Cacace A, Cousins J, Parnes S, et al. Cutaneous-evoked tinnitus. I. Phenomenology, psychophysics and functional imaging. *Audiol Neurootol*. 1999;4:247–257.
15. Phillips J, Baguley D, Patel H, et al. Tinnitus evoked by cutaneous stimulation. *Neurology*. 2004;63:1756.
16. Lockwood A, Salvi R, Burkard R. Tinnitus. *N Engl J Med*. 2002;347:904–910.
17. Tinetti M, Williams C, Gill T. Dizziness among older adults: A possible geriatric syndrome. *Ann Intern Med*. 2000;132:337–344.
18. Tang P, Woollacott M. Balance control in older adults. In: Bronstein A, Brandt T, Woollacott M, Nutt J, eds. *Clinical disorders of balance, posture and gait*. London: Arnold; 2004.
19. Rose D, Allison L. *Identifying and managing elderly fallers*. Portland, OR: NeuroCom International; 1995.
20. Shepard N. Evaluation and management of balance system disorders. In: Katz J, ed. *Handbook of clinical audiology*, 5th ed. Baltimore, MD: Lippincott Williams & Wilkins; 2002.
21. Shepard N, Telian S. Programmatic vestibular rehabilitation. *Otolaryngol Head Neck Surg*. 1995;112:173–182.

SUGGESTED READINGS AND RESOURCES

Contact Information for Self-Help Groups

Self Help for Hard of Hearing People (SHHH)
7910 Woodmont Aven, Suite 1200
Bethesda, MD 20814
(301) 657–2248
(301) 657–2249
(301) 913–9413 (fax)
http://www.shhh.org/
info@hearingloss.org

American Tinnitus Association
PO Box 5
Portland, OR 97207-0005
(503) 248–9985
(503) 248-0024 (fax)
http://www.ata.org/
tinnitus@ata.org

Vestibular Disorders Association
PO Box 4467
Portland, OR 97208-4467
(503) 229–7705
(800) 229–8064
(503) 229–8064 (fax)
http://www.vestibular.org
veda@vestibular.org

13 Dizziness, Syncope, and Falls in the Elderly

Richard Brunader *Janet Leah Retke*

CLINICAL PEARLS 147

NORMAL GAIT AND BALANCE 148

DIZZINESS IN THE ELDERLY 148
Differential Diagnosis 148
Pathophysiology 150
Incidence and Prevalence 151
Signs and Symptoms 151
Impact on Function 152
Workup/Keys to the Diagnosis 152
Management 152

SYNCOPE IN THE ELDERLY 153
Differential Diagnosis 153
Pathophysiology 153
Incidence and Prevalence 153
Course/Timeline 154
Workup/Keys to the Diagnosis 154

FALLS IN THE ELDERLY 154
Pathophysiology 154
Incidence and Prevalence 154
Impact on Function 154
Etiology and Risk Factors 154
Medications 155
Activity and Environmental Causes of Falls 155
Workup/Keys to the Diagnosis 155
Management 158

CLINICAL PEARLS

- Dizziness is the result of a dysfunction in the sensory, central integrative, or motor systems affecting the orienting mechanisms and resulting in a perception of disequilibrium.
- With rare exceptions, dizziness is a benign, self-limited condition not associated with excess mortality.
- Dizziness can be subclassified as vertiginous, lightheadedness, disequilibrium, or "other."
- Brain imaging in patients with dizziness without focal neurological findings is generally not helpful.
- Vestibular rehabilitation therapy is based on central nervous system compensation for the dysfunctioning labyrinth.
- The etiology of syncope may remain undiagnosed in up to 40% of cases.
- Because elderly patients may be amnesic for a syncopal event and recall only having fallen, the history obtained from the patient may be misleading.
- Patients with a normal 12-lead electrocardiogram are extremely unlikely to have an arrhythmia causing syncope and have a very low risk of sudden death.
- Four percent of patients undergoing prolonged ambulatory cardiac monitoring as part of a syncopal evaluation have arrhythmias that are associated with symptoms.
- The fifth leading cause of death in persons older than 65 is accidents. Falls constitute two thirds of these accidents.
- Each year, at least one third of community-dwelling persons who are 65 and older fall.
- Most falls result from the accumulated effects of multiple impairments of the sensory, central integrative, cardiovascular, and musculoskeletal systems, any one of which alone might not have caused falling.

- Multifactorial interventions can reduce the incidence of falls between 12% and 37%.
- All older persons who report a single fall should be evaluated with the "Timed Up and Go Test."

Dizziness, syncope, and falls are often frustrating to physicians because of the frequent vagueness of the complaints and the difficulty in determining a diagnosis. Most causes are benign, but the possibility of the rare life-threatening cause often drives a medical evaluation to be more extensive than necessary. Dizziness, syncope, and falls are combined into a single chapter because of the considerable overlap in their symptoms and etiologies.

NORMAL GAIT AND BALANCE

Decline of gait and balance begins well before the rise in prevalence of falling. Already beginning in the second decade of life and greatly accelerating after the age of 40, balance and gait decline well before attention is generally paid to testing of balance or considering strategies to maintain or improve the balance.[1]

CASE ONE

C.H. is an 84-year-old woman who presents complaining of at least five falls that occurred over the last 12 months. Two weeks ago, while working in her garden, as she extended her neck, she felt a swimming sensation and fell backwards. She relates that she often feels unsteady with neck extension. Approximately 3 months ago, while in the kitchen, she made a sudden turn to answer the telephone, lost her balance and fell. She notices that she becomes unsteady when she makes sudden turns. She is unable to provide any further specifics about her other falls, except to say she believes they occurred in a manner similar to the two that she described, and that she experiences frequent periods of unsteadiness with ambulation. She denies any orthostatic symptoms, true vertigo, or hearing difficulty.

Approximately 6 months ago she suffered a severe upper respiratory infection. As she arose from the dinner table and went into the bathroom, she suddenly fell forward on her face. She suffered a laceration to her forehead and was unresponsive for approximately 1 minute. She was taken by ambulance to a nearby hospital where she stayed overnight. She was informed that all her test results were normal. There has been no reoccurrence of the syncope.

On evaluation, asymptomatic orthostatic hypotension is found. Her screening audiogram and 12-lead electrocardiogram are unremarkable. Her physical examination is otherwise normal except for osteoarthritic changes of her hands and feet. Gait and balance assessment confirm a fall risk and suggest vestibular dysfunction. A cervical x-ray reveals severe osteoarthritis.

You order physical therapy for vestibular rehabilitation and desensitization of cervical-induced dizziness. In terms of her asymptomatic orthostasis, you note in her medical records to titrate her blood pressure medication to standing blood pressure and inform her to be extra cautious at times of illness.

DIZZINESS IN THE ELDERLY

Dizziness is the result of a dysfunction in the sensory, central integrative, or motor systems affecting the orienting mechanisms, resulting in a perception of disequilibrium.[2]

Although the symptoms of dizziness may represent life-threatening conditions such as cardiac arrhythmia, seizure, transient ischemic attack, stroke, hypotension, or pericarditis, these are the unusual presentations. Most cases are benign, self-limited, and not associated with excess mortality.[3]

Differential Diagnosis

Conditions that lead to dizziness, syncope, and falls in the elderly are shown in Table 13.1.

Benign Positional Vertigo

Benign positional vertigo (BPV) is felt to be caused by otoconia that have come loose from the utricle or saccule and have moved to the posterior semicircular canal. BPV is manifested by a sudden onset of vertigo caused by head turning, which resolves within a minute. The diagnosis can be confirmed by the Dix-Hallpike maneuver.[4]

With the Dix-Hallpike maneuver, the patient's head is rapidly shifted from an upright position to a head-down position and tilted 30 degrees to the left. The maneuver is then repeated on the right. In BPV, the side toward which the head is turned when symptoms are induced is the side of dysfunction. Characteristics of a peripheral lesion such as BPV include: Vertiginous symptoms brought on by a rapid change in head position; vertiginous symptoms that subside within 60 seconds; rotatory nystagmus associated with vertiginous symptoms; dizziness and nystagmus occurring after a 2- to 10-second latency following a change in head position; and repetitive induction of the provocative maneuver causing extinction of the symptoms.[3]

In patients with central integrative pathology, such as mass lesions, or demyelinating or other pathology of the posterior fossa, nystagmus onset is immediate, fatigue of nystagmus does not occur, and subjective vertigo is minimal or absent.[2] Patients slowly improve and are generally back to normal within 4 to 6 weeks.[3]

Other Types of Vestibular Dysfunction

Severe vertigo of abrupt onset, which then decreases over the next 1 to 3 weeks is either due to labyrinthitis (if

TABLE 13.1
CONDITIONS THAT LEAD TO DIZZINESS, SYNCOPE, AND FALLS IN THE ELDERLY

Dizziness Condition (ICD-9)	Syncope Condition (ICD-9)	Falls Condition (ICD-9)
Vestibular (780.4)	Arrhythmias (427.9)	Accident/Environment
BPV (386.11)	Heart block (426.9)	Gait/Balance problems (781.2/780.4)
Labyrinthitis (386.10)	Aortic stenosis (424.1)	Muscle weakness (728.9)
Neuronitis (386.12)	Myocardial infarction (410.9)	Dizziness/Vertigo (780.4)
Acoustic neuroma (225.1)	Carotid sinus syndrome (337.0)	Drop attack (780.2)
Postural hypotension (458.0)	Cardiac ischemia (414.9)	Confusion (298.9)
Cervical	Miscellaneous cardiac[a]	Postural hypotension (458.0)
Deconditioning	Postural hypotension (458.0)	Visual disorders (369.9)
Cerebrovascular (386.2)	Vasovagal response (780.2)	Syncope (780.2)
Sensory impairments	Drug induced	Medication (963.9)
Psychiatric (300.11)	Situational[b]	Other specified causes[d]
Hyperventilation (306.1)	Cerebrovascular event (437.1)	
	Seizure disorder (780.39)	
	Postprandial hypotension (458.8)	
	Miscellaneous[c]	
	Unknown	

[a]Includes cough, micturition, and defecation syncope.
[b]Includes pulmonary embolism, pulmonary hypertension, aortic aneurysm.
[c]Includes psychiatric causes, bleeding or anemia, subclavian steal, trigeminal neuralgia, vertigo, drop attack, volume depletion.
[d]This category includes: Arthritis, acute illness, drugs, alcohol, pain, epilepsy, and falling from bed.
BPV, benign positional vertigo.
From references 2–7.

hearing is affected) or vestibular neuronitis (if hearing is not affected). When vestibular dysfunction occurs, the central nervous system is eventually able to compensate to some degree. However, recovery in the elderly may be prolonged because central nervous system compensation is slower, and patients are left with unsteadiness if the compensation is incomplete. A viral infection is felt to be the etiology in younger individuals. In the elderly, infarction is more often the cause. Ménière disease is the likely diagnosis when vertigo is accompanied by tinnitus and gradual development of unilateral low-frequency hearing loss. Recurrent vestibulopathy is the diagnosis when auditory symptoms are absent. The typical patient has an attack about once a year, which lasts a day, and has a more benign prognosis than those with Ménière disease.[4]

An acoustic neuroma grows so slowly that the disruption in brainstem input from the side affected by the tumor is compensated for by central mechanisms. Therefore, the vertigo is generally absent or minimal.[5]

Postural Dizziness

Postural dizziness is generally due to postural hypotension. However, the elderly with symptoms of postural dizziness do not always meet the criteria for orthostatic hypotension, defined as a reduction of systolic blood pressure by at least 20 mm Hg and diastolic blood pressure by at least 10 mm Hg within 3 minutes of standing.[6] It is not uncommon that the sensation of postural dizziness occurs without postural blood pressure changes. Some older patients pool enough blood in their lower extremities to compromise cerebral perfusion without lowering their blood pressure. Sometimes, marked blood pressure declines do not occur until 10 to 30 minutes following standing. Finally, in some patients, the sensation of postural dizziness without postural blood pressure changes is caused by the same conditions as those causing dysequilibrium (see section "Subtypes of Dizziness").[3]

Cervical Dizziness

Pathology in the neck is a frequent cause of dizziness in the elderly. Cervical dizziness may be either proprioceptive or vascular induced. Proprioceptive cervical dizziness occurs when osteoarthritis of the facet joints of the cervical spine impair somatosensory information coming from the neck, which can lead to lightheadedness or vertiginous sensations. Vascular cervical dizziness typically occurs when turning the head or looking up causes an osteoarthritic spur to pinch the vertebral artery.[4]

Physical Deconditioning

Deconditioning is the consequence of physiologic changes following a period of inactivity or low activity that result in functional losses, including loss of muscle strength, third spacing of fluid with development of postural dizziness, and reduced coordination. Similar changes are seen when patients with dizziness restrict their activities because of fear of falling. The inactivity leads to physiologic changes that actually worsens the dizziness and increases the risk of falling.[3]

Therefore, exercise is one of the most useful therapies for chronic dizziness in the elderly. Exercise in the elderly can reverse the orthostasis brought on by lack of movement, rebuild muscle strength, recover joint mobility, and improve vestibular function.[3]

Stroke

The abrupt onset of vertigo can be seen in vertebrobasilar stroke. Because of damage to adjacent brainstem structures, however, vertigo due to cerebral ischemia rarely occurs in isolation without other associated neurological deficits.[2]

Severe vertigo, ataxia, and vomiting can be findings in cerebellar infarction. Because brainstem signs are often absent, it can be mistaken for labyrinthitis; within 24 to 96 hours however, cerebellar edema may lead to progressive brainstem dysfunction.[3]

Unexplained dizziness in the elderly is often attributed to lacunar strokes.[3] The diagnosis, however, can be quite difficult, as revealed in a study comparing magnetic resonance imaging (MRI) scanning of the head and neck in dizzy and nondizzy elderly patients. There were no significant differences found in the prevalence of cerebral atrophy, the number of white matter lesions, the number of cerebral infarcts, or disease of the semicircular canals or cerebellopontine angle in subjects with and without dizziness. The only difference in MRI between them was that midbrain white matter lesions (whose clinical significance is uncertain) were more common in patients with dizziness.[8]

Multiple Sensory Impairments

The visual, proprioceptive, vestibular, cerebellar, and neuromuscular systems must all work in an integrated manner to keep the body balanced and free of dizziness. In multiple neurosensory impairments, separate lesions in more than one area of this postural control system combine to induce dizziness. Because of impaired physiologic function in several systems associated with aging (peripheral neuropathy, impaired visual acuity, reduced labyrinthine function), older persons are particularly susceptible to this type of dizziness.[3]

Medication-Associated Dizziness

A wide variety of medications have been associated with dizziness, including multiple cardiovascular drugs as well as medications with anticholinergic effects. In addition, a number of medications are potentially ototoxic and can cause labyrinthine damage with resultant disequilibrium (see Table 13.2).[3]

TABLE 13.2
DRUG-ASSOCIATED DIZZINESS

Medications Associated with Dizziness	Ototoxic Agents
Diuretics	Aspirin
Calcium blockers	Cisplatin
β-Blockers	Aminoglycosides
α-Blockers	
Vasodilators	
Psychotropic medications	
Antianxiety agents	
Antipsychotics	
Antidepressants	
Sedative–hypnotics	
Muscle relaxants	
Anticonvulsants	
NSAIDs	
Anticholinergic agents[3]	

NSAIDs, nonsteroidal anti-inflammatory drugs.

Hyperventilation Syndrome

Although frequently associated with psychiatric disorders, hyperventilation by itself can produce lightheadedness secondary to reflex decreased cerebral blood flow. However, this finding is more common in younger individuals as opposed to the elderly.[2]

Psychologic Factors

Anxiety and depression lead to a continuous dizziness that is a common etiology in younger adults. This is in contrast to the elderly in whom psychological disorders are rarely the primary cause of dizziness. Most patients have other associated somatic symptoms and dizziness is often present for years.[3]

Pathophysiology

The vestibular labyrinth, and the ocular and proprioceptive systems interact to maintain equilibrium. Any disturbance in either the function or interrelationships of these structures can lead to a loss of equilibrium. When loss of function occurs in one system, the other two systems may gradually compensate so that balance and gait in most situations are maintained.[9]

With advancing age, function of the body's balance control system is affected by a combination of disease, deconditioning, and age-related changes. Aging is associated with a loss of vestibular sensory epithelial cells and vestibular nerve fibers. In addition, hypertension and atherosclerosis affect vestibular pathways in the central nervous system.[10] Presbyopic changes, a decline in contrast sensitivity, along with cataracts, glaucoma, and macular degeneration affect the visual system. Finally, peripheral neuropathy affects more than 25% of persons aged 65 to 75, and 54% of patients older than 85 in the United States.[11] Though these changes are often subclinical with respect to balance control, they do lower the threshold of imbalance. In addition, cardiovascular factors, cognitive impairment, muscle weakness, and medications also contribute.[9,12] All this results in older persons walking more slowly, turning more carefully, and being more susceptible to dizziness, imbalance, and falls.[3] Superimposed upon this functional decline, minor stresses such as anemia, medication effects, electrolyte disturbances, and glucose or thyroid imbalance may cause dizziness and falling.[9,12]

Incidence and Prevalence

Dizziness is reported in approximately 30% of people 65 years and older, and is the third most common cause of falls in the community-dwelling elderly. It is the most common presenting complaint in primary care office practices among patients 75 years and older.[13] Annually, 18% of older persons experience dizziness severe enough to result in a physician visit, use of medication, or interference with daily activities.[3]

There is wide variability in the reported prevalence of many diagnoses causing dizziness in published clinical studies.[14] Vestibular disease has been reported in 4% to 64% of cases of dizziness. Cerebrovascular causes were identified in 0% to 70% of cases, psychiatric causes in 0% to 40%, and cervical spondylosis in 0% to 66%. The frequency with which no diagnosis could be made has ranged from 8% to 22% of cases, and multiple diagnoses in 0% to 85% of cases. Carotid hypersensitivity was diagnosed in 48% of patients in one study.[15]

Reasons for such wide variability in prevalence of findings have been attributed to different populations studied, nonuniform criteria in assigning diagnoses,[12] and bias caused by investigators tending to diagnose conditions in their specialty.[14] However, realizing that dizziness is a syndrome often caused by more than one of several interrelated and interacting conditions, leads to an approach of evaluating each patient with dizziness for multifactorial causes as opposed to looking for discrete conditions.[15]

Signs and Symptoms

To assist in determining an etiology, categorizing dizziness into one of the following four subtypes as well as whether the dizziness is continuous or intermittent is helpful.

Subtypes of Dizziness

Vertigo

An imbalance of the vestibular signals arising from the inner ear, middle ear, brainstem, or cerebellum can lead to vertigo. The vestibular imbalance leads to a misleading sensation of spinning or motion of either the individual or the environment. Causes of vertigo in older persons include BPV, cerebrovascular disease, acute labyrinthitis/vestibular neuronitis, panic disorder, cervical spine disease, serous otitis media, sinusitis, and, in some, drug toxicities.[3]

Presyncopal Lightheadedness

Presyncopal lightheadedness is due to diffuse cortical or brainstem ischemia from vascular or cardiac causes. It is a sensation of impending loss of consciousness. Common causes include vasovagal episodes, postural hypotension, and cardiac disease (arrhythmias, conduction disorders, and low-output states) and are outlined in the syncope section.[3]

Dysequilibrium

Dysequilibrium is an ill-defined sensation of unsteadiness and being off balance. The body is felt to be disoriented as opposed to the head. It can be due to almost any disturbance of neurosensory structures related to the body's balance control system (visual, vestibular, proprioceptive, cerebellar, or motor function). It has been commonly attributed to lacunar strokes, multiple neurosensory deficits, severe unilateral or bilateral vestibular dysfunction, peripheral neuropathy, cerebellar disease, and deconditioning.[3]

Other

Symptoms of floating or nonpresyncopal lightheadedness, or other ill-defined sensations related to balance are placed in this category. Psychological disorders, such as conversion reaction, panic disorder, depression, and generalized anxiety with related somatic symptoms are most often attributed as the cause.[3]

Episodic or Continuous Dizziness. Unfortunately, many dizziness symptoms in older persons cannot be reliably assigned to a single category, and often older persons with dizziness describe several of the above subtypes.[14] Because certain diagnoses produce dizziness continuously, whereas other diagnoses cause symptoms only intermittently with symptom-free periods, this lends to another classification scheme.[2]

Continuous Dizziness. Conditions in this category include psychiatric disorders; deconditioning; certain medications (Table 13.2); and structural damage from stroke, cerebellar atrophy, aminoglycoside-induced vestibular damage, residual labyrinthitis, and peripheral neuropathy.[2]

Episodic Dizziness. Episodic dizziness is the result of diseases causing temporary disruption of the body's balance control system. The three most common causes in this category are BPV, transient ischemic attacks, and Ménière disease. Other causes include recurrent vestibulopathy and migraine.[2]

Impact on Function

Dizziness does not independently predict an increased probability of death or becoming disabled when cofounding factors, such as age and diseases, are controlled for. Instead, dizziness is a marker for other conditions that increase a patient's risk of becoming disabled. These conditions include advanced age, nonwhite race, vascular disease, sensory impairment, and level of morbidity from arthritis, hypertension, and diabetes.[16] However, many patients with dizziness do report great impairment of functional activities, depression, or fear secondary to dizziness.[14]

Workup/Keys to the Diagnosis

A clinical history and focused physical examination will establish the diagnosis in most cases of dizziness.[3] In terms of the physical examination, concentrating on the cardiac and neurologic assessment, neck range of motion, Dix-Hallpike maneuver, and otologic examination are most helpful.

Laboratory tests should be ordered to confirm suspected etiologies. In patients with unclear diagnoses or in whom multiple etiologies are suspected, obtaining thyroid function studies, assessing renal and liver function, blood glucose, calcium, complete blood count, and syphilis serologies can be considered.[3,4]

To screen for acoustic neuroma, audiometry with speech discrimination is best. Other tests useful in select cases include electronystagmography, the Saccade test, rotational testing, posturography, Doppler examination of the carotid and vertebral arteries, brainstem auditory-evoked potentials, electroencephalography, and brain imaging, though with the limitations outlined in the preceding text.[4]

Management

General Measures

The overall prognosis for dizziness is generally good. Anemia, cardiac arrhythmias, adverse drug effects, systemic infections, cerumen against the tympanic membrane, acoustic neuroma, and serous (or acute) otitis media will respond to specific treatments. Migraine, neck osteoarthritis, physical deconditioning, and psychological diagnoses, while not curable, can be improved with therapy. Viral illnesses, labyrinthitis, and BPV are generally self-limited and will often self-resolve.[3]

However, patients whose dizziness is multifactorial are often impossible to cure. These are patients with multiple chronic medical problems, are often depressed or suffer from chronic anxiety, may have sustained falls secondary to the dizziness and thereby are limiting their activity, have visual and functional impairments, and are on multiple medications. In addition, these patients may have peripheral neuropathy, vestibular dysfunction, lacunar infarcts, and disorders of circulation causing orthostasis.[3]

Such patients with chronic disabling dizziness may benefit from a multifactorial approach aimed at identifying and managing contributing conditions. A combination of treating visual impairment, improving muscle strength, adjusting medication regimens, treating anxiety or depression,[14] and balance and gait training can be offered, depending on the preexisting impairments (Evidence Level B). The home should be made as safe as possible (see section "Home Modifications"). Finally, the patient should understand that lack of mobility leads to an ultimate worsening of dizziness[3] (Evidence Level C).

Vestibular Rehabilitation

The primary principle of vestibular rehabilitation is based upon central nervous system compensation to the altered signals from the damaged labyrinth. It is a program of repetitive eye, head, and body movements designed to provoke vertigo and imbalance. Over the course of therapy, the number of repetitions is slowly increased as the patient's tolerance for the exercises increases with a corresponding decrease in symptoms. The exercises stimulate the vestibular system and promote adaptive mechanisms within the central nervous system. These exercises help regain skills and confidence in balance (Evidence Level B).[17]

An example of central adaptation is when an individual obtains new glasses. For a day or so, visual perception is often slightly off, but then adjustment occurs. Another example is a gymnast's or tight-rope walker's finely tuned sense of balance. Their fine balance skills develop because of repetitive stimulation of their balance control mechanism. In the same manner, vestibular rehabilitation exercises stimulate central compensation for peripheral and central neurological deficits. These exercises may consist of a progression of eye and head movements done in progressively more challenging positions from lying down, sitting up, standing, and walking. Examples include moving the eyes up and down and side to side, and moving the head forward and backward, and side to side. Gaze stabilization exercises include focusing on a single stationary target while moving the head side to side or up and down. The response to these exercises is often a marked improvement over a very short period. Once central nervous system adjustment has occurred, the improvement will last for weeks.[12,18]

Treatment of Benign Positional Vertigo

There are two conservative treatments of BPV. One involves a maneuver, the other an exercise. The Epley maneuver involves sequential movement of the head through four positions, staying in each position for roughly 30 seconds. The patient's head is turned 45 degrees toward the side that provokes the symptoms, and then the patient is lowered into a supine position with the head still turned 45 degrees and approximately 30 degrees in extension. In the next position, the head is turned 45 degrees to the opposite side, while maintaining the neck in extension. For the third position, the patient rolls onto the nonprovocative side. Finally, the patient slowly sits up. The maneuver allows the otoconia to be moved out of the posterior canal. Although this treatment has been shown to be very effective with an 80% cure rate, the recurrence rate for BPV after the maneuver is approximately 30% at 1 year, and 50% at 5 years. In some instances, a second treatment may be necessary. Patients can also be instructed to do the maneuver themselves (Evidence Level B).[18]

The exercise used to treat BPV is called the *Brandt-Daroff exercise*. Patients are told to sit on the edge of a bed or the couch, turn their head 45 degrees to one side, then lie down quickly onto the opposite side, with the head still turned 45 degrees. Patients stay in that position until symptoms subside plus 30 seconds, then sit up. The movement is then repeated on the other side. This exercise should be performed three times a day for just over 2 weeks, or two times a day for 3 weeks, for a total of 52 sets. In most persons, complete relief from symptoms is obtained after 30 sets, or approximately 10 days (Evidence Level B).[18]

Medications

Several antihistamines, benzodiazepines, and anticholinergics are commonly used to manage symptoms of dizziness.[4] However, no current medication has well-established efficacy or is suitable for long-term use.[19] Meclizine is a widely used vestibular suppressant in doses of 12.5 to 25 mg orally three times a day as needed. Diazepam, prescribed in doses of 2.5 mg to 5 mg orally three times a day as needed, also has reported efficacy. Both of these medications should be used with caution in older adults to avoid sedation. In addition, anticholinergics such as scopolamine should also be used with prudence in the elderly because of the side effects of visual changes, mucosal dryness, urinary retention, and confusion. All of these medications should be used in low doses, and only for short durations, because they reduce physiologic central nervous system compensation.[4]

SYNCOPE IN THE ELDERLY

Syncope occurs when there is a transient loss of consciousness that causes a fall. Its occurrence is generally unpredictable and with a sudden, rapid onset. Typically, there is complete recovery. Spontaneous remission is frequent, which adds to the diagnostic challenge of syncope.[20]

Differential Diagnosis

Historically, syncope and falls have been considered as separate entities, each with their own unique differential diagnosis and natural history (Table 13.1). However, evidence indicates a complex interrelationship between falls, syncope, and dizziness. Syncope is simply a more severe form of presyncopal lightheadedness,[20] one of the four dizziness subtypes described.[2] Both syncope and presyncopal lightheadedness can lead to falls. Therefore, the separation of falls and syncope into distinct syndromes is artificial. In addition, the history of the event is crucial to the diagnosis.[3] Not only is retrograde amnesia to a syncopal event not uncommon,[21] but up to one third of patients do not even remember they had sustained a fall 3 months after the event.[22]

Finally, older patients experiencing syncope frequently have multiple potential contributing causes. Multiple interventions for possible attributable etiologies are often necessary. This is not only because of an inability to determine which of the attributable causes led to the syncopal event but also the likelihood that a single condition may not have been responsible.[20]

Even after a complete evaluation, the etiology of syncope may remain undiagnosed in up to 40% of cases.[23] Thirty-eight percent of cases are felt to be noncardiac in etiology. Orthostatic hypotension, vasovagal reactions, and medication-induced syncope are felt to be the most common causes in this category. Cardiac etiologies, arrhythmias and heart block being the most common, are felt to account for approximately 25% of all cases of syncope.[7]

Pathophysiology

As one ages, physiologic changes occur in heart rate, blood pressure, and cerebral blood flow. Along with comorbid conditions and concomitant medications, this leads to an increasing prevalence of syncope with age. Changes associated with age include a dampening of the baroreceptor reflex leading to a decreased heart rate and blood pressure response to hypotensive events. Because of a decline in plasma rennin and aldosterone, a rise in atrial natriuretic peptide, and frequent diuretic therapy, the geriatric population is susceptible to a decline in intravascular volume owing to undue salt loss through the kidneys. Low intravascular volume along with age-related cardiac diastolic dysfunction can lead to compromised cardiac output with stress. This predisposes to orthostatic hypotension and other circulatory compromising conditions. Finally, sustained hypertension alters cerebral autoregulation that is needed to maintain a constant cerebral circulation over a wide range of blood pressures.[20]

Incidence and Prevalence

Because many fall studies excluded patients with syncope, and as mentioned many patients with syncope have retrograde amnesia and therefore do not remember specifics surrounding a fall, the frequency of syncope may be underestimated.[21] In studies looking at the etiology of falls, the percentage of falls felt to be due to syncope ranges from 0.5% to 3.0%. However, because syncopal patients were often not evaluated in the studies from which fall statistics were obtained, these percentages may be misleading.[7]

Therefore, the prevalence of cardiovascular causes of falls in the general population is currently unknown.[21]

Course/Timeline

It is unclear whether mortality and sudden death are directly due to syncope or whether syncope reflects the underlying pathophysiology that is responsible. In studies of hospitalized patients with an episode of syncope, 1-year mortality rates range between 13% and 33%.[7] There is a >50% 5-year mortality rate for syncope caused by cardiac disease. This compares with a 30% 5-year mortality for syncope due to noncardiac causes. Patients with unexplained syncope have a 24% 5-year mortality.[23]

Workup/Keys to the Diagnosis

Because elderly patients may be amnesic for a syncopal event and only recall having fallen, the history obtained from the patient may be vague or misleading.[23]

When considering a heart block or an arrhythmia, the 12-lead electrocardiogram is critical. Up to 11% of patients with syncope are diagnosed from their electrocardiogram. However, those with a normal 12-lead electrocardiogram (no QRS or rhythm disturbance) are extremely unlikely to have a conduction disturbance or an arrhythmia causing syncope and a very low risk of sudden death. Often, prolonged ambulatory cardiac monitoring is ordered as part of the initial evaluation. However, detecting a causative arrhythmia during monitoring is rare. Only 4% of patients have arrhythmias that are associated with symptoms. Thirteen percent of patients have arrhythmias without symptoms, and symptoms without arrhythmias occur in up to 17%. Increasing the duration of monitoring from 24 to 72 hours increases the diagnostic yield from 15% to 29%; however, most increased diagnostic yields are arrhythmias unrelated to symptoms.[23] Therefore, unless the history is strongly suggestive or the 12-lead electrocardiogram is abnormal, obtaining prolonged ambulatory monitoring is not useful.

FALLS IN THE ELDERLY

Pathophysiology

Falling has been defined as an event that results in a person unintentionally coming to rest on the ground, floor, or other lower level.[24] To maintain upright stability, the central nervous system must continually and almost instantaneously integrate sensory information from the visual, vestibular, and somatosensory systems. Signals must then be sent to generate complex motor and cardiovascular responses.[19]

Falling occurs at all ages. However, as age brings about impairments to the balance control system, the ability of an individual to compensate for a destabilizing situation declines. Therefore, as one ages, the risk of experiencing a fall due to a given perturbation increases because of a progressive decline in an individual's balance control.[19]

Incidence and Prevalence

In 1948, a landmark study on a random sample of elderly residents in England was performed. Among a number of health-related items was the question, "Are you liable to fall?" Forty-three percent of the women and 21% of the men answered "Yes".[25] Several studies since then have addressed fall rates in the community. Each year, at least one third of community-dwelling persons who are 65 and older fall;[26] of these, one half suffer multiple falling episodes. After age 65, the incidence steadily rises until the age of 80 and older,[7] at which time the incidence increases to almost 50%.[27]

Impact on Function

In the United States, the fifth leading cause of death in persons older than 65 is accidents, and falls constitute two thirds of these accidents.[7] One percent of falls result in hip fracture, 2% result in hospitalization, 5% result in other fractures, 5% result in serious soft tissue injuries, and 50% result in minor injuries such as abrasions or contusions.[28] Of the patients who are hospitalized for a fall, 43% are discharged to a nursing facility,[25] and only 50% are alive 1 year later.[23]

Once they have fallen, between 14% and 50% of community-dwelling elderly are unable to get up without help. Up to 3% of the elderly who fall remain on the ground for 20 minutes or more. Delays increase their risk of dehydration, pressure sores, rhabdomyolysis, and pneumonia.[28]

Unrelated to physical injury, fear of falling is another source of fall-related morbidity, which leads to self-imposed activity restriction. Between 10% and 25% of persons who have fallen admit to avoiding activities such as shopping or housekeeping because of their fears of additional falls or injuries.[29]

It is not just the high incidence of falls that poses a threat to the elderly, because children and athletes have a higher fall rate than all but the frailest older adults. Instead, it is the combination of high incidence with high susceptibility to injury that makes falls a major geriatric health concern.[7] In men and women aged 65 to 69 years, falls result in 24.5 and 36.5 per 1,000 fall-injury events respectively. In patients older than 85 years, the incidence increases to 148.5 and 158.5 per 1,000 fall-injury events in men and women respectively.[23]

Etiology and Risk Factors

Most falls result from the accumulated effect of multiple impairments of the sensory, central integrative, cardiovascular, and musculoskeletal systems, any one of which alone might not have caused a fall.[29] Table 13.1 lists the causes of falls in

TABLE 13.3

RISK FACTORS FOR FALLS IDENTIFIED IN 16 STUDIES THAT EXAMINED MULTIPLE RISK FACTORS

Summary of Univariate Analysis Risk Factor	Significant/Total[a]	Mean RR–OR[b]	Range
Muscle weakness (728.9)	10/11	4.4	1.5–10.3
History of falls	12/13	3.0	1.7–7.0
Gait deficit (781.2)	10/12	2.9	1.3–5.6
Balance deficit (780.4)	8/11	2.9	1.6–5.4
Use assistive device	8/8	2.6	1.2–4.6
Visual deficit (369.9)	6/12	2.5	1.6–3.5
Arthritis (716.9)	3/7	2.4	1.9–2.9
Impaired ADL	8/9	2.3	1.5–3.1
Depression (311)	3/6	2.2	1.7–2.5
Cognitive impairment (294.8)	4/11	1.8	1.0–2.3
Age >80	5/8	1.7	1.1–2.5

[a]Number of studies with significant odds ratio or relative risk ratio in univariate analysis/total number of studies that included each factor.
[b]Relative risk ratios (RR) calculated for prospective studies. Odds ratios (OR) calculated for retrospective studies.
ADL, activities of daily living.
With permission from Rubenstein LZ, Josephson KR. The epidemiology of falls and syncope. *Clin Geriatr Med.* 2002;18:141–158.

community-dwelling elderly patients. The most common causes are environmentally related accidents followed by gait/balance disorders or muscle weakness, and dizziness.

Only approximately 10% of falls in elderly patients occur because of acute illness such as pneumonia, urinary tract infection, or congestive heart failure.[30]

Table 13.3 provides a summary of fall risk factors obtained from 16 studies. There is a four- to fivefold increase in the risk of falls in patients with lower extremity weakness, and a threefold increase in individuals with impaired gait or balance. There is about a 2.5-fold increased risk in persons with general functional impairment, visual deficits, arthritis, and having a prior history of falls. There is a twofold increased risk of falls in patients with depression, cognitive impairment, and age >80 years. Finally, use of psychoactive medication increases the fall risk 1.7 times.[7]

As the number of fall risk factors increases, the risk of falling significantly increases. Annual risks of falling have ranged from 10% to 27% for community-dwelling elderly with no fall risk factors to 69% to 100% for community-dwelling elderly with three or more fall risk factors, depending upon the study.[21]

Medications

Patients taking four or more prescription medications have a threefold increased risk of falling. Falling may be a side effect of the medications. Alternatively, the medications may be markers for underlying illnesses predisposing to falls.[25]

Specific classes of medications found to increase the risk of falling in nursing home patients include psychotropic drugs (OR = 1.7) and cardiac drugs (Class IA antiarrhythmics OR = 1.6; digoxin OR = 1.2; diuretics OR = 1.1).[7] Use of corticosteroids and nonsteroidal anti-inflammatory agents is also associated with an increased fall risk.[25]

Activity and Environmental Causes of Falls

Over 75% of falls in the elderly occur in their own home. Objects tripped over and stairs or steps are the most frequently identified contributors within the home.[30]

Only 10% to 15% of falls in community-dwelling elderly persons occur during high-risk actions such as standing on a chair or climbing a ladder. Most falls occur during commonplace activities such as walking or turning, taking a shower or bath, walking in the garden or entering the home.[30]

Workup/Keys to the Diagnosis

The U.S. Preventive Services Task Force recommends that all persons 75 years of age or older, as well as those 70 to 74 years who have a known risk factor, be counseled about specific measures to prevent falls (Evidence Level C).[31]

In 2001, the American Geriatrics Society, the British Geriatrics Society, and the American Academy of Orthopedic Surgeons published consensus guidelines on fall prevention for the elderly. Older patients (age not defined) should be asked annually whether they have suffered a fall. All older persons who report a single fall should be evaluated with the "Timed Up and Go test" (TUG) (see section "Gait and Balance Assessment Tools"). Those patients successfully completing the test require no additional evaluation. Persons who have difficulty with the test require further assessment. If an elderly patient seeks medical attention because of a fall, reports recurrent falls (defined as two or more in 6 months), or has abnormal gait or balance, they should have a complete fall evaluation performed (Evidence Level C).[21]

Fall Evaluation

Because most falls are due to the accumulated effect of multiple impairments, any one of which alone might not have caused it, a fall evaluation requires a thorough assessment of potential contributing causes.[21]

The history should concentrate on the specific circumstances surrounding each fall the patient is able to recall. The specifics of the event(s) are helpful to focus the evaluation. Unfortunately, 3 months after a fall, a significant number of individuals do not recall the event,[22] and the details surrounding the falls that are remembered are often poor. In addition, all medications should be reviewed, all acute and chronic medical problems should be noted, the patient's functional status assessed, and the living situation along with assistive devices reviewed.[21]

Vital signs should include an assessment of visual acuity as well as orthostatic measurements: heart rate and blood pressure should be obtained after 2 minutes supine, and then standing both at 1 and 3 minutes.[6]

The physical examination should focus on an assessment of basic cardiovascular status and lower extremity joint function. The neurologic examination should include an assessment of mental status; muscle strength; lower extremity peripheral nerves; proprioception; reflexes; and tests of cortical, extrapyramidal, and cerebellar function.[21]

Gait and balance can be assessed by a number of balance and gait assessment instruments discussed in the subsequent text.

The role of laboratory and ancillary testing in the evaluation of falls is not well defined.[31] The history and physical examination, as part of a postfall evaluation, have been shown to reveal most fall-contributing diagnoses.[29] Suggested laboratory tests that might be obtained on all persons undergoing a fall evaluation include a complete blood count, electrolytes, renal function, glucose, vitamin B_{12}, and thyroid function.[31] There is some evidence that vitamin D measurements may be useful in individuals with muscle weakness[32] (see in the subsequent text). Neuroimaging should be obtained only if there is head injury, new focal neurologic findings, or if a central nervous system process is suspected.[31] Indiscriminately obtained, neuroimaging can lead to misleading results.[8] Electroencephalography is hardly ever helpful and indicated only if there is a high degree of clinical suspicion of seizure. Similarly, ambulatory cardiac monitoring only rarely leads to a diagnosis, and can lead to a misdiagnosis if a nonrelated arrhythmia is detected and diverts the evaluation from the true cause(s). Ambulatory cardiac monitoring should be obtained only if there is high-clinical suspicion of arrhythmia by history or if there is an abnormal electrocardiogram (see section "Syncope in the Elderly").[31]

Gait and Balance Assessment Tools

Test Selection

There are a number of gait and balance assessment instruments available to assess an individual's risk of falling (see Table 13.4). The tests are not equivalent. Certain tests may miss pathology in patients with one set of fall-predisposing impairments, and yet detect fall risk in individuals with different predispositions. Assessments geared toward assessing fitness of young people are inappropriate for the frail elderly. Tests geared for the frail older person may not be challenging enough for the more active, higher functioning senior citizen. Assessments that were developed for the population to be tested, and whose measures have been shown to provide meaningful information should be selected.[33]

Specific Tests

Timed Up & Go (TUG):

The TUG test is designed to measure agility, dynamic balance, and rapid maneuvering. It requires little equipment and is relatively quick to administer. An individual is required to rise from a chair, walk 3 m, return, and sit down in the chair. To conduct the test, subjects are seated in a chair with their back against the chair. An assistive device, such as a walker or a cane, if used, is placed within reach. Subjects are given one practice run. On the word "go," the subject stands up, walks at a comfortable, safe speed to a cone placed on the floor 3 m away. They walk around the cone, come back and sit all the way back in the chair. Time starts as soon as the subject's back leaves the chair and stops as soon as it touches it again. Data are averaged from two trials with a rest between the two trials.

Results:

<10 seconds	freely mobile
10 to 19 seconds	mostly independent
20 to 29 seconds	variable mobility
>29 seconds	impaired mobility[33]

The Functional Reach Test:

The Functional Reach Test was developed to assess margin of stability. It is easy to administer and requires little equipment. In this test, the subject stands with his/her feet at a comfortable distance apart, behind a line perpendicular and adjacent to a wall. The subject's arm closest to the wall is raised to shoulder height and the position of the knuckle of the middle finger is measured. The subject is then instructed to keep the feet flat on the floor and lean forward as far as possible without losing balance, touching the wall or taking a step. The position of the knuckle is recorded at the point of farthest reach. The functional reach is the difference

TABLE 13.4
BALANCE AND GAIT ASSESSMENT TOOLS

Test	Equipment	Time	Indications	Limitations
Up and go	Standard height chair, stopwatch, cone	<3 min	Frail, community-dwelling older adult To determine ability to perform basic, independent mobility skills	Ceiling effect with more active older adult
POMA (Tinetti)	An armless standard height chair	15 min	Frail, community-dwelling older adult	Ceiling effect with more active older adult
Berg	A stopwatch, two chairs (one with armrests, one without) a 12-inch ruler, a slipper, and a 6-inch bench	10–15 min	Frail older adult To determine whether therapy intervention is appropriate	Ceiling effect with more active older adult. Lacks sensitivity to identify sensory impairments
DGI	Room to walk 20 feet Shoe boxes Cones	5 min	Higher functioning, community-dwelling older adult; suspected vestibular weakness	Patients using assistive devices automatically considered fall risk
Functional reach	A wall and a yard stick	3 min	Moderately active older adult	Orthopaedic conditions/pain Fear-of-fall
mCTSIB	4- to 6-inch foam pad and stop watch	5–10 min	Suspected vestibular weakness	Patients with diagnosed peripheral neuropathy
"Walkie-Talkie"	Room to walk 50 feet	<5 min	Ability to multitask	None
FAB	Stopwatch, 12-inch and 36-inch rulers, 6-inch high bench, masking tape, foam pad, metronome	10 min	Higher functioning older adults	Floor effect with frail older adults

POMA, Performance-Oriented Mobility Assessment; DGI, Dynamic Gait Index; mCTSIB, Modified Clinical Test of Sensory Interaction and Balance; FAB, Fullerton Advanced Balance Scale.
From references 33–36.

between the two measures. Three measures are recorded on each side and a mean score for each is calculated.[34]

In a study of elderly male veterans over a 6-month period, Duncan et al. found that healthy individuals could reach ≥10 inches. If functional reach is 0 inches, the individual is eight times more likely to have two falls. If functional reach is ≤6 inches, the individual is four times more likely to have two falls. If functional reach is >6 inches but <10 inches, the individual is two times more likely to have two falls.[34]

Performance-Oriented Mobility Assessment (POMA):
POMA is a widely used clinical measure of gait and balance in community-dwelling older adults. Little equipment is required (an armless, standard height chair) and with experience, it is quick to complete. The gait subtest can easily be completed while walking the patient from the waiting area back to the treatment area.[33]

The POMA has been used to describe and monitor balance and gait and to identify individuals who are at risk for falling. There are at least five different versions of the POMA, with versions differing in the items included in the gait and balance subscales, and the scoring of the subscales. One of the more commonly used versions of the POMA has a 25-point balance score and a 12-point gait score. Total scores >31 imply normal gait and balance; scores between 26 and 31 imply moderate fall risk; scores <25 are indicative of high fall risk.[33]

Dynamic Gait Index (DGI):
The DGI was initially developed by Shumway-Cook and Woolacott to assess fall risk in the elderly (>60 years of age). It requires little equipment and minimal time to complete. The test consists of eight tasks with varying demands, such as walking at different speeds, walking while turning the head, ambulating over and around obstacles, ascending and descending stairs, and making quick turns. Each item is scored on a four-level ordinal scale with a maximum possible score on the entire DGI of 24. A score of 19 or less indicates an increased risk of falling in older adults and in patients with vestibular disorders.[35]

Modified Clinical Test of Sensory Interaction and Balance (mCTSIB):
This test is used to evaluate an individual's ability to use the three primary sensory inputs contributing to balance (i.e., vision, somatosensory, and vestibular). It can be used to identify whether the use of sensory information in different sensory environments is normal or abnormal. It requires very little equipment and can be done in <5 minutes. Participants are required to stand quietly for 30 seconds

with shoes off, feet shoulder width apart, and arms folded across the chest in each of four different conditions: Eyes open, standing on a firm surface; eyes closed on a firm surface; eyes open on a foam surface; and eyes closed on a foam surface. For safety, the tests can be conducted with the individual standing in (but not touching) a corner. Each test is repeated three times, with scores averaged. The total score possible is 120 seconds. The test is stopped if arms are lifted from the chest, eyes are opened prematurely, the individual falls into or touches the wall, or the feet move.[36]

The test measures how well a person is able to use sensory inputs when one or more sensory systems are compromised. It attempts to isolate the various contributions of the visual, vestibular, and somatosensory systems to balance. The firm support surface allows accurate information from the somatosensory system. The foam surface decreases or alters somatosensory input. Eyes open allows accurate input from vision, and eyes closed eliminates vision as a sensory cue.[36]

Fullerton Advanced Balance Scale (FAB):
The FAB Scale is a relatively new test specifically designed to assess the older, more active, community-dwelling adult. Inexpensive equipment is required, and the test takes approximately 10 minutes to administer. The test is composed of ten items that are scored using a 4-point scale with a maximum score of 40. The ten items include static and dynamic balance activities performed in various sensory-controlled environments, specifically standing on foam, eyes open and closed, walking with head turns, stepping over obstacles, and jumping.[36]

"Walkie-Talkie:"
The purpose of the "walkie-talkie" test is to determine an individual's ability to divide his/her attention between multiple tasks. The test is extremely easy to conduct and requires very little equipment. While walking 50 feet, the individual is engaged in an open-ended conversation, requiring more than a yes or no response. Results of the test are either negative (able to converse without stopping) or positive (stops walking to respond). A negative score indicates the individual needs to concentrate on balancing and is unable to perform additional tasks at the same time.[36]

No one test provides all of the information needed to determine risk of falling and appropriate intervention. The walkie-talkie test can be performed while escorting a patient from the waiting to the examination room. The mCTSIB requires very little time, equipment, or training, and is especially effective in helping the clinician isolate which sensory systems may be impaired. The DGI requires some training and time, and is useful in determining balance issues if the vestibular system is suspected.

The POMA also requires some training and time, but is relatively easy to administer and is effective in determining multisystem balance issues.

Management

The Multifactorial Approach to Preventing Falls

The corollary to the concept that cumulative deficits lead to instability is that intervention strategies must address multiple deficits to reduce the risk of falling.[26]

Because people fall for a variety of reasons, no single assessment tool can measure all the possible underlying causes related to mobility problems and falls. In addition to the medical and physical activity history, it is also critical to assess a patient's physical impairments, functional limitations, risk of falls, and disability status before designing a fall prevention balance and mobility intervention. Instead of focusing on trying to identify a single cause, performing an evaluation looking for multiple additive insults may be a more appropriate and fruitful approach.[26]

Multifactorial Fall-Intervention Trials

There is now good evidence that multifactorial interventions can prevent falls. Three recent large meta-analyses[26,27,37] agree that multifactorial risk assessment and management programs are effective, although it is not possible to say which components of the multifactorial interventions are the most effective. Overall, it has been possible to achieve reductions of between 12% and 37%, depending upon the study (Evidence Level A).

A meta-analysis by the RAND Corporation for the Centers for Medicare and Medicaid Services. It concluded that when effective intervention programs are provided to individuals at high fall risk, they have the potential to be cost effective. Program costs are more than offset by savings in reduced acute and long-term care. When looking at the medical costs of fall-related injuries, almost 8% of persons older than 70 years annually seek emergency medical attention for fall injuries. Thirty percent to 40% of these elderly patients are subsequently hospitalized with an average cost of $10,000 to $12,000 per stay.[28] This does not include the cost of the roughly 43% of patients subsequently discharged to a skilled nursing facility.[25] Looking only at hip fractures, Medicare expenditures in 1991 were estimated to be $2.9 billion. Because of the demographics of the aging US population, the projected costs of hip fractures in the year 2040 are expected to increase by 100-fold.[26]

Specific Interventions

Exercise
Because lower extremity muscle weakness or poor balance predisposes the elderly to falling, exercise programs designed to strengthen lower extremity muscles and improve balance have been a major focus of investigation.

Most exercise programs that have been studied have had sessions between 3 and 7 days per week. Although the exact type, intensity and duration of exercise to prevent falls remain unclear, most successful programs have been more than 10 weeks in extent. However, the elderly at risk for falls should be offered life-long exercise and balance training.[21]

Most of the randomized controlled trials studied by RAND[26] had a follow-up period of 1 to 2 years with the actual intervention lasting between 3 and 12 months. The RAND meta-analyses found that exercise reduced the number of falls by 19%.

- *Frailty and Injuries: Cooperative Studies of Intervention Techniques (FICSIT) trials.* The FICSIT trials were the most wide-ranging evaluation of the effectiveness of exercise for fall prevention.[38] Pooled results revealed a statistically significant 10% reduction in falls due to exercise. Those trials that involved balance training rather than strength or endurance training showed the largest effect, with a 17% relative risk reduction.
  The above trials found that only some types of exercise are effective. Simply advising older people to be more physically fit is inadequate.[39] It is currently unclear as to what the optimal exercise programs for fall prevention are.
  While the Chang[27] and RAND reviews[26] confirmed the overall benefit of exercise programs, the Cochrane review[37] divided exercise programs into those individually designed for a given patient versus group interventions. The conclusion was that individualized home-based programs of muscle strengthening, balance training, and walking, targeted at high-risk patients, are effective (Evidence Level A). Community-based group exercise interventions however, have not been shown to reduce fall risk.
- *The Tai Chi Trials.* The initial Tai Chi trial reported by Wolf et al did not specifically target people who were at high risk for falls. The subjects were 70 years or older and ambulatory. They were randomized to Tai Chi (biweekly classes for 15 weeks), balance training (weekly sessions for 15 weeks), or the control group. The balance-training group individuals were taught to shift their center of gravity without moving their feet. Tai Chi resulted in a 49% relative risk reduction for falls, whereas balance training was ineffective.[40]

Because of the significant benefit seen in the above Tai Chi study, the authors performed a follow-up study of Tai Chi. As opposed to the vigorous elderly of the first study, patients in the latter study were elderly individuals who met the criteria for transitional frailty. This study was a prospective, single blinded, randomized trial comparing an intensive 48-week Tai Chi exercise program with a wellness program of similar duration on fall occurrences. Surprisingly, the results of the study did not show a significantly decreased risk of falling.[41] Therefore, as opposed to being a universal therapy for all fall risk patients, until additional studies bring forth further evidence, Tai Chi may be most appropriate for the more vigorous elderly, and especially those who have a significant balance disorder as a cause for their falling.

Home Modifications

Although environmental risks are mentioned as the most common cause of falls in community-dwelling elderly, and home modifications have been included in most multifactorial fall-prevention trials, direct research on this topic has been limited.[39]

The Cochrane review (3 trials, 374 participants) provided evidence that home assessment and modification that are prescribed by professionals may be effective for older people with a history of falls in the previous year. Specifically, benefit is seen when home modifications are recommended by occupational therapists who visit the house (Evidence Level B). Interventions whose effectiveness is unknown include home risk modification in association with advice on optimizing medication (1 trial, 658 participants) or in association with an education package on exercise and reducing fall risk (1 trial, 3182 participants) and home risk modification for older people without a history of falling (1 trial, 530 participants).[37]

According to the overall consensus from the RAND meta-analysis,[26] the best approach is to include home modifications as part of a multifactorial strategy of fall prevention specifically performed by an occupational therapist.

The Web site www.homemods.org contains extensive information about home modifications and links to other websites.

Medications

As mentioned, patients on four or more medications are found to be at increased risk of falling. However, almost all patients with chronic heart disease are taking more than four medications. Medication reduction in such cases is generally not appropriate or possible. As previously mentioned, some falls are directly attributable to medication effects; in other cases, the medications are markers of underlying diseases that are predisposing to falls. Therefore, simply decreasing the number of medications is not always the solution. Rather appropriate medication management is more important.

The largest relative risk reduction in any fall-prevention trial reported to date occurred in association with a reduction in psychotropic medication use. The risk of falling was reduced 66% (Evidence Level B). Unfortunately, 81% of patients resumed their pretrial psychotropic medication use within a month of the end of the trial.[39]

Fall-Prevention Education

The Cochrane,[37] RAND,[26] and Chang[27] meta-analyses reviews concluded that patient education given as part of multifactorial fall-prevention programs did not show a significant independent effect (Evidence Level A).

Assistive Devices

Evaluating the effect of assistive devices as an intervention for preventing falls has not had extensive investigation. Demonstrated benefit has been shown in multifactorial intervention studies that have included assistive devices (including bed alarms, canes, walkers, and hip protectors). However, there is no direct evidence linking the use of an assistive device alone with fall prevention. Therefore, while assistive devices may be effective as part of a multifactorial intervention program, the benefit of their use alone without addressing other fall risk factors is unclear (Evidence Level C).[21]

In several studies, hip protectors had been shown to be very effective in reducing the incidence of hip fractures associated with falls. However, a 2004 Cochrane meta-analysis[42] concluded that their effectiveness in community-dwelling elderly is unclear, compliance is poor, and cost effectiveness is uncertain (Evidence Level A). Therefore, while the initial enthusiasm for hip protectors has been somewhat dampened by the most recent Cochrane analysis, they might still be offered to a motivated elderly patient who is at high risk for fall-associated hip fracture. Sources of hip protectors include: http://www.hipprotector.com or http://www.hipsaver.com or www.safehip.com.

Improving Vision

Impaired vision has long been associated with falls and fractures in the elderly. Vision testing has been part of several multifactorial fall-prevention trials, but because of the study design, the effect of vision testing and intervention as an independent outcome could not be determined.[39]

Vitamin D Supplementation

Recent literature has suggested that vitamin D may have a role in preventing falls among the elderly. A meta-analysis was performed on the basis of five randomized controlled trials involving 1,237 subjects, assessing the effectiveness of vitamin D in preventing falling in the elderly. The meta-analysis found that vitamin D reduced the risk of falling by 22% as compared to patients receiving only calcium or placebo; the number needed to treat was 15 (Evidence Level B).[32]

Wearing Safer Footwear

The shoes a patient wears have long been felt to be a potential risk factor in falling. The coefficient of friction on the walking surface, which may influence the risk of slipping, is affected by a shoe's sole material and tread design. A shoe's tendency to tip sideways on an uneven surface can be affected by the height and width of the heel. Foot proprioception can be affected by the thickness of the sole and shoe collar height.[43]

Gait laboratory studies have raised concerns that athletic shoes may be associated with increased risk of falling in the elderly. The thick soles of athletic shoes have been hypothesized to interfere with proprioception. In contrast to the laboratory studies however, a case-controlled study on community-dwelling elderly patients experiencing falls found that athletic shoes were actually associated with a lower fall risk than various other shoe types.[43]

In addition, a significantly increased fall risk was found in those who were barefoot or wearing only stockings. This finding was again in contrast to what had been observed in gait laboratories where being barefoot has been associated with good balance and gait performance. It is hypothesized that without shoes, the foot is more vulnerable to the pain potentially inflicted by the trauma of unexpected obstacles.[43] Therefore, for the elderly patient at risk, a well-fitting athletic shoe is recommended.

REFERENCES

1. Isles RC, Choy NL, Low S, et al. Normal values of balance tests in women aged 20–80. *J Am Geriatr Soc.* 2004;52:1367–1372.
2. Drachman DA, Hart CW. An approach to the dizzy patient. *Neurology.* 1972;22:323–334.
3. Sloane PD. Evaluation and management of dizziness in the older patient. *Clin Geriatr Med.* 1996;12:785–801.
4. Isaacson JE, Rubin AM. Otolaryngologic management of dizziness in the older patient. *Clin Geriatr Med.* 1999;15:179–191.
5. Brandt T, Daroff RB. The multisensory physiologic and pathological vertigo syndromes. *Ann Neurol.* 1980;7:195–203.
6. Mukai S, Lewis LA. Orthostatic hypotension. *Clin Geriatr Med.* 2002;18:253–268.
7. Rubenstein LZ, Josephson KR. The epidemiology of falls and syncope. *Clin Geriatr Med.* 2002;18:141–158.
8. College N, Lewis S, Mead G, et al. Magnetic resonance brain imaging in people with dizziness; a comparison with non-dizzy people. *J Neurol Neurosurg Psychiatry.* 2002;72:587–589.
9. Belal A, Glorig A. Dysequilibrium of aging (presbyastasis). *J Laryngol Otol.* 1986;100:1037–1041.
10. Droler H, Pemberton J. Vertigo in a random sample of elderly people living in their homes. *J Laryngol Otol.* 1953;67:689–695.
11. Mold JW, Vesely SK, Keyk BA, et al. The prevalence, predictors, and consequences of peripheral sensory neuropathy in older patients. *J Am Board Fam Pract.* 2004;17:309–318.
12. Dieterich M. Easy, inexpensive, and effective: Vestibular exercises for balance control. *Ann Intern Med.* 2004;141:641–643.
13. Colledge NR, Barr-Hamilton RM, Lewis SJ, et al. Evaluation of investigations to diagnose the cause of dizziness in elderly people: A community based controlled study. *BMJ.* 1996;313:788–792.
14. Sloane PD, Coeytaux RR, Beck RS. Dizziness: State of the science. *Ann Intern Med.* 2001;134:823–832.
15. Tinetti ME, Williams CS, Gill TM. Dizziness among older adults: A possible geriatric syndrome. *Ann Intern Med.* 2000;132:337–344.
16. Boult C, Murphy J, Sloane P, et al. The relation of dizziness to functional decline. *J Am Geriatr Soc.* 1991;39:858–861.
17. Yardley L, Donovan-Hall M, Smith HE, et al. Effectiveness of primary care-based vestibular rehabilitation for chronic dizziness. *Ann Intern Med.* 2004;141:598–605.
18. Hain Timothy C. *Benign paroxysmal positional positional vertigo.* Last edited: 2/2003. http://www.tchain.com/otoneurology/disorders/bppv/bppv.html
19. Maki BE, McIlroy WE. Postural control in the older adult. *Clin Geriatr Med.* 1996;12:635–658.
20. Kenny RA. Neurally mediated syncope. *Clin Geriatr Med.* 2002; 18(2):191–210.
21. American Geriatrics Society, British Geriatrics Society, and American Academy of Orthopedic Surgeons Panel on Fall Prevention. Guideline for the prevention of falls in older persons. *J Am Geriatr Soc.* 2001;49:664–672.
22. Cummings SR, Nevitt MC, Kidd S. Forgetting falls. The limited accuracy of recall of falls in the elderly. *J Am Geriatr Soc.* 1988;36(7):613–616.
23. O'Shea Diarmuid. Setting up a falls and syncope service for the elderly. *Clin Geriatr Med.* 2002;18:269–278.
24. Buchner DM, Hornbrook MC, Kutner NC, et al. Development of the common data base for the FICSIT trials. *J Am Geriatr Soc.* 1993;41:297–308.

25. Monane M, Avorn J. Medications and falls. Causation, correlation, and prevention. *Clin Geriatr Med.* 1996;12:847–858.
26. Shekell P, Maglione M, Chang J, et al. *Falls prevention interventions in the medicare population.* RAND-HCFA. Evidence Monograph, Baltimore, MD: HCFA; Publication #HCFA 2003;500:98–0281.
27. Chang JT, Morton SC, Rubenstein LZ, et al. Interventions for the prevention of falls in older adults: Systematic review and meta-analysis of randomized clinical trials. *BMJ.* 2004;328:680–683.
28. King MB, Tinetti M. A multifactorial approach to reducing injurious falls. *Clin Geriatr Med.* 1996;12:745–759.
29. Studenski S, Rigler SK. Clinical overview of instability in the elderly. *Clin Geriatr Med.* 1996;12:679–688.
30. Tinetti ME, Speechley M, Ginter SF. Risk factors for falls among elderly persons living in the community. *N Engl J Med.* 1988; 319:1701–1707.
31. Tinetti ME. Preventing falls in elderly persons. *N Engl J Med.* 2003;348:42–49.
32. Bischoff-Ferrari HA, Dawson-Hughes B, Willett WC, et al. Effect of vitamin D on falls: A meta-analysis. *JAMA.* 2004;291:1999–2006.
33. Van Swerington JM, Brach JS. Making geriatric assessment work: Selecting useful measures. *Phys Ther.* 2001;81:1233–1252.
34. Duncan PW, Studenski S, Chandler J, et al. Functional reach: Predictive validity in a sample of elderly male veterans. *J Gerontol Med Sci.* 1992;47:M93–M98.
35. Shumway-Cook A, Baldwin M, Polissar NL, et al. *Phys Ther.* 1997;77:812–819.
36. Rose DJ. *Fall proof! A comprehensive balance and training program.* Champaign, IL: Human Kinetics; 2003.
37. Gillespie LD, Gillespie WJ, Robertson MC, et al. Interventions for preventing falls in elderly people. (Cochrane review). *The Cochrane library*, Issue 2. Chichester: John Wiley and Sons; 2004.
38. Ory MG, Schechtman KB, Miller P, et al. Frailty and injuries in later life: The FICSIT trials. *J Am Geriatr Soc.* 1993;41:283–296.
39. Cumming RG. Intervention strategies and risk-factor modification for falls prevention. A review of recent intervention studies. *Clin Geriatr Med.* 2002;18:175–189.
40. Wolf SL, Barnhart HX, Kutner NG, et al. Reducing frailty and falls in older persons: An investigation of Tai Chi and computerized balance training. *J Am Geriatr Soc.* 1996;44:489–497.
41. Wolf SL, Sattin RW, Kutner M, et al. Intense Tai Chi exercise training and fall occurrences in older, transitionally frail adults: A randomized, controlled trial. *J Am Geriatr Soc.* 2003;51:1693–1701.
42. Parker MJ, Gillespie LD, Gillespie WL. Hip protectors for preventing hip fractures in the elderly (Cochrane review). *The Cochrane library*, Issue 1, Chichester: John Wiley and Sons; 2004.
43. Koepsell TD, Wolf ME, Buchner DM, et al. Footwear style and risk of falls in older adults 2004. *J Am Geriatr Soc.* 52:1495–1501.

SUGGESTED READINGS AND RESOURCES

American Geriatrics Society
www.americangeriatrics.org/education/forum

Centers for Disease Control
www.cdc.gov/ncipc/pub-res/toolkit/toolkit.htm

Centers for Disease Control
www.cdc.gov/ncipc/duip/spotlite/falls.htm

Department of Public Health
San Francisco
www.dph.sf.ca.us/PHP/CHIPPS.htm
Community and home injury prevention program for seniors

National Institute on Aging
www.nia.nih.gov

American Academy of Orthopedic Surgeons
www.orthoinfo.aaos.org

Vestibular Disorders Association
http://www.vestibular.org

Low Back Pain in the Elderly

14

Kim Edward LeBlanc

CLINICAL PEARLS 162

NORMAL AGING OF THE BACK 163

THE ANATOMY OF PAIN IN THE LUMBAR SEGMENT 163

HISTORY 163

PHYSICAL EXAMINATION 164

SPECIFIC CAUSES OF LOW BACK PAIN—DIFFERENTIAL DIAGNOSES 165

Low Back Sprain/Strain—ICD-9 Code: 847.2 165
Degenerative Disc Disease—ICD-9 Code: 722.52 (Low Back Pain: 724.2) 166
Herniated Nucleus Pulposus (Disc)—IDC-9 Code: 722.10 167
Spinal Stenosis—ICD-9 Code: 724.02 169
Compression Fracture—ICD-9 Code: 805.4 170
Metastatic Disease—ICD-9 Code: 198.5 171
Infection 172
Abdominal Aortic Aneurysm—ICD-9 Code: 441.4 173

CONCLUSION 174

CLINICAL PEARLS

- The L4 nerve root is evaluated by the patellar tendon reflex. Afflictions of the L5 nerve root are noted in the great toe. Diseases that affect the S1 nerve root are manifested by changes in the little toe.
- During the side-bending maneuver, pain that is made worse by bending toward the contralateral side suggests muscular disease. Pain that is made worse by bending toward the ipsilateral side suggests disc disease.
- Asymptomatic patients may have abnormal findings on computed tomography (CT) scan and magnetic resonance imaging (MRI). A patient's complaints and symptoms must correlate with the actual findings on the scan.
- A patient with lumbar spinal stenosis will find relief while leaning forward pushing a shopping cart, placing the lumbar spine in a flexed position.
- Compression fractures are a fairly common event in the elderly and, in the lumbar spine, usually involve L1 or L2.
- Approximately 50% of patients with solid tumors will have metastatic disease to the vertebral column.
- In a patient complaining of back pain who has no abnormal findings on lumbosacral examination, the clinician should be alert that the pain may be emanating from an abdominal aortic aneurysm.

Low back pain is one of the most common ailments that afflict the population. In fact, this complaint is second only to an upper respiratory infection as the symptom that most often results in a visit to a physician's office.[1,2] In the United States, approximately 90% of all adults will have at least one episode of back pain in their lifetime.[3] Furthermore, at least 50% of the working population of this country experiences back pain every year.[4] This has significant impact on the well-being of not only the entire population, but the entire workforce as well.

The elderly population has been a relatively underrepresented and underreported group as a whole, but estimates are that the prevalence of pain, in general, may be as high as 67% to 80%.[5] Although the pain may occur in many different areas, similar to that experienced in their younger counterparts, back pain in the elderly has a high rate of occurrence. Back pain has been reported to be the third most common symptom in patients older than 75 years.[6] However, in a systematic review of the literature, the frequency of low back pain in this population has been underestimated.[7]

Low back pain may originate from a wide array of spinal structures, including muscles, fascia, ligaments, facet joints, vertebral periosteum, nerve roots, blood vessels, and the annulus fibrosis. Most commonly, the pain is associated with an age-related degenerative process, intervertebral disc herniation, or a musculoligamentous etiology.

Among patients older than 65, the more common diagnostic possibilities have a different emphasis as compared to those of a younger population. Although a so-called low back strain may occur in the older patient, osteoarthritis, compression fractures, carcinoma, spinal stenosis, and aortic aneurysms become much more frequent. This chapter will focus on some of the more common causes of back pain in the elderly, their diagnoses and treatments.

NORMAL AGING OF THE BACK

Some of the most notable changes associated with aging occur in the musculoskeletal system. Changes that have a direct impact on back stability and motion include the degenerative processes involving the intervertebral discs and joints, loss of bone mineralization, diminution of joint motion, decreased ligament flexibility, and the decline of muscle strength, endurance, and work capacity.

The lumbar spine and its supporting structures undergo degenerative changes with the aging process. The water and proteoglycan content of the nucleus pulposus decreases. This deterioration of the disc allows the vertebrae to move closer together. As this occurs, there is wearing of the articular cartilage of the apophyseal joints. Accompanying this is the formation of osteophytes, which may eventually begin to encroach on the vertebral spinal canal and foramina.

THE ANATOMY OF PAIN IN THE LUMBAR SEGMENT

Although there may be a variety of causes of back pain, a very important consideration in determining the cause is whether it is a mechanical etiology. In the elderly population, a nonmechanical cause should be considered prominently (e.g., primary or metastatic disease, infectious process, vascular disease) and ruled out when necessary.

However, regardless of age, the most common cause is related to a mechanical problem, with the pain emanating from a pain-sensitive structure. The most prominent of these include the vertebral periosteum, the spinal dura, the posterior longitudinal ligament, the outer third of the annulus fibrosis, and the associated vascular structures. These structures have a delicate nerve supply that produces pain whenever it is irritated.

In addition, each lumbar vertebra has a disc, which is pain-sensitive, and two facet joints, which are covered by a synovial membrane that is also pain-sensitive. There are many mechanical stresses placed on these structures that occur during flexion, extension, and rotation, particularly when supporting the body's weight.

As degenerative changes progress, there may be encroachment on the nerve roots as they come off the spinal cord and exit through the intervertebral foraminal opening. Initially, this pain may be localized, but with advancing encroachment the pain may take on a radicular pattern specific to that nerve root.

The vertebrae are separated by intervertebral discs. The discs consist of the gelatinous nucleus pulposus that is surrounded by the annulus fibrosis. The major supporting structures of the vertebrae and discs are the paraspinal muscles and the ligamentous structures. The posterior elements of the vertebrae form the neural foramina, encase the spinal canal with bony protection, and interlock to form the facet joints. The main purpose of the facet joint is to allow motion of the bony segments.

There are several organs that are in close proximity to the lumbar spine lying anteriorly in a retroperitoneal location. These organs include the kidneys and ureters, the aorta and inferior vena cava, pancreas, and the periaortic lymph nodes. Any disease that affects any of these retroperitoneal structures could result in referred pain to the lumbar spine.

HISTORY

A complete and thorough history should allow an accurate working diagnosis in most patients. The history is particularly helpful in the geriatric patient as it aids in determining the effect the pain has on normal daily functioning.

The history should include the usual questions concerning past medical history, particularly comorbid conditions such as diabetes, cardiovascular disease, hypertension, carcinoma, and arthritic conditions. Past family and surgical histories should be obtained as well as questions on smoking, allergies, and present medications.

Specifically, the history should focus on the aspects of the low back pain, such as pain onset, the intensity of the pain, and specific location. Pain diagrams are helpful in allowing the patient to accurately display the location and radiation of the pain. Is there any associated trauma such as a fall or relationship to a particular inciting event or activity? What makes the pain worse? What makes the pain better? In what position is the pain most noticeable? Are there any associated neurologic symptoms or weakness, or bladder or bowel dysfunction? Are the symptoms rapidly progressive? A review of symptoms should be undertaken with questions directed toward underlying causes that may suggest other organic problems, such as uterine leiomyomata, gastrointestinal diseases, aortic aneurysm, or carcinoma.

In the initial evaluation of a patient with acute low back pain it is important to keep in mind that certain positive findings in the history should raise "red flags." These red flags should heighten the clinician's suspicion that this may represent a significant disease process, something other than a simple musculoskeletal problem. For example, pain that begins following significant trauma or a fall should raise the suspicion of spinal fracture. If there is associated weight loss, presence of fever, or pain at rest, this suggests the possibility of a cancerous or infectious process. Pain that increases at night during sleep is quite suggestive of a neoplastic or infectious process as well. Lastly, the presence of bladder or bowel dysfunction, significant motor weakness of a limb, or saddle anesthesia suggests the possibility of cauda equina syndrome. More specific details will be provided in the subsequent text that describe each particular entity in detail.

PHYSICAL EXAMINATION

As in all phases of medicine, the physical examination should be both general and focused toward a specific diagnosis that is suggested by the history. Often overlooked is how the patient actually arrives in the office. The gait should be observed as well as how the patient sits. For example, a patient sitting in a chair and leaning back with an outstretched leg (to avoid stretching the sciatic nerve) should be suspected of having a significant disc problem. It is also important to observe directly and indirectly how the patient dresses and undresses. Indirectly observing a patient dressing and undressing while appearing to be "distracted" will allow the examiner to note inconsistencies in the complaints and movements. Palpation should be performed over specific areas of the lumbar region while noting muscle spasm, generalized and/or point tenderness of bone and soft tissue areas, and the alignment of spinous processes. Specific areas include the supraspinal ligaments, lumbar spinous processes, paraspinal musculature, sacroiliac joints, and coccyx. Localized soft tissue tenderness may be found with tumor, infection, or fracture (particularly point tenderness of bone).

Continuing in an orderly process, range of motion should be determined. The lumbar segment has six cardinal ranges of motion: Flexion, extension, lateral bending (both left and right), and rotation (both left and right). Each of these should be observed. Although the actual range of motion is important, the more pertinent findings should focus on the actual symmetry and quality of the motion. Biomechanical abnormalities and asymmetrical areas of flexibility may be noted during this phase of the examination. Considerable attention should be paid to the L4-5 and L5-S1 lumbar levels. Most of the motion of the lumbar segment occurs at these levels.

One of the most critical areas of the examination involves testing of neurologic function. This includes both the deep tendon reflexes and evaluation of muscle strength and sensation.

The L4 nerve root innervates the medial side of the foot (sensory) and the quadriceps muscle (motor). Consequently, impairment of the L4 nerve root will result in motor weakness during resisted quadriceps extension and difficulty when rising from a squatting position. L4 also has some role in ankle and great toe dorsiflexion. The knee jerk evaluates this nerve root at the patellar tendon level. Without nerve impingement, this deep tendon reflex will be asymmetrical when compared to the normal side.

The L5 nerve root innervates the dorsum of the foot (sensory) and the dorsiflexors of the ankle and great toe (motor). As a result, malfunctioning of this nerve root will result in motor weakness during heel walking and dorsiflexion of the ankle and great toe. There is no deep tendon reflex for the L5 nerve root.

The S1 nerve root innervates the lateral side of the foot and little toe (sensory) and the gastrocnemius muscle, soleus muscle, and toe flexors (motor). Impairment of S1 will result in weakness or inability to toe walk and plantar flex the foot and great toe. The S1 nerve root will be evaluated by the Achilles tendon reflex and noting any asymmetry when compared to the unaffected side.

The straight leg raise is a well-known maneuver that places the sciatic nerve on stretch and may be performed in a supine or sitting position. With impingement of a nerve root secondary to a herniated nucleus pulposus (disc), the resulting stretch will produce pain in a pattern specific to the nerve root. L4 will extend to the anterior thigh and leg; L5 down the leg to the great toe. S1 impingement will extend the pain down the lateral side of the leg to the little toe. A positive finding is reproduction or intensification of the pain that extends below the knee and not just in the back, buttocks, or posterior thigh. An age-related phenomenon must be noted. Older patients often have less disc volume due to desiccation. Therefore, these patients may not have a frankly positive nerve root.

There are occasions when the physical findings may not suggest pathology in the lumbar area and other physical testing should be employed. Most notable, pathology of the hip or sacroiliac joints may pose diagnostic conundrums. The flexion, abduction, and external rotation (FABER) maneuver should be utilized in this situation as it is a provocative maneuver specifically isolating the hip and sacroiliac joints. FABER stands for flexion, abduction, and external rotation and may also be referred to as the "figure-of-4" test. In performing this maneuver, the patient should be in the supine position. The affected lower extremity (hip) is placed in FABER and then the foot is placed on the opposite knee or proximal tibia (essentially producing a figure-of-4). If this maneuver is painful on the ipsilateral side, then hip or sacroiliac joint pathology should be considered, depending on where the patient indicates the pain is located. Pain reproduced on the contralateral side or increased pain caused by the maneuver is a nonspecific finding and may not be helpful.

Abdominal and rectal examinations should be performed for findings that may suggest a cause for the complaints of back pain such as prostate or rectal carcinoma.

Gynecologic examinations should be performed when appropriate.

SPECIFIC CAUSES OF LOW BACK PAIN—DIFFERENTIAL DIAGNOSES

Back pain has a wide array of causes, as noted in Table 14.1.[8] The most common etiologies in the elderly can usually be divided into mechanical causes, pain related to osteoporosis, or systemic entities such as tumor and infection. In determining the cause, the age of the patient does direct the physician to certain diagnoses that occur with higher frequency at that particular time of life.

The next section of this chapter will discuss some of the most common causes of back pain in the elderly population, along with the proper workup, including keys in making the diagnosis, as well as management and treatment of each entity.

Low Back Sprain/Strain—ICD-9 Code: 847.2

CASE ONE

A 66-year-old man presents to your office complaining of low back pain that began while lifting several lawn chairs a few days ago. Although these chairs were not heavy, he noted pain within a few minutes in the lower back, with discomfort also noted in the buttocks and upper posterior thigh regions. He is active and healthy, with no prior history of back problems, weight loss, fever, or prostatic symptoms.

A sprain refers to injury to a ligamentous structure while a strain refers to injury to a muscle. When referring to the low back, sprain may be used in reference to injury to the paraspinal muscles. However, this term is also frequently used when referring to ligamentous injury of the annulus fibrosis or vertebral facet joints. The terms sprain and strain are often used interchangeably because of the deep location of the soft tissues of the lumbar region, rendering a precise location virtually impossible most of the time. Fortunately, a precise determination is usually not required as the management is virtually identical.

TABLE 14.1
DIFFERENTIAL DIAGNOSES OF LOW BACK PAIN

Mechanical Causes (ICD-9)	Nonmechanical Causes (ICD-9)	Visceral Disease (ICD-9)
Lumbar sprain/strain[a] (847.2)	Neoplasia[a] (170.2)	Disease of pelvic organs
Degenerative processes of discs and facets, usually age-related[a] (722.52)	Multiple myeloma (203)	Prostatitis (601.9)
Herniated disc[a] (722.10)	Metastatic carcinoma (170)	Endometriosis (617.9)
Spinal stenosis[a] (724.02)	Lymphoma (202.8) and leukemia (208.9)	Chronic pelvic inflammatory disease (614.9)
Compression fracture[a] (805.4)	Spinal cord tumors (192.2)	Renal disease (593.9)
Spondylolisthesis (738.4)	Retroperitoneal tumors (228.04)	Nephrolithiasis (592)
Traumatic fracture (805.4)	Primary vertebral tumors (170.2)	Pyelonephritis (590.10)
Congenital disease	Infection[a]	Perinephric abscess (590.2)
Severe kyphosis (737.1)	Osteomyelitis (730.00)	Aortic aneurysm[a] (441.4)
Severe scoliosis (737.9)	Septic discitis (722.93)	Gastrointestinal disease
Transitional vertebrae (724)	Paraspinous abscess (324.9)	Pancreatitis (577)
Spondylolysis (738.4)	Epidural abscess (324.1)	Cholecystitis (575)
Internal disc disruption or discogenic back pain (722.2)	Herpes zoster (053.9)	Penetrating ulcer (533.1)
Presumed instability (718.8)	Inflammatory arthritis	
	Ankylosing spondylitis (720)	
	Psoriatic spondylitis (696.0)	
	Reiter syndrome (099.3)	
	Inflammatory bowel disease (555.1)	
	Scheuermann disease (osteochondrosis) (732.8)	
	Paget disease of bone (731)	

[a]Topics covered in this chapter.
Adapted with permission from: Deyo RA, Weinstein JN. Primary care: Low back pain. *N Engl J Med.* 2001;344(5):363–370.

Workup/Keys to Diagnosis

Physical Examination

The patient may have subtle or obvious discomfort, with difficulty standing erect. Sitting may be uncomfortable or require frequent changes in position. Palpation reveals diffuse tenderness in the lower back and perhaps the sacroiliac area. Range of motion will be limited, particularly flexion. Side bending may worsen the pain when bending toward the contralateral side as a result of the stretching of the tissues. Neurologic examination is normal, including both sensory and motor function.

Imaging

In patients with a typical presentation, no studies are necessary. Beyond the age of 30, plain radiographs typically show a varying degree of degeneration such as disc space narrowing with or without spurring. Therefore, plain films are not helpful in this setting. However, in a patient with atypical symptoms or in one who fails to show improvement in 2 weeks, obtaining lumbosacral films should be considered. The overriding reason for obtaining radiographs at this point is to further evaluate the atypical symptoms or lack of significant symptomatic improvement. The radiographs will help confirm the diagnostic suspicions or suggest other causes of back pain, such as malignancy or infections.

Management

Initially, the focus should be on symptomatic relief. A brief period of bed rest (1 to 2 days) may be considered, depending on the functional ability of the patient. Prolonged periods of bed rest are not recommended as they are detrimental to the patient's return to former level of activity (Evidence Level A). In addition, studies have indicated that patients continuing ordinary activities within the limits of their pain have a similar or more rapid recovery than those taking bed rest.[9,10] Acetaminophen or nonsteroidal anti-inflammatory agents may be considered if there are no contraindications for their use and proper precautions are taken (Evidence Level A). These drugs should be used for a period of 7 to 14 days, preferably on a regular basis as opposed to on an as-needed regimen. Although muscle relaxants may be helpful in some cases, current data do not allow a clear recommendation for their use. In addition, there are significant side effects that should be avoided in this population. Narcotic analgesics and sedatives should be avoided. The application of ice or heat may be recommended if the patient finds this helpful. However, patients with vascular insufficiency or decreased sensation should avoid this modality. While in the acute phase, usually up to a week, the patient should avoid any activities that may place stress on the lower back.

Exercise should be recommended and initiated once the acutely painful phase has diminished (Evidence Level C). Low-stress activities may begin with a gradual increase in walking or other aerobic activities such as biking or swimming. Physical therapy may be recommended for instruction on proper back mechanics and instruction on stretching and strengthening exercises for the lumbosacral region (this should include abdominal and hamstring muscles) (Evidence Level C). Stretches should include movements that extend the muscles and tendons to the longest comfortable level. First, this should include forward flexion to try to touch the toes, and then hyperextension by bending backward while keeping the waist still (this maneuver should be omitted if it causes undue pain or discomfort). Side bending should be done by standing erect while allowing one hand to run down the side of the leg until "tight." This should be done on both sides. Next is a twisting maneuver, with the pelvis held stationary and the upper torso twisted to one side and then to the next. These stretches encompass the six cardinal movements—forward, backward, left and right bending, left and right side twisting—of the lumbar spine. These should be held for 30 seconds initially, increasing to 60 to 120 seconds as the patient becomes more flexible. These should be performed two to three times per day.

Follow-up

A follow-up visit is usually not necessary as most low back sprains/strains resolve within 4 to 6 weeks. However, the patient should be instructed to return if the symptoms have not resolved in this time frame. In addition, the patient should return if there is development of neurologic signs or symptoms, worsening symptoms, or significant change in symptoms.

Degenerative Disc Disease—ICD-9 Code: 722.52 (Low Back Pain: 724.2)

CASE TWO

A patient presents complaining of recurring, intermittent low back pain for 4 months. He is not able to relate a singular precipitating event but he had a few episodes of "back pain" when he was younger. Although retired, his former occupation was as a construction worker. The pain does radiate at times into his buttocks and is worsened by bending, lifting (particularly out in the front of the body), twisting, or stooping. There is no radiation of pain, when he is resting. The pain is improved or relieved by a night's rest or simply lying down. Occasionally, he experiences some associated muscle spasm.

Workup/Keys to Diagnosis

Physical Examination

The patient may walk into the room with a "stiff back" or may be found to have a side or forward "list" (trunk shift to one side) secondary to muscle spasm, if present. Tenderness of the lumbar spine and sacroiliac regions may be noted. Range of motion will be limited due to the discomfort, generally in all directions. Sensory and motor functions are intact. Deep tendon reflexes are unaffected. Straight leg raising may be mildly positive; however, the radiation of the pain will not usually be anatomical to any particular dermatome and will be confined to areas proximal to the knee.

Imaging

Anteroposterior (AP) and lateral radiographs of the lumbosacral spine will reveal age-related changes such as narrowing of the disc space on the lateral view and anterior osteophytes. Virtually all lumbar discs will show some degenerative change after the age of 65 years. Other findings that may be noted in these films are reactive sclerosis on the vertebral endplates and the so-called vacuum sign. The vacuum sign is considered to represent a definite sign of disc degeneration and may be described as a dark line seen in the space between two vertebrae on the lateral view (suggesting apparent air in the disc space). There is no need for further imaging studies at this point unless changes are noted that suggest more ominous diagnoses.

Management

Relative rest should be employed. This means avoiding any activities that may exacerbate or contribute to the pain. If analgesics are used, the clinician should recommend the intermittent use of acetaminophen or nonsteroidal anti-inflammatory drugs, provided there are no contraindications to their use (Evidence Level A). Applications of local moist heat may be recommended as long as there are no sensory problems. Similar to most causes of back pain, bed rest should be avoided or only allowed for 1 to 2 days at the most (Evidence Level A). Prolonged periods of bed rest are quite detrimental to all forms of back pain. Once the pain has subsided sufficiently, physical activity may resume and should be encouraged. Physical activity should include stretching and strengthening exercises for the lower back, abdominal muscles, and hamstrings (Evidence Level A). Aerobic exercise and weight reduction should be strongly recommended. The best aerobic exercise is the one that the patient will agree to perform and do three to five times per week for at least 30 minutes (e.g., walking, biking, swimming). As in all patients, the use of tobacco should be strongly discouraged.

Follow-up

If the patient does not respond, the pain is slow to resolve, or the pain recurs, it is prudent to reevaluate the patient within 3 to 4 weeks of treatment to investigate other more serious causes of the back pain. In particular, "red flags" should be noted, such as fever, chills, nighttime pain, weight loss, or pain lasting >6 to 12 months. Other worrisome signs are the onset of neurologic symptoms, such as decreasing sensation or loss of motor function, bladder or bowel dysfunction, or bone pain or tenderness.

Herniated Nucleus Pulposus (Disc)—IDC-9 Code: 722.10

> **CASE THREE**
>
> A 65-year-old patient presents to your office with a history of low back pain that recurs once or twice a year for the past several years. This pain has always been localized to the lumbar region until the last few days. The character of the pain changed after he lifted a heavy trunk in his attic. The back pain seems to be less problematic at this time as the pain is now lancinating and radiating down the posterolateral side of his right leg into the little toe. The pain is quite severe and is worsened by coughing, sneezing, bowel movements, walking, sitting, or standing. Twisting maneuvers also intensify the pain. The patient indicates that relief is found only when he is lying on his side in the fetal position or lying on his back with a pillow beneath his knees. When sitting, he is able to lessen the pain by sitting at the edge of the chair while leaning back into the chair with his leg extended.

While discussing a herniated disc, it is important to remember the structure of the disc itself. The intervertebral disc is composed of the nucleus pulposus, which is a gel-like substance that serves to cushion axial compression. The nucleus pulposus is surrounded by a specialized ligamentous structure called the *anulus fibrosus*. The anulus fibrosus serves to stabilize the spine during bending and lifting. During these activities, increased pressure is applied to the nucleus pulposus, which may bulge or herniate into the lumbar canal through the weaker parts of the anulus fibrosus, most commonly the posterolateral component. If the herniation results in compression of a nerve root, symptoms may ensue causing pain in one or both lower extremities corresponding to the level of nerve root impingement. There may be associated numbness and/or weakness. Although the pain is a direct result of nerve root compression by the herniated disc, a portion of the pain is due to chemical irritation of the nerve root by substances contained within the nucleus pulposus.

The most commonly affected levels for disc herniation are the L4-5 and L5-S1. As disc herniations most commonly compress the nerve that exits the vertebral level below, the corresponding affected nerves would be the L5 or S1 nerve roots, comprising most herniated disc syndromes (>95%). Lumbar disc herniations occurring at more proximal levels are very infrequent and would not produce symptoms below the knee.

Workup/Keys to Diagnosis

Physical Examination

The patient will have decreased range of motion, particularly with flexion. There may be splinting of the back and a noticeable list. Lateral bending may worsen the pain when bending to the ipsilateral side because of the increased compression on the nerve root. A highly reliable sign for herniated disc is the so-called flip sign. While the patient is in the seated position, perform a straight leg raise bringing the body and leg position to 90 degrees. The test result is positive for reproduction of the pain while causing the patient to lean back to extend the spine for reduction of the stretch on the sciatic nerve. This is especially helpful when the supine straight leg raise is also positive (i.e., reproduction of pain at approximately 45 degree of leg extension). Another very helpful test is the Lasègue test. This is another method to place the sciatic nerve on stretch while confirming the straight leg-raise findings. The patient is in the supine position, and a straight leg raise is performed. Once the pain is reproduced, the outstretched leg is lowered slowly until the pain is relieved. While continuing to hold the leg in this position, the foot is dorsiflexed, which will once again place the sciatic nerve on stretch. Reproduction of the pain is a positive sign. All of the straight leg tests place the L5 and S1 nerve roots on stretch. Another test that is highly specific for lumbar nerve root compression is the crossed straight leg–raising test. This test simply means performing a straight leg raise on the uninvolved side. If pain occurs in the involved leg or buttock, this is a positive test and very meaningful.

The next part of the physical examination involves evaluation of sensory and motor functions and the testing of the deep tendon reflexes. Impairment of the L4 nerve root would be the result of disc herniation at the L3-4 level. This would produce numbness of the anterior lower leg, thigh pain, and weakness of the quadriceps muscles. There will be asymmetry or absence of the patellar tendon reflex. Disc herniation at the L4-5 level will produce symptoms involving the L5 nerve root with resultant numbness on the dorsum of the foot and into the first web space. In addition, there will be weakness of the great toe extensors and pain in the posterolateral thigh and calf, extending to the great toe. Heel walking will be difficult, and in extreme cases a foot drop may be present. There is no deep tendon reflex for the L5 nerve root. The S1 nerve root will be affected by herniation of the disc at the L5-S1 level and will result in numbness of the lateral foot and little toe. Motor function will be noted by weakness of plantar flexion of the great toe and weakness of the gastrocsoleus muscle complex as exhibited by an inability to sustain toe walking. Further confirmation will be provided by changes noted in the Achilles tendon reflex.

Imaging

The initial diagnosis of a herniated disc may normally be made on the basis of the history and physical examination. Plain radiographs add little to the diagnosis but should be obtained to view age-appropriate changes as well as to rule out other possible sources of the pain, such as an unsuspected tumor or infectious process.

Other imaging studies, such as computed tomography (CT) scan or magnetic resonance imaging (MRI), are important but their limitations should be recognized and appreciated. CT scan is performed immediately and is able to accurately detect disc herniation or bulging, vertebral end-plate sclerosis, soft tissue calcification, and fractures. However, the CT scan is inferior to MRI for the study of soft tissue structures. In addition, MRI is better suited for the evaluation of internal disc structure because of its superior contrast discrimination. Therefore, it would seem that if further studies are required, the MRI would be appropriate. This, however, is not always the case, and in fact, the MRI and/or CT scan may provide information that is not helpful and may cause some confusion. It has been documented that MRI and CT scan may demonstrate abnormalities in normal, asymptomatic individuals.[11,12] Consequently, positive findings must be properly correlated to the patient's symptoms and physical findings. In one study, MRI revealed herniated discs in approximately 25% of asymptomatic people younger than 60 years and in 33% of those older than 60 years.[11] It should be readily apparent that the simple presence of abnormalities does not imply symptomatic disease. Specific correlations should be made to determine the significance of abnormal findings. Moreover, one study found that the early use of imaging did not appear to affect treatment overall, and observations indicated that decisions about the use of imaging should depend on judgments concerning whether the observed small improvement in outcome justifies the additional cost.[13]

Although not an imaging study, nerve conduction studies and electromyography studies may be quite useful in differentiating peripheral neuropathy from radiculopathy. In addition, they may be helpful in identifying the presence of a previous injury, confirming the diagnosis, localizing a lesion, and determining the extent of that lesion and correlating lesions with radiographic studies. However, these tests are limited by their dependency on patient cooperation and the examiner's skill. Furthermore, abnormal findings may not be apparent until 2 to 4 weeks after the onset of symptoms. Therefore, electrodiagnostic studies have only a limited role in the evaluation of patients with low back pain, particularly those of an acute nature. These studies, similar to the results of MRI and CT scan, require correlation with the patient's symptoms.

Management

Patients with herniated nucleus pulposus often present in severe pain, and any physician would want to provide prompt relief. This, of course, is to be recommended. However, the natural history of herniated discs is actually quite favorable, with the vast majority improving with conservative therapy. Only approximately 10% of patients will have sufficient pain after 6 weeks, which demands surgery as a consideration.[8] In fact, sequential MRI studies reveal that herniations regress with time, with partial or complete resolution in two thirds of cases within 6 months.[8,14,15] With this in mind, it would seem quite prudent to treat all such patients with nonsurgical means for a minimum of 4 to 6 weeks.

As noted earlier, bed rest is to be recommended for only brief periods (1 to 2 days) and only in the acute phase, if it appears to be of benefit, as this adds little to recovery time. Prolonged periods of sitting, standing, or walking should be avoided. Frequent rests should be taken. In this population, the mainstay of treatment remains acetaminophen and/or nonsteroidal anti-inflammatory agents, provided there are no gastrointestinal, renal, or liver diseases that would preclude their use. For relief of significant pain, the use of narcotics may be advisable but should be considered only for a short-term approach. In younger patients, some physicians would use a short course of oral steroids (5 days) (Evidence Level C). This may be considered in the elderly but with much reservation. Epidural steroid injections do not seem to alter the natural course of this disease entity (Evidence Level B).

Once the acute phase has subsided, exercise may be recommended. This is important because it will serve to reverse deconditioning that has occurred, both before and after this ailment, as well as serving to increase the activity and ability of the patient. Additionally, improved fitness will help stave off recurrent attacks. The prior activity level and lifestyle should be kept in mind when making these recommendations. Employing the services of a physical therapist may be helpful. Nonimpact aerobics (e.g., aquatic exercise), gentle back-extension exercises, back-strengthening exercises, and partial sit-ups with knees bent (for the abdominal muscles) should be included for all patients with back pain. For patients with discogenic pain, these exercises should be followed by ones that emphasize joint mobility and flexibility. Limit any lifting to items that weigh no more than the Sunday paper. If overweight, instructions on weight reduction should be included.

Follow-up

Patients should return within 2 to 3 weeks for reevaluation, and perhaps again at 6 weeks. The patient needs to be monitored for progressive improvement with no neurologic deterioration and emergence of "red flags." Patients who have not improved will require imaging studies, if not done before. They should be evaluated for the development of urinary retention, motor or sensory loss, perianal numbness, intractable leg pain, fever, chills, weight loss, progressive neurologic deficits, and abdominal symptoms.

Patients who are improving appropriately should be reminded that time is needed for treatment to take effect. As stated in the preceding text, most symptoms with disc herniation improve. The clinician and patient should not be hurried into proceeding toward any surgical approaches. Not only are they fraught with complications at any age but the outcome may also not be any different from that of a conservative approach.

Spinal Stenosis—ICD-9 Code: 724.02

CASE FOUR

A 77-year-old moderately overweight woman presents to your office complaining of a gradual onset of lower back and upper leg pain (painful paresthesias), numbness, and weakness. Although this has been troubling her for several months, it seems to have worsened over the last week while baby-sitting her great-granddaughter. She notes that she had to frequently pick up the 18-month old, which worsened the discomfort. The pain was worsened by extending the spine and with prolonged standing and walking, yet relieved by sitting. There is no change with coughing or sneezing. She has noted that while pushing a shopping cart, the pain is worsened by standing straight up, but is relieved by leaning forward on the cart. She also states that her legs feel heavy when walking variable distances and will reproduce the pain as a dull ache. Although it is improved by stopping, the pain resolves very slowly. The patient has noted that if she sleeps on her back with her spine extended, she will be awakened by back and leg pain.

Lumbar spinal stenosis is narrowing of the spinal canal of one or more levels, with subsequent compression of the nerve roots. In the older population, it is typically a degenerative process. The stenosis is the result of the slow, progressive development of osteoarthritis with its attendant loss of articular cartilage and the development of osteophytes. When these changes occur in the apophyseal or facet joints of the lumbar spine, there may be encroachment on the lumbar spinal canal and the nerve roots. The levels most commonly affected differ somewhat from those of a herniated disc. The most commonly affected level is the L4-5, with the next most common being the L3-4, followed by L1-2. Therefore, with the exception of the L4-5 level, radicular symptoms would correspond to more proximal nerve roots than that seen with discogenic disease.

The symptoms seen with lumbar spinal stenosis are related to the changes in spinal dynamics. Movements that extend the spine will decrease the volume within the spinal canal and produce symptoms, while movements that flex the spine will increase this volume and relieve the symptoms. Extension of the spine will cause the disc and ligaments to protrude into the spinal canal, narrowing the space within.

Workup/Keys to Diagnosis

Physical Examination

Range of motion may not be affected markedly during flexion; however, extension may be limited by both mechanical causes and symptoms. Lateral bending may be limited and lumbar scoliosis may be noted in some patients. Muscle weakness may be present but may not be apparent unless the patient is examined after walking a distance of approximately 300 feet or until the symptoms appear. Sensory changes may be present following this effort even without activity. Decreased sensation and motor changes may involve more than just one spinal level. Deep tendon reflexes may be asymmetric later in the disease course. Straight leg-raising tests are usually negative in most patients.

Imaging

Plain radiographs are often sufficient to make the diagnosis with the following views: AP, lateral, and obliques. These views should include the lower thoracic vertebrae as well. Degenerative changes, osteophytes, narrowing of the intervertebral disc spaces, and spondylolisthesis may be seen. In addition, evidence of osteopenia or osteoporosis may be seen, as might an old compression fracture. CT scan and/or MRI may be ordered but are frequently not necessary unless surgical intervention is contemplated.

Management

The course of this illness has a wide degree of variability. Approximately 15% of patients improve over a period of 4 years, 70% remain stable, and 15% have deterioration.[8] No specific treatment is necessary in the asymptomatic patient. When a patient does have symptoms, mild analgesics such as acetaminophen may be utilized. Narcotic analgesics should be reserved for those patients with severe pain and who are not surgical candidates. An exercise regimen that focuses on flexing the spine should be initiated to allow for increases in intraspinal volume within the bony canal. These exercises might include arching the back, remaining in a fetal position, or being on all fours while arching the back. Any activity that extends the spine should be avoided. Strengthening the abdominal muscles will aid in lifting the pelvis anteriorly and assist in flexing the lumbar spine. Reducing the amount of intra-abdominal fat is critical in keeping the spine in a more flexed position. Patients who are unable to find relief may be candidates for epidural corticosteroid injections, but there are no clear data to support their use.

Follow-up

Patients should return in 4 to 6 weeks for reevaluation and to reinforce the prior instructions and recommendations. Most patients will improve and be able to tolerate their condition. Red flags such as night pain, chills, fever, weight loss, progressive neurologic deterioration, gait disturbance, or bladder/bowel dysfunction should be noted. Neurologic changes may not be reversed following surgery; therefore, the goal of treatment is to prevent disease progression. Once conservative measures have been tried and failed, surgical management with decompressive laminectomy is an option (Evidence Level C). It should be remembered that surgery is elective, and the patient should have a major role in the decision-making process.

Compression Fracture—ICD-9 Code: 805.4

CASE FIVE

A patient presents complaining of upper lumbar back pain after slipping and falling to a sitting position on her porch steps 3 days ago after a light rain. The patient states that she has never had any back pain but the discomfort is nearly intolerable. She notes that sitting and leaning forward intensifies the nearly constant pain. It is also worsened by walking, trunk motion, and at times by a very hard cough or sneeze. She denies any numbness, tingling, weakness, or bladder or bowel dysfunction.

Fractures of the lumbar spine may occur as a result of significant trauma such as a motor-vehicle accident or fall from a height. They also occur more frequently in susceptible individuals, such as patients who have a history of long-term corticosteroid use, osteoporosis, metastatic disease, or certain endocrine disorders. Most commonly, lumbar compression fractures are seen in the elderly as a result of a relatively minor event and are usually simple fractures involving only the anterior half of the vertebral body. Compression fractures, including most fractures extending into the posterior half, are quite stable. The presenting symptom is usually the pain related to the traumatic event. Nerve root or spinal cord injury is suggested by symptoms such as tingling, numbness, motor weakness, or bowel and bladder dysfunction.

Compression fractures are a fairly common event in the elderly and, in the lumbar spine, usually involve L1 or L2. They usually result from a flexion injury that compresses the anterior portion of the vertebral body. Patients who have compression fractures should be suspected of having osteoporosis. Approximately one third of all vertebral compression fractures are an incidental finding noted on radiographs taken for other reasons.

Workup/Keys to Diagnosis

Physical Examination

The chest, trunk, abdomen, and lumbar regions should be inspected for other signs of trauma, such as swelling and ecchymoses. Bony tenderness at the site of injury is common in the acute phase of the injury. Motion of the lumbar spine will exacerbate the pain, especially with flexion, and therefore range of motion testing is best avoided at this point. In the very acute setting, muscle spasm may be present. Evaluation of sensory and motor functions should be undertaken to be certain that there is no evidence of an associated neurologic injury, particularly distal to the injured level. Signs that suggest spinal cord injury would include weakness, diffuse numbness, asymmetric or loss of deep tendon reflexes, clonus of the ankle, or a positive Babinski sign. If a spinal cord injury is suspected, it is important to test perianal sensation and sphincter function. It is unusual for neurologic or radicular symptoms to be found in an area distant from the fractured vertebra. Therefore, should this be noted, another cause should be sought on physical examination.

Imaging

Plain radiographs are clearly indicated and should be obtained. It is not unusual for the AP view to be normal while the vertebral fracture is easily visible on the lateral view. This view should reveal compression or wedging of the affected vertebra. Rotation of one vertebral body in relation to the one below indicates instability of the vertebral column. These films should be carefully examined so as not to miss other injuries that may have occurred with the trauma. Further imaging studies are generally not required, as the diagnosis is made with the plain films. However, CT scan may be indicated for compression fractures >20%, as this should arouse the suspicion of an unstable burst fracture. In addition, CT scan or MRI may be indicated if there is a possibility of injury to the spinal cord.

Bone scans are usually not indicated. However they may be useful in determining whether there is more than one fracture. If a bone scan is ordered, it should be kept in mind that it may remain abnormal for up to 2 years because of continued remodeling of the bone, although the bone appears healed on plain films.

Management

The major goal of treatment is the prevention of neurologic damage, followed by the restoration of normal function. Once it has been adequately determined that there is no possible injury to the spinal cord, secondary management may begin. Bed rest may be recommended if the patient feels that this is needed. Adequate analgesia may include the use of short-term oral narcotics. Most fractures will have enough fibrous union after 2 weeks so that there is little motion around the fracture site, reducing the pain considerably. However, the pain from this type of fracture may persist for several months, and the patient should be advised accordingly. Gradual ambulation may be encouraged once the severe pain has subsided, and consideration may be given to the use of a lumbosacral supporting brace. Bending, stooping, twisting, and lifting >15 to 20 pounds should be restricted. Once the brace is no longer needed, the patient should be encouraged to strengthen the extensor muscles of the spine to enhance muscular support. Some of the newer therapies such as vertebroplasty may be effective in the control of pain and in obtaining stability of the spine.[16] More research and evaluation are needed in this area of possible treatment for this entity.

Follow-up

The patient should return in 2 to 3 weeks for reevaluation. Assessment of the improving nature of the pain should be undertaken. If the patient has been using a brace, determination should be made if the brace is still necessary and to be certain that there is no skin breakdown as a consequence of its use. In addition, the neurologic status should be assessed to be certain that there is no evidence of compromise or deterioration. Prevention of further falls should be stressed. Evaluation should be made of the effect this injury has had on the patient's independence and the ability to handle normal activities of daily living. Reinforcement that bed rest is not recommended is prudent. Repeat radiographs may be taken at this time if deemed necessary. These films may be viewed to be certain that there are no missed fractures or developing rotational abnormalities and that proper healing is taking place. Further evaluation should be undertaken if the patient's symptoms are not improving or are worsening. Finally, some evaluation for the possibility of osteoporosis should be considered in these patients. This is further discussed in Chapter 23.

Metastatic Disease—ICD-9 Code: 198.5

CASE SIX

A 78-year-old woman presents to your office complaining of a new onset of low back pain that began 2 weeks ago. The pain began when she stooped over to pick up her laundry bag. She is known to have been diagnosed with lung cancer approximately 9 months ago and has been undergoing chemotherapy ever since. The pain is a throbbing, dull ache that is moderately severe, virtually constant, and has been worsening progressively over the last 2 weeks. The pain is relieved by lying down and worsened by weight-bearing activities such as sitting or standing. Over the last 10 days, the pain persists through the night and is preventing sleep. There is no history of any neurologic deficit or bladder or bowel dysfunction.

Metastatic disease to the spine is a common occurrence. Primary malignant tumors are quite rare. Approximately 50% of patients with solid tumors will have metastatic disease to the vertebral column. The carcinomas with the highest probability of metastasis to the spine are the breast, lung, prostate, colon, thyroid, and kidney. Most often, this metastasis involves the bone of the vertebrae with much less common involvement of the neural elements or dura. Fortunately, the rate of progression is typically slow in all but the more aggressive tumors.

Workup/Keys to Diagnosis

Physical Examination

The clinician should start the examination by seeking an area of tenderness to palpation or percussion along the lumbar spine in the site as noted by the patient. If the tumor involves any of the posterior elements such as the lamina or spinous process, a mass may be palpable. Sensory and motor functions of all the nerve roots distal to the lesion should be evaluated. Deep tendon reflexes should be assessed for asymmetry or absence.

Imaging

The initial radiographic evaluation begins with AP and lateral radiographs to include from T10 to the tip of the coccyx. It is helpful to place a radiopaque marker on the area of tenderness that helps localize the area of concern. The AP view often shows the first radiographic sign of tumor involvement, which is loss of the integrity of the pedicles. The lateral view should reveal lytic or blastic lesions with bony destruction and/or loss of height and collapse of the vertebral body.

CT scan or MRI studies are usually not necessary unless there is concern over compromise of the spinal cord or other neural structures. A bone scan may be utilized for evaluation of the extent of metastatic disease in all areas of the bony skeleton.

Management

The treatment of metastatic disease is directed toward the tumor of origin and the status of the patient. Metastatic lesions that have a known primary do not usually require bone biopsy. However, in a newly discovered malignancy or in cases with an unknown primary, bone biopsy may be necessary to make a definitive diagnosis. Treatment would be further dictated by patient preference, extent of neurologic complications, symptom severity, and degree of bony involvement. Asymptomatic tumors that are found during a metastatic workup may be treated by radiation, chemotherapy, and/or hormonal therapy. Metastatic disease that does not have neural compromise or serious deformity may be treated with radiation. If the tumor is not radiation-sensitive or causing severe pain or neurologic deficit, the most appropriate therapy would be a surgical approach with decompression.

Follow-up

The primary care physician should assist the patient in arranging proper therapy and pain management. Return visits should be patient-centered and focused as determined by the patient and physician. Specialty care will be of paramount importance in this situation.

Infection

CASE SEVEN

A 72-year-old patient with diabetes presents with complaints of fairly severe pain and restriction of spinal motion in the lumbar area. This began a few days ago and is described as a sharp, aching pain. The patient has also had generalized malaise with chills and fever as high as 39.44°C (103°F). The pain may be worsened by recumbency. There is no prior history of back problems, malignancies, or neurologic deficits.

Infection is an uncommon clinical entity involving the lower back and is usually a diagnostic challenge. However, it is an important consideration in any patient who may have suppression of their immune system. Patients at such risk would include those with diabetes mellitus, rheumatoid disease, collagen vascular disease, human immunodeficiency virus, and vascular disease or insufficiency. Not uncommonly, this is a particularly difficult diagnosis to make because of the fact that it mimics mechanical problems of the lumbar region. Fever may be absent in the elderly patient, so a high index of suspicion is required.

Workup/Keys to Diagnosis

Physical Examination

The patient may appear acutely ill and quite toxic or may simply seem to have a rather indolent illness. As the infection progresses, the patient will become increasing ill. Fever may or not be apparent in the elderly patient. There will be a markedly decreased range of motion of the lumbar region with associated pain during attempts at movement. The patient may be able to localize the area of the most discomfort, which may have tenderness to palpation but will usually have percussive tenderness. In most cases, there are few neurologic abnormalities. However, this may change in the face of an aggressive infection. A careful neurologic examination of the lumbar neural elements should be undertaken to detect any subtle findings. These may become important later in the course of the disease as part of a monitoring device.

Although not part of the physical examination, laboratory testing should be employed to aid in making the diagnosis. Initially, the complete blood count and white blood cell count may be normal. However, the sedimentation rate of inflammatory markers such as erythrocytes will be markedly elevated and play a key role in raising the level of suspicion for this diagnosis.[17] Blood cultures should be obtained and treatment directed accordingly. The immunocompromised patient may be at risk for the development of tuberculosis, for which a tuberculin skin test should be applied. As the patient may have an anergic response, this should be verified by another skin test.

Imaging

Plain radiographs (AP and lateral views) may show vertebral end-plate erosion, decreased intervertebral disc height, bony erosion, and reactive bone formation. In the early stages of infection, there may be no associated changes noted on plain film evaluation. In this setting, CT scan should be obtained, which will confirm clinical suspicions.[17] Bone infection, such as osteomyelitis, would be readily confirmed by bone scans and further confirmed by CT scan evaluation. MRI may be important for further evaluation of the soft tissues that may be involved, particularly if there is any neurologic compromise or disc space involvement.

Management

The first phases of treatment should be focused on adequately addressing the infectious agent. The patient may be symptomatically treated, while the major emphasis should be on identifying the organism and using the appropriate antimicrobial agent. Antibiotics should be administered after appropriate specimens, including blood sample, have been obtained for culture. However, obtaining the best specimen may require undergoing a bone biopsy to acquire the material for culture and sensitivity testing. Specific intravenous therapy should be based on the *in vitro* susceptibility of the identified organism that is isolated from the blood or bone. While awaiting culture results, empiric antibiotic therapy may be initiated pending definitive results. The choice of the appropriate antibiotic should be based on the most likely organism(s). Typically, the duration of antibiotic therapy is 4 to 6 weeks, which could include the use of intravenous antibiotics administered at home or appropriate oral therapy (Evidence Level B). Surgical consultation should be sought if the patient begins to show signs of neurologic involvement, such as loss of motor or sensory function, bladder or bowel dysfunction, or intractable pain.

Follow-up

This will be dictated by the patient's hospital course. If the patient does not require surgical intervention, the primary care physician will be able to continue with care of the patient. However, if a surgeon is required, comanagement of the patient may be appropriate.

Once the patient is able, activity should progress gradually. This should include stretching and strengthening exercises of the lower back and aerobic exercise. Warm compresses may be applied to the area. By the time the patient returns home, the use of analgesics should be minimal and may be confined to acetaminophen and nonsteroidal anti-inflammatory drugs. Attention should also be focused on any underlying process that has weakened the patient's immune function.

Abdominal Aortic Aneurysm—ICD-9 Code: 441.4

CASE EIGHT

A hypertensive elderly man presents to your office complaining of a rather nonspecific back pain. The pain began gradually approximately 1 week ago but is progressively getting worse. There is no history of trauma, previous back pain, or inciting event. This discomfort is described as a dull ache and does not restrict his motion or activities. There is no radiation of the pain or any loss of sensation or motor function. It does not seem to keep him from sleeping or interfere with his appetite.

There are a number of intra-abdominal problems that may present with complaints of low back pain. The presentation is usually quite dissimilar to the other causes of back pain as previously described. The pain usually begins without a trauma or inciting event, is not usually severe without rupture or tearing of the intima, and is progressive. The pain is not relieved or worsened by changes in position or movement.

Workup/Keys to Diagnosis

Physical Examination

There are none of the usual findings associated with the aforementioned causes of back pain. There is no restriction of motion (which must be viewed in light of the patient's previous functional ability), sensory deficits, or motor weakness. The deep tendon reflexes are unaffected. There is no fever, muscle atrophy, or signs of weight loss.

When there are no abnormal findings noted on the lumbosacral examination, this should alert the clinician that this might be pain emanating from another source. Attention should then be directed toward the abdominal examination and cardiovascular system. Palpation for a pulsatile mass should be made and auscultation for an abdominal bruit should be done. In addition, the peripheral pulses should be evaluated to detect any asymmetry or diminution.

Imaging

Plain films may be more confusing than helpful in this situation. The elderly population will have normal age-dependent degenerative changes in the lumbar spine. Furthermore, the severity of these changes may not correlate to the patient's complaints. In other words, the patient may have severe degenerative disease yet have no complaints related to them. The clinician may be lulled into a false sense of security by attributing the back pain to these findings. A cross-table lateral radiograph may show calcifications of the abdominal aortic wall confirming the presence of an aortic aneurysm. However, if calcifications are not seen and there is clinical suspicion, an ultrasonography of the abdomen should be obtained.

Management

This should be dictated by the size of the aneurysm, the patient's overall health status, and consultation with a cardiovascular surgeon. Surgery is recommended for an aneurysm once it reaches 5 cm in size or if the patient experiences pain from the aneurysm (Evidence Level A). At this point, the risk of rupture rises significantly. With current minimally invasive techniques, the success rate of aneurysm repair is 99%, and patients generally go home the day after the surgery. The key to management of this problem is timely recognition and proper referral.

Follow-up

Proper follow-up should also be dictated by the patient's overall health status and the cardiovascular surgeon. Attention should be directed to the proper treatment of any comorbid conditions.

CONCLUSION

Many of the complaints of low back pain in the elderly patient are simply manifestations of the aging process. It is a normal physiologic occurrence and cannot be prevented. Although physicians are aware that certain changes do occur, such as changes in proteoglycan and water content of the discs and development of osteophytes and their encroachment on the spinal canal, there is no intervention that can be employed to avert this inevitability.

Regardless of age, the usual cause of back pain is a mechanical one. Although we cannot alter the aging process, we can slow its effects by maintaining stability and mobility of the lumbar spine. This may be accomplished by exercise to strengthen both the back and abdominal musculature. Regular exercises may delay some of the normal deteriorating and deleterious effects of aging.

Physicians are well equipped and trained to make an accurate diagnosis. However, no diagnosis should be overlooked, particularly in the elderly population. Therefore, the astute clinician should always be vigilant and aware of other diagnostic possibilities and treat them accordingly.

REFERENCES

1. Andersson GBJ. Epidemiological features of chronic low-back pain. *Lancet*. 1999;354:581–585.
2. Hart LG, Deyo RA, Cherkin DC. Physician office visits for low back pain: Frequency, clinical evaluation, and treatment patterns from a U.S. national survey. *Spine*. 1995;20:11–19.
3. Frymoyer JD. Back pain and sciatica. *N Engl J Med*. 1988;318: 291–300.
4. Nachemson AL. Newest knowledge of low back pain. A critical look. *Clin Orthop*. 1992;279:8–20.
5. Weiner DK, Hanlon JT. Pain in nursing home residents: Management strategies. *Drugs Aging*. 2001;18(1):13–29.
6. Koch K, Smith MC. National Center for Health Statistics. *Office-based ambulatory care for patients 75 years old and over. National Ambulatory Medical Care Survey, 1980 and 1981. no. 110. DHHS pub. no. PHS 85–1250*. Hyattsville, MD: Public Health Research Service; 1985:110:1–14.
7. Bressler HB, Keyes WJ, Rochon PA, et al. The prevalence of low back pain in the elderly: A systematic review of the literature. *Spine*. 1999;24(17):1813–1918.
8. Deyo RA, Weinstein JN. Primary care: Low back pain. *N Engl J Med*. 2001;344(5):363–370.
9. Malmivaara A, Häkkinen U, Aro T, et al. The treatment of acute low back pain—bed rest, exercises, or ordinary activity? *N Engl J Med*. 1995;332(6):351–355.
10. Hofstee DJ, Gijtenbeek JMM, Hoogland PH, et al. Westeinde sciatica trial: Randomized controlled study of bed rest and physiotherapy for acute sciatica. *J Neurosurg Spine*. 2002;96: 45–49.
11. Jensen MC, Brant-Zawadzki MN, Obuchowski N, et al. Magnetic resonance imaging of the lumbar spine in people without back pain. *N Engl J Med*. 1994;331:69–73.
12. Wiesel SW, Tsourmas N, Feffer HL, et al. A study of computer-assisted tomography. The incidence of positive CAT scans in an asymptomatic group of patients. *Spine*. 1994;9:549–551.
13. Gilbert FJ, Grant AM, Gillan MGC, et al. Low back pain: Influence of early MR imaging or CT on treatment and outcome—multicenter randomized trial. *Radiology*. 2004;231(2): 343–351.
14. Komori H, Shinomiya K, Nakai O, et al. The natural history of herniated nucleus pulposis with radiculopathy. *Spine*. 1996;21: 225–229.
15. Benoist M. The natural history of lumbar disc herniation and radiculopathy. *Joint Bone Spine*. 2002;69:155–160.
16. Papaioannou A, Watts NB, Kendler DL, et al. Diagnosis and management of vertebral fractures in elderly adults. *Amer J Med*. 2002;113(3):220–228.
17. Goel V, Young J, Patterson C. Case report: Infective discitis as an uncommon but important cause of back pain in older people. *Age Ageing*. 2000;29(5):454–456.

Urinary Disorders

15

Richard J. Ackermann

CLINICAL PEARLS 175
Urinary Incontinence 175
Urinary Tract Infections 175
Benign Prostatic Hyperplasia 175
Prostate Cancer 176

URINARY INCONTINENCE 176
Normal Aging 176
Pathophysiology 177
Reversible Causes of Urinary Incontinence 178
Established Urinary Incontinence 179
Workup 180
Management 181

URINARY TRACT INFECTIONS 183
Disease Background 183
Workup 183
Management 184
Asymptomatic Bacteriuria 185
Infections in Catheterized Patients 186

BENIGN PROSTATIC HYPERPLASIA 187
Workup 188
Management 188
Choice of Treatment 191

PROSTATE CANCER 191
Workup 191
Management 193

CLINICAL PEARLS

Urinary Incontinence

- Loss of frontal lobe inhibition is the major reason why patients with dementia develop urinary incontinence.
- Normal aging never causes urinary incontinence.
- Detrusor hyperactivity is the most common cause of urinary incontinence in elderly men and women, accounting for 50% to 65% of cases.
- Urinary incontinence is a late finding in patients with dementia; its early appearance should lead to suspicion of other causes.
- In most cases, the diagnosis is made from the history.
- Baseline laboratory tests include a urinalysis, urine culture, and serum blood urea nitrogen (BUN) and creatinine level.
- Absolute dryness may not be a realistic goal.
- For patients with dementia, prompted voiding can be helpful.
- For women with severe stress urinary incontinence, early surgical referral may be indicated.
- For excessive urine ammonia odor, chlorophyllin 100 mg daily may be prescribed.

Urinary Tract Infections

- *Enterococcus* should be suspected in instrumented men and in patients with long-term indwelling catheters.
- The diagnosis of urinary tract infection requires symptoms plus a positive urine culture.
- Reports of "cloudy" or "smelly" urine do not count as symptoms.
- Parenteral antibiotics need to be continued only until the patient is clearly improving, afebrile, and able to take an oral antibiotic.
- Asymptomatic bacteriuria is not associated with the development of either hypertension or renal failure.
- Urinary catheters may be a reasonable and compassionate choice for elders who are terminally ill or functionally very impaired.
- Long-term catheters should be changed when obstructed or every 1 to 3 months.

Benign Prostatic Hyperplasia

- Histologic prostatic hyperplasia affects up to 90% of men older than 85 years.

- The most important part of the history is to quantitate the severity of the symptoms, using the American Urological Association Symptom Index (AUA-SI).
- Therapy is chosen to address the patient's predominant symptoms, not just to reduce the size of the prostate.
- Tamsulosin is the clearly preferred α-blocker because it does not cause hypotension and is equal in efficacy to the nonselective α-blockers.
- A few older men are not fit for operative intervention and would be best served by long-term urinary catheterization.
- A single episode of urinary retention due to prostate hyperplasia does not mandate surgical treatment.

Prostate Cancer

- More than two thirds of men older than 80 years have histologically proven prostate cancer, although only a tiny portion of these men die of this disease.
- Prostate-specific antigen (PSA) is very prostate-specific but not cancer-specific.
- Most older men choosing watchful waiting will do well, particularly if the Gleason grade is favorable and there is no evidence of metastatic disease.
- Select men older than 70 or 75 years may occasionally be candidates for radical prostatectomy, although there is no clear evidence that the benefits outweigh the risks in this group.
- Approximately 50% to 80% of men with prostate cancer treated with hormonal treatment will have a substantial benefit.

Urinary disorders are among the most common conditions faced by the geriatrician. This chapter examines the following: (i) Urinary incontinence, (ii) urinary tract infection, (iii) benign prostatic hyperplasia, and (iv) prostate cancer.

URINARY INCONTINENCE

Urinary incontinence is the involuntary loss of urine severe enough to cause social or health problems. The problem is often undiagnosed because patients may not voluntarily disclose their disability, clinicians may not ask or be comfortable with an evaluation, or multiple other serious conditions consume the attention of the clinician. However, most elders with urinary incontinence can be managed with a straightforward evaluation. Urinary incontinence is one of the fundamental syndromes of geriatrics. It is often caused by something remote from the bladder, such as dementia, pneumonia, or medications.[1,2] As many as 15% to 30% of community-dwelling elders have some degree of urinary incontinence—the rate is always higher in women. The prevalence rises to more than 50% in nursing home patients. In fact, urinary incontinence is commonly a precipitating reason for nursing home placement. Families may tolerate wandering and providing support for feeding and dressing but urinating on the sofa may not be well tolerated.

Normal Aging

Normal aging never causes incontinence. Put another way, urinary incontinence is always pathologic and deserves evaluation. However, several aspects of normal aging of the genitourinary (GU) tract do predispose susceptible elders to developing incontinence. First, uninhibited bladder (detrusor) contractions become increasingly common as one ages. So if an elder with incontinence undergoes urodynamic testing and is found to have detrusor hyperactivity, this may not be the cause of the incontinence, but rather part of normal aging.

Second, fluid excretion through the kidneys is highest during the hours of recumbency at night because of high atrial natriuretic peptide levels, depressed antidiuretic hormone levels, and mobilization of dependent edema. This could lead to filling of the bladder and a need to urinate (nocturia), but it would not be a direct cause of incontinence.

Third, bladder capacity diminishes with age. Bladder capacity, defined as the amount of urine in the bladder when the person feels he or she cannot possibly hold another drop, progressively falls with aging.

Fourth, in men, the prostate grows with aging. This benign growth can encroach on the urinary sphincters, causing symptoms of outlet obstruction, such as poor urinary stream, dribbling, and a sensation of incomplete bladder emptying. However, if prostate growth is the cause of incontinence, it is not normal aging—it is benign prostatic hyperplasia, prostate cancer, or some other pathologic cause.

Fifth, also in men, urinary flow rate falls with advancing age. Normal flow rates in elderly men should exceed 20 mL per second. Urinary flow rates <10 mL per second are clearly abnormal and those between 10 and 20 mL per second are borderline. With hyperplasia of the median lobe of the prostate, the velocity of flow through the urethra decreases. This can be measured with a urine velocity meter, a piece of equipment normally found in a urologist's office. A "poor man's" flow estimate is described later in this chapter.

Urinary incontinence is not just a nuisance; it causes substantial morbidity, including rash, skin infections, urinary tract infection (UTI), restriction of activity, depression, social isolation, decreased sexual function, and falls. Pressure sores are not independently associated with urinary incontinence, once one controls for comorbidities. Probably the most important complication of incontinence is social isolation. For example, an elder may stop going to church and civic clubs because of the embarrassment of becoming wet in a public place. Although urinary incontinence can cause substantial morbidity, it is not independently linked to mortality risk.[3]

It is easy to overlook urinary incontinence, especially in elders with multiple medical problems. For example, an 83-year-old woman with congestive heart failure, renal insufficiency, and poorly controlled diabetes will be on numerous medications and require substantial monitoring. Despite this, her major functional problem may be urinary incontinence—this may be the one thing that is really limiting her life. As part of every comprehensive geriatric assessment, ask a screening question about incontinence. A good question is: "Do you have accidents, or leak, when you urinate?"

Pathophysiology

The bladder has two major functions—it needs to fill and it needs to empty[3] (see Figure 15.1).

The bladder fills through relaxation of the detrusor muscle, with contraction of the bladder sphincters. The detrusor muscle is innervated by the muscarinic parasympathetic nervous system, which proceeds as a defined nerve from the second, third, and fourth sacral nerve roots. Any drug that is cholinergic will therefore contract the bladder (few drugs are cholinergic—e.g., bethanechol); any drug that is anticholinergic would relax the bladder (examples are legion and include antihistamines, antipsychotics, tricyclic antidepressants, and directly anticholinergic drugs).

The bladder sphincter is made up of two parts—the internal and external sphincters. The internal sphincter is innervated by the α part of the sympathetic nervous system. The sympathetic nerves to the internal sphincter arise from the thoracolumbar spinal cord (T11 through L2) and travel along blood vessels, ending in a well-defined bladder neck muscle. Any drug with α-agonist effect will therefore contract the internal sphincter. Examples of this are cold remedies such as pseudoephedrine (Sudafed) or the herb *Ephedra*. Any drug that is an α-antagonist will relax the sphincters. Examples of these drugs include the nonspecific α-blockers phentolamine or phenoxybenzamine and the α_1-blockers prazosin, doxazosin, and tamsulosin.

The external sphincter is under voluntary muscle control. Therefore, it is innervated by a somatic nerve, with acetylcholine as the neurotransmitter. But this acetylcholine receptor is not a muscarinic (autonomic) cholinergic receptor but a nicotinic receptor. The typical anticholinergic drugs mentioned previously have no effect on this sphincter. Unfortunately, the voluntary sphincter cannot maintain continence for long because it requires constant active stimulation. It is mainly used to back up the internal sphincter (as when the bladder is very full and you must consciously "hold" your urine) or when the internal sphincter has been damaged (e.g., after prostate surgery).

So when the bladder is in filling mode, the sympathetic (α) system is on, keeping the sphincters contracted, and the parasympathetic (cholinergic) system is off, keeping the bladder relaxed. Actually, both systems are on, just to different degrees. When the bladder is filling, the sympathetic system dominates. This domination occurs at the level of the brainstem micturition center. This brainstem center regulates the balance of the autonomic nervous system—during the bladder's filling phase, the micturition center turns up the adrenergic, sympathetic tone to the bladder's neck and turns down the cholinergic, parasympathetic tone to the wall of the bladder, the detrusor muscle.

After the bladder fills to a significant extent, it switches to emptying mode. In this case, the brainstem makes a switch in autonomic tone—it revs up cholinergic transmission through parasympathetic nerves to the detrusor, to contract the bladder, and ramps down adrenergic transmission through sympathetic nerves to the internal sphincter. Therefore, the bladder contracts, the sphincters relax, and urine flows.

Note that the brainstem can do this without control by the cortex. In newborn infants, before the cerebral cortex becomes fully developed, the micturition center switches from filling to emptying mode as many as 20 times per day—therefore, 20 wet diapers. As the cortex develops, the final important part of the control of micturition develops—frontal lobe inhibition. The frontal lobes learn to tonically inhibit the micturition center, essentially

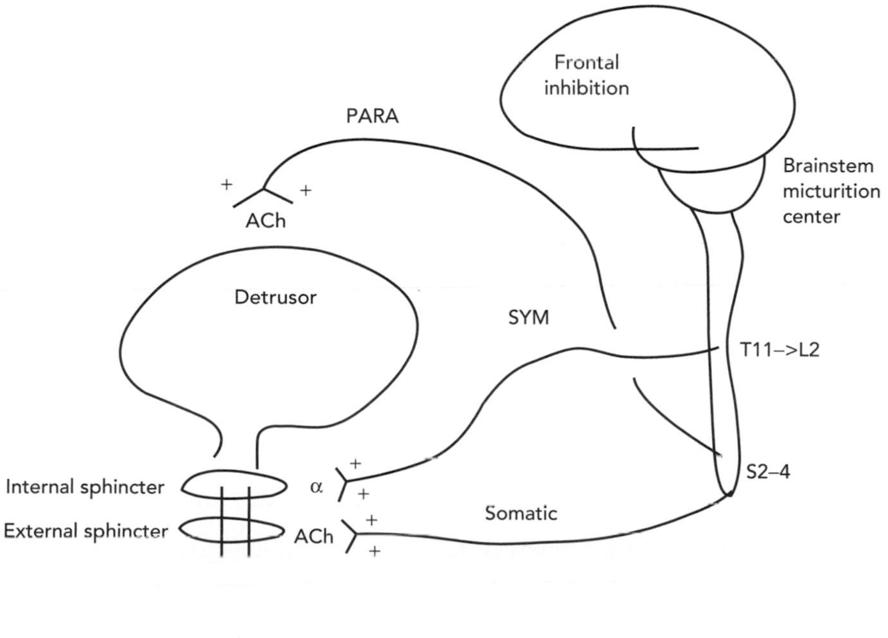

Figure 15.1 Functional anatomy of urination. PARA, parasympathetic; SYM, sympathetic; ACh, acetylcholine.

keeping it in filling mode. Some readers of this text may at the moment have enough urine in the bladder to switch from filling to emptying mode, but their frontal lobes, below the level of consciousness, are telling the bladder not to because this would be socially inappropriate.

Loss of frontal inhibition is the major reason why patients with dementia and other neurodegenerative diseases develop urinary incontinence. In these patients, there is generally nothing wrong with the bladder, its innervation, the spinal cord, or the brainstem, but the frontal lobe loses function. Therefore, the patient loses the tonic frontal inhibition, and the body reverts to its primitive reflex form of urination—the micturition center simply switches from filling to emptying mode whenever an adequate amount of urine has been sensed in the bladder.

Remembering this functional anatomy makes the workup and treatment of urinary incontinence fairly straightforward.

Reversible Causes of Urinary Incontinence

After establishing the presence of incontinence, it is worthwhile to check for acute, reversible, transient causes of this condition. Table 15.1 lists several common causes, using the mnemonic "DIAPPERS."[3]

Elders with delirium frequently have urinary incontinence. For example, a vigorous 86-year-old man, with no prior history of incontinence, is admitted to the hospital with lobar pneumonia, accompanied by fever, hyponatremia, mild dehydration, and urinary incontinence. In this case, the incontinence is almost surely due to the acute illness. An appropriate response would be to treat the underlying infection and reassess the incontinence after he has gone home and fully recovered.

Urinary incontinence is a common symptom in elders with symptomatic UTI. However, both asymptomatic bacteriuria and incontinence are very common, especially in frail, institutionalized elders, so their occurrence in the same patient is very likely to be a coincidence, not cause and effect. In new-onset urinary incontinence, or when incontinence suddenly worsens, it is reasonable to check for infection. One can generally wait for the urine culture and sensitivity, pick a simple antibiotic, and see whether clearing the infection helps the incontinence. If it does not, then the two are not related. Do not get in the endless game of treating every positive urine culture in incontinent patients—this does not help the incontinence and leads to predictable complications of chronic antibiotic therapy.

Atrophic vaginitis/urethritis in elderly women can present with urinary incontinence, especially the stress or outlet incompetence type. Consider treatment with vaginal, transdermal, or oral estrogens, taking care to assess the overall appropriateness of hormone replacement in the woman (Evidence Level B). Even in an older woman with a uterus, however, intermittent vaginal estrogen (e.g., once or twice per week) to treat atrophy and incontinence is very unlikely to cause endometrial hyperplasia or other important side effects. However, the only large clinical trial of oral estrogens (Premarin) in postmenopausal women suggested that estrogen is ineffective (or even harmful) in all types of urinary incontinence.[4]

Many drugs can worsen urinary incontinence. Drugs with centrally acting sedative effect can remove the normal frontal inhibition. Examples include narcotics, sleeping medicines, alcohol, and antidepressants. Anticholinergic medications, including antihistamines and antipsychotics, may cause urinary incontinence by relaxing the detrusor muscle and causing bladder distension and overflow incontinence. Diuretics do not directly cause incontinence, but they can certainly make it worse through direct pharmacologic effects. Most diuretics should be dosed in the morning, so nocturia and nighttime incontinence is less of a problem. α-Agonists or blockers may interfere with proper functioning of the sphincters. Some chemotherapy agents (e.g., cyclophosphamide and vincristine) are toxic either to the bladder or the nerves supplying the bladder.

Depression is a major cause of urinary incontinence, as are other primary psychiatric disorders. Sometimes, incontinence can even be a tool used by patients to manipulate caregivers.

Rarely, polyuria is so excessive, usually from uncontrolled diabetes or hypercalcemia, that it may provoke

TABLE 15.1
CAUSES OF TRANSIENT INCONTINENCE IN THE ELDERLY

D	*D*elirium
I	Symptomatic urinary tract *i*nfection—asymptomatic bacteriuria has poor correlation with incontinence
A	*A*trophic vaginitis/urethritis
P	*P*harmaceuticals—diuretics, anticholinergics, psychotropics, narcotics, α-blockers or agonists, calcium blockers, alcohol, vincristine
P	*P*sychological—especially depression
E	*E*xcessive urine output—hyperglycemia, hypercalcemia, treatment of CHF
R	*R*estricted mobility—musculoskeletal problems, inability to get to the toilet
S	*S*tool impaction

CHF, congestive heart failure.
Reprinted with permission from Resnick NM. Geriatric incontinence. *Urol Clin N Am.* 1996;23:55–74.

urinary incontinence. And in hospitalized patients who receive several liters of intravenous hydration per day, one can expect incontinence, particularly when the patient is tethered to the bed with heart monitors, antithromboembolism leg pumps, oximetry devices, and so on.

A very common cause of acute (and chronic) urinary incontinence is impairment of mobility. A patient with severe osteoarthritis may simply not be able to move fast enough to get from the bed across the room to the bathroom and toilet. In cases like this, placing a portable commode next to the bed is a logical step, if the underlying disease cannot be adequately managed.

Finally, stool impaction can induce or exacerbate urinary incontinence. This is a particular problem in elders who take opiates for long term and in patients with dementia. The enlarging rectal ampulla may mechanically obstruct the bladder outlet and compress the bladder, causing detrusor overactivity.

Established Urinary Incontinence

Once the presence of urinary incontinence is verified, and transient causes have been eliminated, it is helpful to subdivide the incontinence into one of four major categories:

- Detrusor hyperactivity (the bladder is too strong)
- Detrusor underactivity (the bladder is too weak)
- Outlet obstruction (the sphincter is too strong)
- Outlet incompetence (the sphincter is too weak).

Combinations of these subtypes can also occur.

Detrusor hyperactivity (bladder too strong) is the most common cause of urinary incontinence in both elderly men and women, accounting for 50% to 65% of cases. Other common names for this type are urge incontinence, overactive bladder, or bladder spasms. Patients describe an abrupt sensation that urination is imminent. In many cases, no clear cause is found. The most commonly identified causes of detrusor hyperactivity are neurodegenerative diseases that affect the frontal lobes, thereby reducing or eliminating the normal frontal inhibition of the brainstem–spinal cord urinary reflex. Therefore, Alzheimer disease, Parkinson disease, and cortical stroke can cause urinary incontinence by reducing frontal inhibition, leading to uncoordinated detrusor hyperactivity. Incontinence should be a late finding in patients with dementia; its early appearance should lead to suspicion of other causes.

Other rare causes of detrusor hyperactivity are the "normal" increase in bladder contractions in patients who have urethral obstruction. Chronic cystitis, induced by radiation, interstitial disease, or chemotherapy, can cause bladder spasms. Finally, bladder stones or bladder cancer are irritating to the detrusor muscle, leading to detrusor hyperactivity.

Not all patients with an overactive bladder are incontinent. Many patients, especially women, have the intense sensation of urinary urgency, but they still have the mental and physical capacity to get to the bathroom in time. These patients can be assessed and treated like patients with actual urge incontinence.

Elders with detrusor hyperactivity have frequent moderate- or large-volume urine leakage, with leakage at night. The patient describes an intense desire to urinate, followed by a wet episode within a few seconds. Patients with dementia, of course, will not present with this sensation of urge but will simply have reflex incontinence. And in some cognitively intact patients, the urge is not felt, but incontinence still follows uninhibited bladder contraction. A neurologic examination should be normal, except perhaps for signs of frontal lobe release or other focal signs of cortical brain disease. The residual volume, if measured, should be normal.

A subset of patients with detrusor hyperactivity also has impaired bladder contractility, leading to incomplete emptying of the bladder. These patients may have an elevated residual volume.

Detrusor underactivity (bladder too weak) is uncommon. It is usually due to a neurogenic cause, such as disc compression, spinal cord tumor, surgical damage to nerves, or autonomic neuropathy (such as that caused by diabetes, alcohol, vitamin B_{12} deficiency, or syphilis). It can also result as the end stage of chronic outlet obstruction—initially the bladder would hypertrophy and be overactive, but as time progresses, the bladder stretches too far and becomes weak and dilated, with ineffectual contractions.

Elders with detrusor underactivity have frequent small-volume leaks (overflow, hard to distinguish from primary outlet obstruction), rare nocturnal leakage, and possible loss of sacral reflexes or anal sphincter control, depending on the cause. Residual volume is high, and there are clinical symptoms of hesitancy, straining, and a sense of incomplete emptying. These obstructive symptoms are usually caused by outlet obstruction, but keep in mind rare causes of primary detrusor underactivity.

Outlet obstruction (sphincter too strong) is the second most common cause of urinary incontinence in elderly men, after urge incontinence. It is rare in women. It produces characteristic overflow incontinence, with dribbling, incomplete emptying, straining, and hesitancy. By far the most common cause of outlet obstruction is prostatism, either benign or malignant. Urethral strictures in men and, occasionally, a very large cystourethrocele or cervical or ovarian cancer in women are causes. Urinary leakage is nearly continuous and of low volume. Residual volume will be high, but neurologic tests should be normal.

Outlet incompetence (sphincter too weak) is the second most common cause of urinary incontinence in elderly women, after urge incontinence. It is usually of the stress incontinence type caused by intrinsic weakness, vaginal delivery, estrogen deficiency, or surgical damage. From 1% to 2% of men who undergo prostatectomy are left with wide-open outlet incompetence. Rarely, diabetes can be a primary cause of outlet incompetence. Hysterectomy and postmenopausal state may be weakly linked to an increased risk of outlet incompetence.

The characteristic pattern is daytime small leaks with any increase in abdominal pressure, such as with coughing, laughing, or straining. Leakage at night is rare. Residual volume should be low, unless urine pools in a large cystocele, and the neurologic examination is normal.

Workup

Evaluation of urinary incontinence in the elderly relies heavily on history. Indeed, in most cases, the diagnosis is made from history alone. Ask about the pattern of voiding, including onset of urinary incontinence, frequency, severity, and any precipitating or palliating factors. Use a 2- to 3-day voiding record (see Table 15.2) to quantitate and individualize this information. The patient urinates into a measuring cup inserted beneath the toilet seat. Ask about urine leakage at night and about any symptoms of outlet obstruction (hesitancy, dribbling, incomplete emptying).

As in all geriatric conditions, look at the big picture. Look for signs and symptoms of delirium, dementia, stroke, parkinsonism, cord or nerve root compression, and peripheral or autonomic neuropathy. Assess for evidence of functional impairment, and look at the patient's general medical illnesses and medications. The history will usually lead to one of these major categories:

URGE: large-volume leakage preceded by brief warning (seconds to minutes) → detrusor hyperactivity
STRESS: leakage only with increases in abdominal pressure → outlet incompetence
REFLEX: leakage without warning ("I am suddenly wet for no reason.") → detrusor hyperactivity
OVERFLOW: continuous small-volume leakage → outlet obstruction or rarely detrusor underactivity

Note: When urinary incontinence occurs immediately with an increase in abdominal pressure, this strongly suggests outlet incompetence and stress incontinence. When the increase in abdominal pressure is followed several seconds later by urinary leakage, urge incontinence is suggested. In this case, the abdominal pressure secondarily causes bladder spasm (detrusor hyperactivity), which then causes leakage.

Physical examination should be completed but rarely adds any information. One might confirm a distended bladder. Stress leakage can be duplicated by asking the patient to stand with a full bladder and then perform maneuvers increasing abdominal pressure. Rectal examination may demonstrate a fecal impaction, which

TABLE 15.2

BLADDER RECORD, OR VOIDING DIARY

Name: ____________________

Date ________/________/________
month day year

INSTRUCTIONS:

1. In the column "urinated in toilet," make a mark every time during the 2-hour period you urinate into the toilet.
2. Use the next column "amount" to record the amount you urinate (or simply use a check mark if you are not measuring).
3. In the column marked "accident," make a mark every time you accidentally leak urine.
4. In the last column, describe the reason for the accident. For example, if you coughed and leaked a small amount, write "cough—small amount." If you had a large accident after a strong urge to urinate, write "urge—large amount."

Time Interval	Urinated in Toilet	Amount	Accident (YES/NO)	Reason for Accident
6–8 AM				
8–10 AM				
10 AM–Noon				
Noon–2 PM				
2–4 PM				
4–6 PM				
6–8 PM				
8–10 PM				
10 PM–Midnight				
Overnight				
Number of pads used today: ________				

Reprinted with permission from Agency for Healthcare Quality and Research. *Urinary incontinence in adults. Clinical practice guideline*, AHCPR Pub. No. 92–0038, Rockville, MD: AHRQ; March 1992.

itself can worsen urinary incontinence. In men, the prostate can be palpated, but prostate size correlates poorly with obstruction. One can also ask the elderly patient to voluntarily contract the anal sphincter, but at least 15% of normal elders cannot do this, so a negative result for this test is not helpful.

Pelvic examination can demonstrate laxity, such as a cystocele or rectocele, but these findings are rarely the cause of incontinence. Occasionally, a large cystocele may kink the urethra and cause outlet obstruction in women. Signs of atrophic vaginitis suggest estrogen deficiency and outlet incompetence. Finally, there is the Bonney (or Marshall) test—the bladder is pushed up, stabilizing the bladder base and preventing leakage caused by outlet incompetence. This test predicts whether surgery may cure the outlet incompetence.

Laboratory is also of limited usefulness, but in most cases, one should order a urinalysis, urine culture, and serum blood urea nitrogen (BUN) and creatinine level determination. If the urinalysis shows sterile hematuria, then one should move out of the incontinence algorithm and perform a structural workup, usually cystoscopy and some kind of upper tract imaging, such as spiral computed tomography (CT) scan. Urine cytology is only necessary if transitional cell carcinoma is suspected, such as in patients with hematuria. A positive urine culture may indicate UTI or asymptomatic bacteriuria; in select cases, give a trial of antibiotics and assess their effect on continence.

In suspected cases, a postvoid residual volume should be measured. Normal residual volume is <100 mL, and >200 mL is clearly abnormal. If the residual volume is abnormal, order a renal ultrasound to check for hydronephrosis. In men, it is usually safer and easier, although more expensive, to measure residual volume by ultrasonography than by urethral catheterization.

Men with obstructive symptoms should complete the American Urological Association Symptom Index (AUA-SI) (see Table 15.7). An ancillary test in these patients is a urinary flow rate, which is generally done in the urologist's office. If polyuria is present, it is prudent to check the serum glucose and calcium levels to evaluate for causes of osmotic diuresis.

The diagnosis is generally clear from history, physical examination, and basic laboratory tests. If not, then the physician might consider referring the patient to a gynecologist or urologist who specializes in urinary incontinence. Unfortunately, even in severe cases, urodynamic testing is not likely to provide more precise diagnostic and therapeutic information.

Following these diagnostic suggestions leads to a diagnosis in most cases. Consider referral to a surgical specialist in the following cases: Marked pelvic prolapse, severe stress incontinence, marked prostate enlargement, suspicion of cancer, inability to pass a urinary catheter, residual volume >100 to 200 mL, recent pelvic surgery or radiation, sterile hematuria, recalcitrant symptomatic UTIs, and severe obstructive symptoms.

Management

In all cases, try to correct the underlying problem or precipitating factors. Accept that absolute dryness may not be a realistic goal, but a reduction in the number and severity of incontinent episodes is generally possible. Reducing the number of episodes by one or two per day can have a substantial impact on the daily lives of patients and their caregivers.

Realize that drugs have not been adequately tested in the elderly, particularly the sick elderly. Be very careful of drug side effects, and if a drug is not clearly effective, stop it.

Bladder training (habit training) can be useful in most causes of urinary incontinence, except in cognitively impaired elders (Evidence Level B). Ask the patient to void every 30 to 60 minutes; then progressively increase the duration between voids to every 3 to 4 hours. A night schedule is optional.[5]

For detrusor hyperactivity, start with pelvic muscle exercises (Kegel exercises; see Table 15.3). Although these were originally designed for outlet incompetence, when they are done correctly, the sphincter muscles contract and the bladder reflexively relaxes. However, if the exercises are done incorrectly (as is often the case), they can make the situation worse. Referral to a urinary incontinence therapist, usually in the occupational therapy department, can often help. These professionals will place a probe in the vagina of the patient and teach her how to contract and relax the correct muscles, using biofeedback. Several sessions of this training may substantially reduce or even cure incontinence[6,7] (Evidence Level B).

Avoidance of caffeinated beverages, alcohol, and artificial sweeteners may improve symptoms.[8]

TABLE 15.3 KEGEL PUBOCOCCYGEUS MUSCLE EXERCISES FOR DETRUSOR HYPERACTIVITY OR OUTLET INCOMPETENCE

- Pull in or "squeeze" your pelvic muscles as if you were trying to stop urine flow or keep from passing gas
- To better feel the muscles to be contracted, attempt to stop the flow of urine while urinating
- Hold the contraction for several seconds
- Relax completely for a period as long as the contraction was held, then repeat
- Perform at least three sets of eight to ten contractions every day.
- Try to hold contractions for progressively longer times (from 1–2 s to 10 s, if possible)
- Improvement in bladder control may not be evident for 3 mo; keep exercising!

The most commonly used drugs are the bladder smooth muscle relaxants oxybutynin (Ditropan) or tolterodine (Detrol). Oxybutynin comes in immediate-release preparations (5 and 10 mg tablets) that are dosed twice daily. There is also a sustained-release product, oxybutynin (Ditropan XL) (5, 10, and 15 mg), which is dosed once per day. Finally, there is a transdermal oxybutynin product (Oxytrol patch, 3.9 mg) that is dosed twice per week.

Tolterodine (Detrol) may be slightly more bladder specific. It comes as immediate-release (1 and 2 mg) tablets, which are dosed twice daily, and a sustained-release product (Detrol LA, 2 and 4 mg), which is dosed once per day.[9]

There are three newer bladder relaxants: Trospium (Sanctura, 20 mg twice daily),[10] darifenacin (Enablex, 7.5 to 15 mg daily),[11] and solifenacin (VESIcare, 5 mg daily).[12] These newer drugs may be more bladder specific, but there is no convincing evidence of increased efficacy. All the anticholinergic drugs for overactive bladder are only modestly more effective than placebo (Evidence Level A).

If these drugs do not clearly decrease the number and severity of incontinent episodes, they should be discontinued. If the physician is unsure whether the drug will be helpful, a limited trial is indicated. If, on the other hand, the physician is unsure whether the drug is really doing any good, then a trial off the drug is a good idea. Common side effects include dry mouth, constipation, blurred vision, and gastroesophageal reflux. Patients with dementia may become more confused. Side effects may be less common with the sustained-release products. All anticholinergic drugs can rarely precipitate urinary retention, especially if there is any degree of underlying outlet obstruction.

For patients with dementia, prompted voiding can be helpful.[13] In this approach, the caregiver first completes a voiding diary to understand the pattern of incontinence episodes. Then, he or she approaches the patient at the appropriate time and asks, "Do you need help in going to the bathroom?" If the patient says yes, then the caregiver calmly helps. If the patient says no, the caregiver lets the patient know he or she is available if needed. If the patient still wets himself or herself, then calm cleaning, without scolding or belittling is needed. This "simple" maneuver may reduce the number of incontinent episodes by 50% or more. A randomized trial in nursing home patients with detrusor hyperactivity associated with dementia found that adding oxybutynin to a schedule of prompted voiding added no extra benefit in reducing incontinent episodes.[14]

A few other drugs have been suggested to help with detrusor hyperactivity, but their side effects generally preclude their use in the elderly, particularly the frail elderly. Drugs with doubtful efficacy include imipramine (Tofranil), dicyclomine (Bentyl), flavoxate (Urispas), and the strongly anticholinergic drug propantheline (Pro-Banthine).

An indwelling catheter, although it immediately prevents wetting, is not recommended. In addition to a substantially increased risk of urosepsis, the underlying bladder spasms often worsen because there is a foreign body in the bladder. Eventually in some of these patients, spasms increase to the extent that urine leaks around the catheter, leading to placement of a larger catheter and a vicious cycle.

Detrusor underactivity can be overcome with the Credé maneuver (physically pushing on the abdominal wall to encourage bladder emptying) or Valsalva maneuvers. In patients who are dexterous enough or who have capable caregivers, intermittent catheterization is an option. Another choice is to place an indwelling catheter for 2 to 4 weeks and then attempt discontinuation of the catheter to see whether the bladder has contracted down and regained some muscular tone. The cholinergic drug bethanechol (Urecholine) or the α-blocker phenoxybenzamine (Dibenzyline) often have too many side effects to be useful.

In patients with outlet obstruction, usually men, the appropriate first step is relief from the obstruction. This usually means surgery, as with a transurethral resection of the prostate (TURP) or dilation of a urethral stricture. In some patients, surgical repair is not possible or the patient may be at too high a risk for surgery. In these cases, long-term drainage of the bladder by an indwelling catheter is indicated. Choices include urethral or suprapubic catheters. The catheter should be meticulously maintained to avoid mechanical and infectious complications.

Drugs have little role in incontinence caused by outlet obstruction. An α-blocker such as phenoxybenzamine (Dibenzyline) or terazosin (Hytrin) or tamsulosin (Flomax), although indicated for obstructive symptoms of benign prostatic hyperplasia (BPH), are usually inappropriate if incontinence is present.

Finally, there are several effective treatments for patients with incontinence caused by outlet incompetence. For women with severe stress incontinence, early surgical referral may be indicated, either to urologists or to gynecologists with a special interest in this area. Short of surgery, pelvic floor exercises (Table 15.3), perhaps with a referral to an incontinence therapist who can use biofeedback, weight loss, and intravaginal weighted cones, are possibilities. In men, urinary incontinence following prostatectomy can be treated with a penile clamp, penile sheath, or condom catheter. In some women, pessaries may be helpful, but these must be changed frequently. Other possibilities for women include an artificial sphincter and polytetrafluoroethylene (Teflon) injections of the sphincter.

The major drug (for women only!) for outlet incompetence is estrogen. This can be given orally, transdermally, or vaginally, with the usual precautions. Some women may benefit from relatively low doses of vaginal cream given two or three nights per week (Evidence Level B). Paradoxically, recent studies suggest that estrogen replacement in postmenopausal women may actually increase the risk of urinary incontinence.[4,15] Wide-open stress incontinence does not usually respond to estrogens and may require surgery.

Other drugs are not generally recommended in the elderly with outlet incompetence. α-Agonists (ephedrine or pseudoephedrine) may strengthen the urinary sphincter, but these drugs have too many vascular side effects. Anticholinergic drugs have been used to weaken bladder contractions, but this does not address the underlying problem.

In many cases, there will be treatment failures. For most elders, the incontinence will not be cured; it will be managed. Patients, families, and caregivers may need access to adult diapers such as Depends or Attends. These cost less than a dollar each, but if several are used per day, costs can be considerable. Patients may need launderable bed pads, and men may consider using external collection devices such as the sheath or condom catheters.

For excessive urine ammonia odor, chlorophyllin 100 mg daily may be prescribed. This does nothing for the incontinence, but it masks the smell. It also turns stool green. Patients with urinary incontinence need special attention to skin care and prevention of pressure sores. Do not treat bacteriuria in patients with incontinence unless the patient is symptomatic.

URINARY TRACT INFECTIONS

UTIs are the most common bacterial infections in the elderly, as well as the most common cause of bacteremia in this age-group. Nosocomial UTIs are usually secondary to catheters, are common and very serious, and may be caused by organisms resistant to first-line antibiotics. UTI in the elderly presents a range of severity, from asymptomatic bacteriuria, which requires no treatment, to bacteremia, which has a 15% to 35% mortality.[16]

Aging contributes to an increased risk of UTI. Estrogen deficiency probably explains the higher rates in women. Older men have less bactericidal secretions in their prostatic secretions than younger men. Increased residual volume, prostate growth in men, incomplete voiding, a higher rate of diabetes, and central nervous system diseases such as Alzheimer disease or Parkinson disease also contribute.

Disease Background

The most common organism causing UTI is *Escherichia coli*, but this accounts for only 40% to 60%, unlike in younger patients, when *E. coli* may cause up to 85% of cases. There are many other gram-negative rods, especially *Pseudomonas, Proteus, Klebsiella, Providencia, Serratia, Citrobacter, Morganella*, and others. *Proteus* may be more common than *E. coli* in institutionalized men.[16] Also, the incidence of one particular gram-positive organism, *Enterococcus*, is also increased. This coagulase-negative organism should be suspected in instrumented men and in patients with long-term indwelling catheters. *Staphylococcus aureus* is not a common pathogen; when isolated from urine, its source is usually found to be from another site, such as bacteremia from a skin infection.

TABLE 15.4
SECONDARY CAUSES OF URINARY TRACT INFECTION IN THE ELDERLY

Urethral stricture
Neurogenic bladder—diabetes, spinal cord disease, etc.
Dementia
Instrumentation, catheters, stones
Prostate disease
Perineal soiling due to fecal incontinence—e.g., in women who are bedridden and cannot make it to the toilet

Table 15.4 lists common secondary causes of UTI in the elderly. Late in dementia, elderly women are particularly prone to UTI because of perineal soiling from fecal incontinence.

Workup

The diagnosis of UTI requires symptoms plus a positive urine culture. The latter alone is inadequate; this would be called *asymptomatic bacteriuria*. Most elders present with the typical symptoms of fever, dysuria, frequency, and so on, but atypical manifestations are increasingly common as the patient ages and develops more comorbidities. A change in mental status (e.g., lethargy or increased confusion) or an abrupt decline in function may signal UTI, even without fever. Other nonspecific symptoms include abdominal pain, anorexia, nausea, vomiting, new or worsening urinary incontinence, dizziness, falls, or fatigue. Patients with non-GU symptoms need a comprehensive geriatric assessment.

In nursing home patients, only 10% to 15% of fevers in patients with a positive urine culture are attributable to a urinary source. Making a diagnosis of UTI on the basis of fever and a positive urine culture should therefore be provisional; the clinician should search for other causes of fever, and the patient needs close follow-up.[17]

The leucocyte esterase test is useful in excluding UTI, but there are too many false-positives for a positive test to be useful. Pyuria is also of limited significance: 90% of elders with positive urine cultures have pyuria, but it is also present in more than 30% of patients with negative cultures.[17] The leucocyte esterase test, the presence of pyuria, or the nitrite test cannot replace a carefully collected urine culture. From 10% to 25% of UTIs in the elderly are polymicrobial, particularly in patients with long-term catheters.

Hematuria in the elderly is rarely due simply to a urinary infection (hemorrhagic cystitis). However, the condition causing hematuria may weaken the mucosal barrier and be associated with infection and fever. When appropriate, elders with hematuria should undergo a structural workup.

Reports of "cloudy" or "smelly" urine do not qualify as symptoms, even with a positive culture.

Before treatment of UTI, obtain an adequate urinalysis and culture. Get the specimen by clean-catch procedure or by in/out catheter. In elderly men who cannot obtain a clean-catch, it is appropriate to clean the meatus, place a new condom catheter, and take the urine culture from the leg bag. In/out catheterization in elderly men is often difficult and can lead to infections or other complications; it should rarely be used. Elderly women often cannot obtain a clean-catch; in this population, if clinical judgment indicates, it is acceptable to obtain a urine culture by in/out catheterization.

If there is a long-term catheter, remove the old catheter, insert a new one, and take the urine sample from the new catheter, else organisms simply growing in the contaminated collection bag that may not represent the organism actually causing the infection may be sampled.

Management

In general, do not use single-dose therapy. There is preliminary evidence that 3-day therapy in vigorous elderly women may be effective, but more studies are needed. Treat elderly women for 7 to 14 days and men for 2 to 6 weeks (Evidence Level B).

A urine Gram stain can help tailor antibiotic therapy; however, it is underused. A common strategy is to simply cover all likely organisms with initial antibiotic coverage and then to reassess once the culture and sensitivity report become available. In younger, healthier populations, one can treat low-risk patients on the basis of a urinalysis or even a report of symptoms, but in the elderly, obtain a culture before initiating antibiotics.

There are few relevant clinical trials comparing one antibiotic (or combination of antibiotics) with another in frail elders with suspected UTI. Therefore, clinicians should use local epidemiologic data in making the initial choice of antimicrobial therapy.

Table 15.5 provides suggestions for initial antibiotic choices in various clinical situations. Choice and dose of antibiotics are not really different in the elderly. Clinicians should know the antibiotic susceptibility of organisms in their region/hospital and prescribe accordingly. Potent combinations of antibiotics should be used if the patient is hypotensive or immunosuppressed or has recently been on antibiotics. Antibiotics need to be given without delay if bacteremia is likely because early appropriate antibiotic therapy reduces mortality.

Single-agent empiric antibiotic treatment is often appropriate for both uncomplicated and complicated UTIs in the elderly; add ampicillin (to cover *Enterococcus*) in patients with long-term catheters. If a gram-positive organism is suggested on Gram stain, it would also be reasonable to use vancomycin initially, which would cover both *Enterococcus* and methicillin-resistant *S. aureus*.[18]

In terminal patients, including those with advanced dementia, it may be appropriate to withhold antibiotic therapy and provide comfort, with neither laboratory workup nor antibiotic treatment.

Can the clinician predict which patient with UTI will have bacteremia? In general, the answer is no. Pfitzenmeyer et al. examined 558 suspected episodes of bacteremic in very old patients in a Swiss hospital.[19] No combination of clinical factors or initial laboratory tests was able to predict the risk of bacteremia accurately enough to be clinically useful. Fontanarosa et al. studied 750 persons (mean age 81 years) admitted to a hospital for possible sepsis.[20] Eleven percent of these persons were found to be bacteremic, most commonly from the urinary tract. Again, no combination of markers was reliable enough to influence decision making. Several series of bacteremic UTIs have found that up to 15% of elders with this condition present with neither fever nor elevated white blood cell count. The most consistent finding of these studies is that advanced age itself did not predict mortality; however, comorbidities do increase the risk of death.[16,21]

Mortality rates remain increased in elders who experience bacteremic UTI, even after they are discharged from the

TABLE 15.5

INITIAL ANTIBIOTIC CHOICES IN ELDERLY PATIENTS WITH URINARY TRACT INFECTION

Clinical Situation	Initial Antibiotic Choices
Ambulatory, stable, no catheter or prior antibiotics	Trimethoprim/sulfamethoxazole, cephalosporin, amoxicillin/clavulanate, nitrofurantoin, quinolone
Debilitated but stable, no catheter or antibiotics	As above, especially quinolone, or ceftriaxone IM
Long-term catheter, stable	As above
Unstable—high fever or toxic, no catheter	Parenteral ticarcillin/clavulanate, ampicillin/sulbactam, quinolone, third-generation cephalosporin, aztreonam, aminoglycosides (often combinations)
Unstable, with long-term catheter	Parenteral ampicillin + third-generation cephalosporin, or ampicillin + aminoglycoside

hospital. In one study of 1,991 patients (median 72 years) with bacteremia from a wide variety of sources, 1-year mortality was 48%, with 63% dead by 4 years.[22]

Hospitalized patients should have a blood culture, chemistry panel, and chest x-ray performed, as well as a thorough search for other sources of infection. Fluid resuscitation and hemodynamic monitoring may be necessary. Avoid placing a urinary catheter unless it is clearly necessary, and remove the catheter as soon as possible. Parenteral antibiotics need be continued only until the patient is clearly improving, afebrile, and able to take an oral antibiotic (Evidence Level A).

In the nursing home, it is common to evaluate an elderly person with substantial fever (more than 101°F [38°C]) without finding a clear source. In this case, after thorough history and physical examination, a reasonable strategy is to obtain a complete blood count, blood culture, urinalysis, and culture and then give oral or parenteral antibiotics for 1 to 2 days. Reexamine the patient and check the culture results. If the febrile illness resolves without a clear diagnosis being made, discontinue the antibiotics (Evidence Level C). In other cases, a definitive diagnosis becomes apparent. Avoid the temptation to initiate antibiotics, without appropriate workup, for febrile elders.

Complicated UTIs include patients who are very ill or hemodynamically unstable and those with structural GU abnormalities, poorly controlled diabetes or immunosuppression, and recent urologic manipulation, such as cystoscopy. These patients and those with bacteremia should generally undergo more evaluation, at least a renal ultrasonography, especially if they do not respond quickly to appropriate antibiotics. For slow responders, check for antibiotic resistance and also consider renal CT scan, which is more sensitive than ultrasonography for focal renal infections.

Follow-up urine cultures are generally not necessary, unless the patient is bacteremic, has difficult recurrent infections, or has a high-risk condition such as urinary obstruction or struvite stones. As asymptomatic bacteriuria is not treated, prolonged sterile urine cultures are not the goal when treating UTI in the elderly.

There is a markedly higher mortality in patients with bacteremia who had a long-term urethral catheter—in this group, mortality rates as high as 30% to 35% are reported.[21] Some of these bacteremic episodes and deaths could probably have been prevented if the catheter had not been placed. Bacteremia associated with urinary catheterization is more likely to involve non–*E. coli* gram-negative rods than bacteremia in patients not exposed to these devices.

Most serious UTIs in the elderly are likely to be treated in the hospital. However, if adequate evaluation and follow-up can be managed in the nursing home or even the patient's home, these are acceptable places to manage these infections. The ability to treat serious infections in long-term care settings depends on many factors, including the frequency of physician visits, availability of registered nurse support, and intravenous therapy. It may be appropriate to treat with an intramuscular antibiotic such as ceftriaxone for 1 to 2 days. After this period, the patient and the bacterial cultures can be reassessed.[23]

Recurrent UTI may be defined as more than two episodes in 1 year. These are divided into two types—relapse and reinfection. A relapse is defined as a UTI with the same organism within 2 weeks. In this case, one can treat with an antibiotic of known sensitivity for 6 weeks. If sensitivity is not known or prostatitis may be present, consider using trimethoprim/sulfamethoxazole or a quinolone, both of which penetrate prostate tissues reasonably well (Evidence Level A).

The second type of recurrence is reinfection, which is defined as a new organism causing infection. In this case, one should consider anatomic workup, with renal ultrasonography and cystoscopy. If no cause is identified, some of these patients may benefit from antibiotic prophylaxis.

Although most UTIs resolve easily, there may be occasional life-threatening complications. These include sepsis, multisystem failure, bacteremia with metastatic infection, perinephric abscess, papillary necrosis (especially in diabetics), and gram-negative lumbar osteomyelitis.

There are interventions that may reduce the incidence of UTI in noncatheterized patients. Estrogen, either topical or systemic, in older women is generally not effective, although a subset of women with frequent recurrences may benefit.[24] Middle-aged women with recurrent cystitis have fewer recurrences with low-dose antimicrobial prophylaxis, but it is not clear whether this is effective in elderly women. No data exist to support antimicrobial prophylaxis of UTI in institutionalized elders. There are unusual cases in which prolonged (months to years) antibiotic treatment is indicated, but these should be carefully assessed. Suppressive therapy may be indicated in patients with infected stones that cannot be removed or in patients with recurrent serious UTIs, especially if there is underlying obstruction that cannot be resolved.[25]

Asymptomatic Bacteriuria

Asymptomatic bacteriuria is defined as a positive urine culture in the absence of symptoms. Technically, this is not an accurate term, because virtually all bacteriuria in elders elicits a host inflammatory response and, therefore, is an infection.

Asymptomatic bacteriuria is very common in the elderly, with a prevalence of 10% to 20% in ambulatory elders and 20% to 50% in patients living in the nursing home. The prevalence rises as patients become more frail and disabled, eventually reaching essentially 100% of patients who have a long-term indwelling catheter for more than a month. Women have higher rates than men.

Asymptomatic bacteriuria does not progress to renal insufficiency or hypertension in elders in the absence of obstruction. It frequently resolves spontaneously, with replacement by different organisms, or the same organism with different antibiotic susceptibilities. Persistence of a single organism is unusual. Earlier studies suggested an increased mortality in elders with asymptomatic bacteriuria, but better investigations, which have controlled for age and the presence of serious disease, show no association. Debilitated patients are simply more apt to be bacteriuric.[26]

There is an increased risk of UTI (i.e., positive urine cultures with symptoms) in elders with asymptomatic bacteriuria, but this rarely progresses to pyelonephritis. Antibiotic therapy can transiently eradicate bacteriuria in most cases but does not improve survival or prevent recurrence. Antibiotics can select for resistant organisms, cause superinfections such as *Clostridium difficile* colitis, and may have serious side effects. In general, do not treat asymptomatic bacteriuria in the elderly.[27]

If vague symptoms (e.g., more confusion, decline in function) might be attributable to bacteriuria, try a single course of a sensitive antibiotic. If the clinical situation is not urgent, wait for the culture and sensitivity report and pick a simple antibiotic such as nitrofurantoin or cephalexin. If treatment of bacteriuria fails to improve the target symptom, then stop treating. Do not endlessly repeat cultures and rounds of increasing powerful antibiotics.[28]

Do not obtain routine urine cultures or screening urinalyses in the frail elderly, particularly in those living in nursing homes. If a positive culture is obtained, there is often irresistible pressure to treat with antibiotics, and if you do not treat personally, the nurses may get the on-call doctor to prescribe antibiotics. Therefore, screening for asymptomatic bacteriuria is not recommended, except in high-risk states, such as patients with structural renal abnormalities, obstruction, or recurrent symptomatic infections.

Definitely treat if there is urinary tract obstruction. This is a dangerous situation—essentially an infection in a closed space, an abscess. Also consider treatment for patients with asymptomatic bacteriuria who also have uncontrolled diabetes (but not most patients with diabetes), immunosuppression, or prosthetic heart valves. Consider antibiotic prophylaxis for women with recurrent symptomatic infections, patients who undergo urologic or gynecologic procedures, and men with chronic bacterial prostatitis (Evidence Level C). Also consider treatment of asymptomatic bacteriuria if the patient has structural abnormalities such as urolithiasis, polycystic kidney disease, or medullary sponge kidney.

Do try to clear bacteriuria before urinary tract manipulation or surgery. For example, if a patient with a new hip fracture is found to have asymptomatic bacteriuria, give a standard antibiotic course. In situations like this, one would want to eliminate any small risk of transient bacteremia (Evidence Level C). It is not necessary to give antibiotics simply for a urethral catheterization.

There are several ways to prevent asymptomatic bacteriuria, although because the condition is generally benign, prevention may not be high priority. The most effective ways to reduce bacteriuria are to avoid urinary catheters and ensure good fluid intake. Urinary acidification may have a minor role. Some evidence suggests that cranberry juice reduces the frequency of bacteriuria, but it probably does not substantially alter the rate of symptomatic infection.

Infections in Catheterized Patients

Strive to not use long-term indwelling catheters. In studies of hospitalized adults, initial indications and continued use of catheters were unjustified in more than half of the patients.[29]

From 5% to 10% of long-term care patients have long-term urinary catheters, and the most common reasons for these catheters are urinary incontinence and retention. Table 15.6 lists the clear indications for long-term catheters. A frail, demented 92-year-old man with diffuse vascular disease who has prostate-induced urinary retention is probably best treated with a suprapubic catheter rather than surgery of the prostate.

Patients with sacral or trochanteric pressure wounds should not routinely have urinary catheters placed—this intervention probably increases the risk of sepsis. However, if the wounds have been debrided, pressure removed, nutrition addressed, and underlying medical conditions stabilized, it is possible that presence of urine in the wound for a long period may be a contributor to poor healing. In this case, a trial of a catheter may be indicated. If this is done, place the catheter for several weeks and objectively measure whether the wound gets better.

Catheters may be a reasonable and compassionate choice for elders who are terminally ill or functionally very impaired. For example, an elderly woman with end-stage dementia may have contractures and lie in a fetal position; in such cases, keeping the perineum clean may be difficult. A urinary catheter would be a reasonable choice to manage the incontinence. Similarly, an 80-year-old man with prostate cancer metastatic to bone may have severe pain getting up to urinate. Palliation with a catheter makes good sense.

Avoid catheters simply to treat incontinence. For example, a 90-year-old woman with moderate dementia begins to have intermittent incontinence because of the loss

TABLE 15.6
INDICATIONS FOR LONG-TERM URETHRAL CATHETERIZATION IN THE ELDERLY

1. Urinary retention that cannot be managed medically, surgically, or by condom or intermittent catheterization
2. Pressure sores or other chronic wounds in which urinary incontinence is impairing healing (not just for a pressure sore)
3. Care of terminally ill or severely impaired patients
4. Preference of a patient (or their caregiver) who has urinary incontinence

of frontal lobe inhibition. A catheter will "cure" the wetting but at a substantial price. She will likely not understand and repetitively pull out the catheter, which may eventually lead to inappropriate mechanical or chemical restraints. The risk of infection is increased. Finally, if the underlying cause of the incontinence is detrusor hyperactivity, placing a catheter in a twitchy bladder worsens the problem. Eventually, a large number of such patients will start leaking around the catheter. This may lead to placement of successively larger catheters, and then you have two reasons for incontinence—detrusor hyperactivity plus a damaged sphincter.

In select cases, patients or their surrogates may choose bladder catheterization to manage incontinence, with informed consent. For example, urinary incontinence in patients with dementia is a frequent cause ("last straw") of nursing home placement. If standard behavioral or pharmacologic treatment does not help an elder with dementia who has typical urge incontinence, the family may opt for a trial of catheter management to keep the patient at home longer. Virtually all patients with long-term bladder catheters develop bacteriuria and remain colonized. From 3% to 10% become bacteriuric per day, 20% to 50% are bacteriuric within 1 week, and almost 100% are bacteriuric by 4 weeks. Symptomatic UTIs are also common. There are intermediate rates of bacteriuria and symptomatic UTI with the condom catheter or intermittent catheterization. Despite the universal occurrence of bacteriuria in patients catheterized for long term, the risk of actual UTI and sepsis is remarkably low. Febrile episodes occur only about once per 100 patient-days, and a large number of these resolve spontaneously, without any antibiotic treatment.[30]

There are no randomized trials comparing complication rates between urethral (Foley) catheters and suprapubic catheters. In general, rates of infection are similar, except that suprapubic catheters are much more likely to lead to gram-positive infections, such as *S. aureus* or *Enterococcus*. Of course, placement of a suprapubic catheter requires the expertise of a urologist, and it is sometimes difficult to place urethral catheters in men.

Several commonly employed interventions have been shown to be ineffective in preventing UTIs in patients with long-term catheters. These include topical antibiotics to the meatus, antiseptics in the drainage bag, chronic low-dose antibiotics, and antibiotic-impregnated catheters.

On the other hand, there are two methods that have clearly been shown to reduce infections and transmission of infections in the patients catheterized for long term: Gravity drainage and removing the catheter. Maintain strict integrity of the closed gravity drainage system and empty the collection bag frequently. When the Foley bag is thrown on top of the gurney to transport the patient, the drainage system is violated. Aides who drain the bags need to use proper technique—a clean container should be used, and the drainage tube should not touch the edge of the container. And do not forget to remove the catheter as soon as medically indicated.

Other methods seem reasonable but have less evidence behind them:

- Emphasize hand washing between patients.
- Secure the catheter to the abdomen or thigh; however, in men, be careful not to apply traction on the penis or it may be filleted open over time from simple pressure.
- Do not order "surveillance" cultures or antibiotic prophylaxis.
- Treat only symptomatic infections.

Catheterized patients who do develop an actual infection (UTI) will generally not have GU symptoms such as dysuria or suprapubic pain. Their symptoms will be more general and vague, such as fever, cognitive impairment (or worsening of a baseline cognitive impairment), functional change, tachycardia, or tachypnea. Ammonia-smelling urine does not constitute an infection. Sediment in the urine bag also does not constitute an infection and should not lead to a urine culture or antibiotic treatment.

Long-term catheters should be changed when obstructed, or every 1 to 3 months. If catheter obstruction occurs frequently and cultures grow *Providencia stuartii* or *Proteus mirabilis*, antibiotics may reduce the frequency of obstruction. In the absence of urea-splitting organisms, consider acidification. If frequent blockage persists, consider using a silicon catheter.

If a catheterized patient develops urosepsis, the indication for the catheter should be critically reassessed. Men are more likely to have unusual organisms, but this may be due to higher use of catheters in this population. UTIs in catheterized patients should be treated with broad-spectrum antibiotics. For nontoxic patients, an oral quinolone or cefoperazone would be a reasonable choice. For toxic patients, use parenteral combinations, including a drug that will cover *Enterococcus*. Remember that *Enterococcus* is uniformly resistant to cephalosporins.

Candiduria is also common in patients catheterized for long term, related to the duration of the catheter. Simply removing the catheter may eliminate candiduria in at least one third of the cases. It is unclear whether asymptomatic candiduria should be treated—one strategy is to treat with oral fluconazole if the candiduria is persistent or symptomatic.

BENIGN PROSTATIC HYPERPLASIA

The prostate gland lies at the base of the bladder. This walnut-sized gland adds nutrients and fluid to sperm during ejaculation. The normal prostate gland begins its inexorable hyperplastic growth (BPH) after the age of 40 years in nearly all men. Histologic BPH affects 50% of 60-year-old men and up to 90% of men older than 85 years. Most of these patients can be managed by the primary care clinician. Only 1% of patients with BPH will develop obstruction severe enough to cause renal failure.

Besides age, the major cause of BPH is the androgen testosterone. This hormone is secreted by both the testes and adrenal glands and is converted by the enzyme 5α-reductase to form the much more active dihydrotestosterone (DHT), which is responsible for stimulating prostate glandular tissue to hyperplasia.

From 50% to 80% of the prostate gland is made up of stromal (muscle) tissue, with the remainder being glandular. The prostate gland has two major anatomic zones—the peripheral zone (70% of prostate volume), where most prostate cancers arise, and the periurethral zone (15%), which is not palpable by digital rectal examination (DRE) and where BPH occurs. Growth of the prostate is both mechanical and dynamic. Prostate glands physically enlarge, as do the stroma and smooth muscle of the prostate. In addition, α-sympathetic activity constricts the bladder neck, accentuating obstructive symptoms. This explains why the size of the prostate gland correlates so poorly with flow obstruction.

Workup

Gradual prostate enlargement causes a host of symptoms. There can be lower urinary tract symptoms, either obstructive (i.e., hesitancy, straining, weak stream, postvoid dribbling, and a sensation of incomplete emptying) or irritative (e.g., frequency, urgency, and nocturia). Men with prostate disease often have erectile dysfunction. If dysuria is a prominent symptom, expand the differential diagnosis to include urethral stricture, bladder neck contracture, neurogenic bladder, infections, and interstitial cystitis. If irritative symptoms are prominent, order urine cytology to look for transitional cell carcinoma or carcinoma *in situ*. In up to 10% of cases, the presenting symptom of BPH is urinary retention.

Initial evaluation of the patient with symptoms of prostate enlargement includes a history, DRE and focused physical examination, serum BUN and creatinine, and urinalysis. All patients should undergo a comprehensive geriatric assessment, with particular attention to past GU infections or instrumentation and neurologic disorders. Look carefully at medications, particularly those with anticholinergic (relaxes the bladder) and α-adrenergic (contracts the sphincter) effects and anabolic steroids (promotes prostate growth).

The most important part of the history is to quantitate the severity of the symptoms, using the AUA-SI (see Table 15.7).[31] This score also helps with progression of disease, as well as suggesting whether therapy is working. The AUA-SI varies from 0 to 35, with higher numbers indicating severity: 0 to 7 indicates mild symptoms, 8 to 19 moderate, and 20 to 35 severe. In addition to the numerical score, there is a quality-of-life question.

DRE and palpation of the lower abdomen comprise the essential physical examination of patients with prostate symptoms. A normal prostate is soft and the size of a walnut. BPH generally feels enlarged and rubbery, often with loss of the median furrow. Features suggesting malignancy would be hardness or a discrete nodule.

The urinalysis is mainly used to screen for hematuria and UTI. If the urinalysis shows hematuria, further anatomic workup (cystoscopy and some imaging of the upper tract such as spiral CT scan) is indicated. Prostate-specific antigen (PSA) level is appropriate in select patients (see section "Prostate Cancer"). PSA level can be elevated in both benign and malignant diseases of the prostate, and the level is correlated with prostate size. If the BUN or creatinine level is elevated, order renal ultrasonography to evaluate the possibility of obstruction.

Urinary flow rates are commonly measured in the urologist's office. A normal flow rate is >20 mL per second, clearly abnormal rate is <10 mL per second, and borderline rate is 10 to 20 mL per second. Men with decreased urine flow rates should undergo further evaluation for urinary obstruction. A simple way to estimate urinary flow rate is to ask the patient to begin urinating; when the stream is going, ask the man to urinate into a container for 5 seconds. More than 100 mL of urine in 5 seconds (>20 mL per second) is normal, <50 mL is abnormal, and 50 to 100 mL is borderline.

Measurement of the postvoid residual is not routinely indicated. Residual volume can be measured either by catheterization or by ultrasonography. The latter method is safer and easier, although more expensive and less available. Most urology offices have a portable ultrasonography scanner for this purpose. A residual volume <100 mL is clearly normal, 100 to 200 mL is borderline, and >200 mL is clearly abnormal. Men with an elevated residual volume need close monitoring for progression of upper tract dysfunction.

In select cases, the urologist may use other tests, such as transurethral ultrasonography or prostate biopsy, but these are not part of the initial evaluation of BPH symptoms.

In follow-up, repeat the DRE and AUA-SI at periodic intervals. Advise patients against taking cold or allergy medicines that contain anticholinergic or sympathomimetic activity. Warn patients of the rare complication of urinary retention, which requires prompt medical attention.

Patients with obstruction due to BPH are at risk for several serious complications, in addition to progressive renal insufficiency. Infection in an obstructed bladder can lead to severe pyelonephritis and sepsis. Chronic obstruction can also lead to bladder stones and persistent hematuria of prostatic origin.[32]

Management

Treatment is generally indicated with moderate or severe symptoms (AUA-SI $\geq$8) or if the patient is bothered by the symptoms. Therapy is chosen to address the patient's predominant symptoms, not just to reduce the size of the prostate.

TABLE 15.7
THE AMERICAN UROLOGIC ASSOCIATION SYMPTOM INDEX (AUA-SI)

Over the Past Month,	Not at All	Less than One Time in Five	Less than Half the Time	About Half the Time	More than Half the Time	Almost Always
1. how often have you had the sensation of not emptying your bladder completely after you finished urinating?	0	1	2	3	4	5
2. how often have you had to urinate again <2 hours after you finished urinating?	0	1	2	3	4	5
3. how often have you found that you stopped and started again several times when you urinated?	0	1	2	3	4	5
4. how often have you found it difficult to postpone urination?	0	1	2	3	4	5
5. how often have you had a weak urinary stream?	0	1	2	3	4	5
6. how often have you had to push or strain to begin urination?	0	1	2	3	4	5
7. how many times did you most typically get up to urinate from the time you went to bed at night until the time you got up in the morning?	0	1	2	3	4	≥ 5

	Delighted	Pleased	Mostly Satisfied	Mixed	Mostly Dissatisfied	Unhappy	Terrible
If you were to spend the rest of your life with your urinary condition just the way it is now, how would feel about that?	0	1	2	3	4	5	6

Reprinted with permission from McConnell JD, Barry MJ, Bruskewitz RC. Benign prostatic hyperplasia: Diagnosis and treatment. Agency for Health Care Policy and Research. *Clin Pract Guidel Quick Ref Guide Clin.* 1994;(8):1–17.

There are three major choices of therapy:

1. Watchful waiting
2. Medications
3. Surgery

Watchful Waiting

As many as 40% of men with BPH will show no progression of their symptoms, without any intervention, over the long run[33] (Evidence Level B). Although no lifestyle changes clearly alter this natural history, it is reasonable to suggest that patients consider reducing fluid intake, and decrease salt, alcohol, caffeine, and spicy foods, particularly if irritative symptoms are prominent. Voiding every 1 to 2 hours ("timed voiding") may also reduce the need for further intervention.

Consider referring patients to a urologist if symptoms progress rapidly, if the AUA-SI becomes high and if there is recurrent urinary retention, gross hematuria, or an elevated creatinine level.

Generally, for patients with mild symptoms (AUA-SI 0 to 7) and whose quality of life is not impaired, watchful waiting is indicated because medical or surgical therapy probably provides more risk than benefit.

Medications

There are three major classes of drugs that benefit men with obstructive6 BPH:

1. α-Blockers
2. 5α-Reductase inhibitors
3. Saw palmetto

Medications are generally well tolerated, and if they are not effective, surgery can be considered.[34]

The neck of the bladder is innervated by α-adrenergic receptors, which cause closure of the urinary sphincter. There are several subsets of α-receptors, with the prostate responding mainly to α_1-receptors. Therefore, blocking the α_1-receptor can lead to prompt relaxation of the urinary sphincter and relief from obstructive symptoms, often within hours of the first dose. Monitoring the AUA-SI score before and after a 6-week course of α-blocker therapy is appropriate.

Each of the available α-blockers is equally effective, so there is little reason to switch from one to another if the first choice does not work. However, side effects vary substantially. The nonselective α-blockers can cause severe orthostatic hypotension, especially when first used ("first-dose effect"). Other side effects include retrograde ejaculation, dizziness, headache, nasal congestion, and lethargy. Give the medications at bedtime and start with low doses, titrating slowly.

Tamsulosin (Flomax) has pharmacologic selectivity because it specifically blocks the α_{1a}-receptor, which is specific to the bladder neck and prostate. This selectivity has made tamsulosin the clearly preferred α-blocker because it does not cause hypotension and is equal in efficacy to the nonselective α-blockers (Evidence Level B).

The drug alfuzosin (Uroxatral) is very slowly released and therefore causes less first-dose hypotensive effect. Neither tamsulosin nor alfuzosin needs dose titration; one can start with the optimal dose.

Even patients with concomitant hypertension should generally be given tamsulosin because α-blockers have less evidence for reduction of cardiovascular outcomes in patients with hypertension than alternatives. The original α-blocker, prazosin, should not be used because of its high incidence of hypotension. All the α-blockers, including tamsulosin, can cause retrograde ejaculation (see Table 15.8 for suggested dosing).

The 5α-reductase inhibitors inhibit the conversion of testosterone to the active form of this hormone, DHT. Two of these agents are currently available—finasteride (Proscar) and dutasteride (Avodart). These compounds cause profound androgen deprivation, which causes regression of prostate epithelium and a 20% to 30% reduction in prostate volume. They work more slowly than α-blockers and by a different mechanism. One should counsel patients to give these agents at least 6 months before making a decision on effectiveness (compared with 6 weeks for an α-blocker trial). Men who have larger prostates are more likely to have reduction of symptoms. Approximately 50% of patients with BPH benefit from 5α-reductase inhibitors (Evidence Level A).

From 10% to 20% of men taking 5α-reductase inhibitors experience sexual side effects such as reduced libido, decrease in erectile rigidity, and decrease in ejaculate volume, but all of these are reversible. Remember that PSA level decreases to 50% of its initial value after approximately 3 months of therapy (reflecting a reduction in prostate volume), so if PSA is being used to evaluate for the possibility of prostate cancer, the value should be doubled. It is also wise to have a pretreatment PSA level available for comparison.[35]

TABLE 15.8

USUAL OPTIMAL DOSES OF PRESCRIPTION MEDICATIONS USED TO TREAT BENIGN PROSTATIC HYPERPLASIA

Drug	Usual Optimal Dose
α-Blockers	
Alfuzosin (Uroxatral)	10 mg/d
Doxazosin (Cardura)	4–8 mg/d
Terazosin (Hytrin)	5–10 mg/d
Tamsulosin (Flomax)	0.4–0.8 mg/d
5α-Reductase Inhibitors	
Dutasteride (Avodart)	0.5 mg/d
Finasteride (Proscar)	5 mg/d
Natural Products	
Saw palmetto	320 mg/d

Finasteride may actually prevent some prostate cancers, but one recent study suggested an increased risk of high-grade prostate cancer.[36] Combination therapy—an α-blocker plus a 5α-reductase inhibitor—is more effective than either drug alone in treating BPH[37] (Evidence Level A).

Finally, there is weak evidence to support the use of saw palmetto (*Serenoa repens*), a plant extract.[38] A meta-analysis suggested that a standard dose of 160 mg twice daily (Table 15.8) caused minor improvements in the AUA-SI, nocturia, and peak urinary flow rates but a recent randomized trial showed no benefit in either symptoms or objective measurements[2,39] (Evidence Level A). It is likely that saw palmetto is less effective than either α-blockers or 5α-reductase inhibitors, but the medication is safe and is an option for patients with mild symptoms. Saw palmetto can worsen the symptoms of gastroesophageal reflux. There is little evidence to support other alternative therapies, including bark of the *Pygeum africanum* tree, *Cucurbita pepo* seeds, *Echinacea purpurea*, or pollen extracts.

Surgery

Immediate surgical intervention is indicated in men with renal insufficiency and bilateral hydronephrosis due to BPH, recurrent UTIs, recurrent gross hematuria, bladder stones, and refractory urinary retention.

The standard surgery is TURP; this option is actually needed in fewer and fewer patients because of available medications and new, much less invasive procedures. Some patients may have symptoms of BPH for 20 years before a surgical procedure becomes necessary.

TURP is still the most effective and long-lasting surgical option for BPH; indeed, it is the single most effective of all the treatments for BPH. It is still indicated for the serious medical conditions outlined in the preceding text. This procedure is performed in an operating room, and risks of bleeding and hyponatremia have been dramatically reduced with newer techniques. Patients can often leave the hospital without a catheter on the day following surgery. Open prostatectomy is reserved for unusual cases, such as very large prostates or when cancer is strongly suspected.

There are many less invasive options available now, and men may opt for one of these rather than take medications for many years. These procedures are not as effective as TURP, but they also have fewer complications, and some can be performed in the urologist's office. Transurethral microwave hyperthermia, transurethral needle ablation, visual laser ablation of the prostate, and interstitial laser coagulation use controlled heating to destroy deep prostatic tissue. Most of these patients will have a urethral catheter for several days because of prostate swelling and possibility of abrupt retention. Symptoms start improving within 2 weeks and are usually maximal by 6 weeks (Evidence Level A).

Finally, there are a few older men who are not fit for operative intervention and who would be best served by long-term urinary catheterization. In some cases, such as soon after a myocardial infarction, catheterization may solve the immediate problem, and surgery can be reconsidered later.

Choice of Treatment

Base treatment on the severity of symptoms. Some elderly men are mainly worried about the possibility of prostate cancer; evaluation and reassurance may be all that is necessary. Other considerations in elderly men include the patient's overall fitness for surgery and quality of life. Unfortunately, we do not know much about the natural history of BPH in elderly men, although most patients will have mild, nonprogressive symptoms.

For patients with mild symptoms (AUA-SI 0 to 7) and whose quality of life is not impaired, watchful waiting is indicated because medical or surgical therapy probably provides more risk than benefit. Some urologists recommend that men with PSA levels >1.5 ng per mL, even if they have minimal symptoms, be treated with medications to reduce the risk of progression and complications, but this strategy has not been tested in a clinical trial.[5]

Most men evaluated for BPH symptoms will have mild to moderate symptoms (AUA-SI 8 to 19), with some impact on the quality of life. The physician should review treatment options with these patients—including watchful waiting, medical therapy, minimally invasive surgery, or the standard TURP.

A single episode of urinary retention due to BPH does not mandate surgical treatment. In this case, place a urinary catheter and discontinue any drugs with anticholinergic or α-adrenergic effect. After several days or weeks, the catheter can be removed, and most patients will not have a recurrence.

PROSTATE CANCER

Prostate cancer is the most common nonskin malignancy in elderly men and the second most common cause of cancer death (after lung cancer). Risk of prostate cancer is strikingly age related, with the prevalence of this disease doubling every 5 years beyond the age of 60 years. Mainly because of the PSA test, the incidence of diagnosed disease has also increased over the last two decades. Although most prostate cancer is indolent, even asymptomatic, a small minority of men with the disease has substantial morbidity from metastatic disease.

More than two thirds of men older than 80 years have histologically proven prostate cancer, although only a tiny portion of these men die of this disease. Older African American men have more incidence of prostate cancer and advanced prostate cancer and a higher death rate from prostate cancer. Asian men probably have lower rates of prostate cancer. Approximately 25% of men diagnosed with prostate cancer will die from it, but most men with prostate cancer are asymptomatic and never diagnosed. The lifetime risk of an American man dying of prostate cancer is only 3%. More than half of the men with newly diagnosed prostate cancer in the United States are older than 70 years.[40]

Other than increasing age, African American heritage, and family history, there are no clear risk factors for prostate cancer. Cadmium intake, a history of androgen use, a history of vasectomy, and smoking are not clearly linked as causes of prostate cancer. A high fat diet has been inconsistently linked to prostate cancer, and dietary green tea and soy may be protective.

Workup

Screening for prostate cancer by either DRE or serum PSA test remains disappointing. There is virtually no evidence that DRE, an honored part of the annual physical examination, has any impact on prostate cancer mortality. The American Academy of Family Physicians recommends that physicians have a frank and thorough discussion of the pros and cons of prostate cancer screening in men aged 50 to 60 years.[41] The American Cancer Society and the American Urological Association have recommended annual DRE and PSA test from age 40 to 70 years in black men and from age 50 to 70 years in other men. The U.S. Preventive Services Task Force concludes that the evidence is insufficient to recommend for or against routine screening for prostate cancer using PSA testing or DRE for any age-group.[42] No expert groups routinely recommend screening for men older than 70 years.

TABLE 15.9

AGE-SPECIFIC NORMAL RANGE FOR SERUM PROSTATE-SPECIFIC ANTIGEN LEVEL IN MEN

Age (y)	Normal Range (ng/mL)
40–50	0–2.5
51–60	2.5–3.5
61–70	3.5–4.5
71–80	4.5–6.5

Reprinted with permission from Oesterling JE, Jacobsen SJ, Chute CG, et al. Serum prostate-specific antigen in a community-based population of healthy men. Establishment of age-specific reference range. *JAMA*. 1993;270:860–864.

Prostate cancer is frequently diagnosed in the elderly. Early symptoms may include hematuria, obstructive symptoms, or new voiding problems. Many older men present with symptoms suggestive of advanced disease, such as complete urinary obstruction, back pain, or other signs of metastasis. The possibility of metastatic disease can be evaluated by bone scan or serum acid phosphatase level.

PSA is prostate specific, but it is not cancer specific. All the following nonmalignant conditions can raise the PSA level: Urinary retention, prostatitis, prostate massage, recent ejaculation, recent urethral catheter placement or cryoscopy, or prostate biopsy. If one of these is present, PSA test should be repeated in 6 weeks before proceeding to workup of cancer. For patients on 5α-reductase inhibitors, the PSA level may be falsely low because these drugs can depress the PSA level by 50% after 6 months of use.

Normal PSA ranges have been published, adjusted for age (see Table 15.9),[43] and may be helpful to the urologist in deciding who needs to be biopsied. However, recent evidence suggests that 15% of men with PSA levels clearly in the normal range have prostate cancer on biopsy and that approximately 80% of men with elevated levels do not have cancer on biopsy. This leads to substantial problems with both false-positive and false-negative results. Suggestions to improve diagnostic accuracy have included PSA velocity, free PSA level, and PSA density, but none of these have been rigorously evaluated.[44]

Recently, the accuracy of age-adjusted PSA level ranges has been challenged. A large group of 2,950 men with PSA level <4.0 ng per mL and normal DRE underwent prostate biopsy.[45] Of these "normal" men, 15% had prostate cancer. Among men with PSA level above 4.0 ng per mL, 25% had prostate cancer on biopsy. This study leads to at least three concerns: First, PSA screening of the general population is certain to result in overdiagnosis of cancer. Second, use of PSA level <4.0 ng per mL as normal value misses a large number of cancers (underdiagnosis). Third, the fact that most detected tumors have high Gleason grades, combined with the low (3%) lifetime risk of prostate cancer death, suggests that our ability to predict the future of any individual cancer is very poor. PSA should not be used as a routine screening tool in asymptomatic elderly men (Evidence Level B).

With the development of the PSA test and transrectal ultrasound (TRUS), the incidence of prostate cancer increased dramatically in the United States. However, annual increases in incidence of 10% to 20% have recently leveled off. These tests, along with improvement in surgical techniques, also led to a dramatic increase in the number of radical prostatectomies, which peaked in 1993.

Interestingly, mortality from prostate cancer has steadily but slowly fallen since the early 1990s. It may be that the reductions in prostate cancer death being seen now are the result of more aggressive surgical treatments 5 to 10 years ago. A Scandinavian study comparing men (mean age 65 years, all younger than 75 years) with localized prostate cancer who underwent radical prostatectomy or watchful waiting showed that those undergoing surgery were half as likely (4.6% vs. 8.9%) to die of prostate cancer. However, overall mortality was identical in the two groups. Another point is that these men were all nearly symptomatic at the time of diagnosis, unlike most American men in the PSA era, who have asymptomatic disease. So the controversy continues.[46]

The widespread use of PSA testing also dramatically changed the typical stage of disease at diagnosis. PSA test probably detects disease 5 to 10 years earlier than DRE. The natural history of PSA-detected prostate cancer is not well known. At least 30% of these asymptomatic, PSA-detected tumors are very small and well differentiated; treating these tumors would almost surely lead to no benefit for the patient.

Prostate cancer is histologically graded using the Gleason system. Gleason grades vary from 2 to 10, with higher numbers indicating more aggressive disease. The pathologist assigns a grade (1 through 5) on the most prevalent and the second most prevalent grade of cancer seen in the specimen(s); the sum of these is the Gleason grade.

In general, an elevated PSA level is further evaluated by urologic referral and TRUS. These studies may lead to one or more biopsies. If a patient is to undergo prostate biopsy, anticoagulants should be held. Warfarin (Coumadin) should generally be held for 4 days, and aspirin and other nonsteroidal anti-inflammatory drugs should be held for 10 days.

Patients with a diagnosis of prostate cancer undergo a staging workup, which traditionally includes a whole body bone scan and CT scan or magnetic resonance imaging (MRI) of the abdomen and pelvis. One large study suggested that men with low total PSA levels and Gleason scores did not need these staging tests. Other routine tests include alkaline and acid phosphatase levels, BUN and creatinine levels, as well as cystoscopy and some kind of imaging of the upper GU tract. Prostate cancer can be staged using the TNM (tumor, node, metastasis) or ABCD (asymmetry, border, color, and dimension) systems.

Management

There are four major options for treating early prostate cancer:

1. Watchful waiting
2. Radical prostatectomy
3. Radiation therapy
4. Hormone ablation (medications or orchiectomy)

Patients and their spouses will need detailed information from their primary care clinician, urologist, and perhaps others to make an informed decision. Some factors that may influence the choice of therapy include the age and vigor of the patient, aggressiveness of the tumor (Gleason grade), cancer stage, and PSA level.

For the very old and frail (i.e., those with a limited life expectancy), watchful waiting or radiation therapy may be acceptable.[47] The term *watchful waiting* is actually a misnomer because many men who opt for this will eventually receive some sort of treatment, so a better name might be *delayed treatment*. In one community-based database, 30% of men older than 75 years who chose watchful waiting began some treatment by 2 years, with 50% on treatment at 5 years.[48] Other candidates who may consider watchful waiting include those with metastatic disease beyond cure or those with low-grade, small-volume cancer.

However, most men do not have well-differentiated (low-grade) cancer, and in the United States, these men are generally considered for curative treatments. Studies from England and Scandinavia indicate that most older men choosing watchful waiting will do well, particularly if the Gleason grade is favorable and there is no evidence of metastatic disease.[49,50] However, life-long follow-up is necessary, and the risk of metastasis persists even after a decade or more. Older men with at least a 10-year life expectancy could reasonably consider curative treatments.

For vigorous men at younger ages with disease limited to the prostate on staging workup, radical prostatectomy may offer the best chance for cure, although this recommendation is not based on randomized clinical trials. Mortality from radical prostatectomy is as low as 0.2%. Over the last two decades, the surgical technique has improved and complication rates have decreased, so more men are likely to be eligible for surgery. Urinary incontinence occurs in 10% to 15% of men, although it is severe and incapacitating in only 1% to 2%. Erectile dysfunction occurs in 30% to 50% of men who were potent preoperatively. Men who experience erectile dysfunction will often benefit from pharmacologic treatment or vacuum devices.

In decision models, men with at least a 10-year life expectancy may benefit from radical prostatectomy. The average 70-year-old man has a life expectancy of 13 years; a 75-year-old man can expect to live for an average of 10 years. Select men older than 70 or 75 years may occasionally be candidates for radical prostatectomy, although there is no clear evidence that the risks outweigh the benefits in this group. Older men who undergo radical prostatectomy should probably have a thorough cardiovascular evaluation before surgery.

Radiation therapy is generally well tolerated for early prostate cancer, although the cancer recurrence rate is probably higher than that for radical prostatectomy. Choices include external beam radiation therapy (usually 50 cGy to the pelvis with a 20 cGy boost to the prostate) or radioactive implants with either iodine (^{125}I) or palladium (^{103}Pd). It appears that men with lower grade prostate cancer do equally well with radical prostatectomy or radiation therapy, whereas men with higher Gleason grade or higher pretreatment PSA levels have less recurrence after surgery than after radiation. There are differences of opinion in this area, and the primary care clinician may suggest that an individual patient get opinions from both a urologist and a radiation oncologist. There are several contraindications to radiation therapy: Large prostate (>60 mL in size), prominent median lobes, previous TURP, and previous pelvic radiation. Erectile dysfunction occurs in up to 50% of patients treated with radiation.

Hormone treatment (androgen deprivation) is not curative, but it does have two major roles. In younger, more vigorous men, it is generally reserved for treatment of advanced disease or when curative procedures (surgery or radiation) have failed. However, in the very old or frail, it may also be a primary treatment. All hormonal treatments attempt to decrease the level of testosterone, thereby hindering growth of malignant prostate cells.

Choices include using monotherapy with either testicular blockade or adrenal blockade, or dual therapy with both agents. Diethylstilbestrol (a synthetic estrogen) should not be used, even at the low dose of 1 mg per day because of cardiovascular toxicity. Approximately 50% to 80% of men with prostate cancer treated with hormonal treatment will have a substantial benefit; whether this response rate declines with increasing age is not clear.

Side effects of all hormonal treatments include erectile dysfunction, decreased libido, hot flashes, fluid retention, breast enlargement, and insomnia. Over the long-term, low testosterone levels can cause or worsen osteoporosis, so bone mineral density should be measured for long-term prostate cancer survivors on antiandrogens, and they should be treated with bisphosphonates if osteoporosis is documented. Many patients get gastrointestinal side effects such as nausea, diarrhea, or constipation, and liver functions should be periodically monitored.

Orchiectomy can be performed as an office procedure and has very few surgical complications. It also has the advantage of low cost. It obviates the need for monthly injections and may be psychologically advantageous in that patients are more likely to perceive themselves as free of cancer.

Gonadotropin-releasing hormone analogs are increasingly used—they are given as periodic intramuscular injections. This therapy is very expensive, and it should not be used if immediate control of metastatic disease is necessary because there is a transient increase in the concentration of serum testosterone. For example, a patient with impending spinal cord compression should not receive this therapy alone.

Most patients who undergo androgen deprivation treatment, of whatever type, will have a response for 18 to 24 months, sometimes even longer. If the patient fails the first attempt at hormonal treatment, one can try the other methods, or combinations. Ketoconazole, which reduces the production of adrenal androgens, or another antiandrogen, such as bicalutamide, may be used. An herbal mixture called PC-SPES, which was touted to have anti-cancer efficacy, was withdrawn because it was shown to contain substances with estrogenic activity.[51]

If diffuse bony metastasis is found, hormonal therapy should be initiated, even if the patient is asymptomatic. A British controlled trial showed that delaying therapy in patients with asymptomatic metastatic disease until symptoms appeared led to substantially worse morbidity than immediate androgen deprivation.[52]

If a bony metastasis is discovered in a weight-bearing bone, the patient should be made non–weight bearing and should be promptly referred for consideration of radiation or surgical options. If there are symptoms of cord compression, refer the patient promptly for MRI or CT myelogram. Often, hormonal therapy does not completely relieve the pain of bony metastasis, and local radiation therapy may be helpful.

Prostate cancer had formerly been considered to be relatively chemotherapy resistant, but newer multiagent regimens are in clinical trials. Adjuvant chemotherapy or adjuvant hormone therapy for patients at high risk for recurrence is not clearly indicated. Chemotherapy is generally reserved for metastatic disease that is hormone refractory. The most commonly used agents are mitoxantrone, cyclophosphamide, doxorubicin, mitomycin C, and the taxanes.

Follow-up of prostate cancer usually entails DRE and PSA surveillance, although there is no clear evidence that regular testing reduces complications. Most clinicians order monthly to every 3-month PSA test and DRE and then space out the examinations as time passes. If the patient recurs within 6 months after local therapy (prostatectomy or radiation), he is likely to have metastatic disease that simply was not discovered before the local therapy.

Patients who have a more typical local recurrence at 1 to 3 years after prostatectomy may be salvaged with radiation therapy. Salvage prostatectomy after definitive radiation therapy is usually not possible. Patients whose PSA levels have short doubling times after definitive treatment (e.g., a doubling time <6 months) have a much higher likelihood of metastatic disease.[40]

REFERENCES

1. Agency for Healthcare Quality and Research. *Urinary Incontinence in Adults. Clinical Practice Guideline, AHCPR Pub. No. 92-0038*, Rockville, MD: AHRQ; 1992.
2. Ouslander JG, Palmer MH, Rovner BW, et al. Urinary incontinence in nursing homes: Incidence, remission, and associated factors. *J Am Geriatr Soc*. 1993;41:1083–1089.
3. Resnick NM. Geriatric incontinence. *Urol Clin North Am*. 1996;23:55–74.
4. Hendrix SL, Cochrane BB, Nygaard IE, et al. Effects of estrogen with and without progestin on urinary incontinence. *JAMA*. 2005;293:935–948.
5. Fantl JA, Wyman JF, McClish DK, et al. Efficacy of bladder training in older women with urinary incontinence. *JAMA*. 1991;265:609–613.
6. Burgio KL, Locher JL, Goode PS, et al. Behavioral vs drug treatment for urge urinary incontinence in older women: A randomized controlled trial. *JAMA*. 1998;280:1995–2000.
7. Khan IJ, Tariq SH. Urinary incontinence: Behavioral modification therapy in older adults. *Clin Geriatr Med*. 2004;40:499–509.
8. Arya LA, Myers DL, Jackson ND. Dietary caffeine intake and the risk for detrusor instability: A case-control study. *Obstet Gynecol*. 2000;96:85–89.
9. Malone-Lee JG, Walsh JB, Maugourd MF. Tolterodine: A safe and effective treatment for older patients with overactive bladder. *J Am Geriatr Soc*. 2001;49:700–705.
10. Zinner N, Gittelman M, Harris R, et al. Trospium chloride improves overactive bladder symptoms: A multicenter phase III trial. *J Urol*. 2004;171:2311–2315.
11. Haab F, Stewart L, Dwyer P. Darifenacin, an M3 selective receptor antagonist, is an effective and well-tolerated once-daily treatment for overactive bladder. *Eur Urol*. 2004;45:420–429.
12. Chapple CR, Rechberger T, Al-Shakri S, et al. Randomized, double-blind placebo- and tolterodine-controlled trial of the once-daily antimuscarinic agent solifenacin in patients with symptomatic overactive bladder. *BJU Int*. 2004;93:303–310.
13. Skelly J, Flint AJ. Urinary incontinence associated with dementia. *J Am Geriatr Soc*. 1995;43:286–294.
14. Ouslander JG, Schnelle JF, Uman G, et al. Does oxybutynin add to the effectiveness of prompted voiding for urinary incontinence among nursing patients? A placebo-controlled trial. *J Am Geriatr Soc*. 1995;43:610–617.
15. Fantl JA, Bump RC, Robinson D, et al. Efficacy of estrogen supplementation in the treatment of urinary incontinence. The Continence Program for Women Research Group. *Obstet Gynecol*. 1996;88:745–749.
16. Ackermann RJ. Treatment and outcome of bacteremic urinary-tract infection in the older patient. *Clin Geriatr*. 1996;4(13): 18,21–24,28,29.
17. Orr PH, Nicolle LE, Duckworth H, et al. Febrile urinary infection in the institutionalized elderly. *Am J Med*. 1996;100:71–77.
18. Yoshikawa TT, Nicolle LE, Norman DC. Management of complicated urinary tract infection in older patients. *J Am Geriatr Soc*. 1996;44:1235–1241.
19. Pfitzenmeyer P, Decrey H, Auckenthaler R, et al. Predicting bacteremia in older patients. *J Am Geriatr Soc*. 1995;43:230–235.
20. Fontanarosa PB, Kaeberlein FJ, Gerson LW, et al. Difficulty in predicting bacteremia in elderly emergency patients. *Ann Emerg Med*. 1992;21:842–848.
21. Ackermann RJ, Monroe RW. Bacteremic urinary infection in older people. *J Am Geriatr Soc*. 1996;44:927–933.
22. Leibovici L, Samra Z, Konigsberger H, et al. Long-term survival following bacteremia or fungemia. *JAMA*. 1995;274:807–812.
23. Ackermann RJ. Nursing home care. Strategies to manage most acute and chronic illnesses without hospitalization. *Geriatrics*. 2001;56:37–48.
24. Raz R, Stamm WE. A controlled trial of intravaginal estriol in postmenopausal women with recurrent urinary tract infections. *N Engl J Med*. 1993;329:753–758.
25. Stamm WE, Hooton TM. Management of urinary tract infection in adults. *N Engl J Med*. 1993;329:1328–1334.
26. Abrutyn E, Mossey J, Berline JA, et al. Does asymptomatic bacteriuria predict mortality and does antimicrobial treatment

reduce mortality in elderly ambulatory women. *Ann Intern Med.* 1994;120:827–833; Erratum in : *Ann Intern Med.* 1994;121: 901.
27. Boscia JA, Kobasa WD, Knight RA, et al. Therapy vs. no therapy for bacteriuria in elderly ambulatory nonhospitalized women. *JAMA.* 1987;257:1067–1071.
28. Ouslander JG, Schapira M, Schnelle JF, et al. Does eradicating bacteriuria affect the severity of chronic urinary incontinence in nursing home residents? *Ann Intern Med.* 1995;122:749–754.
29. Jain P, Parada JP, David A, et al. Overuse of the indwelling urinary tract catheter in hospitalized medical patients. *Arch Intern Med.* 1995;155:1425–1329.
30. Warren JW, Damron D, Tenney JH, et al. Fever, bacteremia, and death as complications of bacteriuria in women with long-term urethral catheters. *J Infect Dis.* 1987;155:1151–1158.
31. Barry MJ, Fowler FJ Jr, O'Leary MP, et al. The American Urological Association symptom index for benign prostatic hyperplasia. The Measurement Committee of the American Urological Association. *J Urol.* 1992;148;1549–1557.
32. McConnell JD, Barry MJ, Bruskewitz RC. Benign prostatic hyperplasia: Diagnosis and treatment. Agency for Health Care Policy and Research. *Clin Pract Guidel Quick Ref Guide Clin.* 1994;(8):1–17.
33. Jacobsen SJ, Girman CJ, Lieber MM. Natural history of benign prostatic hyperplasia. *Urology.* 2001;58(6 Suppl 1):5–16.
34. Marks LS. Treatment of men with minimally symptomatic benign prostatic hyperplasia—PRO: The argument in favor. *Urology.* 2003;62:781–783.
35. McConnell JD, Roehrborn CG, Bautista OM, et al. The long-term effect of doxazosin, finasteride, and combination therapy on the clinical progression of benign prostatic hyperplasia. *N Engl J Med.* 2003;349;2387–2398.
36. Thompson IM, Goodman PJ, Tangen CM, et al. The influence of finasteride on the development of prostate cancer. *N Engl J Med.* 2003;349:215–224.
37. McConnell JD, Bruskewitz R, Walsh P, et al. The effect of finasteride on the risk of acute urinary retention and the need for surgical treatment among men with benign prostate hyperplasia. Finasteride Long-Term Efficacy and Safety Study Group. *N Engl J Med.* 1998;338:557–563.
38. Wilt TJ, Ishani A, Stark G, et al. Saw palmetto extracts for treatment of benign prostatic hyperplasia: A systematic review. *JAMA.* 1998;280:1604–1609; Erratum in : *JAMA.* 1999;281:515.
39. Bent S, Kane C, Shinohara K, et al. Saw palmetto for benign prostatic hyperplasia. *N Engl J Med.* 2006;354:557–566.
40. Raghavan D, Skinner E. Genitourinary cancer in the elderly. *Semin Oncol.* 2004;31:249–263.
41. O'Dell KJ, Volk RJ, Cass AR, et al. Screening for prostate cancer with the prostate specific antigen test: Are patients making informed decisions? *J Fam Pract.* 1999;48:682–688.
42. U.S. Preventive Services Task Force. Screening for prostate cancer: Recommendations and rationale. *Originally published in Ann Intern Med.* 2002;137:915–916; Rockville, MD: Agency for Healthcare Research and Quality; Available from: http://www.ahrq.gov/clinic/3rduspstf/prostatescr/prostaterr.htm.
43. Oesterling JE, Jacobsen SJ, Chute CG, et al. Serum prostate-specific antigen in a community-based population of healthy men. Establishment of age-specific reference range. *JAMA.* 1993;270:860–864.
44. Hernández J, Thompson IM. Prostate-specific antigen: A review of the validation of the most commonly used cancer biomarker. *Cancer.* 2004;101:894–904.
45. Thompson IM, Pauler DK, Goodman PJ, et al. Prevalence of prostate cancer among men with a prostate-specific antigen level > or = 4.0 ng per milliliter. *N Engl J Med.* 2004;350:2239–2246; Erratum in : *N Engl J Med.* 2004;351:1470.
46. Holmberg L, Bill-Axelson A, Helgesen F, et al. A randomized trial comparing radical prostatectomy with watchful waiting in early prostate cancer. *N Engl J Med.* 2002;347:781–789.
47. Khan MA, Partin AW, Carter HB. Expectant management of localized prostate cancer. *Urology.* 2003;62:793–799.
48. Koppie TM, Grossfeld GD, Miller D, et al. Patterns of treatment of patients with prostate cancer initially managed with surveillance. Results from the CaPSURE database. Cancer of the Prostate Strategic Urological Research Endeavor. *J Urol.* 2000;164:81–88.
49. Johansson JE, Andren O, Andersson SO, et al. Natural history of early, localized prostate cancer. *JAMA.* 2004;291:2713–2719.
50. George NJ. Natural history of localised prostate cancer treated by conservative therapy alone. *Lancet.* 1988;1(8584):494–497.
51. DiPaola RS, Morton RA. Proven and unproven therapy for benign prostatic hyperplasia. *N Engl J Med.* 2006;354:632–634.
52. The Medical Research Council Prostate Cancer Working Party Investigators Group. Immediate versus deferred treatment for advanced prostatic cancer: Initial results of the Medical Research Council Trial. *Br J Urol.* 1997;79:235–246.

SUGGESTED READINGS AND RESOURCES

Sears Catalog
A useful health care catalogue of continence aids
1-800-326-1750
National organizations dedicated to assisting patients and families suffering from urinary incontinence:

National Association for Continence
Box 8310, Spartanburg, SC 29305-8310
(864)-579-7900
www.nafc.org

The Simon Foundation for Continence
Box 835-F, Wilmette, IL 60091
(800)-237-4666
www.simonfoundation.org

Sexual Function and the Older Adult

16

Fran E. Kaiser

CLINICAL PEARLS 196

MYTHS OF AGING AND SEXUALITY 197
Myth 1: Loss of Sexual Function and Interest is a Natural Part of Aging 197
Myth 2: Sexuality is the Province of the Young 197
Myth 3: Physicians Obtain Sexual Histories and are Comfortable Discussing Sexual Issues 197
Myth 4: Older Adults are Not at Risk for Sexually Transmitted Diseases and Human Immunodeficiency Virus 198

PREVALENCE OF SEXUAL ACTIVITY WITH AGING 198

CLASSIFICATION OF SEXUAL DISORDERS 199
Sexual Desire Disorders 199
Sexual Arousal Disorders 201
Orgasmic Disorders 203
Sexual Pain Disorders 203

HISTORY TAKING AND EVALUATION 203

SEX AND ENVIRONMENTAL ISSUES 205

CONCLUSION 205

CLINICAL PEARLS

- There is no age at which expressions of sexuality and intimacy end.
- In men, vascular disease is the major pathogenetic factor for erectile dysfunction (ED), with other risk factors being hypertension, hypercholesterolemia, diabetes, and smoking. ED may presage other signs of arterial insufficiency.
- Age is not a barrier for sexually transmitted diseases, including human immunodeficiency virus/acquired immunodeficiency syndrome (HIV/AIDS).
- The psychogenic overlay that exists despite organic etiologies of sexual dysfunction should not be negated or neglected.
- The best predictors of sexual distress in women are lack of general emotional well-being and intimacy with a partner during sexual experiences.

"…. Brief is life, but love is long…."

Alfred, Lord Tennyson

Aging and sexuality (i.e., sexual attitudes, behaviors, practice, and activity) are not dichotomous entities. Sexuality can be conceptualized as a complex interplay of needs for intimacy, affection, connection, self-pleasure, and self-image, as well as the individual's context related to his or her biology, physiology, psychology, emotion, gender, interpersonal interactions, ethnicity, and community.[1] Not a simple subject indeed. In the 21st century, with greater focus on quality-of-life issues for the aging population and the advances in knowledge related to sexual function from the molecular level to psychosocial and cultural change, as well as novel and emerging pharmacotherapies to enhance sexual function in both men and women, attention is being paid as never before to maintenance and/or enhancement of sexual function in the aging population. Recognition of the impact of sexuality and sexual function as part of sense of self and its impact on every facet of health and well-being is an area of continued and needed exploration. Indeed, the advent of newer therapies for sexual dysfunction in men has spurred greater attention and focus on sexuality and sexual function in women, which had not previously occurred, although some have railed against what has been termed as *corporate sponsorship of new diseases*. Often, it is only the emergence of potential interventions that prompts further study of basic physiologic and pathophysiologic mechanisms. Although our society has often labeled sexual activity in older adults with pejorative terms—*inappropriate, bizarre*, and *limited to "dirty" old men and women*—these labels are far from reality.[2,3]

As the older than 65 population doubles, and one of five people in the United States will be older than 65 by the year 2030, sexual myths and barriers about aging are likely to be shattered. The World Health Organization defined sexual health as:

> "the state of physical, emotional, mental, and social well-being in relation to sexuality; it is not merely the absence of disease, dysfunction, and infirmity. Sexual health requires a positive, respectful approach to sexuality and sexual relationships, as well as the possibility of having pleasurable and safe sexual experiences, free of coercion, discrimination, and violence. For sexual health to be attained and maintained, the sexual rights of all persons must be respected, protected and fulfilled."[4]

The constituents of normative sexual functioning must be defined by individuals themselves on the basis of experience, expectation, opportunity, relationship, culture, choice, and lack of coercion. Similarly, what can be considered sexual dysfunction—the persistent impediment to a normal pattern of sexual interest, activity, or response—must be individually and personally judged to be a problem by that person, not necessarily by the health care provider.

Despite the numerous studies that focus on coitus as *the* measure of sexual function, it must be recognized that sexual activity is not just intercourse. Most reports of sexual function have not examined kissing, hugging, touch, orogenital activity, and masturbation, and the myriad other forms of sexual activity people choose to engage in. Few data are available on age-related issues and/or alterations in sexual function for gay, lesbian, and transgender older adults. Masturbation remains a viable alternative for many individuals, and with many in an unpartnered situation as they age, sexual activity for one becomes an increasingly important issue. Environmental issues such as living in nursing homes may also pose challenges to sexual expression. The desire for pleasure, intimacy, affection, connection, and love does not end at any age.

MYTHS OF AGING AND SEXUALITY

A variety of stereotypic myths that still abound regarding aging and sexuality are discussed in the subsequent text.

Myth 1: Loss of Sexual Function and Interest is a Natural Part of Aging

Conditions such as atherosclerosis, diabetes, pain, arthritis, menopause, and male hypogonadism increase with age, and as such they play a role in the etiology of sexual dysfunction. In one of the largest global studies to date, with 27,500 men and women aged 40 to 80, utilizing a questionnaire on sexual attitudes and behavior, 28% of men and 39% of women said they were affected by at least one sexual dysfunction.[5] Turning that about, it means the majority did not have sexual dysfunction. The health status of individuals and their previous level of sexual function in younger years were the best reflection of sexual functioning in their older years. If sexual relations were not important, not frequent, and/or not enjoyed for an individual in earlier years, it will not be enhanced with the aging process. If an individual was very sexually active and enjoyed sex in his or her earlier years, he or she is more likely to wish to maintain sexual function with age.

When asked at what age older people should stop having sex, Alex Comfort noted that "old folk stop having sex for the same reason they stop riding a bicycle: general infirmity, thinking it looks ridiculous and lack of a bicycle."[6] For the coming cohort of aging Americans, remaining vital (and this includes intimate relations or sex, even for one) may be an important component of well-being, sense of self, and self-esteem. For others, this may not be the case.

Myth 2: Sexuality is the Province of the Young

Media attention to youth-oriented sexuality (except for erectile dysfunction [ED]) leaves the image of aging Americans as asexual or dysfunctional and is a concept yet to be shaken from American culture. This may still change with the coming tsunami of baby boomers, but the change has not occurred at this time. Over two decades ago, Starr and Weiner noted that sexuality is the quality of the person, an energy force that is expressed in every aspect of the person's being,[7] that is, a spark that does not go out until death, despite lack of media attention on it.

Myth 3: Physicians Obtain Sexual Histories and are Comfortable Discussing Sexual Issues

Little attention is paid to the teaching of sexuality and sex-oriented issues in medical schools and postgraduate training. Although this has certainly improved within the recent years in relation to ED and the new therapeutic options that have became available, little attention is paid to other parameters of sexual functioning. Further, the lack of good and proven therapeutic options for sexual dysfunction in women may pose a barrier to even raising issues about sexual dysfunction by the health care provider. Physicians may perceive discomfort, offense, and/or embarrassment by themselves and/or the patient regarding sexual topics; there may be a belief that a sexual history is not relevant to the chief complaint, and the limited time spent with the patient precludes what is perceived to be extremely time consuming; and sexual history taking is often felt to be someone else's (e.g., other physicians such as an obstetrician–gynecologist or urologist, social worker, or nurse) responsibility. Additionally, physicians may feel that they have had inadequate preparation and training in this aspect of care. Sex education, from a quantitative, qualitative, and efficacy standpoint in medical school training, is difficult to ascertain, and even more difficult to assess, especially about gay, lesbian, bisexual, and transgender issues.

In a telephone poll of 500 adults older than 25, conducted in 1999, 71% of respondents thought the physician would dismiss concerns about sexual issues brought up by the patient.[8] Despite this, 85% would talk to their physician about a sexual problem even if they thought they might not receive treatment for it. Sixty-eight percent of the respondents felt their doctor would be uncomfortable talking about sexual issues with them.

Myth 4: Older Adults are Not at Risk for Sexually Transmitted Diseases and Human Immunodeficiency Virus

More than 10% of new acquired immunodeficiency virus (AIDS) cases in the United States occur in people older than 50, with most caused by sexual transmission.[9] Although many AIDS cases are the result of infection at an earlier age, many are also due to infections at older ages. Undertesting and underreporting of human immunodeficiency virus (HIV)/AIDS in older adults is likely, with many older adults only diagnosed at later stages of disease after fatigue and weight and memory alterations/dementia have gone unrecognized as potential HIV/AIDS symptoms. Little AIDS information is targeted at older adults, and their knowledge of condom use to prevent AIDS may be lacking or felt to be unnecessary at their age. A recent cross-sectional survey of 514 women in geographic areas at high risk for HIV/AIDS found that only 13% (all older than 50) knew that condoms were effective in preventing HIV, and 76% felt oral sex was a high-risk activity.[10] Older men and women may not always reveal sexual preferences, for being gay or bisexual, to their health providers or admit to indulging in risky behaviors such as utilizing prostitutes or using illicit drugs, and they may not be queried about sexual encounters beyond what appear to be stable relationships. Data on condom use in individuals older than 65, even those with high-risk behaviors, are hard to find. Sexually transmitted diseases (STDs) such as herpes, hepatitis B, HIV, gonorrhea, and syphilis, and those caused by human papilloma virus, *Chlamydia*, and *Trichomonas* affect >65 million people in the United States. Health care professionals and patients alike appear to think this is the purview of the young. It is unclear whether patients older than 65 who have new or multiple sex partners ever receive advice or information about STD screening.

PREVALENCE OF SEXUAL ACTIVITY WITH AGING

Data from the pioneering studies of Kinsey et al. involved relatively few older adults, but even so, 70% of married women older than 60 remained sexually active, and in men older than 80, the frequency of intercourse was approximately once every 10 weeks.[11,12] The presence or absence of a partner certainly makes a difference when activity is measured as intercourse. The American Association of Retired Persons (AARP) reported that 84% of men aged 45 to 59, 79% of men aged 60 to 74, and 58% of men older than 75 were currently partnered.[13] In contrast, 78% of women aged 45 to 59, 53% of women aged 60 to 74, and 21% of those women older than 75 were partnered. The most recent data from the U.S. Census 2000 on the ratio of women to men can be found in Table 16.1. Partnership, the relationship with that partner, and partner's health and self-health have a clear effect on sexual activity. The National Council on Aging study noted that 82% of partnered men aged 60 and older and 77% of partnered women older than 60 were sexually active.[14] Data from the AARP study noted that weekly intercourse was reported by 54.8% of men aged 45 to 59, 30.9% of men aged 60 to 74, and 19.1% of men older than 75. For women, the prevalence of weekly intercourse went from 49.6% for those aged 45 to 59 to 24.2% for those aged 60 to 74 and 6.6% for those older than 75.[13] The Association of Reproductive Health Professional survey conducted in 1999 (1,000 telephone interviews with those older than 18 to older than 70), found that 61.6% of men in their fifties versus 35.5% of men aged 70 or older were sexually active.[15] Among women of the same age-groups, sexual activity went from 50.2% of those in their fifties to 18.1% of those aged 70 and older (sexual activity was not defined for this aspect of the survey). The presence of a partner or spouse appeared to be part of the defining issue for activity in all the studies. Optimism about quality of life is helpful with aging, and 67% of men and 57% of women aged 45 and older said a sexual relationship was important

TABLE 16.1
U.S. CENSUS 2000 DATA ON THE RATIO OF WOMEN TO MEN IN RELATION TO AGE

Age (y)	Number of Women Per One Man
65–69	1.23
70–74	1.34
75–79	1.58
80–84	1.89
85–89	2.41
90+	3.10

Social Service Data Analysis Network (SSDAN), Frey W. For: Public Data Queries (PDQ). Elderly Populations in the United States. A guided investigation of US Census Data using PDQ Explore. *Census 2000*.

as part of that quality of life. Aging appeared to improve viewing a partner as being romantic and/or physically attractive. However, population-based evaluations indicate that sexual activity tends to decline with age.

AARP did query respondents about particular sexual activities.[13] Kissing, hugging, and sexual touching at least weekly was common in both men and women older than 45, but the frequency of oral sex and self-stimulation was low. However, in those older than 75, the percentage of patients with no activity in the form of kissing or hugging over the past 6 months was 22.3% in men and 67.4% in women, a marked rise in inactivity from previous years. Frequency of sexual touching or caressing, oral sex, intercourse, and masturbation was also found to decrease with age. The National Council on the Aging survey (1998) found that 35% of men in their seventies and 38% in their eighties were satisfied with how often they had sex.[14] Thirty-eight percent of women in their seventies and 26% older than 80 were satisfied with their sexual frequency. Approximately 60% of men and women aged 60 and older who had partners felt their sex life was physically unchanged or even more satisfying than in their forties. The National Health and Social Life Survey of 1,749 women and 1,410 men aged 18 to 59 found 31% of men and 43% of women noted sexual problems.[16]

Population-based studies have generally indicated that a decline in sexual function occurs with age. Information from the Massachusetts Male Aging study (a longitudinal examination of some parameters of sexual function in 1,085 men aged 40 to 80 at baseline) found that a decline in erection frequency, desire, intercourse frequency, and masturbatory ejaculation occurred in men aged 40 to 70 over the 9-year period of follow-up.[17] In a Pfizer-sponsored cross-sectional study, 27,500 men and women aged 40 to 80 in 29 countries were queried by questionnaire to assess the prevalence of sexual dysfunction and the importance of sex for the individuals and their relationships.[5] Eighty percent of the men and 65% of the women aged 40 to 80 had sexual intercourse in the past year. In men, premature ejaculation (14%), erectile difficulties (10%), lack of sexual interest (9%), and anorgasmia (7%) tended to rise with age, whereas in women lack of sexual interest (21%), anorgasmia (16%), and lubrication difficulties (16%) were noted in this global population.

Sexual interest represents the confluence of hormonal and other physiologic changes with age, such as lower testosterone levels for both men and women, as well as the influence of other concurrent phenomena, such as illness, stress, relationship issues, body image, cultural issues, and self and partner values, which form some aspects of sexual desire. ED is truly a "rising problem" with age in men. It has been estimated that one in ten men worldwide have ED and that it is the most common chronic disorder affecting men older than 40.[18] The probability of severe ED in the 1,290 men in the Massachusetts Male Aging Study tripled from 5.1% to 15% in men between age 40 and 70. In men between age 40 and 70, the overall prevalence of ED is 52% and nearly 70% for those older than 70. Other sexual disorders, such as loss of or hypoactive sexual desire (libido), and ejaculatory disorders, such as decreased volume of ejaculate, can also be found with increasing age in men. It is not clear whether premature ejaculation prevalence increases with age.

In women, a recent small cross-sectional study of those aged 18 to 82 found no differences in female sexual disorders (using the International Consensus Classification) between older and younger women but a high prevalence of problems such as orgasmic disorders, sexual arousal disorders, and dyspareunia in both groups.[19] In fact, cross-sectional data tend to not find age-related increments in sexual problems in women, but the problem is still a relative lack of good prospective data for women (and men) well into their older years, such as those older than 80, and measures that may be independent of partner issues.[20,21]

CLASSIFICATION OF SEXUAL DISORDERS

A variety of classification formats exists for sexual dysfunction but most rely on the *Diagnostic and Statistical Manual of Mental Disorders, Fourth Edition* (DSM-IV) (see Table 16.2) or the American Urologic Association/International Consensus Development Conference on Female Sexual Dysfunction.[22,23]

Some revisions in the classification of sexual dysfunction in women are still being undertaken but can be broken down into the areas noted in the subsequent text. Many of the categories in classification systems are artificial because the psychologic/emotional relationship overlay onto organic disease makes the separation into these categories less distinct than we often feel comfortable with in medicine. Not everyone can fit into the neat boxes we (or a consensus conference) design. Further, this classification system, based predominantly on symptoms rather than diagnostic or disease-oriented factors, has some inherent problems. It is also likely that regardless of erectile problems, which can be remedied with a variety of therapies, there remain levels and layers related to sexuality and function in men that also need to be considered. All of the sexual disorders noted in the subsequent text can be lifelong or acquired, generalized, or situational, having single or multiple etiologies. Further, it is imperative not to place values and/or judgments on "normative" function for a given individual. One person's normal or excess is another's deficiency state.

Sexual Desire Disorders

Sexual Aversion Disorder

Sexual aversion disorder has been defined as distress or interpersonal difficulty resulting from the "persistent or

TABLE 16.2
DIAGNOSTIC AND STATISTICAL MANUAL OF MENTAL DISORDERS, FOURTH EDITION CLASSIFICATION OF SEXUAL AND GENDER IDENTITY DISORDERS

- Sexual desire disorders 302.71
  - Aversion and hypoactive sexual desire disorders
- Sexual arousal disorders 302.72
  - Female sexual arousal disorder
  - Male erectile disorder
- Orgasmic disorders 607.84
  - Female orgasmic disorders 302.73
  - Male orgasmic disorders 302.74
  - Premature ejaculation 302.75
- Sexual pain disorders
  - Dyspareunia 625.0
  - Vaginismus 625.1
- Sexual dysfunction due to a general medical condition
  - Female dyspareunia 625.0
  - Female hypoactive sexual desire disorder
  - Male erectile disorder 607.84
  - Male hypoactive sexual desire disorder 302.72
  - Male dyspareunia 608.9
  - Other female sexual dysfunction
  - Other male sexual dysfunction
  - Substance-induced sexual dysfunction
- Sexual dysfunction NOS (302.70)
- Paraphilias
  - Exhibitionism 302.4
  - Fetishism 302.81
  - Frotteurism
  - Pedophilia 302.2
  - Masochism 302.83
  - Sadism 302.84
  - Transvestic fetishism 302.85
  - Voyeurism 302.82
  - Paraphilia NOS (302.9)
- Gender identity disorder:
  - Children 302.6
  - Adolescents or adults 302.6
  - Gender identity disorder NOS (302.6)
- Sexual disorder NOS (302.9)

Each disorder can be subtyped: Lifelong versus acquired, generalized versus situational, and etiology—organic, psychogenic, mixed, or unknown.
NOS, not otherwise specified.

recurrent extreme aversion to, and avoidance of, all (or almost all) genital sexual contact with a sexual partner."

Again, as with all sexual disorders, it can be lifelong, or acquired, generalized, or situational, having single or multiple etiologies. This disorder may be more associated with fear about sexual activity and the wish to avoid it. This may relate to etiologies such as sexual trauma, rape, incest, or abuse but may also be associated with partner-related issues such as fear of causing harm (e.g., heart attack or angina during intercourse) or partner behaviors before or during sexual activity that the individual wishes to avoid, or fears.

Hypoactive Sexual Desire Disorder

Hypoactive sexual desire disorder has been defined as the persistent or recurrent deficiency or absence of sexual fantasies and desire for sexual activity, causing marked distress or interpersonal difficulty.

A proposal to redefine hypoactive or absent sexual desire disorders for women has been put forward, with the definition as: Absent or diminished feelings of sexual interest or desire, absent sexual thoughts or fantasies, and a lack of responsive desire. Motivations (reasons/incentives) for becoming sexually aroused are scant or absent. The lack of interest is considered to be beyond normative lessening with life cycle and relationship duration.[23] For this to be a disorder, it must cause personal distress to the individual. Hypoactive or absent sexual desire disorder can be lifelong, acquired, generalized, or situational, having single or multiple etiologies.

The contextual issues of sexual hypoactive disorder (such as but not limited to age, culture, religious and social background, past history of trauma, past sexual experiences, partner issues, level of expectation, stressors, medical and psychiatric conditions, body image issues, and medication [legal and otherwise]) all factor into what needs to become an expanded definition, but final clarification and consensus await. Hypoactive sexual desire has been linked (but not limited) to conditions as varied as testosterone deficiency, depression, the use of selective serotonin reuptake inhibitors (SSRIs), chronic illness, anxiety, fatigue (for both men and women), and menopause. The ability to parse out the myriad effects of menopause can be difficult—menopausal symptoms may affect well-being, in turn influencing desire, responsiveness, and activity. Variance exists in reports of parameters of libido, response, and sexual satisfaction in postmenopausal women, with some studies noting no change and others noting a decrease in these elements of sexual function.[24,25]

It is likely that additional attention will be paid to this area of sexual disorders as additional pharmacologic interventions continue to be evaluated and considered for both men and women. It is clear from cross-sectional and longitudinal studies that men are likely to have a decrease in testosterone levels as a function of age, with an even greater decrement in bioavailable testosterone.[26–28] As testosterone is bound to proteins such as sex hormone–binding globulin (SHBG) and albumin, a measure of total testosterone level is not all that helpful, just as a total thyroid hormone level is less helpful than a free thyroxine index. SHBG level tends to rise with age. Testosterone bound to albumin can easily come off albumin to be utilized by tissues. Free testosterone measures non–SHBG- and non–albumin-bound testosterone, whereas bioavailable (weakly bound testosterone) measures non–SHBG-bound testosterone. Unlike in women, where menopause is a universal event, partial androgen (testosterone) deficiency, although common, does not exist in all men with aging. Symptoms and findings of testosterone deficiency in men may be similar to those associated with aging. They include loss of energy, depressed mood, decreased libido, ED, lethargy, sleep disturbance, inability to concentrate, decreased muscle mass and strength, increased fat mass, frailty, osteopenia, osteoporosis, and regression of secondary sex characteristics. The role of testosterone in erectile ability is less clear-cut and may depend more on its effect on libido.[29,30] Incidence rates of androgen deficiency based on both signs/symptoms of hypogonadism and biochemical parameters of hypogonadism (total testosterone and free and/or bioavailable testosterone) increase with age.[31] In postmenopausal women, both estrogen (diminished estradiol and estrone levels, with estrone higher than estradiol) and testosterone levels (both stromal ovarian cell and adrenal production) diminish, and these hormone levels undergo drastic immediate reduction in premenopausal women who have bilateral oophorectomies. Steroid use and chronic illness are also associated with lower testosterone levels. As a consequence of the greater loss of estrogen than testosterone with aging, the estrogen-to-testosterone ratio decreases. Difficulty in ascertaining what constitutes female androgen insufficiency disorder is compounded by poor standardization of normal testosterone (or bioavailable testosterone levels) in pre- and postmenopausal women and by the uncertainty whether any threshold levels exist that may aid in diagnosis. Clinical evidence of androgen deficiency in postmenopausal women is also difficult to distinguish from many symptoms seen with aging: fatigue, diminished sense of well-being, decreased muscle mass, and decreased libido. The effects of estrogen (and/or testosterone) on sexual function have been studied in relatively few randomized controlled trials, with small numbers of subjects for the most part. This is further complicated by differing regimens of estrogen and testosterone therapy and by the use of various validated and unvalidated questionnaires. Androgen administration in women increases arousal, sexual fantasy, and libido (Evidence Level B).[32,33] However, the potential long-term adverse effects of testosterone administration—fluid retention, sleep apnea, liver enzyme abnormalities (with α-alkylated testosterone preparations), polycythemia, lipid abnormalities, aromatization of androgen to estrogen that may impact breast hyperplasia or neoplasia—as well as the fact that testosterone is not approved by the U.S. Food and Drug Administration to treat sexual dysfunction in either men or women, and the pressing need for carefully done large-scale randomized controlled trials makes use of testosterone problematic at present.

Sexual Arousal Disorders

Erectile Dysfunction

In men, ED is classified as a male sexual arousal disorder. In its broadest sense, ED historically had, from an etiologic standpoint, been divided into organic and psychogenic causes, but it has become apparent that the two are interlinked. The organic form can be differentiated according to vascular, neurogenic, anatomic, endocrinologic, drug/medication, and systemic disease–related causes.[34] With the psychogenic form, a distinction is made between generalized and situational-dependent ED. In addition to purely organic or purely psychological origin, mixed forms combining both causes frequently exist, and although most causes are indeed organic, one can never discount the overlay of psychogenic issues that accompanies ED. Erection disorders are subdivided into mild, moderate, or severe ED, according to the severity of the symptoms. Risk factors for ED include vascular disease, diabetes, hypertension, hypogonadism, smoking, hyperlipidemia, alcohol use, surgery or trauma to pelvis/spine, Peyronie disease, stroke, Parkinson disease, medications, depression, and partner/relationship issues (see Table 16.3).

The balance between contraction and relaxation of muscles, and therefore arterial inflow and venous outflow, determines penile functional status. Sympathetic, parasympathetic, sensory, and motor nerves supply the penis. Nitric oxide (NO)—and likely many other neurotransmitters yet to be identified—is released from both the nonadrenergic noncholinergic nerves that supply the penis and the endothelial cells that line the sinusoids of the corpora cavernosa. Relaxation of smooth muscle, and therefore enhanced arterial filling, can be produced by neurotransmitters such as vasoactive intestinal peptide, neuropeptide Y, acetylcholine, calcitonin gene–related peptide, and prostaglandin E_1 (PGE_1). Detumescence occurs when neurotransmitter release ceases—phosphodiesterases (PDEs) break down cyclic guanosine monophosphate (cGMP), and other neurotransmitters such as prostaglandin F_{2a}, norepinephrine, substance P, and histamine are released, causing smooth muscle contraction and constricting arterial inflow, with enhanced venous outflow.

TABLE 16.3
DRUGS ASSOCIATED WITH SEXUAL DYSFUNCTION

Anticancer agents
Antiandrogens
Anticholinergics
Antihistamines
Antiarrhythmics
Antihypertensives
Diuretics
Hormones—steroids, progestins
Illicit and nonprescription drugs—alcohol, amphetamines, cocaine, heroin, marijuana, nicotine
Opiates
Psychotropic agents—antianxiety agents, anticonvulsants, antidepressants, antipsychotics, sedatives, hypnotics

Assessment

The use of questionnaires to assess sexual function and level of satisfaction or dissatisfaction (history and assessment) are quite helpful. Medication use (e.g., prescription, nonlegal, and over the counter) should be carefully ascertained. Physical examination should include assessment for fibrous bands or plaques in the penis, suggestive of Peyronie, assessment of neurologic function, and pulses and bruits. Depending on history, assessment for hypogonadism, hypo/hyperthyroidism, diabetes (glucose level), and hyperlipidemia may be helpful.[35]

Treatment

Treatment options for ED[36,37] have been revolutionized by the use of PDE 5 inhibitors sildenafil, vardenafil, and tadalafil (Evidence Level A), with the likelihood of additional drugs in this class and others to come. Although PDE 5 inhibitors are cGMP specific, there are at least seven PDE classes with a variety of subtypes that may be variably affected by these agents. (All are contraindicated in the face of nitrate use, and the use of α-blockers with vardenafil and tadalafil is also contraindicated, whether the α-blocker is for the treatment of hypertension or symptoms of benign prostatic hyperplasia.) These antihypertensive drugs, in combination with PDE 5 inhibitors, can be associated with marked drops in blood pressure. Cardiovascular risks with these PDE 5 inhibitors include sudden death and myocardial infarction, and they may reduce pre- and afterload in patients with hypertrophic cardiomyopathy, resulting in an unstable hemodynamic state. Table 16.4 compares the three drugs in this class that are presently approved for the treatment of ED. There is an overall improvement in approximately 70% of patients. It is important to assess the sexual goals of the patient (and their partner) such that mismatch of expectations and lack of successful outcomes can be minimized.

Vacuum tumescent devices are also a tried and true method (Evidence Level B) of enhancing erections, creating a negative pressure that draws blood into the penis, with a band or ring placed at the base of the penis to restrict venous outflow. The technique is effective in 60% to 90% of patients, and the erection lasts approximately 30 minutes, when the band or ring must be removed. Intracavernosal injections (Evidence Level A) or intraurethral insertion of alprostadil (Evidence Level B) (PGE_1) have been superseded by oral agents but remain standbys if needed. Adverse events (including injections) include burning sensation and priapism. Adverse events are less common in the urethral form of alprostadil. Randomized controlled trials do not exist to assess penile prostheses, but this therapeutic measure is generally a last resort for patients. Future therapies including the use of other neurotransmitters; other nitric oxide donors, neuropeptide Y, apomorphine, and melanocortin receptor agents; other delivery systems for presently utilized drugs (PGE_1); and even gene therapy will continue to keep this area one of growing interest.

Sexual Arousal Disorder in Women

Another definition that may undergo significant change is that of sexual arousal disorder in women, defined as the persistent or recurrent inability to attain or maintain sufficient sexual excitement, causing personal distress. It may be expressed in women as a lack of subjective excitement, genital response (e.g., lubrication, vulval/clitoral swelling), or other somatic responses. A different way of viewing this has been put forward to better distinguish types of problems within disorders of sexual arousal.[38] Combined sexual arousal disorder is the absence or markedly diminished feeling of sexual arousal (i.e., sexual excitement and sexual pleasure), as well as absent or impaired genital sexual arousal (i.e., vulval swelling and lubrication). Subjective arousal disorder is the absence or decrease in feelings of sexual arousal but the maintenance of vaginal lubrication or other signs of physical response. Genital arousal disorder involves absent or impaired genital sexual arousal but maintenance of subjective sexual excitement still occurring from nongenital sexual stimuli. There is difficulty in ascertaining this aspect of sexual health and the specific role of hormones, genital vascular response, and subjective sexual arousal, given the multitude of physical, emotional, and cognitive factors that are integrated into a woman's sexual response. Estrogen status has been called into question as a factor because a recent study noted higher levels of

TABLE 16.4
PHOSPHODIESTERASE INHIBITORS

	Sildenafil (Viagra)	Vardenafil (Levitra)	Tadalafil (Cialis)
Onset of Action	30–60 min	40 min	16 min
Duration	4 h	4 h	36 h
Starting dose in the Elderly (mg)	25–50	5	10
Contraindications	Nitrates	Nitrates, α-blockers	Nitrates, α-blockers
Adverse Effects	Headache, flushing, dyspepsia, abnormal vision	Headache, flushing, rhinitis, change in vision, color vision	Headache, dyspepsia, back pain, change in color vision

vaginal atrophy in postmenopausal women compared to premenopausal women but found no differences in vaginal atrophy between postmenopausal women with and without female sexual arousal disorder as a *Diagnostic and Statistical Manual* (DSM) definition. Unlike the situation in men with ED, it has not yet been clearly shown that vascular alterations mean that this organic factor is the complete etiology of sexual dysfunction. There is however a treatment option to increase blood flow to the clitoris, the Eros clitoral therapy device. Although urogenital atrophy is very common in postmenopausal women, most of them do not have dyspareunia due to vaginal dryness, and vaginal lubrication (i.e., increased interstitial fluid in vaginal capillaries moving from the epithelium into the vaginal lumen) can occur despite estrogen depletion.[39,40]

Orgasmic Disorders

Premature ejaculation is an orgasmic disorder in men and is defined in DSM-IV as persistent or recurrent ejaculation with minimal sexual stimulation before, on, or shortly after penetration and before the person wishes it, which is associated with marked distress or interpersonal difficulty. Although generally not thought of as a disorder in older men, because the orgasmic latency period tends to increase with aging, it may occur, and prevalence estimates range from 4% to 39% of men in the general community. Three aspects of antegrade ejaculation are recognized—emission, ejection, and orgasm—and they have different control mechanisms. Both organic and psychogenic factors appear to play a role, with glans penis hypersensitivity and serotonergic and genetic factors, as well as anxiety, frequency of intercourse, and control techniques, also involved. It is known that SSRIs significantly retard ejaculation, and they have been utilized to treat premature ejaculation (Evidence Level A).[41] SSRIs enhance 5-HT neurotransmission and activate 5-HT receptors. Topical anesthetics have also been used as therapeutic options but may result in penile loss of sensitivity or vaginal numbness for the female partner.[42]

It also has been suggested that the DSM-IV definition of orgasmic disorder in women should be modified. The existing definition is persistent or recurrent difficulty, delay in, or absence of attaining orgasm following sufficient sexual stimulation and arousal, causing personal distress. The suggested new definition is a lack of orgasm, markedly diminished intensity of orgasmic sensations, or marked delay of orgasm from any kind of stimulation despite self report of high sexual arousal/excitement.[38] This alteration in definition allows one to distinguish between arousal and orgasmic disorder. Interestingly, women on SSRIs may experience orgasmic delay or anorgasmia. Although some patients develop tolerance or spontaneous improvement of SSRI-induced orgasmic delay/anorgasmia, there are some suggestions that "antidotes" such as antiserotonergic agents (e.g., cyproheptadine, trazodone, and others), dopamine agonists (e.g., amantadine and methylphenidate), bupropion (Evidence Level B), and buspirone and sildenafil (Evidence Level B) may ameliorate this problem.[43]

Sexual Pain Disorders

Dyspareunia (recurrent or persistent genital pain associated with intercourse) is the more common of the sexual pain disorders, occurring in approximately 46% of women with a sexual pain disorder in primary care practices. It has also been modified to "persistent or recurrent pain with attempted or complete vaginal entry and/or penile–vaginal intercourse."[38] Dyspareunia can be associated with vaginal atrophy, but in women who maintain such regular sexual activity as intercourse or vaginal insertion of dildo/vibrator, these changes are less marked. Regular use of vaginal moisturizers (e.g., Astroglide, Replens, Glide, and others) has an efficacy equivalent to local hormone replacement for the treatment of local urogenital symptoms such as vaginal itching, irritation, and dyspareunia and can be offered to women wishing to avoid the use of hormone replacement therapy (Evidence Level A). Women experiencing vaginal atrophy can utilize effective vaginal estrogen replacement therapies: Conjugated equine estrogen cream (Evidence Level A), a sustained-release intravaginal estradiol ring (Evidence Level A), or a low-dose estradiol tablet (Evidence Level A).

Vaginismus is the recurrent or persistent involuntary spasm of the musculature of the outer third of the vagina when penetration with penis, finger, tampon, or speculum is attempted. The disturbance causes marked distress or interpersonal difficulty. This definition has also been modified as the persistent or recurrent difficulty in allowing vaginal entry of a penis, a finger, and/or any object despite the woman's expressed wish to do so. There is often (phobic) avoidance, anticipation/fear, and pain, along with variable and involuntary pelvic muscle contraction. Structural or other physical abnormalities must be ruled out or addressed.[38] Treatment directed at gaining control and developing a sense of comfort, such as anatomic education, relaxation techniques, cognitive therapy, and the use of vaginal dilators help in controlling the degree of spasm (Evidence Level C).[41,44]

HISTORY TAKING AND EVALUATION

Health care providers rarely discuss sexual health proactively. Thirty-five percent of primary care clinicians have noted that they took a sexual history 75% or more of the time.[45] Patients may also sense discomfort and lack of empathy on the part of physician providers. The most important aspect of history taking is to ask questions in a nonjudgmental manner, not interject personal opinions and create an environment where the patient feels comfortable raising any concerns. Reminding the patient that sexual health is part of overall health and taking a sexual history is part of the standard of care that should be provided to the individual that may help ease the discussion. When physicians increase sexual history taking, the rate of reported sexual problems can increase dramatically (sixfold in one study).[46] Raising the topic of sexual function, or dysfunction, self-image and self-esteem, and partner issues as part of the overall state of health of the individual; reassurances of confidentiality; and assessment of patient (and/or partner goals) can make the discussion easier.[47]

It is important to find out from the patients whether they are comfortable with the physician having a separate interview with the partner.

Table 16.5 lists some of the basics that should be covered in a sexual history, with the nature of the problem leading to more specific questioning about the particular area of distress.[48–50] When a patient comes in to address a sexual problem, it is an excellent time to address other health issues such as diabetes, cardiovascular risk factors, hypertension, the need for medication, or medication reduction. Especially for men seeking a solution to a sexual problem, this may be a rare opportunity to look at some known risk factors for ED: Hypercholesterolemia, smoking, diabetes, hypertension, and hypogonadism. Assessment screening tools such as the Geriatric Depression Scale or the Beck Depression Inventory may help diagnose unrecognized depression. It is also important to obtain not only a medication use history and its relation to any sexual dysfunction but also a careful assessment of the use of herbal and over-the-counter remedies. The use of the fewest medications at the lowest doses possible for adequate therapy for a condition has always been part of geriatric care. A thorough physical examination for both men and women is critical to evaluate anatomic abnormalities, assess vascular and neurologic status, and detect any evidence of comorbidities that may impact sexual function.

Patients with loss of libido should have an endocrine evaluation (e.g., testosterone, bioavailable testosterone, and luteinizing hormone [LH]). Instruments such as the Androgen Deficiency in the Aging Male questionnaire, which has an 88% sensitivity and 60% specificity, are reasonable ways of identifying those for whom laboratory assessment of bioavailable and total testosterone, as well as LH and follicle stimulating hormone, may be appropriate.[51] A screening laboratory examination for risk factors such as diabetes, hyperlipidemia, and renal failure may be of assistance.

TABLE 16.5
ABBREVIATED GENERAL AREAS COVERED IN A SEXUAL HISTORY

1. What is the nature of the problem or concern? Could the problem also involve gaps in knowledge, or unrealistic expectations?
2. Duration of the problem
3. Is it a problem that relates to time, place, or partner? Are there factors that ameliorate or exacerbate the problem(s)? Is there more than one sexual partner presently? Is the partner having sex with other individuals?
4. Has sex drive or interest diminished or is there dislike of sexual contact?
5. Are there problems in the relationship including health issues for the partner? Is communication with the partner about sexual issues comfortable?
6. Is there other anxiety, guilt, or anger not expressed?
7. Is there any pain during sexual encounters? Is there a sense of coercion or any present/past history of trauma associated with sex?

Short history taking for erectile dysfunction:
Do you have any difficulty with sexual function or performance? Please describe
Do you have a current partner interested in a sexual relationship?
Number of attempts at intercourse per week ____
Number of successful attempts per week ____
Do you masturbate? Can you get an erection with masturbation?
Do you have any difficulty getting or maintaining an erection?
Number of erections per week ____
Best erection is ___% of normal for you
Is the erection maintained during attempts to penetrate?
Can you ejaculate (come)? Has the amount of fluid increased, decreased, or remained the same?
Has your desire for sex (libido or sex drive) increased, decreased, or remained the same?
On a scale of 1–10, with 10 being the best, what is your overall quality of life?
On a scale of 1–10, with 10 being the best, what is your sexual quality of life?
Do you think your partner is interested in maintaining sexual activity? More, the same, or less than you? Have you had more than one partner in the past decade?
Do you consider yourself heterosexual, bisexual, or gay?
Do you use condoms?

Adapted from Kaiser FE, Morley JE. *Health assessment: Taking charge of your health.* Missouri, MO: Missouri Gateway Geriatric Education Center; 1997:37–39.

SEX AND ENVIRONMENTAL ISSUES

Having the most intimate of relations is often a difficult concept for health providers, administrators, and family members of the individuals involved to come to grips with in nursing home living. Institutional living, by itself, should not negate the need for those who wish to carry on relations as long as they do not involve coercion and assent is freely given by the individuals involved. Nearly one of five people older than 85 resides in a nursing home. Although sexual activity may be relatively low compared to the community-dwelling elderly, interest remains strong, with lack of opportunity cited as the major reason for inactivity.[52,53] A variety of barriers exist in a nursing home setting: Lack of privacy, lack of partner, illness (physical and/or mental), and again the attitude of staff/family members and concerns about liability. Although the Patient Bill of Rights has mandated the right of a patient "to associate and communicate privately with persons of his or her choice, including other patients," privacy and access to protective items such as condoms, lubricants, and educational material may not be on the top of the list for a nursing home. Patients with dementia pose a special challenge, and whether a sexual relationship is consensual may be difficult to ascertain.[54,55] Sexual hyperexpression can be addressed by ascertaining whether conduct is in fact sexual in nature (does the patient need something as simple as toileting) and by diverting techniques, elimination of precipitating causes, or shifts in personnel, and as a last resort pharmacologic intervention. The use of pharmacologic agents such as SSRIs, estrogen in men, anticonvulsants, and neuroleptics are limited to case-based anecdotal data[56,57] (Evidence Level C).

CONCLUSION

Maintaining and enhancing the ability of older adults to realize and express their needs for sexual expression, affection, intimacy, connection to others, and self-pleasure—whether they are dwelling in the community or in other settings such as nursing homes—can go a very long way as part of their quality of life and overall health and well-being. Sexual health must become part of our process of care for all older adults.

REFERENCES

1. Kaiser FE. Sexual function and the older woman. *Med Clin North Am*. 2003;19:463–472.
2. Deacon S, Minichiello V, Plummer D. Sexuality and older people: Revisiting the assumptions. *Educ Gerontol*. 1995;21:497–513.
3. Hall A, Selby J, Vanclay FM. Sexual Ageism. *Aust J Aging*. 1982;1: 29–34.
4. World Health Organization. *Challenges in sexual and reproductive health: Technical consultation on sexual health*. 28–31 January, 2002, http://www.who.int/reproductive-health/gender/sexual_health.html, 2002.
5. Nicolosi A, Laumann EO, Glasser DB, et al. Sexual behavior and sexual dysfunctions after age 40: Global study of sexual attitudes and behaviors. *Urology*. 2004;64:991–997.
6. Comfort A, Dial LK. Sexuality and Aging. An overview. *Clin Geriatr Med*. 1991;7:1–7.
7. Starr BD, Weiner MB. *The Starr-Weiner report on sex and sexuality in the mature years*. New York, NY: Stein and Day; 1981.
8. Marwick C. Survey says patients expect little physician help on sex. *JAMA*. 1999;281:2173–2174.
9. Centers for Disease Control and Prevention. *HIV/AIDS surveillance report*. 1997;8:15.
10. Henderson SJ, Bernstein LB, George DM, et al. Older women and HIV: How much do they know and where are they getting their information? *J Am Geriatr Soc*. 2004;52:1549–1553.
11. Kinsey AC, Pomeroy WB, Martin CE. *Sexual behavior in the human male*. Philadelphia, PA: WB Saunders; 1948.
12. Kinsey AC, Pomeroy WB, Martin CE, et al. *Sexual behavior in the human female*. Philadelphia, PA. WB Saunders; 1953.
13. NFO Research Inc. *AARP/Modern maturity sexuality study*. Washington, DC: AARP; 1999.
14. National Council on the Aging (NCOA). *Sex after 60: A natural part of life*. Washington, DC; 1998, http://www.ncoa.org/content.cfm?sectionID=109&detail=134#survey.
15. Association of Reproductive Health Professionals (ARHP). *Mature sexuality*. Washington, DC: ARHP; 1999, http://www.arhp.org/healthcareproviders/onlinepublications/clinicalproceedings/maturesexualitypatprocp/02.cfm?ID=196.
16. Laumann EO, Gagnon JH, Michael RT, et al. *The social organization of sexuality. Sexual practices in the United States*. Chicago, Ill: University of Chicago Press; 1994.
17. Araujo AB, Mohr BA, McKinlay JB. Changes in sexual function in middle-aged and older men: Longitudinal data from the Massachusetts Male Aging Study. *J Am Geriatr Soc*. 2004;52: 1502–1509.
18. Carson CC. Erectile dysfunction in the 21st century: Whom we can treat, whom we cannot treat and patient education. *Int J Impot Res*. 2002;14(Suppl 1):S29–S34.
19. Geiss IM, Umek WH, Dungl A, et al. *Prevalence of female sexual dysfunction in gynecologic and urogynecologic patients according to the international consensus classification Urology*. 2003;62:514–518.
20. Laumann EO, Paik A, Rosen RC. Sexual dysfunction in the United States. Prevalence and predictors. *JAMA*. 1999;281:537–545.
21. Simons JS, Carey MP. Prevalence of sexual dysfunctions: Results from a decade of research. *Arch Sex Behav*. 2001;30:177–219.
22. American Psychiatric Association. *DSM-IV TRDC*. American Psychiatric Press; 2000.
23. Basson R, Berman J, Burnett A, et al. Report of the International Consensus Development conference on female sexual dysfunction: Definitions and classification. *J Urology*. 2000;163:888–893.
24. Dennestein L, Smith AMA, Morse CA, et al. Sexuality and the menopause. *J Psychosom Obstet Gynecol*. 1994;12:59–66.
25. Cawood EH, Bancroft J. Steroid hormones, the menopause: Sexuality and well being of women. *Psychol Med*. 1996;26:926–936.
26. Kaiser FE, Viosca SP, Morley JE, et al. Impotence and aging: Clinical and hormonal factors. *J Am Geriatr Soc*. 1988;36:511–519.
27. Morley JE, Kaiser FE, Perry HM III, et al. Longitudinal changes in testosterone, luteinizing hormone, and follicle stimulating hormone in healthy older men. *Metabolism*. 1997;46:410–413.
28. Nahoul K, Roger M. Age-related decline of plasma bioavailable testosterone in adult men. *J Steroid Biochem*. 1990;35:293–299.
29. Hajjar RR, Kaiser FE, Morley JE. Outcomes of long-term testosterone replacement in older hypogonadal males: A retrospective analysis. *J Clin Endocrinol Metab*. 1997;82:3793–3796.
30. Morales A, Johnston B, Heaton JP, et al. Testosterone supplementation for hypogonadal impotence: Assessment of biochemical measures and therapeutic outcomes. *J Urol*. 1997;157:849–854.
31. The Endocrine society. *2001 summary from the 2nd annual andropause consensus meeting*. Chevy Chase, MD: The Endocrine Society; 2001.
32. Shifren JL, Braunstein GD, Simon JA, et al. Transdermal testosterone in women with impaired sexual function after oophorectomy. *N Engl J Med*. 2000;343:682–688.
33. Davison SL, Davis SR. Androgens in women. *J Steroid Biochem Mol Biol*. 2003;85(2–5):363–368.

34. Lizza E, Rosen R. Definition and classification of erectile dysfunction: Report of the Nomenclature Committee of the International Society of Impotence Research. *Int J Impot Res*. 1999; 11:141–143.
35. Earle CM, Stuckey BG. Biochemical screening in the assessment of erectile dysfunction: What tests decide future therapy? *Urology*. 2003;62:727–731.
36. Kaiser FE. Erectile dysfunction in the aging man. *Med Clin North Am*. 1999;83:1267–1278.
37. Morales A. Erectile dysfunction: An overview. *Clin Geriatr Med*. 2003;19:529–538.
38. Basson R, Leiblum SL, Brotto L, et al. Definitions of women's sexual dysfunctions reconsidered: Advocating expansion and revision. *J Psychosom Obstet Gynecol*. 2003;24:221–229.
39. Laan E, van Driel E, van Lunsen RHW. Sexual responses of women with sexual arousal disorder to visual sexual stimuli. *Tijdschr Seksuol*. 2003;27:1–13.
40. van Lunsen RHW, Laan E. Genital vascular responsiveness and sexual feelings in midlife women: Psychophysiologic, brain and genital imaging studies. *Menopause*. 2004;11:741–748.
41. Chia S. Management of premature ejaculation—a comparison of treatment outcome in patients with and with erectile dysfunction. *Int J Androl*. 2002;25:301–305.
42. Henry R, Morales A. Topical lidocaine-prilocaine spray for the treatment of premature ejaculation: A proof of concept study. *Int J Impot Res*. 2003;15:277–281.
43. Hensley PL, Nurnberg HG, Slonimski CK. Selective serotonin reuptake inhibitors and sexual dysfunction in women. *Female Patient*. 2004;29:14–22.
44. Butcher J. ABC of sexual problems II: Sexual pain and sexual fears. *Br Med J*. 1999;318:110–112.
45. McCance KL, Moser R Jr, Smithg KR. A survey of physicians' knowledge and application of AIDS prevention capabilities. *Am J Prev Med*. 1991;7:141–145.
46. Bachmann GA, Leiblum SR, Grill J. Brief sexual inquiry in gynecologic practice. *Obstet Gynecol*. 1989;73(3 part 1):425–427.
47. Nusbaum MRH, Hamilton CD. The proactive sexual health history. *Am Fam Physician*. 2002;66:1705–1712.
48. Rosen RC, Riley A, Wagner G, et al. The International Index of Erectile Function (IIEF): A multidimensional scale for assessment of erectile dysfunction. *Urology*. 1997;49:822–830.
49. Rosen RC, Lobo RA, Block BA, et al. Menopausal Sexual Interest Questionnaire(MSIQ): A unidimensional scale for the assessment of sexual interest in postmenopausal women. *J Sex Marital Ther*. 2004;30:235–250.
50. McHorney CA, Rust J, Golombok S, et al. Profile of female sexual function: A patient-based, international, psychometric instrument for the assessment of hypoactive sexual desire in oophorectomized women. *Menopause*. 2004;11:474–483.
51. Morley JE, Charlton E, Patrick P, et al. Validation of a screening questionnaire for androgen deficiency in aging males. *Metabolism*. 2000;49:1239–1242.
52. White CB. Sexual interest, attitude, knowledge and sexual history in relation to sexual behavior in the institutionalized aged. *Arch Sex Behav*. 1983;22:11–21.
53. Mulligan T, Palguta RF. Sexual interest, activity, and satisfaction among male nursing home residents. *Arch Sex Behav*. 1991;20: 199–204.
54. Kaiser FE, Morley JE. Sexuality and dementia. In: Morris JC, ed. *Handbook of dementing illnesses*. New York, NY: Marcel Dekker; 1994:539–548.
55. Hajjar RR, Kamel HK. Sex and the nursing home. *Clin Geriatr Med*. 2003;19:575–586.
56. Higgins A, Barker P, Begley CM. Hypersexuality and dementia: Dealing with inappropriate sexual expression. *Br J Nurs*. 2004;13: 1330–1334.
57. Alkhalil C, Tanvir F, Alkhalil B, et al. Treatment of sexual disinhibition in dementia: Case reports and review of the literature. *Am J Ther*. 2004;11:231–235.

ADDITIONAL QUESTIONNAIRE REFERENCES

Rosen RC, Fisher WA, Niederberger C, et al. The multinational men's attitudes to life events and sexuality (MALES) study: 1. Prevalence of erectile dysfunction and related health concerns in the general population. *Curr Med Res Opin*. 2004;20:607–617.

Rosen RC, Lobo RA, Block BA, et al. Menopausal sexual interest questionnaire (MSIQ); a unidimensional scale for the assessment of sexual interest in postmenopausal women. *J Sex Marital Ther*. 2004;30:235–250.

Morley JE, Charlton E, Patrick P, et al. Validation of a screening questionnaire for androgen deficiency in aging males. *Metabolism*. 2000;49:1239–1242.

17

Evaluation and Treatment of Depression

Robin R. Whitebird   Richard L. Heinrich   Patrick J. O'Connor   Leif I. Solberg

CLINICAL PEARLS 207

DEPRESSION DEFINED 208
Major Depression 208
Minor Depression 209
Dysthymia 209
Seasonal Affective Disorder 209
Bipolar Disorder 209

DIAGNOSING DEPRESSION 210
Signs and Symptoms of Depression 210
Cultural Considerations 211
Screening Tools 211
Diagnosis 212
Differential Diagnosis 213

TREATMENT OF DEPRESSION 214
Acute-Phase Management 215
Duration of Treatment: Set Expectations from the Beginning 215
Antidepressant Medications 215
Management of Other Symptoms 219
Monitoring in Acute-Phase Management (First 3 Months) 219
Continuation Phase Management (3 to 6 Months) 219
Maintenance Phase of Treatment 220
Failure to Respond to Initial Treatment 220
When to Refer to a Mental Health Specialist 220

CAUSES OF DEPRESSION 221
Retirement 221
Declining Health and Function 221
Chronic Illness 221
Bereavement 222
Informal Caregiving 222
Gender Differences 223

CONCLUSIONS 223

CLINICAL PEARLS

- Depression is not a normal part of aging.
- Depression is not a normal response to or consequence of chronic or acute illness.
- Depression may be a side effect of medications used to treat other chronic conditions; when in doubt try a substitute medication or discontinue it briefly.
- Symptoms of depression in the elderly may differ from those in younger adults and often present as physical complaints.
- The elderly are at greatest risk for depression related to significant changes, such as moving to a new environment or experiencing bereavement or losses in their life.
- Men are far less likely to admit depression than are women, and doctors are less likely to suspect it in men.
- The presence of an understandable reason for depression should not mitigate the need for treatment.
- Minor depression and dysthymia should be treated in elderly patients.

- The risk of suicide increases over age 65. More women attempt suicide, but men are four times more likely to complete a suicide.
- Treat an initial episode of depression for at least 6 months, and monitor proactively for subsequent relapse.
- Depression can be a chronic condition and lifetime treatment with antidepressants should be considered after two or more occurrences.

Depression is one of the most common, significant, and unrecognized health problems of advancing age, and fortunately one of the most treatable. It affects up to 10% of older adults seen in primary care, with community studies showing up to 25% of the elderly reporting symptoms of depression.[1] Depression is underdiagnosed in the elderly; however, only an estimated 20% to 50% of those with depression are diagnosed across a broad range of care settings.[2] Many factors contribute to the underdiagnosis of depression, including a widespread belief that depression is a normal response to aging, disability, or serious illness. Depression, however, is not a normal part of aging or illness, and if left untreated it is often associated with severe morbidity or mortality, functional impairment, poor quality of life, increased health care costs, and a great deal of potentially preventable human suffering.[3]

Depression in clinical settings is likely overlooked in part, because of the many competing demands that occur during a clinic visit, where other conditions and needs vie for the limited available time. Physicians typically focus on established chronic diseases, presenting symptoms, or preventive care measures. Depression and mental health issues are often seen as secondary concerns that will be addressed only as time allows. The effects of depression, however, are not limited to emotional symptoms but instead intersect with every aspect of a patient's life, including their physical, emotional, and mental well-being. Depression may exacerbate the severity of many other medical illnesses, lead to poor adherence to medication, and amplify somatic symptoms associated with other chronic conditions.[4] By treating depression, physicians improve their ability to help patients manage comorbid chronic conditions and improve quality of life.

The elderly are particularly at risk for depression because of the many changes and losses associated with the process of aging. Elderly patients who are experiencing depression are more likely to seek help from their regular primary care physician than from a mental health specialist. Older adults are often reluctant to discuss emotional problems or difficulties, and may resist referral to mental health providers, partly because of social stigma related to mental health disorders. Depression may be seen by the patient or associates as a sign of weakness in character and failure to manage one's life. Elderly patients, however, most often have long-standing and trusting relationships with their physicians, who they may hold in high esteem. With appropriate encouragement from their physician, more elderly patients may accept treatment for depression and a referral to a mental health clinician when needed.

DEPRESSION DEFINED

Depression is a widely experienced human psychological and emotional reaction to social and interpersonal circumstances, characterized by sadness, disappointment, frustration, unhappiness, or despair. Feelings such as sadness or frustration may occur frequently in relation to stress related to day-to-day work, home situations, or other factors. However, when such feelings become overwhelming, pervasive, increase in intensity and frequency, impair functioning, and last for >2 weeks, a diagnosis of depression should be seriously considered along with appropriate treatment options.[5]

Depressive disorders are classified along a continuum, with variations in their degree of persistence and severity of symptoms; from short-term, minor or subclinical depression or elation, to severe delusional depression or delirious mania. Specific disorders include major depression, minor or subsyndromal depression, dysthymia, seasonal affective disorder (SAD), and atypical depression. Depression combined with mania often signifies bipolar disorder, whereas cyclothymia represents a milder form of bipolar disorder.[5] Depression with mania can be quite complex to treat and manage, and is usually best referred to a mental health specialist or team of mental health providers. The referring physician can then work collaboratively with the mental health provider to rule out other possible medical problems that might cause or exacerbate an episode of depression with mania, such as dementia or medication problems (see section "Differential Diagnosis").

Major Depression

Major depression is defined as at least 2 weeks of a depressed mood or loss of interest in usual activities, accompanied by at least four additional symptoms from the list in Table 17.1.[6] A wide range of symptoms may be present with a major depressive disorder including feelings of sadness, irritability, or tension; loss of interest or pleasure in most activities or hobbies; anorexia or hyperphagia; hopelessness and the inability to envision a future; change in sleeping patterns including insomnia, early morning waking, or too much sleep; difficulty concentrating and making decisions; and thoughts of suicide or death. In extreme cases, patients can exhibit psychotic symptoms, with severe impairment in social and personal functioning, loss of contact with reality, and delusions.

Elderly patients also often present with physical complaints, such as persistent headaches, stomachaches, or chronic pain, and they may be reluctant to discuss emotional concerns.[7] Elderly patients may also show impaired memory and disorientation not related to illness or disease, or may show an exaggerated indifference or apathy to their surroundings.

TABLE 17.1
CRITERIA FOR MAJOR DEPRESSION

Present for at least the previous 2 wk and represent a change from previous functioning
Must include either symptom 1 or 2 and four or more additional symptoms
1. Depressed mood—reports feeling sad or empty nearly every day
2. Loss of interest or pleasure in all, or almost all, activities (anhedonia)
3. Change in appetite or weight (either gain or loss when not dieting)
4. Sleep disturbances (nearly every day—insomnia most common)
5. Restlessness, agitation, or being slowed down (observable by another)
6. Fatigue or loss of energy (nearly every day)
7. Feelings of worthlessness or guilt (nearly every day—not just self-reproach or guilt over being sick)
8. Difficulty thinking, concentrating, or making decisions (nearly every day, by self account or observed by others)
9. Recurrent thoughts of death or suicidal ideation with or without plans or attempts

Major depression often begins insidiously and therefore can be difficult to diagnose. There can be a prodromal period that lasts for weeks to months with minor depressive symptoms or anxiety. An episode of major depression can last for 6 months or longer. Major depression tends to be recurrent or chronic, with more than 50% of people who experience one episode of major depression eventually experiencing another.

Minor Depression

Minor depression, also called subsyndromal or subthreshold depression, differs from major depression in the degree of severity and number of symptoms present. Minor depression is thought to be far more common among the elderly than major depression and is often precipitated by physical health problems and stress.[8] There is currently no firm agreement on diagnostic criteria for minor depression—it is often seen as clinically relevant depression that does not fulfill the diagnostic criteria for major depression.[9,10] Minor depression, however, can still have significant health and personal consequences for the elderly, with recent research indicating that even mild chronic depression can impair immune response in older adults and is associated with increased risk of death.[11,12]

Dysthymia

CASE ONE

Mrs. A. visited her doctor every other month with persistent complaints of low energy, sleeping problems, various aches and pains, and poor appetite. Although a workup years earlier had revealed no physical causes for her problems, at that time, her doctor suggested increased exercise and social activity. Mrs. A. continued with complaints about her husband and children, and felt that no one cared for her. She would lament her inability to go out to activities, and then focus on how poor her health was. Mrs. A.'s husband confided to her doctor that she had always been "a sort of depressed person" who was unwilling to do anything about it but complain.

Mrs. A. probably has dysthymia. Dysthymic disorder is defined as a chronically depressed mood that occurs for most of the day and for most days over at least 2 years. It is far more prevalent in women than in men. The symptoms are the same as those for other depressive disorders, but especially include poor appetite or overeating, insomnia or excessive sleepiness, low energy or fatigue, poor self-esteem, poor concentration and difficulty making decisions, and feelings of hopelessness. Dysthymia is very similar to minor depression in that it is a milder version along the continuum of mood disorders, with less severe symptoms, both in degree of severity and number of symptoms present.

The difference between dysthymic disorder and minor depression is that dysthymia is a chronic long-term condition, which often begins in early life. It was previously called depressive personality, because of the long-term course and features that include low self-interest and self-criticism, with the dysthymic person often seeing himself or herself as uninteresting and incapable.[6] People with dysthymic disorder can also experience episodes of major depression at some time in their life.

Seasonal Affective Disorder

SAD is not a specific diagnosis in itself, but rather a term used to add additional specification to an identified depressive disorder, and can be part of either unipolar or bipolar depression. It indicates that the depression is related to temporal or seasonal changes that occur at particular periods of the calendar year. It is believed that these changes are related to the changing patterns of dark and light, because in most cases the disorder begins in the fall or winter and then recedes with spring. It is far more prevalent in higher latitudes and winter seasons, with younger people and women the most at risk. A diagnosis of depression with seasonal pattern can be made if patients report a regular relationship between the onset and improvement of depression and a particular time of year (unrelated to seasonal psychosocial stressors) for at least 2 years.

Bipolar Disorder

Bipolar disorder, also called manic depressive illness, is characterized by cyclic mood changes, alternating between the highs of mania and the lows of depression. Mood changes can be dramatic and rapid or mild and gradual.

Mania is characterized by excessive elation, unusual irritability, decreased need for sleep, grandiose notions, increased talking, racing thoughts, increased energy and sexual desire, poor judgment, and inappropriate behavior.[7] Left untreated, it can progress to a psychotic state. Episodes of mania can result in serious consequences for the patient with bipolar disorder and his or her family. Manic behavior often leads to unwise financial decisions, social embarrassment, and deteriorating family relationships.

Bipolar depression is a recurrent disorder, and over 90% of people experience multiple episodes.[6] It is thought to have a strong genetic component, but all members of a family with genetic predisposition to the disorder will not develop it. Environmental factors such as stress and life circumstances often appear to trigger the onset of bipolar disorder, or lead to episodic relapses that sometimes require hospitalization. Bipolar disorder most often represents a long-term chronic illness and is usually best managed by mental health specialists with appropriate experience and expertise.

DIAGNOSING DEPRESSION

There are no specific laboratory tests or findings that are diagnostic of depression, despite the fact that a number of neurotransmitters that produce chemical changes in the brain are the source of depressive symptoms. These neurotransmitters include norepinephrine, serotonin, acetylcholine, dopamine, and γ-aminobutyric acid. Because we cannot measure these changes directly, a diagnosis of depression is instead made through assessment and interview, using standardized screening criteria to assess symptoms of depression and potential causes, and then using the standard diagnostic criteria in the Diagnostic and Statistical Manual of Mental Disorders Fourth Edition (DSM-IV) to determine the presence or absence of specific depressive disorders.[6]

The U.S. Preventive Services Task Force (USPSTF) now recommends "screening adults for depression (Evidence Level B) in clinical practices that have systems in place to assure accurate diagnosis, effective treatment, and follow-up."[13,14] The task force notes that the benefits of screening and treatment are unlikely to be realized unless such clinical systems are in place. The recommendations for screening and diagnosis presented here are based on the assumption that the physician has such systems in place to assure consistent management and follow-up of depression in elderly patients. Follow-up and management over time are key to successful treatment of depression in the elderly (see section "Treatment of Depression").

Assessment may be best regarded as a two-stage process, with (a) a brief screen for the two primary symptoms of depression and (b) a more extensive screening process for depression if the brief assessment is positive (Evidence Level B). This two-stage process saves time during brief clinic visits, identifying those who may require more in-depth evaluation for both major and minor depressive disorders.[15] It is also important to remember during the screening process that the expression of depressive symptoms among the elderly is often strongly influenced by cultural norms and expressions and may vary dramatically across cultures. A complete assessment for diagnosing depression should include the components listed in Table 17.2 (Evidence Level C).[16]

TABLE 17.2
ASSESSMENT FOR DEPRESSION

1. A brief screen consisting of two questions related to depressed mood and loss of pleasure
2. If the screen is positive, a full assessment using standardized criteria or a standardized depression screening instrument
3. Review of the medical history to rule out and treat symptoms that may be related to ongoing chronic medical conditions or past history of depressive episodes
4. Review of medications to rule out side effects of current medication use
5. An assessment of current mental, physical, and functional status to rule out the development of new conditions such as dementia, delirium, thyroid disorders, or anemia
6. Assessment of psychosocial concerns such as recent bereavement, alcohol use, or significant changes in the social environment
7. Assessment of suicide risk

Signs and Symptoms of Depression

Two major symptoms can be used as criteria to screen for the presence of depression in adults: (i) A frequently depressed mood, and (ii) a loss of pleasure or interest in most or all activities (anhedonia). One or both of these symptoms must be present for at least 2 weeks to meet the criteria for a diagnosis of major depression. These questions are incorporated in the Patient Health Questionnaire 2 (PHQ2) and can be used as a formal instrument for this purpose (see Table 20.4).[17] The PHQ2 questions are drawn from a larger scale, and can also be used for screening for depression (see Table 17.3). Physicians may best incorporate these two questions into practice by making them part of the rooming system in which nurses ask them as part of vital sign collection. A positive response to either question should prompt the physician to ask additional questions about other symptoms of depression.

There are nine symptoms commonly associated with depression (including the two mentioned above) and are considered the gold standard for diagnosing depression. These symptoms are listed as the diagnostic criteria for depression in the DSM-IV.[16] For a diagnosis of major depression, at least five of the nine symptoms must be present for at least 2 weeks, and must include symptom 1 or 2 from the list (Table 17.1). For a diagnosis of minor depression, at least two, but less than five of the symptoms should be present for at least 2 weeks and represent a change from

TABLE 17.3
STANDARDIZED SCREENING INSTRUMENTS FOR DEPRESSION IN THE ELDERLY

Instruments	Type of Response Format	Long Form Number of Questions	Short Form Number of Questions	Minutes to Fill Out	Note
Patient Health Questionnaire (from the PRIME MD) PHQ9—long version PHQ2—short version	Ordinal	9	2	5–10	Developed from the DSM-IV symptoms list for ease in office administration—good validity and reliability[18]
Geriatric Depression Scale (Brink 1982)	Yes/no	30	15	8–10	Good reliability, specificity, and sensitivity with the elderly
Center for Epidemiologic Studies Depression Scale (NIMH)	Ordinal	20	10	8–10	Adequate reliability and validity; can generate high false-positives
Beck Depression Inventory (Beck, 1961)	Ordinal	10		10–15	Good reliability and validity; high sensitivity, but low specificity
The Self-Rating Depression Scale (Zung, 1965)	Ordinal	20		10–15	Adequate reliability and validity; focuses on frequency rather than severity of symptoms

PRIME MD, Primary Care Evaluation of Mental Disorders; PHQ, Patient Health Questionnaire; DSM-IV, Diagnostic and Statistical Manual of Mental Disorders Fourth Edition; NIMH, National Institute of Mental Health.

previous functioning; one of the symptoms must be either symptoms 1 or 2 from the list (see Table 17.1).

Symptoms of depression in the elderly may also vary from those in the general adult population, creating difficulty in the assessment process. Elderly patients often focus on physical symptoms as their presenting complaint (e.g., headaches, stomach, or bowel problems). This often leads to other tests to rule out physical causes of depression. The presence of multiple unexplained physical symptoms is highly suggestive of the presence of depression. Elderly patients may also agree that they are depressed, but blame their depression on physical conditions such as pain from arthritis or back pain. Older patients may also present with apathy or a severe lack of motivation; in this case, careful assessment is indicated to rule out other causes such as dementia, pseudo dementia, or a new condition such as anemia. Additional symptoms that may be present in the elderly are included in Table 17.4.

TABLE 17.4
ADDITIONAL SYMPTOMS THAT MAY BE PRESENT IN THE ELDERLY

Increased somatic complaints—headaches, stomach problems, pain (unrelated to a known physical cause)
Apathy toward environment
Diminished self-care
Irritability
Confusion (unrelated to illness or dementia)
Psychomotor retardation
Distractibility
Hopelessness, the inability to envision a future

Cultural Considerations

Each culture has unique forms of expression to communicate feelings; this is particularly true in the expression of symptoms related to mental health problems. How patients express and communicate depressive symptoms will be strongly influenced by what are acceptable expressions of depression within their culture. The DSM-IV notes that patients may refer to problems related to their "nerves" (Latino), or "weakness" or "imbalance" (Asian), or heart or being "heartbroken" (Middle Eastern cultures).[6] Cultures will also differ in how seriously depression is viewed, presenting significant treatment issues. When cultural differences are present between the patient and the physician, it is particularly important to listen to and question patients carefully, and to express in clear medical terms why treatment of depression is important.

Screening Tools

There are many standardized screening tools available to assess the symptoms of depression, some of which can be used in primary care settings with older adults. Screening tools for depression vary in length and response criteria; the more complex the screen, the more difficult it will be to use with the elderly. Many instruments have also been modified as short forms that are easier and less time-consuming to complete. Table 17.3 contains a brief overview of validated screening tools that can be self-administered in primary care settings as part of the intake or rooming processes. Other screening tools for depression that are used primarily for

Scoring: One point for each response in capital letters.

Scoring cutoff: Normal (0–5), above 5 suggests depression.

Choose the best answer for how you have felt over the past week:

1. Are you basically satisfied with your life?	yes	NO
2. Have you dropped many of your activities and interests?	YES	no
3. Do you feel that your life is empty?	YES	no
4. Do you often get bored?	YES	no
5. Are you in good spirits most of the time?	yes	NO
6. Are you afraid that something bad is going to happen to you?	YES	no
7. Do you feel happy most of the time?	yes	NO
8. Do you often feel helpless?	YES	no
9. Do you prefer to stay at home, rather than going out and doing new things?	YES	no
10. Do you feel you have more problems with memory than most?	YES	no
11. Do you think it is wonderful to be alive now?	yes	NO
12. Do you feel pretty worthless the way you are now?	YES	no
13. Do you feel full of energy?	yes	NO
14. Do you feel that your situation is hopeless?	YES	no
15. Do you think that most people are better off than you are?	YES	no

Figure 17.1 The Geriatric Depression Scale—Short Form.

research or that must be administered by a mental health practitioner are not included here.

There has been some question in the literature as to whether standard instruments for assessing depression take into account features such as sleep disturbance or weight loss that may occur in the elderly as a result of the normal effects of aging rather than from depression per se. The Geriatric Depression Scale (GDS) is the only instrument from the list in Table 17.3 that is specifically designed to assess depression in the elderly; the instrument does not rely on somatic symptoms and is simple and clear in ease of administration. The GDS has been found to perform just as well as other measures of depression, with good reliability and validity (see Fig. 17.1).[19]

Screening instruments can be helpful in clinical practice if they are short, reliable, can be self-administered, and are readily available when needed. Focusing on a two-stage screening system that incorporates a brief two-question screen into regular clinical practice has many benefits. First, even if depression is not present, it provides an opening for the patient to talk about their mental health concerns. Many elderly are reluctant to discuss emotional concerns, but may be willing if a trusted physician raises the question first. Second, the brief screen will clarify who needs more in-depth assessment for depression, rather than spending time during limited visits on a more extensive screening process, especially with the elderly who are likely to have many physical concerns that need to be addressed. The brief screen also demonstrates to patients on a regular basis that good mental health is as important as good physical health. Finally, a brief assessment done regularly may identify many of the estimated 50% of cases of depression that go unrecognized in clinical practice every year.[20]

Diagnosis

Once a screening test for depression is positive, further questioning will be needed to establish a diagnosis and determine whether a treatment course is needed. The diagnosis is based not only on the number of symptoms present, but also on the degree of persistence and severity, and the change represented in the patient's ability to function in his or her daily life. For a diagnosis of major depression, five of the nine symptoms listed in Table 17.1 must be present for the past 2 weeks and must include the two primary symptoms of depressed mood and anhedonia. The episode should also be accompanied by clinically significant distress, or impairment in other important areas of functioning and should represent a change from previous functioning for the patient.

For a diagnosis of minor depression, two to four of the symptoms listed in Table 17.1 should be present for at least 2 weeks and represent a change in previous functioning, with one of the symptoms being either depressed mood (symptom 1) or anhedonia (symptom 2). The distinguishing feature between minor depression and dysthymic disorder is chronicity, with dysthymia characterized by a chronically depressed mood that occurs for most days over a period of at least 2 years.

The standard ICD-9 code that has long been used in primary care settings for a diagnosis of depression is the code 311 (depression not otherwise specified). This code does not distinguish between major and minor depression or dysthymia, nor does it specify recurrence or additional features, as is the case with ICD-9 coding using the DSM-IV. There has been some movement in recent years toward more accurate coding of major depression using the DSM-IV code 296.*xx* for major depression. Unless the physician can clearly distinguish between major and minor depression and dysthymia, the standard ICD-9 coding of 311 is recommended.

Differential Diagnosis

Once a diagnosis of depression is made, a review of the patient's medical history and current medications should be conducted to rule out other causes of depressive symptoms. Serious medical conditions can be primary or secondary to depression, with some symptoms of medical conditions mimicking symptoms of depression, including problems with sleep, changes in appetite, or changes in normal energy levels (see Table 17.5). A review of past episodes of depression will help in clarifying recurrent or chronic depression. Major depression is recurrent or chronic in at least 50% of people and a past history of depression should guide treatment decisions for the current episode.

An assessment of current mental, physical, and functional status should also be done to rule out the development of new conditions whose symptoms could be mistaken for the onset of depression (e.g., dementia, delirium, or anemia). A more complete discussion of mental status screening for dementia is available in Chapter 20, and for delirium in Chapter 18. Recent clinical guidelines for the management of depressive disorders suggest considering the following laboratory studies to rule out medical disorders that may cause symptoms of depression: A complete blood count, chemistry profile, thyroid studies, toxicology screen, and possibly an electrocardiogram.[16]

Substance-Induced Depression

Depression can be caused by either the use or abuse of certain substances, such as exposure to toxins, medications, and alcohol or drugs. Heavy metals and toxins that can produce depressive symptoms include volatile substances such as gasoline and paint, organophosphate insecticides, nerve gases, carbon monoxide, and carbon dioxide.[6] Many commonly prescribed medications also produce depressive-like symptoms as a side effect. Careful evaluation of both prescribed and over-the-counter medications is important. Some of the medications that can cause depression are angiotensin-converting enzyme inhibitors, anabolic steroids, antihyperlipidemics, benzodiazepines, cimetidine, ranitidine, clonidine, cycloserine, digitalis, glucocorticoids, gonadotropin-releasing agonists, interferons, levodopa, methyldopa, metoclopramide, pimozide, propranolol (β-blockers), reserpine, topiramate, and verapamil (calcium channel blockers).[16] In addition, patient compliance with medication use should be assessed to ensure that patients are taking medications as prescribed.

TABLE 17.5
DIFFERENTIAL DIAGNOSIS FOR DEPRESSION

	Depressive Disorders Related to Other Medical Conditions	
Taxonomy of Primary Depressive Disorders	**Conditions that are Primary Causes of Depression (Correct Underlying Cause)**	**Depression Secondary to a Medical Condition (293.83) (Treat Symptoms)**
Depression NOS (311)	Anemia (285.xx)	Alzheimer disease (331.0)
Major depression (296.xx)	B_{12} deficiency (281.0)	Dementia with depression (290.21)
Minor depression (311)	Substance abuse—alcohol (291.8)	Diabetes (250)
Dysthymia (300.4)	Substance abuse—drug (292)	Coronary heart disease (410–414)
Bipolar disorder (296.xx)	Adverse drug effects (995.2)	Congestive heart failure (428)
Cyclothymic disorder (301.13)[a]	Nutritional abuse (305.00)	Parkinson disease (332)
	Hypothyroidism (244)	Stroke (434.91/436)
	Delirium (780.09, 293)	Cancer–neoplasm
		Rheumatoid arthritis (714)
		Macular degeneration (362.5)[b]

[a]See DSM-IV for further clarification of depressive disorders.
[b]Many chronic medical conditions are associated with depression, especially those conditions resulting in significant physical symptoms and/or associated with significant life changes.
NOS, not otherwise specified.

Problems with memory or finances can lead to over- or underuse of medications.

An assessment for alcohol or substance abuse is particularly important. Substance abuse disorders in the elderly have been described as a hidden epidemic, unnoticed because the elderly are not in the public view as are younger adults in the work force. Alcohol and drug use, either prescribed or illicit, are often an attempt to self-medicate for a variety of problems including depression. A quick screen for alcohol abuse often used in clinical settings is the four-item CAGE (cutting down, annoyed, guilty, and eye-opener) questionnaire that asks about whether a patient has thought about cutting down on their drinking, been annoyed by criticism of their drinking, felt guilty about their drinking or had a morning drink as an "eye-opener." It should be noted that the CAGE screen was developed for detecting the presence of alcoholism and does not pick up abuse patterns well, so additional questions should be asked if alcohol or substance abuse is suspected. Depression in men is more often masked by alcohol and drug use than in women. Men are also more likely to present with anger, irritability, and discouragement as symptoms of depression.

Social Support and Environment

Last, an assessment of significant changes in the patient's social support and environment can alert the physician to potential causes of depression not related to health, as well as assist in developing a plan for the treatment and management of depression. Recent bereavement, for instance, may present as depression (see section "Bereavement"). Normal bereavement, however, will subside with time, and if treatment is needed grief counseling or support groups are usually indicated rather than antidepressants. Moving to a new living situation, especially if the patient feels he or she had little choice in the decision, can also trigger a depressive episode. Issues related to personal autonomy and control often increase with age, especially when mental or functional status decreases. Careful probing in this area can alert the physician to social or support problems that will help in choosing and managing a treatment course as well as provide helpful information regarding referrals to community services.

Changing family dynamics with adult children or grandchildren can also be a challenge to an elderly patient, leading to an episode of depression. Role reversal with adult children is not uncommon, especially around issues of failing health or functional status. Well-meaning adult children can appear controlling and demeaning to their parents if issues of mental status or competence are at question. These issues can severely stress family relationships and the patient's social support system; this is particularly true if the issue revolves around the elderly patient's ability to continue living in their current home setting. Involving family when appropriate in the process of diagnosis and treatment can assist in strengthening the patient's social support system and family relationships.

Suicide

Every diagnosis of depression should include screening for the risk of suicide or self-harm. Suicide has a bimodal curve in the US population, with high levels in the very old and the very young. People older than 65 accounted for 12% of the US population in the year 2000, but 18% of all suicides in that year. Women are far more likely to attempt suicide than are men, but men are more likely to complete a suicide attempt, often choosing more lethal methods such as guns. The physician should always ask a depressed patient about thoughts of suicide. If there is any indication of suicide risk, probing is needed to see if the patient has worked out a plan for it. If suicide is thought to be a serious risk, the physician will need to develop a specific plan with the patient and the patient's caregivers; this plan may include hospitalization if indicated.

A suicidal patient is a medical and psychiatric emergency. Recent studies have found that 45% of victims of suicide had seen their primary care physician within one month of their suicide, and out of patients aged 55 and older who committed suicide, 58% had visited their primary care physician about 1 month prior to their suicide.[21–23] Depending on the primary care physician's practice, there are a range of actions the physician can take. Potential actions include immediate referral and transport to a mental health specialist, or to an emergency room where psychiatric evaluation can then take place. The physician may also consider release to a family member or caregiver who will agree to supervise the patient and ensure adherence to an antidepressant medication trial and referral to a mental health professional for ongoing treatment, as well as removal of guns or other potentially lethal weapons from the house.

TREATMENT OF DEPRESSION

The treatment of depression in the elderly may include the use of antidepressant medications, various types of psychotherapy, lifestyle changes, or environmental changes. The choice of initial treatment should be guided by a full assessment and address not only the symptoms but also the potential sources of depression. Referrals for psychosocial therapies to a social worker or mental health specialist, as well as changes in lifestyle such as increased physical activity, social interaction, improved nutrition, and the support of family and friends can play a vital role in treating depression (Evidence Level A). Treatment with antidepressants will address the symptoms of depression, but the use of other therapeutic modalities that help address the source of the depression is often indicated.

Antidepressant use has increased dramatically in the past decade as newer antidepressant medications with fewer adverse side effects have come into the market. All medications however, have potential adverse side effects and drug–drug interactions. Therefore, treatment with antidepressants needs to be monitored carefully, with appropriate follow-up and management to ensure that the treatment is safe and effective. The best outcomes for treatment of depression in the elderly have been achieved through a combination of psychosocial therapy and antidepressant medication (Evidence Level A).[24–27]

Depending on the severity of the depression, treatment with antidepressants may or may not be indicated. A diagnosis of minor depression, for instance, in an elderly patient who has recently relocated to a new environment and is having difficulty adjusting or is feeling socially isolated may not be a first-line treatment consideration. A referral to a social worker or psychotherapist who could facilitate social interaction or help the patient address their feeling regarding the move may be more beneficial. Increased family involvement may also help the patient as he or she is adjusting to the new environment.

An initial episode of major depression may herald the onset of depression as a chronic condition. Evidence-based, effective management of the initial episode may prevent or minimize subsequent illness and suffering from this condition. In order to address the acute and long-term consequences of depressive illness the physician should conceptualize the management of depressive illness in three distinct phases: Acute, continuation, and maintenance (Evidence Level C, expert opinion).[28]

Acute-Phase Management

Management in the acute phase of depression first includes a review of treatment options with the patient and possibly a family member or caregiver. Treatment options can include talk therapy with a counselor, use of support groups, lifestyle changes including improved diet and exercise, decreased alcohol use, recreation or hobbies, social support, and treatment with antidepressant medications (Evidence Level B). For depression that includes SAD, treatment with full-spectrum light therapy may be beneficial (Evidence Level A).[29] Family understanding and support are also important factors in the treatment of depression. Providing family members with access to educational materials about depression can help them develop a better understanding of depression and its treatment and how they can support the patient through the treatment process. There are many available resources on the Internet regarding depression and its treatment. The physician should emphasize that depression is a treatable illness, and that the treatment plan is developed in partnership with the patient and family.

Duration of Treatment: Set Expectations from the Beginning

Most depressive episodes have an average duration of 6 to 9 months, so treatment with antidepressants should be maintained for at least 6 months (Evidence Level A). In elderly patients who may have a more brittle course, longer treatment is probably better than a shorter treatment period, and patients should be prepared by the physician for an extended, open-ended treatment course that may be lifelong. Premature termination of treatment can lead to relapse and potentially preventable suffering. Psychotherapies and environmental therapies may have a duration based on other considerations, for example, family and interpersonal issues, social and environment issues, and work-related stresses.

As noted in the preceding text, a combination of treatment with medication and psychosocial therapies has the best documented outcomes for depression in elderly patients.[24] Developing a working relationship with a counselor or therapist who is comfortable collaborating with a primary care physician will enhance outcomes and lead to fewer unnecessary medical visits, as well as achieve better adherence to the medication regimen.

CASE TWO

Mrs. J. is a 90-year-old, living in an assisted-living facility. The assisted-living staff have noticed that the patient has not been eating well, is reluctant to come into the dining room for meals and has been losing weight. The family have also noted that she is calling frequently in the evening and sometimes in the middle of the night complaining that the staff are not letting her visit her mother. The patient is known to have a mild dementia secondary to Alzheimer disease. She is evaluated by her primary care physician, who determines that she has a urinary tract infection, which is then treated successfully. However, her symptoms continue. The primary care physician diagnoses the patient with dementia with depression and begins her on mirtazapine 7.5 mg at night. This is eventually increased to 15 mg at night and the patient begins sleeping better, her appetite improves and she reengages in the activities and meals in the assisted-living facility.

Antidepressant Medications

The medication choices available for the treatment of depression in the elderly are presented in Table 17.6, grouped by general class: Heterocyclics (that include tricyclics), selective serotonin reuptake inhibitors (SSRIs), dual agents (venlafaxine and mirtazapine), and atypical antidepressants. In general, for a primary care physician working with elderly depressed patients, the SSRIs are initial, safe and effective choices. This is especially true for medically ill patients who are on multiple medications where drug–drug interactions and side effect profile are important considerations.[30]

The general suggestions in this section for the use of antidepressant medications in elderly patients are applicable to relatively uncomplicated, mild to moderate depressive illness. For a complex depressive episode that is

TABLE 17.6
CHOICE OF INITIAL PHARMACOTHERAPY

Drug		Pill Size Available (mg)	Dose Level 1	2	3	4
Heterocyclic Antidepressants						
Elavil	Amitriptyline HCl	10, 25, 50, 75, 100, 150	≤50	51–100	101–199	200+
Nortriptyline	Nortriptyline HCl	10, 25, 50, 75	—	—	—	—
Desipramine	Desipramine HCl	10, 25, 50, 75, 100, 150	≤50	51–100	101–199	200+
Doxepin	Doxepin HCl	10, 25, 50, 75, 100, 150	≤50	51–100	101–199	200+
Tofranil	Imipramine HCl	10, 25, 50	≤50	51–100	101–199	200+
Vivactil	Protriptyline HCl	5, 10	—	—	—	—
Surmontil	Trimipramine maleate	25, 50, 100	≤50	51–100	101–199	200+
Selective Serotonin Reuptake Inhibitors						
Prozac	Fluoxetine HCl	10, 20, 40	≤10	11–20	21–40	>40
Paxil	Paroxetine HCl	10, 20, 30, 40	≤10	11–20	21–40	>40
Lexapro	Escitalopram oxalate	5, 10, 20	≤5	6–10	11–20	>20
Celexa	Citalopram HBr	10, 20, 40	≤10	11–20	21–40	>40
Zoloft	Sertraline HCl	25, 50, 100	≤50	51–100	101–150	>150
Dual Agent AD						
Effexor	Venlafaxine HCl	25, 37.5, 50, 75, 100	≤50	51–75	76–100	>100
Remeron	Mirtazapine	15, 30, 45	≤15	16–30	31–45	>45
Atypical AD						
Wellbutrin	Bupropion HCl	75, 100	≤75	76–150	151–200	>200
Trazodone	Trazodone HCl	50, 100, 150	≤50	51–100	101–199	>200

complicated by recurrent and bipolar depressive disorders, severe medical illness, suicidality, drug–drug interactions, or for patients with personality disorders that may influence their adherence to medical treatments, we strongly encourage a collaborative approach to care that includes a mental health professional.

Selective Serotonin Reuptake Inhibitors

CASE THREE

Mrs. A. is a recently widowed 75-year-old woman. She has lost 15 pounds over the past month, finds it difficult to get out of bed in the morning, has no energy, and thinks she would be better off joining her dead husband. Her adult children are quite worried about her. Her primary care physician, who knows her well, starts her on fluoxetine 10 mg in the morning. He also refers the patient to a grief counselor and develops a plan with the patient's family to check on her regularly until her depression resolves. Over a period of 6 weeks the patient's symptoms diminish and she returns to her usual active and involved baseline. Approximately 2 months later the daughter calls the primary care physician to share a concern that her mother's behavior has been strange. She is not sleeping well and calls in the middle of the night, seeing men in her apartment. She is also complaining of excessive fatigue during the day. Laboratory tests reveal a very low sodium level. He corrects the sodium level and switches the patient to venlafaxine, to which she responds well.

SSRIs are safe and effective choices for the treatment of elderly patients with depression and have a spectrum of actions from activating to calming (Evidence Level A). There are some differences in the SSRIs that can influence the choice among them. Fluoxetine and sertraline are thought to be the most activating SSRIs, whereas paroxetine is the most calming. Citalopram and escitalopram are somewhere in the middle of the activation and calming spectrum. Patients who have a depressive illness with predominant withdrawal, hypersomnia, and other vegetative signs may do well with either sertraline or fluoxetine. Patients who are highly agitated with significant sleep disturbance may respond better with paroxetine. With mixed patterns of agitation and withdrawal, patients may do well initially with citalopram or escitalopram.

Special Considerations

SSRIs are an excellent choice in patients with post-myocardial infarction (MI) depression because of the antithrombotic effects on platelets, as well as the beneficial effects on depression that otherwise may increase the risk of post-MI mortality.

Selective Serotonin Reuptake Inhibitors and Drug–Drug Interactions and Half-lives

Citalopram and escitalopram have the least effect on the cytochrome P-450 enzymes and are good choices when patients have complex medical illnesses and are taking many medications. Fluoxetine has an extremely long half-life that can be a benefit if patients occasionally forget to take their medications, but can also be problematic as it has a more significant suppression of cytochrome P-450 enzymes, a profile that it shares with paroxetine.

Dosing

Many physiologic changes occur with aging, some of which affect the pharmacokinetics and/or pharmacodynamics of medications. The physiologic changes include, but are not limited to, declines in renal and hepatic function, decreased total body water, increased proportion of body fat, decreased proportion of body weight as lean muscle, decreased gastrointestinal motility and body flow, and increased end-organ sensitivity to central nervous system–active drugs. All of these changes can require drug dosage adjustment. To further complicate the situation, elderly patients usually have more comorbidities and use more medications, placing them at higher risk for toxicity and adverse drug–drug interactions. For all of the above reasons, the adage "start low and go slow" is apt for antidepressants as well. Patients may not need higher doses to achieve a therapeutic benefit because of the decreased muscle mass and buffering capacity, but if there are no improvements at lower dosing, they should receive a full therapeutic trial at the highest doses tolerated.

Side Effects: Educating and Preparing Patients

The common side effects of SSRIs include sexual dysfunction, gastric distress, nausea, loose and frequent stools, and headache (see Table 17.7). It is important to educate and prepare patients for these side effects. Many of the undesired effects dissipate with time and can be treated symptomatically, for example, using acetaminophen for headache and taking medications with food. Sexual dysfunction, which often presents as ejaculatory delay in men, may be managed by use of sildenafil (Viagra) or related medications (if there is no contraindication present), or by concomitant use of bupropion. Rare but serious side effects that can occur at any stage of the treatment include hyponatremia and bleeding. SSRIs may cause a mild syndrome of inappropriate antidiuretic hormone secretion (SIADH) leading to decreased sodium and possible mental status changes. Bleeding or bruising may be attributable to SSRI interference with platelet aggregation.

In addition to the side effects, it is important to prepare patients and family members for the length of time it takes to observe and experience therapeutic improvements. It can be a month or two before the full effects of the medications are noticed. An interesting aspect of the improvement process is that family, caregivers, and friends may notice the improvement in the patient long before the patient actually reports feeling better. Patients may be more active, sleep better, and have more expression in their face and voice, but still do not see themselves as improving. Let the patients know that they may be the last to know when and how they are improving and that they should check out what others are observing.

Dual Agents

Mirtazapine, a dual action antidepressant (norepinephrine and serotonin reuptake inhibitor) is an excellent choice for elderly patients with agitation, weight loss, and insomnia. It is a dual action antidepressant, blocking reuptake of both serotonin and norepinephrine. At lower doses it is calming, helps with sleep, and stimulates appetite. At high doses, it becomes more activating. In at least one randomized control comparison, mirtazapine had a more rapid onset of action, was more effective in agitation and insomnia, and was better tolerated than paroxetine. Because of its long half-life, single day dosing is adequate and should be given at night to target sleep disturbance. The starting dose is 7.5 mg and can be increased to 15 mg within a few days. If sedation is a problem during the day a more rapid increase to higher doses may help, as it becomes more activating at higher doses. Compared to the SSRIs as a class, mirtazapine and venlafaxine are thought to have fewer effects on the cytochrome P-450 enzyme systems and therefore less impact on drug–drug interactions.

Special Considerations

- Mirtazapine may be a better choice in patients with Parkinson disease because it is less likely to affect the dopamine system.
- Appetite stimulation is frequently an important aspect of treatment in frail, elderly patients; therefore, it can be helpful in overall management of anorexia that may have causes other than the depressive episode.
- Venlafaxine is also a dual action antidepressant and is an excellent choice for patients with depressive episodes characterized by social withdrawal, decreased energy, and hypersomnia. It also has minimal impact on the cytochrome P-450 enzyme systems, which makes it a good choice for medically ill, frail elderly patients. It can cause some increase in blood pressure, so that patients with hypertension and related stroke risks may not be good candidates for this particular antidepressant. There is a withdrawal syndrome associated with sudden cessation of the medication. When terminating venlafaxine, it should be tapered gradually. One disadvantage is the need for multiple dosing, but there are now long acting preparations that can be taken once a day. Because of its activating properties in general, it should be given in the morning.

TABLE 17.7
SYMPTOMS AND SIDE EFFECTS OF ANTIDEPRESSANT MEDICATIONS

The Good	The Bad	The Ugly
Heterocyclic Antidepressants		
Effective	Sedation	Cardiac arrhythmia
Good for neuropathic pain	Orthostatic hypotension	Urinary retention
	Constipation	Lethal in overdose
	Heartburn	
	Anticholinergic	
SSRIs		
Safe	GI upset	Hyponatremia and delirium
Generally well tolerated	Sexual dysfunction	Increased bleeding diathesis
Effective	Headaches	Dopamine blocking and tardive dyskinesia
Simple dosing schedules	Drug–drug interactions	
Dual Agents		
Mirtazapine		
Rapid onset of action	Sedation	
Well tolerated	Delirium	
Effective for sleep, increased appetite and agitation	Dizziness	
Simple dosing schedule	Falls	
Minimal drug–drug interactions		
Venlafaxine		
Broad-spectrum efficacy including melancholia	Nausea	Serotonin syndrome
Minimal drug–drug interactions	Dizziness	Withdrawal symptoms
	Sedation	
	Sweating	
	Tremor	
	Increased blood pressure	
Atypical ADs		
Bupropion		
Safe	Activating, causing agitation	Increased risk of seizures at doses >450 mg/d
Well tolerated	Some GI distress	
No sexual side effects	Headaches	
No decreased REM sleep		
May help with smoking cessation		
Trazodone		
Effective for sleep disturbance	Orthostatic hypotension	Priapism
Helpful for agitation	Cardiotoxicity	
	Sedation	

SSRIs, selective serotonin reuptake inhibitors; GI, gastrointestinal; ADs, antidepressants; REM, rapid eye movement.

Heterocyclic Antidepressants

This class of antidepressants is one of the oldest groups, so there is a significant amount of information on their effectiveness and disadvantages. The side effect profile of this class is not as desirable as the newer antidepressants, especially in older patients, and unlike the SSRIs, these medications can be lethal in overdose. The side effects of concern in an elderly group of patients include: Dry mouth, cognition problems, urinary retention, constipation, sinus tachycardia, prolonged PR interval with increased risk of *torsade de pointes*, orthostatic hypotension, heartburn, and sedation (Table 17.7) (Evidence Level A). They do have a niche as second-line antidepressants when other antidepressants are not effective. They are also helpful in the treatment of neuropathic pain. The preferred choices within this group that have the least problems are the secondary amines nortriptyline and desipramine. Nortriptyline is especially good for patients with agitated depression and desipramine for patients who are withdrawn and anergic.

Atypical Antidepressants

Bupropion is useful in treating elderly patients with depression. It is generally well tolerated, has activating properties, and may be quite helpful in frail, elderly patients who complain of no energy and are withdrawn. It was originally taken off the market because of an increased incidence of seizures. It was extensively studied and then brought back into clinical use when the studies revealed that the increased incidence of seizures occurred only if the daily dosing was >450 mg per day. It has generally weak effects on the norepinephrine, serotonin, and dopamine systems, and its antidepressant mechanism of action is not known.

Trazodone has not been in use as a first-line treatment for depression over the past decade or so. It was found to be too sedating for many patients, and priapism was a concern for men. More recently, it has reentered the treatment arena as an adjunctive treatment for sleep and agitation, especially in elderly patients with dementia. It often has an immediate positive impact on sleep problems at low doses, 25 to 50 mg at night.

Management of Other Symptoms

Sleep disturbance is a common symptom of depression and patients are often desperate to receive some relief. Trazodone at low doses, 25 mg with a repeat, and increases up to 150 mg orally at night can provide immediate relief when another antidepressant is being increased to a therapeutic level and eventually resets the sleep-cycle disturbance.

CASE FOUR

Mr. S. is a 69-year-old married executive who recently retired. He suffered an acute MI and had become increasingly depressed despite excellent progress in his cardiac rehabilitation program. He reported sleep difficulties, constant worrying about having another heart attack, lack of interest in his usual activities, and lack of interest in having sex with his wife. He was started on paroxetine 10 mg at night, along with some low-dose trazodone 25 mg on a p.r.n. basis for sleep. He initially reported some problems of mild headache and loose stools after starting on the paroxetine. Acetaminophen was effective for the headache, and the loose stools resolved after several days without treatment. Sleep gradually improved with occasional use of trazodone at night. After 2 weeks paroxetine was increased to 20 mg because of continuing symptoms and social withdrawal. By 4 weeks his wife noticed a significant improvement, as did the patient. He was also referred for counseling where some of his fears were explored and he was able to express some concerns about resuming sex because of his concerns that it might cause another heart attack.

Monitoring in Acute-Phase Management (First 3 Months)

With elderly patients who are depressed, the early acute-phase management requires frequent monitoring to address possible side effects, to identify and address the reluctance of some patients to take the medication on a regular basis, and to impress upon patients how important the physician regards adherence to the medication protocol. Patients should be scheduled for a follow-up appointment in the first month following the beginning of treatment with antidepressants, with office visits supplemented with brief but frequent phone contacts by the physician or office nurse. A follow-up visit is also recommended 4 to 8 weeks following the first visit, supplemented again with brief phone contact during that period (Evidence Level B). Many patients have problems with side effects of medications, are reluctant to go to therapists or return to the doctor, or simply stop the medication because it did not seem to help. Others stop prematurely (before 6 months) because they feel better. A major obstacle to better depression care is the failure of a patient to have follow-up visits and evaluation. Evidence suggests the importance of two office strategies to maximize patient follow-up: (i) Schedule a specific follow-up appointment time, and (ii) active outreach to patients with depression who do not return for scheduled visits, using a tracking system of some kind (Evidence Level A).

At each follow-up visit, a depression screening questionnaire like the GDS or PHQ9 should be used to assess and document changes in depression symptoms. Families or caregivers providing care for elderly and frail patients should be encouraged to contact the physician with any concerns regarding symptoms or adherence to medications. If a counselor or psychotherapist is making regular weekly visits, they should also be integrated into the monitoring process.

The goal of acute-phase management is to ameliorate symptoms and decrease duration of the episode.

- Some patients improve within the first week, but most do not until 6 to 8 weeks of treatment.
- Continue starting dose of antidepressants for 4 weeks.
- Patient needs to make office visit within first 4 weeks to assess (GDS or PHQ9) symptom severity and treatment; plan active outreach if patient fails to come in.
- If there is <25% improvement in depression symptoms after 4 weeks, double the dose (or increase slowly if side effects) for 4 more weeks.
- If there is <50% improvement in depressive symptoms after 8 weeks, switch to another SSRI.

Continuation Phase Management (3 to 6 Months)

Continuation phase management and follow-up are important components to the successful treatment of depressive disorders. Patients' adherence to medications should be monitored, dosage adjustments made as needed to achieve optimal therapeutic success, and side effects of medications addressed. Elderly patients who achieve remission of depressive symptoms often decide they no longer need medications or additional therapies that were started during acute-phase management. The physician should encourage patients to maintain their antidepressant treatments for a minimum of 6 months, and up to a full year to achieve complete remission and decrease the likelihood of a reoccurrence of depression (Evidence Level A). If the episode of depression was a second reoccurrence, evidence suggests treatment with medication for 3 years, and for a third episode of depression lifetime treatment is recommended.[31]

If a counselor or psychotherapist is involved with the patient, continued coordination and a collaborative approach to treatment planning are needed, with periodic communication between the physician and therapist. If environmental or lifestyle changes were begun during the acute-phase management, the patient should be encouraged to maintain those changes as an ongoing part of maintaining good mental and physical health. Monitoring during the continuation phase should include a follow-up visit or phone call at least every 4 weeks during the first 6 months to address medication decisions and decide on continued treatment.

The goals of continuation phase management are to stabilize initial response, to convert to full remission, and to prevent relapse.

- Once remission is achieved, keep the patient on the full dose of antidepressant for a minimum of 6 to 12 months for the patient who is being treated for the first episode.
- Treatment with antidepressants should be considered for up to 3 years if the episode represents the first reoccurrence of depression.
- Lifetime treatment with antidepressants should be considered after two or more reoccurrences.
- Visits should be made at least every 6 months to assess depression status and address treatment options.

Maintenance Phase of Treatment

The maintenance phase of depression treatment focuses on the prevention of relapse. Because depression in many cases is a chronic illness, the more episodes of depression a patient has had, the higher the likelihood that depression will reoccur. If this is the case, lifetime treatment with antidepressants should be considered (Evidence Level A). Involvement of a counselor or therapist is also strongly recommended for patients with recurrent depressive disorders. Collaborative management between mental health and primary care will ensure that the patient is receiving optimum long-term management for depression and that both the symptoms and any remediable causes of depression are being addressed.

The goal of maintenance phase treatment is to prevent recurrence.

- For many patients depression is a chronic, relapsing, recurrent disorder (50% to 85%), especially when there is a history of three or more episodes.
- Consider continuous life-long prophylactic treatment with antidepressant at the same therapeutic dose.
- Annual visits should include full depression evaluation, with additional visits as needed during the year for optimum long-term management.

Failure to Respond to Initial Treatment

Although many patients respond to initial therapy for depression as outlined above, new evidence indicates that nearly half of patients may not respond to initial treatment with SSRIs or other modalities. In such a clinical scenario, it is important first to address issues of treatment adherence, to review and confirm the accuracy of a unipolar, nonpsychotic depression diagnosis, and to consider alternative diagnoses such as bipolar disorder, grief, or anxiety disorder. Assuming that these issues have been addressed and a unipolar, nonpsychotic depression diagnosis confirmed, there is growing evidence to suggest that treatment with either (a) augmentation of therapy with second agent such as bupropion, be considered when not contraindicated and when agreeable to the patient, or (b) initial SSRI therapy be stopped and replaced with an alternative pharmacologic agent such as bupropion, venlafaxine, or another SSRI.[32,33]

When to Refer to a Mental Health Specialist

Referral to a mental health counselor or therapist should be discussed with most elderly patients as a part of their initial treatment plan. The elderly are often reluctant to speak to mental health specialists because of the stigma attached to issues of mental health, viewing the problem as a personal failure or sign of weakness in character. Therefore, discuss this frankly but carefully, acknowledging any concerns they might have. It may be helpful for the patient to know that the best outcomes in the treatment of depression are often achieved through a combination of medication and psychosocial therapy.

Other reasons to encourage a referral to mental health are if there is diagnostic uncertainty, a history of bipolar disorder or manic depression, symptoms suggestive of bipolar disorder, psychotic symptoms, high levels of anxiety or panic in addition to depression, alcohol, or substance abuse, or if there is known or suspected domestic violence. In cases of suicidal or homicidal ideation, with or without a plan, the physician should immediately refer the patient to a mental health specialist (see section "Suicide").

Consider a referral to mental health counselor if no remission in depressive symptoms has been achieved by 12 weeks of treatment with antidepressants, or if only minor improvement is seen following treatment for 2 months. Additionally, if two different antidepressant medications have been tried without success, a referral to a mental health professional should be considered.

CAUSES OF DEPRESSION

As noted earlier the causes of depression are still not well understood, although a combination of biologic or genetic factors combined with environmental stresses and life events appear the most likely explanation for most cases. For the elderly, however, most depressive disorders appear to be a reactive response to life events and circumstances related to the process of aging, illness, and physical decline. This is especially true in cases of minor depression, which is believed to be far more prevalent among elderly adults. The aging process brings with it significant changes for the older adult in role functioning, financial status, physical health, and social networks; for some, the magnitude of these changes can be overwhelming and result in depression. Some of the precipitating causes of depression in older adults are retirement, declining physical health and functioning, chronic illness, bereavement, and informal caregiving. Women are also at greater risk for depressive episodes than are men.

CASE FIVE

Mrs. N. had been seeing the same physician for much of her life for health problems including diabetes and arthritis. On recent visits her physician noted that she seemed withdrawn and presented a number of persistent minor complaints such as headaches, inability to sleep, and stomach problems, which he had initially attributed to arthritis and difficulty in managing diabetes. At her next visit, her doctor, noting her sad and withdrawn mood, asked if she had been feeling sad or depressed. Mrs. N. nodded "yes" and then tearfully explained how difficult things had become for her. She and her husband had worked and saved much of their lives believing that after they both retired they would have time for all of the activities they had long talked about yet put off, such as travel and hobbies. But in his early sixties Mr. N. was beset by increasing health problems, including heart disease and progressive forgetfulness. Mrs. N. now suddenly found herself becoming a full-time caregiver for her husband who had recently been diagnosed with Alzheimer disease. All of their dreams for long and happy retirement were lost and as she told her doctor "the future holds nothing for me now."

Retirement

A major late-life transition comes with retirement from work or career. When employment ceases, a number of major changes are set into motion that can have both beneficial and detrimental effects on well-being. First, there can be significant shifts in economic well-being and financial security. Depending on work, career, and financial history, seniors may experience a large decline in their income, with ongoing financial distress and worry. Next, social interactions and relationships can also change dramatically, especially for older adults with major social interactions in the work setting. For seniors without well-established hobbies, interests, or activities, retirement can become a lonely time that requires redefining concepts of self and relationships with others. Onset of depression following retirement is common, especially for men whose primary focus in life has been work and career. The impact on a spouse who is a homemaker may also be pronounced, and can sometimes increase relationship conflict and distress.

Declining Health and Function

An overall decline in physical functioning also occurs with age, resulting in reduced stamina and strength, declines in hearing and vision, and greater risk for multiple health problems. Declining physical health can also result in impaired functional status including the ability to perform independent activities of daily living such as cooking, cleaning, and shopping, as well as more basic activities including walking and performing self-cares such as bathing and dressing. These declines are accompanied not only by reduced levels of physical activity, but also by decreased social contact and involvement, resulting in social isolation and loneliness. The association of physical decline and chronic disease with depression is a hallmark of late-life depression. It is not surprising, therefore, that rates of depression peak in the elderly at 80 years of age, when declines in physical function may lead to feelings of lowered personal control and perceptions of status loss, especially in a society that is focused primarily on the young and healthy.[34]

Chronic Illness

Depression often co-occurs with other serious chronic conditions such as heart disease, diabetes, Alzheimer disease, stroke, cancer, macular degeneration, and neurologic conditions such as Parkinson disease. Because of the seriousness of most of these conditions, both physicians and patients often mistakenly conclude that depression is a normal response or consequence of the condition. Depression, however, is not a normal response to chronic illness and can worsen the symptoms of many chronic conditions, delay recovery, and increase mortality. It is not yet clear whether depression is a psychological response to illness, or whether physical changes in the body are accompanied by mental changes as well.

There is a significant body of research accumulated over the past decade establishing strong links between depression and coronary heart disease (CHD), with the prevalence of major depression in adults with heart disease estimated to be from 18% to 23% and depressive symptoms in up to 65% of patients following a significant cardiac event.[35-39] Depression is linked to increased complications related to cardiac events, and to increased mortality in patients with CHD. Depressive disorders may also be predictive of heart attacks or MI—some studies suggest that adults with a history of depression are four times more likely to have an MI than those with no depression.[40]

There is also a strong relationship between stroke and depression, with estimates of the prevalence of depression following a stroke ranging from 26% to 54%.[41] The risk for depression is the highest in the first two years following the stroke and it is increased if the left cerebral cortex is affected or the stroke damage is closer to the frontal pole.[41] Depression following a stroke can be mistaken for a functional disorder and left unrecognized, especially if verbal expression is impaired. There is also evidence that as with heart disease, depression may also be predictive of stroke.

Recent studies of the relationship between diabetes and depression find that adults with diabetes have higher rates of depression, more severe depression symptoms, and longer episodes of depression than adults without diabetes.[42-45] It is believed that biological mechanisms, and other factors (the intrusiveness of the illness, diabetes complications, and ability to adapt to the illness) are involved in explaining this relationship. However, the biological mechanisms through which this might occur are not clear. Possible explanations include the complex metabolic derangements that characterize both type 1 and type 2 diabetes and that may directly affect neurophysiologic pathways and predispose patients with diabetes to depression. Excessive fluctuations in glucose levels associated with diabetes and its treatment have also been shown to affect many aspects of neurologic functioning. In addition, metabolic changes in glucose, insulin, glucagon, and other factors associated with diabetes may also affect adrenal function and impact neuropsychologic function through changes in levels of cortisol, epinephrine, norepinephrine, or other humoral factors.[46]

There is also a strong relationship between cancer and depression, with estimates of depression in patients with cancer ranging from 25% to 50%, depending on the type and the clinical stage of the cancer. A diagnosis of cancer significantly interrupts the life course, bringing tremendous emotional upheaval including changes in lifestyles, social roles, body image, and fear of death. Symptoms of depression may sometimes be mistaken for those of cancer or side effects of treatment. Careful inquiry about the type, severity, and duration of symptoms is important in distinguishing treatment-related effects from depression.

The recognition of a relationship between depression and various chronic diseases is not new, but the value of more clearly identifying and treating depression in those with chronic disease is. There has long been a common misperception that depression is a natural response to chronic and acute illness, and because it is seen as a natural response treatment can be overlooked. Depression, however, is not a normal response to illness and if left untreated will increase the burden of illness, as well as the likelihood for poor outcomes. Depression may also not be strictly a psychological response to the illness, but may be the result of biologic changes that are taking place as a result of the illness.

Bereavement

There are few life events that are as emotionally stressful and as personally traumatic as the death of a family member or a close friend. Bereavement, the state of mourning or suffering the death of a loved one, is often accompanied by significant psychological and emotional distress. Bereavement can also precipitate events of acute crisis and major life transitions and is believed to exacerbate underlying physical conditions and emotional problems, even in the presence of supportive social networks.[47] Normal bereavement is self-limiting, gradually subsiding with time as adjustments are made to accommodate the significant changes that result from death and accompanying losses. The closer the relationship, the more difficult the period of mourning that will follow. Bereavement can also become complicated, and in this instance major depression is often the result.

Elderly persons inevitably experience the death of family and friends as they age. Perhaps the most significant of these events is the death of a spouse. Widowhood is far more common at advanced ages and has been associated with impaired physical, psychological, and social functioning, as well as increased mortality.[48] The death of a spouse may be one of the most significant life-changing experiences that occur in old age, especially for long-term marriages.[49] During marriage, every daily habit and most social exchanges involve the married partner. Tasks and duties are split up, often creating a dependence between individuals that permeates all aspects of daily living. The losses that accompany the death of a spouse are significant and long lasting. Depression that does not abate in the year following the death of a spouse is indicative of complicated bereavement and should be treated with medication and referral for grief counseling.

Informal Caregiving

Informal caregiving is the act of one member of a family or social group providing significant personal care and assistance to another. Older spouses and adult children are the most likely to become caregivers in response to the declining health, chronic illness, or onset of cognitive difficulties or dementia in a loved one. Providing care for another, especially if the care needs are significant, can become an all-consuming task, turning into a 24 hour-a-day job. Providing care for another is also emotionally and physically stressful, bringing isolation from normal physical and social activities as well as feelings of anger, resentment, sadness, anxiety, guilt, and exhaustion. It is not unusual for caregivers to experience depression as a result of the constant demands they face.

Gender Differences

Gender differences have long been reported in rates of depressive illness, with studies indicating that depression occurs twice as often in women than in men. Women are also two to three times more likely to develop dysthymic disorder than are men. Research on this difference indicates that the higher rate of depression among women is not a result of women's willingness to report their symptoms, or related to their willingness to engage in help-seeking behavior, but instead reflects a real gender difference in mental health.[50] One unfortunate result of this difference is that physicians can often overlook depressive symptoms in men. Men may also experience depression differently, and are more likely to report symptoms of fatigue, irritability, loss of interest in work or hobbies and sleep disturbances, rather than feelings of sadness, loneliness, or excessive guilt. Men are also more likely to deny or minimize symptoms of depression than are women.

CONCLUSIONS

Depression is a serious condition that is chronic or recurrent for most patients and increases in prevalence with advancing years. At a time when many elderly are already struggling to address the changes that are a normal part of the aging process, depression can compromise their ability to adapt to these changes and significantly reduce quality and even length of life.[51] Fortunately, early diagnosis and effective treatment can significantly improve outcomes if physicians are sensitized to this problem and its often occult presentations in this age group. New medications combined with lifestyle changes and counseling have shown impressive results in treating depression in older adults. However, the most important requirement for the effective use of these treatments is having reliable office systems in place to ensure accurate diagnosis, effective treatment, and ongoing follow-up. Without such systems, the USPSTF found little benefit to case finding and identification for depression given that proper diagnosis, treatment and follow-up are not assured. The most significant benefits for elderly patients will be realized in clinical practices with systems in place that coordinate the results of screening with effective follow-up procedures and ongoing treatment.

REFERENCES

1. Unutzer J, Katon W, Callahan CM, et al. Depression treatment in a sample of 1,801 depressed older adults in primary care. *J Am Geriatr Soc Apr*. 2003;51:505–514.
2. Stewart JT. Why don't physicians consider depression in the elderly? Age-related bias, atypical symptoms, and ineffective screening approaches may be at play. *Postgrad Med*. 2004;115: 57–59.
3. van Marwijk H, Hoeksema HL, Hermans J, et al. Prevalence of depressive symptoms and depressive disorder in primary care patients over 65 years of age. *Fam Pract*. 1994;11:80–84.
4. Himelhoch S, Weller WE, Wu AW, et al. Chronic medical illness, depression, and use of acute medical services among medicare beneficiaries. *Med Care*. 2004;42:512–521.
5. Rowe CJ. *An outline of psychiatry*, 9th ed. Dubuque, Iowa: Wm. C. Brown Publishers; 1989.
6. American Psychiatric Association. *Diagnostic and statistical manual of mental disorders*, 4th ed. Washington, DC: American Psychiatric Association; 1994.
7. National Institute of Mental Health, National Institutes of Health (NIMH). *Depression*. Bethesda, MD: US Department of Health and Human Services; (NIH Publication #02-3561); 2000.
8. Blazer DG. Epidemiology of late-life depression. In: Schneider LS, Reynolds CF III, Lebowitz BD, et al. eds. *Diagnosis and treatment of depression in late life: Results of the NIH consensus development conference*. Washington, DC: American Psychiatric Press; 1994:9–21.
9. Beekman AT, Deeg DJ, Braam AW, et al. Consequences of major and minor depression in later life: A study of disability, well-being and service utilization. *Psychol Med*. 1997;27:1397–1409.
10. Papassotiropoulos A, Heun R. Detection of subthreshold depression and subthreshold anxiety in the elderly. *Int J Geriatr Psychiatry*. 1999;14:643–650.
11. McGuire L, Kiecolt-Glaser JK, Glaser R. Depressive symptoms and lymphocyte proliferation in older adults. *J Abnorm Psychol*. 2002;111:192–197.
12. Penninx BW, Geerlings SW, Deeg DJ, et al. Minor and major depression and the risk of death in older persons. *Arch Gen Psychiatry*. 1999;56:889–895.
13. Pignone MP, Gaynes BN, Rushton JL, et al. Screening for depression in adults: A summary of the evidence for the US Preventive Services Task ForceScreening for depression: Recommendations and rationale. *Ann Intern Med*. 2002;136(10):765–776.
14. U.S. Preventive Services Task Force. Screening for depression: Recommendations and rationale. *Ann Intern Med*. 2002;136(10): 760–764.
15. Nease DE Jr, Maloin JM. Depression screening: A practical strategy. *J Fam Pract*. 2003;52(2):118–124.
16. VHA/DOD. *Clinical practice guidelines for the management of major depressive disorder in adults*. Washington, DC: Department of Veterans Affairs; 2000.
17. Thibault JM, Steiner RW. Efficient identification of adults with depression and dementia. *Am Fam Physician*. 2004;70(6): 1101–1110. Sep 15.
18. Lowe B, Unutzer J, Callahan CM, et al. Monitoring depression treatment outcomes with the patient health questionnaire-9. *Med Care*. 2004;42(12):1194–1201.
19. McDowell I, Newell C. *Measuring health: A guide to rating scales and questionnaires*, 2nd ed. New York, NY: Oxford University Press; 1996.
20. Katon WJ, Simon G, Russo J, et al. Quality of depression care in a population-based sample of patients with diabetes and major depression. *Med Care*. 2004;42(12):1222–1229.
21. Luoma JB, Martin CE, Pearson JL. Contact with mental health and primary care providers before suicide: A review of the evidence. *Am J Psychiatry*. 2002;159(6):909–916.
22. Pirkis J, Burgess P. Suicide and recency of health care contacts. A systematic review. *Br J Psychiatry*. 1998;173:462–474.
23. Schulberg HC, Bruce ML, Lee PW, et al. Preventing suicide in primary care patients: The primary care physician's role. *Gen Hosp Psychiatry*. 2004;26(5):337–345.
24. Lebowitz BD, Pearson JL, Schneider LS, et al. Diagnosis and treatment of depression in late life. Consensus statement update. *JAMA*. 1997;278(14):1186–1190.
25. Ciechanowski P, Wagner E, Schmaling K, et al. Community-integrated home-based depression treatment in older adults: A randomized controlled trial. *JAMA*. 2004;291:1569–1577.
26. Blazer DG. The treatment of late-life depression. *Clin Geriatr*. 1996;4:16–24.
27. Blazer DG. Depression in late life: Review and commentary. *J Gerontol A Biol Sci Med Sci*. 2003;58:249–265.
28. Institute for Clinical Systems Improvement (ICSI). *Major depression in adults for mental health care*. Bloomington, MN: ICSI; 2004.
29. Leppamaki SJ, Partonen TT, Hurme J, et al. Randomized trial of the efficacy of bright-light exposure and aerobic exercise on depressive symptoms and serum lipids. *J Clin Psychiatry*. 2002;63(4): 316–321.

30. Salzman C. *Clinical geriatric psychopharmacology*. Baltimore, MD: Lippincott Williams & Wilkins; 1998.
31. Institute for Clinical Systems Improvement (ICSI). *Health care guideline: Major depression, panic disorder and generalized anxiety disorder in adults in primary care*. Bloomington, MN: ICSI; 2001.
32. Rush AJ, Trivedi MH, Wisniewski SR, et al. Bupropion-SR, sertraline, or venlafaxine-XR after failure of SSRIs for depression. *N Engl J Med*. 2006;354(12):1231–1242.
33. Trivedi MH, Fava M, Wisniewski SR, et al. Medication augmentation after the failure of SSRIs for depression. *N Engl J Med*. 2006;354(12):1243–1252.
34. Mirowsky J, Ross CE. Age and depression. *J Health Soc Behav*. 1992;33:187–205;discussion206–112.
35. Appels A. Depression and coronary heart disease: Observations and questions. *J Psychosom Res*. 1997;43:443–452.
36. Carney RM, Freedland KE, Miller GE, et al. Depression as a risk factor for cardiac mortality and morbidity: A review of potential mechanisms. *J Psychosom Res*. 2002;53:897–902.
37. Carney RM, Freedland KE, Sheline YI, et al. Depression and coronary heart disease: A review for cardiologists. *Clin Cardiol*. 1997;20:196–200.
38. Sirois BC, Burg MM. Negative emotion and coronary heart disease. *A Review. Behav Modif*. 2003;27:83–102.
39. Valkamo M, Hintikka J, Niskanen L, et al. Depression and associated factors in coronary heart disease. *Scand Cardiovasc J*. 2001;35:259–263.
40. Chapman DP, Perry GS, Strine TW. The vital link between chronic disease and depressive disorders. *Prev Chronic Dis*. 2005;2:A14.
41. Raj A. Depression in the elderly. Tailoring medical therapy to their special needs. *Postgrad Med*. 2004;115:26–28,37–42.
42. Anderson RJ, Freedland KE, Clouse RE, et al. The prevalence of comorbid depression in adults with diabetes: A meta-analysis. *Diabetes Care*. 2001;24:1069–1078.
43. Eaton WW, Armenian H, Gallo J, et al. Depression and risk for onset of type II diabetes. A prospective population-based study. *Diabetes Care*. 1996;19(10):1097–1102.
44. Talbot F, Nouwen A. A review of the relationship between depression and diabetes in adults: Is there a link? *Diabetes Care*. 2000; 23(10):1556–1562.
45. Peyrot M, Rubin RR. Levels and risks of depression and anxiety symptomatology among diabetic adults. *Diabetes Care*. 1997; 20(4):585–590.
46. de Groot M, Jacobson AM, Samson JA, et al. Glycemic control and major depression in patients with type 1 and type 2 diabetes mellitus. *J Psychosom Res*. 1999;46(5):425–435.
47. McHorney CA, Mor V. Predictors of bereavement depression and its health services consequences. *Med Care*. 1988;26(9):882–893.
48. Umberson D, Wortman CB, Kessler RC. Widowhood and depression: Explaining long-term gender differences in vulnerability. *J Health Soc Behav*. 1992;33(1):10–24.
49. Wray NP, DeBehnke RD, Ashton CM, et al. Characteristics of the recurrently hospitalized adult. An information synthesis. *Med Care*. 1988;26(11):1046–1056.
50. Sherbourne CD, Weiss R, Duan N, et al. Do the effects of quality improvement for depression care differ for men and women? Results of a group-level randomized controlled trial. *Med Care*. 2004;42(12):1186–1193.
51. Blazer D. The diagnosis of depression in the elderly. *J Am Geriatr Soc*. 1980;28(2):52–58.

Delirium

18

Sidney T. Bogardus, Jr.

CLINICAL PEARLS 225

EPIDEMIOLOGY OF DELIRIUM 226
Incidence and Prevalence 226
Adverse Consequences 226

PATHOPHYSIOLOGY OF DELIRIUM 226

CLINICAL FEATURES OF DELIRIUM 227
Definition 227
Symptoms and Signs 227
Differential Diagnosis 228
Evaluation of the Patient with Delirium 228

RISK FACTORS FOR DELIRIUM 229
Predisposing and Precipitating Risk Factors 230
Postoperative Delirium 230

PREVENTION OF DELIRIUM 231

TREATMENT OF DELIRIUM 232
Nonpharmacologic Approaches to Management 233
Pharmacologic Approaches to Management 233

CONCLUSION 234

CLINICAL PEARLS

- Delirium is an acute change in attention and cognition. The acuteness of the mental status change helps differentiate delirium from dementia.
- Inattention is one of the hallmarks of delirium and also helps differentiate delirium from dementia.
- Delirium occurs in 10% to 65% of hospitalized older patients but is diagnosed in only 33% to 66% of cases.
- Delirium represents a medical emergency and is associated with substantial in-hospital and posthospital morbidity and mortality, persistent cognitive and functional decline, institutionalization, and high economic costs.
- According to the Confusion Assessment Method (CAM), delirium is present when there is an acute change and fluctuating course to the mental status, inattention, and either disorganized thinking or altered level of consciousness.
- Predisposing risk factors include age, dementia, prior delirium, and visual or hearing impairment.
- In-hospital or precipitating risk factors include medications, infection, congestive heart failure, metabolic derangements, restraints and catheters, immobility, and other noxious insults.
- Interventions targeting known risk factors (e.g., cognitive impairment, immobility, vision impairment, hearing impairment, dehydration, and poor sleep) prevent 40% of delirium cases.
- Evaluation of a patient with delirium should include a search for offending medications, infection, congestive heart failure, metabolic derangements, or another adverse clinical development.
- Medications are implicated in approximately half of delirium cases.
- Treatment should focus on mitigating existing risk factors and underlying illnesses, and on creating an environment that emphasizes cognitive and social engagement and mobility.
- Use of antipsychotic medications, such as haloperidol, should be reserved for the patient with acute delirium who is a danger to himself/herself or to others.
- Antipsychotic mediation should ideally be tapered beginning by the second day of use.
- Medications used to treat delirium, including antipsychotics, can worsen delirium.

Delirium, defined as an acute change in attention and cognition, is a serious and common complication of hospitalization among older patients. Delirium is associated with a wide range of adverse consequences, including in-hospital morbidity, cognitive and functional decline, prolonged hospital length-of-stay, institutionalization, increased costs, and substantial mortality. Many, if not most, cases of delirium go unrecognized in the hospital. However, efforts to prevent delirium by focusing on risk factors have recently proved successful and cost effective.

EPIDEMIOLOGY OF DELIRIUM

Incidence and Prevalence

Delirium is very common among hospitalized older patients. Estimates suggest that approximately 15% to 30% of older patients are delirious on arrival at the hospital and that the incidence of delirium during hospitalization is approximately 15% to 60%, depending on the setting.[1–6] In certain settings, such as the intensive care unit, the incidence of delirium may reach 70%.[7] Delirium is also encountered in the emergency department (10%)[8] and in hospice units (42%).[9] Given that people older than 65 years account for approximately 35% of hospital stays and almost 50% of hospital days, nearly 30% of the entire older hospital population will experience delirium at some point during hospitalization.[10,11] However, although it is one of the most common adverse occurrences in the hospital, delirium is substantially under-recognized, with only 33% to 66% of cases diagnosed.[12] Some studies suggest that 84% to 95% of cases are not detected by attending physicians.[13,14]

Adverse Consequences

Delirium is often thought of as a temporary and reversible period of confusion associated with acute illness, and clinicians may assume that the confusion will resolve as the acute illness is treated. This is a misconception. Delirium is associated with substantial morbidity and increased mortality (see Table 18.1).[1,3,11,15–27] Patients with delirium have longer hospitalizations, prolonged cognitive and functional decline, greater risk of institutionalization, increased caregiver burden, and higher costs. Patients with delirium may be at risk for other adverse outcomes, including falls with injury, malnutrition, pressure sores, and infection. The cognitive symptoms of delirium can persist for months following hospitalization, with some estimates indicating that in fewer than half of the patients with delirium all symptoms attributable to the condition resolve 6 months after hospitalization.

Delirium is associated with excess mortality.[3,11,16,17,19–21,25,27] In-hospital mortality rates range from 25% to 33%. Mortality 1 month following hospitalization is approximately 14% and 6 months following hospitalization is approximately 22%.[15] Other studies have confirmed that patients with delirium in the hospital are more likely to die during the year following hospitalization than those without delirium, with one study finding a hazard ratio of 2.11 after adjusting for dementia and other confounding factors.[16] In a multisite study by Inouye et al. delirium was shown to be an independent predictor of poor outcomes after controlling for health status, age, dementia, and functional status.[11]

TABLE 18.1
ADVERSE OUTCOMES ASSOCIATED WITH DELIRIUM

Category	Example
In-hospital morbidity	Falls
	Pressure ulcers
	Incontinence
	Restraint use
	Unnecessary medication use
Health status	Cognitive decline (often persisting after hospital discharge)
	Functional decline (impairment in activities of daily living)
Health services utilization	Longer length of stay
	Rehospitalization
	Increased health care utilization
	Increased nursing home placement
Death	

PATHOPHYSIOLOGY OF DELIRIUM

The pathophysiology of delirium is not well understood but appears to be complex.[28–30] The variety of clinical settings in which delirium occurs would seem to suggest common pathways, anatomic regions, or neurotransmitters that could be involved in the development of delirium. Unfortunately, neuroimaging studies, which could provide useful information, are very difficult to perform in patients with active delirium. Attention deficits, which are one of the hallmarks of delirium, are found in a range of conditions, such as strokes, in which there is damage to the brainstem, prefrontal region, and right parietal lobe.[28] Infarctions of the middle cerebral artery affecting the frontostriatal and basal ganglia regions can also cause deficits in selective attention and cognition.

Anticholinergic drugs are often associated with delirium[31–33] that can be reversed by the cholinesterase inhibitor physostigmine. Furthermore, elevated serum anticholinergic activity has been correlated with delirium. These findings have led to a cholinergic hypothesis of delirium. Dopaminergic drugs can also lead to delirium. Hypoxia, which can precipitate delirium, increases extracellular dopamine concentration and reduces acetylcholine release. Dopamine also exists in a balance with acetylcholine. Serotonin, which impacts mood, wakefulness, and cognition, is increased in hepatic encephalopathy and septic delirium. Other suspect neurotransmitters include γ-aminobutyric acid (GABA), glutamate, endorphins, and cortisol.

Under the "final common pathway" theory, many different illnesses or causes lead to the same ultimate defect in brain chemistry, resulting in a set of core symptoms (e.g., disorientation, cognitive deficits, sleep–wake cycle disturbances, disorganized thinking, and language abnormalities). The exact nature of the final defect remains to be firmly identified. Other investigators suggest that delirium is more likely to be a "final common symptom," or set of symptoms, caused by a variety of different brain defects. Cognitive function is a high-order function and may be especially likely to fail in the face of mounting stresses on the equilibrium of a frail or vulnerable patient.

CLINICAL FEATURES OF DELIRIUM

Definition

Delirium is broadly defined as an acute decline in attention and cognition. Numerous other terms are often used interchangeably with delirium, including acute confusional state, acute confusional episode, toxic-metabolic encephalopathy, acute brain syndrome, acute brain failure, intensive care unit (ICU) psychosis, and others. The American Psychiatric Association's Diagnostic and Statistical Manual, Fourth edition (DSM-IV)[34] lists four central features of delirium (see Table 18.2).

Symptoms and Signs

Patients with delirium are usually sick. Many are frail to begin with, having multiple chronic illnesses. However, it is also possible that delirium may be the only sign of new or worsening illness in a hospitalized patient. For example, a patient with impending sepsis may not present with fever or a localizing symptom or sign, and delirium may be the only clue to the presence of infection. Likewise, a patient with myocardial infarction or congestive heart failure may develop delirium without other conventional localizing symptoms. In older patients with dementia, delirium may be the only sign suggesting the presence of new acute illness. Consequently, any patient with new delirium should be evaluated medically for new or worsening illness.

The development of delirium is relatively rapid over a period of hours to days but it then persists for days or even months, even after the patient's acute illness or illnesses has/have resolved. The course of delirium for an individual patient tends to fluctuate during the course of the day. Many patients have worse symptoms in the evening or at night, with lucid periods in the morning or during the day. If a patient is seen only during a lucid period, delirium may be missed; history from family or nursing staff who have been with the patient at other times may provide the clues to the diagnosis by documenting the presence of mental status change.

Inattention is one of the hallmarks of delirium. Patients with delirium have difficulty focusing, sustaining or shifting attention. Distractibility can be noticed in casual conversation but may be easier to miss than more prominent findings of tangentiality, disorganization, or frank confusion. Lack of attention can sometimes be subtle and may be attributed to illness or fatigue or dementia.

Patients with delirium generally have altered levels of consciousness. At one end of the spectrum, perhaps a third of patients have a reduced level of consciousness and may be drowsy, or even lethargic and difficult to arouse. At the other end of the spectrum, approximately a third of patients may be hypervigilant. The remaining patients may have periods of a reduced level of consciousness alternating with periods of a heightened level of consciousness. A common picture of the patient with delirium is of a hyperactive person who is agitated and confused, often vocalizing inappropriately, and with behavioral problems complicating patient care (e.g., pulling out intravenous lines). The diagnosis of delirium in these patients is usually straightforward because the behavioral problems are brought to the attention of treating clinicians. However, the patients who have hypoactive delirium with a slightly reduced level of consciousness may not be recognized as delirious precisely because the lack of agitation may not cause any overt problems in their day-to-day care. If the patient's level of consciousness is reduced enough, it may make it difficult to discern the problems in cognition that are another common feature of delirium.

Patients with delirium present with a variety of cognitive and perceptual disturbances, including disorientation to time and location, memory deficits, and comprehension or language problems. Perceptual problems may include

TABLE 18.2

***DIAGNOSTIC AND STATISTICAL MANUAL, FOURTH EDITION,* (DSM-IV) FEATURES OF DELIRIUM**

A. Disturbance of consciousness (e.g., reduced clarity of awareness of the environment) with reduced ability to focus, sustain, or shift attention
B. A change in cognition (e.g., memory deficit, disorientation, language disturbance) or the development of a perceptual disturbance that is not better accounted for by a preexisting, established, or evolving dementia
C. The disturbance develops over a short period of time (usually hours to days) and tends to fluctuate during the course of the day
D. There is evidence from the history, physical examination, or laboratory findings that the disturbance is caused by the direct physiologic consequences of a general medical condition
D. (alternative) There is evidence from the history, physical examination, or laboratory findings that the delirium has more than one etiology (e.g., more than one etiologic general medical condition) or a general medical condition plus substance intoxication or medication side effect

American Psychiatric Association. *Diagnostic and statistical manual of mental disorders*, 4th ed. text revision. Washington, DC: American Psychiatric Association; 2000.

misidentification, visual misperception and illusions, and delusions of harm. Occasionally, patients may have frank hallucinations, but these are uncommonly reported.

Differential Diagnosis

The diagnosis of delirium is established on clinical grounds on the basis of an evaluation of patient history and findings. There are no laboratory or radiologic tests that establish the diagnosis. Simple observation while interacting with the patient may reveal an abnormality in level of consciousness, often somnolence or lethargy but sometimes also hyperalertness. It is tempting to attribute an abnormal level of consciousness to fatigue, illness, or lack of sleep, but the clinician should keep in mind the possibility of delirium. Distractibility or an inability to focus or sustain attention during conversation or while attempting to obtain a history may suggest the presence of inattention but can be easy to miss if subtle. Conversation may also reveal disorientation, memory problems, abnormal speech, or even frank confusion.

Formal mental status testing, while often not performed in older patients in the hospital, can confirm the presence of cognitive deficits in patients with delirium. One of the most commonly used brief bedside tests of cognitive function is the Mini-Mental State Examination, a 30-point screening test originally described by Folstein that evaluates different domains of cognitive function, including memory, orientation, attention and calculation, language, and visuospatial skills.[35] It is important to keep in mind that the tests of cognitive function do not differentiate between causes of cognitive dysfunction, such as dementia or delirium.

History from people who know the patient often provides the most useful data when assessing the possibility of delirium. Family members or friends can describe the patient's prehospital functional and cognitive state, including the presence of preexisting dementia. Family members may also be able to describe whether a patient's current state represents a change from baseline. Simply by noticing that a patient seems "different," family members can provide the first clue to the presence of subtle delirium. Clinical updates should also be sought from nurses and other clinical staff, who may be in a better position than physicians to notice subtle cognitive or perceptual changes in patients by virtue of their more frequent patient interactions. Moreover, because the course of delirium tends to fluctuate frequently, physicians may miss delirium if they happen to see the patient during a lucid interval; nurses, who generally see patients multiple times during a shift, may have more opportunities to observe patients during both lucid and nonlucid periods.

One of the most useful and efficient diagnostic algorithms is the Confusion Assessment Method (CAM).[36] By interviewing and examining the patient, and by incorporating history from other informants, clinicians can use the CAM criteria to make the diagnosis of delirium in a few minutes. There are four CAM criteria for delirium (see Table 18.3).

TABLE 18.3
CONFUSION ASSESSMENT METHOD FEATURES OF DELIRIUM

1. Acute onset and fluctuating course
2. Inattention
3. Disorganized thinking
4. Altered level of consciousness

Diagnosis of delirium requires features 1 and 2, and either 3 or 4.

Inouye SK, van Dyck CH, Alessi CA, et al. Clarifying confusion: The confusion assessment method. A new method for detection of delirium. *Ann Intern Med.* 1990;113:941–948.

Delirium is diagnosed on the basis of the presence of the first two CAM criteria and one or both of the second two criteria. The CAM criteria emphasize the temporal course of the change in mental status and the presence of inattention. Because it may be difficult to discern the presence of disturbed cognition when a patient has a substantially reduced level of consciousness, only one of the last two criteria must be present. The CAM has excellent test characteristics, with a sensitivity of 94% to 100% and a specificity of 90% to 95%. It has become a standard tool in both clinical and research settings. Moreover, because delirium is so common in the ICU, where it may be difficult to assess mechanically ventilated patients, the CAM-ICU instrument has been developed.[37] The CAM-ICU incorporates observed behaviors and simple questions with nonverbal responses.

Delirium is sometimes confused with other conditions, such as dementia, depression, or other psychiatric illness. It is usually fairly easy to distinguish delirium from other conditions because of the cardinal features of acute onset and fluctuating course, inattention, and altered level of consciousness. Dementia, for example, tends to have an insidious onset, does not fluctuate significantly, and is characterized neither by inattention nor by an altered level of consciousness. It is important to keep in mind, however, that delirium may coexist with dementia, depression, or other psychiatric illness. Preexisting dementia, for example, is one of the more common and potent risk factors for the development of delirium. If the diagnosis of delirium is not clear in the face of other neuropsychiatric illness, the safest course is to assume that delirium is present, both because delirium may be the only indication that serious illness is present and because the presence of delirium implies that it may be possible to improve the patient's mental status by identifying and treating delirium risk factors.

Evaluation of the Patient with Delirium

Once delirium has been diagnosed, it is critically important to evaluate the patient for the presence of serious illness and other risk factors that might contribute to the development of delirium. This is most often a multifactorial condition, with multiple risk factors potentially implicated in an individual patient. Identifying and treating these risk factors may not only help resolve the delirium but also improve the patient's overall health status. Almost any medical condition may contribute to delirium, but the most commonly implicated conditions and factors in the hospital include medications, infections, fluid and electrolyte disorders, metabolic disorders, congestive heart failure, postoperative state, and drug/alcohol toxicity or withdrawal. Risk factors are described in greater detail in the following text.

The history should seek recent changes in clinical condition, new treatments and interventions, and environmental alterations. Moreover, the history can provide clues about important patient characteristics not previously identified, such as prior cognitive and functional status, history of depression, dementia, or alcohol and/or substance abuse, the presence of pain, adequacy of oral intake, lack of mobility, use of restraints or catheters, and other features. In addition, the history may suggest specific medical causes of altered mental status, such as uremia or hepatic encephalopathy.

The physical examination may reveal abnormal vital signs, evidence of dehydration, congestive heart failure, pneumonia, an intra-abdominal process, or new focal neurologic signs. Clinicians should keep in mind, however, that serious illness may be present even without impressive clinical findings on examination. For example, fever may be absent even in the face of serious infection. Pulmonary and abdominal findings may be subtle in spite of significant disease. Moreover, the physical examination may be difficult to perform if the patient is agitated and confused or if the patient's level of consciousness is substantially abnormal. In particular, it may be difficult to perform a satisfactory screening neurologic examination if the patient is uncooperative. Features such as visual field cuts, cranial nerve findings, and motor deficits may be easier to evaluate and may be more informative than sensory findings.

Medication review is particularly important for the patient with delirium. Medications are implicated in approximately 40% of cases of delirium.[5,12] Potential culprits might include narcotics, psychoactive medications including benzodiazepines, and medications with anticholinergic properties.[33] It is important to keep in mind the fact that some medications used to treat delirium, including antipsychotics such as haloperidol, can also worsen confusion. In addition, many medications not typically considered as anticholinergic may in fact have measurable anticholinergic activity, and it is useful to consider the total cognitive burden of the patient's medications even if no single medication presents itself as an obvious offender. Moreover, previous work has identified the addition of more than three medications in the hospital, regardless of type or name, as a potent independent risk factor for delirium.

Laboratory evaluation should generally be performed but may be targeted depending on the patient's underlying conditions. It is reasonable to check blood counts, serum electrolytes, blood urea nitrogen (BUN) and creatinine, glucose, and calcium in most patients. In patients taking medications that can cause delirium, such as digoxin or lithium, it may be appropriate to check drug levels. Other tests, such as thyroid function tests, may be considered. Lumbar puncture with analysis of cerebrospinal fluid (CSF) may be appropriate in a febrile or septic-appearing patient with delirium if another focus of infection is not obvious. Older patients with bacterial meningitis may present with delirium and without classic signs of meningitis.

Neuroimaging with head CT scan or MRI is not required in every patient with delirium but should be considered for patients who have new focal neurologic findings or diminished responsiveness. Responsive patients with obvious non-neurologic conditions contributing to the delirium and without trauma or focal neurologic signs may not need neuroimaging. MRI may be more sensitive for acute stroke, but head CT scan is often quicker and easier to obtain. The overall yield of neuroimaging tests among hospitalized older patients is low for lesions that alter management.

RISK FACTORS FOR DELIRIUM

Most of the conditions that are often called *causes* of delirium, such as severe illness, use of certain medications, infection, metabolic abnormalities, and others, are probably better viewed as risk factors because some patients with these conditions do not develop delirium. Moreover, conceptualizing delirium as a multi–risk factor condition has important advantages. Many risk factors can be identified before delirium develops, and many of these risk factors can potentially be modified.

A number of studies have evaluated risk factors for the development of delirium.[5,6,24,38–40] The most consistently identified independent risk factors for delirium in hospitalized older patients include preexisting cognitive impairment, severe illness, advanced age, abnormal serum chemistries (e.g., abnormal BUN-to-creatinine ratio and abnormal sodium or potassium levels), alcohol abuse, sensory impairment, and medications.[38]

A useful way to remember risk factors may be to consider the following four categories: Intrinsic patient-risk factors, illness-related risk factors, pharmacologic risk factors, and environmental risk factors (see Table 18.4).[41] Intrinsic patient-risk factors include age, preexisting cognitive impairment, depression, and comorbidity. Illness-related risk factors include severe illness, postoperative state, infection, congestive heart failure, dehydration, and metabolic abnormalities. Pharmacologic risk factors include the use of psychoactive medications, narcotics, or medications with anticholinergic properties. Environmental risk factors include unfamiliar or inappropriate environments (e.g., excessive noise or light) or anything that alters the ability

TABLE 18.4
DIFFERENTIAL DIAGNOSIS: DELIRIUM RISK FACTORS

Intrinsic patient factors	Age Preexisting cognitive impairment Previous delirium Extensive or severe comorbidity
Illness-related factors	Postoperative state (particularly for emergency operations, long operations, orthopaedic or thoracic operations) Infection Congestive heart failure Hypoxemia Metabolic/electrolyte disturbance Dehydration, malnutrition
Pharmacologic factors	Addition of more than three new medications Alcohol or illicit drug use Use of specific medications (e.g., anticholinergic agents, narcotics, benzodiazepines, and psychoactive medications)
Environmental factors	Sensory extremes (i.e., too hot or too cold) Vision or hearing impairment Immobility, including use of mobility-restricting devices (e.g., bladder catheter, physical restraints) Social isolation Unfamiliar environment

Categories adapted from Meagher D. Delirium: Optimizing management. *BMJ.* 2001;322:144–149.

TABLE 18.5
DELIRIUM RISK FACTOR PNEUMONIC

*D*ementia
*E*lectrolyte abnormalities
*L*ung, liver, heart, kidney, or brain illness
*I*nfection
*R*x—multiple medications, psychoactive medications
*I*njury, pain, or stress
*U*nfamiliar environment, inability to interact with environment (hearing or vision loss)
*M*etabolic disturbance

to interact with the environment (e.g., sensory impairment due to hearing or vision impairment or immobility due to use of catheters or restraints). An alternative way of remembering risk factors is to use a pneumonic such as that contained in Table 18.5.

Predisposing and Precipitating Risk Factors

Sharon Inouye has published important studies identifying separate predisposing[6] and precipitating[5] risk factors for delirium. Predisposing risk factors are present before hospitalization and alter a patient's baseline vulnerability. In effect, they "set the patient up" for delirium by making the patient more vulnerable to noxious insults in the hospital. The four independent predisposing risk factors identified by Inouye include vision impairment (adjusted relative risk 3.5), severe illness (adjusted relative risk 3.5), cognitive impairment (adjusted relative risk 2.8), and dehydration (adjusted relative risk 2.0). Precipitating risk factors are the noxious insults happening in the hospital that may precipitate delirium in vulnerable hosts. The five independent precipitating risk factors identified by Inouye include use of physical restraints (adjusted relative risk 4.4), malnutrition (adjusted relative risk 4.0), addition of more than three new medications (adjusted relative risk 2.9), placement of a bladder catheter (adjusted relative risk 2.4), and any iatrogenic event (adjusted relative risk 1.9). Table 18.6 lists the predisposing and precipitating risk factors identified in Inouye's studies.

One of the implications of the interaction of predisposing and precipitating risk factors is that a highly vulnerable patient (e.g., an 80-year-old patient with mild cognitive impairment, presbycusis, macular degeneration, mobility-limiting arthritis, and multiple medications) may require only a trivial insult in the hospital (e.g., use of certain medications or development of a urinary tract infection) to trigger delirium. Conversely, a patient who is not very vulnerable (a 60-year-old patient who is fit and physically active, without cognitive impairment, and not on medication) may require a substantially noxious insult before delirium develops.

Postoperative Delirium

Marcantonio et al. and others have identified risk factors for postoperative patients.[42–44] These risk factors include age >70 years; history of self-reported alcohol abuse; poor cognitive status; poor functional status; abnormal preoperative

TABLE 18.6
PREDISPOSING AND PRECIPITATING RISK FACTORS

Predisposing risk factors	Visual impairment	Adj RR 3.5
	Severe illness	Adj RR 3.5
	Cognitive impairment	Adj RR 2.8
	Dehydration	Adj RR 2.0
Risk of delirium with	0 Predisposing risk factors	3%–9%
	1–2 Predisposing risk factors	16%–23%
	3–4 Predisposing risk factors	32%–83%
Precipitating risk factors	Physical restraints	Adj RR 4.4
	Malnutrition	Adj RR 4.0
	More than three new medications	Adj RR 2.9
	Bladder catheter	Adj RR 2.4
	Any iatrogenic event	Adj RR 1.9
Risk of delirium with	0 Precipitating risk factors	3%–4%
	1–2 Precipitating risk factors	20%
	3–5 Precipitating risk factors	35%–59%

Adj RR, adjusted relative risk.
Inouye SK, Charpentier PA. Precipitating factors for delirium in hospitalized elderly persons. Predictive model and interrelationship with baseline vulnerability. *JAMA*. 1996;275:852–857; Inouye SK, Viscoli CM, Horwitz RI, et al. A predictive model for delirium in hospitalized elderly medical patients based on admission characteristics. *Ann Intern Med*. 1993;119:474–481.

sodium, potassium, or glucose level; noncardiac thoracic surgery; and aortic aneurysm surgery.[45] As with other sets of risk factors, the risk of postoperative delirium increases substantially as the number of risk factors possessed by an individual patient increases.

PREVENTION OF DELIRIUM

The first large, controlled clinical trial to demonstrate conclusively that it is possible to prevent delirium was published in 1999 by Inouye et al.[46] This study was based on previous clinical epidemiologic studies identifying common and potentially modifiable risk factors for delirium and on the notion, already demonstrated in preventing falls, that a targeted multicomponent intervention is the appropriate strategy for preventing complex multi–risk factor conditions such as delirium. The Delirium Prevention Trial focused on six specific risk factors for delirium: Cognitive impairment, sleep deprivation, immobility, visual impairment, hearing impairment, and dehydration. Each of these risk factors was chosen because, in addition to being common and potentially modifiable, the requisite interventions were feasible, did not require expensive or complex technology, and were plausibly transportable. Interventions were performed by a team of nurses and staff and specially trained volunteers.

For each risk factor in the Delirium Prevention Trial, a standardized intervention protocol was developed. For cognitive impairment, the protocol contained two components: An orientation protocol (use of a board with names of care-team members and the day's schedule and communication to reorient to surroundings) and a therapeutic activities protocol (cognitive stimulation activities such as current events discussion or structured reminiscence). For sleep deprivation, the protocol also contained two components: A nonpharmacologic sleep protocol (including warm noncaffeinated drink, relaxation tapes or music, and a back massage) and a unit-wide sleep-enhancement protocol (including silent pill crushers, vibrating beepers, quiet hallways, and rescheduling of medications and procedures). For immobility, the protocol focused on early mobilization with ambulation whenever possible and range-of-motion exercises when not, as well as active attempts to minimize use of mobility-restricting devices such as catheters or restraints. For visual impairment, the protocol focused on provision of visual aids (e.g., glasses or magnifying lenses) and adaptive equipment (e.g., large illuminated telephone keypads) with reinforcement of their use. For hearing impairment, the protocol focused on provision of portable amplifying devices, earwax removal, and communication techniques, with reinforcement of their use. And for dehydration, the protocol focused on early recognition of dehydration and volume repletion, with encouragement of oral fluid intake when appropriate. Each intervention component was targeted at patients with the specified impairment (e.g., patients without visual impairment would not receive the visual impairment protocol). All patients received cognitive and mobility attention at least once daily, with impaired patients receiving the protocols three times daily.

The results of the Delirium Prevention Trial (see Table 18.7) demonstrated a clinically and statistically significant reduction in the incidence of delirium, with an odds ratio of 0.60 ($p = 0.02$). Moreover, the trial resulted in fewer total days of delirium ($p = 0.02$) and

TABLE 18.7
TARGETED INTERVENTIONS FROM THE DELIRIUM PREVENTION TRIAL

Risk Factor	Intervention	Description
Cognitive impairment	Reorientation	Board with names of care-team members and daily schedule; reorienting communication
	Therapeutic activities	Cognitively stimulating activities (e.g., current events discussion, structured reminiscence, word games)
Mobility impairment	Early mobility	Ambulation or active range-of-motion exercises; minimal use of immobilizing equipment (e.g., bladder catheters, restraints)
Sleep deprivation	Unit-wide noise reduction	Unit-wide noise-reduction strategies (e.g., silent pill crushers, vibrating beeper, quiet hallways) and schedule adjustments (e.g., rescheduling of medications and procedures)
	Nonpharmacologic sleep promotion	Warm drink at bedtime, relaxation tapes or music, back massage
Vision impairment	Vision enhancement	Visual aids (e.g., glasses or magnifying lenses) and adaptive equipment (e.g., large illuminated telephone, large-print books, and fluorescent tape on call bell), with daily reinforcement on use
Hearing impairment	Hearing enhancement	Portable amplifying devices, earwax disimpaction, special communication techniques, with daily reinforcement on use
Dehydration	Rehydration	Early recognition of dehydration and volume repletion (i.e., encouragement of oral fluid intake)

From Inouye SK, Bogardus ST, Charpentier PA, et al. A multicomponent intervention to prevent delirium in hospitalized older patients. *N Engl J Med.* 1999;340:669–676.

fewer total episodes of delirium ($p = 0.03$). However, the trial did not reduce the severity of delirium in patients who developed the condition. Further work has since demonstrated that the intervention is cost effective.[47] Interestingly, most of the effect of the intervention was found in patients at intermediate risk for delirium, not high risk (low-risk patients were not enrolled in the trial). This suggests that it is possible to change the clinical course of delirium in patients who have elevated risk for an adverse outcome such as delirium but that patients at high risk may be so vulnerable to delirium that a successful intervention must be extraordinarily potent to prevent delirium.

The intervention has expanded into a program, the Hospital Elder Life Program (HELP), focused broadly on preserving cognitive and functional status in hospitalized older patients.[48] The HELP program, which has gained wide distribution, has demonstrated beneficial effects on cognitive status (as measured by decline in Mini-Mental State Examination scores) and functional status (as measured by activities of daily living) (Evidence Level B).

Two other recent trials have evaluated strategies to prevent delirium after hip fracture, occurring in 35% to 65% of such patients. A study by Marcantonio et al.[49] using a proactive geriatrics consultation intervention, demonstrated a clinically and statistically significant reduction in delirium, with a relative risk of 0.64 (95% confidence interval 0.37 to 0.98). One case of delirium was prevented for every 5.6 patients in the intervention group. Moreover, this study appeared to show an especially large reduction in cases of severe delirium, with a relative risk of 0.40 (95% confidence interval 0.18 to 0.89). Subgroup analyses suggest that the intervention was most effective for patients without preexisting cognitive or functional impairment. The intervention in this study consisted of daily geriatrician visits, with targeted recommendations made on the basis of a structured protocol. The protocol contained ten standardized modules addressing the following clinical issues: (i) Oxygenation, (ii) fluid/electrolyte balance, (iii) pain treatment, (iv) elimination of unnecessary medications, (v) bowel/bladder function, (vi) nutritional intake, (vii) early mobilization and rehabilitation, (viii) major postoperative complications, (ix) appropriate environmental stimulus, and (x) treatment of agitated delirium. An average of ten recommendations per intervention patient were made during the course of hospitalization. (Evidence Level B)

A second study by Milisen et al.,[50] employed a nurse-led interdisciplinary intervention program. The intervention in this study relied on staff resource nurses for delirium, who were specially trained in identification and management of older patients with hip fracture who were at risk for delirium. In addition, the intervention carried a special emphasis on appropriate pain control. This study did not demonstrate a reduction in the incidence of delirium but did show a reduction in its duration and severity for the intervention group, as well as suggesting higher cognitive functioning and a shorter length of stay.

TREATMENT OF DELIRIUM

Unlike studies of prevention, trials of delirium treatment have not demonstrated substantially positive results. Some

TABLE 18.8
ENVIRONMENTAL INTERVENTIONS FOR PATIENTS WITH DELIRIUM

Provide support and orientation	Communicate clearly and frequently Provide signposts (e.g., clock, calendar, and chart) Provide familiar objects from home Ensure consistency of staff Involve family and caregivers
Provide unambiguous environment	Remove unnecessary objects Consider single room near nursing station Provide adequate lighting Control excess noise Keep room temperature appropriate
Maintain competence	Identify/correct hearing/vision impairment Encourage self-care Allow uninterrupted sleep Maintain activity and ambulation

Adapted from Meagher D. Delirium: Optimizing management. *BMJ.* 2001;322:144–149.

limited studies have suggested a role for antipsychotic medication in certain patients. A recent randomized clinical trial of a multidisciplinary intervention by Cole et al.[13] failed to demonstrate greater benefit than usual care in terms of time to cognitive improvement or other outcomes. This trial employed an intervention based on systematic detection and multidisciplinary care of delirium in older patients admitted to a general medical service. The negative results of this trial, in contrast to the positive results of some prevention trials, suggest that the most effective strategy in dealing with delirium may be to prevent it in the first place.

Nonetheless, there are several reasons why it is important to treat delirium once it occurs. The first is that delirium may be the only indication of serious underlying illness, and recognition and treatment of delirium may lead to recognition and treatment of underlying illness. The second is that the type of care employed for patients with delirium is, as Rockwood has pointed out,[51] the type of care most of us would like to see for our older relatives. This care is attentive and addresses a number of cross-cutting geriatric issues such as mobility, functional status, cognitive status, sensory impairment, and social interaction.

Nonpharmacologic Approaches to Management

Once the patient has been examined for causes of delirium and the proper interventions have been undertaken to correct medical or metabolic derangement, adjust medication regimens, or intervene in other risk factors, attention should be turned to the management of the delirium itself. Nonpharmacologic approaches should be used for all patients with delirium and should include a number of relatively straightforward and common approaches to provide a suitable environment, frequent orientation, familiarity, clear communication, and suitable activity (see Table 18.8).[41]

For example, the patient should be in a calm, quiet environment with adequate light. Consider moving the patient close to the nursing station and use sitters. Encourage family members to bring in familiar objects and stay with the patient. Provide frequent orientation, with clear, calm communication and face-to-face contact. Keep tasks simple and avoid multiple or confusing stimuli. Try to allow as much uninterrupted time for sleep as possible at night. Use clocks and calendars. Encourage the use of eyeglasses and hearing aids if needed. Encourage mobility and self-care as much as possible and avoid physical restraints (which carry risks of injury and immobility). If a patient does something dangerous such as trying to climb out of bed at night when they have impediments, for example, physical impairment or intravenous lines, consider placing the mattress on the floor rather than using restraints (or use one of the newer hospital beds that are able to descend close to the floor). Try nonpharmacologic approaches for relaxation in the agitated patient, such as music, relaxation tapes, or massage.

Pharmacologic Approaches to Management

In patients in whom the delirium may adversely affect the delivery of important medical therapies or in whom the delirium endangers either the patient or others, it may be necessary to use pharmacologic approaches. There is no ideal drug, so drug choice may be guided by issues such as required route of administration.

Antipsychotic agents are generally preferred to benzodiazepines, which may lead to oversedation or increased confusion. Benzodiazepines should be reserved for various withdrawal syndromes, such as alcohol withdrawal. The traditional agent of choice has been haloperidol, which can be given orally or parenterally. The initial dose of 0.5 to 1.0 mg can be repeated every 20 to 30 minutes until the patient is awake but calm and not oversedated; seldom does one need more than 5.0 mg in the first 24 hours for an elderly patient, and usually less is needed. Efforts should be made to taper the medication over the next several days (Evidence Level C).

There are several newer antipsychotic agents available (e.g., risperidone, olanzapine, and quetiapine), which may also be used depending on the comfort and familiarity of the physician, availability of the medication, and administration routes. Some medications may be available in forms that are easier to use in a patient with delirium. Haloperidol, for example, in addition to being available in parenteral and standard tablet forms, is also available as an oral solution. Olanzapine is available in an orally disintegrating tablet. Keep in mind that any of these agents can cloud mental status, making it difficult to follow the patient's course.

CONCLUSION

Delirium is very common among hospitalized older patients and causes substantial morbidity and increased mortality. Delirium may be particularly common among certain patient populations (e.g., in the ICU and among postsurgical patients). Adverse outcomes linked to delirium include persistent cognitive and functional decline, longer length of stay, increased rates of institutionalization, and higher costs. Mortality in patients with delirium is increased both during hospitalization and after hospitalization. The management of delirium remains challenging and is made more difficult by the fact that delirium is often unrecognized.

Clinical epidemiologic studies have identified risk factors for delirium, many of which are potentially modifiable. Moreover, clinical trials have demonstrated that interventions targeting delirium risk factors can successfully reduce the incidence of delirium, both among older general medical patients and among those with hip fracture. Prevention strategies are closely linked to high-quality hospital care for older patients and are both feasible and cost effective. Although efforts to prevent delirium may stand the best chance of reducing the morbidity associated with delirium, it is important to remember that delirium may be the only indication that a patient has or is developing a serious and urgent medical illness.

Once delirium is recognized, clinicians should perform a targeted evaluation, focusing on treatable medical issues such as inappropriate medication use, infection, congestive heart failure, and metabolic disturbances. All patients with delirium should be placed in a therapeutically appropriate environment, and medications may be used for agitated patients who present a danger to themselves or others. Future research should continue to investigate novel strategies to treat delirium once it occurs.

REFERENCES

1. Inouye SK. Delirium in hospitalized older patients. *Clin Geriatr Med.* 1998;14:745–764.
2. Inouye SK, Schlesinger J, Lydon TJ. Delirium: A symptom of how hospital care is failing older persons and a window to improve quality of hospital care. *Am J Med.* 1999;106:565–573.
3. Francis J, Martin D, Kapoor WN. A prospective study of delirium in hospitalized elderly. *JAMA.* 1990;263:1097–1101.
4. Rockwood K. Acute confusion in elderly medical patients. *J Am Geriatr Soc.* 1989;37:150–154.
5. Inouye SK, Charpentier PA. Precipitating factors for delirium in hospitalized elderly persons. Predictive model and interrelationship with baseline vulnerability. *JAMA.* 1996;275:852–857.
6. Inouye SK, Viscoli CM, Horwitz RI, et al. A predictive model for delirium in hospitalized elderly medical patients based on admission characteristics. *Ann Intern Med.* 1993;119:474–481.
7. McNicoll L, Pisani MA, Zhang Y, et al. Delirium in the intensive care unit: Occurrence and clinical course in older patients. *J Am Geriatr Soc.* 2003;51:591–598.
8. Elie MK, Rousseau F, Cole M, et al. Prevalence and detection of delirium in elderly emergency department patients. *Can Med Assoc J.* 2000;163:977–981.
9. Lawlor PG, Gagnon B, Mancini IL, et al. Occurrence, causes and outcomes of delirium in patients with advanced cancer: A prospective study. *Arch Intern Med.* 2000;160:786–794.
10. Francis J. Delirium in older patients. *J Am Geriatr Soc.* 1992; 40:829–838.
11. Inouye SK, Rushing JT, Foreman MD, et al. Does delirium contribute to poor hospital outcomes? A three-site epidemiologic study. *J Gen Intern Med.* 1998;13:234–242.
12. Inouye SK. The dilemma of delirium: Clinical and research controversies regarding diagnosis and evaluation of delirium in hospitalized elderly medical patients. *Am Jour Med.* 1994;97: 278–288.
13. Cole MG, McCusker J, Bellavance F, et al. Systematic detection and multidisciplinary care of delirium in older medical inpatients: A randomized trial. *Can Med Assoc J.* 2002;167:753–759.
14. McCusker J, Cole M, Dendukuri N, et al. The course of delirium in older medical inpatients: A prospective study. *J Gen Intern Med.* 2003;18:696–704.
15. Cole MG, Primeau FJ. Prognosis of delirium in elderly hospital patients. *Can Med Assoc J.* 1993;149:41–46.
16. McCusker J, Cole M, Abrahamowicz M, et al. Delirium predicts 12-month mortality. *Arch Intern Med.* 2002;162:457–463.
17. Francis J, Kapoor WN. Prognosis after hospital discharge of older medical patients with delirium. *J Am Geriatr Soc.* 1992;40: 601–606.
18. Murray AM, Levkoff SE, Eetle TT, et al. Acute delirium and functional decline in hospitalized elderly patients. *J Gerontol.* 1993;48:M181–M186.
19. Levkoff SE, Evans DA, Liptzin B, et al. Delirium. The occurrence and persistence of symptoms among elderly hospitalized patients. *Arch Inter Med.* 1992;152:334–340.
20. O'Keefe S, Lavan J. The prognostic significance of delirium in older hospital patients. *J Am Geriatr Soc.* 1997;45:174–178.
21. Milbrandt EB, Deppen S, Harrison PL, et al. Costs associated with delirium in mechanically ventilated patients. *Crit Care Med.* 2004;32:955–962.
22. Franco K, Litaker D, Locala J, et al. The cost of delirium in the surgical patient. *Psychosomatics.* 2001;42:68–73.
23. Rabins PV, Folstein MF. Delirium and dementia: Diagnostic criteria and fatality rates. *Br J Psych.* 1982;140:149–153.
24. Pompei P, Foreman M, Rudberg MA, et al. Delirium in hospitalized older persons: Outcomes and predictors. *J Am Geriatr Soc.* 1994;42:809–815.
25. Lin SM, Liu CY, Wang CH, et al. The impact of delirium on the survival of mechanically ventilated patients. *Crit Care Med.* 2004;32:2254–2259.
26. Edelstein DM, Aharonoff GB, Karp A, et al. Effect of postoperative delirium on outcome after hip fracture. *Clin Orthop.* 2004; 422:195–200.
27. Rockwood K, Cosway S, Carver D, et al. The risk of dementia and death after delirium. *Age Ageing.* 1999;28:551–556.

28. Trzepacz PT. The neuropathogenesis of delirium: A need to focus our research. *Psychosomatics*. 1994;35:374–341.
29. Trzepacz PT. Update on the neuropathogenesis of delirium. *Dement Geriatr Cogn Disord*. 1999;10:330–334.
30. Flacker JM, Lipsitz LA. Neural Mechanisms of delirium: Current hypothesis and evolving concepts. *J Gerontol*. 1999;54A: B239–B246.
31. Tune L, Carr S, Hoag E, et al. Anticholinergic effects of drugs commonly prescribed for the elderly: Potential means for assessing risk of delirium. *Am J Psychiatry*. 1993;149: 1393–1394.
32. Mach JR, Dysken MW, Kuskowski M, et al. Serum anticholinergic activity in hospitalized older persons with delirium: A preliminary study. *J Am Geriatr Soc*. 1995;43:491–495.
33. Moore AR, O'Keeffe ST. Drug-induced cognitive impairment in the elderly. *Drugs Aging*. 1999;15:15–28.
34. American Psychiatric Association. *Diagnostic and statistical manual of mental disorders*, 4th ed. text revision, Washington, DC: American Psychiatric Association; 2000.
35. Folstein MF, Folstein SE, McHugh PR. "Mini-mental state." A practical method for grading the cognitive state of patients for the clinician. *J Psychiatr Res*. 1975;12:189–198.
36. Inouye SK, vanDyck CH, Alessi CA, et al. Clarifying confusion: The confusion assessment method, a new method for detection of delirium. *Ann Intern Med*. 1990;113:941–948.
37. Ely EW, Inouye SK, Bernard GR, et al. Delirium in mechanically ventilated patients: Validity and reliability of the confusion assessment method for the intensive care unit (CAM-ICU). *JAMA*. 2001;286:2703–2710.
38. Elie M, Cole MG, Primeau FJ, et al. Delirium risk factors in elderly hospitalized patients. *J Gen Med*. 1998;13:204–212.
39. McCusker J, Cole M, Abrahamowicz M, et al. Environmental risk factors for delirium in hospitalized older people. *J Am Geriatr Soc*. 2001;49:1327–1334.
40. Schor JD, Levkoff SE, Lipsitz LA, et al. Risk factors for delirium in hospitalized elderly. *JAMA*. 1992;267:827–831.
41. Meagher D. Delirium: Optimizing management. *Brit Med Jour*. 2001;322:144–149.
42. Marcantonio ER, Goldman L, Mangione CM, et al. A clinical prediction rule for delirium after elective noncardiac surgery. *JAMA*. 1994;271:134–139.
43. Marcantonio ER, Goldman L, Orav EJ, et al. The association of intraoperative factors with the development of postoperative delirium. *Am J Med*. 1998;105:380–384.
44. Pompei P, Foreman M, Rudberg MA, et al. Delirium in hospitalized older persons: Outcomes and predictors. *J Am Geriatr Soc*. 1994;42:809–815.
45. Williams-Russo P, Urquhart RN, Sharrock ME, et al. Postoperative delirium: Predictors and prognosis in elderly orthopedic patients. *J Am Geriatr Soc*. 1992;40:759–767.
46. Inouye SK, Bogardus ST, Charpentier PA, et al. A multicomponent intervention to prevent delirium in hospitalized older patients. *N Engl J Med*. 1999;340:669–676.
47. Rizzo J, Bogardus ST, Leo-Summers L, et al. Multicomponent targeted intervention to prevent delirium in hospitalized older persons. *Med Care*. 2001;39:740–752.
48. Inouye SK, Bogardus ST, Baker DI, et al. The hospital elder life program: A model of care to prevent cognitive and functional decline in older hospitalized patients. *J Am Geriatr Soc*. 2000; 48:1697–1706.
49. Marcantonio E, Flacker J, Wright RJ, et al. Reducing delirium after hip fracture: A randomized trial. *J Am Geriatr Soc*. 2001; 49:516–522.
50. Milisen K, Foreman M, Abraham I, et al. A nurse-led interdisciplinary intervention program for delirium in elderly hip-fracture patients. *J Am Geriatr Soc*. 2001;49:523–532.
51. Rockwood K. Out of the furrow and into the fire: Where do we go with delirium? *Can Med Assoc J*. 2002;167:763–764.

Chronic Memory Impairment

19

Thomas C. Rosenthal

CLINICAL PEARLS 236

NORMAL MEMORY AGING 237
Screening 239

SYMPTOMS AND SIGNS OF DEMENTIA 239

DIFFERENTIAL DIAGNOSIS 241
Depression 242

ALZHEIMER DISEASE 242
Definition 242
Pathophysiology 243
Incidence and Prevalence 243
Genetics 244
Time Course of Alzheimer Disease 244
Workup/Keys to Diagnosis 244
Laboratory 245
Management 245

NON-ALZHEIMER DISEASE DEMENTIA 247
Vascular Dementia 247
Lewy Body Dementia 248
Dementia Associated with Parkinson Disease 248
Frontotemporal Dementia 248
White Matter Dementia 249
Mixed Dementia 249

OTHER CAUSES OF DEMENTIA 249

BEHAVIORAL PROBLEMS IN DEMENTIA 250

CAREGIVERS 251

CONCLUSION 252

CLINICAL PEARLS

- The prevalence of dementia doubles every 5 years over 60 years of age, accounting for half of all skilled nursing facility admissions.
- Forgetting what things are used for, becoming unable to understand simple instructions or getting lost in familiar surroundings represent thresholds for the diagnosis of dementia.
- Performance of novel tasks recruits larger areas of the frontal lobe and hippocampus than does repetition of activities such as counting.
- Using formal inventories such as the Mini-Mental State Examination (MMSE), Pfeiffer Short Portable Mental Status Questionnaire and the clock test to score patients can reveal dementia earlier.
- As scores on the MMSE drop below 24, nonroutine functions become impaired.
- Alzheimer disease is characterized by gradual loss of memory that is serious enough to interfere with social function.
- One secretase subtype cleaves the amyloid precursor proteins to form insoluble β-amyloid, which clings to the cell wall as a barnacle-like plaque and generates an inflammatory response.
- β-amyloid plaques activate enzymes that damage intracellular microtubules through hyperphosphorylation of tau protein. The tubules twist into compact neurofibrillary tangles that act like foreign bodies within the cell.
- Gene typing is commercially available, but variable expression limits its use as a prognostic indicator.
- A computed tomography (CT) scan or a magnetic resonance imaging (MRI) study of the head should be obtained in most patients once during the workup,

TABLE 19.1
THE DIFFERENTIAL DIAGNOSIS OF DEMENTIA

Structural (ICD-9)	Metabolic (ICD-9)	Infectious (ICD-9)
Alzheimer disease (331.0)[a]	B_{12} deficiency (281.0)	Endocarditis (421.0)
Amyotrophic lateral sclerosis (335.20)	Chronic drug/alcohol nutritional abuse (305.00)	Creutzfeldt-Jakob disease (046.1)
Brain trauma (854)	Hyperparathyroidism (252.0)	HIV-related disorders (042)
Brain tumor (191)	Hypothyroidism (244.0)	Neurosyphilis (090)
Cerebellar degeneration (331.9)	Hepatic encephalopathy (572.2)	Tuberculous and fungal meningitis (322.9)
Communicating hydrocephalus (331.0)	Uremic encephalopathy (585)	Viral encephalitis (049.9)
Dementia with depression (290.21)[a]	Respiratory encephalopathy (496)	Dementia NOS (290.0)
Huntington disease (333.4)	Pellagra (265.2)	
Irradiation to frontal lobes (990)		
Lewy body dementia (294.8)[a]		
Multiple sclerosis (340)		
Parkinson disease (332.0)		
Pick disease (331.1)[a]		
Supranuclear palsy (333.0)		
Vascular disease (290.4)[a]		
White matter dementia (349.9)[a]		
Wilson disease (275.1)		

[a]Subjects covered in this chapter.
HIV, human immunodeficiency virus; NOS, not otherwise specified.

particularly if the dementia is associated with rapid onset or focal neurologic signs.

- Cholinesterase inhibitors are the principal pharmacologic therapy available today but they have a low therapeutic index and a wide variation of individual response.
- Lewy body dementia frequently presents with parkinsonian signs, visual hallucinations, and verbal difficulty.
- Vascular dementia is associated with focal neurologic signs and gait instability.
- Frontotemporal dementia presents as word-finding problems and loss of social prudence.
- Low-pressure hydrocephalus presents with blunting of personality, shuffle gait, and urinary incontinence.
- Two thirds of patients have multiple causes for dementia on autopsy.
- Trazodone is a commonly used agent for elderly patients requiring nighttime sedation.

Dementia is cognitive brain failure. The cognitive deficits are manifested by memory impairment (inability to learn new information) and associated with a disturbance in language (aphasia), impaired motor ability (apraxia), inability to identify objects (agnosia), and/or a disturbance in executive functioning (planning, organizing, sequencing, abstracting). To be classified as dementia these defects must impair social or occupational function and represent a decline from a previous level of functioning. Forty percent of people older than 80 years suffer dementia.

Some decline in recall is a normal part of aging, as is a decline in taste, olfaction, vision, and hearing. Healthy elderly people compensate for forgetfulness by writing reminders, putting everything back in its place, and creating other memory aids. Forgetting what things are used for, becoming unable to understand simple instructions, or getting lost in familiar surroundings are often the thresholds for unmasking dementia.

The prevalence of dementia doubles every 5 years after 60 years of age, accounting for half of all skilled nursing facility admissions.[1] Home care for patients with dementia costs $3,000 per year.[2] Alzheimer disease is the most common cause of dementia in the elderly but it accounts for only 65% of cognitive failure. A number of diseases, listed on Table 19.1, can damage the cerebral cortex and subcortical gray matter, and cause cognitive decline. Optimism for future intervention lies in the plasticity exhibited by the human brain. Today's treatments supplement brain chemistry; tomorrow's will protect or rebuild structure. This chapter focuses on the differential diagnosis of dementia leading to appropriate choice of management options for patients at risk for progressive dementia.

NORMAL MEMORY AGING

Memory and cognition are dependent on adequate, responsive growth in brain structure. Positron emission tomography (PET) studies of regional cerebral blood flow in subjects learning new tasks demonstrate that memory and recall require frontal lobe and hippocampal activity. Performing novel tasks recruits larger areas of the frontal lobe and hippocampus than does repetition, as demonstrated by London cab drivers who show enlargement of the hippocampus on magnetic resonance imaging (MRI) during their first year of learning the city's

TABLE 19.2
MINI-MENTAL STATE EXAMINATION (TO BE COMPLETED BY A TRAINED CLINICIAN)

PATIENT NAME: ____________ DATE: ________ TIME (24hr): ________

Birthdate (mm): (dd): (yyyy):

Sex: [ ] Male [ ] Female Enter education (years):

Race: [ ] Caucasian [ ] Black [ ] Hispanic [ ] Asian [ ] Other

Orientation Questions: Ask the following questions:

right/ wrong

[ ] [ ] 1. What is today's date?
[ ] [ ] 2. What is the month?
[ ] [ ] 3. What is the year?
[ ] [ ] 4. What day of the week is today?
[ ] [ ] 5. What season is it? DATE
[ ] [ ] 6. What is the name of this clinic (place)?
[ ] [ ] 7. What floor are we on?
[ ] [ ] 8. What city are we in?
[ ] [ ] 9. What county are we in?
[ ] [ ] 10. What state are we in? PLACE

IMMEDIATE RECALL: Ask the subject if you may test his/her memory. Then say "ball", "flag", "tree" clearly and slowly, about 1 second for each. After you have said all 3 words, ask him/her to repeat them. The first repetition determines the score (0–3), but keep saying them until he/she can repeat all 3, up to 6 tries. If he/she does not eventually learn all 3, recall cannot be meaningfully tested:

[ ] [ ] 11. BALL
[ ] [ ] 12. FLAG
[ ] [ ] 13. TREE Note # trials: IMMEDIATE RECALL:

ATTENTION

A) Ask the subject to begin with 100 and count backwards by 7. Stop after 5 subtractions. Score the correct subtractions.

[ ] [ ] 14. "93"
[ ] [ ] 15. "86"
[ ] [ ] 16. "79"
[ ] [ ] 17. "72"
[ ] [ ] 18. "65" SERIAL 7's TOTAL:

B) Ask the subject to spell the word "WORLD" backwards. The score is the number of letters in correct position. For example, "DLROW" is 5, "DLORW" is 3, "LROWD" is 0.

[ ] [ ] 19. "D"
[ ] [ ] 20. "L"
[ ] [ ] 21. "R"
[ ] [ ] 22. "O"
[ ] [ ] 23. "W" "DLROW" TOTAL: Greater score of A or B:

DELAYED VERBAL RECALL: Ask the subject to recall the 3 words you previously asked him/her to remember.

[ ] [ ] 24. BALL?
[ ] [ ] 25. FLAG?
[ ] [ ] 26. TREE? DELAYED VERBAL RECALL:

NAMING: Show the subject a wrist watch and ask him/her what it is. Repeat for pencil.

[ ] [ ] 27. WATCH
[ ] [ ] 28. PENCIL
[ ] [ ] 29. REPETITION (Ask patient to repeat items in 24, 25 and 26)

3-STAGE COMMAND: Give the subject a plain piece of paper and say, "Take the paper in your hand, fold it in half, and put it on the floor."

[ ] [ ] 30. TAKES
[ ] [ ] 31. FOLDS
[ ] [ ] 32. PUTS

(continued)

TABLE 19.2
(continued)

READING: Hold up a card reading, "Close your eyes", so the subject can see it clearly. Ask him/her to read it and do what it says. Score correctly only if the subject actually closes his/her eyes.

[ ] [ ] 33. CLOSES EYES

WRITING: Give subject a piece of paper and ask him/her to write a sentence. It is to be written spontaneously. It must contain a subject and verb and be sensible. Correct grammar and punctuation are not necessary.

[ ] [ ] 34. SENTENCE LANGUAGE:
[ ] [ ] 35. DRAW PENTAGONS

TOTAL MMSE:________________

(MMSE maximum score = 30; 24–30 normal, depending on age, education, complaints; 20–23 mild; 10–19 moderate; 1–9 severe; 0 profound.)

MEDAFILE.COM

(calculation derived from Ashford et al., 1995; Mendiondo et al., 2000)

(forms are in public domain; HTML scripted by Ashford, JW, copyright 2000)

streets.[3] Elderly subjects with mild memory loss and MRI evidence of depleted hippocampal volume are most likely to progress to dementia.

New memory is associated with an increase in the thousands of dendritic synapses each neuron already projects. Healthy elderly people, especially those with high intellectual achievement, have a greater number of memory dendrites available for alternate pathways and recall. When a processing deficiency arises, their brain networks compensate. The velocity of function is biochemical and under the influence of fatigue, nutrition, and mood.

The ability to memorize decreases with age but other cognitive functions remain relatively intact in the healthy individual. Recall may be more labored and the names of familiar persons may not leap to the lips but they are usually recovered with time. In fact, given time, the intellectual performance of healthy elderly people is usually equivalent to earlier years.

Mild cognitive impairment is common. A quarter of community-based elderly demonstrate abnormal scores on a mental state examination without previous evidence of dementia. Most patients who score 24/30 or better on the Mini-Mental State Examination (MMSE) are able to carry out activities of daily living with acceptable adjustments. Family members may first perceive a disability when the patient fails to appear for appointments arranged over the telephone. Progression of mild cognitive impairment is highly variable, and many patients will not progress. Those most likely to progress are older, suffer coexisting cardiovascular disease, have fewer years of education, are undernourished, or have hippocampal atrophy.

Screening

The U.S. Preventive Services Task Force does not recommend for or against routine screening for dementia in older adults because of insufficient evidence of benefit. Early recognition of dementia will become more important as effective pharmacologic agents become available in the future. At present we must rely on family reports of subtle changes in function or behavior. Six items derived from the MMSE can be used to screen patients. The patient who can recall three items (e.g., ball, flag, tree) in 1 minute and correctly state the day of week, month, and year will likely score 24 or above on the MMSE (sensitivity 88.7; specificity 88).[4] The MMSE (see Table 19.2), Pfeiffer's Short Portable Mental Status Questionnaire (see Table 19.3), and the clock-drawing test (see Fig. 19.1) are validated examinations that are generally accepted by patients.[5–7] The clock test is more sensitive than the others but less precise in scoring. (The Original Folstein Mini-Mental State Exam is protected by copyright and available from Psychological Assessment Resources, Inc., 16204 North Florida Avenue, Lutz, Florida 33549, or by calling (800) 331-8378. A modified version is available online at www.medafile.com.)

Adults with mental retardation and other chronic intellectual disabilities live longer and create unique challenges as they age. On an average these patients may experience dementia 10 years earlier than the general population. Several screening tools using informant observation have been developed that can assist in recognizing dementia in this special group of adults.[8]

SYMPTOMS AND SIGNS OF DEMENTIA

The earliest sign of dementia, especially the Alzheimer disease type, may be loss of imagination, emotional lability, and eventual withdrawal as the patient becomes frustrated with the challenge of recalling recent events. The family may notice that the patient forgets phone calls or those present at dinner the previous night. A high functioning person ritualistically replaces keys and writes

TABLE 19.3
SHORT PORTABLE MENTAL STATUS QUESTIONNAIRE—SPMSQ-PFEIFFER

Instructions: Ask questions 1–10 in this list and record all answers. Ask question 4A only if the patient does not have a telephone. Record the number of errors based on ten questions.

+	−		
___	___	1.	What is the date today? Month Day Year
___	___	2.	What day of the week is it?____________
___	___	3.	What is the name of this place?____________
___	___	4.	What is your telephone number?____________
___	___	4A.	What is your street address?____________ (Ask only if the patient does not have a telephone.)
___	___	5.	How old are you?____________
___	___	6.	When were you born?____________
___	___	7.	Who is the President of the United States now?____________
___	___	8.	Who was President before him?____________
___	___	9.	What was your mother's maiden name?____________
___	___	10.	Subtract 3 from 20 and keep subtracting 3 from each new number, all the way down

________ Total number of Errors

To Be Completed by Interviewer

Patient's Name:____________________ Date:

____

Sex: ________ Male
________ Female

Years of Education: ________
________ Grade school
________ High school
________ Beyond high school

Race: ______ White
______ Black
______ Other

Interviewee's Name: ____________________

Instructions for Completion of the Short Portable Mental Status Questionnaire

All responses to be scored as correct must be given by the subject without reference to the calendar, newspaper, birth certificate, or other aids to memory.

Question 1 is to be scored as correct only when the exact month, date, and year are given correctly.
Question 2 is self-explanatory.
Question 3 should be scored as correct if any correct description of the location is given. "My home", correct name of the town or city of residence, or the name of hospital or institution if the subject is institutionalized are all acceptable.
Question 4 should be scored as correct when the correct telephone number can be verified, or when the subject can repeat the same number at another point in the questioning.
Question 5 is scored as correct when stated age corresponds to the date of birth.
Question 6 is to be scored as correct only when the month, exact date, and year are all given.
Question 7 requires only the last name of the President.
Question 8 requires only the last name of the previous President.
Question 9 does not need to be verified. It is scored as correct if a female first name plus a last name other that subject's last name is given.
Question 10 requires that the entire series must be performed correctly to be scored as correct. Any error in the series or unwillingness to attempt the series is scored as incorrect.

Scoring of the Short Portable Mental Status Questionnaire

The data suggest that both education and race influence performance on the Mental Status Questionnaire and they must accordingly be taken into account while evaluating the score attained by an individual.

For purposes of scoring, three educational levels have been established:
1. Persons who have had only a grade school education
2. Persons who have had any high school education or who have completed high school
3. Persons who have had any education beyond the high school level, including college, graduate school, or business school.

(continued)

TABLE 19.3
(continued)

For white subjects with at least some high school education but not more than high school education, the following criteria have been established:
0–2 errors—Intact intellectual functioning
3–4 errors—Mild intellectual impairment
5–7 errors—Moderate intellectual impairment
8–10 errors—Severe intellectual impairment

Allow one more error if subject has had only a grade school education.
Allow one less error if subject has had education beyond high school.
Allow one more error for black subjects, using identical educational criteria.

From Pfeiffer E. A short portable mental status questionnaire for the assessment of organic brain deficit in elder patients. *J Am Geriatric Soc.* 1975;23:433–41.

notes, and when they are forced to forgo a ritual they become anxious. Conversation becomes blunted as abstract thinking wanes. The patient begins to rely on the bank to balance their checkbook, avoiding the embarrassment of disputed arithmetic.

As dementia progresses and scores on the MMSE drop below 24, daily function becomes impaired. The patient may get lost in familiar territory, and wandering may become a problem. Recall of remote events is compromised, but not completely lost. As the MMSE drops below 19, personal hygiene suffers and the anxiety created by confusion may express itself as aggression.

As the MMSE drops below 12, the patient is unable to perform activities of daily living and becomes incontinent, at least intermittently. The patient becomes mute because recall is severely compromised. Walking becomes unbalanced and less spontaneous. Sleep patterns become fragmented and haphazard. Expected sensations of hunger and later thirst seem to fail. Below an MMSE score of 9, a blunted febrile and leukocyte response to infection further complicates diagnosing pneumonia or cystitis.

While this linear depiction of Alzheimer disease progression is overly simplified and individually variable, in the terminal phase Alzheimer disease and other structural dementia look much alike. They are terminal illnesses with predictable patterns and should be managed with the support and attention appropriate to any terminal illness. Seizures, coma, and death are common final pathways, often accompanied by sepsis from pneumonia or urinary tract infection.

DIFFERENTIAL DIAGNOSIS

The late stages of dementia are hard to differentiate by clinical examination. The clinician's challenge is to make the correct diagnosis in the early stages when specific intervention may be possible (Table 19.1 lists conditions associated with dementia in the elderly). Alzheimer disease is characterized by gradual loss of memory. Lewy body dementia frequently presents with parkinsonian signs, and upon questioning many patients describe visual hallucinations. Vascular dementia is associated with focal neurologic signs and falling. Frontotemporal dementia starts earlier, with loss of social prudence. Many, if not most, elderly patients will have a dementia of multiple causes, blurring the diagnostic distinctions.

Causes of delirium are discussed in Chapter 18. Delirium develops rapidly and characteristically impacts the patient's

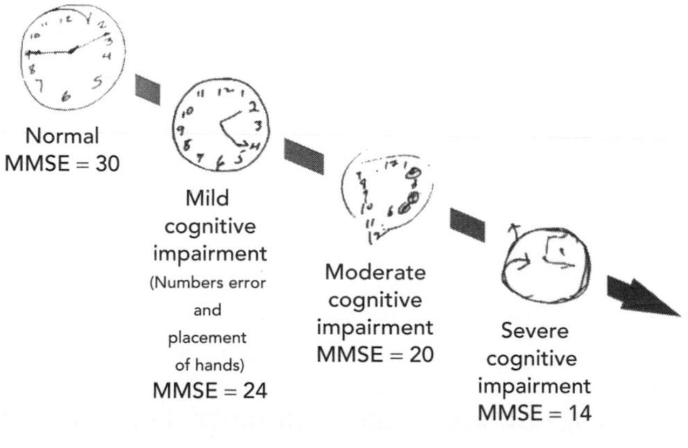

Figure 19.1 Clock drawing. Instructions: "Draw a clock with all the numbers on it. Then put hands on the clock to make it read 2:45."

TABLE 19.4
BRIEF DEPRESSION SCREEN

Over the past 2 weeks, how often have you been bothered by any of the following problems?

1. Little interest or pleasure in doing things
   0: Not at all
   1: Several days
   2: More than half the days
   3: Nearly every day
2. Feeling down, depressed, or hopeless
   0: Not at all
   1: Several days
   2: More than half the days
   3: Nearly every day

Score Interpretation

Score	Probability of Major Depressive Disorder (%)	Probability of Any Depressive Disorder (%)
1	15.4	36.9
2	21.1	48.3
3	38.4	75.0
4	45.5	81.2
5	56.4	84.6
6	78.6	92.9

From Thibault JM, Steiner RW. Efficient identification of adults with depression and dementia. *Am Fam Physician.* 2004;70(6):1101–1110.

attention. The course is fluctuating and usually reversible. Delirium may be because of a systemic medical disease or drugs, and should elicit urgent evaluation and treatment.

Depression

Patients should be screened for depression, a condition difficult to recognize in a brief visit. A quick and effective way to screen patients is with the two questions in Table 19.4, drawn from the Patient Health Questionnaire-9 (PHQ-9).[9] If the patient answers yes to either question or scores at risk for depression, another depression scale, such as the PHQ-9 or the Beck Depression Inventory, can be used to confirm the diagnosis. The two-question screen has a sensitivity of 96% but a specificity of only 57%. Specificity is improved to 90% if a more detailed follow-up depression inventory is used (Evidence Level B).[9] Treatment includes adjustment of the patient's environment, exercise, and carefully titrated serotonin reuptake inhibitors. A more complete discussion of the management of depression is available in Chapter 17.

ALZHEIMER DISEASE

CASE ONE

Mr. G. is an 81-year-old retired engineer you have cared for over the past 8 years. His son accompanies him today because they want you to fill out an application for skilled nursing home placement. Two weeks ago they moved Mr. G. to the son's home because he had gone for a drive and had gotten lost. Mr. G. is talkative, bright, and alert, as he has been at previous visits, but you ask him to perform a clock test and are surprised that he cannot arrange the numbers on the face. He scores 19/30 on the MMSE. You recommend a workup and a trial course of a cholinesterase inhibitor. The family agrees to delay placement for a few weeks. When Mr. G. returns in 4 weeks he has lost 3 pounds but scores 24/30 on the MMSE. The family has returned him to his home but taken away his car. You gradually increase his medication to the maximum tolerable amount. Fourteen months later Mr. G. moves into a nursing facility.

This patient scenario represents an outstanding response. More often patients demonstrate little clinically relevant response or stop drugs due to gastrointestinal side effects. Mr. G. was a "responder."

Definition

Alzheimer disease is a progressive, inexorable loss of cognitive function associated with a large number of β-amyloid plaques in the cerebral cortex (and subcortical gray matter) and neurofibrillary tangles of tau protein. The diagnosis requires that symptoms be associated with cognitive loss in at least two domains including language, calculations, orientation, or judgment. The impairment must be severe enough to cause disability in social or occupational

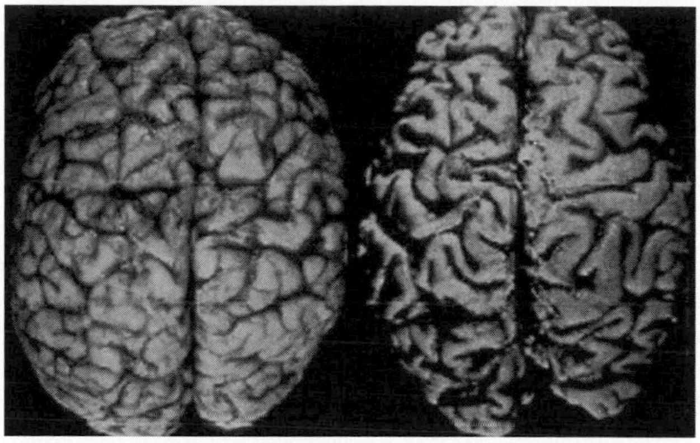

Figure 19.2 Structural neuronal loss in Alzheimer disease (AD).

function.[10] Attention is preserved until late in the course of the illness. In 1906, Alois Alzheimer, correlated the autopsy findings in a 55-year-old patient with dementia who he had followed up for several years. He described the plaques, stringy tangles, and empty spaces we have come to associate with Alzheimer disease. Table 19.5 compares the common types of dementia with Alzheimer disease.

Pathophysiology

Most elderly patients will have β-amyloid plaques, but the prevailing theory is that in those patients distinguished by Alzheimer disease a large burden of these plaques acts much like a barnacle, destroying the neuron. β-Amyloid is a breakdown product of a repair protein (amyloid precursor protein) in the cell membranes of neurons. Several enzymes on the cell surface cleave amyloid precursor proteins but one secretase subtype splits it to form insoluble β-amyloid. This sticky protein fragment clings to the cell wall. An inflammatory response is initiated by the release of cytokines and complement, attracting glial cells to form a plaque. Research is in pursuit of drugs to selectively block secretase activity.

β-Amyloid plaques result in activation of kinase (Cdk5 and Csk-3β) that damages intracellular microtubules through hyperphosphorylation of tau protein, the microtubular skeleton. The tubules twist into dysfunctional filaments that act like foreign bodies within the cell. These neurofibrillary tangles are also pathognomonic for Alzheimer disease.[11]

It is generally agreed that plaques and tangles alter ionic homeostasis and calcium transport, causing neuronal dysfunction, pruning of dendrites, loss of synapses, decreased neurotransmitter release (especially acetylcholine), and cell death. The load and distribution of plaques formed from β-amyloid correlate directly with the severity and manifestation of Alzheimer disease (see Fig. 19.2).

Incidence and Prevalence

Approximately 1% of 60-year-olds and 30% of 85-year-olds have dementia. Alzheimer disease accounts for >60% of dementia in the older-than-60 age-group. Women are at

TABLE 19.5
COMMON DEMENTIA DIAGNOSES

Dementia Diagnosis (Percentage of Dementia)	Clinical Characteristics	Pathology	Treatment
Alzheimer disease (50%–65%)	Progressive loss of cognitive function expressed as memory loss plus disturbances in aphasia, apraxia, agnosia, or executive functioning	β-Amyloid plaques in cerebral cortex Neurofibrillary tangles consisting of tau protein Decreased dopamine	Nutrition Vitamin E Cholinesterase inhibitors Memantine
Diffuse Lewy body dementia (15%–20%)	Hallucinations Fluctuation Parkinsonism	Cytoplasmic inclusion bodies	Cholinesterase inhibitors Antipsychotics, or anti-parkinsonian medications
Frontotemporal dementia (Pick disease) (15%)	Poor hygiene Disinhibition Inability to refrain from touching	Atrophy of the frontal and temporal lobes	Palliative only
Vascular dementia (10%–20%)	Step deterioration Physical signs of neurologic deficit Evidence of atherosclerosis Frequent falls	Lack of blood supply to the brain related to multiple infarcts	Management of hypertension, hyperlipidemia, carotid disease, arrhythmias, diabetes mellitus, polycythemia, and smoking Antiplatelet agents
White matter dementia (5%)	Mood disorders Apathy Perseveration	A complication of diseases of the myelinated white brain matter	Identify underlying condition

greater risk for developing Alzheimer disease type dementia than men, even when adjusted for their longer life span. A patient with an affected first-degree relative has a 50% risk of developing Alzheimer disease by age 90. Other risk factors include low intellectual achievement and a history of head trauma. Superior intellect, associated with larger brain size, more rapid nerve conduction, more dendritic connections, and cognitive reserve, decreases the risk of Alzheimer disease. Many patients with Alzheimer disease have a mixed dementia and coexisting etiologies of dementia.

Genetics

Only 10% to 20% of Alzheimer disease cases suggest a familial mode of transmission, but understanding phenotypes produced by these mutations has contributed to understanding Alzheimer disease. Mutations in four genes are known to increase the risk for Alzheimer disease and other mutations are under study.

The amyloid precursor protein gene, found on chromosome 21, results in increased production of precursor proteins and may explain the prevalence of Alzheimer disease in Down syndrome. Another mutation of the presenilin 1 gene, located on chromosome 14, accounts for 4% of Alzheimer disease cases starting below the age of 50. A third mutation, presenilin 2, is on chromosome 1 and accounts for 1% of early onset Alzheimer disease cases. The presenilin mutations increase levels of a secretase enzyme and result in a rapidly progressive form of Alzheimer disease.[12]

The fourth, and the most common form of inherited Alzheimer disease, is associated with one of several mutations on chromosome 19, the apolipoprotein E alleles. These mutations cause enhanced aggregation of β-amyloid in the brain. Their expression is variable but accounts for 50% of early Alzheimer disease and 20% of late onset disease. The presence of the $\varepsilon 4$ allele mutation is associated with increased risk in whites, and $\varepsilon 2$ and 4 alleles with increased risk in African Americans.

Routine genetic testing is not recommended at this time. While identification of a specific mutation is possible in 70% of families with a pattern of autosomal dominant Alzheimer disease and the apolipoprotein gene typing is commercially available, the prognostic value is limited. Female carriers have a 45% probability of developing Alzheimer disease by age 73 but men have only a 25% probability.[12] Testing is expensive, may result in insurance denials, or lead to deterministic behavior, and patients may have limited conceptual understanding of risk.

Time Course of Alzheimer Disease

It is difficult to define the onset of Alzheimer disease. Many patients with mild cognitive dysfunction do not progress to Alzheimer disease, but for those who do the transition to dementia is vague. Several years of compensation and decline precede a pattern diagnosable as Alzheimer disease. Table 19.6 displays the typical but highly variable time line for Alzheimer disease to progress to death. Alzheimer disease is a terminal illness and will result in death in all patients.

The skills of life deteriorate in a predictable pattern. The patient first has problems with shopping because of the complexity of choices and money management. Personal hygiene wanes. Later the patient becomes incontinent, has difficulties with meals and requires full-time care. Death is from aspiration pneumonia, urinary tract infection, sepsis from decubiti, or complications of concomitant medical illnesses.

Workup/Keys to Diagnosis

Studies suggest that 97% of patients with mild dementia and 50% with moderate dementia are stimulated by the clinical encounter and avoid detection. Patients who miss medication, forget appointments, live alone, or are otherwise at risk for dementia can be screened with a tool

TABLE 19.6
TIME COURSE OF ALZHEIMER DISEASE

Prediagnosis (Mild Cognitive Impairment?)	Mild Dementia	Moderate Dementia	Severe Dementia	Death
MMSE = 24–30 May be present for 5 y or more Mild memory loss Normal function	MMSE = 20–23 Clinical phase: 5–10 y Survival can be 2–20 y Forgetfulness Repeats questions Daily function impaired.	MMSE = 10–19 Clinical phase: 5–10 y Survival can be 2–20 y Short-term memory loss Word-finding difficulties Cannot shop on own	MMSE = 0–9 Clinical phase: 5–10 y Survival can be 2–20 y Agitation Altered sleep pattern Dependence: dressing, feeding, bathing	Alzheimer disease is a terminal condition Aspiration pneumonia Urinary tract infection Sepsis from decubiti Concomitant medical illness

Time frames reported here reflect a population of patients and may vary for individuals.

such as an MMSE or the clock test. Any patient who cannot give the correct day, date, month, year and season, and cannot remember three objects for 1 minute should be scored using one of the validated instruments described in the preceding text.

The American Psychiatric Association Fourth Edition criteria for the clinical diagnosis of Alzheimer disease define the cognitive deficits as memory impairment (inability to learn new information) associated with one or more of the following: Disturbance in language (aphasia), impaired motor ability (apraxia), inability to identify objects (agnosia) and/or a disturbance in executive functioning (planning, organizing, sequencing, abstracting). The cognitive deficits must result in a progressive decline in social or occupational function not due to other central nervous system conditions affecting memory and cognition nor due to systemic conditions known to cause dementia (e.g., hypothyroidism, vitamin B_{12} or folic acid deficiency, niacin deficiency, hypercalcemia, neurosyphilis, human immunodeficiency virus [HIV] infection) or substance-induced conditions.

Clinical examination has limited specificity, leading to common use of the term Alzheimer disease-like dementia. Brain biopsy would confirm the presence of β-amyloid plaques but it is not indicated in uncomplicated dementia. Biopsy would only be considered if there is reason to suspect herpes encephalitis or a condition that may respond to treatment.

If the physical examination reveals coexisting conditions, the clinician should assess how these conditions affect, exacerbate, or interfere with cognition and be alert for opportunities to improve the dementia by treatment.

Laboratory

The goal of laboratory workup in a patient with dementia is to accurately diagnose the disorder responsible for the dementia. In a study of patients referred to a neurology clinic, laboratory workup changed management in 13% of the patients.[13]

Most patients should have a complete blood count; electrolyte panel; comprehensive metabolic panel; thyroid-stimulating hormone, vitamin B_{12}, and folate levels; syphilis screening; prealbumin test; and urinalysis. If there is profound weight loss, thrush, or atypical neurologic findings, other screening procedures to be considered include erythrocyte sedimentation rate, HIV, chest x-ray, toxicology, and lead screening.

A computed tomography (CT) scan or MRI of the head should be considered in most patients. Imaging is particularly important if the dementia is associated with rapid onset, focal neurologic signs, abnormal gait, cancer, systemic disease, trauma, or seizures. The expected finding is diffuse atrophy but a focal assessment of the hippocampal volume may assist in assessing prognosis.

Functional imaging by PET or single photon emission computed tomography (SPECT) is 86% sensitive and 86% specific. Meta-analysis suggests that a PET or SPECT scan rarely alters the treatment of dementia and should be ordered only when the diagnosis is in question.[14]

The cerebrospinal fluid (CSF) in patients with Alzheimer disease demonstrates higher levels of tau protein. Measures of tau protein are not commercially available and would not alter treatment. A free radical breakdown of arachidonic acid is elevated in the urine of many patients with Alzheimer disease. Arachidonic acid analysis is commercially available but the overlap between affected and nonaffected groups makes it clinically useless.[15]

Management

All patients should be scored using one of the standardized and validated dementia instruments. Repeating the MMSE every 3 to 6 months will (i) quantify mental status, unmasking the degree of disability and guiding medication use; (ii) evaluate executive function; and (iii) guide recommendations for level of supervision needed.

Competency to manage daily social and personal activities, also called executive function, requires a capacity to make and communicate reasonably stable choices and appreciate their consequences. The patient needs to rationally accept or reject information and compare benefits and risks. Executive function declines in somewhat predictable patterns starting with financial skills (math and decision making), bathing, dressing, toileting, and finally feeding and continence. Deficiency in any of these areas should lead to an evaluation of the current living situation.

Almost a third of patients with cognitive impairment have evidence of malnutrition. Low levels of vitamins C, B_{12}, riboflavin, and folic acid are associated with lower cognitive scores. Prealbumin is a sensitive test for protein malnutrition. It identifies patients at risk for decompensation and can be used to assess response to improved nutrition.[16]

Lifestyle

Physical activities such as walking, dancing, and even board games decrease the incidence of falls, improve peak pulmonary expiratory flow rate, reduce depression, and delay cognitive decline in community-based persons older than 65 years[17–22] (Evidence Level A). Cognitive exercises focusing on memory, reasoning, or thought processing (e.g., crossword puzzles) have been shown to slow the progression of dementia.[23] Functional improvement, as observed on PET scans, is as good after cognitive exercises as it is after cholinesterase inhibitors[24,25] (Evidence Level B). These studies support the assertion that a stimulating environment leads to a sense of engagement and usefulness that sustains cognitive function longer.

Medications

Cholinesterase inhibitors are the principal palliative pharmacologic therapies available today (see Table 19.7).

TABLE 19.7
AGENTS APPROVED FOR USE IN DEMENTIA

Medication Mechanism	Documented Response	Percentage Drop-outs	Length of Response Documented	Dosing	Monitor
Donepezil[55] Cholinesterase inhibitor	23% respond 6.3% improvement in function, stabilization	16%	50 wk	5 mg/d for 4 wk, then 10 mg/d for duration of response Not affected by food	Nausea and vomiting, weight loss, muscle cramps, bradycardia
Rivastigmine[56,57] Cholinesterase inhibitor	25% respond 4.1% improvement in function, stabilization.	29%	40 wk	Start 1.5 mg b.i.d., increase every 4 wk to 6 mg b.i.d. to maximum improvement	Nausea and vomiting, anorexia, weight loss
Galantamine[58] Cholinesterase inhibitor	37% respond 2.3% improvement in function, stabilization	16%	52 wk	Start 4 mg b.i.d. After 4 wk increase to 8 mg b.i.d. After 4 more wk increase to maintenance dose of 12 mg b.i.d.	Nausea and vomiting, anorexia, weight loss, urinary retention
Memantine[59] NMDA-receptor antagonist	15% respond Treated group declined slower than placebo group	23%	28 wk	Start 5 mg q.d. for 1 wk, then 5 mg b.i.d. for 1 wk, then 10 mg AM and 5 mg PM for 1 wk then 10 mg b.i.d.	Agitation, headache, confusion, insomnia, and diarrhea similar to placebo Often used with cholinesterase inhibitors

Tacrine (Cognex) is now a second line agent due to high incidence of gastrointestinal (GI) side effects and liver toxicity. Hepatotoxicity has not been directly attributed to the agents listed in the table.
NMDA, *N*-methyl-D-aspartate.

Acetylcholine production by neurons in the cortex and hippocampus correlates inversely with dementia. Cholinesterase inhibitors reduce the enzymatic degradation of acetylcholine in the synapse, thereby enhancing neuron-to-neuron communication. They have a low therapeutic index and wide variation of individual response. Only a third of patients with moderate Alzheimer disease respond with improved performance on mental state evaluations. Mood disorders such as depression, anxiety, or agitation do not generally respond. However, cholinesterase inhibitors may improve apathy, appetite, sleep, and motor skills while decreasing hallucinations. As a result, families may report a response when none is obvious to the clinician.

Studies generally demonstrate a one-point increase in MMSE score and inconsistent delays in institutionalization between cholinesterase inhibitors and placebo.[26] Lack of clinical improvement and gastrointestinal side effects such as nausea, vomiting, and diarrhea, as well as liver toxicity, weight loss, and bradycardia are the most common reasons cholinesterase inhibitors are discontinued. Pharmacologic effects may persist 6 weeks after discontinuation. Costs range from $120 to $140 per month.

Donepezil is a piperidine-based cholinesterase inhibitor selective for brain cholinesterase. A long plasma half-life (50 to 70 hours) allows for once-a-day dosing, and absorption is not affected by food. Start patients on 5 mg per day for 4 to 6 weeks, and then increase to 10 mg per day. Rivastigmine offers somewhat more flexibility in dosing and has an indication in Lewy body dementia, but it has a greater incidence of gastrointestinal side effects. Galantamine may be considered in patients who have not tolerated donepezil or rivastigmine.

Cholinesterase inhibitors are palliative treatment. In practice they are equally effective and may delay progression of dementia for 6 to 18 months in some patients. Once a clinical diagnosis of Alzheimer disease is established and depression, if present, is stabilized, it is reasonable to consider a trial of cholinesterase inhibitor in most patients. Apply a standardized mental state instrument and begin the starting dose of the medication of choice. Advise patients on the use of antacids or antidiarrhea agents and evaluate side effects in 2 weeks. At 4 weeks, rescore the patient and increase the dose. Push the drugs to the maximum dose unless side effects are problematic. If there is no response or the patient develops significant side effects, try another cholinesterase inhibitor (Evidence Level C).[1] If the patient demonstrates benefits by the mental status examination or family report, reevaluate the patient every 8 weeks and check aspartate and alanine aminotransferase regularly.

It is unclear when to discontinue cholinesterase inhibitors when there has been a clinical response. Early trials focused on patients with mild to moderate disease, but there is limited evidence that patients with severe dementia may be more manageable on cholinesterase inhibitors.[1]

Memantine, an *N*-methyl-D-aspartate receptor antagonist is approved for the treatment of moderate to severe

Alzheimer disease. Memantine interferes with glutamatergic toxicity, particularly in hippocampal neurons. It is a well-tolerated drug when administered to patients receiving stable doses of a cholinesterase inhibitor and may ameliorate some of the gastrointestinal effects. Adding memantine to a cholinesterase inhibitor produces a modest improvement in cognitive function, activities of daily living, and behavioral symptoms (Evidence Level B).[27]

Research is under way to develop drugs that impact on the enzymatic reactions that create β-amyloid and neurofibrillary tangles. Excitement about vaccine-induced immunologic clearing of β-amyloid has waned because of encephalitis experienced by patients in an early trial but efforts in this arena continue.

Alternative Treatments

The free radical scavengers, antioxidants, have been promoted for the prevention and treatment of Alzheimer disease. A 2-year study using vitamin E (alphatocopherol) at doses of 800 to 2,000 IU daily demonstrated slower progression of cognitive dysfunction over placebo, but concern has been raised on the safety of using over 400 IU long term (Evidence Level B). Vitamin C and selegiline (a monoamine oxidase [MAO] inhibitor/antioxidant) have limited or inconsistent effects.[28] Estrogen has a weak antioxidant effect but has failed to demonstrate a cognitive benefit. The Women's Health Initiative has removed any hope that estrogen would be protective.[29]

Ginkgo biloba is a flavonoid with antioxidant effect. While a number of limited design trials suggest ginkgo biloba is effective, at least one randomized crossover study showed no effect.[30] Two percent of patients will have adverse effects such as gastrointestinal symptoms, headache, allergic reactions, and bleeding. The benefits, if any, are modest.

Huperzine A is a potent cholinesterase inhibitor derived from the herb Chinese Club Moss. It is marketed by itself or combined with vitamin E and ginkgo. Side effects include nausea, sweating, and blurred vision. It is effective but is less predictable than pharmaceutical grade medications.[31]

Observational studies have associated the long-term use of nonsteroidal anti-inflammatory drugs with a lower risk of dementia and slower rate of decline. The proposed mechanism has been blockade of the inflammatory cyclooxegenase-2 cascade initiated by neuritic plaques. Unfortunately, prospective studies have not demonstrated a protective effect.[1,32] Aspirin and acetaminophen also have no demonstrable effect.

There is considerable optimism that the use of statins in controlling hyperlipidemia and folic acid in controlling homocysteine will delay the onset of Alzheimer disease. Whether the important role of these agents in cardiovascular disease has a crossover impact on Alzheimer disease will require further research.

NON-ALZHEIMER DISEASE DEMENTIA

Vascular Dementia

CASE TWO

The patient's wife complains that her husband has been forgetful for 2 months. He stopped reading the paper and now wears only slip-on shoes because he finds it "annoying" to tie a bow. On one occasion he started mowing the lawn but left the mower running and abandoned before he was done. He has fallen twice in the last month. On physical examination, he has hyperactive reflexes on his right side and weakness in the right hand.

Vascular dementia results from diminished blood supply to multiple areas of the brain due to thromboembolism, hemorrhage, or ischemia. It accounts for 10% to 20% of dementia. Large artery occlusion results in a multi-infarct dementia often associated with focal neurologic findings on examination. Small vessel disease, including conditions known as lacunar state, ischemic vascular dementia, and Binswanger disease, presents with apathy, dementia, and urinary incontinence in patients with other stigmata of arteriosclerosis.[33] The clinical hallmark of the dementia due to vascular disease is a decline in competency or executive function (disorganized thought or emotion), gait disturbance, and apathy brought on by disruption of frontal–subcortical connections. Patients have trouble completing tasks and poor problem solving before obvious memory loss.

Alois Alzheimer devoted considerable attention to atherosclerotic dementia and argued that it was distinct from dementia caused by plaques and tangles. Modern treatment of hypertension delays the impact of vascular disease as a common cofactor in dementia from other causes in the older-than-65 age-group. The Nun Study demonstrated that patients with lacuna infarcts require fewer β-amyloid plaques to exhibit cognitive decline.[33] Whether caused by a single infarct or multiple small infarcts, a decrease of brain volume by 50 mL is associated with dementia.[33] Risk factors include hypertension, diabetes mellitus, hyperlipidemia, vasculitis, and tobacco use.

Clock drawing is disrupted early in vascular dementia because it requires coordination, spatial organization, and frontal-lobe-driven task completion. Patients with pure vascular dementia may not be able to follow directions to draw a clock face but may do quite well if asked to copy a clock face.[33] CT scan or MRI confirms brain infarcts in 80% of patients with clinically suspected vascular dementia.[34]

Prevention is more effective than treatment and is directed at arresting arteriosclerosis, particularly in small vessels, before brain infarcts occur. In one study, the lowering of systolic blood pressure by 7 mm Hg over 3 years halved the incidence of dementia. This is an absolute reduction of 3 cases for every 100 treated.[35] Statins have been shown to lower the incidence by 1 per 100.[35]

Treatment is focused on comprehensive management of hypertension, hyperlipidemia, carotid disease, arrhythmia, diabetes mellitus, polycythemia, and nicotine addiction. Antiplatelet agents may have a role (Evidence Level B).[33] Cholinesterase inhibitors and memantine have demonstrated limited improvement in vascular dementia.

Binswanger disease is a subcortical atherosclerotic encephalopathy involving multiple infarcts deep in the white matter of the brain. It is associated with severe hypertension. The clinical course is rapid, months not years, and the MRI and CT scan demonstrate leukoencephalopathy in the cerebrum. Treatment, as with other forms of vascular dementia, is directed at controlling hypertension.

Lewy Body Dementia

> **CASE THREE**
>
> "The other morning I lay in bed and all of a sudden, this yellow object appeared on the wall. It would flit away and another one, different size, shape, all jagged would appear and this thing kept going back and forth. I was wide awake. It was a light show projected on the wall. All this stuff, and then it stopped. That's one of the more pleasant things to have happened, a light show." Statement by Mr. B. on a lucid day.

Diffuse Lewy body dementia is characterized by hyaline cytoplasmic inclusion bodies in the gray matter neurons and a combined dopaminergic and cholinergic deficit. It is more common than generally recognized, accounting for 15% to 20% of dementia. It is the most common dementia presenting with parkinsonian features and is often confused with parkinsonism.

Clinical characteristics include visual and auditory hallucinations, attention deficit, wide fluctuations in cognition, and motor features of parkinsonism. While survival is similar to Alzheimer disease, patients with Lewy body dementia maintain performance on memory tasks until later in their disease.[36] Lewy body dementia is differentiated from Parkinson disease by cognitive failure, which is not present until late in Parkinson disease. The fluctuating cognition can suggest transient ischemic attacks of vascular dementia; progression, however, is not stepwise and focal neurologic signs are not typical. Fluctuations can cycle over several days or less than half an hour, and they can span from near normal cognition to disorientation and inattention. Typically, patients do not seem threatened by their hallucinations, which often involve lights, little people, children, or animals.

Treatment is directed at the major complaints and problems, but balancing side effects can be difficult. Because the hallucinations are seldom troublesome they may be left untreated. If control is desired, clonazepam is the drug of choice. Unfortunately, antipsychotic medications can aggravate the motor symptoms. Motor symptoms may respond to dopaminergic drugs but these drugs may worsen the psychosis. The cholinesterase inhibitor rivastigmine has been found to improve hallucinations, delusions, anxiety, apathy, and fluctuations in attention when given to patients with Lewy body dementia. The other cholinesterase inhibitors may also be beneficial (Evidence Level B).[37]

Dementia Associated with Parkinson Disease

Dementia will develop in half of all patients with Parkinson disease. If dementia develops in the first 2 years of the onset of motor symptoms, the diagnosis of Lewy body dementia should be entertained. Some debate exists as to whether these are variations of the same process, as Parkinson disease dementia is also characterized by visual and auditory hallucinations, attention deficit, and wide fluctuations in cognition. Cholinesterase inhibitors may be beneficial for patients with Parkinson disease dementia but the results are limited. Functional improvement equates to approximately one point on the MMSE for approximately 6 months at the expense of increased tremor.[38]

Frontotemporal Dementia

> **CASE FOUR**
>
> "Jim does not swear as much as he did. Much of his day now is spent flipping TV channels. He laughs in a high squeaky voice and says '___ off!' to most everything. He chews an unlit cigar constantly. He will steal magazines and hitchhike if I let him out of my sight. I convince him to shower daily but he then wanders around naked. We still love to snuggle in bed and he sleeps most of the night, thank God. He approaches strangers, usually young women, and introduces himself." The wife of a 52-year-old radio announcer with Pick disease.

Frontotemporal dementia, originally described by Pick in 1892, is caused by asymmetric degeneration of the gray matter marked by atrophy of the frontal and temporal lobes of the brain. It accounts for 15% of dementia and is characterized by behavioral disturbances affecting personal conduct and interpersonal interactions. Disinhibition (especially sexual) is common. Patients inappropriately touch objects and people, and personal hygiene suffers. Memory and calculation are relatively preserved until later stages. Onset is typically before age 65, with a course of 2 to 6 years. Speech can be fluent but empty of meaning and eventually becomes disorganized and stuttering. Amyotrophic lateral sclerosis is occasionally accompanied by a frontotemporal dementia.

The key to clinical diagnosis is progressive deterioration of behavior associated with almost secondary memory difficulties. The deterioration of normal social behavior in a patient who seems not to care about consequences frequently results in accusations of alcohol or drug abuse. Unprecedented shoplifting and indecent exposure can be presenting features. Impulsivity is common but patients may also present with apathy misdiagnosed as depression. Brain imaging confirms frontal lobe atrophy.[39]

There are three patterns of frontotemporal lobar degeneration determined by the distribution of lesions in the frontal and anterior temporal lobes. Frontotemporal dementia (Pick disease) is the most common subtype and most likely to be confused with early onset Alzheimer disease. In the "primary progressive aphasia" subtype, patients present with a nonfluent aphasia and word-finding difficulty that impairs speech antecedent to obvious behavioral problems. The "semantic degeneration" subtype presents with impaired recognition of previously familiar objects or people. The patient may describe an object's function but be unable to name it. Progression of the aphasia subtypes results in speech that becomes vague and incomprehensible as the patient substitutes "it" or "thing" for all objects.[39]

Impaired social judgment reflects right frontal damage. Nonfluent speech results from left frontal hemisphere degeneration. Left temporal lobe atrophy causes naming difficulties and right temporal lobe atrophy is reflected in the behavioral changes. Neurofibrillary tangles of tau protein dominate pathologic findings.

Three mutations on chromosome 17 where tau protein is encoded were initially identified in genetic studies of 13 families with autosomal dominant dementia. Since then, 20 different mutations related to tau protein production have been described, accounting for a third of familial frontotemporal dementia.

Treatment is unsatisfactory. Patients with frontotemporal degeneration actively deny there are any problems, but the absence of inhibition is such a burden to the caregiver that institutional care is common. Limited studies have suggested that selective serotonin reuptake inhibitors (SSRIs) may improve behavior, depression, and compulsions (Evidence Level B).[40] MAO inhibitors such as selegiline may improve depression, irritability, mental rigidity, and perseveration (Evidence Level B). Risperidone may improve sleep.[39]

White Matter Dementia

> **CASE FIVE**
>
> "When Lida's multiple sclerosis immobilized her, she became my eyes and ears. She answered the phone and balanced the checkbook. We would talk a lot, especially while I fed her. She was company. In the last year she has become easily confused. At first I agreed with you and attributed it to depression, but it's worse now. She cries at the least suggestion, and stares into space. She is just plain miserable." Lida's husband.

White matter dementia is a complication of diseases of the myelinated white brain matter, such as multiple sclerosis, ischemic demyelination (Binswanger dementia), acquired immunodeficiency syndrome dementia, B_{12} deficiency, normal pressure hydrocephalus, and atrophy of aging. It accounts for 5% of dementia. The arcuate fasciculi, the occipitofrontal fasciculi and the uncinate fasciculi of the brain's white matter form the network between the frontal, parietal, temporal, and occipital lobes. White matter is necessary for complex, multifocal brain functions such as attention, memory, language, visual–spatial perception, abstract reasoning, and emotional competence. The blood supply is through long penetrating arterioles originating from large vessels at the base of the brain.

Toluene, inhaled as a drug of abuse or as a component of spray paints and other products, causes a leukoencephalopathy affecting myelin, with devastating neurobehavioral consequences. Toluene inhalation can lead to a dementia resembling white matter degeneration from other causes.

In the elderly, white matter degeneration results in difficulty sustaining attention or vigilance, and in depression. Symptoms vary greatly and include attention problems, mood disorder, apathy, and perseveration. Language skills are relatively spared. Remissions, particularly in multiple sclerosis, are common because the nerves may recover after brief episodes of demylenation.[41] MRI has greatly enhanced the ability to identify lesions within the white matter.

Treatment is directed at the underlying disorder. Modest improvement of cognitive function with interferon β 1b had been reported in multiple sclerosis.

Mixed Dementia

Only one third of elderly patients will have a pure form of dementia. Nearly a quarter of patients diagnosed with Alzheimer disease will be found, on autopsy, to also have enough vascular lesions to cause dementia. Different pathologies synergistically contribute to the severity of cognitive impairment.[42]

OTHER CAUSES OF DEMENTIA

Normal pressure hydrocephalus is a rare cause of dementia characterized by a triad of gait disorder, urinary incontinence, and cognitive decline. The gait is characterized by short steps and poor turning. Patients report feeling like their feet are glued to the floor. The cognitive dysfunction is usually mild. The possibility of normal pressure hydrocephalus is most commonly raised after an MRI or a CT scan of the head has been ordered for other reasons. Imaging studies show an increase in ventricular size and compression of cerebral parenchyma. A spinal tap reveals normal protein and glucose levels, a white blood cell count of fewer than 5 cells per mm^3, and an opening pressure of <200 mm H_2O. Removal of 60 cc of CSF may improve symptoms and suggests that the patient may respond to ventriculoperitoneal shunting. Shunting is used to relieve ventricular fluid buildup thought to cause the disorder, but there are no controlled studies to confirm its effectiveness. Only 30% of patients will have sustained improvement after shunting. The differential diagnosis should include alcoholism, multi-infarct dementia, Parkinson disease, and subdural hematoma. Patients with ataxia and incontinence who only recently demonstrated mild dementia (not due to other causes) are the best candidates for shunting (Evidence Level B).[43]

Viral encephalopathies, such as herpes simplex, usually have a course characterized by systemic illness. Fungal infections, in particular *Cryptococcus*, are rare causes of dementia and more common in patients who are immunocompromised. Parasites such as toxoplasmosis can cause dementia and are generally discovered by brain imaging. HIV infection is also associated with dementia.

Creutzfeldt-Jakob disease (CJD) is caused by transmissible proteins called prions. The classic features of CJD include dementia, myoclonus, visual disturbance, and a distinctive pattern on electroencephalogram. Patients exhibit rapid changes from month to month, with most patients becoming akinetic and mute within 6 months.

Syphilis dementia occurs 15 to 30 years after acute exposure and is associated with behavioral disturbances, especially delusions. A CSF white blood cell count of >5 per mm^3 and positive spinal fluid serology are necessary to make the diagnosis. Antibiotic treatment may slow progression of dementia but not resolve it.

B_{12} deficiencies can present with cognitive and behavioral changes, usually in the context of peripheral neuropathy and degeneration of the posterior and lateral columns of the spinal cord. Numbness and tingling in the extremities is the most frequent neurologic symptom. Twenty-eight percent of patients will not have anemia or macrocytosis. With treatment the dementia can completely resolve.[44]

Severe hypothyroidism leads to lethargy, inattention, apathy, and depression, but frank dementia is uncommon. Most patients will demonstrate classic features of hypothyroidism. Hyperthyroidism results in irritability, emotional lability, and inability to concentrate. Poor performance on cognitive testing may result from reduced ability to focus. Tremor is often present. Cognition improves with treatment.

Alcohol abuse is often considered a cause of dementia but there is no distinctive pattern. Alcohol-related nutritional deficiencies can lead to Korsakoff syndrome, with amnesia, confabulation, and a disabling limited memory span. Korsakoff is linked to acute Wernicke encephalopathy and thiamine deficiency. Pellagra, due to nicotinic acid deficiency, also leads to cognitive impairments in alcohol abusers.[44]

Medications and depression are common causes of pseudodementia and should be considered in all patients with cognitive failure.

BEHAVIORAL PROBLEMS IN DEMENTIA

One third of patients with mild to moderate dementia will demonstrate behavioral symptoms at least once a week.[45] Table 19.8 summarizes several approaches to behavioral problems in elderly patients with dementia. Behavior generally has a trigger. Caregivers must seek out triggers using their own insight about the patient's perceptions and reactions. Gentle touching or massage and soothing vocalization are likely to calm an agitated patient, whereas instructions usually do not. Removing aggravating stimuli decreases aggressive behavior better than pharmacology. Consider patterns in timing, as well as surroundings, clothing, others who are involved, and the possibility of abuse. Think of things such as missing glasses, hearing aids, teeth, or medications.

A good rule for agitation management is, "They cannot resist if you do not insist."[46] Almost no controlled research exists to guide the management of wandering, pacing, continuous talking, or constant picking, but drugs are rarely effective. Maximum freedom in a safe environment is more effective than restraints, which often generate more agitation. Although "geriatric chairs" are often tolerated, appropriate use of fencing and a "child proof" environment can improve physical health and avoid confrontation.

SSRIs are safe, efficacious, and well tolerated in elderly patients with depression. Observational studies have suggested they also improve irritability and mood reactivity in patients with dementia without depression. Citalpram (10 to 40 mg at bedtime) or sertraline (25 to 100 mg every morning) are well studied in the elderly and may have fewer drug interactions than other SSRIs. Trazodone (25 to 200 mg at night) is the most popular non-neuroleptic medication in England for treatment of agitation and may be as effective as antipsychotic medications, with fewer side effects. Mirtazapine (15 mg to 45 mg at night), a tetracyclic, also has a good safety profile and has a tendency to promote appetite, weight gain, and sleep (Evidence Level B).[46]

Sixty percent of nursing home elders demonstrate some psychotic symptoms, often associated with agitation, delusions, or hallucinations.[47] Conventional antipsychotics are modestly effective (Evidence Level A). Haloperidol (1 to 3 mg per day) remains the most commonly used neuroleptic for the treatment of behavioral and psychologic symptoms associated with dementia. Extrapyramidal signs are common. Atypical antipsychotics such as risperidone, olanzapine, and quetiapine have been associated with increased mortality in the elderly.[53] Several studies confirm that risperidone (1 mg per day) modestly improves symptoms of psychosis, decreases aggression, and decreases nursing burden (Evidence Level A).[48,49]

Anticonvulsants are an alternative to control agitation associated with dementia. Valproic acid, divalproex, and carbamazepine are established for treating agitation in dementia and are well tolerated. Side effects include reversible parkinsonism and cognitive decline (Evidence Level B).[46] Benzodiazepines are commonly used as needed to calm patients, but are associated with mental dulling, falls, and disinhibition. Intramuscular medroxyprogesterone acetate

TABLE 19.8
TREATING BEHAVIORAL PROBLEMS[60]

Behavior	Investigation	Treatment
Aggression	Seek out triggers	Remove aggravation stimuli Benzodiazepines Carbamazepine Valproic acid
Hypersexuality	Staff counseling	SSRI antidepressants Suppress testosterone: Cimetidine Medroxyprogesterone Leuprolide
Wandering, pacing, continuous talking, picking	Assure patient safety Geriatric chairs	Maximize freedom Restraints increase agitation Cholinesterase inhibitors
Insomnia	Check for sources of pain Leg cramps, arthritis, constipation Diuretic effects Shortness of breath Fear of darkness	Adjust medications Night lights Daytime activity Cholinesterase inhibitors Trazodone Short-acting sedatives
Anorexia	Likes and dislikes Rule out depression	Doxepin Avoid feeding tubes
Orthostatic hypotension	Review medications Rule out: Parkinson disease, B_{12} deficiency, diabetes mellitus, or syphilis	Treat hypertension conservatively Add salt to diet Fludrocortisone Compression stockings Frequent small feedings
Incontinence	Urinalysis, culture Review medications Define urge vs. stress incontinence	Frequent toileting Pessary placement Treat urge or stress incontinence if defined Diapers
Hallucinations, delusions	Investigate triggers Often an end-stage sign	Treat if unpleasant Haloperidol

SSRI, selective serotonin reuptake inhibitor.
From Trinh NH, et al. Efficacy of cholinesterase inhibitors in the treatment of neuropsychiatric symptoms and functional impairment in Alzheimer disease: A meta-analysis. *JAMA.* 2003;289(2):210–216.

at 150 mg every 2 weeks has proved effective for sexual aggression in elderly men (Evidence Level A).[46]

Nutrition is challenging in a confused patient. Caregivers should attempt to make mealtime as appealing as possible, even repeating favorite foods over and over if that is necessary to achieve calorie targets. Unfortunately, the more confused the patient the more likely that presenting high-calorie supplements between meals will simply result in fewer calories at mealtime, rather than more overall calories.[50] Improving nutrition may not improve dementia for patients with severe dementia.[51]

Over 40,000 gastrostomy tubes are inserted in elderly patients with dementia each year, but tube feeding seldom achieves the intended medical aims. Feeding tubes can cause reflux, pneumonia, and increased suffering in patients with terminal dementia. The Supreme Court has ruled that artificial nutrition and hydration constitutes medical intervention. As a medical intervention it can be withheld.[52]

CAREGIVERS

The number of Americans afflicted with Alzheimer disease will triple to 14 million by 2050. Their caregivers, limited by resources and options, will face a life of round-the-clock vigils in an act of stoic devotion. Two thirds of patients are cared for at home throughout their illness, turning family ties upside down and challenging individual capacity to care. Most families benefit from logistical help offered by community social services, lawyers to arrange wills and power of attorney, support groups, and respite care.

TABLE 19.9
CAREGIVER BURDEN SCREEN[61]

For each of the following statements, please circle the answer that indicates the degree to which you believe the experience or event has caused you distress (such as being upset or nervous). If the event has not occurred, indicate "did not occur." (Internal consistency: $\alpha = 0.86$)

Key: 0 = Did not occur
1 = Occurred but did not cause distress
2 = Mild distress
3 = Moderate distress
4 = Severe distress

Question	Response
1. I feel so alone, as if I have the world on my shoulders	
2. I have little control over my relative's behavior	
3. I have to do too many jobs/chores (feeding, shopping) that my relative used to do	
4. I am upset that I cannot communicate with my relative	
5. My relative is constantly asking the same questions over and over	
6. I have little control over my relative's illness	
7. My relative does not cooperate with the rest of our family	

Score: 3s or 4s to any question indicate a caregiver at risk

From Hirschman KB, et al. The development of a rapid screen for caregiver burden. *J Am Geriatr Soc.* 2004;52(10):1724–1729.

It is difficult to assess the amount of stress the caregiver experiences. Caregiver mortality risk is 60% higher than peers but returns to normal after the death of the patient.[54] If the caregiver is also a patient he/she should be monitored for worsening of hypertension, diabetes, and other chronic conditions of their own. Table 19.9 presents a rapid caregiver burden screen to assist in quantifying the continuing capacity of a caregiver. Results correlate with depression, so the screen can be used to assess how the caregiver's burden is impacting their mood as well as their level of distress.

CONCLUSION

There have been many advancements in our understanding of dementia in the elderly over the past decade. Unfortunately treatment still produces modest benefits, often <1 point on the MMSE. While statistically significant, the impact on daily function may be so small as to not be worth the cost or the side effects. The clinical quandary is whether the effects are so small that treatment may not be useful, or whether treatment should be tried on every patient and continued on those who respond. As this chapter describes, there are many modalities to delay dementia and manage dysfunction, and in the end they all rely on supportive, safe environments.

REFERENCES

1. Cummings JL. Alzheimer's disease. *N Engl J Med.* 2004;351(1): 56–67.
2. Langa KM, et al. Out-of-pocket health care expenditures among older Americans with dementia. *Alzheimer Dis Assoc Disord.* 2004;18(2):90–98.
3. Maguire EA, et al. Navigation-related structural change in the hippocampi of taxi drivers. *Proc Natl Acad Sci U S A.* 2000;97(8):4398–4403.
4. Callahan CM, et al. Six-item screener to identify cognitive impairment among potential subjects for clinical research. *Med Care.* 2002;40(9):771–781.
5. Folstein MF, Folstein SE, McHugh PR. "Mini-mental state". A practical method for grading the cognitive state of patients for the clinician. *J Psychiatr Res.* 1975;12(3):189–198.
6. Pfeiffer E. A short portable mental status questionnaire for the assessment of organic brain deficit in elderly patients. *J Am Geriatr Soc.* 1975;23(10):433–441.
7. Sunderland T, et al. Clock drawing in Alzheimer's disease. A novel measure of dementia severity. *J Am Geriatr Soc.* 1989;37(8):725–729.
8. Strydom A, Hassiotis A. Diagnostic instruments for dementia in older people with intellectual disability in clinical practice. *Aging Ment Health.* 2003;7(6):431–437.
9. Thibault JM, Steiner RW. Efficient identification of adults with depression and dementia. *Am Fam Physician.* 2004;70(6): 1101–1110.
10. Kawas CH. Clinical practice. Early Alzheimer's disease. *N Engl J Med.* 2003;349(11):1056–1063.
11. Rosenthal TC, Khotianov N. Managing Alzheimer dementia tomorrow. *J Am Board Fam Pract.* 2003;16(5):423–434.
12. Selkoe DJ. Alzheimer's disease: Genes, proteins, and therapy. *Physiol Rev.* 2001;81(2):741–766.
13. Chui H, Zhang Q. Evaluation of dementia: A systematic study of the usefulness of the American academy of neurology's practice parameters. *Neurology.* 1997;49(4):925–935.
14. Patwardhan MB, et al. Alzheimer disease: Operating characteristics of PET-a meta-analysis. *Radiology.* 2004;231(1):73–80.
15. Tuppo EE, et al. Sign of lipid peroxidation as measured in the urine of patients with probable Alzheimer's disease. *Brain Res Bull.* 2001;54(5):565–568.
16. Beck FK, Rosenthal TC. Prealbumin: A marker for nutritional evaluation. *Am Fam Physician.* 2002;65(8):1575–1578.
17. Albert MS, et al. Predictors of cognitive change in older persons: MacArthur studies of successful aging. *Psychol Aging.* 1995;10(4):578–589.

18. Barnes DE, et al. A longitudinal study of cardiorespiratory fitness and cognitive function in healthy older adults. *J Am Geriatr Soc.* 2003;51(4):459–465.
19. Teri L, et al. Exercise plus behavioral management in patients with Alzheimer disease: A randomized controlled trial. *JAMA.* 2003;290(15):2015–2022.
20. McCurry SM, et al. Training caregivers to change the sleep hygiene practices of patients with dementia: The NITE-AD project. *J Am Geriatr Soc.* 2003;51(10):1455–1460.
21. Abbott RD, et al. Walking and dementia in physically capable elderly men. *JAMA.* 2004;292(12):1447–1453.
22. Weuve J, et al. Physical activity, including walking, and cognitive function in older women. *JAMA.* 2004;292(12):1454–1461.
23. Ball K, et al. Effects of cognitive training interventions with older adults: A randomized controlled trial. *JAMA.* 2002;288(18):2271 2281.
24. Scarmeas N, et al. Cognitive reserve-mediated modulation of positron emission tomographic activations during memory tasks in Alzheimer disease. *Arch Neurol.* 2004;61(1):73–78.
25. Heiss WD, et al. Long-term effects of Phosphatidylserine, pyritinol and cognitive training in Alzheimer's disease. *Dementia.* 1994;5:88–98.
26. Courtney C, et al. Long-term donepezil treatment in 565 patients with Alzheimer's disease (AD2000): Randomised double-blind trial. *Lancet.* 2004;363(9427):2105–2115.
27. Tariot PN, et al. Memantine treatment in patients with moderate to severe Alzheimer disease already receiving donepezil: A randomized controlled trial. *JAMA.* 2004;291(3):317–324.
28. Morris MC, et al. Dietary intake of antioxidant nutrients and the risk of incident Alzheimer disease in a biracial community study. *JAMA.* 2002;287(24):3230–3237.
29. Shumaker SA, et al. Conjugated equine estrogens and incidence of probable dementia and mild cognitive impairment in postmenopausal women: Women's Health Initiative Memory Study. *JAMA.* 2004;291(24):2947–2958.
30. van Dongen MC, et al. The efficacy of ginkgo for elderly people with dementia and age-associated memory impairment: New results of a randomized clinical trial. *J Am Geriatr Soc.* 2000;48(10):1183–1194.
31. Skolnick AA. Old chinese herbal medicine used for fever yields possible new Alzheimer disease therapy. *JAMA.* 1997;277(10): 776.
32. Aisen PS, et al. Effects of Rofecoxib or Naproxen vs Placebo on Alzheimer disease progression: A randomized controlled trial. *JAMA.* 2003;289(21):2819–2826.
33. Roman GC. Vascular dementia: Distinguishing characteristics, treatment, and prevention. *J Am Geriatr Soc.* 2003;51(5 suppl Dementia):S296–S304.
34. Chui H. Vascular dementia, a new beginning: Shifting focus from clinical phenotype to ischemic brain injury. *Neurol Clin.* 2000;18(4):951–978.
35. Bowler JV. Vascular cognitive impairment. *Stroke.* 2004;35(2): 386–388.
36. Heyman A, et al. Comparison of Lewy body variant of Alzheimer's disease with pure Alzheimer's disease: Consortium to establish a registry for Alzheimer's disease, Part XIX. *Neurology.* 1999;52(9):1839–1844.
37. McKeith IG, et al. Consensus guidelines for the clinical and pathologic diagnosis of dementia with Lewy bodies (DLB): Report of the consortium on DLB international workshop. *Neurology.* 1996;47(5):1113–1124.
38. Emre M, et al. Rivastigmine for dementia associated with Parkinson's disease. *N Engl J Med.* 2004;351(24):2509–2518.
39. Hou CE, Carlin D, Miller BL. Non-Alzheimer's disease dementias: Anatomic, clinical, and molecular correlates. *Can J Psychiatry.* 2004;49(3):164–171.
40. Lebert F, et al. Frontotemporal dementia: A randomised, controlled trial with trazodone. *Dement Geriatr Cogn Disord.* 2004;17(4):355–359.
41. Filley CM. The behavioral neurology of cerebral white matter. *Neurology.* 1998;50(6):1535–1540.
42. Riekse RG, et al. Effect of vascular lesions on cognition in Alzheimer's disease: A community-based study. *J Am Geriatr Soc.* 2004;52(9):1442–1448.
43. Verrees M, Selman WR. Management of normal pressure hydrocephalus. *Am Fam Physician.* 2004;70(6):1071–1078.
44. Geldmacher DS. Differential diagnosis of dementia syndromes. *Clin Geriatr Med.* 2004;20(1):27–43.
45. Gruber-Baldini AL, et al. Behavioral symptoms in residential care/assisted living facilities: Prevalence, risk factors, and medication management. *J Am Geriatr Soc.* 2004;52(10):1610–1617.
46. Gray KF. Managing agitation and difficult behavior in dementia. *Clin Geriatr Med.* 2004;20(1):69–82.
47. Schneider LS, Dagerman KS. Psychosis of Alzheimer's disease: Clinical characteristics and history. *J Psychiatr Res.* 2004;38(1):105–111.
48. Lee PE, et al. Atypical antipsychotic drugs in the treatment of behavioural and psychological symptoms of dementia: Systematic review. *BMJ.* 2004;329(7457):75.
49. Frank L, et al. The effect of risperidone on nursing burden associated with caring for patients with dementia. *J Am Geriatr Soc.* 2004;52(9):1449–1455.
50. Young KW, et al. Providing nutrition supplements to institutionalized seniors with probable Alzheimer's disease is least beneficial to those with low body weight status. *J Am Geriatr Soc.* 2004;52(8):1305–1312.
51. Lauque S, et al. Improvement of weight and fat-free mass with oral nutritional supplementation in patients with Alzheimer's disease at risk of malnutrition: A prospective randomized study. *J Am Geriatr Soc.* 2004;52(10):1702–1707.
52. Gillick MR. Rethinking the role of tube feeding in patients with advanced dementia. *N Engl J Med.* 2000;342(3):206–210.
53. Schneider LS, Dagerman KS, Insel P. Risk of death with atypical antipsychotic drug treatment for dementia: Meta-analysis of randomized placebo-controlled trials. *JAMA.* 2005 Oct 19:294(15):1934–1943.
54. Schulz R, et al. End-of-life care and the effects of bereavement on family caregivers of persons with dementia. *N Engl J Med.* 2003;349(20):1936–1942.
55. Mayeux R, Sano M. Treatment of Alzheimer's disease. *N Engl J Med.* 1999;341(22):1670–1679.
56. Jann MW. Rivastigmine, a new-generation cholinesterase inhibitor for the treatment of Alzheimer's disease. *Pharmacotherapy.* 2000;20(1):1–12.
57. Rosler M, et al. Efficacy and safety of rivastigmine in patients with Alzheimer's disease: International randomised controlled trial. *BMJ.* 1999;318(7184):633–638.
58. Scott LJ, Goa KL. Galantamine: A review of its use in Alzheimer's disease. *Drugs.* 2000;60(5):1095–1122.
59. Reisberg B, et al. Memantine in moderate-to-severe Alzheimer's disease. *N Engl J Med.* 2003;348(14):1333–1341.
60. Trinh NH, et al. Efficacy of cholinesterase inhibitors in the treatment of neuropsychiatric symptoms and functional impairment in Alzheimer disease: A meta-analysis. *JAMA.* 2003;289(2): 210–216.
61. Hirschman KB, et al. The development of a rapid screen for caregiver burden. *J Am Geriatr Soc.* 2004;52(10):1724–1729.

SUGGESTED READINGS AND RESOURCES

Organizations that can assist in finding local support for caregivers include:

The Alzheimer's Disease and Related Disorders Association
www.alz.org
The Alzheimer's Association also sponsors a national, government-funded program called Safe Return that assists in the identification and safe return of individuals with dementia who become lost. Their phone number is 888-572-8566.

The National Family Caregivers Association
www.nfcacares.org

Garegiving Online
www.caregiving.com

Caregiverzone
www.caregiverzone.com.

Sleep Disorders

20

Tarannum Alam   *Cathy A. Alessi*

CLINICAL PEARLS 254

OVERVIEW OF SLEEP ARCHITECTURE AND SLEEP STAGES 255

CHANGES IN SLEEP WITH NORMAL AGING 255

DIAGNOSTIC APPROACH/ASSESSMENT OF POTENTIAL SLEEP DISORDERS 255

CLASSIFICATION OF SLEEP DISORDERS 256

SPECIFIC SLEEP DISORDERS 257
Insomnia 257
Sleep-Disordered Breathing 261
Periodic Limb Movement Disorder and Restless Legs Syndrome 262
Circadian Rhythm Sleep Disorders 263
Rapid Eye Movement Sleep Behavior Disorder 263
Narcolepsy 264

CHANGES IN SLEEP WITH DEMENTIA 264
Treatment 264

SLEEP IN THE NURSING HOME 264

CONCLUSION 265

CLINICAL PEARLS

- Sleep complaints must be interpreted with respect to the normal age-dependent changes in sleep.
- Age-related changes in sleep include decreased sleep efficiency, increased sleep latency, earlier bedtime, earlier morning awakenings, more nighttime arousal, more daytime sleepiness, and a decrease in deep sleep.
- Psychiatric disorders, particularly depression, are the most common etiology of sleep problems in community-dwelling elders presenting with insomnia.
- Treatment for insomnia in older people requires careful consideration of the underlying causes because secondary insomnia accounts for 80% to 95% of cases in the geriatric population.
- It is not appropriate to start an older patient on sedative–hypnotic agents without an assessment of the sleep complaints.
- Sleep hygiene and cognitive behavioral therapy can reduce use of hypnotics in patients with insomnia.
- Obstructive sleep apnea is a cause of excessive daytime sleepiness in older people.
- Respiratory depressants, such as sedatives and alcohol, can worsen sleep apnea.
- Sleep changes in dementia include frequent nighttime arousals, further decrease in stages 3 and 4 sleep, disturbances of the sleep–wake cycle, and "sundowning."
- Impaired sleep in nursing home residents is caused by medical illnesses, incontinence, neurodegenerative conditions, depression, certain medications, lack of physical activity, lack of bright light exposure, environmental factors, and frequent primary sleep disorders.
- Referral for polysomnography is indicated if a primary sleep disorder such as sleep apnea or periodic limb movement disorder is suspected or for chronic insomnia where etiology is unclear.

Sleep complaints and disorders are common in the older population. More than half of community-dwelling older people have reported sleeping problems.[1] In a 2003 National Sleep Foundation survey, approximately two thirds of older adults reported experiencing sleep problems at least a few nights a week. Fifty percent of community-dwelling older people use over-the-counter and/or prescribed sleeping medications. The magnitude of sleep problems is even higher in residents of long-term care facilities.[2]

Sleep is an active state that is as complex as wakefulness. It is hypothesized that sleep is caused by reciprocal interactions between sleep- and wake-promoting brain regions, which produces a flip–flop switch.[3] Notable wake-promoting brain regions include serotonergic and noradrenergic cell groups in the pontine and midbrain reticular formation, histaminergic and hypocretinergic neurons in the posterior and lateral hypothalamus, and cholinergic cell groups in the basal forebrain. The preoptic region of the hypothalamus promotes sleep and predominantly contains sleep-active γ-aminobutyric acid (GABA)ergic neurons.[4]

The exact biologic function(s) of sleep is still a mystery, although it is well established that sleep is essential and that its deprivation leads to neurologic, autonomic, and biochemical changes. Sleep is believed to have restorative, conservative, adaptive, thermoregulatory, and consolidative functions. Disrupted sleep is a sign of several significant illnesses of old age, including depression, physical problems, and primary sleep disorders. Problems with sleep can adversely affect the quality of life in older people and can be associated with increased morbidity and mortality.[5] Primary care clinicians caring for older patients should have a high index of suspicion for early recognition and intervention of sleep disorders. Also, the primary care provider must be able to distinguish age-related changes in sleep pattern from changes that are associated with medical illnesses and/or sleep disorders.

OVERVIEW OF SLEEP ARCHITECTURE AND SLEEP STAGES

Within sleep, two separate states have been defined, including nonrapid eye movement (NREM) sleep and rapid eye movement (REM) sleep. NREM sleep is further subdivided into four stages on the basis of electroencephalographic (EEG) criteria. These stages roughly parallel a depth-of-sleep continuum, with stages 1 and 2 considered as light sleep and stages 3 and 4 considered as deep sleep. Stage 1 sleep is characterized by relatively fast EEG frequencies in the theta range (4 to 7 Hz). During stage 2 sleep, there is slowing of EEG frequency and an increase in EEG amplitude with appearance of sleep spindles and K complexes. Stages 3 and 4 of NREM sleep are defined by high-amplitude, low-frequency (1.5 to 3 Hz) delta EEG waves. Stages 3 and 4 together are also referred to as *delta or slow-wave sleep*. REM sleep, also referred to as *paradoxical sleep*, is a period of active sleep with EEG activation, complete atonia of muscles, and bursts of REM. Unlike NREM sleep, REM sleep is also marked by increased oxygen requirements, increased autonomic activity, and dreaming.

Sleep is normally entered through NREM, and both NREM and REM stages alternate with a period near 90 minutes in normal young adults. NREM sleep comprises 75% to 80% of the total sleep time. The remaining 20% to 25% of sleep is spent in REM sleep that occurs in four to six discrete episodes during the night. REM sleep predominates in the last third of night and is linked to the circadian rhythm.

CHANGES IN SLEEP WITH NORMAL AGING

Age-dependent changes in sleep architecture (stages of sleep) and pattern (the amount and timing of sleep) have been well described in the literature.[6,7] The most notable change in sleep structure with aging is a decrease in slow-wave sleep (stages 3 and 4), with stages 1 and 2 sleep increasing or remaining unchanged. In persons older than 90 years, stages 3 and 4 may disappear completely. Other findings include an earlier onset of REM sleep and decreased total REM sleep but no change in the percentage of REM sleep. There is also a more equal distribution of REM sleep throughout the night in older people.

Changes in sleep pattern include decreased sleep efficiency (time asleep over time in bed), increased sleep latency (time to fall asleep), more nighttime arousals, earlier morning awakenings, and more daytime napping. The 24-hour total sleep time remains similar or slightly decreased. The significance of all these changes is unclear. Recent evidence suggests that certain age-related changes in sleep reflect a decrease in the ability to sleep rather than a decrease in the need for sleep.

Circadian rhythmicity also changes with age. Neuronal loss in the suprachiasmatic nucleus in the hypothalamus, which serves as the "body clock," as well as decreased production of melatonin by the pineal gland with aging, weakens circadian rhythmicity in older people, resulting in less sleep at night but more during the day.

DIAGNOSTIC APPROACH/ASSESSMENT OF POTENTIAL SLEEP DISORDERS

Diagnosis of sleep disorders in older persons can be challenging. Patients may not report sleep complaints unless specifically asked for the symptoms. To aid in screening older patients for sleep problems, the National Institutes of Health Consensus Statement on the Treatment of Sleep Disorders of Older People (1991) suggested three simple questions for the clinician, which are as follows:

1. Is the person satisfied with his or her sleep?
2. Does sleep or fatigue intrude with daytime activities?
3. Does the bed partner or others complain of unusual behavior during sleep, such as snoring, interrupted breathing, or leg movements?

In one representative sample, the most common sleep complaints among community-dwelling older people included difficulty falling asleep (37% of the sample), nighttime awakenings (29%), and early morning awakenings (19%).[8] Daytime sleepiness is also common. Transient sleep problems (<2 to 3 weeks) are usually situational. Persistent sleep problems require more detailed evaluation.

A sleep diary may be helpful in clarifying sleep habits. Each morning, in a sleep diary, the patient records his/her time in bed, estimated amount of sleep, number of awakenings, time of morning awakening, and any symptoms that occurred during the night. The physician should try to obtain corroborating evidence from the bed partner, if available.

Initially, it is important to rule out an underlying medical condition, substance abuse, or another mental health problem contributing to sleep complaints. A careful psychosocial history is essential to evaluate the potential role of depression and anxiety. A mental status examination to rule out dementia is also indicated. Changes in social and environmental circumstances such as relocation and bereavement should be addressed. A careful review of systems including questions about pain, nocturia, nocturnal cough, orthopnea, and other symptoms should be performed to seek treatable medical conditions contributing to sleep problems. A full medication history, including over-the-counter and herbal medications, is absolutely essential (see Table 20.1).

A focused physical examination based on positive findings from the history should also be performed. The history and physical examination should guide laboratory testing. On the basis of this initial assessment, further studies or objective evaluation may be indicated.

Polysomnography (PSG) is the gold standard for the evaluation of sleep.

During PSG, several physiologic variables are simultaneously recorded; the parameters include EEG, electromyogram (EMG), electrooculogram (EOG), electrocardiogram (EKG), airflow at the nose and mouth; respiratory effort; and oxygen saturation. The EEG, EOG, and EMG recordings are scored for stages of sleep, total sleep time, sleep-onset latency, and percentage of time in NREM versus REM sleep.

According to the recommendations of the American Academy of Sleep Medicine (1997), PSG is primarily indicated when a sleep-related breathing disorder, periodic limb movement disorder (PLMD), narcolepsy, or REM sleep behavior disorder (RBD) is suspected.[9] PSG is also commonly used when the initial diagnosis is uncertain or treatments fail in patients with chronic insomnia. Some sleep experts recommend PSG before embarking on the treatment of chronic insomnia because primary sleep disorders are common in older people. However, PSG is not indicated for routine evaluation of transient insomnia or insomnia secondary to psychiatric disorders.

The multiple sleep latency test (MSLT) is primarily used in the diagnosis of narcolepsy. During this test, the individual is polygraphically monitored during five scheduled daytime naps. The MSLT records the latency (i.e., time to fall asleep) for each nap, the mean sleep latency, and the presence or absence of REM sleep during any of the naps.

Other methods for the assessment of sleep include wrist actigraphy, which is a relatively low-cost method. A wrist actigraph is a portable device about the size of a wristwatch, which estimates sleep–wake amount on the basis of wrist activity. It is particularly valuable for studying individuals who might have difficulty sleeping in a sleep laboratory, such as those with insomnia and the elderly. Patients are studied in their own environment for multiple nights. Although this method cannot be used to determine the cause of insomnia, it can help in the evaluation of its severity. It also provides information about daytime napping. Actigraphy on nursing home residents has documented the extreme fragmentation of sleep in this population, leading to ongoing studies to improve the quality and quantity of sleep in this vulnerable group of patients.

Referral to a sleep specialist for PSG is indicated in the evaluation of suspected primary sleep disorders. A sleep specialist can also be helpful in the evaluation and management of chronic sleep complaints, even if PSG is not indicated. The key points to be considered while evaluating sleep disorders in older patients are summarized in Table 20.2.

TABLE 20.1

DRUGS THAT INTERFERE WITH SLEEP

Common Drugs Associated with Insomnia

Alcohol
Caffeine
Nicotine
Antidepressants (e.g., MAOIs; occasionally SSRIs, venlafaxine, and bupropion)
Asthma/COPD medications (e.g., theophylline)
Corticosteroids (e.g., oral prednisone and dexamethasone, IV hydrocortisone)
Decongestants (e.g., pseudoephedrine)
H_2-blockers (e.g., cimetidine)
Antihypertensives (e.g., β-blockers that cross the blood–brain barrier, such as propranolol, pindolol, metoprolol)

Common Drugs Associated with Daytime Sleepiness

Analgesics (e.g., narcotics)
Antidepressants (e.g., imipramine, trazodone)
Antihypertensives (e.g., clonidine)
Antihistamines

MAOIs, monoamine oxidase inhibitors; SSRI, selective serotonin reuptake inhibitor; COPD, chronic obstructive pulmonary disease.

CLASSIFICATION OF SLEEP DISORDERS

Sleep disorders have been classified in various ways. The International Classification of Sleep Disorders (ICSD)[10] is the most widely used. The *ICSD Diagnostic and Coding Manual* lists 88 sleep disorders with their diagnostic criteria. It also includes a differential diagnosis listing of sleep disorders that cause the two main sleep symptoms,

TABLE 20.2
KEY POINTS IN THE EVALUATION OF OLDER PATIENTS WITH SLEEPING DIFFICULTIES

1. Perform a focused history and physical examination
2. Review sleep hygiene
3. Is there a potentially causative medical condition (e.g., pain from arthritis, symptoms of gastroesophageal reflux, nocturia)?
4. Is there a potentially causative medication?
5. Has the patient been using sedatives/hypnotics chronically?
6. Is there evidence of depression?
7. Is there evidence of dementia?
8. Is there evidence of an alcohol-induced sleep problem?
9. Is there evidence of a primary sleep disorder, such as sleep apnea, periodic limb movement disorder, or circadian rhythm abnormality?
10. Does the patient need referral to a sleep specialist for overnight polysomnography or other evaluation/testing?

insomnia and excessive daytime sleepiness, and those that produce other symptoms.

The ICSD has classified sleep disorders into four major categories: (i) The *dyssomnias,* which are disorders of initiating and maintaining sleep and the disorders of excessive sleepiness; (ii) the *parasomnias,* which are disorders of arousal, partial arousal, and sleep-stage transition that intrude into the sleep process; (iii) *disorders associated with medical or psychiatric disorders;* and (iv) the *proposed sleep disorders for which there is insufficient information to confirm their acceptance as a definitive sleep disorder.*

The *Diagnostic and Statistical Manual of Mental Disorders Fourth Edition* (DSM-IV) lists another system of classifying sleep disorders, which is mainly used by psychiatrists and shows considerable overlap with ICSD.[11] Table 20.3 classifies some of the sleep disorders commonly encountered by primary care clinicians.

TABLE 20.3
COMMON SLEEP DISORDERS, THEIR CLASSIFICATION AND ICD-9 CODES

I. Primary sleep disorders
   A. Dyssomnias
      1. Idiopathic (780.52) and psychophysiologic (307.42-4) insomnias
      2. Obstructive (780.53) and central (780.51) sleep apnea syndrome
      3. Periodic limb movement disorder (780.52-4)
      4. Restless legs syndrome (780.52-5)
      5. Narcolepsy (347)
      6. Circadian rhythm sleep disorders (e.g., jet lag [307.45], shift-work syndrome [307.45-1], delayed or advanced sleep-phase syndrome [780.55])
   B. Parasomnias
      1. Sleepwalking (307.46) and sleeptalking (307.47-3)
      2. Parasomnias associated with REM sleep (e.g., nightmares [307.47], and sleep paralysis [780.56-2])
      3. REM sleep behavior disorder (780.59)
      4. Sleep bruxism (306.8)
II. Sleep disorders associated with medical and psychiatric conditions
   A. Associated with mental disorders (290–319) (e.g., psychosis, mood disorders, anxiety disorders, and panic disorders)
   B. Associated with neurologic disorders (320–389) (e.g., dementia, parkinsonism, and cerebral degenerative disorders)
   C. Associated with other medical disorders (e.g., chronic obstructive pulmonary disease, congestive heart failure, gastroesophageal reflux disease, peptic ulcer disease, and fibromyalgia)
III. Sleep disorders associated with extrinsic factors
   A. Inadequate sleep hygiene (307.41-1)
   B. Hypnotic- (780.52-0)/stimulant-dependent sleep disorders (780.52-1)
   C. Alcohol-dependent sleep disorder (780.52-3)

SPECIFIC SLEEP DISORDERS

Insomnia

CASE ONE

A 78-year-old woman reports trouble sleeping. She takes a long time to get to sleep at night, wakes up frequently during the night, and wakes up early in the morning. Her husband died 1 year ago. Since then, she stopped going to the local senior center and dropped many other interests and activities.

CASE TWO

A 65-year-old man reports frequent nighttime awakenings. He is not well rested the next day but does not nap or fall asleep during the day. He reports burning chest discomfort at night.

Insomnia is a complaint of inadequate or nonrestorative sleep characterized by one or more of the following: Difficulty falling asleep, repeated awakening, inadequate total sleep time or poor quality of sleep, as reflected in daytime functioning. The definition of insomnia must also include a complaint of daytime dysfunction in the form of a change in alertness, energy, cognitive dysfunction, behavior, or emotional state. In contrast, people who are normal "short sleepers" may complain of decreased total sleep time, but there are no significant daytime consequences associated with the complaint.

The prevalence of insomnia increases with age. Epidemiologic studies have found that insomnia is the most common sleep disturbance in the older population, with up to 40% of those older than 60 complaining of difficulty falling asleep and/or maintaining sleep, and >20% reporting severe insomnia.[1] There is a clear gender difference, with insomnia being more prevalent in women. A 1995 survey found that almost 70% of patients with chronic insomnia never discuss the problem with their physicians. Even when physicians are aware of the problem and prescribe medication, adequate evaluation is often lacking.

Depending upon the time course, insomnia can be acute, subacute, or chronic. The ICSD defines acute or transient insomnia as persisting for no more than 1 week and subacute or short-term insomnia as lasting from 1 week to 3 months. Both transient and short-term insomnias are almost universal experiences and are categorized under the diagnosis of adjustment sleep disorder. Although situational insomnia often resolves spontaneously, it must be recognized that it can also represent the foundation of a long-term condition. Chronic insomnia frequently begins as a stress-related phenomenon. Therefore, early identification and intervention may play an important role in the prevention of chronic insomnia.

Insomnia can also be classified as primary or secondary. When insomnia is not related to other specific medical, psychiatric, or medication-associated conditions, it may be considered primary (i.e., psychophysiologic, idiopathic, or sleep-state misperception). Psychophysiologic insomnia predominantly involves somatized tension and learned sleep-preventing associations that result in the complaint of insomnia and associated decreased functioning during wakefulness. When the insomnia is related to a specific medical, neurologic, or other sleep disorder, substance abuse, or psychiatric condition, it is considered to be secondary insomnia. Secondary insomnia accounts for 80% to 95% of cases in the geriatric population. For example, the patient in Case One presents with symptoms suggestive of insomnia secondary to depression, whereas Case Two suggests insomnia secondary to gastroesophageal reflux disease.

When a complaint of insomnia is identified, a detailed, skilled sleep history obtained in a systematic manner is the foundation of initial evaluation. Sleep questionnaires and at-home sleep logs can also provide important information. Bed partners/roommates/caregivers are potential sources of information about the quantity and quality of sleep, daytime consequences, and occurrence of nocturnal events. Patients should be questioned about abnormal events occurring during sleep, including periodic limb movement, respiratory distress, panic attack, pain, headache, or gastroesophageal reflux. Recent stressors and symptoms of depression, anxiety, and other psychiatric disorders need to be identified. Inquiry about previous interventions and outcomes can reveal important information. The clinician should also determine whether previous interventions have received a fair trial and what factors may have accounted for treatment failures. Medical history and a complete list of medications, including over-the-counter and herbal remedies, should be reviewed.

The American Academy of Sleep Medicine does not recommend routine PSG in the evaluation of insomnia unless there is a diagnostic uncertainty or when treatment interventions have proved unsuccessful. In addition, PSG is indicated when a sleep-related breathing disorder, narcolepsy, PLMD, or unusual parasomnias are suspected.[9] Wrist actigraphy is also not indicated for routine diagnosis of insomnia but may be useful as an adjunct to other assessment procedures or in evaluating response to therapy.

Differential Diagnosis of Insomnia

The etiologies of insomnia are commonly psychiatric/psychological problems, symptoms related to underlying medical illness, effects of medications, or problems in the sleep–wake cycle. In fact, multiple factors may contribute to insomnia in the older patient.

Psychiatric Disorders

Most studies report that psychiatric disorders are the etiology of sleep problems in more than half of the patients presenting with disorders of initiating or maintaining sleep. This is particularly true for depression, where early morning awakening is the most characteristic pattern, along with increased sleep latency and more nighttime wakefulness. In fact, sleep disturbance in older people who are not currently depressed can be an important predictor of future depression. Bereavement, anxiety, and stress can also affect sleep, usually resulting in difficulty initiating sleep.

Medical Problems

Medical problems can be the cause or aggravating factor in sleep difficulties. Chronic pain at night is a very common medical cause, particularly in older patients with rheumatologic disorders, neuropathy, and cancer. Other common etiologies include cough, dyspnea of cardiac or pulmonary origin, gastroesophageal reflux, and nocturia.

Drug and Alcohol Dependency

Drug and alcohol use are thought to account for 10% to 15% of cases of insomnia. Chronic use of sedatives can lead to fragmented sleep. Most sleeping medications, when used chronically, can lead to tolerance and are associated with rebound insomnia when stopped abruptly.

The use of medications to treat medical problems can also lead to insomnia. Commonly prescribed medications that may cause insomnia include corticosteroids, bronchodilators, decongestants, theophylline, β-blockers, diuretics, central nervous system (CNS) stimulants, and antidepressants such as fluoxetine, paroxetine, sertraline, and venlafaxine. Some antidepressants can cause insomnia or somnolence depending upon the dose (e.g., nortriptyline, trazodone, and imipramine). Many over-the-counter medications produce side effects that are either sedating or stimulating. Older patients often take multiple medications, which may be prescribed by multiple providers, compounding the situation.

Caffeine also causes insomnia. In addition to coffee, caffeine is an ingredient in many nonprescription medications (e.g., headache medications and dietary supplements), chocolate, and beverages. Caffeine increases sleep latency (i.e., time to fall asleep) and sleep fragmentation and decreases total sleep time.

Alcohol abuse is often associated with fragmented sleep. Many people attempt to self-treat sleeping difficulties with alcohol. Although it does reduce sleep latency, it also causes sleep fragmentation, decreased REM, REM rebound, and early morning awakenings. The use of alcohol combined with hypnotics may further exacerbate sleep difficulties.

Primary Sleep Disorders

Restless legs syndrome (RLS), PLMD, sleep-disordered breathing, circadian rhythm disturbance, partial arousal disorders, and RBD can also cause insomnia. These conditions are discussed in the subsequent text.

Poor Sleep Hygiene

Poor sleep hygiene includes maladaptive practices that interfere with normal sleep and contribute to insomnia complaints. It can be one of the factors that lead a stress-related short-term insomnia to become chronic insomnia.

Management

Because insomnia is a symptom of a wide variety of medical, psychological, and psychiatric conditions, it is crucial to identify the underlying causes, which can lead to specific treatments such as analgesics for nocturnal pain, treatment for depression, and stabilization of underlying medical problems such as heart failure or chronic obstructive pulmonary disease. Treating insomnia without addressing the underlying cause(s) can result in treatment failure and even exacerbation of the problem. All drugs that have the potential to cause sleep disturbance should be eliminated or substituted, if possible. For chronic insomnia, after underlying problems have been addressed, behavioral therapy should be initiated, with sedatives–hypnotics as the last resort. However, it is appropriate to use sedative–hypnotics early in cases of stress-related transient insomnia, such as during acute hospitalization.

Nonpharmacologic Treatment

Sleep Hygiene Education

Sleep hygiene is an educational approach to make patients more aware of health practices (e.g., diet, exercise, and substance abuse) and environmental factors (e.g., light, noise, temperature, and mattress) that may be either detrimental or beneficial to sleep. Patients with sleep problems should be routinely educated about good sleep hygiene (see Table 20.4).

Stimulus Control

The objective of stimulus control is to retrain the patient with insomnia who has developed a conditioned response associating the bed and bedroom with resultant poor sleep. For example, the patient may be instructed to use the bed only for sleeping and to leave the bed if he or she is awake for >15 to 30 minutes.

TABLE 20.4

EXAMPLES OF SLEEP HYGIENE MEASURES TO IMPROVE SLEEP

- Maintain a regular morning rising time
- Avoid daytime naps or limit napping to the early afternoon for less than an hour
- Exercise or increase activity level in the afternoon but not in the evening or immediately before bedtime
- Increase exposure to bright light during the day or early evening
- Take a hot bath within 2 h of bedtime
- Avoid caffeine, nicotine, and alcohol in the evening
- Avoid excessive food or fluid intake at night
- Practice a bedtime routine, minimize light and noise exposure in the bedroom, and use bedroom only for sleep

Sleep Restriction Therapy

Sleep restriction therapy involves curtailing the amount of time in bed to the actual amount of time spent asleep and then lengthening sleep time after sleep efficiency improves. The restriction of time in bed may initially create sleep deprivation, which in itself produces more consolidated sleep. Prescribed time in bed is based on individual sleep diaries. Implementation of this technique requires a high level of motivation and compliance on the patient's part and close follow-up by the clinician.

Progressive Muscle Relaxation

Progressive muscle relaxation involves a method of tensing and relaxing different muscle groups throughout the body and has been observed to be useful in patients with insomnia who often display high levels of arousal both at night and during the daytime. Unfortunately, this method may not be as effective in older people.

Multicomponent Behavioral Therapy

Multicomponent behavioral therapy includes various combinations of both psychological and behavioral interventions, such as changing the patient's beliefs and attitudes about insomnia, stimulus control, sleep restriction, and progressive muscle relaxation.

Bright Light Therapy

Bright light therapy is used to correct circadian rhythm causes of sleeping difficulty. The patient is exposed to sunlight or a commercially available light box. The duration and intensity of bright light exposure has varied considerably between studies. The patient sits in front of a 10,000-lux light for 30 to 40 minutes either early in the morning or evening, depending on whether the patient has difficulty falling asleep or is bothered by early morning awakenings. Response is generally evident

TABLE 20.5
SOME COMMONLY USED SEDATIVES/HYPNOTICS IN OLDER PEOPLE

Generic Name (Trade Name)	Class	Usual Dose Range in Older People (mg)	Half-life (h)
Lorazepam (Ativan)	Intermediate-acting benzodiazepine	0.25–2	8–12
Temazepam (Restoril)	Intermediate-acting benzodiazepine	15–30	8–10 (up to 30 h in older people)
Estazolam (ProSom)	Intermediate-acting benzodiazepine	0.5–2	12–18
Zolpidem (Ambien)	Nonbenzodiazepine, imidazopyridine (short-acting)	5–10	1.5–4.5 (10 h in cirrhosis)
Zaleplon (Sonata)	Nonbenzodiazepine, pyrazolopyrimidine (short-acting)	5–10	1
Trazodone (Desyrel)	Sedating antidepressant	25–150	2–4

after 2 to 3 weeks of treatment. Potential side effects include transient headache, eyestrain, and photosensitizing effects for patients on medications such as amiodarone and hydrochlorothiazide. A routine eye examination is recommended before treatment.

Pharmacologic Treatment

Use of sleep medications is extremely common in older adults. They are also likely to continue therapy for extended periods. The decision to initiate drug therapy for insomnia should be based on the presence and severity of daytime symptoms and their impact on functioning and quality of life. Short-term hypnotic therapy may be appropriate in conjunction with improved sleep hygiene in some cases of transient, situational insomnia, particularly during bereavement, acute hospitalizations, and other periods of temporary acute stress. However, in patients with chronic insomnia, sedative–hypnotic agents should be considered cautiously because of the complications associated with long-term use of these agents.

An ideal hypnotic agent in older people should have a rapid onset of action to reduce sleep latency, a duration of action that lasts throughout the night with no residual effects, and no adverse effects. However, none of the available agents fulfill all the above criteria. Altered metabolism of drugs, high rate of polypharmacy, and increased sensitivity to the depressant effects of some medications on the CNS in older people have to be taken into account. Sedatives/hypnotics should be used as briefly as possible, and essentially all agents are approved for short-term use only (i.e., 2 to 3 weeks only). For patients with chronic insomnia, treatment is best accomplished by using hypnotics on an "as-needed basis," but time to onset of action for many agents can make "p.r.n." use problematic. Extreme care should be taken to avoid dependence with these medications because continued use results in tolerance to therapeutic effects with most hypnotics and may result in escalation of dose. The sedative–hypnotics commonly used and those to be avoided in older people are listed in Tables 20.5 and 20.6, respectively.

TABLE 20.6
SLEEP MEDICATIONS TO AVOID IN OLDER PEOPLE

Benzodiazepines
Quazepam (Doral): Active metabolite half-life is 70 h
Flurazepam (Dalmane): Active metabolite half-life may exceed 100 h
Triazolam (Halcion): Anterograde amnesia, agitation, confusion reported in elderly
Nonbenzodiazepine CNS Depressant
Chloral hydrate (Noctec): Drug interactions, GI discomfort
Sedating Antihistamine
Diphenhydramine (e.g., Benadryl): Potent anticholinergic effects

CNS, central nervous system; GI, gastrointestinal.

Benzodiazepine receptor agonists (including benzodiazepines such as temazepam and nonbenzodiazepine hypnotics such as zolpidem and zaleplon) remain the most preferred drugs for the treatment of insomnia in older people (Evidence Level A). The use of sedating antidepressants in patients with concomitant diagnosis of mood disorders is also widespread.

Short-acting benzodiazepines are recommended for problems initiating sleep, and intermediate-acting agents are recommended for problems with sleep maintenance. Short-acting agents have fewer daytime effects and are less likely to be associated with falls and hip fractures. However, agents with rapid elimination also produce the most pronounced rebound and withdrawal syndromes after discontinuation. Drug dose and half-life are important factors in rebound insomnia. Using the lowest effective dose and tapering the dosage before discontinuation of the drug can reduce the potential for rebound insomnia.

When used for insomnia, the benzodiazepines decrease sleep latency, increase total sleep time, and decrease nocturnal awakenings. However, the sleep architecture is different from natural sleep because benzodiazepines prolong stage 1 and 2 sleep and reduce both slow-wave and REM sleep.

Intermediate-acting drugs have less association with daytime drowsiness as compared to long-acting agents. Temazepam has an intermediate half-life and no known active metabolites. Also, its metabolism is not affected by aging. Its onset of action is 45 to 60 minutes.

Estazolam is a benzodiazepine with rapid onset and intermediate duration of action, so it may be effective in initiating and maintaining sleep.

Long-acting agents such as quazepam and flurazepam should not be used in older people because these agents are transformed into clinically active metabolites with a half-life of >100 hours. These metabolites accumulate substantially and have been associated with significant hangover effects, such as sedation, drowsiness, incoordination, and cognitive and psychomotor impairment. Triazolam is a short-acting benzodiazepine that should not be used in older people because it has been associated with nocturnal confusion, amnesia, and psychotic reactions.

Zaleplon and zolpidem are two newer short-acting nonbenzodiazepine hypnotics. They are structurally different from traditional benzodiazepine agents; however, they act on the GABA–benzodiazepine receptor complex, binding selectively and mainly to the benzodiazepine-1 receptor subtype. This selective subtype affinity makes pharmacologic actions of zaleplon and zolpidem different from the actions of agents that bind nonselectively to benzodiazepine receptors. Both these agents reduce the time to onset of sleep and increase the duration of sleep and may be less likely to disturb the architecture of sleep.

In placebo-controlled trials, zaleplon had no adverse effect on daytime performance in psychomotor testing and did not produce rebound insomnia or withdrawal effects. Because of rapid onset of action, zolpidem and zaleplon should only be taken immediately before bedtime or after the patient has gone to bed and has been unable to fall asleep. No evidence of tolerance has been observed with either drug. However, as with other sedatives–hypnotics, these agents are labeled for short-term use only and, if used longer, for only two or three nights per week.

Eszopiclone, a $GABA_A$ receptor agonist, has been recently approved by the U.S. Food and Drug Administration (FDA) for treatment of insomnia. In elderly patients, eszopiclone has been shown to produce significant improvement in sleep maintenance and a reduction in the number and duration of naps (Evidence Level B). The recommended initial dosage is 1 mg immediately before bedtime.

Low doses of sedating antidepressants such as trazodone, doxepin, and mirtazapine at bedtime may be used as a sleeping aid, particularly in patients with depression. Efficacy of these agents as hypnotics in nondepressed patients remains unknown. Other situations to consider off-label use of low-dose sedating antidepressants for sleep include patients who have had problems with benzodiazepine receptor agonists and in people with sleep apnea, fibromyalgia, or a history of substance abuse.

Over-the-counter sleep medications are often self-prescribed by older people. The most frequently used products are sedating antihistamines and analgesics marketed for nighttime use, which combine an analgesic (e.g., acetaminophen) with a sedating antihistamine. Diphenhydramine is a long-acting antihistamine, which has potent anticholinergic effects and can also lead to daytime sedation and cognitive impairment. There are no data to show that antihistamines either improve insomnia or prolong sleep. Their use as a sleeping aid should be strongly discouraged, especially in frail older people.

Melatonin is a hormone that helps control circadian rhythms. It is also a popular over-the-counter nutritional supplement marketed as a sleeping aid. Evidence is mixed about the effectiveness of melatonin in the treatment of insomnia. However, melatonin is not FDA regulated. It is sold in health food stores usually as 3-mg tablets. Because of mixed results and the lack of regulatory control of the currently available melatonin products, routine use of melatonin is not recommended for insomnia. However, there may be some role for melatonin in jet lag, shift-work adaptation, and sleep problems in blind people.

Valerian is an herbal product with several active compounds, which is also marketed as a sleeping aid. Its use should probably not be recommended because of lack of studies and regulation and because of evidence of its minimal effectiveness as a sleep aid.

Sleep-Disordered Breathing

CASE THREE

A 75-year-old man falls asleep in your office waiting room. He has hypertension, weighs 130 kg, and is 175 cms. He admits to feeling sleepy during the daytime. His wife reports he snores loudly at night.

This case is suggestive of sleep-disordered breathing, which is (commonly referred to as *sleep apnea*) characterized by repeated episodes of either cessation or marked decrease of airflow during sleep. Complete cessation of airflow for >10 seconds with a 2% to 4% drop in oxygen saturation is referred to as an *apnea* (generally associated with sleep fragmentation) and partial cessation of respiration during sleep is referred to as a *hypopnea*. The apnea–hypopnea index (also known as the *respiratory disturbance index*) refers to the total number of apneas and hypopneas per hour of sleep. Apneas and hypopneas during sleep can result from obstruction of the upper airway (obstructive apnea), loss of ventilatory efforts (central apnea), or a combination of the two. However, central and obstructive events are rarely seen in isolation.

Obstructive sleep apnea (OSA) is the most common sleep disorder diagnosed in sleep laboratories, probably because of referral patterns by primary providers to these centers. OSA is characterized by recurrent episodes involving the collapse of the upper airway and a reduction or cessation of airflow despite persistent ventilatory efforts during sleep. When this is associated with symptoms such as daytime somnolence, the term *OSA syndrome* is applied.

The prevalence of sleep apnea increases with age. The reported prevalence of sleep apnea among older persons varies from 20% to 70%, depending on the population studied. Obesity is the strongest risk factor for OSA. Neck circumference or the hip-to-waist ratio may exhibit an even better correlation with presence of OSA than body mass index.

OSA may be aggravated by alcohol ingestion (especially before bedtime), sedatives, sleep deprivation, nasal congestion, and supine sleeping posture. Also, there appears to be a higher prevalence of OSA in patients with dementia.

The clinical consequences of sleep apnea are many, including hypertension, cardiac arrhythmia, heart failure, memory impairment, and increased mortality. Recently, endothelial dysfunction has been implicated in patients with OSA, which likely predisposes to atherosclerosis and development of cardiovascular disease.

Clinical Symptoms

Excessive daytime sleepiness is the most common complaint in OSA. Sleepiness may range from subtle symptoms (such as midafternoon drowsiness) to severe (such as falling asleep while driving). Loud snoring, nocturnal gasping, and witnessed apneas may be reported by bed partners. Apneic episodes are usually terminated by gasps, chokes, snorts, or brief awakenings. Patients complain of morning headache, daytime fatigue, and impaired dexterity, attention, memory, or judgment. Personality changes such as irritability, anxiety, or depression may be observed.

Clinical examination of a patient suspected of having OSA should include an evaluation of body habitus with measurements of height, weight, and neck circumference and a careful upper airway examination to identify structures or abnormalities that potentially narrow the airway.

Laboratory Evaluation

Thyroid disorders should be ruled out because hypothyroidism predisposes to OSA. Patients suspected of having sleep apnea should be referred to a sleep laboratory for overnight PSG, from which an apnea–hypopnea index is calculated.

Treatment

Nasally applied continuous positive airway pressure (CPAP) is the established treatment of choice for sleep apnea (Evidence Level A). It requires the patient to wear a sealed mask over the nose during sleep. Regardless of the mechanism, nasal CPAP has been documented to eliminate both mixed and obstructive apneas. Split-night studies are often used in sleep laboratories, in which the first half of the night PSG is used for diagnosis and the second half of the night is used for CPAP titration to establish the patient's CPAP prescription. Recently, auto-CPAP machines have been introduced, which automatically titrate pressure needed to keep the upper airway open.

Use of CPAP in patients with dementia is a challenge. Treatment of sleep apnea does not seem to affect the progression of dementia. However, if a patient with sleep apnea and dementia is somnolent during daytime, treatment of sleep apnea may be useful in increasing quality of life. Ethical considerations should be weighed carefully before instituting treatment with CPAP.

Other general measures consist of avoiding sedatives, hypnotics, and alcohol, which can worsen OSA. In obese patients, reduction of body weight is recommended. In a few severe cases, surgical treatments such as uvulopalatopharyngoplasty or hyoid suspension may be considered. Laser and radio frequency uvulopalatopharyngoplasty have been tried. Oral and dental appliances that reposition the jaw or tongue are also available. The best evidence for use of these oral and dental devices is in mild cases of OSA.

Periodic Limb Movement Disorder and Restless Legs Syndrome

> **CASE FOUR**
>
> An 80-year-old man with diabetes, anemia, and peripheral vascular disease reports that he is doing well "except for those darn legs." He describes an uncomfortable sensation in his legs at night that keeps him from falling asleep. He thinks his mother "had the same thing."

Periodic limb movements of sleep (PLMS) are episodes of repetitive and highly stereotyped movements (primarily of the legs) during sleep. When PLMS is associated with a complaint of insomnia and/or excessive sleepiness with no other disorder to explain the symptoms, it is referred to as *PLMD*. The leg movements may occur as much as every 20 to 40 seconds during sleep and last approximately 0.5 to 5.0 seconds. Intense movements may lead to brief arousals from sleep, causing nonrestorative sleep.

The occurrence of PLMS seems to increase with age and may or may not be associated with sleep impairment in different individuals. In a sample of community-dwelling adults older than 65 years, the prevalence of PLMS was found to be 45%.[12] The diagnosis of PLMD is established by

PSG. The number of leg jerks per hour is termed the *PLMS index*. A clinical diagnosis of PLMD is made when a patient complaining of insomnia and/or excessive sleepiness has five or more leg kicks per hour of sleep, each causing an arousal, and other sleep disorders have been excluded. Two consecutive nights of PSG have been recommended because the PLMS index shows night-to-night variability, but this can be a costly approach.

RLS is an awake phenomenon characterized by an irresistible urge to move the legs, usually associated with sensory complaints such as paresthesia or dysesthesia at night. The dysesthesia may be described by patients as a sensation of pins and needles, internal itching, or a creeping or crawling sensation. There is usually worsening of symptoms at rest and relief with motor activity. Symptoms are worse later in the day or at night. Patients usually have difficulty in initiating sleep. Some patients wake up in the middle of the night with paresthesias, which force them to walk around to relieve the discomfort. Prevalence of RLS also increases with age. The diagnosis of RLS is made on history alone. There may be a family history of the condition and, in some cases, an underlying medical disorder, such as uremia, iron deficiency, or peripheral neuropathy, that predisposes to the condition. The symptoms in Case Four are suggestive of RLS.

RLS and PLMD are distinct syndromes that may coexist. Approximately 80% of individuals with RLS have evidence of PLMS on PSG. Symptoms from RLS and PLMD may have a major impact on the patient and bed partner, including severe insomnia, anxiety, depression, and social dysfunction.

Treatment

Pharmacologic treatment should be limited to patients who meet specific diagnostic criteria. The presence of secondary forms and comorbid conditions indicate the need for treatment of the underlying disorders. RLS in association with low ferritin levels may respond to iron replacement therapy.

In older patients with PLMD and RLS, dopaminergic agents are the initial agents of choice for both conditions (Evidence Level B). A nighttime dose of carbidopa/levodopa can be used on an "as-needed basis" for infrequent symptoms. Chronic symptoms are best treated with a dopamine agonist such as pramipexole or ropinirole. Benzodiazepines (e.g., clonazepam) and opioids (e.g., oxycodone) may also be effective but because of risks of side effects, optimal dosage, and misuse potential in older people, these agents are not first-line therapy. Periodic reevaluation to monitor the overall risk–benefit ratio for individual patients is required when these agents are being used. There is limited evidence about the use of carbamazepine, gabapentin, and clonidine in the treatment of PLMS and RLS. Quinine has been a folk remedy for generations, but there is limited evidence to support its effectiveness.

Circadian Rhythm Sleep Disorders

> **CASE FIVE**
>
> An 84-year-old woman falls asleep early (about 7 PM) and gets up early (approximately 3 AM). She feels rested during the day and has no other complaints, other than concern about missing family activities because of her sleeping habits.

In circadian rhythm sleep disorders, patients have difficulty sleeping as a result of desynchronization between their endogenous circadian clock and external environmental cycles. The suprachiasmatic nucleus in the anterior hypothalamus is responsible for the generation of circadian rhythmicity. These rhythms are entrained to periods close to 24 hours in duration by time cues or "zeitgebers," the most important of which is the light–dark cycle.[13] The most common circadian rhythm sleep disorders are jet lag (associated with high-speed air travel across time zones) and shift-work sleep disorder. Evidence for age-associated decrement in entrainment ability to circadian rhythm comes from studies of shift work and jet lag, which show that older adults have more sleep disturbance as compared to younger people.

Older adults often exhibit the advanced sleep-phase syndrome (ASPS) in which they go to sleep early in the evening and wake up early in the morning, as described in Case Five. Often, individuals with ASPS try to stay up late, yet their biologic clock still causes them to awaken in the early morning hours. As a result they do not get enough sleep and are sleepy during the day. Sleep diaries and activity monitoring can be used to detect early evening sleepiness, as well as early morning awakenings, which may indicate ASPS. In contrast, people with the delayed phase syndrome have difficulty sleeping early in the evening. They fall asleep late and wake up late in the morning.

Treatment

Behavioral treatments to entrain the sleep–wake cycle are the most appropriate forms of treatment. Problems related to ASPS may respond to appropriately timed bright light exposure (e.g., evening bright light therapy for 30 to 60 minutes). Some studies suggest that melatonin replacement therapy improves sleep efficiency in this population.[14] Patients with a significant sleep-phase cycle disturbance should be referred to a sleep laboratory for evaluation.

Rapid Eye Movement Sleep Behavior Disorder

> **CASE SIX**
>
> A 72-year-old man is referred to you for evaluation of falls. His falls occur only at night, when he falls out of bed during sleep. He also reports frightening dreams in which

he is fighting off monsters or large animals. His wife says that he "thrashes about" while asleep, sometimes resulting in injury to himself and/or her.

The symptoms in Case Six suggest RBD, which is a REM sleep parasomnia characterized by excessive motor activities during sleep, with the pathologic absence of the normal muscle atonia that should occur during REM sleep. The presenting symptoms are usually vigorous sleep behaviors associated with vivid dreams. These behaviors may result in injury to the patient or bed partner. There may be a family history of this condition. Acute transient RBD has been associated with toxic-metabolic abnormalities, primarily drug or alcohol withdrawal or intoxication. Certain medications, such as selective serotonin reuptake inhibitors and related antidepressants, and other agents have been implicated. The chronic form of RBD is usually idiopathic or is often associated with other neurologic disorders, such as dementia, Parkinson disease, and multiple system atrophy.

Treatment

The diagnosis of RBD is suspected on clinical grounds and established by PSG. Clonazepam is reported to be highly effective in the treatment of RBD, with little evidence of tolerance or abuse over long periods of treatment. Environmental safety interventions are essential, such as removing potentially dangerous objects from the bedroom, putting cushions around the bed, and in some cases, placing the mattress on the floor. The safety of the bed partner should also be ensured.

Narcolepsy

Narcolepsy is a chronic sleep disorder characterized by excessive daytime sleepiness, cataplexy (attacks of weakness on emotional arousal), sleep paralysis, hypnagogic hallucinations, and REM sleep at sleep onset. Recently, narcolepsy has been linked to the loss or malfunction of hypocretin neurons in the hypothalamus.[15]

Patients with narcolepsy tend to fall asleep rapidly at night but experience poor nocturnal sleep with frequent awakenings. In older people with narcolepsy, the cataplexy is less severe, although excessive daytime sleepiness remains similar to that experienced by younger people with this disorder. Narcolepsy rarely develops in old age, but many patients may remain undiagnosed for decades. Older patients with narcolepsy are often misdiagnosed as having epilepsy or schizophrenia. Patients with onset of symptoms of narcolepsy after the age of 50 should undergo neuroimaging to exclude structural lesions in the brain.

Treatment

Patients suspected of having narcolepsy should be referred to a sleep specialist for overnight PSG and multiple sleep latency testing. Once the diagnosis is confirmed, treatment of narcolepsy includes CNS stimulants such as modafinil for excessive daytime sleepiness, as well as anticholinergic and antidepressant drugs for cataplexy. People with narcolepsy should also ensure that they get an adequate amount of nocturnal sleep. Scheduled naps are another important adjunct to drug therapy.

CHANGES IN SLEEP WITH DEMENTIA

Most studies examining sleep in dementia have focused on Alzheimer disease (AD). Unfortunately, the waking EEG of patients with dementia typically shows diffuse slow-wave activity, which makes discrimination between sleep and wakefulness, as well as among various sleep stages, difficult during PSG. The population of patients with dementia studied in the sleep laboratory is also biased by selection factors because most patients with dementia cannot tolerate the procedure.

Patients with dementia have frequent sleep disruption and arousals, lower sleep efficiency, a higher percentage of stage 1 sleep, and a decrease in stages 3 and 4 sleep.[7,16] Changes in REM pattern are of particular interest in patients with AD because integrity of cholinergic systems may be related to both induction of REM sleep and the pathophysiology of AD. REM sleep has been reported to be decreased with dementia in some studies. Disturbances of sleep–wake cycles are common with dementia, resulting in daytime sleep and nighttime wakefulness.

Many patients with dementia "sundown" during the evening hours or during the night (experience a worsening of confusion and/or agitation). Primary care providers are often asked treatment recommendations about such cases.

Treatment

Nonpharmacologic management of sundowning includes enhanced daytime bright light exposure, restriction of daytime napping, and institution of structured social and physical activity protocols. Once medical causes such as infection, polypharmacy, and fecal impaction are excluded, newer antipsychotics such as risperidone, quetiapine, or olanzapine may be used to improve sleep disturbance related to severe nocturnal agitation in patients with dementia.

SLEEP IN THE NURSING HOME

Sleep disturbance and resulting behavioral consequences are a common reason for nursing home placement. Up to 70% of caregivers report that nighttime difficulties played a role in their decision to institutionalize their family member.[17] Studies of sleep in nursing home residents have shown marked disruption in sleep, with frequent arousal during the night. One study reported average duration of sleep episodes of only 20 minutes at a time during the night.[2] Multiple factors affect sleep in this population, including medical illnesses and geriatric syndromes such as incontinence, neurodegenerative conditions, depression, certain medications, lack of physical activity, lack of bright light exposure during the day, and a high prevalence of primary sleep disorders. Nursing home environmental factors, such as nighttime noise, light, and nursing care activities can also have a disruptive influence on sleep.[18] Some interventional studies suggest that improvement in the nursing home environment is an important aspect of the management of sleeping difficulties, in addition to comprehensive assessment and treatment of the multiple conditions that can interfere with sleep in this setting. Residents who fail these interventions can be considered for limited treatment with sleep medications. There is, however, little data on the effectiveness of sleep medications and specific management of sleep disorders in nursing home settings,[19,20] and side effects of sedative–hypnotics can be significant in these frail older people.

CONCLUSION

Sleep disorders are very common in older people and can significantly affect their daytime function, quality of life, and well-being. Unfortunately, problems in clearly expressing sleep complaints can lead to the underdiagnosis or misdiagnosis of sleep disorders. In some cases, inappropriate treatment can aggravate symptoms. Most sleep disturbances in older adults are caused by specific problems, which should be properly evaluated. Obtaining a good sleep history is absolutely essential. Referral should be made when appropriate. Accurate diagnosis and appropriate therapy of sleep disorders may substantially improve sleep and quality of life in older people.

REFERENCES

1. Foley DJ, Monjan AA, Brown SL, et al. Sleep complaints among elderly persons: An epidemiologic study of three communities. *Sleep.* 1995;18(6):425–432.
2. Ancoli-Israel S, Parker L, Sinaee R, et al. Sleep fragmentation in patients from a nursing home. *J Gerontol.* 1989;44(1):M18–M21.
3. Saper CB, Chou TC, Scammell TE. The sleep switch: Hypothalamic control of sleep and wakefulness. *Trends Neurosci.* 2001;24(12):726–731.
4. McGinty D, Szymusiak R. Hypothalamic regulation of sleep and arousal. *Front Biosci.* 2003;8:s1074–s1083.
5. Manabe K, Matsui T, Yamaya M, et al. Sleep patterns and mortality among elderly patients in a geriatric hospital. *Gerontology.* 2000;46(6):318–322.
6. Prinz PN, Vitiello MV, Raskind MA, et al. Geriatrics: Sleep disorders and aging. *N Engl J Med.* 1990;323(8):520–526.
7. Bliwise DL. Sleep in normal aging and dementia. *Sleep.* 1993;16(1):40–81.
8. Ganguli M, Reynolds CF, Gilby JE. Prevalence and persistence of sleep complaints in a rural older community sample: The MoVIES project. *J Am Geriatr Soc.* 1996;44(7):778–784.
9. Standards of Practice Committee of the American Academy of Sleep Medicine. Practice parameters for using polysomnography to evaluate insomnia: An update for 2002. *Sleep.* 2003;26:754–760.
10. American Sleep Disorders Association. *International classification of sleep disorders, revised: Diagnostic and coding manual.* Rochester, MN: American Sleep Disorders Association; 1997:177–180
11. American Psychiatric Association. Diagnostic and statistical manual of mental disorders. *Sleep disorders.* Washington, DC: American Psychiatric Association; 1994:551–607.
12. Ancoli-Israel S, Kripke DF, Klauber MR, et al. Periodic limb movements in sleep in community-dwelling elderly. *Sleep.* 1991;14(6):496–500.
13. Duffy JF, Kronauer RE, Czeisler CA. Phase-shifting human circadian rhythms: Influence of sleep timing, social contact and light exposure. *J Physiol.* 1996;495(Pt 1):289–297.
14. Garfinkel D, Laudon M, Nof D, et al. Improvement of sleep quality in elderly people by controlled-release melatonin. *Lancet.* 1995;346(8974):541–544.
15. Siegel JM. Hypocretin (orexin): Role in normal behavior and neuropathology. *Annu Rev Psychol.* 2004;55:125–148.
16. Bliwise DL. Sleep disorders in Alzheimer's disease and other dementias. *Clin Cornerstone.* 2004;6(Suppl 1A):S16–S28.
17. Pollak CP, Perlick D. Sleep problems and institutionalization of the elderly. *J Geriatr Psychiatry Neurol.* 1991;4(4):204–210.
18. Schnelle JF, Sowell VA, Hu TW, et al. Reduction of urinary incontinence in nursing homes: Does it reduce or increase costs? *J Am Geriatr Soc.* 1988;36(1):34–39.
19. Schnelle JF, Alessi CA, Al-Samarrai NR, et al. The nursing home at night: Effects of an intervention on noise, light, and sleep. *J Am Geriatr Soc.* 1999;47(4):430–438.
20. Alessi CA, Schnelle JF. Approach to sleep disorders in the nursing home setting. Review article. *Sleep Med Rev.* 2000;4(1):45–56.

SUGGESTED READINGS AND RESOURCES

American Academy of Sleep Medicine
http://www.aasmnet.org

National Institutes of Health, National Center on Sleep Disorders Research
http://www.nhlbi.nih.gov/sleep

National Sleep Foundation
http://www.sleepfoundation.org
Kryger MH, Roth T, Dement WC. *Principles and practice of sleep medicine,* 3rd ed. Philadelphia, PA: WB Saunders; 2000.

Sleep Research Society
http://www.srs.org

21 Schizophrenia and Anxiety in Late Age

Kim S. Griswold

CLINICAL PEARLS 266

EPIDEMIOLOGY AND SIGNIFICANCE TO AGING 267

SCHIZOPHRENIA 267
- Description 267
- Pathophysiology in Late-age Schizophrenia 267
- Genetics 268
- Differential Diagnosis 268
- Workup 269
- Management 270
- Disease Course 271

ANXIETY 272
- Description 272
- Pathophysiology and Late-age Anxiety 272
- Genetics 272
- Differential Diagnosis 272
- Workup 273
- Management 273
- Disease Course 274

SUMMARY 274

CLINICAL PEARLS

- Older individuals with mental health problems receive most of their health care in primary care settings.
- Women in late age are more likely than men to present with anxiety disorders or late-onset schizophrenia.
- Phobias may become more pronounced with aging, and can represent generalized anxiety or posttraumatic stress disorder.
- The fragility of the autonomic nervous system in late age may enhance the anxiety response.
- A late-onset delusional disorder unrelated to dementia may be a variant of schizophrenia.
- Benzodiazepines have been overused in this population, and are often the cause of falls and confusion in the elderly.
- Benzodiazepines with shorter half-lives are safer in older persons because they do not produce active metabolites, and are inactivated by direct conjugation in the liver.
- Buspirone is well tolerated in the elderly.
- Anxiety comorbidity in schizophrenia is often underdiagnosed.
- Before prescribing and during the course of use with atypical antipsychotics, monitor for weight gain, and abnormal lipid and glucose levels.
- In the management of anxiety and psychotic disorders, patient and family support and education are crucial.

A consensus statement has declared a national crisis in geriatric mental health care, because the current health care system appears inadequate to meet the demands of the expected increase in numbers of elderly individuals with mental health problems.[1] In the Surgeon General's Report, disorders that will cause major disability for individuals over age 65 include dementia, depression, and schizophrenia.[2] Older persons with mental health disorders are more likely to have unmet needs and suffer from an "expertise gap" in care, meaning failure to incorporate research findings into practice.[3]

Mental health problems (excluding dementia) occur in approximately 13% of individuals over age 65, and the effects of aging on mental health may represent changes in behavior as a consequence of organic disease, acute or chronic illness, medications, or alterations in the socio-environmental milieu.[4,5] Most older individuals with a psychiatric disorder present initially to their primary care physician rather than to a mental health professional.[6,7] Primary care clinicians who are informed about the presentation and treatment of the more common mental health problems in this age-group will be better able to provide both the mental health and medical care so often needed. This chapter will discuss the primary care presentation and management of schizophrenia and anxiety disorder in the geriatric population. The goals are to provide an understanding of and an evidence-based approach to the presentation, recognition, and management of anxiety and schizophrenia in later life, and the effects of these conditions on health, behavior, and functional status.

EPIDEMIOLOGY AND SIGNIFICANCE TO AGING

The prevalence of psychiatric disorder among individuals over age 65 is approximately 12.3% to 16%, with a higher prevalence rate among women (13.6% for women, versus 10.5% among men).[1,8] Due to increased life span and better treatment of psychiatric illnesses, it is predicted that over the next three decades the number of elderly with mental illness will more than double, reaching 15 million in 2030.

Table 21.1 presents the current community prevalence rates for older versus younger persons per the Epidemiological Catchment Area study.[1] As shown in the table, the 1-year prevalence rate in groups over age 65 is approximately 2.2% for generalized anxiety disorder (GAD) and 0.3% for schizophrenia. However, one study suggests that for patients over age 60, the annual incidence of schizophrenia-like psychoses increases by 11% with each 5-year age increase.[9] Specific figures for older persons indicate a prevalence rate of 4.8% for phobias (agoraphobia, social, and simple phobia), 0.1% for panic disorder, and 4.6% for GAD; although these rates should be viewed with caution because of the lack of dedicated research focusing on anxiety disorders in late age.[10] Anxiety may present as a comorbid condition with a physical illness or other psychiatric disorders; the prevalence of GAD in elderly persons may demonstrate a temporal increase.[11]

Several sources indicate that among individuals over age 65, the prevalence rate for anxiety disorders in urban and rural primary care practices range from 6% to 10%; and approximately 30% of older patients may present with anxiety symptoms.[12] Even these numbers may be an underrepresentation. For example, one study found low rates of psychiatric diagnosis and treatment in an older population even when an appropriate screening tool was used.[13]

SCHIZOPHRENIA

Description

Schizophrenia is a disturbance of thought and behavior, and probably represents a variety of disorders with heterogeneous causes and variable expressions.[14] An early classification of "dementia precox" proposed by Emil Kraeplin described a deteriorating course marked by delusions and hallucinations, although cognitive abilities were less affected—making the term *dementia* somewhat misleading in this historical context. Eugen Bleuler was the first to use the word "schizophrenia," and he also categorized symptoms into the "4 A's" of looseness of associations, affective symptoms, autism, and ambivalence. Kurt Schneider proposed diagnostic signs and symptoms that are the basis of the Diagnostic and Statistical Manual criteria.

Pathophysiology in Late-age Schizophrenia

Etiology is seldom known. In later ages, symptom occurrence may be associated with sensory impairments and social isolation, although not with progressive dementia.[15] In several studies, when compared to patients with an earlier age onset, patients with late-age schizophrenic-like symptoms were more likely to be women, had higher functioning in areas of learning and abstraction, and required lower doses of neuroleptic medications.[16]

Magnetic resonance imaging (MRI) examination of patients with late-age onsets of schizophrenia demonstrate either no increase in structural abnormalities, or larger thalami.[16] *Paraphrenia* is a term that has been used to describe an apparent form of schizophrenia with initial presentation in late life marked by hallucinations and delusions, but with less significant affective disturbance.[14] Due to ambiguity about the presentation and epidemiology of this later onset schizophrenia-like syndrome, an international group formed to review the literature agreed that diagnoses of late-onset (after age 40) and very–late-onset (after age 60) schizophrenia-like psychoses have "face validity and clinical utility."[15] Like its earlier age counterpart, the very late age presentation of schizophrenia-like symptoms is presumed to represent a group of heterogeneous disorders, characterized by delusional thinking, hallucinations, variable degrees of social–environmental dysfunction, and some cognitive impairment; in contrast to early-age onset schizophrenia, late-age symptoms include a higher prevalence of visual hallucinations, and a lower rate of affective flattening and formal thought disorder.[15]

Schizophrenia may be the most expensive psychiatric disorder.[17] In one community-based study, the health-related quality of life was worse in middle-aged and older persons with schizophrenia than it was for patients with acquired immunodeficiency syndrome.[17,18]

TABLE 21.1
PREVALENCE OF PSYCHIATRIC DISORDERS AMONG YOUNGER VERSUS OLDER ADULTS

	Younger Adults (Aged 30–44 y), ECA		Older Adults (Aged ≥65 y), ECA		Older Adults
DSM-III **Diagnostic Category**	**1-y Prevalence**	**Lifetime Prevalence**	**1-y Prevalence**	**Lifetime Prevalence**	**Prevalence of Clinically Significant Symptoms**
Affective disorders					
Any	2.7 (Men) 7.9 (Women)	6.6 (Men) 15.3 (Women)	0.6 (Men) 1.5 (Women)	1.6 (Men) 3.3 (Women)	15–25[7,8]
Major depression	3.9	7.5	0.9	1.4	
Dysthymia	—	3.8	—	1.7	
Bipolar I	1.2	1.4	0.1	0.1	
Bipolar II	0.3	0.6	0.1	0.1	
Anxiety disorders					17–21[9]
Panic disorder	0.7 (Men) 1.9 (Women)	1.8 (Men) 3.1 (Women)	0.04 (Men) 0.4 (Women)	0.1 (Men) 0.7 (Women)	
Phobic disorder	6.1 (Men) 16.1 (Women)	10.5 (Men) 22.6 (Women)	4.9 (Men) 8.8 (Women)	7.8 (Men) 13.7 (Women)	
Generalized anxiety disorder	3.6	4.9–6.8	2.2	2.6–4.3	
Obsessive-compulsive disorder	2.1	3.3	0.9	1.2	
Alcohol abuse/dependence	14.1 (Men)	27.9 (Men)	3.1 (Men)	13.5 (Men)	7–8 community-dwelling elderly persons who consume 12–21 drinks per wk[10]
	2.1 (Women)	5.5 (Women)	0.5 (Women)	1.5 (Women)	10–15 older primary care patients may have alcohol-related problems[11,12]
Other drug abuse/dependence	—	6.7	—	0.1	—
Schizophrenia	1.5	2.3	0.2	0.3	—
Antisocial personality disorder	1.5	3.7	0.0	0.3	—
Cognitive impairment					
Severe[a]	0.3 (Aged 35–54 y)	—	1.0 (Aged 55–74 y)	—	—
			5.0 (Aged ≥75 y)	—	—
	3.1 (Aged 35–54 y)		7.5 (Aged 55–74 y)	—	—
Mild	—	—	19.1 (Aged ≥75 y)	—	—
Any psychiatric disorder (excluding cognitive impairment)	23	39	13	21	—

[a]Although not a psychiatric disorder *per se*, suicide is generally secondary to a major mental illness such as depression or schizophrenia. Suicide rates increase with advancing age (especially in white men) and seem to be increasing among more recent cohorts of older persons. Among older patients in primary care, the prevalence of suicidal ideation is 0.7% to 1.2%. Data are presented as percentages.
ECA, Epidemiologic Catchment Area study (which used DSM-III criteria).
Reprinted from Jeste DV, et al. Consensus statement on the upcoming crisis in geriatric mental health: Research agenda for the next two decades. Arch Gen Psychiatry. 1999;56(9):848–853.

Genetics

There is no concrete evidence of familial aggregation in the later-age onset of schizophrenia, although some evidence exists that families of these patients may have a greater prevalence of affective disorders.[15] The later onset schizophrenia-like disorder more commonly occurs in women, raising the possibility of an estrogenic protective effect in some women prior to menopause.[16]

Differential Diagnosis

In Table 21.2, the differential diagnosis for schizophrenia-like illness is presented. Kaplan and Sadock have proposed guidelines for diagnosis that include careful investigation for identifiable organic disease, a reevaluation at each episode of symptoms for possible organic etiology, and a complete family history. One example of an organic cause is epitomized by the now defunct term *general paralysis of*

TABLE 21.2
DIFFERENTIAL DIAGNOSIS OF SCHIZOPHRENIA-LIKE SYMPTOMS AND ICD CODES

Medical	Neurologic	Psychiatric
Drug-induced (amphetamine, hallucinogens, belladonna, alkaloids, alcohol hallucinosis, barbiturate withdrawal, cocaine, PCP)	Epilepsy (345.90) (particularly temporal lobe epilepsy)	Atypical psychosis (298.9) Brief reactive psychosis (298.8)
Delirium (780.09) AIDS (042) Acute intermittent porphyria (277.1)	Neoplasm (191.9) CVA (434.91) Cerebral lipoidosis (330.1) Head trauma (959.01) Creutzfeldt-Jakob disease (046.1)	Malingering (V65.2) Mood disorder (296.90) Paranoid disorder (297.9) Personality disorder (301.9) Schizoaffective disorder (295.70) Schizophreniform disorder (295.4)
B_{12} deficiency (266.2) Fabry disease (272.7) CO poisoning (986) Heavy metal poisoning (984.9) Homocystinuria (270.4) Pellagra (265.2) Systemic lupus (710.0)	Fahr-Volhard disease (403.00) Hallervorden-Spatz disease (333.0) Herpes encephalitis (054.3) Huntington chorea (333.4) Metachromatic leukodystrophy (330.0) Neurosyphillis (094.9) Normal pressure hydrocephalus (331.4) Wernicke-Korsakoff syndrome (291.1) (alcoholic) (294.0) (nonalcoholic) Wilson disease (275.1)	

AIDS, acquired immunodeficiency syndrome; CVA, cerebrovascular accident; CO, carbon monoxide; PCP, Phencyclidine.
Reprinted from Kaplan HI and Sadock BJ: *Synopsis of psychiatry*, 7th ed, with permission.

the insane, which referred to schizophrenia-like symptoms and was due to tertiary syphilis.[19]

CASE ONE

Ms. F. is 65 years old and was diagnosed with paranoid schizophrenia as a young woman. When you first started caring for her 5 years ago, she would not let you examine her and exhibited paranoid delusional thinking. Three years ago, she allowed you to begin physical exams, and began to follow through with her mammograms and other preventive care visits. She was stable on her psychiatric medications, until she was moved from one assisted living home to another. At that time, she began to lose weight and became more withdrawn—with an increase in the negative symptoms of schizophrenia. Her family noted that she seemed depressed. Medical workup was benign, except for ill-fitting dentures, causing pain when she ate. She was able to discuss some of her feelings of sadness with you. With an adjustment of her medication, family support, and new dentures, Ms. F. was able to integrate into her new home and her symptoms stabilized. At her last visit with you, she showed you pictures of her niece and nephew with real satisfaction.

Workup

Older patients who have been treated for chronic schizophrenia over the course of years may exhibit signs of tardive dyskinesia or other extrapyramidal symptoms. If an older patient begins to display unusual symptoms indicative of psychosis or other behavioral disturbance, a complete history and physical examination might include a laboratory evaluation of endocrine function, including thyroid testing, metabolic abnormalities, dietary deficiencies, infection such as tertiary syphilis, and trauma.[20] Patients should be queried about medication compliance, usual prescription, and over-the-counter (OTC) medications, homeopathic preparations, and use of alcohol and recreational drugs. Sensitive inquiries should be made about the patient's living situation, and the possibility of elder abuse or domestic violence.

The mental status examination and/or use of a screening tool can help to clarify a diagnosis.[21] If a schizophrenia-like illness is suspected, the mental status examination should focus on the American Psychiatric Association criteria found in the *Diagnostic and Statistical Manual,* presented in Table 21.3.[22] Key diagnostic findings include delusions or hallucinations, disorganized speech or behavior, and social dysfunction. Negative symptoms are flattening of affect, social withdrawal, and/or alogia (poverty of speech, blocking, increased latency of response). If behavioral symptoms predominate, an evaluation for coexisting cognitive impairment can assist in diagnosis and management.[5] Psychiatric comorbidity with schizophrenia includes anxiety and depression, and a mental status examination can elucidate symptomatology of these coexisting disorders.[23] Assessment of suicide attempt history, family suicidal history, suicidal ideation, and intent should be ascertained during

TABLE 21.3
DIAGNOSTIC CRITERIA FOR SCHIZOPHRENIA

A. *Characteristic symptoms:* Two (or more) of the following, each present for a significant portion of time during a 1-month period (or less if successfully treated):
   1. Delusions
   2. Hallucinations
   3. Disorganized speech (e.g., frequent derailment or incoherence)
   4. Grossly disorganized or catatonic behavior
   5. Negative symptoms, i.e., affective flattening, alogia, or avolition

B. *Social/occupational dysfunction:* For a significant portion of the time since the onset of the disturbance, one or more major areas of functioning such as work, interpersonal relations, or self-care are markedly below the level achieved prior to the onset (or when the onset is in childhood or adolescence, failure to achieve the expected level of interpersonal, academic, or occupational achievement).

C. *Duration:* Continuous signs of the disturbance persist for at least 6 months. This 6-month period must include at least 1 month of symptoms (or less if successfully treated) that meet Criterion A (i.e., active-phase symptoms) and may include periods of prodromal or residual symptoms. During these prodromal or residual periods, the signs of the disturbance may be manifested only by negative symptoms or two or more symptoms listed in Criterion A present in an attenuated form (e.g., odd beliefs, unusual perceptual experiences).

D. *Schizoaffective and mood disorder exclusion:* Schizoaffective disorder and mood disorder with psychotic features have been ruled out because either (i) no major depressive, manic, or mixed episodes have occurred concurrently with the active-phase symptoms; or (ii) if mood episodes have occurred during active-phase symptoms, their total duration has been brief relative to the duration of the active and residual periods.

E. *Substance/general medical condition exclusion:* The disturbance is not due to the direct physiologic effects of a substance (e.g., a drug of abuse, a medication) or a general medical condition.

F. *Relationship to a pervasive developmental disorder:* If there is a history of autistic disorder or another pervasive developmental disorder, the additional diagnosis of schizophrenia is made only if prominent delusions or hallucinations are also present for at least a month (or less if successfully treated).

Classification of longitudinal course (can be applied only after at least 1 year has elapsed since the initial onset of active-phase symptoms):

Episodic with inter-episode residual symptoms (episodes are defined by the reemergence of prominent psychotic symptoms); also specify if with prominent negative symptoms
Episodic with no inter-episode residual symptoms
Continuous (prominent psychotic symptoms are present throughout the period of observation); also specify if with prominent negative symptoms
Single episode in partial remission; also specify if with prominent negative symptoms
Single episode in full remission
Other or unspecified pattern

Only one Criterion A symptom is required if delusions are bizarre or hallucinations consist of a voice keeping up a running commentary on the person's behavior or thoughts, or two or more voices conversing with each other.
Reproduced with permission from the American Psychiatric Association. *Diagnostic and statistical manual of mental disorders*, 4th ed. Washington, DC: American Psychiatric Association; 2000.

the initial and subsequent interviews. Risk factors for suicidal attempt or completion include medical comorbidity, use of alcohol, other substances, and tobacco, and number of psychiatric hospitalizations.[24,25]

Specific health concerns that may occur include a high prevalence of tobacco use among people with schizophrenia,[26] anxiety symptoms with or without depression, and an association between anxiety and urinary incontinence.[27] Increasing evidence supports a relationship between the use of second-generation antipsychotics, weight gain, abnormal lipid profiles and diabetes, as well as other physical health concerns.[28] For persons using the atypical antipsychotics, several studies indicate a prevalence rate for obesity and diabetes twice that of the general population.[29]

Management

The mainstay of treatment is the use of antipsychotic medications, with appropriate family involvement and use of ancillary supports such as case managers as important treatment components.

For late-age schizophrenia, few Level A evidence-based randomized control studies or meta-analyses were found, although (Evidence Levels B and C) consensus expert statements and published reviews support the effectiveness of antipsychotic medications.[30]

Atypical antipsychotics appear to be safer in terms of motor side effects (Evidence Level B).[30] One study has shown a potential benefit of combined psychosocial and behavioral skills training (Evidence Level B).[31] Additional (Evidence Level A) evidence is found in a randomized control study on nurse case management in the community for individuals with severe psychiatric illness.[32]

Comprehensive guidelines for the treatment of schizophrenia are contained in the American Psychiatric Association's Practice Guidelines[33] and in the Schizophrenia Patient Outcomes Research Team (PORT) guidelines.[34]

Pharmacologic management of the psychotic symptoms of schizophrenia involves the choice between typical and atypical preparations. Tardive dyskinesia rates are less with the use of atypical antipsychotics, although these results are for individuals aged 36 to 50.[35] When any psychotropic agent is used, recommendations are for lower dosing, frequent monitoring, and very slow dosage increments.

Atypical or second-generation agents include clozapine, risperidone, quetiapine, olanzapine, aripiprazole, and ziprasidone. These drugs produce lower rates of extrapyramidal side effects, improve the negative symptoms of schizophrenia and have less effect on prolactin levels; the mechanism appears to be a higher ratio of serotonin 5-HT_2 to dopamine D_2 receptors.[36]

Most of the atypical medications can produce weight gain, neuroleptic malignant syndrome, dry mouth, sexual dysfunction, and dizziness, among other effects. Specific side effects of these atypical antipsychotics include:

Aripiprazole (Abilify): Anxiety, orthostatic hypotension, blurred vision
Clozapine (Clozaril): Agranulocytosis, myocarditis, and seizure risk
Olanzapine (Zyprexa): Abdominal pain, cough, pharyngitis, joint pain, peripheral edema
Quetiapine (Seroquel): Agitation, syncope, increased alanine transaminase
Risperidone (Risperdal): Rhinitis, tachycardia, unusual dreams, visual disturbances, cerebrovascular accident
Ziprasidone (Geodan): QT prolongation, somnolence, priapism.

Metabolic abnormalities occur most prominently with clozapine and olanzapine; weight gain and the risk of diabetes is less for the second-generation antipsychotics aripiprazole and ziprasidone—although there are limited long-term data on these newer medications.[37]

Several excellent reviews provide further guidance on prescribing, dosages, and side effects.[38,39] Medications for anxiety and depression may be important adjuncts for persons with comorbid presentations. It is important to remember that changes in Medicare over upcoming years may increase out-of-pocket medication costs for elderly consumers; this in turn could influence medication adherence.

Psychological management is a crucial component, and begins with a therapeutic alliance between the patient and primary care and psychiatric provider. It is important to try to offset the possible isolation a patient may experience, through peer support, case management, pet-assisted therapy, or community services such as meals on wheels.[40] One study showed that of the older patients with psychotic disorders surveyed, 92% tended to use community services, such as for counseling, assistance through social services programs, and daily assistance support.[41] Assertive Community Treatment (ACT) teams provide an integrated team approach toward caring for seriously mentally ill patients in the community, and ACT teams often either provide or connect to physical health providers for their clients. Another promising approach to the treatment and follow-up of community-dwelling elderly patients with psychiatric illness is the use of nurse case managers; a prospective randomized study found that a nurse mobile outreach program was more effective than usual care in reducing psychiatric symptoms.[32]

Specific recommendations for physical health care, particularly in patients on second-generation antipsychotics, include monitoring for body mass index, glucose and lipid levels, and electrocardiograms (EKGs) to look for QT prolongation and ophthalmologic exams.[42,43]

For persons with schizophrenia, the continuity of a long-term patient-provider relationship is crucial in maintaining patient trust and anticipating changes over time—whether in primary care or psychiatric settings. Strategies that bridge gaps between mental health sectors and primary care are providing important dimensions of care.[44,45] Integrated models of care are demonstrating improved patient outcomes.[46] Initiating a therapeutic alliance and maximizing psychosocial interventions are key ingredients of the treatment and rehabilitative plans.

Disease Course

There is evidence that sustained remission can occur among community-dwelling elders with schizophrenia, but at a low prevalence rate.[47] Some older patients with schizophrenia have reported and been found to have greater functional disability, and expressed a need for physical health services and education about their illness.[48,49]

Coexisting anxiety symptoms in some older outpatients with schizophrenia negatively affected their quality of life.[50] In general, the course of early-onset schizophrenia in later ages appears relatively stable, with some chronic disability.[51] The true course and treatment outcomes of later-age presentations have not been sufficiently studied.

Among persons with schizophrenia, mortality rates are higher when compared to the general population.[42] This is in part due to an increased rate of suicide, but also may reflect the burden of chronic medical illness. The course of both the psychiatric symptomatology and comorbid medical conditions is affected by the adherence rates to medication treatment. In one study, 24% of Medicaid enrollees were nonadherent, and 16% only partially to the use of antipsychotic medication.[52] An evaluation of adherence rates to nonpsychiatric medications among older persons with psychotic disorders showed that patients filled their prescriptions only about half the time in a 12-month period; the medications included agents for diabetes, hypertension, and hyperlipidemia.[53] The use of community support, nurse outreach, and improved education may be interventions that can make a difference in adherence rates and help to improve morbidity and mortality rates.

ANXIETY

Description

Although anxiety disorders in the elderly have not been extensively studied, evidence suggests that the prevalence rates are twice that of depression in older age-groups; the most common disorders are GAD and phobias.[10] Anxiety may present differently at a later age, expressed through behavioral changes and physiologic symptoms or as part of depressive episodes, at times making anxiety syndromes a diagnostic challenge, particularly in primary care.[54] Late age anxiety disorders are also almost twice as common in women than in men, although the gender difference may become equivalent at very late ages.[55] The DSM-IV-R criteria for GAD are found in Table 21.4.

Pathophysiology and Late-age Anxiety

A specific etiology of anxiety disorders is not known; it is hypothesized that neurotransmitter systems in the frontal lobe and limbic systems are involved, with either up- or down-regulation of the autonomic nervous system.[14] Presentations of anxiety in later ages are tempered by coexisting factors such as medical comorbidity, adaptive responses over time, psychiatric comorbidity, medications, and their side effects, and social, and environmental milieus.[10,54] There may be differences in the character of anxiety in late age in contrast to younger cohorts. Studies have looked at "genuine" fears, such as reaction to fear of death or losing loved ones, fear of medical illness, loss of autonomy and fear of dependence, as well as "the content of worry (reflecting) developmentally appropriate themes across the lifespan."[10]

Genetics

There may be inherited links—up to one fourth of first degree relative women may exhibit anxiety disorder, with male relatives more often having an alcohol-use disorder.[14] Although anxiety disorders most often present early in life, a bimodal distribution has been described with occurrence in later life in response to a stressor.[10]

Differential Diagnosis

Anxiety can be a component or the result of a multitude of medical problems and diagnoses. An organic differential list is shown in Table 21.5.

Additional medical and physiologic factors that may play a more prominent role in the elderly include poor vision and hearing, leading to isolation and fear of falling, dizziness and postural imbalance, and decreased physical mobility.[10,54]

> **CASE TWO**
>
> Mrs. V. is 70 years old and lives alone in an inner city apartment. She says she has always been somewhat of a "worrier." Her medical problems are hypertension and

TABLE 21.4
DIAGNOSTIC CRITERIA FOR 300.02 GENERALIZED ANXIETY DISORDER (GAD)

A. Excessive anxiety and worry (apprehensive expectation), occurring more days than not for at least 6 months, about a number of events or activities (such as work or school performance)
B. The person finds it difficult to control the worry
C. The anxiety and worry are associated with three (or more) of the following six symptoms (with at least some symptoms present for more days than not over the past 6 months) (Note: Only one item is required in children)
   1. Restlessness or feeling keyed up or on edge
   2. Being easily fatigued
   3. Difficulty concentrating or mind going blank
   4. Irritability
   5. Muscle tension
   6. Sleep disturbance (difficulty falling or staying asleep, or restless unsatisfying sleep)
D. The focus of the anxiety and worry is not confined to the features of an axis I disorder, (e.g., the anxiety or worry is not about having a panic attack [as in panic disorder]), being embarrassed in public (as in social phobia), being contaminated (as in obsessive-compulsive disorder), being away from home or close relatives (as in separation anxiety disorder), gaining weight (as in anorexia nervosa), having multiple physical complaints (as in somatization disorder), or having a serious illness (as in hypochondriasis), and the anxiety and worry do not occur exclusively during posttraumatic stress disorder
E. The anxiety, worry, or physical symptoms cause clinically significant distress or impairment in social, occupational, or other important areas of functioning
F. The disturbance is not due to the direct physiologic effects of a substance (e.g., a drug of abuse, a medication) or a general medical condition (e.g., hyperthyroidism) and does not occur exclusively during a mood disorder, a psychotic disorder, or a pervasive developmental disorder

Reproduced with permission from the American Psychiatric Association. *Diagnostic and statistical manual of mental disorders*, 4th ed. Washington, DC: American Psychiatric Association; 2000.

TABLE 21.5
DIFFERENTIAL DIAGNOSIS FOR ANXIETY

Cardiovascular	Pulmonary	Neurologic	Endocrine
Hypertension (401.9) Atrial fibrillation (427.31) CHF (428.0) Angina (413.9)	COPD (496) Hypoxia (799.0) Asthma (493.90) PE (415.10)	CVA (434.91) Epilepsy (345.90) Ménière (386.00) MS (340) TIA (435.9) Parkinson (332.0)	Thyroid disease (246.9) Carcinoid Addison (255.4) DM (250.00)
Medication	**Hematologic**	**Psychiatric**	**Oncologic**
Any drug effect/side effect Polypharmacy Illicit drugs Alcohol Drug therapy	Microcytic anemia (280.9) Macrocytic anemia (281.9) Leukemia (208.90)	Delirium (780.9) Sepsis (995.91) Meningitis (322.9) UTI (599.0) Depression (311) Dementia (294.8) Schizophrenia (295.90) Elder abuse (995.80) Intimate partner abuse	Initial diagnosis of cancer[62] Ongoing therapy

COPD, chronic obstructive pulmonary disease; CVA, cerebrovascular accident; PE, pulmonary embolism; MS, multiple sclerosis; CHF, congestive heart failure; TIA, transient ischemic attack; DM, diabetes mellitus; UTI, urinary tract infection.
Reproduced from Kaplan HI, Sadock BJ. *Synopsis of psychiatry*. Baltimore, MD: Williams and Wilkins; 1998:399.

osteoporosis. She was recently the victim of an attack on the street by a purse snatcher. She resisted the attack, trying to protect her purse. As a consequence she suffered a broken arm and bruises. She now does not come to see you very often, because she is afraid to leave her home. She also says sometimes she now hears "voices in the night." A short course of a selective serotonin reuptake inhibitor (SSRI), and a longer course of buspirone helps her symptoms of worry and fear, but she remains traumatized by the event.

Workup

When an older primary care patient presents with signs and symptoms of anxiety or behavioral disturbances, medical comorbidity should be considered. If the patient has a known history of anxiety disorder and presents with exacerbated symptoms, an inquiry can examine changes in the patient's medication regimen, environmental influences, and family support. After the history and physical examination, the laboratory analysis might include thyroid testing, B_{12}/folate, calcium, complete blood count, blood urea nitrogen/creatinine, electrolytes, and glucose. A complete mental status examination should include emphasis on signs and symptoms of coexisting depression, cognitive impairment, and suicidal ideation. Anxiety may be a prominent component of psychosis, as mentioned earlier. Screening instruments may aid in the diagnosis of anxiety and assessment of its severity, as well as in the assessment of worry.[11,56,57]

Management

There are few extensively researched recommendations for treating anxiety disorders in elderly people. Bartels et al. report that although anxiety disorders are common among the elderly, only general reviews (Evidence Level C) examine effective treatments.[3] Benzodiazepines are the most commonly prescribed agents, particularly in institutions, but there is no solid evidence that these medications are effective in the long-term when used in elderly patients.

Case reports (Evidence Level B) suggest that the use of SSRIs is efficacious in the elderly, although newer SSRIs have not been adequately researched in this group.[55] Regarding cognitive behavioral therapy (CBT), one controlled study looking at GAD found that CBT was more effective than supportive psychotherapy (Evidence Level A) in 48 older persons;[58] however, there was a 33% attrition rate. A Nordhus and Pallesen study also found that psychosocial interventions produced short-term improvements in function (Evidence Level A).[59]

The treatment for late-life anxiety combines correction of underlying contributing factors, use of targeted medications, psychological support, and psychosocial interventions. Benzodiazepines are the most frequently prescribed medication for anxiety symptoms but can have significant side effects, as shown in Table 21.6. Furthermore, there are issues of drug dependence and withdrawal when used in the longer term. The use of benzodiazepines with a shorter half-life is preferable, as they do not produce metabolites.[60] The SSRIs have been used to treat GADs, and recent work

TABLE 21.6
COMPLICATIONS OF BENZODIAZEPINES[60]

Excessive drowsiness
Cognitive impairment and confusion
Psychomotor impairment and risk of falls
Depression
Intoxication (even on therapeutic doses)
Paradoxical reactions
Amnesic syndromes
Respiratory problems
Abuse and dependence
Breakthrough withdrawal reactions

Reproduced from Sheikh JT, Cassidy EL. Treatment of anxiety disorders in the elderly: Issues and strategies. *J Anxiety Dis.* 14(2):173–190.

demonstrates their efficacy when compared to placebo.[61] Another double-blind study has revealed the superior effect of venlafaxine versus placebo in the treatment of anxiety.[60] However, controlled studies have not been conducted in elderly populations. Buspirone is a representative of the azaspirodecanediones, which are selective antagonists of the 5-HT_{1A} neurotransmitter receptor. Buspirone is an effective agent for anxiety, does not produce sedation, and appears to be well tolerated in older persons (Evidence Level C).[55]

Disease Course

The course depends on the particular etiology of the anxiety, and the duration of symptoms. In the elderly population, comorbid medical illness, living arrangements, family support, and issues of safety are concerns that may assume a larger role in outcome. Work by Wetherell et al.[50] suggests that when compared to asymptomatic individuals, GAD in the elderly is associated with significant decrements in the quality of life. One empirical review of nonpharmacologic treatment in late-life anxiety[59] reports that "psychosocial interventions produce significant improvements in self-reported, as well as diagnosed, anxiety in older patients at posttreatment." However, in the Nordhus study, the length of follow-up varied and there is little information on the long-term outcome.

SUMMARY

There is emerging consensus in the published literature that more controlled studies are urgently needed on treatment choices and outcomes for elderly persons with schizophrenia and anxiety disorders. The primary care site is an ideal venue for establishing the kind of sustained partnerships with patients that form the framework of trust and communication that are so important for the management of mental illness.

For older persons with chronic schizophrenia, or for those persons exhibiting signs of schizophrenia for the first time at a late age, appropriate treatment includes antipsychotic medications, as well as patient and family education and support. Comprehensive treatment guidelines are available. In cases of anxiety, medications might include a short course of a benzodiazepine, although the side effects must be carefully monitored. Buspirone and SSRIs are other excellent choices. Psychosocial and behavioral treatments are extremely efficacious, often as first-line therapies.

The continuity of care and therapeutic relationships formed in primary care support the treatment of late-age schizophrenia and anxiety. Although the management of these conditions can be challenging, older patients with these disorders are appropriately managed by primary care providers, often in ongoing collaborative arrangements with psychiatric and other mental health providers.

Family and community support as well as psychosocial interventions are critically important components of optimum care.

REFERENCES

1. Jeste DV, Alexopoulos GS, Bartels SJ, et al. Consensus statement on the upcoming crisis in geriatric mental health: Research agenda for the next 2 decades. *Arch Gen Psychiatry.* 1999;56(9):848–853.
2. *Older adults and mental health: Issues and opportunities*: Department of Health and Human Services. Administration on Aging; January 2001.
3. Bartels SJ, Dums AR, Oxman TE, et al. Evidence-based practices in geriatric mental health care. *Psychiatr Serv.* 2002;53(11): 1419–1431.
4. Robins LN, Regier DA. *Psychiatric disorders in America: The epidemiologic catchment area study.* New York, NY: The Free Press; 1991.
5. Gruber-Baldini AL, Boustani M, Sloane PD, et al. Behavioral symptoms in residential care/assisted living facilities: Prevalence, risk factors, and medication management. *J Am Geriatr Soc.* 2004;52(10):1610–1617.
6. Woolley DC. Geriatric psychiatry in primary care. A focus on ambulatory settings. *Psychiatr Clin North Am.* 1997;20(1):241–260.
7. Thompson TL, Mitchell WD, House RM II. Geriatric psychiatry patients' care by primary care physicians. *Psychosomatics.* 1989;30(1):65–72.
8. Hybels CF, Blazer DG. Epidemiology of late-life mental disorders. *Clin Geriatr Med.* 2003;19(4):663–696.
9. Vas Os J, Howard R, Takei N, et al. Increasing age is a risk factor for psychosis in the elderly. *Soc Psychiatry Psychiatr Epidemiol.* 1995;30(4):161–164.
10. Stanley MA and Beck JG. Anxiety disorders. *Clin Psychol Rev.* 2000;20(6):731–754.
11. Krasucki C, Howard R, Mann A. Anxiety and its treatment in the elderly. *Int Psychogeriatr.* 1999;11(1):25–45.
12. Zung WW. Prevalence of clinically significant anxiety in a family practice setting. *Am J Psychiatry.* 1986;143(11):1471–1472.
13. Valenstein M, Kales H, Mellou A, et al. Psychiatric diagnosis and intervention in older and younger patients in a primary care clinic: Effect of a screening and diagnostic instrument. *J Am Geriatr Soc.* 1998;46(12):1499–1505.
14. Kaplan HI, Sadock BJ. Synopsis of psychiatry. *Behavioral sciences/clinical psychiatry.* 6th ed. Baltimore, MD: Williams & Wilkins; 1991.
15. Howard R, Rabins PV, Seeman MV, et al. The International Late-Onset Schizophrenia Group. Late-onset schizophrenia and very-late-onset schizophrenia-like psychosis: An international consensus. *Am J Psychiatry.* 2000;157(2):172–178.
16. Palmer BW, Heaton SC, Jeste DV. Older patients with schizophrenia: Challenges in the coming decades. *Psychiatr Serv.* 1999;50(9):1178–1183.
17. Cuffel BJ, Jeste DV, Halpain M, et al. Treatment costs and use of community mental health services for schizophrenia by age cohorts. *Am J Psychiatry.* 1996;153(7):870–876.

18. Jeste DV, Unutzer J. Improving the delivery of care to the seriously mentally ill. *Med Care*. 2001;39(9):907–909.
19. Green B. *A review of schizophrenia, in psychiatry on line*. Retrieved November 4, 2004; from http://www.prior.com/psych.htm.
20. Woo BK, Daly JW, Allen EC, et al. Unrecognized medical disorders in older psychiatric inpatients in a senior behavioral health unit in a university hospital. *J Geriatr Psychiatry Neurol*. 2003;16(2):121–125.
21. Carlat DJ. The psychiatric review of symptoms: A screening tool for family physicians. *Am Fam Physician*. 1998;58(7):1617–1624.
22. American Psychiatric Association. *Diagnostic and statistical manual of mental disorders,*. 4th ed. Text Revision. Washington, DC: American Psychiatric Association; 2000.
23. Evins E, Lieberman JA, Meltzer HY. Schizophrenia: More than classical symptoms. *Clin Psychiatry News*. 2004;(suppl).
24. Potkin SG, Alphs L, Hsu C, et al. Predicting suicidal risk in schizophrenic and schizoaffective patients in a prospective two-year trial. *Biol Psychiatry*. 2003;54(4):444–452.
25. Brown S, Inskip H, Barraclough B. Causes of the excess mortality of schizophrenia. *Br J Psychiatry*. 2000;177:212–217.
26. McEvoy JP, Brown S. Smoking in first-episode patients with schizophrenia. *Am J Psychiatry*. 1999;156(7):1120–1121.
27. Mehta K, Simonsick EM, Penninx BW, et al. Prevalence and correlates of anxiety symptoms in well-functioning older adults: Findings from the health aging and body composition study. *J Am Geriatric Soc*. 2003;51(4):499–504.
28. Rosenheck R, Perlick D, Bingham S, et al. Effectiveness and cost of olanzapine and haloperidol in the treatment of schizophrenia: A randomized controlled trial. *JAMA*. 2003;290(20):2693–2702.
29. Barrett EJ, et al. Consensus development conference on antipsychotic drugs and obesity and diabetes: Response to holt, citrome and volevka, isaac and isaac, and boehm. *Diabetes Care*. 2004;27(8):2089–2090.
30. Jeste DV, Okomoto A, Napolitano J, et al. Low incidence of persistent tardive dyskinesia in elderly patients with dementia treated with risperidone. *Am J Psychiatry*. 2000;157(7):1150–1155.
31. Granholm E, McQuaid JR, McClure FS, et al. A randomized controlled pilot study of cognitive behavioral social skills training for older patients with schizophrenia. *Schizophr Res*. 2002;53(1–2):167–169.
32. Rabins PV, Black BS, Roca R, et al. Effectiveness of a nurse-based outreach program for identifying and treating psychiatric illness in the elderly. *JAMA*. 2000;283(21):2802–2809.
33. Treating schizophrenia. A quick reference guide. Based on Practice Guideline for the Treatment of Patients with Schizophrenia.
34. Lehman AF and Steinwachs DM. Patterns of usual care for schizophrenia: Initial results from the Schizophrenia Patient Outcomes Research Team (PORT) client survey. *Schizophr Bull*. 1998;24(1):11–20; discussion 20–32.
35. Kane JM. Tardive dyskinesia rates with atypical antipsychotics in adults: Prevalence and incidence. *J Clin Psychiatry*. 2004;65(suppl 9):16–20.
36. Hamner M. The new antipsychotic agents: Guidelines for primary care physicians. *Fam Pract Recertif*. 1998;20(9):39–56.
37. Consensus development conference on antipsychotic drugs and obesity and diabetes. *J Clin Psychiatry*. 2004;65(2):267–272.
38. Arenson C, Wender R. *Newer psychotropics and the older patient, in patient care*; 1999.
39. Amadio PB, Cross LB, Amadio P Jr. New drugs for schizophrenia: An update for family physicians. *Am Fam Physician*. 1997;56(4):1149–1156,1159–1160.
40. Aguera-Ortiz L, Reneses-Prieto B. Practical psychological management of old age psychosis. *J Nutr Health Aging*. 2003;7(6): 412–420.
41. Shaw WS, Paterson TL, Semple SJ, et al. Use of community support services by middle-aged and older patients with psychotic disorders. *Psychiatr Serv*. 2000;51(4):506–512.
42. Marder SR, Essock SM, Miller AL, et al. Physical health monitoring of patients with schizophrenia. *Am J Psychiatry*. 2004;161(8):1334–1349.
43. *Advanced studies in nursing. Nursing strategies for the prevention and management of antipsychotic-induced metabolic abnormalities*. Baltimore, MD: The Institute for John Hopkins Nursing; 2004.
44. Michaelides T, Stout C. *Integrating primary care and mental health*. Mental Health Issues Today;2004.
45. Griswold K, Servoss TJ, Leonard KE, et al. Connections to primary medical care after psychiatric crisis. *J Am Board Fam Pract*.2005;18(3):166–172.
46. Druss BG, Rohrbaugh RM, Levinson CM et al. Integrated medical care for patients with serious psychiatric illness: A randomized trial. *Arch Gen Psychiatry*. 2001;58(9):861–868.
47. Auslander LA, Jeste DV. Sustained remission of schizophrenia among community-dwelling older outpatients. *Am J Psychiatry*. 2004;161(8):1490–1493.
48. McKibbin C, Patterson TL, Jeste DV. Assessing disability in older patients with schizophrenia: Results from the WHODAS-II. *J Nerv Ment Dis*. 2004;192(6):405–413.
49. Patterson TL, Klapow JC, Eastham JH, et al. Correlates of functional status in older patients with schizophrenia. *Psychiatry Res*. 1998;80(1):41–52.
50. Wetherell JL, Palmer BW, Thorp SR, et al. Anxiety symptoms and quality of life in middle-aged and older outpatients with schizophrenia and schizoaffective disorder. *J Clin Psychiatry*. 2003;64(12):1476–1482.
51. Jeste DV, Twamley EW, Eyler Zorilla LT, et al. Aging and outcome in schizophrenia. *Acta Psychiatr Scand*. 2003;107(5):336–343.
52. Gilmer TP, Dolder CR, Lacro JP, et al. Adherence to treatment with antipsychotic medication and health care costs among Medicaid beneficiaries with schizophrenia. *Am J Psychiatry*. 2004;161(4):692–699.
53. Dolder CR, Lacro JP, Jeste DV. Adherence to antipsychotic and nonpsychiatric medications in middle-aged and older patients with psychotic disorders. *Psychosom Med*. 2003;65(1):156–162.
54. Palmer BW, Jeste DV, Sheikh J. Anxiety disorders in the elderly: DSM-IV and other barriers to diagnosis and treatment. *J Affect Disord*. 1997;46:183–190.
55. Sable JA, Jeste DV. Anxiety disorders in older adults. *Curr Psychiatry Rep*. 2001;3(4):302–307.
56. Fifer SK, Mathias SD, Patrick DL, et al. Untreated anxiety among adult primary care patients in a Health Maintenance Organization. *Arch Gen Psychiatry*. 1994;51(9):740–750.
57. Spitzer RL, Kroenke K, Linzer M, et al. Health-related quality of life in primary care patients with mental disorders. Results from the PRIME-MD 1000 Study. *JAMA*. 1995;274(19):1511–1517.
58. Stanley MA, Beck JG, Glassco JD. Treatment of generalized anxiety in older adults: A preliminary comparison of cognitive behavioral and supportive approaches. *Behav Ther*. 1996;27:565–581.
59. Nordhus IH, Pallesen S. Psychological treatment of late-life anxiety: An empirical review. *J Consult Clin Psychol*. 2003;71(4):643–651.
60. Sheikh JI, Cassidy EL. Treatment of anxiety disorders in the elderly: Issues and strategies. *J Anxiety Disord*. 2000;14(2):173–190.
61. Kapczinski F, Lima MS, Souza JS, et al. Antidepressants for generalized anxiety disorder. *Cochrane Database Syst Rev*. 2003;2:CD003592.
62. Stark D, Kiely M, Smith A, et al. Anxiety disorders in cancer patients: Their nature, associations, and relation to quality of life. *J Clin Oncol*. 2002;20(14):3137–3148.

Musculoskeletal Problems in the Elderly

22

Kim Edward LeBlanc

CLINICAL PEARLS 276

CHANGES IN MUSCULOSKELETAL TISSUE WITH AGING 277

GENERAL AREAS OF INJURY 277
Tendon Injuries 278
Ligamentous Sprains 278
Articular Cartilage Injuries 278
Muscle Strains 278

HISTORY 278

CERVICAL SPRAIN—ICD-9 CODE 847.0 279
Workup/Keys to Diagnosis 279

CERVICAL SPONDYLOSIS (WITHOUT MYELOPATHY)—ICD-9 CODE 721.0 281
Workup/Keys to Diagnosis 281

OSTEOARTHRITIS OF THE SHOULDER—ICD-9 CODE 715.11 282
Workup/Keys to Diagnosis 282

ADHESIVE CAPSULITIS OF THE SHOULDER—ICD-9 CODE 726 283
Workup/Keys to Diagnosis 283

IMPINGEMENT SYNDROME—ICD-9 CODE 726.10 284
Workup/Keys to Diagnosis 284

ROTATOR CUFF RUPTURE/TEAR—ICD-9 CODE 727.61 285
Workup/Keys to Diagnosis 285

BICEPS TENDON RUPTURE—ICD-9 CODE 840.8 286
Workup/Keys to Diagnosis 286

OLECRANON BURSITIS—ICD-9 CODE 726.33 287
Workup/Keys to Diagnosis 287

DUPUYTREN CONTRACTURE/ DISEASE—ICD-9 CODE 728.6 287
Workup/Keys to Diagnosis 288

OSTEOARTHRITIS OF THE HIP—ICD-9 CODE 715.15 288
Workup/Keys to Diagnosis 288

OSTEOARTHRITIS OF THE KNEE—ICD-9 CODE 715.16 289
Workup/Keys to Diagnosis 289

PLANTAR FASCIITIS—ICD-9 CODE 728.71 290
Workup/Keys to Diagnosis 290

CORNS AND CALLUSES OF THE FOOT—ICD-9 CODE 700.00 291
Workup/Keys to Diagnosis 291

CONCLUSION 291

CLINICAL PEARLS

- Between age 20 and 40, both men and women attain their highest level of muscular strength. Strength loss in the elderly is directly related to their decreasing mobility and declining fitness level.

- The mechanism of injury will provide the clinician with the critical information needed to proceed in making the diagnosis and formulating a treatment plan.
- The Spurling maneuver is helpful in assessing encroachment on a cervical nerve root by disc pathology.
- Impingement syndrome of the shoulder is diagnosed by positive Neer and/or Hawkins signs and a painful arc.
- Nighttime shoulder pain is characteristic of rotator cuff pathology.
- The sudden appearance of a bulge in the lower arm on strenuous use, causing the arm to have a "Popeye" appearance, is usually diagnostic of biceps tendon rupture.
- Symptomatic or markedly swollen olecranon bursitis may be aspirated, followed by corticosteroid instillation and a 48-hour compression dressing.
- Dupuytren contracture will cause flexion contractures of fingers, which must be surgically treated if the disease significantly impairs the function of the hand.
- When evaluating osteoarthritis of the knee, anteroposterior radiographs are much more valuable when accompanied by weight-bearing views.
- One of the historic hallmarks of the diagnosis of plantar fasciitis is the severe pain on taking the first few steps in the morning.

Musculoskeletal problems are one of the most common complaints in the aging population. Although these problems are often thought of as part and parcel of the normal aging process, musculoskeletal disease is not necessarily part of the inevitable consequences of increasing birthdays. The proper management of these injuries is critical. Seemingly minor injuries, if neglected or improperly treated, will result in significantly negative effects on the quality of life or, worse, significant disability that will only worsen with time.

Perhaps a bit surprisingly, age does not appear to affect the incidence of injury, even in those who exercise.[1] Therefore, fear of injury should not deter anyone from exercising at any age. Furthermore, although all measures of physiologic performance typically decline with age, this decline does not occur at a uniform rate. For example, aerobic capacity declines at a faster rate than nerve-conduction velocities. Continued activity will slow decline significantly and afford an improved quality of life and maintenance of independence.

This chapter begins with a discussion on changes in connective tissues, followed by patterns of injury common to the elderly. The remainder of the chapter covers the common musculoskeletal problems and how to manage them.

CHANGES IN MUSCULOSKELETAL TISSUE WITH AGING

Connective tissue becomes stiffer as we age as a result of the thickening of the basement membrane and a decrease in elastin. Collagen stiffens as a consequence of an increase in the number of cross-links within its framework. Because collagen is the major component of tendons and ligaments, these structures become weaker and stiffer with age. These microscopic structural alterations may be manifested on a macroscopic level by a decrease in the range of motion. This would only be worsened by injury or decreased use.

There are many factors that influence the degenerative changes. Some of them are related to genetics but much is related to activity. It has been demonstrated that the range of motion of a joint and musculotendinous flexibility may be maintained and/or increased by activity and stretching.[2] Simply stated, an individual's tissues may stiffen with time, but the deterioration may be attenuated by activity regardless of the genetic background.

Generally speaking, between the age of 20 and 40, both men and women attain their highest level of muscular strength. Subsequently, muscle strength begins to decline, slowly at first, but more rapidly after middle age. Strength loss in the elderly is directly related to their decreasing mobility and declining fitness level. Decreased activity coupled with the aging process results in loss of muscle motor units and in muscle fiber atrophy, culminating in the reduction of strength. However, the elderly maintain remarkable plasticity in structural, physiologic, and performance characteristics. Muscles have the ability to respond to training and conditioning with marked improvements in strength, even into the ninth decade of life.[3,4] Consequently, continued activity will allow strength maintenance and/or gains. This will allow improved function such that the ability to rise out of a chair, maintain balance, and climb stairs will be preserved.

Articular cartilage lines the bony ends of the joints. It is a thin layer of deformable tissue with the ability to support and distribute forces that are generated during the loading of the joint. In addition, it provides a lubricating surface that assists in preventing the wear and tear of the joint surface. Although cartilage is a metabolically active tissue, it has a limited capacity for self-restoration. Injuries to this tissue due to trauma or degenerative joint disease will impair the mechanical properties of the cartilage, leading to loss of joint function and pain. With aging and as a consequence of erosive loss, the thickness of the joint cartilage will decrease. In addition, water content decreases while collagen content and cross-linking increases. Changes in the pattern of glycosylation of the protein, sulfation of chondroitin, alteration of proteoglycan components, and decreases in chondroitin concentration contribute to the processes occurring in the aging cartilage.

GENERAL AREAS OF INJURY

Although there are a multitude of examples of injury, any discussion of injury patterns may be divided into four basic categories: Tendon injuries, ligamentous sprains, injuries to the articular cartilage, and muscle strains, which are the most common of these maladies. It should always be remembered that, regardless of the pattern of injury, prolonged immobility will lead to a lengthy recovery and great difficulty in returning to the previous level of functioning. A gradual return to activity should be initiated as soon as feasible to avoid disabling or other negative ramifications from a relatively minor problem.

Tendon Injuries

Nearly all clinicians are familiar with tendinitis, but as commonly used to imply symptomatic inflammation of a tendon, the term is a misnomer. Most of these conditions are truly tendinosis. Tendinitis refers specifically to symptomatic degeneration with vascular disruption and an inflammatory response. Tendinosis, on the other hand, refers to intratendinous degeneration commonly due to aging, microtrauma, and/or vascular compromise. Furthermore, tendinosis implies tendon degeneration without clinical or histologic signs of intratendinous inflammation and is not necessarily symptomatic.[5,6] The use of the term *tendinosis* appropriately suggests the chronicity of the condition, which is much more common in the elderly patient.

Elderly patients with a chronic tendinosis are particularly prone to eventual rupture of the affected tendon. Therefore, a proper diagnosis and treatment plan must be initiated to effect proper recovery and avoid tendon rupture. The most commonly affected tendons in this population are the Achilles and rotator cuff tendons. Other less commonly affected tendons are the wrist extensors of the elbow and adductor muscles of the thigh, particularly in very active individuals. The Achilles and rotator cuff tendons are particularly prone to weakening and tendon rupture.

Ligamentous Sprains

Ligamentous sprains are injuries that are usually seen as a result of repetitive overuse or in the early phases of a new activity. It may also occur in someone who is physically active but forgets to do proper warm-up or begins the activity too vigorously. These scenarios may result in ligamentous injury or injury to the joint capsule. Differentiating between the two may be difficult, but joint capsular injuries usually hurt at the extremes of motion, and the tenderness is located directly over the joint capsule as opposed to the specific ligament. Many of these injuries are related to a decreased range of motion of the joint due to stiffness of the surrounding supporting structures, regardless of whether it is due to aging or previous injury or surgery. Lack of flexibility of a joint, for example, the ankle, will not allow compensation for a misstep. As a result, the person will "roll the ankle" and cause subsequent sprain of the lateral ankle ligaments.

Articular Cartilage Injuries

The knee joint is the most commonly affected when speaking of cartilaginous problems. Because of all the weight bearing in a lifetime, it is not surprising that degeneration of this cartilage surface would ensue. When joints are subjected to activity, problems may occur even in someone without previous injury because of the normal cartilage aging process. It should be noted that there is no direct correlation between the extent of radiographic evidence of cartilaginous degeneration and osteoarthritis and the amount of pain that the individual patient may experience. Some patients with extensive osteoarthritic changes on radiographs will have only minimal discomfort, whereas others with minimal changes have significant pain. Furthermore, it should be noted that osteoarthritic changes may begin to appear after the age of 30 in many individuals, so clinical correlation must always be considered.

Muscle Strains

Any muscle group may be affected by muscle strains, the most common musculoskeletal problem. These injuries may be a consequence of a single traumatic event (e.g., straining to move a heavy sofa) or a result of chronic use (e.g., daily working in the garden). In active older individuals, the most commonly affected muscles are the back, abdomen, hamstrings, and quadriceps. In less active individuals, it may also be the back, but upper extremity muscles will be affected frequently as well. Muscle strains may be seen in someone who is beginning an activity for the first time. Muscles that are unaccustomed to such an endeavor will fatigue quickly and be prone to injury. In addition, even muscles that are used frequently for a specific activity may become injured by repetitive overuse or increased intensity or duration of use. Generally speaking, the treatment of these strains is similar to that in the younger population. However, prolonged rest or immobilization in the elderly is detrimental. Rest should be relative, and alternative activity should be encouraged. Gentle stretching and gradual return to activity is critical in the recovery of muscle injuries.

HISTORY

It is not unusual for the patient to present with a known event that has resulted in his or her discomfort or problem. The patient may be able to specifically identify the offending activity that led to the injury. Determination of the mechanism of injury is crucial to making the proper diagnosis. By knowing the mechanism of injury, the practitioner is better able to determine what structure is most likely injured, which is critical in formulating the appropriate treatment plan.

Certain questions should be asked to elicit the best information. If it can be identified, the offending activity should be described. How often is the activity performed? How intense is the patient's participation in this activity? Is this a new activity? Is it being done more often? Has there been a sudden increase in the level of activity? What specific movement was the patient doing when the injury occurred? When was the problem first noted? Was it a single event or has it developed gradually over time? Has it been present for some time and then suddenly worsened (implying that this is an acute event superimposed on a chronic condition)? What makes the pain worse? Have there been any similar problems in the past? What medications are you taking? What is the past medical and surgical history?

Because of the potential to harbor an occult malignancy, this possibility should always be considered. If there is unexplained weight loss or fever, pain that is suddenly severe with no apparent reason, or an unusual presentation of a particular complaint, more immediate diagnostic studies should be performed.

CERVICAL SPRAIN—ICD-9 CODE 847.0

CASE ONE

A 78-year-old woman presents to your office complaining of a gradual onset of posterior neck pain for the past 3 days. She can relate no specific trauma but states that the pain began when she was going to sit in her easy chair and fell "heavily" into the chair in the sitting position when her grandson unexpectedly jumped into her lap. She denies any previous problems with her neck. There is no headache or dizziness and no numbness or radiation of the pain. The discomfort is made worse by motion of the neck and is causing sleep difficulties. She is also having difficulty performing some of her usual activities because of her discomfort and reduced neck mobility.

A sprain refers to an injury to a ligamentous structure. A cervical strain should refer to an injury to the paraspinal muscles. However, in neck injuries these terms are commonly used interchangeably because of the deep location of the soft tissues of the cervical region. It is not uncommon that rendering a precise location of the problem is very difficult. As long as one does not suspect serious cervical injuries, such as an unstable fracture or potentially damaging neurologic problems, these soft tissue injuries are diagnosed and managed in a similar manner.

Workup/Keys to Diagnosis

Physical Examination

There will usually be areas of tenderness such as the paraspinal muscles, interspinous ligaments, or spinous processes of the vertebrae. At times, depending on the severity, there may be tenderness along the medial aspects of the scapulas. Range of motion should be assessed in all directions, including rotation, lateral bending, flexion, and extension. Not infrequently, pain may be noted at the extremes of motion. Limited motion is a very common occurrence with this entity. It is helpful to know whether there was limited motion before this event. Decreased cervical range of motion is not uncommon in the elderly, particularly extension. In addition, symmetry of rotation (left compared to right) should be assessed because this may be decreased even in the healthy older individual, but it should be fairly close to symmetrical. Flexion is usually fairly well maintained. There is no deformity noted on visual inspection. Neurologic examination is normal. The differential diagnosis (see Table 22.1) includes cervical sprain, cervical spondylosis, cervical disc herniation, arthritic conditions of the spine, vertebral spinal fracture, tumor, and infection.

Imaging

No specific studies are warranted initially. It is reasonable to treat this patient with conservative management and reevaluate in 2 weeks. If the pain has not improved or has worsened by this point, radiographs should be obtained.

If warranted, three standard radiographs should be ordered: Anteroposterior, lateral, and odontoid views. All seven vertebrae should be clearly seen. Although cervical fracture is unlikely in this patient, it should be noted that the width of the prevertebral soft tissue at C3 should not exceed 7 mm in healthy adults. If there is significant spasm, the normal lordotic curve may be straightened or reversed; however, this may not be readily apparent in the elderly patient with significant degenerative changes. Degenerative changes will usually be noted that would predate the diagnosis of a simple cervical sprain. These are age related and most are commonly seen at levels C5-6 and C6-7.

Management

The use of a soft cervical collar will aid the patient significantly, although there are no randomized outcome studies of this approach. However, this device should be used for no longer than 1 to 2 weeks (Evidence Level C). Beyond this period, muscular atrophy will begin to occur and further stiffness of the ligamentous structures will follow. The use of heat, either dry or moist, may be of benefit but should not be used for an extended period (20 to 30 minutes) nor should it be too hot (Evidence Level B). If a heating pad is used, it should not be placed higher than medium heat. The use of balms that provide warmth combined with wet or dry heat should be disallowed because burns may result if left on for too long. The use of heat may provide relief from symptoms but does not speed recovery.

Acetaminophen and/or nonsteroidal anti-inflammatory agents may be used as analgesics (Evidence Level A). If necessary, mild narcotic analgesics may be used during the first week or so. Activity should be allowed but in a limited manner. Gentle stretches that could be suggested include trying to touch the chin to the chest, extending the head backward, and trying to touch the ear to the shoulder on each side, as well as trying to place the chin on each shoulder. These stretches should be done without pain and each held for approximately 15 to 30 seconds at first. This

TABLE 22.1
DIFFERENTIAL DIAGNOSES FOR MUSCULOSKELETAL/SOFT TISSUE CONDITIONS (ICD-9)

Cervical Sprain (847)	**Cervical Spondylosis, Without Myelopathy (721.0)**	**Osteoarthritis of the Shoulder (715.11)**
Cervical sprain (847) Cervical spondylosis (721.1) Cervical disc herniation (722.0) Arthritic conditions of the spine (721.0) Vertebral spinal fracture (805) Tumor (170) Infection	Cervical sprain (847) Cervical spondylosis (721.1) Cervical disc herniation (722.0) Arthritic conditions of the spine (721.0) Vertebral subluxation, particularly in patients with rheumatoid arthritis (839.0) Vertebral spinal fracture (805) Tumor, metastatic or of spinal cord (170) Infection	Adhesive capsulitis ("frozen shoulder") (726) Rotator cuff tear (727.61) or tendinitis (726.10) Bicipital tendinitis (726.12) Rheumatoid disease (714.0) Cervical disc herniation (722.0) Subacromial/subdeltoid bursitis (726.19) Recurrent or chronic dislocation (831.0) Referred cardiac pain (413.9) Metastatic tumor (170) Infection
Adhesive Capsulitis of the Shoulder (726.0)	**Impingement Syndrome (726.10)**	**Rotator Cuff Rupture/Tear (727.61)**
Glenohumeral arthritis (715.1) Impingement syndrome (726.10) Chronic posterior glenohumeral dislocation (731.2) Posttraumatic shoulder stiffness (719.5) Subacromial bursitis (726.19) Rotator cuff tear (727.61) or tendinitis (726.10) Tumor (170)	Adhesive capsulitis (726) Glenohumeral arthritis (715.1) Rotator cuff tear (727.61) or tendinitis (726.10) Subacromial/subdeltoid bursitis (726.19) Acromioclavicular arthritis (715.1) Bicipital tendinitis (726.12)	Adhesive capsulitis (726) Glenohumeral arthritis (715.1) Rotator cuff tendinitis (726.10) Subacromial/subdeltoid bursitis (726.19) Impingement syndrome (726.10) Cervical spondylosis (721.1) Acromioclavicular arthritis (715.1) Bicipital tendinitis (726.12) Pancoast tumor (162.3)
Biceps Tendon Rupture (840.8)	**Olecranon Bursitis (726.33)**	**Dupuytren Contracture/Disease (728.6)**
Rupture of distal biceps tendon (841.8) Dislocated biceps tendon (840.9) Rotator cuff tendinitis (726.10) or tear (727.61) Rupture of pectoralis major muscle (840.8) Impingement syndrome (726.10) Glenohumeral arthritis (715.1)	Gout (274.0) Infectious bursitis (726.39) Olecranon process fracture (813.01) Rheumatoid disease (714.0) Synovial cyst of elbow joint (727.40)	Trigger finger that is locked (727.03) Flexion contracture due to previous injury (727.8)
Osteoarthritis of the Hip (715.15)	**Osteoarthritis of the Knee (715.16)**	**Plantar Fasciitis (728.71)**
Inflammatory arthritis of the hip (714.9) Osteonecrosis of the femoral head (733.42) Lumbar disc herniation (722.1) Degenerative lumbar disc disease (722.5) Trochanteric bursitis (727.3) Tumor of spine or pelvis (170)	Meniscal tear (836.2) Osteonecrosis of the knee joint (733.40) Rheumatoid arthritis (714.0) Pathology of the hip (referred pain) (729.5) Lumbar disc disease (722.5) Bursitis (727.3)	Calcaneal stress fracture (825.0) or tumor (239.2) Atrophy of the fat pad of the heel (924.20) Tarsal tunnel syndrome (355.5) Lumbar radiculopathy (722.1)
Corns and Calluses of the Foot (700.00)		
Plantar wart (078.10) Foreign body (729.6) Synovitis (727) Morton neuroma (355.6)		

should be gradually increased to 60 seconds as flexibility increases. Physical modalities may be added if the patient is in severe discomfort; these would include massage, ultrasound, and/or phonophoresis (Evidence Level B). Manipulation of the spine is contraindicated.

Follow-up

This is a self-limited condition; however, it is not unusual for discomfort to persist for up to 6 weeks. The patient may be seen within 2 weeks if necessary. If the patient is worsening, radicular symptoms have developed, or the patient has not substantially improved within 6 weeks, further studies may be ordered such as computed tomography (CT) scan or magnetic resonance imaging (MRI). Subsequently, referral may be considered, but this is rarely, if ever, necessary.

CERVICAL SPONDYLOSIS (WITHOUT MYELOPATHY)—ICD-9 CODE 721.0

CASE TWO

An active 83-year-old man presents complaining of stiffness of his neck. He states that he has been having neck pain for at least 3 years, which worsens with upright activity. It has been affecting his ability to tend his garden and sleep. His wife says this discomfort makes him irritable as well. He further states that he can frequently hear a grinding or popping noise in his neck when he looks from side to side. He also indicates that, at times, he may have some tingling and weakness of the upper arms, particularly the left one.

The term *cervical spondylosis* is synonymous with cervical arthritis and degenerative disc disease of the cervical spine. It may cause cervical pain, radiculopathy (encroachment on the nerve root), and/or myelopathy (bony encroachment on the spinal cord). Cervical stiffness and chronic neck pain that is exacerbated by upright activity are the most common symptoms of cervical spondylosis. Often patients will complain of grinding or popping with motion of the neck. Headaches, muscle spasms, impaired tolerance to activity, irritability, and sleep disturbances may also be described. As the disease worsens over time, there may be pain in the upper extremities and radicular symptoms such as aching or burning pain following a dermatomal pattern, particularly with lateral stenosis and/or compromise of a particular nerve root. Most commonly this involves the C5-6 and C6-7 disc spaces, which leads to entrapment of the C6 (pain and sensory changes in the thumb and index finger) and/or C7 (pain and sensory changes in the index and middle fingers) nerve roots, respectively.

Workup/Keys to Diagnosis

Physical Examination

Inspection of the musculature is important to detect any asymmetry or atrophy suggesting a longer-standing lesion or more serious nerve root involvement. Palpation along the spinous processes and lateral neck may identify any tender areas. Passive and active range of motion should be assessed to determine any reproduction of pain or limitation of motion, both of which are common. In patients with radiculopathy, the Spurling maneuver is frequently positive. This is performed by asking the patient to extend the neck while tilting the head to the side, with application of a gentle axial load by the examiner. This maneuver causes narrowing of the neural foramen and will reproduce or increase radicular symptoms with either cervical spondylosis or disc herniations. Evaluations of the sensory and motor function of the nerve roots should be performed (see Table 22.2). The differential diagnosis includes cervical sprain, cervical spondylosis, cervical disc herniation, arthritic conditions of the spine, vertebral subluxation (particularly in patients with rheumatoid arthritis), vertebral spinal fracture, tumor (metastatic or of spinal cord), and infection.

TABLE 22.2
EVALUATIONS OF THE SENSORY AND MOTOR FUNCTIONS OF THE NERVE ROOTS

Nerve Root	Disc Level	Findings
C3	C2-3	Pain in posterior cervical region; decreased sensation in the back of neck, mastoid area
C4	C3-4	Pain in back of neck, upper anterior chest, levator scapula with sensory changes in these areas
C5	C4-5	Pain in neck, upper shoulder, and bicipital area with sensory changes over the deltoid muscle; decreased strength of deltoid and biceps muscles; diminution of the biceps reflex
C6	C5-6	Pain in neck, shoulder, medial scapula, dorsal forearm, and lateral arm; sensory changes of thumb and index finger; weakness of biceps muscle; diminished biceps reflex
C7	C6-7	Pain in neck, shoulder, medial scapula, dorsal forearm, and lateral arm; sensory changes of index and middle finger; weakness of triceps muscle; diminution of triceps reflex
C8	C7-T1	Pain in neck, medial scapula, medial arm, and forearm; sensory changes in ring and little fingers; weakness of intrinsic muscles of the hand

Imaging

Anteroposterior and lateral radiographs of the cervical spine are essential. Degenerative changes are most commonly noted at the C5-6 and C6-7 disc spaces. These changes may be represented as disc space narrowing, narrowing of the foramina, facet joint degeneration, instability, or the development of osteophytes. Osteophytes may be commonly seen projecting anteriorly, with associated sclerosis of the intervertebral disc areas. Osteophytes may cause stenosis of the cervical canal if they are directed posteriorly. The possibility of cervical stenosis with associated neurologic deficits is increased with any anterior subluxation of a vertebra onto the one below. These plain films also serve to rule out the possibility of tumors or infection. Further studies, such as CT scan or MRI, are usually not necessary because they will add little to the diagnosis or treatment of cervical spondylosis unless serious neurologic compromise is encountered on physical examination and surgical intervention is being considered.

Management

Treatment is most commonly supportive and conservative. However, the patient must be informed that the symptoms may last several months and, in fact, may become chronic. Relative rest is prescribed depending on the severity of the symptoms, but prolonged restriction of activity is more detrimental than beneficial. Immobilization of the neck by using a soft cervical collar may be considered until acute pain subsides (Evidence Level B). Continued use of a soft collar is helpful at night, when the neck is unprotected and may be subjected to awkward positions or movements. Non-narcotic pain medication, such as acetaminophen or nonsteroidal anti-inflammatory drugs, may be sufficient for pain relief (Evidence Level A). The use of amitriptyline, particularly at night, may be helpful (Evidence Level C). It is usually prudent to avoid narcotic analgesics, particularly for long-term use. When reclining, the use of a cervical pillow is recommended, although there are no randomized outcome studies evaluating the use of this modality.

Physical therapy modalities are particularly helpful for those with atrophic or weakened cervical muscles, which is all too common in this age-group (Evidence Level B). The physical therapist should instruct the patient on proper exercises to stretch and strengthen the muscles of both the upper extremities and cervical regions.

Follow-up

Fortunately, cervical spondylosis will respond to conservative measures most of the time. However, the patient and clinician should be mindful that this may take many weeks or months. Moreover, it should be remembered that conservative modalities do nothing to change the natural course of the disease. Neurosurgical consultation for decompression and fusion should be considered when patients have intractable pain, progressively deteriorating neurologic findings, or symptoms of spinal cord compression. Radicular symptoms that seem to worsen with neck motion are another indication for further assessment.

OSTEOARTHRITIS OF THE SHOULDER—ICD-9 CODE 715.11

CASE THREE

A 66-year-old man presents to your office complaining of a diffuse pain in his shoulder. He has been having this pain for approximately 5 years or more. Initially, it bothered him only with strenuous activity and mostly in the posterior shoulder. Over the last year or so, nearly all movements of the shoulder cause discomfort. Over the last few months, the pain is present at rest and at night. He has also noted that certain movements are becoming restricted, particularly overhead activities.

Osteoarthritis is manifested by loss of joint space and destruction of joint cartilage. Glenohumeral arthritis is fairly common and usually affects patients older than 50 years. Patients usually present complaining of a diffuse pain in the shoulder often localized to the posterior aspect. The pain usually has an insidious onset and is worsened by strenuous activity. With time, the disease may worsen and become associated with pain with any motion, at rest, and at night. As the joint deteriorates, the pain may increase and the range of motion will become progressively limited. Normal activities of daily living will be affected, especially activities that require overhead movement such as combing the hair and dressing. There does not appear to be any correlation between previous level of activity and the development of osteoarthritis. Osteoarthritis of the shoulder may develop as a result of rotator cuff pathology, which is detailed later in this chapter.

Workup/Keys to Diagnosis

Physical Examination

Inspection of the shoulder should be done to evaluate for muscular atrophy. Palpation of the entire joint should be performed to check for tenderness, swelling, increased warmth, or crepitus. Quite commonly, there is bone-on-bone crepitus with flexion and/or rotation of the humeral head. All ranges of motion should be assessed, including forward flexion, extension, internal and external rotation, adduction, abduction, and circumduction. The motion should be compared to that of the opposite side, bearing in mind that the contralateral shoulder may be similarly affected. Patients with rotator cuff tears typically have more passive range of motion than active. The differential diagnosis includes adhesive capsulitis ("frozen shoulder"), rotator cuff tear or tendinitis, biceps tendinitis, rheumatoid disease, herniated cervical disc, bursitis (subacromial or subdeltoid), recurrent or chronic dislocation, referred cardiac pain, metastatic tumor, or infection.

Imaging

Anteroposterior and lateral views are usually taken. However, the most reliable position to evaluate the joint space is the axillary view, which allows a fairly clear determination of the destruction within the cartilage and joint space. Certain radiographic findings are consistent with a diagnosis of osteoarthritis, such as inferior osteophyte formation, posterior erosion of the glenoid, and flattening of the humeral head. Superior migration of the humeral head suggests a rather large tear of the rotator cuff. Other imaging studies are usually not required because they add little to the management of these conditions unless diseases other than arthritis are suspected.

Management

The major focus of treatment should be directed toward conservative management. Gentle stretching and strengthening exercises should be recommended along with mild heat (Evidence Level B). This will help in preserving strength and range of motion. Modification of activities may be of benefit in the reduction of pain and symptoms. Nonsteroidal anti-inflammatory drugs and/or acetaminophen may be utilized (Evidence Level B). Although definitive studies are underway and results are not yet available, a trial of glucosamine and/or chondroitin sulfate may be considered (Evidence Level B). A frequently employed modality is the intra-articular injection of corticosteroids combined with local anesthetic. As adjunctive therapy, these injections are beneficial to many patients, particularly those who are unable to tolerate oral medications[7,8] (Evidence Level C). Despite many randomized controlled trials of corticosteroid injections for the treatment of shoulder pain, their small sample sizes, variable methodology, and quality do not provide definitive evidence to guide this treatment for undiagnosed shoulder pain.

Follow-up

Most patients should be given at least 3 to 4 months of conservative therapy to evaluate their response. However, after this period, those patients who continue to have intolerable pain, especially if associated with progressive loss of motion, should be considered for surgical intervention. The elderly patient may benefit from such procedures as a hemiarthroplasty or total shoulder replacement. Patients who are considered for such procedures should be fairly active and in need of joint motion and pain relief.

ADHESIVE CAPSULITIS OF THE SHOULDER—ICD-9 CODE 726

CASE FOUR

A 65-year-old female patient presents with complaints of shoulder stiffness. This has been progressively worsening over the last several months. She describes an insidious onset and diffuse pain and stiffness. She is unable to comb her hair and has difficulty fastening and unfastening her brassiere because of the discomfort and restricted motion. Initially, the pain was quite noticeable, but it has subsided somewhat. However, the stiffness has remained. She is unable to relate any specific history of trauma.

Adhesive capsulitis of the shoulder is also commonly known as a *frozen shoulder*. The etiology is uncertain but certain diseases seem to be a risk factor, such as diabetes mellitus, hypothyroidism, cervical disc disease, parkinsonism, and Dupuytren disease. Usually, the disease progresses slowly over time, beginning with pain followed by progressive stiffness, the pain eventually decreases and there is slow improvement in the limitation of motion. This process may take up to 2 years or more to evolve. Many patients will be left with some discomfort and restriction of motion.

Workup/Keys to Diagnosis

Physical Examination

Early on, there may be some tenderness about the shoulder, which gradually subsides as the inflammation wanes or is controlled. Initially, passive range of motion may be less affected; however, over time there will be quite noticeable reduction of motion of the shoulder, both actively and passively. Most commonly, the motions that are most affected are abduction and external rotation. Motion is usually painful, particularly at the extremes of motion. The arm is held close to the patient's side, usually in a neutral position. If the pain is long standing, there may be noticeable atrophy of the musculature secondary to disuse, most notably in the deltoid muscles. The differential diagnosis includes osteoarthritis of the glenohumeral joint, impingement syndrome, chronic posterior glenohumeral dislocation, posttraumatic shoulder stiffness, subacromial bursitis, rotator cuff tear or tendinitis, and tumor.

Imaging

Customarily, the only radiographs that are required are anteroposterior and axillary views. The physician should rule out osteophytes, calcium deposits, loose bodies, or tumors. The glenohumeral joint should be examined to be certain that the joint space is intact, with a smooth and concentric joint surface. If the plain films are normal, there is usually no need for further studies such as CT scan, MRI, or arthrography.

Management

One of the most important aspects of treatment is the institution of a gentle stretching and range-of-motion exercise program (Evidence Level C). These exercises should be increased as the pain subsides and done to the patient's tolerance level. Initially, the patient should be instructed by a physical therapist. Subsequently, the exercises may be continued at home but must be done three to four times a day without fail.

Acetaminophen and/or nonsteroidal anti-inflammatory drugs may be used. Moist low heat may also be of benefit, if not contraindicated. Intra-articular corticosteroid injections may assist in pain control and assist the patient in improving shoulder mobility (Evidence Level C). Injection of an anesthetic agent alone into the glenohumeral joint may result in improved pain control but does not aid in improving range of motion.

Follow-up

The patient should be advised from the outset that recovery from adhesive capsulitis is a slow process. Significant recovery may occur over 1 to 2 years, but full recovery—defined as full range of motion and being completely pain free—may never be achieved. Therapy should never be too aggressive because this could aggravate the symptoms and deter the patient from continuing the activities. Shoulder manipulation under general anesthesia should be reserved only for those patients who have failed all attempts at conservative management and continue to have severe pain and significantly restricted motion (Evidence Level C). The time factor here is quite variable but will involve several months. This should be individualized, allowing pain and limitation to serve as benchmarks on how to proceed.

IMPINGEMENT SYNDROME—ICD-9 CODE 726.10

CASE FIVE

A 70-year-old male farmer presents complaining of pain in the lateral and anterior shoulder. This pain began approximately 3 to 4 weeks ago and was quite severe but has been subsiding somewhat. The patient says he is having nighttime pain that wakens him and prevents him from sleeping on the affected side. He has noted that the pain is worsened by overhead activity, but all movements are painful at times. He has also noted some limitation of motion when performing overhead activities. The pain and this limitation have affected his ability to work around the farm as he is accustomed. There is no specific history of trauma or previous injury.

Impingement syndrome is commonly overlooked and frequently associated with rotator cuff tendinitis and subacromial bursitis. In fact, some clinicians think of them as one entity. As these entities are closely related, this discussion encompasses all of them, with specific reference to each one when appropriate.

A coracoacromial arch is formed within the shoulder by the following structures: The acromioclavicular joint capsule, the acromion, the coracoacromial ligament, and the coracoid process of the scapula. The muscle of the rotator cuff, made up of the supraspinatus, infraspinatus, teres minor, and subscapularis, resides beneath this arch.

In addition, between the rotator cuff and the coracoacromial arch is the subacromial bursa. Under normal circumstances, this bursa serves to allow smooth tendinous motion along the bony structures. When the rotator cuff becomes injured or inflamed and/or the subacromial bursa becomes inflamed, this leads to edema and swelling beneath the arch. This space becomes narrowed and leads to pain and discomfort with certain motions.

Workup/Keys to Diagnosis

Physical Examination

Inspect the shoulder to assess for any evidence of muscular atrophy. Significant atrophy is usually indicative of a rotator cuff tear. Palpation over the subacromial bursa and the greater tuberosity frequently uncovers tenderness in this area. Crepitus may be noted with shoulder motion. Pain may be reproduced by having the patient slowly lower the abducted arm against resistance. Patients with impingement will have positive Neer and Hawkins impingement signs. In the Neer impingement test the patient's scapula is stabilized and depressed while the arm is elevated. The test elicits pain caused by the compression of the greater tuberosity against the anterior acromion. This indicates the presence of a rotator cuff tear or impingement syndrome. The Hawkins impingement sign is a confirmatory test for the Neer sign. The patient's shoulder and arm are elevated to 90 degrees, and the elbow flexed at 90 degrees with the forearm in neutral position (thumbs pointing to chest). Support the arm while internally rotating the humerus. Pain that is elicited has the same implications as the Neer sign.

Another test that may be performed to confirm impingement is the subacromial injection of an anesthetic followed by testing for impingement. The diagnosis of impingement syndrome is supported by complete relief from pain with this injection.

The rotator cuff muscles may be tested, in particular, the supraspinatus muscle. This is the most superior muscle of the four and is the most commonly affected because of its anatomic location. The supraspinatus muscle is tested by positioning the arm in 90 degrees elevation and rotating internally (thumbs down). The examiner pushes down on the arm while the patient resists this attempt. When compared to the other side, weakness suggests a rotator cuff tear. However, if this weakness is eliminated by a subacromial injection, the likely cause of the weakness is not a tear but rather an inflammation.

Another common finding with rotator cuff tendinitis is a painful arc sign. From the standing position, the patient is asked to abduct the arm from the resting position at his side. At approximately 45 degrees, the inflamed/injured tissues are forced underneath the acromion, and the patient will begin to feel the pain. As the patient continues abduction, the pain will continue until the 120-degree point. Beyond 120 degrees, the tissues are moved away from under the acromion and the pain subsides. There is usually no pain from 120 to 180 degrees. The differential diagnosis includes adhesive capsulitis, glenohumeral arthritis, rotator cuff tear/tendinitis, subacromial/subdeltoid bursitis, acromioclavicular arthritis, and bicipital tendinitis.

Imaging

Anteroposterior and axillary radiographs are commonly normal. Degenerative changes should be observed beneath the acromion and over the greater tuberosity of the humerus. An MRI may be advisable to determine the extent of a possible rotator cuff tear. Initially, this may not be warranted because the patient's response to treatment is important. A long-standing rotator cuff tear may be suspected on the plain films. Normally, the space between the humeral head and the undersurface of the acromion is >7 mm. Narrowing of this space suggests a long-standing tear of the rotator cuff.

Management

Any offending activities should be avoided. The use of nonsteroidal anti-inflammatory drugs will be helpful as an analgesic, as well as an anti-inflammatory agent (Evidence Level C). Ice or heat may also be applied cautiously. A program of gentle stretching may be initiated with particular emphasis on the posterior capsule (Evidence Level B). The patient should perform these exercises three to four times a day, every day for at least 6 weeks. Should the above measures fail to provide significant relief, local injection of a corticosteroid with anesthetic is helpful in reducing inflammation and relieving pain (Evidence Level C). Once the shoulder is more agile and less painful, a rotator cuff strengthening program may be added to the stretching regimen (Evidence Level C).

Follow-up

The patient should be seen within 3 to 4 weeks for reassessment, encouragement, and instruction to continue with the previous recommendations. If a local corticosteroid injection has not been attempted previously, this would be useful to try here (Evidence Level C). However, even with these injections, significant weakness of the rotator cuff or failure to improve after 3 to 4 months of rehabilitation/therapy should prompt reevaluation. If not previously obtained, an MRI should be utilized to assess the glenohumeral joint, the coracoacromial arch, and the integrity of the rotator cuff. Surgical interventions may be necessary, depending on the previous level of functioning of the patient.

ROTATOR CUFF RUPTURE/TEAR—ICD-9 CODE 727.61

CASE SIX

An 82-year-old man presents to your clinic complaining of recurrent shoulder pain for the last several months. Although he has been having mild occasional shoulder discomfort, he noted that after moving things in his attic he began to have increased pain. In particular, he began noticing there was significant nighttime pain that was causing difficulty sleeping. He also noticed considerable weakness and "catching" of this shoulder, especially in activities that involved lifting his arm overhead.

Rotator cuff tears are one of the most common problems of the shoulder. There is a strong correlation to the patient's age. Rotator cuff tears are rather rare before the age of 40 but common after 60. However, there is poor correlation between the presence of a rotator cuff tear and clinical symptoms. In fact, most clinical studies have demonstrated that although there is a higher frequency with advancing age, these tears are most often associated with normal, painless, and functional activity.

On presentation, patients commonly report that they have been having recurrent shoulder pain for several months. Usually, they can relate a specific event that set off pain. Characteristically, the patient has difficulty sleeping on the affected side and has significant nighttime pain. Other common symptoms are catching, weakness, and grinding, particularly with overhead activity.

Workup/Keys to Diagnosis

Physical Examination

With a long-standing cuff tear, atrophy of the supraspinatus and infraspinatus muscles will be apparent because the back of the shoulder will appear sunken. Some patients, in spite of large tears, are able to maintain near full range of motion. Other patients will have some degree of limitation of active motion, although passive motion is usually well preserved. A large tear may be suspected if the patient can only shrug the shoulder when attempting to lift the arm. There may be a palpable grating sensation as the patient lifts the arm. There is usually tenderness over the greater tuberosity of the humerus on palpation. The differential diagnosis includes adhesive capsulitis, glenohumeral arthritis, rotator cuff tendinitis, subacromial/subdeltoid bursitis, impingement syndrome, cervical spondylosis, acromioclavicular arthritis, bicipital tendinitis, and Pancoast tumor.

Imaging

Early on, plain radiographs may be normal. With long-standing large tears, the anteroposterior radiographs may reveal superior displacement of the humerus. This would be noted as a high-riding humerus in relationship to the glenoid of the scapula. Treatment may usually be initiated with no other diagnostic studies. However, if the diagnosis is unclear or if operative intervention is being contemplated, MRI is the preferred study. The MRI will provide clear evidence of the status of the glenohumeral joint, the status of the rotator cuff muscles, and the size of the tear itself.

Management

As noted in the preceding text, many patients are able to function very well even with large rotator cuff tears. Therefore, initial treatment should be directed toward nonsurgical therapy. This should include the use of nonsteroidal anti-inflammatory drugs (Evidence Level C). Physical therapy is strongly recommended and should include stretching and strengthening exercises (Evidence Level B). Avoidance of aggravating movements, particularly overhead activities, should be stressed. Corticosteroid injections are considered beneficial in the treatment of rotator cuff disorders (Evidence Level C). They decrease the attendant inflammation and also treat any associated subacromial bursitis. The arm should be rested for approximately 2 weeks following the infiltration. However, it should be remembered that corticosteroids should be used judiciously because they will weaken the tendon. Injections should be limited to no more than three times per year. Corticosteroids should never be injected into the body of the tendon.

Follow-up

Most patients will respond favorably to treatment. Only those patients with severe pain or with significant limitations of motion or of strength and function or those who have simply failed all rehabilitative efforts should be considered for surgery. Nonsurgical therapy should be attempted for at least 6 to 12 weeks before any surgical procedures are considered.

BICEPS TENDON RUPTURE—ICD-9 CODE 840.8

CASE SEVEN

An 81-year-old man presents complaining of a sudden onset of pain in his upper arm, which began 2 days ago. This began when he was helping his wife over a curb and she fell. He states he caught her to break her fall then felt and heard a snap, followed by pain. The pain was not severe. He indicates that he then noticed a bulge in the lower arm and now has bruising. He has also noted that he is weaker in this arm with flexion. Medical history is pertinent because you have treated him in the past for shoulder impingement syndrome.

In the elderly, rupture of the biceps tendon occurs proximally. This rupture involves the proximal long head of the biceps muscle. The position of the long head of the biceps tendon in the bicipital groove predisposes it to attritional changes and subsequent weakening. Ultimately, the tendon may fail in a relatively minor but sudden event. This will occur with an audible snap and subsequent ecchymoses of the upper arm. The sudden appearance of a bulge in the lower arm, which gives the arm a "Popeye" appearance, is usually quickly noted by the patient. These ruptures are frequently seen in older adults, particularly those with a previous history of shoulder problems such as impingement syndrome. Distal tendon rupture is quite rare at any age but is almost unheard of in the elderly.

Workup/Keys to Diagnosis

Physical Examination

In the mid to lower arm a bulge will be readily apparent; this represents the retraction of the biceps muscle after the long head tendon rupture. Because of the distal migration of the biceps, a defect can be palpated proximally. In the acute phase, ecchymoses will be noted in the middle and distal aspects of the arm. As the patient flexes the arm against resistance, the bulge will be accentuated and the diagnosis easily confirmed. Frequently, pain may be elicited by palpation of the bicipital groove of the humerus, with the arm held at 10 to 15 degrees of internal rotation and the elbow at 90 degrees. The differential diagnosis includes rupture of distal biceps tendon, dislocated biceps tendon, rotator cuff tendinitis or tear, rupture of pectoralis major muscle, impingement syndrome, and glenohumeral arthritis.

Imaging

This is a clinical diagnosis and, accordingly, radiographs and other studies are not helpful in the confirmation. However, anteroposterior and axillary radiographs would be helpful to rule out other pathology, such as tumors and fractures. Other studies, such as an MRI, should be performed only if there is suspicion of a rotator cuff tear and the diagnosis must be made.

Management

The need for surgical repair is rare (Evidence Level C). Rupture of the biceps tendon results in very little loss of function. Most patients only lose approximately 10% to 20% of forearm supination and elbow flexion (i.e., the usual functions of the biceps muscle). Although there may be a cosmetic deformity, most patients find this quite acceptable, and with subsequent atrophy, it will diminish over time. Patients should be encouraged to exercise to maintain or regain strength and range of motion.

Follow-up

There is little need for follow-up because most patients do quite well. In patients who are feeble, reevaluation may be necessary to be certain that they are not adversely affected by even this minimal loss of function. Reevaluation should also be done in patients who are suspected of having an associated rotator cuff tear if this might appear to be a problem for them at a later date.

OLECRANON BURSITIS—ICD-9 CODE 726.33

> **CASE EIGHT**
>
> The patient presents with gradual swelling over the elbow. It has been present for several weeks with little or no tenderness or pain. There is no history of trauma or falling, but the patient does admit to leaning on his elbows most of the day.

Olecranon bursitis may develop acutely because of a direct blow or fall. However, it is not unusual for this to develop in elderly patients who excessively lean on their elbows, causing prolonged irritation and resultant inflammation. If the swelling develops suddenly, it is most often due to trauma or infection. If it develops gradually, it is usually a chronic situation. It may be seen in patients with gout or rheumatoid arthritis.

Workup/Keys to Diagnosis

Physical Examination

Over the tip of the elbow there will be an obvious 5 or 6 cm soft mass. Excess heat or redness suggests infection. Usually, chronic olecranon bursitis is not tender. If there is considerable tenderness (unrelated to recent trauma), the clinician should be highly suspicious of an infectious process. There is usually full range of motion and no associated muscular atrophy. Frequently, there will be palpable lumps on the olecranon itself. These represent scar tissue that is left as the swelling and fluid resolve. The differential diagnosis includes gout, infectious bursitis, olecranon process fracture, rheumatoid disease, and synovial cyst of elbow joint.

Imaging

Usually, the diagnosis is straightforward and no radiographs are necessary. However, if there is associated trauma, anteroposterior and lateral radiographs should be obtained to rule out fracture of the olecranon process or osteomyelitis.

Management

Under most circumstances, there is nothing that is necessary, particularly if the bursal swelling is small and only mildly symptomatic. Modification of activity, avoidance of pressure on the affected elbow, and the use of nonsteroidal anti-inflammatory drugs may be all that is necessary. If the swelling is quite large and symptomatic, aspiration under sterile conditions may be performed using a lateral approach. If indicated, the fluid may be sent for Gram stain and culture. If there is no evidence of infection, a corticosteroid preparation may be instilled followed by the application of a compression dressing. This dressing should remain in place for 48 hours, if possible (Evidence Level C).

Septic olecranon bursitis must be cultured and treated accordingly. The most common offending organism is penicillin-resistant *Staphylococcus aureus*. Oral antibiotics may be used if diagnosis is made early.

Follow-up

Patients should be reevaluated within 2 to 5 days of aspiration. If aspiration was not performed, the patient can decide on returning if necessary. If there is no infection, there is little need for any further treatment unless the swollen bursa becomes chronically inflamed and symptomatic. In such cases, excision may be entertained. However, this is usually discouraged because of the frequent formation of a chronically draining sinus (with or without infection).

DUPUYTREN CONTRACTURE/ DISEASE—ICD-9 CODE 728.6

> **CASE NINE**
>
> An elderly man presents to your office complaining of progressively restricted motion in the ring and little fingers of his hand. This has been developing gradually over several years. Initially, there was minimal discomfort but this has resolved. He has noticed several nodules near the distal palmar crease that are painful whenever he grasps something. There is no loss of sensation. He does mention that he is having difficulty fully extending the affected fingers.

Dupuytren disease affects the palmar fascia of the hand. It involves a nodular thickening and subsequent contracture deformity of the affected fingers, most commonly the ring finger, followed in order of frequency by the little finger, middle finger, thumb, and lastly the index finger.

There seems to be a genetic predisposition because it is more frequently seen in people of northern European descent. Certain conditions seem to be associated with this disease, such as pulmonary disease, diabetes, alcoholism, and repetitive trauma.

Although there may be some initial discomfort and sensitivity, it becomes painless as the disease progresses. As the nodules gradually thicken, they begin to cause contracture deformities, which restrict extension with no adverse effects on finger flexion. Sensation is usually maintained. As the contractures develop, patients may have difficulty with activities that require extension of the fingers, such as putting hands into pockets, putting on gloves, or grasping and holding certain objects.

Workup/Keys to Diagnosis

Physical Examination

In the early stages, examination will reveal palmar nodules that resemble calluses. As the disease progresses, fascial bands develop that extend distally along the tendons and sometimes proximally as well. The bands may eventually cross the metacarpophalangeal (MP) joint and perhaps the proximal interphalangeal joint. This will cause the affected finger to be held in a contracted flexed position, which will limit extension of the finger. Sensation is intact, and there is no discoloration. Tenderness of these bands, or cords, will only be noted in the early stages of the disease. The differential diagnosis includes trigger finger that is locked or flexion contracture due to previous injury.

Imaging

This is strictly a clinical diagnosis. No tests are required.

Management

There is no specific cure for Dupuytren disease or contracture formation. Splinting may allow some slowing of the progression of the disease. As the disease progresses, patients who have significant contractures of the MP joints (usually >30 degrees) that affect finger motion may be candidates for surgical therapy (Evidence Level C). Surgical intervention involves excision of the thickened soft tissue bands and release of the contractures of the joints.

Follow-up

No specific follow-up is required. The contractures may be evaluated on other visits to the physician's office. Usually, there is no need for intervention, and watching and waiting is the most prudent course of action. If the contractures seem to be worsening, documentation of the limitations is useful for following the course of deterioration, which may later direct surgical choices.

OSTEOARTHRITIS OF THE HIP—ICD-9 CODE 715.15

CASE TEN

A 76-year-old woman presents complaining of a gradual onset of knee pain. At the same time, she began experiencing pain in her anterior thigh and hip area. This has been present for more than a year, and initially the pain occurred only with activity. Over the last 2 months, the pain has increased such that it is uncomfortable with no activity and has awakened her from sleep on several occasions. There is no history of prior trauma or injury. There is no history of weight loss or fever.

The loss of articular cartilage of the hip results in osteoarthritis of this joint. There is usually no history of previous injury. Some patients may have had childhood problems, such as slipped femoral capital epiphysis, which would predispose to this problem. The pain may frequently be referred to the knee.

Workup/Keys to Diagnosis

Physical Examination

The earliest manifestation of osteoarthritis of the hip is loss of internal rotation. As the disease progresses, there will be loss of flexion and extension. The gait may eventually be affected because of the development of flexion contractures, weakness of abductor muscles, and alteration of gait to compensate for the pain. The differential diagnosis includes inflammatory arthritis of the hip, osteonecrosis of the femoral head, lumbar disc herniation, degenerative lumbar disc disease, trochanteric bursitis, and tumor of spine or pelvis.

Imaging

The classic radiographic findings are usually seen readily on anteroposterior and lateral films. These consist of narrowing of the hip joint space, formation of osteophyte, formation of bony cysts, and subchondral sclerosis. Usually, the diagnosis is easily made with these plain films and further studies are not necessary. If there is suspected osteonecrosis of the femoral head, CT scan or MRI may be warranted.

Management

This disease is progressive and has no cure. Treatment should be dictated by the age of the patient and the stage of the disease process. Initial pain relief may be achieved by the use of acetaminophen. Nonsteroidal anti-inflammatory drugs may be helpful for analgesia and its effects on inflammation (Evidence Level A). Early use of physical therapy will help in improving and preserving strength and range of motion (Evidence Level B). Later, the use of a cane may provide stability and leverage. It should be noted that the cane should be used by the contralateral hand so that weight may be supported and removed from the affected hip.

Follow-up

The patient may be seen within a few weeks to assess therapeutic results. In addition, pain that progressively worsens at rest should be further evaluated for more serious disease such as carcinoma. As the disease progresses, medications may be altered to provide additional relief. The judicious use of narcotics may be of benefit to some patients. When the pain becomes intolerable or motion becomes limited, a total hip replacement should be considered. Surgery should be considered before muscle atrophy is too advanced.

OSTEOARTHRITIS OF THE KNEE—ICD-9 CODE 715.16

CASE ELEVEN

An active 67-year-old man presents with complaints of right knee pain. He is approximately 27 kg overweight and has gained 12 kg over the last 6 months. You have treated him for minor knee pain in the past but now he states that it is much worse because he gained the extra weight. The patient states that the pain is made worse by walking or prolonged standing. He also states that the knee feels unsteady and wants to "give way." Climbing up or down the stairs is particularly troublesome. He feels like there is increasing stiffness and states that at times it might appear to have a little swelling. He has a family history of "wear and tear" arthritis of the knees.

Osteoarthritis is a very common occurrence and is particularly prevalent in obese patients and those with a genetic predisposition. The disease usually has a gradual and insidious onset and is first noticed because of pain. The pain will be especially noticed on weight bearing. Patients commonly complain of buckling of the knee or a sensation of giving way. This is caused by the increasing contact of bony areas and their subsequent impinging on each other. Stiffness and intermittent swelling of the joint will occur, further limiting the range of motion, particularly at the extremes. Furthermore, the patient will complain of difficulty ascending and descending stairs because of the pain and unsteadiness that accompanies this disorder. As the cartilage deteriorates, there may be further symptoms, such as locking, similar to signs of a meniscal tear. As the patient becomes less and less mobile, muscular atrophy will ensue, which further compromises the normal functioning of the knee joint. The medial compartment of the knee is the most frequently affected portion of the joint, leading to genu varum deformity.

Workup/Keys to Diagnosis

Physical Examination

Inspection of the knee may reveal muscular atrophy, particularly of the vastus medialis obliquus. On weight bearing, the varus (or valgus) deformity will be apparent. Comparison to the contralateral knee is helpful, but it may be similarly affected. A mild joint effusion may be present, as well as tenderness, which may be diffuse but is very often present along the joint line. Osteophytes may be palpable along the femoral condyles. Crepitus should be noted, as well as any loss of range of motion. The differential diagnosis includes meniscal tear, osteonecrosis of the knee joint, rheumatoid arthritis, pathology of the hip (referred pain), lumbar disc disease, and bursitis.

Imaging

Anteroposterior radiographs are quite helpful but are much more valuable when accompanied by weight-bearing views. Typical findings are collapse of the medial compartment (most commonly), joint narrowing, osteophyte formation, and subchondral bony sclerosis. Lateral and patellofemoral views will be useful in assessing these areas of the joint. Osteophyte formation may be found with the tunnel view, which identifies the intercondylar notch. Further studies are usually not necessary because these plain films readily make the diagnosis and reveal the extent of the disease.

Management

Adequate analgesia should be provided, and relief may only require the use of acetaminophen in the early stages (Evidence Level A). Subsequently, the addition of nonsteroidal anti-inflammatory drugs is very helpful (Evidence Level A). Application of ice or heat and topical creams may provide some benefit in reducing the aching and stiffness of the joint (Evidence Level C). The use of elastic bandages or neoprene sleeves as mechanical aids may be of benefit but they should not be placed too tightly, particularly in patients with arterial or venous insufficiency. Mechanical support may assist in controlling the swelling and provide a certain amount of joint stability when walking, although there are no randomized studies of this approach. Physical therapy should be recommended and actively pursued as the pain allows (Evidence Level A). This will support maintenance of muscle tone and forestall the attendant muscular disuse and atrophy that will occur. Assisted devices such as canes and/or walkers are quite useful in keeping the patient mobile and lessening the risk of falling.

The use of intra-articular injections is common and provides significant benefit to many patients (Evidence Level A). Combined injections of corticosteroids and local anesthetics provide substantial, albeit temporary, relief. However, some patients are able to obtain prolonged periods of relief with these injections, depending on their level of activity. In addition, some patients may derive benefit from viscosupplementation with hyaluronic acid (Evidence Level A). A recent meta-analysis found that the intra-articular injection of hyaluronic acid decreased the symptoms of osteoarthritis of the knee. This analysis also found that those treated had significant improvement in terms of reduction in pain and functionality with very few adverse events.[9]

Follow-up

Patients may be seen on an as-needed basis but should be warned that the disease will progress. It is helpful to periodically see these patients to remind them of the importance of remaining active and maintaining muscle tone and strength. These patients will need encouragement to continue their activities, medications, and modalities. The judicious and limited use of narcotic analgesics may be considered in patients who occasionally require more substantial relief from pain (Evidence Level C).

As the disease progresses, many patients may become candidates for full knee-replacement surgery (Evidence Level C). Potential candidates would be those with severe pain, pain at rest, limitations of function, or significantly decreased range of motion. Patients who are rarely ambulatory or immobile are not usually considered for surgical therapy.

PLANTAR FASCIITIS—ICD-9 CODE 728.71

> **CASE TWELVE**
>
> An obese 67-year-old woman presents complaining of a gradual onset of pain in her heel. The pain is localized to the medial side of her foot just anterior to the calcaneus. The pain is very severe when first arising in the morning and beginning to walk. It is also very painful with the first few steps after she has been seated for a while. Once she takes the pressure off of her foot, the pain very quickly resolves. There is no history of trauma or previous complaints.

Plantar fasciitis is the most common cause of heel pain. Although the exact etiology is not known, it is thought to be due to the degeneration of the plantar fascia at its origin from the calcaneus. The symptoms usually begin insidiously and are not related to any specific event. Wearing shoes that provide little support to the foot may be a precipitating factor. It is more common in women and in individuals who are overweight. The characteristic complaint is the pain that begins with the first few steps, particularly when arising from bed in the morning. Similar pain after sitting is characteristic as well. The pain will be exacerbated and reproduced by prolonged standing or walking. Once the pressure is off of the area, such as when seated, the pain is relieved.

Workup/Keys to Diagnosis

Physical Examination

Usually there is no visible abnormality. Palpation reveals a distinct area of tenderness located 1 to 2 cm anterior to the medial calcaneal tuberosity. It may be necessary to apply considerable pressure to reproduce the symptoms to mimic weight-bearing situations. Stretching of the plantar fascia by inversion of the midfoot or passive dorsiflexion of the foot may reproduce symptoms as well. In nearly all patients, the Achilles tendon will be very tight. The differential diagnosis includes calcaneal stress fracture or tumor, atrophy of the fat pad of the heel, tarsal tunnel syndrome, and lumbar radiculopathy.

Imaging

A patient presenting with the classic complaints mentioned in preceding text will not require any radiographs. These are not helpful in the management of the disorder. If radiographs are taken, they should include standing lateral films. Frequently, patients will want x-rays because they want to know whether they have a spur. A calcaneal spur, or osteophyte, may be present in up to approximately 50% of cases. However, even if present, this has little to do with plantar fasciitis. This is a traction spur that has evolved over many years. Moreover, this osteophyte develops at the origin of the flexor brevis muscle, which is not in the same plane as the plantar fascia and lies superior to it. Unless there is suspicion of a stress fracture or tumor, bone scans and MRIs are not necessary.

Management

Nearly all patients will respond to conservative management, but they should be informed that it may take up to a year to resolve. Patients who are very active will need to modify their weight-bearing activities to avoid further undue stress on the plantar fascia. One of the most important elements in treating plantar fasciitis is the stretching of the Achilles tendon. If this is not done, patients will be plagued by symptoms for a much longer period. Proper Achilles tendon stretching should be carefully explained and demonstrated to the patient (Evidence Level C).

Instructions for proper Achilles stretching should be as follows: Lean forward against a wall, keeping one knee straight, and heel flat on the floor. The other knee is moved forward of the body in a bended position. This should be done individually on both sides and held for 60 seconds. The patient should be able to feel the stretch of the Achilles tendon. This stretch should be repeated at least four times a day.

The plantar fascia may be stretched as follows: Have the patient lean forward over a table or chair; spread the feet apart with one foot in front of the other while bending the knees. Squat down slowly while maintaining heel contact with the floor. As the patient squats, the stretch of the plantar fascia and Achilles tendon will be felt. This should be held for 30 to 60 seconds and performed at least four times a day.

If not contraindicated (as in patients with decreased sensation or vascular insufficiency), ice massage should be used. An easy method for this is to freeze water in a Styrofoam coffee cup and then to peel away a small portion of the top of the cup to reveal the ice. The cup becomes an easily manageable tool. Massaging the affected area for 10 to 20 minutes three to four times a day will aid in decreasing inflammation. In addition, nonsteroidal anti-inflammatory drugs may be tried, as well as shoes with good shock-absorbing soles and lateral heel support (Evidence Level C).

Night splints have also been shown to be useful. These splints are designed to hold the ankle and foot in slight extension, which will stretch both the plantar fascia and the Achilles tendon (Evidence Level C).

Follow-up

Patients should be given at least 8 to 12 weeks of the above treatment for improvement to take place. If the symptoms remain unchanged, injecting a corticosteroid plus a local anesthetic into the area of pain may be considered.

Up to three injections may be used. If three injections render no relief, further use will serve no purpose (Evidence Level C).

An alternative to injection is the use of two physical therapy modalities. These are phonophoresis and/or iontophoresis. These should be discussed with the physical therapist and tried for 3 to 4 weeks (Evidence Level C).

Finally, for patients who do not respond to any of these measures and continue to have persistent symptoms, referral to a podiatrist may be in order. Surgical treatment consists of a plantar fascia release but may result in a pes planus deformity and attendant problems associated with it (Evidence Level C).

CORNS AND CALLUSES OF THE FOOT—ICD-9 CODE 700.00

CASE THIRTEEN

A 68-year-old man presents to your office accompanied by his wife. He is complaining of pain under his big toe joint and "thickened skin." Although this has been present for many years, it has not bothered him until recently, when he began a walking regimen after his retirement. During this office visit, his wife says she has a similar complaint. She states that since they started walking, she has begun to have pain in the medial aspect of her second toe. She has also noted a hard "growth" over the middle joint.

The descriptions in the preceding case suggest that the man has a callus while his wife has a corn. A callus represents a hyperkeratotic lesion of the skin that most commonly occurs over a bony prominence in response to excessive pressure. It commonly forms under a metatarsal head. It is not uncommon for a callus to form on a medial or lateral bony prominence of a toe (hard corn) or in the web spaces (soft corn). This is usually precipitated by toe deformities and inappropriately fitting shoes. Typically, pain is noted on walking or wearing shoes.

Workup/Keys to Diagnosis

Physical Examination

Calluses and corns may be readily seen as a soft tissue elevation over a bony prominence or in a web space. They usually have a waxy and uniform appearance. They are tender with direct pressure, whereas a plantar wart is tender when the sides are pinched. The differential diagnosis includes plantar wart, foreign body, synovitis, and Morton neuroma.

Imaging

No tests are required unless there is a potential for a foreign body. In this case, metal and some types of glass may be detected by plain radiographs.

Management

Pressure relief is provided by paring of the callus or corn. This should be accomplished by the use of a scalpel without the need of anesthesia. As much of the avascular keratin tissue as possible should be removed without causing pain or bleeding. This may be easier if the foot is soaked for a few minutes in warm water before paring (Evidence Level C).

Follow-up

Little follow-up is necessary, but patients should be instructed to maintain the paring at home by using a pumice stone or callus file. In addition, less oppressive shoes should be used with a toe box adequate to avoid the offending pressure. Cushions or pads made of silicone or foam may be used to further relieve the pressure.

Should the above measures fail and the patient remains symptomatic, surgical treatment may be warranted. The development of ulcerations or infection requires further evaluation.

CONCLUSION

There are a wide variety of common musculoskeletal and soft tissue problems that may develop in elderly patients. Fortunately, most of them may be handled by primary care clinicians. Most of them are readily recognized and satisfactorily treated. The astute clinician should always be aware of the possibility of more ominous diseases masquerading as benign problems.

REFERENCES

1. Macera CA, Jackson KL, Hagenmaier GW, et al. Age, physical activity, physical fitness, body composition, and incidence of orthopedic problems. *Res Q Exerc Sport*. 1989;60:225–229.
2. Taylor DC, Dalton JD, Seaber AV, et al. Viscoelastic properties of muscle-tendon units: The biomechanical effects of stretching. *Am J Sports Med*. 1990;18:300–309.
3. Fiatarone MA, O'Neill EF, Ryan ND. Exercise training and nutritional supplementation for physical frailty in very elderly people. *N Engl J Med*. 1994;330:1769–1774.
4. Frontera WR, Meredith CN, O'Reilly KP, et al. Strength conditioning in older men: Skeletal muscle hypertrophy and improved function. *J Appl Physiol*. 1988;64:1038–1044.
5. Maffulli N, Khan KM, Puddu GC. Overuse tendon conditions: Time to change a confusing terminology. *Arthroscopy*. 1998;14:840–843.
6. Maffulli N, Wong J, Almekinders LC. Types and epidemiology of tendinopathy. *Clin Sports Med*. 2003;22(4):675–692.
7. Klippel JH, ed. *Primer on the rheumatic diseases*, 12th ed. Atlanta, GA: Arthritis Foundation; 2001.
8. Tallia AF, Cardone DA. Diagnostic and therapeutic injection of the shoulder region. *Am Fam Physician*. 2003;67(6):1271–1278.
9. Wang CT, Lin J, Chang CJ, et al. Therapeutic effects of hyaluronic acid on osteoarthritis of the knee: A meta-analysis of randomized controlled trials. *J Bone Joint Surg Am*. 2004;86(3):538–545.

Metabolic Bone Disease

23

Ailleen Heras-Herzig *Theresa A. Guise*

CLINICAL PEARLS 293

OSTEOPOROSIS 293
Workup/Keys to Diagnosis 295
Management 296

OSTEOMALACIA 299
Workup/Keys to Diagnosis 301
Management 302

PRIMARY HYPERPARATHYROIDISM 303
Workup/Key to Diagnosis 303
Management 304

RENAL OSTEODYSTROPHY 305
Workup/Key to Diagnosis 305
Management 306

ACKNOWLEDGMENT 308

CLINICAL PEARLS

- Screen high-risk populations for osteoporosis.
- Assess clinical risk factors.
- Address lifestyle and dietary modifications.
- Screen for secondary causes of low bone mineral density.
- Correct vitamin D deficiency and insufficiency prior to initiating other treatments for osteoporosis.

As the population in the United States ages, we can expect practitioners to encounter an increasing number of patients with metabolic bone disease and associated low bone mass. These disorders are usually divided into primary and secondary causes of low bone mass (see Table 23.1). The most common types of metabolic bone disease—including (i) osteoporosis; (ii) osteomalacia; (iii) primary hyperparathyroidism; and (iv) renal osteodystrophy—will be discussed in this chapter. Recognizing the presence of these bone disorders is a major challenge for physicians. These abnormalities of the bone and calcium/phosphorus metabolism are usually silent until well advanced and present with complications of the disease, most commonly, fracture. Therefore, a high level of suspicion and a clear plan for the screening of high-risk patients can have a significant impact on quality of life and society's health care costs.

OSTEOPOROSIS

Osteoporosis is defined as a skeletal disorder characterized by low bone density and poor bone quality that lead to an increased risk of fragility fractures. Primary or involutional osteoporosis refers to the normal bone loss that occurs with aging. This can be further subdivided into type I or II osteoporosis syndromes. Type I is characterized by the rapid bone loss observed in the first 15 to 20 years after menopause, with a disproportionate trabecular over cortical bone loss. During this accelerated rate of bone loss, women may lose as much as 20% to 30% of trabecular bone and 5% to 10% of cortical bone and are at increased risk of Colles fractures and vertebral compression fractures. Type II or senile involutional osteoporosis refers to the slow phase of age-related bone loss and leads to equal losses of cortical and trabecular bones. This type of osteoporosis affects the entire population and is progressive throughout aging. This results in an increase in fracture risk in people at the lower end of the age-specific distribution for bone mineral density (BMD). Clinically, this type of osteoporosis presents with predominantly proximal femur and vertebral fractures, but fractures at other sites with a combination of cortical and trabecular bones can also be seen.

Type I osteoporosis has been widely believed to be a result of low estrogen concentration in menopause. While this is certainly a primary factor, estrogen deficiency leads to an increase in certain cytokines such as interleukin-6 and tumor necrosis factor as well as an increase in urinary

TABLE 23.1
SECONDARY CAUSES OF LOW BONE MASS

Endocrine Disorders	**Hematopoietic Disorders**
Hyperparathyroidism (252.00)	Multiple myeloma (203.00)
Vitamin D insufficiency or deficiency (268.9)	Sickle cell disease (282.60)
Hyperthyroidism (242.90)	Thalassemia (282.49)
Cushing syndrome (255.0)	Metastatic carcinoma
Hyperprolactinemia (253.1)	Systemic mastocytosis (202.60)
Hypogonadism—female (256.39) male (257.2)	AIDS/HIV (042)/(V08)
Pregnancy and lactation	Leukemia and lymphoma 10.60/202.80
Nutritional and Gastrointestinal Disorders	Lipidoses: Gaucher disease (272.7)
Malabsorptive syndromes (579.9)	**Drug-Induced**
Bariatric surgery	Alcohol
Total parenteral nutrition	Glucocorticoids
Gastrectomy	Anticonvulsants
Hepatobiliary disease	Heparin
Renal Disorders	Lithium
Renal osteodystrophy (588.0)	Cyclosporine
Renal tubular acidosis (588.89)	Gonadotropin-releasing hormone agonists
Hypercalciuria (275.40)	Aluminum
Connective Tissue Disorders	Smoking
Rheumatoid arthritis (714.00)	**Miscellaneous**
Osteogenesis imperfecta (756.51)	Immobilization
Ehlers-Danlos syndrome (756.83)	Reflex sympathetic dystrophy (337.20)
Homocystinuria (270.4)	Weight loss (783.21)
Lysinuria (270.9)	Multiple sclerosis (340)
Ankylosing spondylitis (720.0)	Porphyria (277.1)
Marfan syndrome (759.82)	

AIDS, acquired immunodeficiency syndrome; HIV, human immunodeficiency virus.

calcium excretion. It is probably the genetically determined susceptibility to these factors in the bone and kidney that determines, to a great extent, the degree of observed bone loss. On the other hand, type II osteoporosis is believed to be the result of a combination of secondary hyperparathyroidism and decreased bone formation rates, and both processes are a consequence of lower estrogen concentration in aging women and men.

While the clinical hallmark of osteoporosis is the presence of low-trauma fractures, this precludes diagnosis in individuals who may be at high risk for fracture and in whom fracture prevention should be the standard of care. Therefore, in 1994, the World Health Organization (WHO) offered a definition of osteoporosis on the basis of bone density measurements and history of fracture (see Table 23.2). These criteria designate osteoporosis as a BMD equal to or <2.5 standard deviations (SDs) below a young mean adult value. On the basis of the WHO criteria, 20% to 30% of postmenopausal women in the United States have osteoporosis, and 1.3 million fractures a year are attributable to this disease. The WHO criteria were originally developed to describe fracture risk in white postmenopausal women. Whether the same criteria can be applied to other populations, particularly in men, is still an area of much controversy. Nonetheless, in recent years, the International Society for Clinical Densitometry (ISCD), in association with an expert panel, determined that it is appropriate to apply the same criteria to men while using a gender-specific database for BMD. Using these established cutoffs, it is estimated that 1 to 2 million men have osteoporosis and 8 to 13 million have osteopenia. The respective age-adjusted prevalence figures are 6% and 47%. If one uses fracture as a clear endpoint, then the estimated lifetime risk is 13% to 25%. Either way, this is a significant health problem for both aging women and men.

Morbidity and mortality following a vertebral or hip fracture are high. Vertebral fractures lead to a progressive decrease in physical activity, kyphotic deformity, height loss, and chronic back pain, all of which, in turn, cause increasing social isolation, depression, and low self-esteem. The 5-year age-matched survival after a vertebral fracture is 72% for men and 84% for women. Similarly, a hip fracture leads to significant disability. One year after a hip fracture, 40% of patients are unable to walk independently and 60% require assistance with activities of daily living. Hip fracture mortality is higher in men than in women. Approximately 8% of men and 3% of women over age 50 die during their initial hospitalization for hip fracture. One year after a hip fracture, the mortality is 36% for men and 21% for women. Therefore, the challenge is to recognize individuals who are at high risk for osteoporotic fractures before the first fracture

TABLE 23.2
DEFINING OSTEOPOROSIS BY BONE MINERAL DENSITY ON THE BASIS OF THE WORLD HEALTH ORGANIZATION CRITERIA

Category	Definition by BMD
Normal	BMD is within 1 SD from a young healthy adult (T-score greater than or equal to −1.0)
Osteopenia	BMD is between 1 and 2.5 SD below that of a young healthy adult (T-score between −1 and −2.5)
Osteoporosis	BMD is 2.5 SD or more below that of a young healthy adult (T-score at or below −2.5)
Severe osteoporosis (established)	BMD >2.5 SD below that of a young adult mean in the presence of one or more fragility fractures

BMD, bone mineral density; SD, standard deviation.
World Health Organization 1994.

occurs. While it is recognized that for every 1 SD decrease in BMD there is an associated two- to threefold increase in fracture risk, 50% of patients who suffer a fragility fracture have a BMD above the osteoporosis threshold as defined by the WHO criteria. Case-finding strategies should therefore incorporate the known risk factors for fracture, and treatment decisions should be based not only on the BMD scores but also on risk factor assessment.

Workup/Keys to Diagnosis

The first step in assessing fracture risk is a thorough assessment of clinical risk factors (see Table 23.3). The most important, readily recognized factor is probably age. It is well known that for any given BMD, the fracture risk increases with aging. For example, the risk of hip fracture increases 30-fold between the ages of 50 and 80, while one would predict a fourfold increase solely on the basis of the average BMD. Other significant risk factors for fracture that capture aspects of risk beyond that assessed by BMD include previous fragility fracture, glucocorticoid therapy, family history of fragility fracture, and low body weight, among others. Utilizing this risk factor assessment, one can therefore identify a subgroup of patients for whom the risk of a future fracture is high enough to warrant therapy, regardless of the baseline BMD. In these patients, BMD may still be utilized to monitor their response to therapy. On the other hand, individuals with a paucity of risk factors may not warrant BMD testing because their fracture risk is low, regardless of bone density measurements. Therefore, the National Osteoporosis Foundation (NOF) has provided a set of guidelines to aid practitioners in identifying patients for whom BMD testing is appropriate (see Table 23.4). These and similar guidelines issued by Medicare and the ISCD are not all encompassing and, therefore, should be used in the context of a patient's particular situation.

TABLE 23.3
RISK FACTORS FOR OSTEOPOROTIC FRACTURES

Major Risk Factors in White Women
- Personal history of fracture as an adult
- History of fragility fracture in a first-degree relative
- Low body weight (<58 kgs)
- Current smoking
- Use of oral corticosteroid therapy for >3 mo

Additional Risk factors
- Premature menopause (<45 y)
- Primary or secondary amenorrhea
- Primary and secondary hypogonadism in men
- Impaired vision
- Prolonged immobilization
- Dementia
- Excessive alcohol consumption (>2 drinks/d)
- Low calcium intake
- Recent falls
- Poor health/frailty

BMD testing remains a cornerstone of osteoporosis diagnosis and assessment of response to treatment. Central dual x-ray absorptiometry (DXA) is the standard for BMD testing. Central DXA has been used extensively in epidemiologic studies and, therefore, its relationship to fracture risk has been best characterized. Fracture prediction at a specific site is most accurate for BMD measurements at that particular site. For instance, BMD at the hip correlates best with hip fracture risk, although a general fracture risk assessment can be estimated from the measurement at any site. Quantitative computed tomography (QCT) of the spine is another central modality for bone density measurement. The greatest advantage of this technology is that it provides a true volumetric assessment of bone density, while DXA only provides an areal density. QCT requires specific software, and it has not been traditionally used in epidemiologic studies or longitudinal studies of treatment effect. Furthermore, QCT results in a high

TABLE 23.4
WHO SHOULD BE TESTED

National Osteoporosis Foundation

1. All women aged 65 and older, regardless of risk factors
2. Younger postmenopausal women with one or more risk factors (other than being white, postmenopausal, and female)
3. Postmenopausal women who are considering therapy if BMD testing would facilitate the decision
4. Postmenopausal women who present with fractures (to confirm the diagnosis and determine the disease severity)

Medicare Coverage for BMD in Individuals Aged 65 and Older—Bone Mass Act

1. Estrogen-deficient women at clinical risk for osteoporosis
2. Individuals with vertebral abnormalities
3. Individuals receiving, or planning to receive, long-term glucocorticoid (steroid) therapy
4. Individuals with primary hyperparathyroidism
5. Individuals being monitored to assess the response or efficacy of an approved osteoporosis drug therapy

BMD, bone mineral density.

radiation exposure, far in excess of that observed with DXA. This technology may best be used in patients at the extremes of size or weight.

Peripheral technologies such as pQCT, pDXA, and quantitative ultrasound (QUS) are increasingly being used for screening purposes. The WHO criteria should not be applied to these measurements and, therefore, it is recommended that anyone with a positive study undergoes central DXA measurement. Furthermore, sites traditionally measured by these methods respond poorly to osteoporosis treatment, and it is recommended that central sites be used to assess response to therapy. On the other hand, peripheral BMD does provide an assessment of global fracture risk, as recently demonstrated in two large prospective studies, and may therefore serve as a cost-effective initial screening tool.

While osteoporosis has few diagnostic signs in physical examination, there are a number of findings that can alert the practitioner to the possibility of disease and/or an increased fracture risk. Poor visual acuity and depth perception, decreased proprioception, decreased proximal muscle strength, and an impaired "get up and go" test are all risk factors for fall and fracture and can be easily assessed in the clinic. Furthermore, kyphotic deformities of the spine are late sequelae of vertebral fractures and should prompt the physician to pursue further diagnosis and treatment.

We recommend that all patients diagnosed with osteoporosis undergo basic laboratory testing for secondary causes of osteoporosis. These tests should include, at a minimum, the measurement of calcium, phosphorus, magnesium, creatinine, parathyroid hormone (PTH), and 25(OH) vitamin D levels. The prevalence of vitamin D deficiency in the elderly population is estimated to be between 25% and 54%. This number is probably even higher for institutionalized or debilitated individuals. Vitamin D deficiency may, in turn, lead to secondary hyperparathyroidism and its associated adverse effects on bone. Therefore, vitamin D deficiency should be routinely screened for and aggressively treated. All men should have a serum testosterone measurement because treatment of hypogonadism may result in increased bone mass. In addition, other tests such as serum and urine protein electrophoresis and screening tests for hypercortisolism or malabsorptive syndromes should be obtained in select patients. Finally, whether to measure 24-hour urine excretion for calcium is controversial. There is high variability in calcium urine excretion from day to day and this is at least partly related to dietary variability. This is useful when calcium malabsorption is a significant issue and may result in a therapeutic change. We have also identified a significant number of patients with idiopathic hypercalciuria, which has been associated with secondary hyperparathyroidism and low BMD. Such patients may benefit from treatment with thiazide diuretics to reduce renal calcium excretion.

As previously outlined, treatment decisions should be based on a combination of clinical risk factor assessment and BMD measurement. NOF recommends that treatment should be considered in postmenopausal women with a T-score of < -2.0 or in women with a T-score of < -1.5 but with other risk factors. These criteria have also been extrapolated to men. However, in the absence of other risk factors, treatment based solely on BMD should be reserved for men older than 65 to 70 years of age, because this is when fracture risk increases in this population (see Fig. 23.1).

Management

The management of osteoporosis is multifactorial and includes a combination of lifestyle modifications, nutritional counseling, and pharmacologic interventions. As described in the preceding text, the first step in osteoporosis management entails screening for secondary causes of osteoporosis and correcting as indicated.

Lifestyle interventions are crucial in the treatment of osteoporosis, but perhaps more importantly, in fracture prevention. All patients should be advised to pursue a combination of weight-bearing exercises and strength training. Exercise serves to decrease osteoporosis and fracture risk in several important ways. Low impact to bone stimulates bone remodeling with the uptake of old, possibly fragile, bone and the deposition of new, stronger bone. In addition, exercise increases balance and muscle strength and, therefore, decreases the risk of falls. Patients with severe mobility impairment should be referred to physical therapy for instruction on appropriate exercises and balance training. All patients should be advised to pursue fall prevention measures at home including (i) proper lighting in all rooms; (ii) removal of area rugs and floor clutter; (iii) use of walking devices as deemed

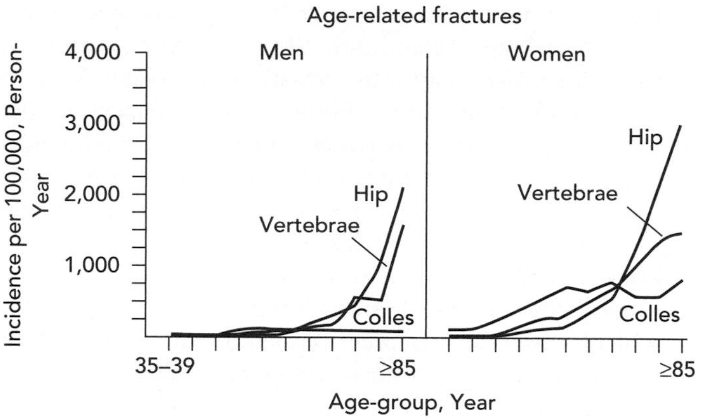

Figure 23.1 Fracture incidence for men and women with aging. (Reproduced from Cooper C. Epidemiology of osteoporosis. In: Favus M, ed. The *Primer on the metabolic bone diseases and disorders of mineral metabolism*, 5th ed. Washington, DC: American Society for Bone and Mineral Research; 2003:307–313 with permission of the American Society for Bone and Mineral Research.)

appropriate; and (vi) avoidance of uneven walking surfaces. In addition, patients should be advised against smoking and excessive alcohol use, because both these have been shown to have detrimental effects on bone metabolism.

Nutritional counseling plays a central role in the treatment of osteoporosis. Most adult Americans do not consume the currently recommended daily allowances of calcium and vitamin D. It is estimated that <1 in 100 women over the age of 70 and <25% of men in any age-group meet the daily dietary calcium requirements. The numbers are similar for vitamin D consumption. In the clinic, we encounter a large number of patients with superimposed osteomalacia due to vitamin D deficiency and consequent bone mineralization defects. The treatment of vitamin D deficiency will be discussed in more detail in the subsequent text, but, in general, the goal is to maintain a 25(OH) vitamin D concentration of 30 ng per mL or greater. The recommended daily intake of calcium and vitamin D in adults varies greatly worldwide. It is the current consensus that all patients with a diagnosis of osteoporosis should be advised to take 1,500 mg of calcium and 800 to 1,000 IU of vitamin D daily. These daily requirements should be met by a combination of foods high in these nutrients and dietary supplements. In general, calcium is poorly absorbed in the gut. It is therefore important to recognize that not all dietary supplements have been tested for absorption efficiency. Calcium carbonate, the most commonly used supplement, is best absorbed with food. Because the calcium-absorbing capacity of the gastrointestinal tract is limited, not more than 500 mg of calcium should be ingested at one time. It is best to spread calcium and vitamin D supplementation throughout the day. Studies of calcium and vitamin D supplementation have shown a reduction of fractures at all sites, including the hip (Evidence Level A).[1,2] In addition, other minerals are known to have both direct and indirect effects on bone. Magnesium deficiency is also a common problem in the US population. Magnesium is important in the regulation of PTH secretion, and, therefore, a goal of the treatment should be to maintain normal magnesium levels.

Finally, pharmacologic therapy remains the mainstay of therapy for osteoporosis. There are several general classes of medications available for both osteoporosis prevention and treatment. These include hormone therapy (HT); selective estrogen receptor modulators (SERMs); calcitonin; bisphosphonates, and recombinant human PTH (hPTH).

HT: This has been shown to be efficacious in trials of both osteoporosis prevention and treatment, with measured increases in BMD at the spine, hip, and forearm (Evidence Level A). Analysis of these trials by estrogen dose have shown persistent increases in BMD with the use of low-dose estrogen (equivalent to Premarin 0.3 mg), albeit more modest than those observed with high-dose therapy.[3] The results of the Women's Health Initiative showed a 23% reduction in all fractures and a 34% reduction in hip and vertebral fractures after an average of 5.2 years of HT.[4] Therefore, HT is currently recommended for osteoporosis prevention in high-risk women who have no known contraindications to HT use. However, given the increasing number of alternative therapies for osteoporosis and the potential side effects of long-term HT, the use of these agents should be approached cautiously with a plan for only short-term use in postmenopausal women.

SERMs: These compounds bind with high affinity to the estrogen receptor and may act as an estrogen agonist or antagonist, depending on the specific type of estrogen-responsive tissue. Tamoxifen has been used for many years for the treatment of estrogen receptor–positive breast cancer. In trials of breast cancer treatment and prevention, tamoxifen was shown to act as an estrogen agonist at the level of the bone, with observed increases in bone density. Raloxifene, as tamoxifen, has been shown to act as an estrogen agonist in bone. Raloxifene has been approved for the treatment and prevention of postmenopausal osteoporosis. The currently approved daily dose of 60 mg has been shown to increase BMD at the spine, hip, and the total body after 2 years of treatment (Evidence Level A).[5] There is also an associated decrease in bone-turnover markers, with restoration to premenopausal levels. Most importantly, in the Multiple Outcomes of Raloxifene Evaluation (MORE) trial, a large placebo-controlled trial including 7,705 postmenopausal women, raloxifene was shown to decrease clinical vertebral fractures by 62% after

1 year of treatment.[6] On the other hand, there was no significant decrease in the rate of nonvertebral fractures after the original 36-month study or after the 1-year extension. The safety profile of raloxifene is quite favorable. However, in the MORE trial, there was an increased risk of thromboembolic disease similar to that observed with HT. On the other hand, given the low incidence of this complication, the attributable risk is still very low.

Calcitonin: This acts as a hypocalcemic factor by its inhibitory effect on osteoclast resorption. This 32-amino acid peptide is secreted by the C cells of the thyroid, but its exact physiologic role in calcium homeostasis is still unknown. Salmon calcitonin is available in a parenteral and a nasal spray formulation for the treatment of women with osteoporosis for more than 5 years postmenopause. While only very modest increases in BMD of 1% to 2% at the lumbar spine have been shown with the use of nasal calcitonin in postmenopausal women, the Prevent Recurrence of Osteoporotic Fractures trial in women with osteopenia ($T < -2.0$) of the spine showed a 33% reduction in vertebral risk when compared to placebo (Evidence Level B).[7] This effect was only observed with a dose of 200 IU a day but not with the doses of 100 or 400 IU. No increase in BMD or decrease in fracture of the hip or other sites has been demonstrated with the use of any calcitonin preparation. Calcitonin is probably unique among osteoporosis treatments in that it has an analgesic effect on bone pain after an acute vertebral fracture, and it is therefore used at times for this indication. The most common side effect with the use of nasal calcitonin is a higher incidence of rhinitis and/or epistaxis. Injectable calcitonin may cause flushing, nausea, and vomiting. In clinical practice, the use of calcitonin has been reserved for the treatment of patients with acute bone pain or those who are intolerant to other approved osteoporosis therapies.

Bisphosphonates: These compounds bind with high affinity to hydroxyapatite crystals in the bone surfaces, particularly of active bones. They lead to osteoclastic apoptosis and, thereby, to a decrease in bone resorption, with a subsequent increase in BMD. Two bisphosphonates—alendronate and risedronate—are approved in the United States for the treatment and prevention of osteoporosis. These are both nitrogen-containing compounds and are available in daily and weekly formulations. The bioavailability of all oral bisphosphonates is poor, and they should therefore be taken on an empty stomach with a large glass of water, and the patient should wait at least 30 minutes before eating.

Alendronate was the first bisphosphonate approved in the United States for the treatment of osteoporosis. It is approved for the prevention and treatment of postmenopausal osteoporosis (Evidence Level A) and also for the treatment of glucocorticoid-induced osteoporosis and for the treatment of osteoporosis in men. BMD has been shown to increase by 9% in the lumbar spine and by 6% in the hip after 3 years of treatment with alendronate.[8] BMD continues to increase after 10 years of therapy, albeit at a slower rate.[9] In addition, BMD gains are maintained for at least 2 years after the cessation of therapy. There is a concomitant decrease in bone-turnover markers of 50% to 70%. These BMD increases translate to a 55% reduction in vertebral fractures and a 51% reduction in hip fractures.[10] Furthermore, in recently menopausal women, a 5-mg daily dose of alendronate was shown to prevent bone loss at the spine and hip over 5 years of treatment. Alendronate is formulated in a 5-mg daily or 35-mg weekly tablet for osteoporosis prevention and in a 10-mg daily or 70-mg weekly tablet for osteoporosis treatment.

Risedronate has been approved by the U.S. Food and Drug Administration (FDA) for the prevention and treatment of postmenopausal osteoporosis and for the prevention and treatment of glucocorticoid-induced osteoporosis (Evidence Level A). This agent increases BMD at the spine by 5% and in the hip by 3% within 3 years. This is associated with decreases of 40% to 60% in bone-turnover markers. Risedronate has been shown to decrease vertebral fractures by 41% and nonvertebral fractures by 39% compared to placebo during 3 years of treatment.[11] In the Hip Intervention Program, which enrolled almost 9,500 women, there was a significant 30% decrease in overall hip fracture risk after 3 years of therapy.[12] Interestingly, in a subset of elderly women who were enrolled on the basis of clinical risk factors but not low BMD, there was no observed decrease in hip fracture risk, thereby emphasizing the importance of a comprehensive approach to fracture prevention. Risedronate has also been shown to either maintain or increase BMD at the lumbar spine, femoral neck, trochanter, and distal radius in men and women on glucocorticoid therapy.[13] Furthermore, after 1 year of therapy with risedronate in these patients, there was a significant 70% reduction in vertebral fracture compared to the placebo-treated group. Risedronate is available in a 5-mg daily and 35-mg weekly tablet for both osteoporosis treatment and prevention.

Ibandronate was recently approved for the treatment and prevention of osteoporosis in postmenopausal women. Studies comparing ibandronate 2.5 mg daily to placebo over a 3-year period demonstrated significant increases in BMD at the lumbar spine and hip in the treatment group compared to the placebo arm. In addition, there was a relative risk reduction of 52% in the incidence of vertebral fractures when compared to placebo. There was no difference noted in the number of nonvertebral fractures among the two groups. Ibandronate is available as a 150-mg tablet once monthly preparation or a 3-mg injection to be given intravenously over 15 to 30 seconds every 3 months. This is the first injectable bisphosphonate approved for the treatment of osteoporosis.

Although combination therapy with two antiresorptive agents has been shown to lead to greater increases in BMD, there have been no studies to demonstrate a greater fracture reduction. As a result, the simultaneous use of two antiresorptive agents is generally not recommended.

The safety profile with all bisphosphonates is quite favorable. With daily alendronate therapy, there appears to be an increased incidence of upper gastrointestinal side effects including heartburn and dysphagia; however, this increased incidence has not been observed with weekly dosing. There have also been concerns that potent bisphosphonates such as alendronate and risedronate may lead to adynamic bone disease (ABD) or "frozen" bone after years of therapy. Long-term biopsy data have not shown this to be the case.

Teriparatide: This is the only anabolic agent currently approved for the treatment of osteoporosis in men and women as well as for glucocorticoid-induced osteoporosis (Evidence Level A). The approved dose of teriparatide is 20 μg subcutaneously once daily for 2 years. This agent is composed of the amino terminal portion of the hPTH molecule (1 to 34). This fragment of the intact molecule binds to the PTH1 receptor and, when given as intermittent daily injections, results in the recruitment of quiescent bone-forming osteoblast cells. In addition, it also prevents the apoptosis of osteoblast cells, prolonging their bone-forming potential. These combined effects of teriparatide result in net bone formation. A study of 1,637 postmenopausal women receiving 20 μg or 40 μg teriparatide or placebo showed increases in BMD with teriparatide of 9% to 13% for the lumbar spine and 2% to 4% for the total hip after 21 months of treatment.[15] In contrast, BMD at the shaft of the radius declined by 2% to 3%, reaching statistical significance only for the higher dose tested (40 μg). The risk of vertebral fracture for both teriparatide groups was decreased by 65% to 69% and that of nonvertebral fractures was decreased by 35% to 40%. Studies of teriparatide in men with idiopathic osteoporosis or in men and women with glucocorticoid-induced osteoporosis have shown a similar response to therapy.

Whether teriparatide should be used concomitant to an antiresorptive drug is an area of much controversy and is being further explored by ongoing studies. A study on the effects of teriparatide alone or in combination with alendronate in men with osteoporosis showed that increases in BMD at the lumbar spine and the femoral neck were greatest for men treated with teriparatide alone when compared to alendronate alone or the combination of alendronate and teriparatide.[16] The diminished effect on bone density acquisition observed with combination therapy may be the result of blunting of teriparatide-induced bone formation by a potent antiresorptive. In contrast, postmenopausal women treated with combination estrogen and teriparatide had increases in BMD similar to those observed with teriparatide alone. Therefore, whether concomitant treatment with teriparatide and a weaker antiresorptive agent is of clinical benefit remains unknown. There are, however, substantial data to suggest a rapid decline in BMD after stopping teriparatide use, which can be abrogated by follow-up treatment with an antiresorptive agent.[17]

At the lower approved dose of teriparatide, there appear to be few clinically significant side effects. A transient mild hypercalcemia and a rise in uric acid levels were noted during the study of postmenopausal women. Neither change in chemistries had any apparent clinical sequelae. There is also a reported higher incidence of dizziness and leg cramps with the use of teriparatide when compared to placebo. In addition, initial clinical studies of teriparatide were terminated early owing to results in Fisher rat studies showing a higher incidence of osteosarcoma with high-dose drug administration to growing rats. In over 2,000 study patients treated with teriparatide, there have been no reported cases of osteosarcoma. Nonetheless, the use of this agent is limited by the FDA to not more than 2 years, and it is not approved for use in children or adolescents or in patients with Paget disease of the bone, hyperparathyroidism, or a history of cancer.

OSTEOMALACIA

Osteomalacia is characterized by a failure of mineralization of newly formed osteoids at the sites of bone turnover. A similar problem of mineralization in growing children has been termed rickets, in which there is poor mineralization of new bone at the growth plates. While both rickets and osteomalacia were recognized as common problems in northern Europe and North America, vitamin D supplementation and the fortification of foods such as milk appeared to lead to a substantial decrease in the incidence of these conditions. Nonetheless, recent studies have shown that nutritional and drug-induced rickets/osteomalacia continue to be a significant problem worldwide. In this chapter, we will focus on the adult version of this disease, which affects a great number of the elderly population.

Nutritional osteomalacia may be caused by deficiencies of vitamin D, calcium, or phosphorus. Most natural foods contain only a very small amount of vitamin D. Most of the vitamin D requirements in humans is fulfilled by the conversion of 7-dehydrocholesterol in the skin to 25(OH) vitamin D by the action of ultraviolet-B irradiation (see Fig. 23.2). Therefore, people living in northern latitudes, those wearing sunscreen or extensive clothing, darkly pigmented individuals, or institutionalized people are at a high risk of developing vitamin D deficiency. In addition, the elderly have poor vitamin D formation in the skin, likely as a result of diminishing substrate. These populations are therefore dependent on vitamin D supplementation. Despite guidelines on adequate vitamin D intake, most adults in the United States and around the world do not consume the recommended daily amounts. The dietary reference intake for vitamin D published by the National Academy of Sciences for healthy, nondeficient individuals is 5 μg of cholecalciferol a day (1 μg cholecalciferol = 40 IU vitamin D) for men and women 50 years of age or younger; 10 μg cholecalciferol for those aged 51 to 70; and 15 μg for those aged 70 or above.

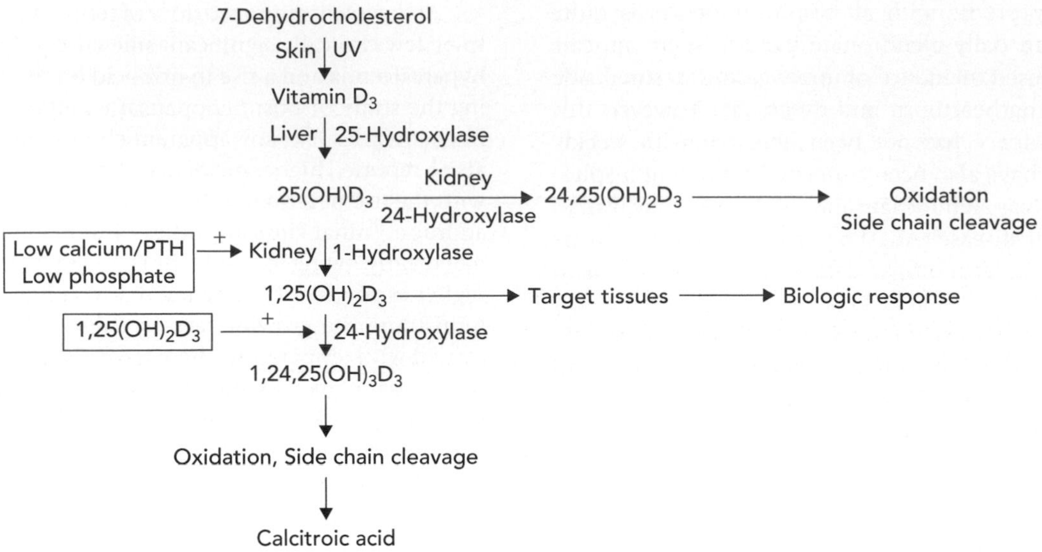

Figure 23.2 Vitamin D metabolism.

Vitamin D, in its active form ($1,25(OH)_2D_3$), is crucial for normal calcium and phosphorus absorption from the gastrointestinal tract. Inadequate vitamin D concentration leads to a decrease in serum calcium levels and a resultant increase in parathyroid secretion. This secondary hyperparathyroidism acts to increase calcium and phosphorus mobilization from bone through osteoclast activation and bone resorption. In addition, PTH acts in the kidney to increase calcium retention and increase phosphorus excretion. The decrease in phosphorus absorption from the gut in addition to the increase in renal phosphorus excretion leads to low serum phosphorus levels. While low vitamin D levels probably have a direct effect on bone, most osseous consequences of vitamin D deficiency are probably mediated through the low calcium and phosphorus levels and the effects of PTH on bone.

Similarly, most adults do not consume the recommended amounts of calcium—1,200 mg daily for adult men and women over the age of 50. It is estimated that 55% of men and 78% of women over the age of 20 do not meet their dietary calcium needs. This, in turn, leads to a picture very similar to that observed in vitamin D deficiency. Poor calcium intake leads to secondary hyperparathyroidism with a resultant increase in renal calcium absorption and bone calcium mobilization, keeping serum calcium levels in the normal range. Nutritional phosphate deficiency is rare because phosphorus is ubiquitous in food. Furthermore, there is rapid renal adaptation with nearly 100% reabsorption of filtered phosphate. Phosphate depletion may be more common in cases of severe oral restriction in association with chronic diarrhea, causing a marked negative phosphate balance. Clinically, low phosphate levels are more likely due to vitamin D deficiency as a result of the mechanisms outlined in the preceding text.

Drug-induced osteomalacia: Drugs that induce the hepatic cytochrome P-450 enzymes may lead to an increase in the metabolism of vitamin D with a resultant vitamin D deficiency and osteomalacia. This presentation is best characterized in patients using anticonvulsants such as phenytoin, carbamazepine, and phenobarbitone. In addition, phenytoin has been shown to have direct deleterious effects on calcium metabolism by decreasing calcium absorption in the gut and direct effects in bone by increasing bone resorption. Therefore, clinically apparent vitamin D deficiency presenting as fractures is common in patients treated long-term with anticonvulsants, particularly those who are institutionalized and may have low sun exposure.

Cholestyramine is an anion exchange resin used to bind bile salts in the gut. It may interfere with the vitamin D absorption in the gut, leading to osteomalacia. Similarly, aluminum- and magnesium-containing antacids bind phosphate in the gut, leading to hypophosphatemia with characteristic muscle weakness and osteomalacia after prolonged use.

Heavy metals such as cadmium and drugs such as ifosfamide and saccharated ferric oxide interfere with renal phosphate reabsorption. Cadmium exposure has been shown to lead to permanent renal glomerular and tubular damage with subsequent phosphaturia, proteinuria, and renal failure. Cadmium may also have direct effects on the osteoclast and osteoblast, worsening the hypophosphatemia-induced osteomalacia. This syndrome was first described in Japan and was named *Itai-Itai* disease. Ifosfamide, a chemotherapeutic agent, can produce a renal Fanconi syndrome and hypophosphatemic osteomalacia. Prolonged use of intravenous ferric oxide for the treatment of anemia can lead to reversible proximal tubular damage with associated phosphate wasting and inadequate $1,25(OH)_2D$ levels owing to impaired 1α-hydroxylation.

Several agents are known to cause direct mineralization defects, leading to osteomalacia. These include aluminum, fluoride, and etidronate therapies. Aluminum-induced osteomalacia is most commonly seen in patients treated with parenteral nutrition, hemodialysis patients, or patients with renal failure on chronic aluminum-containing phosphate binders. Aluminum inhibits PTH release and directly inhibits 1α-hydroxylation of 25(OH)D in the kidney. Furthermore, aluminum leads to decreased osteoblast function with decreased bone formation as well as decreased mineralization of osteoid. The prevalence of aluminum toxicity has significantly declined as a result of decreased contamination by aluminum of hemodialysis baths and by the removal of casein hydrolysates as the protein source in parenteral nutrition. Furthermore, the increasing use of calcium-based phosphate binders in renal failure has significantly decreased the use of aluminum-containing products in these patients.

Fluoride was commonly used for the treatment of low BMD. It binds to newly formed hydroxyapatite crystals, preventing its resorption; however, it also prevents the mineralization of newly formed osteoids. Fluoride use is radiographically associated with increased bone density. In contrast, bone quality and strength are poor, with a resultant increase in fracture risk. Endemic fluorosis due to chronic ingestion of water with high fluoride contents has been observed in countries of sub-Saharan Africa. Affected individuals usually present with progressive bony pain, stiffness, and vertebral deformities. This toxicity is characterized by radiographically apparent osteosclerosis and diffuse osteophyte formation, particularly of the spine.

Etidronate, one of the first bisphosphonates approved for clinical use, was found to lead to impaired mineralization when used in high doses, leading to a syndrome of "frozen" bone. Etidronate is now rarely used in the clinic; however, lower doses of the medication, when given in a cyclic manner, appear to be safe. The newer bisphosphonates have not been shown to lead to mineralization defects even after prolonged use.

Specific disorders: Intestinal malabsorption of vitamin D is becoming increasingly recognized as a common cause of osteomalacia. Studies have shown that approximately 30% of patients with gastrectomy have associated vitamin D deficiency. Those whose status is post-Billroth II procedure with the exclusion of the duodenum appear to be at highest risk. Recently, gastric bypass has also been shown to be a risk factor for vitamin D deficiency. In addition, many patients with celiac sprue, cystic fibrosis, or infiltrative diseases of the gastrointestinal tract, such as amyloidosis or lymphoma, will also present with evidence of malabsorption. Hepatic disease is another common cause of vitamin D deficiency due to impaired 25-hydroxylation of vitamin D in the liver.

Renal phosphate wasting due to genetic mutation, such as that seen in X-linked hypophosphatemic rickets and autosomal dominant hypophosphatemic rickets, leads to hypophosphatemia and osteomalacia. A rare disorder of tumor-induced osteomalacia presents with phosphate wasting similar to that observed with the inherited syndromes. In addition, Fanconi syndrome, with its associated defect in proximal tubular renal reabsorption, leads to hypophosphatemia in association with renal bicarbonate loss, type II renal tubular acidosis, glucosuria, hypouricemia, and aminoaciduria. In adults, the most common etiology of Fanconi syndrome is multiple myeloma.

Hypophosphatasia, a rare autosomal disorder characterized by low alkaline phosphatase levels in the urine and blood, can present in a severe form in childhood or in a milder form in the adult. Patients usually present with osteomalacia and fractures and severe periodontal disease.

Finally, one of the increasingly recognized forms of osteomalacia is that seen in patients with chronic renal failure, particularly those on long-term hemodialysis. This topic will be reviewed in full later in this chapter.

Workup/Keys to Diagnosis

The clinical presentation in osteomalacia is quite varied. Many patients will be asymptomatic; they are recognized by evidence of low BMD in plain radiographs or DXA scan. Others may present with characteristic symptoms of muscle weakness, bone pain, and tenderness or low-trauma fractures. The observed muscle weakness is probably the result of a combination of hypophosphatemia, low vitamin D levels, and increased PTH. It is characteristically proximal in nature and can be associated with muscle wasting and hypotonia. It often results in gait instability, with a higher risk for falls. Bone pain is usually constant and gnawing in nature and most pronounced in the lower back, pelvis, and lower extremities. Pretibial tenderness is also characteristic of this condition, as may be tenderness to palpation of other bony areas. Low fragility fractures are common and may involve the ribs, vertebrae, and long bones. Frank skeletal deformities such as abnormalities in spine curvature or bowing deformities of the lower extremities are rare in individuals presenting as adults.

The gold standard for the diagnosis of osteomalacia is bone biopsy after tetracycline labeling. Tetracyclines are fluorescent and are readily deposited in the newly formed bone at the mineralization front. Two different tetracycline derivatives with different fluorescence when viewed under the microscope are given at set intervals. The growth rate of the skeleton can then be estimated in iliac crest biopsy by measuring the distance between the tetracycline bands. Osteomalacia is characterized by (i) a reduced distance between the bands and (ii) increased osteoid volume ($>$10%) with a widened osteoid seam ($>$15 μm). Nevertheless, given the invasiveness of the procedure, it is rarely used in clinical practice, and the diagnosis of osteomalacia is made by noninvasive means.

Patients with osteomalacia will often present with one or more of the following laboratory abnormalities: Increased alkaline phosphatase, low plasma calcium, low phosphorus, low calcidiol (25(OH)D), increased PTH levels, and low urinary calcium excretion. Therefore, the laboratory evaluation of a patient with suspected osteomalacia should include measurement of calcium, phosphorus, calcidiol, PTH and alkaline phosphatase concentration, and a 24-hour urine for calcium excretion. In patients with evidence of renal insufficiency, a $1,25(OH)_2D$ level should also be obtained.

The laboratory findings will vary depending on the etiology of the osteomalacia. For vitamin D deficiency, patients will usually have hypophosphatemia with or without hypocalcemia, an elevated alkaline phosphatase level, low calcidiol level, and an increased PTH, suggestive of secondary hyperparathyroidism. In patients with low phosphorus level but no other evidence of vitamin D insufficiency, a 24-hour urine for fractional excretion of phosphate should be obtained. This should be <5% in the setting of hypophosphatemia. If elevated, the causes of renal phosphate wasting should be entertained. Isolated calcium malabsorption may present with low or normal calcium levels, increased PTH levels, elevated alkaline phosphatase, and low 24-hour urine calcium excretion. In rare cases of hypophosphatasia, the alkaline phosphatase will be decreased with normal plasma concentrations of calcium and phosphorus.

The most common finding in plain radiographs is that of low bone density with apparent thinning of the cortex. More specific findings of osteomalacia include Looser zones and changes in vertebral bodies. Looser zones are characterized by pseudofractures, fissures, or radiolucent lines approximately 2 to 5 mm in width with sclerotic borders. They usually lie perpendicular to the cortex and are typically bilateral. Most commonly, they are found in the lower extremities in the femoral neck or femoral shaft or immediately underneath the pubic and ischial rami. The term '*Milkman syndrome*' has been used to describe evidence of bilateral, symmetrical, and multiple pseudofractures in patients with osteomalacia. Vertebral bodies may be noted to have a very thin cortex with a concave deformity also known as *codfish vertebrae*.

A bone scan may identify hot spots at the site of Looser zones or may appear as diffuse uptake in long bones. Low bone density may also be detected by DXA scan, and by this modality it is indistinguishable from osteoporosis. Laboratory evaluation is therefore necessary to distinguish osteomalacia from osteoporosis.

Management

The treatment of osteomalacia should be targeted at the underlying cause of the disease. Patients with vitamin D deficiency should be treated with ergocalciferol (vitamin D_2) 50,000 units once or twice weekly until the vitamin D concentration returns to normal. The normal range for vitamin D is quite broad, but studies have shown that a 25(OH)D concentration of 30 ng per mL or higher is necessary for skeletal health (Evidence Level B). As the concentration of 25(OH)D drops below 30 ng per mL, there is a compensatory increase in PTH secretion, suggestive of inadequate vitamin D substrate to keep normal calcium and phosphorus homeostasis. When the goal of 30 ng per mL or higher has been reached, the patients should continue to be treated with 800 to 1,000 units of vitamin D daily. Patients with intestinal malabsorption may require higher doses to maintain normal levels, sometimes as high as 10,000 to 50,000 units a day.

Once vitamin D deficiency has been corrected, assessment for concomitant or primary calcium malabsorption should be pursued. These patients are treated with increasing daily supplementation of calcium. It is important to recognize that calcium is, in general, poorly absorbed and that not all calcium supplements have been tested for absorption. Patients are usually treated with calcium carbonate or calcium citrate. In patients with underlying achlorhydria either from chronic use of H_2 blockers or secondary to gastrectomy, vagal surgery, or autoimmune disease, calcium malabsorption may be of particular concern. Acidity in the gut is required for dissolution of calcium from supplements and food. Therefore, in patients with low acid levels in the gut, the use of calcium citrate, with a higher dissolution, may be indicated. All patients with osteomalacia should have a daily intake of at least 1,500 mg of calcium in order to promote normal bone mineralization. Despite this level of supplementation, many patients continue to have uncorrected secondary hyperparathyroidism and low 24-hour urine calcium excretion, suggestive of abnormal calcium homeostasis. In these patients, calcium intake should be increased until these abnormalities are corrected.

Patients with advanced liver disease and impaired 25-hydroxylation of vitamin D and those with impaired 1α-hydroxylation in the kidney are commonly treated with the active form of the vitamin. Calcitriol (1,25-dihydroxycholecalciferol) is available in 0.25 and 0.5 μg tablets with relatively good absorption and rapid onset of action. The goals of treatment in liver disease include normalization of $1,25(OH)_2D_3$ levels, correction of secondary hyperparathyroidism, and maintenance of normal serum calcium and phosphorus levels. Twenty-four-hour urine calcium excretion and kidney function should be monitored in order to avoid hypercalciuria. Most patients with liver disease will require 0.25 to 1.0 μg of calcitriol daily. The treatment goals in patients with chronic renal insufficiency and abnormal vitamin D metabolism will be discussed later in this chapter.

Hereditary and acquired hypophosphatemic disorders are generally treated with a combination of phosphate and calcitriol supplementation. Treatment goals differ for adults and children. In children, the aim is to provide enough phosphorus and calcium to promote normal bone mineralization and growth. In general, adults are only treated if symptomatic because of the high incidence of renal insufficiency in patients after long-term therapy.

PRIMARY HYPERPARATHYROIDISM

Primary hyperparathyroidism (PHPT) is a common endocrine disorder characterized by inappropriate secretion of PTH by one or more parathyroid glands. This leads to increased renal calcium absorption and phosphorus excretion; increased bone resorption of mineralized matrix with excretion into the serum of calcium and phosphorus; and increased $1,25(OH)_2D_3$ synthesis with resultant increased gut calcium and, to a lesser extent, phosphorus absorption. The net effects of hyperparathyroidism are hypercalcemia and hypophosphatemia. The incidence and prevalence of this disorder are much higher than previously recognized. PHPT is more common in women than in men, and its incidence increases with aging in both sexes with a peak in the sixth decade.

PHPT is most commonly the result of clonal expansion of parathyroid cells to form a single adenoma in over 85% of cases. However, polyclonal parathyroid cell proliferation leads to multiple gland hyperplasia, usually in the setting of inherited PHPT. The defect in PHPT arises not only from an increase in the mass of abnormal parathyroid cells but also from abnormalities in calcium sensing at the level of the parathyroid. Normally, serum calcium levels are tightly regulated by the calcium-sensing receptor (CaSR) in the parathyroid gland that controls PTH release. However, in PHPT the sensing of extracellular calcium concentration is reset, leading to abnormal PTH secretion in the setting of high calcium. The abnormality in calcium homeostasis appears to be related to a decrease in the number of otherwise normal CaSR in the parathyroid gland.

Although uncommon, PHPT can be a manifestation of several inherited syndromes. Multiple endocrine neoplasia type 1 (MEN 1), resulting from a mutation of the *Menin* gene, is characterized by tumors of the parathyroid and anterior pituitary glands and pancreatic islet cells. Ninety-five percent of patients will develop PHPT usually in the second and third decades of life. Management includes resection of $3^1/_2$ of the parathyroid glands with or without autotransplantation of the remaining tissue to the forearm or sternocleidomastoid muscle. MEN 2A is characterized by mutations of the *RET* protooncogene and the familial clustering of medullary thyroid carcinoma, pheochromocytoma, and hyperparathyroidism. However, the incidence of PHPT is only 5% to 20% in contrast with the high incidence observed in MEN 1. The operative management of hyperparathyroidism in MEN 2A is similar to that of MEN 1. Other rare causes of PHPT include hereditary-isolated PHPT, which is characterized by multiple and sometimes malignant parathyroid tumors, and the hyperparathyroidism-jaw tumor syndrome associated with fibrous jaw tumors.

The skeletal involvement in PHPT was first described, in its most severe form, by von Recklinghausen in 1891 and was named *osteitis fibrosa cystica*. The bone changes in PHPT are characterized by increased bone turnover. Endosteal bone resorption leads to an approximately 30% increase in cortical bone porosity and thinning of the cortical bone. On the other hand, trabecular bone density appears to remain unchanged or even improved. However, in severe disease, the cortical bone changes may outweigh any positive changes in trabecular bone, thereby leading to an overall increase in bone fragility and increased fracture risk.

PHPT is also characterized by abnormalities in the kidney, which are predominantly related to renal calcium handling. Receptors to PTH are widespread throughout the renal tubule. In addition, serum calcium affects renal calcium handling through the CaSR. While PTH binding to its receptor leads to increased calcium absorption and increased phosphate excretion, CaSR activation increases renal calcium excretion. Furthermore, calcium handling is regulated by the expression of renal 25-hydroxyvitamin D 1α-hydroxylase, which is stimulated by PTH and is responsible for metabolizing 25-hydroxyvitamin D to $1,25(OH)_2D_3$, the active form of vitamin D. Approximately 97% of calcium filtered in the kidney is reabsorbed. At normal calcium intake, the 24-hour urine excretion is <250 mg in women and 300 mg in men. In PHPT, hypercalciuria is common. In mild forms, the increased calcium renal excretion is, in great part, due to calcium hyperabsorption in the gut mediated by the inappropriately high $1,25(OH)_2D_3$ levels. However, as PHPT becomes more severe, skeletal calcium loss through PTH action contributes to the observed hypercalciuria. In addition, PTH decreases the proximal tubular reabsorption of bicarbonate, leading to mild hyperchloremic acidosis and urine alkalinization. Increased urinary calcium concentration and alkaline urine predisposes patients to nephrolithiasis consisting primarily of calcium-phosphate stones. The incidence of nephrolithiasis in PHPT ranges from 10% to 50%, depending on the clinical setting. In contrast, nephrocalcinosis, which refers to the radiographic appearance of pinpoint diffuse calcification in the renal pyramids, is a rare complication. Glomerular filtration rate (GFR) may be reduced over time and it may be a result of nephrolithiasis, nephrocalcinosis, or severe hypercalcemia. While nephrolithiasis is reversible with parathyroidectomy, chronic decreases in GFR and nephrocalcinosis tend to be irreversible.

Workup/Key to Diagnosis

The frequent use of automated serum-screening chemistry panels has led to an increasing number of patients being diagnosed with PHPT while still asymptomatic. The classic associated kidney and bone morbidities are therefore identified less often at the time of presentation. Classical PHPT is characterized by bone disease; renal disease; neuropsychiatric symptoms including poor concentration, depression, apathy, and psychosis; conjunctival calcifications; band keratopathy; hypertension; and gastrointestinal symptoms such as anorexia, nausea, abdominal pain, and constipation; and neuromuscular weakness. Patients may present with any combination of these symptoms.

The laboratory assessment of patients with suspected PHPT includes measurement of serum calcium, phosphorus, creatinine, alkaline phosphatase, 25(OH)D, and PTH. Twenty-four-hour urine should also be obtained for the measurement of creatinine clearance and calcium excretion. Elevations of calcium, PTH, and alkaline phosphatase (because of high bone turnover) with a parallel decrease in phosphate levels are typical. In patients with more severe hypercalciuria, an increase in serum creatinine may also occur. Determinations of $1,25(OH)_2D_3$ are not usually helpful because these levels may be low, normal, or high, depending on the amount of available substrate (25(OH)D), duration of illness, and underlying renal function. On the other hand, the measurement of 25(OH)D concentration is recommended because many of these patients become vitamin D deplete owing to the prolonged stimulus of 1α-hydroxylation. Vitamin D deficiency should be corrected because this may contribute to the bone loss observed in PHPT.

Radiographs of the abdomen may be obtained to assess for evidence of calcium-containing stones. Although bone radiographs are not routinely obtained for diagnosis, observed bone changes may include generalized osteopenia; subperiosteal bone resorption particularly in the phalanges; bone cysts predominantly in the shafts of the metacarpals, ribs, or pelvis; "brown tumors" composed of multiple multinucleated osteoclasts; or pathologic fractures. Nonetheless, most patients with PHPT will have normal-appearing plain radiographs.

All patients should have a DXA scan to look for evidence of osteoporosis. This study should include the forearm, which has a high proportion of cortical bone, as well as the lumbar spine and the hip. Some patients may present with generalized osteopenia or osteoporosis, while others may manifest a disproportionate loss of bone in the forearm when compared to other sites with a higher proportion of trabecular bone.

Management

The mainstay of treatment for PHPT is surgical resection of an adenoma or hyperplastic glands. The indications for surgery in asymptomatic individuals include (i) serum calcium 1.0 mg per dL above the upper limit of normal; (ii) 24-hour urine calcium >400 mg per 24 hour; (iii) reduction of creatinine clearance by 30%; (iv) T-score < -2.5 at any site (spine, hip, or forearm) as assessed by BMD; (v) <50 years of age; or (vi) patients for whom medical surveillance would not be possible (Evidence Level C). Patients who are not deemed surgical candidates should be followed closely and should have serum calcium measured biannually; serum creatinine measured annually; and BMD at the spine, hip, and forearm measured annually.

Parathyroid surgery should be performed only by surgeons with extensive experience in the operation. The traditional surgical approach requires a full neck exploration and identification of the four parathyroid glands. Approximately 15% to 20% of patients with nonfamilial PHPT will have more than one enlarged parathyroid gland. Preoperative localization is not usually necessary. On the other hand, minimally invasive parathyroid surgery using local anesthesia requires preoperative localization using technetium-99-labeled sestamibi-single photon emission computed tomography (SPECT) imaging. In addition, intraoperative PTH levels are obtained to ascertain the removal of the source of excess PTH. A PTH level is drawn immediately prior to the parathyroidectomy and then a few minutes after. The PTH level should drop by >50%. If the PTH level does not decrease as expected, then full neck exploration should be done to identify other overactive glands.

Apart from SPECT imaging, other noninvasive imaging studies such as magnetic resonance imaging (MRI), computed tomography scan, and ultrasonography might be helpful in the localization of enlarged parathyroid tissue. These may be particularly useful in patients who have had failed exploratory neck surgery. However, the diagnosis of PHPT needs to be confirmed by a standard workup because none of these radiologic studies should be used to make the diagnosis of PHPT.

For those patients in need of treatment but who are not considered surgical candidates owing to substantial comorbidities, or for those who do not opt to proceed with definitive surgery, there are no medical therapies that are considered, at this time, to have proved efficacy and safety. While estrogen, raloxifene, bisphosphonates, and calcimimetics have been proposed as possible therapies, their long-term effect on hyperparathyroidism-associated comorbidities has not been described.

HT has been shown to increase BMD at the lumbar spine and the femoral neck in postmenopausal women with mild PHPT without significant changes in calcium and PTH levels (Evidence Level B).[18] Other studies using higher doses of estrogen have documented decreases in both the serum calcium and hypercalciuria. This therapy is obviously limited to women with no contraindications to HT. However, the recent data on the long-term effects of HT make this a less desirable therapy for long-term treatment of PHPT. A recent study using the oral bisphosphonate alendronate demonstrated increases in the femoral neck and lumbar spine BMD at 48 weeks, which was associated with a decrease in serum calcium, alkaline phosphatase, and bone-turnover markers when compared to placebo (Evidence Level B).[19] A compensatory rise in PTH may occur after prolonged treatment of PHPT with bisphosphonates, which may in turn limit their use. Newer compounds called *calcimimetics* that activate the CaSR, thereby mimicking the effect of extracellular calcium, have shown promise in the treatment of PHPT. In postmenopausal women with PHPT, a single dose of the calcimimetic R-568 resulted in a decrease in PTH and calcium levels.[20] More recently, a 52-week study with the oral calcimimetic cinacalcet hydrochloride showed a reduction in PTH levels and normalization of calcium levels in 73% of patients treated with this drug.[21] Calcimimetics are currently approved for the treatment of parathyroid carcinoma and secondary hyperparathyroidism in chronic kidney disease. Lastly, dietary calcium restriction could lead to increased PTH secretion, thereby enhancing the pathophysiologic process in PHPT. The current recommendation is for adherence to optimal dietary calcium consumption of 1,000 to 1,200 mg per day in adults.

RENAL OSTEODYSTROPHY

As the GFR falls below 60 mL per minute, phosphate is retained owing to a decrease in renal phosphate clearance. This, in turn, leads to a direct stimulation by phosphate for PTH secretion. There is a concomitant decrease in 1α-hydroxylation of 25(OH)D with declining renal function, which leads to a decrease in calcitriol levels. The end result is a decrease in renal phosphate reabsorption as a result of increasing PTH levels and stimulation of $1,25(OH)_2D_3$ formation by PTH helping to maintain normal calcium homeostasis. As GFR falls to 20 to 40 mL per minute, there is a further decrease in $1,25(OH)_2D_3$ levels, and calcium and phosphorus homeostasis cannot be maintained by adaptive mechanisms. The abnormal calcium and phosphorus levels, coupled with the continuing rise in PTH and decrease in calcitriol, contribute to abnormal bone turnover and mineralization defects. In addition, a skeletal resistance to PTH, believed to be at least partly due to a downregulation of the PTH receptor, contributes to the observed changes in bone. Similarly, metabolic acidosis, commonly seen in end-stage renal disease (ESRD), leads to further calcium release from bone as a result of the buffering of hydrogen ions by bone carbonate. Maintenance of normal bicarbonate levels in hemodialysis patients can decrease the rate of progression of uremic bone disease.

Changes in bone biopsy can be apparent when GFR falls below 60 mL per minute. There are four major types of bone disease observed in ESRD, which are collectively termed *renal osteodystrophy*. These include (i) osteitis fibrosa (predominantly hyperparathyroid bone disease); (ii) low turnover osteomalacia (abnormal mineralization with reduced osteoclast and osteoblast activity); (iii) mixed uremic osteodystrophy (hyperparathyroid bone disease with a superimposed mineralization defect); and (iv) ABD (diminished bone turnover).

Osteitis fibrosa is characterized by high bone turnover stimulated by high PTH levels due to secondary hyperparathyroidism. Tetracycline labeling in bone biopsy covers a great extent of the bone surface with no associated mineralization defect. The chronic high PTH concentration leads to marrow fibrosis, increased woven osteoid, increased osteoblast activation, and numerous osteoclast-covered resorptive surfaces. This type of bone disease accounts for approximately 40% of the cases of renal osteodystrophy.

Osteomalacia has become increasingly rare as a result of the decrease in the use of aluminum binders. Characteristically, this disease has markedly widened, unmineralized osteoid seams in bone biopsy. Other contributing factors include chronic acidosis and low $1,25(OH)_2D_3$ levels.

Mixed uremic osteodystrophy has many of the characteristic findings of hyperparathyroid bone disease in bone biopsy; there is, however, evidence of mineralization defects with increased mineralization lag time and absence of tetracycline labeling in some bone-forming surfaces.

ABD characterized by both decreased bone formation and resorption has become increasingly prevalent. It is estimated to be the underlying bone pathology in one third of patients with ESRD predialysis and has been reported in 25% to 60% of biopsy specimens from dialysis patients. It is associated with decreased PTH levels, likely a result of calcium exposure and use of calcitriol. This disorder may be more commonly seen in patients after long-term dialysis, in the elderly and in those on continuous peritoneal dialysis. There is also an association between diabetes and ABD. It is believed that chronic hypoinsulinemia and hyperglycemia may inhibit PTH release. Patients with ABD have an increased risk of fractures (particularly hip fractures), poor calcium control with a propensity for hypercalcemia as a result of decreased calcium deposition in bone, increased vascular calcification, and higher risk of calciphylaxis. In children, ABD is associated with decreased growth rates beyond that observed in other children with ESRD.

Both men and women on dialysis have an increased relative risk of hip fracture of 4.4 and increased mortality following a fracture, with a relative risk of 2.4, when compared to the general population. Patients with low serum intact PTH (iPTH) appear to be at the highest risk. In addition, men on chronic dialysis also have an increased vertebral fracture risk, which is threefold that of the general population. Similarly, men in the lowest tertile of PTH levels appear to be at the highest risk, with the lowest fracture prevalence observed in patients with PTH levels in the midtertile range.

Workup/Key to Diagnosis

The clinical manifestations of renal osteodystrophy are relatively nonspecific but may include muscle weakness, bone pain, skeletal deformities, and metastatic calcifications. Patients may present with a proximal myopathy characterized by proximal muscle weakness and pain. This may be associated with abnormal vitamin D metabolism, severe hyperparathyroidism, or aluminum toxicity. The bone pain of renal osteodystrophy may be diffuse, but when localized it is more likely to affect the lower back and lower extremities. Severe bone pain is characteristic of aluminum-induced bone disease. While skeletal deformities are prominent in children with ESRD, these are less common in adults with renal osteodystrophy. In patients with severe long-standing hyperparathyroidism, deformities of the ribs and pseudoclubbing may develop. Those with aluminum toxicity may develop scoliosis, particularly of the lumbar spine and kyphosis. Metastatic calcifications are most common in the periarticular area and in the vasculature and may be easily visualized in radiographs. In patients with extensive vascular calcification, ischemic necrosis of the skin, muscle, and subcutaneous tissue—a condition called *calciphylaxis*—may occur.

Measurement of serum calcium, phosphorus, calcium-phosphate product, bicarbonate, iPTH, and bone-specific alkaline phosphate (BSAP) are key to the management of renal osteodystrophy. Nevertheless, the underlying bone disease cannot be characterized with complete reliability by any of these measurements, and bone biopsy remains the gold standard for the diagnosis of renal osteodystrophy.[22]

As described in the preceding text, phosphate metabolism is at the root of the metabolic derangements that lead to the development of renal osteodystrophy in patients with ESRD and in those on chronic dialysis.[23] The target phosphorus level in patients with stage 3 to 4 kidney disease (GFR 15 to 59 mL per minute) is 3.0 to 4.6 mg per dL and for stage 5 disease (GFR <15 mL per minute) is 3.5 to 5.5. Lowering of phosphorus levels in moderate renal insufficiency can lead to normalization of calcium and PTH levels and amelioration of calcitriol deficiency. In patients with more advanced disease, correction of the hyperphosphatemia leads to a decrease in PTH, independent of any changes in the calcium and calcitriol levels.

The target for calcium includes normal levels in stage 3 to 4 disease and 8.8 to 9.5 mg per dL in stage 5 renal failure. When the calcium-phosphorus product (obtained by multiplying calcium × phosphorus in mg per dL) exceeds 70, there is an increased risk of metastatic calcification of arteries, joints, and soft tissues and, when most severe, ischemia and calciphylaxis.

Target iPTH levels are 35 to 110 pg per mL in stages 3 to 4 and 150 to 300 in stage 5 disease. PTH levels are commonly measured by the "intact" assay. These sandwich assays have been shown to measure the full-length (1 to 84) active PTH molecule as well as amino-terminally truncated fragments (7 to 84) similar to full-length PTH. Recent evidence has shown a possible antagonizing effect of PTH function by the amino-terminally truncated fragments. While some centers now use polyclonal antibodies to measure full-length PTH and are able to derive levels of the truncated fragments by comparison to iPTH readings, there is, as yet, no widespread use of this technique or clear guidelines for its interpretation.

iPTH levels <100 pg per mL are associated with an increased likelihood of ABD. On the other hand, levels above 450 pg per mL are typically associated with osteitis fibrosa or with mixed uremic osteodystrophy. PTH levels between 100 and 450 pg per mL do not correlate well with any specific type of bone histology and may be associated with normal bone parameters or increased or decreased bone turnover.

Bone-specific alkaline phosphatase, a marker of bone formation, may be helpful when used in combination with iPTH levels. An elevated BSAP (>20 ng per mL), especially in combination with a high PTH, has been shown to be highly sensitive and specific for high turnover bone disease. On the other hand, a low plasma BSAP (<7 ng per mL) in combination with a low iPTH is suggestive of low turnover disease.

While measurement of biochemical markers is helpful clinically, bone biopsy is the gold standard for the diagnosis and characterization of renal osteodystrophy. Prior to bone biopsy of the iliac crest, patients are given two separate courses of tetracycline derivatives at set intervals: One of tetracycline HCL and the other of demeclocycline. This results in tetracycline labeling in areas of bone formation that can be visualized through a fluoroscope. In addition, these specimens are stained for aluminum and iron to rule out evidence of aluminum toxicity. Bone biopsies are not routinely obtained in clinical practice; however, their possible uses include establishing the diagnosis of ABD in symptomatic patients with PTH levels <100 pg per mL; establishing therapy in patients with PTH levels between 100 and 450 pg per mL; determining bone histology and aluminum deposition prior to parathyroidectomy, because low postoperative PTH levels may exacerbate ABD; and determining the extent of aluminum deposition.

Bone x-rays are generally not useful in determining the type of bone disease. However, one may see typical findings of osteitis fibrosa such as subperiosteal bone resorption and patchy osteosclerosis, leading to the "salt and pepper" appearance of the skull or the "rugger jersey" appearance of the spine. Patients with osteomalacia may be identified by the presence of pseudofractures.

Bone density measurement by DXA scan, particularly of the spine, may be falsely elevated because of extensive vascular calcification in patients with ESRD. Bone density measurements of the hip and radius are probably more reliable. In addition, the association between bone density and fracture risk observed in epidemiologic studies does not seem to be applicable to patients with ESRD. In studies of dialysis patients, those with fragility fractures had BMD measurements similar to those without fractures. Therefore, while DXA screening is recommended for all patients with stage 5 kidney disease and patients with stage 3 to 4 with risk factors for disease, the BMD results should be interpreted in the context of biochemical markers and clinical presentation.

Management

Control and prevention of hyperphosphatemia is the mainstay of therapy in ESRD (Evidence Level C). Restriction of dietary phosphate and binding of phosphate in the gut by the use of antacids are at the core of therapy. Limiting phosphate intake to approximately 800 mg daily is reasonable. Most of the phosphate is found in protein-containing foods, particularly dairy products. Complete protein restriction is inadvisable in patients with ESRD, given that malnutrition is common in patients on dialysis. While aluminum-based binders were commonly used to keep phosphate levels normal, the complications of aluminum toxicity have resulted in a shift in clinical management to calcium-based therapy. Both calcium carbonate and calcium acetate are commonly used. Calcium acetate is a more efficient phosphate binder, requiring only about half the amount of calcium when compared to calcium carbonate. In addition, calcium carbonate requires normal gastric acidity for dissolution. However, the incidence of hypercalcemia is equivalent in both treatments and, therefore, both are commonly used. Generally, the dose of calcium binders is increased until phosphate levels are controlled or hypercalcemia develops. Hypercalcemia is more common in patients also being treated with vitamin D preparations. Sevelamer is a calcium- and aluminum-free phosphate binder. Its phosphate-binding capacity is equivalent to that of calcium but it does not cause hypercalcemia. There is also a decreased incidence of low PTH levels and decreased vascular calcification with the use of sevelamer when compared to calcium-containing preparations. In general, calcium-based binders are used as initial therapy because of their lower expense. Sevelamer is generally reserved for patients when they develop hypercalcemia. All phosphate binders work best when taken with meals and snacks.

In stage 3 or 4 kidney disease, 25(OH)D levels should be measured in patients in whom PTH levels are above target. If low, treatment should be initiated with ergocalciferol until the vitamin D deficiency is corrected or hypercalcemia develops. If phosphate levels increase, the dose of phosphate binders can be adjusted. The use of active vitamin D is usually initiated in patients with stage 5 kidney disease in whom PTH levels rise above 300 pg per mL despite the use of phosphate binders. It is generally believed that vitamin D is more effective in treating secondary hyperparathyroidism and in preventing worsening parathyroid hyperplasia. Vitamin D works to decrease PTH by binding to the vitamin D receptor in the parathyroid gland and by decreasing the PTH transcription. In addition, by increasing calcium levels, there is an increased binding of calcium to the CaSR with a decrease in PTH secretion from the parathyroid glands. The main limiting factor of vitamin D therapy is worsening of the phosphate levels owing to the stimulation of calcium and phosphorus absorption in the gut with a resultant increase in the calcium-phosphate product. The ideal route for administration of calcitriol is still unknown. While some studies have shown that intermittent intravenous bolus administration of calcitriol may be more effective in controlling hyperparathyroidism, others have shown no difference in the effectiveness of intermittent oral or intravenous therapy. Calcitriol therapy is usually administered three times a week in doses similar to the normal physiologic levels of $1,25(OH)_2D_3$ (0.5 to 0.75 μg per day). Patients on dialysis are usually treated three times a week by intravenous bolus after dialysis.

Newer vitamin D analogs which appear to have less calcemic and phosphatemic effects but which retain the ability to suppress PTH have been developed. Two such agents are approved for use in the United States—paricalcitol and doxercalciferol. Trials comparing paricalcitol and calcitriol in hemodialysis patients showed a more rapid decrease in PTH levels in the paricalcitol group, but no differences were observed at the end of treatment. Similarly, there were no significant differences in calcium and calcium-phosphate product noted between groups at the completion of study. However, in consecutive blood draws, more patients in the calcitriol group had hypercalcemia or an elevated calcium-phosphate product. A different study showed a possible survival advantage in patients treated with paricalcitol when compared to calcitriol-treated patients. The starting dose of paricalcitol is 0.04 to 0.1 μg/kg/bolus given three times a week with dialysis. The dose is titrated every 2 to 4 weeks until the desired PTH reduction is observed or there is an elevation in calcium or phosphorus levels. Doxercalciferol has been shown to be tolerated well and to effectively lower PTH levels. It is available in both an oral and an intravenous formulation, and starting doses are 5 μg orally or 2 μg intravenously three times a week. There are no studies comparing doxercalciferol with calcitriol use.

More recently, the calcimimetic cinacalcet has been approved for use in patients with secondary hyperparathyroidism treated with dialysis. Cinacalcet allosterically increases the sensitivity of the CaSR in the parathyroid gland to calcium. Studies of dialysis patients who have been given cinacalcet have shown a decrease in PTH levels as well as decreases in calcium, phosphorus, and the calcium-phosphate product.[24] This agent is not currently approved for patients predialysis because of the risk of hypocalcemia. The initial dose of cinacalcet is 30 mg daily. This agent should not be started in patients with calcium levels $<$8.4 mg per dL, and calcium levels should be measured within 1 week of the initiation of therapy. The main side effect noted in studies of cinacalcet was nonrecurrent nausea and vomiting.

Parathyroidectomy is reserved for patients who have severe hyperparathyroidism with PTH $>$800 pg per mL and associated hypercalcemia and/or hyperphosphatemia or symptoms related to elevations in PTH, calcium, or phosphorus such as pruritus unresponsive to medical therapy; progressive extraskeletal calcification; or symptomatic myopathy. Either subtotal parathyroidectomy or four-gland parathyroidectomy with autotransplantation is the procedure of choice.

Although bisphosphonates are commonly used to treat patients with osteoporosis, the use of these agents in patients with ESRD has not been studied. There are therefore no available data on BMD response or fracture rate in patients with ESRD treated with bisphosphonates. There is particular interest in the possible use of antiresorptive agents in renal patients with persistent high bone turnover despite aggressive control of underlying hyperparathyroidism. A common concern is that these agents may trigger ABD in patients with ESRD. To date, no evidence exists to support this concern. However, given the paucity of data, widespread use of bisphosphonate in patients treated with dialysis cannot be recommended.[25]

Recognition of bone disease in high-risk populations remains the cornerstone of fracture prevention. In general, preventive measures to minimize bone loss in the elderly should be aggressively implemented. On the other hand, in patients with established bone disease, timely treatment has been shown to be beneficial in reducing long-term morbidity and mortality.

ACKNOWLEDGMENT

With support from the Aurbach Endowment of the University of Virginia, Charlottesville, Virginia.

REFERENCES

1. Dawson-Hughes B, Harris SS, Krall EA, et al. Effect of calcium and vitamin D supplementation on bone density in men and women 65 years of age or older. *N Engl J Med*. 1997;337(10):670–676.
2. Chapuy MC, Arlot ME, Duboeuf F, et al. Vitamin D3 and calcium to prevent hip fractures in the elderly women. *N Engl J Med*. 1992;327(23):1637–1642.
3. The Writing Group for the PEPI. Effects of hormone therapy on bone mineral density: Results from the Postmenopausal Estrogen/Progestin Interventions (PEPI) trial. *JAMA*. 1996;276(17):1389–1396.
4. Rossouw JE, Anderson GL, Prentice RL, et al. Risks and benefits of estrogen plus progestin in healthy postmenopausal women: Principal results from the Women's Health Initiative randomized controlled trial. *JAMA*. 2002;288(3):321–333.
5. Delmas PD, Bjarnason NH, Mitlak BH, et al. Effects of raloxifene on bone mineral density, serum cholesterol concentrations, and uterine endometrium in postmenopausal women. *N Engl J Med*. 1997;337(23):1641–1647.
6. Ettinger B, Black DM, Mitlak BH, et al. Reduction of vertebral fracture risk in postmenopausal women with osteoporosis treated with raloxifene: Results from a 3-year randomized clinical trial. Multiple Outcomes of Raloxifene Evaluation (MORE) investigators. *JAMA*. 1999;282(7):637–645.
7. Chesnut CH III, Silverman S, Andriano K, et al. PROOF Study Group. A randomized trial of nasal spray salmon calcitonin in postmenopausal women with established osteoporosis: The prevent recurrence of osteoporotic fractures study. *Am J Med*. 2000;109(4):267–276.
8. Liberman UA, Weiss SR, Broll J, et al. The Alendronate Phase III Osteoporosis Treatment Study Group. Effect of oral alendronate on bone mineral density and the incidence of fractures in postmenopausal osteoporosis. *N Engl J Med*. 1995;333(22):1437–1743.
9. Bone HG, Hosking D, Devogelaer JP, et al. Ten years' experience with alendronate for osteoporosis in postmenopausal women. *N Engl J Med*. 2004;350(12):1189–1199.
10. Black DM, Cummings SR, Karpf DB, et al. Fracture Intervention Trial Research Group. Randomised trial of effect of alendronate on risk of fracture in women with existing vertebral fractures. *Lancet*. 1996;348(9041):1535–1541.
11. Harris ST, Watts NB, Genant HK, et al. Vertebral Efficacy with Risedronate Therapy (VERT) Study Group. Effects of risedronate treatment on vertebral and nonvertebral fractures in women with postmenopausal osteoporosis: A randomized controlled trial. *JAMA*. 1999;282(14):1344–1352.
12. McClung MR, Geusens P, Miller PD, et al. Hip Intervention Program Study Group. Effect of risedronate on the risk of hip fracture in elderly women. *N Engl J Med*. 2001;344(5):333–340.
13. Wallach S, Cohen S, Reid DM, et al. Effects of risedronate treatment on bone density and vertebral fracture in patients on corticosteroid therapy. *Calcif Tissue Int*. 2000;67(4):277–285.
14. Rosen CJ, Hochberg MC, Bonnick SL, et al. Treatment with once-weekly alendronate 70 mg compared with once-weekly risedronate 35 mg in women with postmenopausal osteoporosis: A randomized double-blind study. *J Bone Miner Res*. 2005;17(12):2094–2105; 20:141–151.
15. Neer RM, Arnaud CD, Zanchetta JR, et al. Effect of parathyroid hormone (1–34) on fractures and bone mineral density in postmenopausal women with osteoporosis. *N Engl J Med*. 2001;344(19):1434–1441.
16. Finkelstein JS, Hayes A, Hunzelman JL, et al. The effects of parathyroid hormone, alendronate, or both in men with osteoporosis. *N Engl J Med*. 2003;349(13):1216–1226.
17. Kurland ES, Heller SL, Diamon B, et al. The importance of bisphosphonate therapy in maintaining bone mass in men after therapy with teriparatide [human parathyroid hormone (1–34)]. *Osteoporos Int*. 2004;15:992–997.
18. Orr-Walker BJ, Evans MC, Clearwater JM, et al. Effects of hormone replacement therapy on bone mineral density in postmenopausal women with primary hyperparathyroidism: Four-year follow-up and comparison with healthy postmenopausal women. *Arch Intern Med*. 2000;160(14):2161–2166.
19. Chow CC, Chan WB, Li JK, et al. Oral alendronate increases bone mineral density in postmenopausal women with primary hyperparathyroidism. *J Clin Endocrinol Metab*. 2003;88(2):581–587.
20. Silverberg SJ, Bone HG III, Marriott TB, et al. Short-term inhibition of parathyroid hormone secretion by a calcium-receptor agonist in patients with primary hyperparathyroidism. *N Engl J Med*. 1997;337(21):1506–1510.
21. Peacock M, Bilezikian JP, Klassen PS, et al. Cinacalcet hydrochloride maintains long-term normocalcemia in patients with primary hyperparathyroidism. *J Clin Endocrinol Metab*. 2005;90(1):135–141.
22. Elder G. Pathophysiology and recent advances in the management of renal osteodystrophy. [Review]. *J Bone Miner Res*. 2002;17(12):2094–2105.
23. Moe SM, Drueke TB. A bridge to improving healthcare outcomes and quality of life. *Am J Kidney Dis*. 2004;43(3):552–557.
24. Block GA, Martin KJ, de Francisco AL, et al. Cinacalcet for secondary hyperparathyroidism in patients receiving hemodialysis. *N Engl J Med*. 2004;350(15):1516–1525.
25. Fan SL, Cunningham J. Bisphosphonates in renal osteodystrophy. [Review]. *Curr Opin Nephrol Hypertens*. 2001;10(5):581–588.

Hypertension and Lipid Disorders

24

Vinod R. Patel Thomas C. Rosenthal

CLINICAL PEARLS 309

HYPERTENSION 309
History, Symptomatology, and Initial Evaluation 310
Types of Hypertension 310
Complications 311
Workup/Keys to Diagnosis 311
Management 312

LIPID DISORDERS 314
Age-related Cholesterol Metabolism 315
Benefits of Lipid Lowering in the Elderly 315
Definition 315
Screening 315
Primary Prevention 315
Secondary Prevention 316
Management of Hyperlipidemia 316

CLINICAL PEARLS

- Hypertension and lipid disorders are among the most common and asymptomatic problems in the elderly population today.
- Despite apparent benefits, compliance with statin therapy declines substantially with time in elderly patients. This occurs even when cost is not an issue.
- Hypertension is a common problem in elderly subjects, reaching a prevalence of 60% to 80%.
- Isolated systolic hypertension accounts for 60% of cases of hypertension in the elderly.
- In persons older than 50 years, systolic blood pressure (BP) >140 mm Hg is a much more important cardiovascular disease risk factor than diastolic pressure.
- Patient compliance is the factor most associated with successful treatment. Motivation improves when patients have a positive experience with, and trust in the clinician.
- The elderly may have sluggish baroreceptors and sympathetic responsiveness, as well as impaired cerebral autoregulation. Therapy should be gentle and gradual, avoiding drugs that are likely to cause postural hypotension.
- The elderly may ingest more sodium to compensate for a decrease in taste sensitivity.
- The elderly may depend more on processed, prepackaged foods that are high in sodium and fat rather than fresh foods that are low in sodium.
- Lower initial doses of medications (often one half that in younger patients) should be used to minimize the risk of side effects.
- The reduction in BP should be gradual to minimize the risk of ischemic symptoms, particularly in patients with postural hypotension.
- In advancing age, one must consider comorbid treatments of diabetes, renal failure, dementia, arthritis, coronary artery disease, and benign prostatic hyperplasia.
- Nonsteroidal anti-inflammatory drugs (NSAIDs) may adversely impact BP control.
- Despite their proved benefit, lipid-lowering drugs and antihypertensive medications are markedly underutilized in elderly patients.

HYPERTENSION

Aging is associated with an increased prevalence of hypertension, coronary artery disease, and heart failure and a reduction in exercise capacity.[1] Elevated blood

TABLE 24.1
DEFINITION OF HYPERTENSION (JNC 7)

Classification	Systolic	Diastolic
Normal blood pressure	<120 mm Hg	<80 mm Hg
Prehypertension	120–139 mm Hg	80–89 mm Hg
Stage 1 hypertension	140–159 mm Hg	90–99 mm Hg
Stage 2 hypertension	≥160 mm Hg	≥100 mm Hg

Chobanian AV, Bakris, GL, Black HR, et al. The seventh report of the Joint National Committee on prevention, detection, evaluation, and treatment of high blood pressure: The JNC 7 report. *JAMA*. 2003;289:2560.

pressure (BP) and dyslipidemia are the most common and asymptomatic problems in the ambulatory care setting worldwide. The incidence of hypertension is increasing because of increase in awareness, life span, and clarification of the definition of hypertension by the Joint National Committee (JNC) (see Table 24.1). Hypertension will become an epidemic as the baby boomers age.

Although the diastolic BP peaks at age 50, the systolic BP continues to increase with age. It increases in all races. African Americans tend to develop hypertension more often and at younger ages, Mexican Americans tend to develop hypertension later in life, and white Americans show continuous increase to a prevalence of 60% to 80% by late life.[2] Only 34% of the individuals with hypertension have adequate control, defined as a level below 140/90 mm Hg.[3]

Current definitions for hypertension have been established by the seventh report of the JNC.[3] They are based on the average of two or more readings at each of two or more visits after an initial screen. Normal BP is defined as systolic BP of 120 mm Hg and diastolic BP of 80 mm Hg. BP between normal and 139 mm Hg systolic, and 89 mm Hg diastolic is considered prehypertension. High normal BP for over 12 years is associated with a 1.6-fold greater risk of cardiovascular disease in men and 2.5-fold greater risk in women compared with subjects with optimal BP at baseline.[3–5] In the absence of end-organ damage, a patient should not be labeled as having hypertension unless the BP is persistently elevated after three to six visits over a period of several months.

History, Symptomatology, and Initial Evaluation

Hypertension is asymptomatic. Patients may have been told by a health care provider during health screening examinations that they had a high reading. Patients with severe hypertension may present with headache and dizziness. Patients with long-standing hypertension may present with target organ damage, like blindness, loss of visual acuity, floaters in front of the eyes, episodic weakness, chest pain, shortness of breath, and symptoms of peripheral vascular disease like claudication. If the patient presents with muscle weakness, flank pain, thinning of the skin, intermittent tachycardia, sweating, tremors, pedal edema, secondary hypertension should be considered. Some hypertensive patients will report palpitations while taking over-the-counter medication like pseudoephedrine.

Risk factors for developing hypertension are high sodium intake, excess alcohol and saturated fat intake, physical inactivity, smoking, diabetes, dyslipidemias, hormonal medications (estrogens, androgens), and psychological factors including stress, family circumstances, and type A personality.

In essential hypertension there is usually a family history of hypertension. Other family history may include premature cardiovascular death, diabetes, and familial diseases such as pheochromocytoma.

Physical examinations should include accurate measurement of BP, general examinations for distribution of body fat, skin lesions, examination of carotids, cardiac and respiratory auscultation, detection of carotid or abdominal bruits, peripheral edema, and muscle strength.

Types of Hypertension

Essential Hypertension

Essential hypertension is the most common type of hypertension, especially in patients with a family history.[6] Essential hypertension is seen primarily in societies in which salt intake is above 100 mEq per day (2.3 g sodium).[7] Essential hypertension is particularly common in obese patients and is often associated with metabolic syndrome and diabetes mellitus.[8] It is more common and more severe in black populations.

Secondary hypertension is less common and potentially correctable. Renal disease usually presents with pedal edema, abnormal urinalysis, and hypertension. Pheochromocytoma may present with paroxysm of hypertension associated with tachycardia and may have family history. Patients using steroids may have cushingoid faces and central obesity. Other rare causes of hypertension are hyperthyroidism and hyperparathyroidism. Physical findings associated with secondary hypertension are listed in Table 24.2.

Isolated Systolic Hypertension

JNC 7 defines isolated systolic hypertension as a systolic level of 140 mm Hg regardless of age.[3] Isolated systolic hypertension accounts for 65% to 75% of cases of hypertension in the elderly.[9] Isolated systolic hypertension is associated with a two- to fourfold increase in the risk of myocardial infarction, left ventricular hypertrophy, renal dysfunction, stroke, and cardiovascular mortality.[10,11] As the systolic pressure rises and the diastolic pressure falls after age 60 in both normotensive and untreated hypertensive subjects,[12] the pulse pressure becomes widened. The widened pulse pressure has been considered a risk factor

TABLE 24.2
PHYSICAL FINDINGS IN SECONDARY HYPERTENSION

Causes	Findings
Renal disease like glomerulonephritis or secondary renal disease	Hypertension along with other glomerulonephritis symptoms
Pheochromocytoma	Paroxysmal tachycardia and hypertension
Primary hyperaldosteronism	Hypertension, hypokalemia, and metabolic alkalosis
Coarctation of aorta	Bruit in back, decreased/lagging pulsations
Cushing syndrome	Cushingoid features on physical examination

for cardiovascular disease as it may interfere with tissue perfusion. Caution is advised when treating elderly patients with isolated systolic hypertension, who start with lower diastolic pressures. The diastolic BP should not be reduced to <60 mm Hg to attain the target systolic pressure.

Complications

Risk increases as a continuum as the BP rises above 110/75 mm Hg.[13] In older patients, systolic pressure and pulse pressure are more powerful determinants of risk than diastolic pressure.[14,15] Hypertension increases the workload of the cardiac muscle, causing left ventricular hypertrophy,[16] which is associated with heart failure, ventricular arrhythmias, myocardial infarction, and sudden cardiac death.[17] Hypertension is the most important risk factor for stroke and intracerebral hemorrhage, and the incidence of both are markedly reduced by effective antihypertensive therapy.[18] BP reduction as low as a 2 mm Hg fall in mean systolic BP would be associated with 7% lower risk of ischemic heart disease death and a 10% lower risk of stroke death.[19] When compared to diabetes, cigarette smoking, and dyslipidemia, hypertension is the most powerful risk factor for heart disease and stroke death.[20]

Hypertension is also associated with nephrosclerosis secondary to chronic renal injuries and can accelerate the progression of underlying renal diseases, causing chronic renal insufficiency and end-stage renal disease.[21]

Malignant hypertension is an acute, severe elevation of BP that can be a life-threatening emergency.[22] It is associated with papilledema, encephalopathy, subarachnoid hemorrhage, and intracerebral hemorrhage.

Workup/Keys to Diagnosis

There are two goals to working up a patient with hypertension: (i) Establish whether the patient has essential hypertension, white coat hypertension or secondary hypertension, and (ii) determine end-organ damage (see Table 24.3). Once a patient has met the JNC 7 criteria for high BP, they should be examined for curable secondary causes of hypertension. In absence of signs of secondary hypertension, patients need to undergo a relatively limited workup.

Patients with elevated BP in the office and normal pressure at home may have white coat hypertension. In the absence of end-organ damage, a patient with "white coat hypertension" might require 24-hour ambulatory monitoring to establish their mean BP and determine whether treatment is necessary.

Laboratory testing should include complete blood count, urinalysis, urine microalbumin, complete metabolic profile, fasting lipid profile, and thyroid-stimulating hormone. Electrocardiogram (ECG), radiograph of the chest, and echocardiography may be indicated to determine myocardial hypertrophy. If renal artery stenosis is suspected, angiography is indicated. Measurement of plasma renin activity is usually performed only in patients with possible low-renin forms of hypertension, such as primary hyperaldosteronism.

TABLE 24.3
DIFFERENTIAL DIAGNOSIS

Structural (ICD-9)	Metabolic (ICD-9)	Drug Induced (ICD-9)
Aortic dissection (441.0)	Atherosclerosis (440.9)	Cardiomyopathy, cocaine induced (425.4)
Aortic coarctation (747.1)	Malignant hypertension (401.0)	
Sleep apnea (780.57)	Hyperthyroidism (242.9)	
Renal artery stenosis (447.1)	Pheochromocytoma (194.0, 255.6)	
Adrenal adenoma (227.0)	Primary hyperaldosteronism (255.1)	
Essential hypertension (401.1)		

Management

Medication sensitivity, atherosclerosis, renal dysfunction, and aging physiology conspire to potentiate adverse reactions to antihypertensive medication. Cognitive decline and the expense of medications may further challenge treatment. Therefore, all patients should be counseled about salt restriction, weight loss, and exercise (Evidence Level A).

When needed, antihypertensive therapy has been associated with 35% to 40% mean reductions in stroke incidence; 20% to 25% in myocardial infarction; and >50% in heart failure.[23] Controlling hypertension to below 130/80 mm Hg could prevent 37% of coronary artery diseases in men and 56% in women.[24]

Equal if not greater benefits have been shown with the treatment of elderly hypertensive patients (older than 65), most of whom have isolated systolic hypertension. Because the elderly start at such higher overall cardiovascular risk, short-term reductions in their hypertension provide apparently greater benefits than that observed in younger patients.

Lifestyle Modification

Salt and alcohol restriction, weight reduction, calcium and magnesium supplementation, ingestion of a vegetarian diet or fish oil supplements, and possibly increasing potassium intake (40 to 80 mEq per day) have demonstrated benefits in the treatment of hypertension.[3,25] All of these maneuvers tend to induce a small and unpredictable reduction in BP in most patients.[26–28] Dietary modifications may also lower low-density lipoprotein-cholesterol (LDL-C) while raising high-density lipoprotein-cholesterol (HDL-C). The JNC 7 report recommends moderate sodium restriction (100 mEq per day). The easiest way to do this is by lowering intake of processed foods. Elderly patients, particularly those living alone, may depend on processed, prepackaged foods that are high in sodium rather than fresh foods. The elderly may ingest more sodium to compensate for a decrease in taste sensitivity, leading to volume expansion and a rise in BP.

Behavioral modification such as cessation of smoking, regular aerobic exercise and limited alcohol intake are as important as diet. Consumption of one to two drinks per day appears to reduce cardiovascular risk in hypertensive as well as normotensive patients but patients who consume more than two drinks per day have a twofold increase in the incidence of hypertension compared to nondrinkers.[29] Hostile attitudes and impatience should also be discouraged.[30]

Drug Treatment

Antihypertensive medications should generally be started if the systolic pressure is persistently 140 mm Hg and/or the diastolic pressure is persistently 90 mm Hg on three office visits or on home readings. For patients with diabetes or chronic renal failure, antihypertensive therapy is indicated and should be more aggressive when the systolic pressure is persistently above 130 mm Hg and/or the diastolic pressure is above 80 mm Hg. This is particularly true for patients with proteinuria. Some patients will have normal readings at home in spite of consistently elevated reading in the office. Twenty-four-hour ambulatory BP monitoring may establish an accurate mean BP and determine if they are truly hypertensive.

The seventh JNC (JNC 7) report recommends initiating therapy in uncomplicated hypertensive patients with a low-dose thiazide diuretic based on improved outcomes in the Antihypertensive and Lipid-Lowering Treatment to Prevent Heart Attack Trial (ALLHAT) study.[31] In most patients monotherapy will fail to attain goal BP. Then an angiotensin-converting enzyme (ACE) inhibitor, angiotensin II receptor blocker (ARB), β-blocker, or calcium channel blocker can be sequentially added or substituted. Table 24.4 lists the classes of available antihypertensive.

Diuretics are inexpensive, and have been demonstrated to provide better cardioprotection than an ACE inhibitor or calcium channel blocker in patients with diabetes type 2, known cardiovascular disease, hyperlipidemias, left ventricular hypertrophy, or in cigarette smokers.[31] Hydrochlorothiazide or chlorthalidone (12.5 to 25 mg) have been associated with a low rate of metabolic complications, such as hypokalemia, glucose intolerance, and hyperuricemia (Evidence Level A).

ACE inhibitors block the enzyme that converts angiotensin I into angiotensin II, a potent vasoconstrictor. ACE inhibitors also retard the degradation of potent vasodilator-bradykinins. They are broadly effective in all age-groups, and lack metabolic side effects (Evidence Level B). Used long term, they reduce the proteinuria secondary to diabetes or hypertension. ACE inhibitors have been shown to provide survival benefits in patients with heart failure and myocardial infarction and renal benefits in patients with proteinuric chronic renal failure. ACE inhibitors are more effective at reversing left ventricular hypertrophy than β-blockers. Therefore, ACE inhibitors should be chosen first or second line in patients with heart failure, prior myocardial infraction, left ventricular dysfunction, type 1 diabetics with nephropathy, and nondiabetic proteinuric chronic renal failure. Because serum creatinine may transiently increase with the use of ACE inhibitors, they should be avoided in patients with creatinine above 3 mg per dL. Side effect includes cough, hypotension, hyperkalemia, and rarely angioedema.

ARBs have effects similar to those of ACE inhibitors except they do not cause cough or angioedema. Their utility and tolerability are similar to ACE inhibitors. ARBs have shown benefit in severe hypertension with ECG evidence of left ventricular hypertrophy in the Losartan Intervention for Endpoint (LIFE) reduction in hypertension study[32] and in type 2 diabetics with microalbuminuria or nephropathy.[33]

TABLE 24.4
ANTIHYPERTENSIVE MEDICATIONS

Medication Class	Medications	Dosages	Advantages	Side Effects	Contraindications	Special Disease Conditions to Use
Diuretics	Hydrochlorothiazide Chlorthalidone Furosemide Spironolactone (potassium-sparing diuretics)	12.5–25 mg 12.5–25 mg 20–80 mg b.i.d.–t.i.d.	Cheaper Cardioprotective	Hypokalemia Hyperglycemia Hyperuricemia Dyslipidemia Osteoporosis	Gout Diabetes Primary hyperaldosteronism	Systolic heart failure Coronary artery diseases Postmyocardial infarction
ACE inhibitors	Captopril Enalapril Lisinopril	12.5–75 mg b.i.d. 2.5–40 mg q.d. 5–40 mg q.d.	No sexual side effects Shown to have survival benefits	Cough Angioedema Hyperkalemia	Renal artery stenosis Pregnancy	Systolic heart failure Diabetics Coronary artery disease Postmyocardial infarction
ARBs	Losartan Valsartan	25–50 mg/d 80–320 mg/d	No sexual side effects	Hyperkalemia Acute renal failure with renal artery stenosis	Pregnancy Renal artery stenosis	Systolic heart failure
β-Blockers	Metoprolol Atenolol Carvedilol	12.5–200 mg/d 25–100 mg/d 12.5–50 mg/d	Inexpensive	Dizziness Bradycardia Depression Bronchospasm, Dyslipidemias	Congestive heart failure Diabetes Asthma Second- or third-degree heart block COPD	Angina pectoris Atrial fibrillation Atrial flutter
Calcium channel inhibitors	Amlodipine Diltiazem Verapamil	2.5–10 mg/d 180–300 mg/d 120–480 mg/d	Once a day dosing	Headache Tachycardia Edema, can cause heart block Raynaud syndrome	Heart failure Second- or third-degree heart block	Diastolic heart failure Isolated systolic hypertension
α-Blockers	Terazosin Doxazosin Prazosin	1–20 mg/d 1–16 mg/d 1–10 mg/d		Orthostatic hypotension Tachycardia Flushing Sudden syncope	Use with caution in elderly Severe coronary artery disease	Prostatic hypertrophy
Vasodilators	Hydralazine Minoxidil	10–75 mg q.i.d. 2.5–40 mg/d	Inexpensive	Headache Tachycardia Exacerbates angina Abnormal hair growth	Lupus Severe coronary artery diseases	Heart failure, particularly in African Americans
Centrally acting drugs	Methyldopa Clonidine	250–750 mg 0.1–0.3 t.i.d.	Inexpensive	Postural hypotension Drowsiness Rebound hypertension Impaired ejaculation Gynecomastia		

ACE, angiotensin-converting enzyme; ARBs, angiotensin II receptor blockers; COPD, chronic obstructive pulmonary disease.

Recent studies have used ARBs in combination with ACE inhibitors in heart failure.

β-Blockers block the sympathetic effects on the heart; therefore, they reduce cardiac output and lower arterial pressure in patients at risk for cardiac sympathetic nerve activity. For this reason, β-blockers should be reserved for use in elderly patients who will benefit from rate control in atrial fibrillation, control of angina, and in anxiety disorders. Sympathetic hyperactivity is a hallmark of heart failure that explains the recently established role of β-blockers in stable cardiomyopathies. They are contraindicated in chronic obstructive pulmonary disease (COPD), asthma, severe peripheral vascular disease, Raynaud phenomenon, depression, bradycardia, second- or third-degree heart block, and in diabetics prone to hypoglycemia.

Calcium channel blockers modify calcium entry into cells by interacting with specific binding sites on calcium channels, thereby causing vasodilation. They are therefore useful in angina pectoris and atrial fibrillation for rate control, and can be used in patients with COPD. Their effectiveness in patients with low rennin activity, and their lack of metabolic side effects make them useful in elderly patients. Side effects include dizziness, headache, flushing, peripheral edema, constipation, and delayed cardiac conduction. Generally not first-line drugs, calcium channel blockers may be chosen as first line in patients with angina pectoris, recurrent supraventricular tachycardia, migraine headache, diastolic heart failure, and esophageal spasm. Calcium channel blockers are contraindicated with second- or third-degree heart block or systolic heart failure and should be avoided immediately after acute myocardial infarction.

Vasodilators relax the smooth muscle and act mainly on arterial resistance. They are not first-line agents due to reflex tachycardia. Hydralazine can cause a lupus-like syndrome, and minoxidil can cause hypertrichosis and fluid retention. This group can be helpful in treating patients with renal failure where ACE inhibitors are contraindicated.

α-Adrenergic blockers block the action of norepinephrine at α-adrenergic receptor sites. They can cause postural hypotension and should be used cautiously in elderly. They may reduce the symptoms of benign prostatic hypertrophy, but tamsulosin has similar prostatic effect with less risk of orthostasis. α-Blockers also lower low-density lipoprotein (LDL), increase high-density lipoprotein (HDL), and improve insulin sensitivity. Side effects include dizziness, syncope, headache, and weakness.

Centrally acting agents act on the vasomotor center as well as on the peripheral neurons, where they modify catecholamine release. They can cause rebound hypertension on abrupt discontinuation and therefore they are seldom used as first-line agents or in noncompliant patients. This drug does not offer any cardiovascular protective benefit like ACE inhibitors or ARBs but lacks metabolic side effect. Common complaints include dry mouth, sedation, sexual dysfunction, and rebound hypertension.

Combinations

Most patients will require more than one medication to reach target BPs. The clinician may choose to push the first drug to maximum recommended dosage or alternatively may add a second drug after a failed trial of a moderate dose of the first drug. The latter approach may induce fewer side effects. As per JNC 7 guidelines, two drugs should be considered when the BP is >20/10 mm Hg above the goal.[3] Combinations should be based on patient comorbidities, side effects of medications and synergistic effect of the drugs (Evidence Level A). Examples include using ACE in diabetics, α-blockers with benign prostatic hypertrophy, and ACE inhibitors or β-blockers in congestive heart failure. ACE and β-blockers have a synergistic effect with diuretics. Other synergistic combinations include an ACE inhibitor with a calcium channel blocker, and a β-blocker with a vasodilator. Combinations of β-blockers and calcium channel blockers should be avoided because of the danger of complete heart block.

If after some effort, the BP goal is not achieved, the clinician should consider advancing to optimum drug dosages. Consideration must be given to the possibility that the patient is noncompliant, has white coat hypertension, indulges in substance abuse, or is using an over-the-counter medication that can raise the BP.

Treatment of Isolated Systolic Hypertension

When treating isolated systolic hypertension, the clinician must consider the associated fall in diastolic BP. Maintaining a diastolic below 60 mm Hg may lead to paradoxical increase in cardiovascular events due to diminished filling during diastole. Initial choice of therapy is diuretics. Calcium channel blockers and long-acting/sustained-release nitrate formulations have shown to be effective in isolated systolic hypertension (Evidence Level B).

Compliance with the chosen antihypertensive plan requires lifestyle modifications and a lifelong commitment. Hypertension is asymptomatic and not well understood by many patients. In some cases taking medications can limit job performance, insurance availability, and sexuality. Patients must be educated and reeducated about the advantages of treatment while cost of medications, side effects, and dosing schedules must be addressed regularly.

LIPID DISORDERS

Most clinical trials for primary prevention of coronary heart disease (CHD) have excluded elderly patient populations. It is challenging to do a cost–benefit analysis of preventive care in the elderly, who typically have comorbidities, more frequent side effects, polypharmacy, and limited life expectancy. Because the absolute risk for coronary artery disease increases dramatically with age in men and women, benefit from lowering cholesterol could be greatest in the elderly.[34,35] However, the decision whether to treat hypercholesterolemia in an elderly individual should be based on both chronologic and physiologic age. A patient with a limited life span from a concomitant illness will probably not benefit from drug therapy. On the other hand, an otherwise healthy elderly individual should not be denied drug therapy on the basis of age alone (Evidence Level C).

The Third Report of the Expert Panel on Detection, Evaluation, and Treatment of High Blood Cholesterol in Adults (Adult Treatment Panel III [ATP III]) presents the National Cholesterol Education Program (NCEP)'s updated clinical guidelines for cholesterol testing and management.[36] The ATP III guidelines are based on epidemiologic observations that showed a graded relationship between the total cholesterol concentration and coronary risk. ATP III recommends intensive treatment of lipidemias in patients with CHD but adds recommendations on primary prevention in patients with multiple risk factors.

Age-related Cholesterol Metabolism

Lipoproteins are spherical particles and are made up of hundreds of lipid molecules. The major lipids in these lipoprotein complexes are cholesterol, triglycerides, and phospholipids. Triglycerides are an esterified form of cholesterol and are hydrophobic. Phospholipids are soluble in lipid and aqueous environments. Lipoproteins are classified into five major classes: Chylomicrons, very low-density lipoprotein (VLDL), intermediate-density lipoprotein, LDL, and HDL. After age 20, the plasma total cholesterol concentration increases progressively, and in men reaches a plateau between the age of 50 and 60 years, whereas in women, it reaches a peak between 60 and 70 years of age. The LDL-C concentration increases progressively in men and women after age 20, but more rapidly in men, accounting for most of the overall gender difference in total cholesterol. The rate at which the LDL-C concentration increases in women begins to accelerate between 40 and 50 years of age, and the concentration exceeds that in men by 55 to 60 years. HDL-C concentrations decrease in men during puberty and early adulthood, and thereafter remain lower than those in women at all comparable ages. The HDL-C concentrations remain constant in women throughout their lifetime.[37]

Benefits of Lipid Lowering in the Elderly

Several studies have confirmed clinically relevant benefits of lowering cholesterol in as little as 6 months. The 4S trials demonstrated reduction in all-cause mortality, mortality from CHD, major coronary events, and number of revascularization procedures.[38] The Cholesterol and Recurrent Events (CARE) trial included patients between the age of 65 and 75 and showed reduction in cardiovascular hospitalization and events similar to the 4S trials.[39] The Long-Term Intervention with Pravastatin in Ischemic Disease (LIPID) trial also included patients between the age of 65 and 75 with hyperlipidemias and prior infarction or unstable angina. The benefits of lipid lowering were greatest in the older group in this study.[40] The Heart Protection Study with patients from age 40 to 80 years with a history of coronary, cerebrovascular, and peripheral vascular disease; diabetes mellitus; and/or treated hypertension demonstrate similar benefits above and below age 65.[41] And lastly, the Prospective Study of Pravastatin in the Elderly at Risk (PROSPER) study included men and women aged 70 to 82 years with a history of or risk factors for vascular disease. This study also confirmed a significantly reduced risk of coronary death, nonfatal myocardial infarction, and fatal or nonfatal stroke (Evidence Level A).

Definition

Dyslipidemia is total cholesterol, LDL-C, triglyceride, apolipoprotein (apo) B, or Lp(a) levels above the 90th percentile, or HDL-C or apo A-I levels below the 10th percentile for the general population. The primary dyslipidemias may be because of an overproduction and/or impaired removal of lipoproteins brought on by an abnormality in either the lipoprotein itself or in the lipoprotein receptor.

Screening

Annual testing for lipid disorders is recommended in patients with family history of coronary artery disease, patients with diabetes, thyroid dysfunction, obesity, hypertension, or a history of smoking. Patients with no risk factors and normal lipid analysis may be screened every 3 to 5 years (Evidence Level C). A fasting lipid profile is the preferred screening test. Nonfasting samples can only be tested for total cholesterol and HDL, as the value for triglycerides and LDL may be misleading.

Emerging risk factors such as lipoprotein (a), homocystine, prothrombotic, and proinflammatory factors appear to contribute to predicting coronary risk to varying degrees and in the future may help guide the intensity of treatment in select groups of the population.[35]

Primary Prevention

There are limited data to recommend for or against treatment of high cholesterol in primary prevention of CHD in elderly patients with high cholesterol. Intervention should be targeted at reducing weight in obese individuals,

TABLE 24.5
LOW-DENSITY LIPOPROTEIN GOAL FOR PRIMARY PREVENTION

LDL Cholesterol	
<100	Optimal
100–129	Near optimal/above normal
130–159	Borderline high
160–189	High
≥190	Very high
Total Cholesterol	
<200	Desirable
200–239	Borderline high
≥240	High
HDL Cholesterol	
<40	Low
≥60	High

LDL, low-density lipoprotein; HDL, high-density lipoprotein.
Adapted from ATP III Guidelines at http://www.nhlbi.nih.gov/

TABLE 24.6
LOW-DENSITY LIPOPROTEIN GOAL FOR SECONDARY PREVENTION

Risk Category	LDL Goal	LDL Level (Lifestyle Changes)	LDL Level (Drug Therapy)
CHD or CHD risk equivalents	<100 mg/dL Possibly as low as <70 mg/dL	≥100 mg/dL	≥130 mg/dL (100–129 mg/dL drug optional)
2+ risk factors (10-y risk ≤20%)	<130 mg/dL	≥130 mg/dL	10-y risk 10%–20% ≥130 mg/dL 10-y risk <10% ≥160 mg/dL
0–1 risk factor	<160 mg/dL	≥160 mg/dL	≥190 mg/dL (160–189 mg/dL LDL-lowering drug optional)

LDL, low-density lipoprotein; CHD, coronary heart disease.
Adapted from ATP III guidelines and of the National Heart, Lung, and Blood Institute, the American College of Cardiology Foundation, and the American Heart Association.

increasing physical activity, and reducing dietary intakes of saturated fats and cholesterol. If lifestyle changes do not achieve the goal for LDL-C and the patient has a reasonable life expectancy, then they should be started on LDL-lowering agents shown to reduce the risk for major coronary events[42,43] (see Table 24.5).

Secondary Prevention

Patients with established heart disease who do not have survival limiting comorbidities and patients who have multiple risk factors should be treated aggressively according to the guidelines established by the NCEP (see Table 24.6). This recommendation reflects a better understanding of both the high risk conferred by the presence of coronary artery disease and the impact of cholesterol lowering in these patients (Evidence Level B).

Lifestyle modification is important in all patients; those with coronary artery diseases who are significantly above the goal LDL should not have drug therapy delayed.[40,44,45] Patients who require drug therapy should almost always be treated with statins. Fasting lipid should be analyzed every 4 to 6 weeks, with titration of the lipid-lowering drugs to achieve the LDL goal.

Management of Hyperlipidemia

Dietary modifications should include reduced intakes of saturated fats (<7% of total calories) and cholesterol (<200 mg per day). Limited intake of carbohydrate to approximately 50% to 60% of the total calories and limited protein intake of approximately 15% of total calories are recommended. Fiber intake should be approximately 20 to 30 g per day. Patients should also be encouraged to use plant stanols/sterol (2 g per day) to enhance LDL lowering. Patients with low HDL may benefit with ω-3 fatty acids intake. Total consumption of calories should be titrated against the daily requirement to enhance weight loss. Physical activity equivalent to 30 minutes of walking most days should be encouraged. Depending on risk factors, patients should be reevaluated within 3 to 12 months to determine the response of the lifestyle changes. Individual responses vary according to compliance, genetic predisposition, and body mass index. Patients should be started on cholesterol lowering agents if the goal is not met for primary or secondary prevention after 6 to 12 months.

Drug Therapy

Statins are the only class of drugs to demonstrate clear improvements in overall mortality in primary and secondary prevention (Evidence Level A). Large trials of cholestyramine, clofibrate, and gemfibrozil in primary prevention not only failed to show mortality benefits but showed worrisome trends toward an increase in noncardiac deaths. A large trial of gemfibrozil in secondary prevention also failed to show any improvement in overall mortality, although cardiac mortality was reduced.[8] Niacin has shown some mortality benefits in secondary prevention.

Patients should be started on low dosages of statin therapy and reevaluated every 6 to 8 weeks for the response of the medications. Dosages should be titrated to achieve targets in Table 24.7. Liver function test should be obtained at "regular" intervals but these intervals are not well defined. Checking liver function tests at 3 months, 6 months, and yearly thereafter would seem prudent (Evidence Level C).

Patients who develop muscle aches may be given a trial of pravastatin, a hydrophilic statin that appears to have a lower risk of inducing a myopathy. Patients with myositis and elevated creatine phosphokinase (CPK) level should discontinue statin.

In patients who do not tolerate any statin and are being treated for secondary prevention, reasonable options include the use of ezetimibe, bile acid sequestrants,

TABLE 24.7
LIPID-LOWERING AGENTS

Class	Mechanism	Results	Side Effects	Contraindication
HMG-CoA reductase also known as statins, dosages 10–80 mg/d	Decreases cholesterol synthesis Increases LDL receptors	Decreases LDL by 25%–55% Increase HDL by 5%–10%	Hepatic dysfunction Myositis	Risk of myositis increased by impaired renal function
Nicotinic acid Niacin (Niaspan) 1–2 g/d	Decreases synthesis of LDL	Reduces LDL by 15%–25% Increases HDL by 15%–30%	Flushing Hepatic dysfunction Tachycardia Pruritus Glucose intolerance	Peptic ulcer disease Cardiac arrhythmias Hepatic disease Gout
Bile acid-binding resins, cholestyramine 8–12 g/b.i.d., colestipol 10–15 g/b.i.d.	Increases LDL receptors Increases synthesis of new bile acids from cholesterol	Reduces LDL by 20%–30%, Increases HDL by 5%	Constipation Gastric discomfort Nausea	Biliary tract obstruction Gastric outlet obstruction
Fibric acid derivatives Gemfibrozil 600 mg/b.i.d., Fenofibrate 200 mg/d	Increases triglyceride hydrolysis Increases LDL catabolism Decreases VLDL synthesis	Decreases triglyceride by 25%–40% Increases HDL by 5%–15%	Gall stones Nausea Hepatic dysfunction Cardiac arrhythmias	Hepatic or biliary disease Renal insufficiency
Ezetimibe 10 mg/d	Impairs absorption of dietary and biliary cholesterol at the brush border of the intestine	Modestly lowers the LDL when used with statins	Hepatic dysfunction Myopathy	Hypersensitivity to ezetimibe

HMG-CoA, 3-hydroxy-3-methylglutaryl coenzyme A; LDL, low-density lipoprotein; HDL, high-density lipoprotein; VLDL, very low-density lipoprotein.

fenofibrate, and niacin. Referral to a lipid specialist is appropriate in such patients.

If additional agents are needed, the specific pattern of lipoprotein abnormality may influence the choice of second agents. In patients with pure elevation in LDL-C who are being treated for secondary prevention, addition of ezetimibe or a bile acid sequestrate is a reasonable option. Patients with other components of the metabolic syndrome (hypertriglyceridemia and low HDL-C) may benefit from concurrent therapy with a fibrate or nicotinic acid. Patients with low HDL may benefit from addition of niacin along with statin therapy.

Patients with hypertriglyceridemia who also have hypercholesterolemia and/or hypoalphalipoproteinemia should be treated. Because triglyceride-rich lipoproteins also transport cholesterol, hypercholesterolemia often accompanies hypertriglyceridemia. The magnitude of the hypercholesterolemia depends on the composition of triglyceride-rich lipoproteins that are present. Therefore, the presence of hypertriglyceridemia should suggest that any increase in serum total cholesterol is due in part to increased VLDL-cholesterol.

Treatment of isolated hypertriglyceridemia is indicated in the presence of overt heart disease, a strong family history of CHD, or multiple coexisting cardiac risk factors. In addition, subjects with very high triglyceride levels (>500 mg per dL [5.6 mmol per L]) should be treated to avoid pancreatitis. Patients with high triglyceride, high LDL, and low HDL can be treated with nicotinic acid along with statin therapy.

High serum HDL-C (>60 mg per dL [1.6 mmol per L]) is associated with a lower risk of CHD. An elevated LDL-C level may be less important in this setting, although specific guidelines are lacking. This pattern is most likely to occur in women.

Specific Lipid-Lowering Agents

3-Hydroxy-3-methylglutaryl coenzyme A (HMG-CoA) reductase inhibitors, also called *statins*, limit hepatic cholesterol biosynthesis, causing an increase in LDL receptor levels in hepatocytes and enhanced clearance of LDL-C from circulation. Presently available drugs include lovastatin, simvastatin, pravastatin, fluvastatin, atorvastatin, and cerivastatin. They reduce LDL by 20% to 45% at usual doses and as high as 60% at higher doses. Statins increase HDL by 5% to 10% at lower doses but may lower HDL at higher dosages. Atorvastatin and rosuvastatin are more potent statins with the added advantage of lowering triglyceride from 14% to 33%.

Side effects include transient increase in liver enzymes (aspartate aminotransferase [AST] and alanine aminotransferase [ALT]). Patients should be monitored for elevation in liver enzymes, and statins should be discontinued if enzymes rise to more than three times the normal. Other side effects include muscle pain, myositis, and myopathy, causing an increase in CPK level.

Niacin appears to inhibit liver secretion of lipoproteins-containing apo B-100. Niacin increases HDL by 15% to 25% and reduces both total and LDL-C by 15% to 25% and VLDL by 25% to 35%. Side effects include cutaneous flushing with or without pruritus. These side effects can be reduced by giving low-dose aspirin, preferably 30 minutes prior to niacin dosages. Niacin can also increase liver enzymes and uric acid. Niacin should be used cautiously in patients with diabetes, as it can worsen the glucose control.

Fibric acid (fenofibrate, clofibrate) stimulates the activity of a liver transcription factor termed peroxisome proliferator-activated receptor α, which increases production of apo A-I. It can reduce the triglycerides level by 25% to 40% and increase the HDL level by 5% to 15%. Paradoxically LDL level may also rise. Possible side effects are gastrointestinal distress in the form of epigastric pain. There is an increased risk of muscle toxicity in patients taking a fibrate and a statin. They should not be used in combination.

Bile acid-binding resins interfere with reabsorption of bile acids in the intestine. Resin can reduce total cholesterol by 15% to 25% and LDL-C by 20% to 35%, with modest increase in HDL. It can be used in combination with statin or nicotinic acid. Common side effects include gas, bloating, and constipation.

Ezetimibe impairs the absorption of dietary and biliary cholesterol absorption at the brush border of the intestine without affecting the absorption of triglycerides and fat-soluble vitamins. It modestly lowers the LDL-C when used alone but may have its greatest use in combination with statins, particularly when it is desirable to avoid the use of high-dose statins. It can elevate serum transaminase levels, so baseline liver function test should be obtained.

REFERENCES

1. Wei JY. Age and the cardiovascular system. *N Engl J Med.* 1992;327(24):1735–1739.
2. Burt VL, Whelton P, Roccella EJ, et al. Prevalence of hypertension in the US adult population. Results from the Third National Health and Nutrition Examination Survey: 1988–1991. *Hypertension.* 1995;25(3):305–313.
3. Chobanian AV, Bakris GL, Black HR, et al. The seventh report of the Joint National Committee on Prevention, Detection, Evaluation, and Treatment of High Blood Pressure: The JNC 7 report. *JAMA.* 2003;289:2560.
4. Vasan RS, Larson MG, Leip EP. Impact of high-normal blood pressure on the risk of cardiovascular disease. *N Engl J Med.* 2001;345:1291–1297.
5. The sixth report of the Joint National Committee on detection, evaluation, and diagnosis of high blood pressure (JNC VI). *Arch Intern Med.* 1997;157:2413.
6. Staessen JA, Wang J, Bianchi G, et al. Essential hypertension. *Lancet.* 2003;361:1629–1641.
7. Elliott P, Stamler J, Nichols R, et al. Intersalt Cooperative Research Group. Intersalt revisited: Further analyses of 24 hour sodium excretion and blood pressure within and across populations. *BMJ.* 1996;312(7041):1249–1253.
8. Thompson D, Edelsberg J, Colditz GA, et al. Lifetime health and economic consequences of obesity. *Arch Intern Med.* 1999;159(18):2177–2183.
9. Franklin SS, Jacobs MJ, Wong ND, et al. Predominance of isolated systolic hypertension among middle-aged and elderly US hypertensives: Analysis based on National Health and Nutrition Examination Survey (NHANES) III. *Hypertension.* 2001;37(3):869–874.
10. Izzo JLJ, Levy D, Black HR. Clinical advisory statement. Importance of systolic blood pressure in older Americans. *Hypertension.* 2000;35(5):1021–1024.
11. Young JH, Klag M, Muntner PJ, et al. Blood pressure and decline in kidney function: Findings from the Systolic Hypertension in the Elderly Program (SHEP). *J Am Soc Nephrol.* 2002;13(11):2776–2782.
12. Franklin SS, Gustin W, Wong ND, et al. The Framingham Heart Study. Hemodynamic patterns of age-related changes in blood pressure. *Circulation.* 1997;96(1):308–315.
13. Lewington S, Clarke R, Qizilbash N, et al. Age-specific relevance of usual blood pressure to vascular mortality: A meta-analysis of individual data for one million adults in 61 prospective studies. *Lancet.* 2002;360(9349):1903–1913.
14. Franklin SS, Larson MG, Khan SA, et al. Does the relation of blood pressure to coronary heart disease risk change with aging? The Framingham Heart Study. *Circulation.* 2001;103(9):1245–1249.
15. Psaty BM, Furberg CD, Kuller LH, et al. Association between blood pressure level and the risk of myocardial infarction, stroke, and total mortality: The cardiovascular health study. *Arch Intern Med.* 2001;161(9):1183–1192.
16. Lorell BH, Carabello BA. Left ventricular hypertrophy: Pathogenesis, detection, and prognosis. *Circulation.* 2000;102(4):470–479.
17. Vakili BA, Okin PM, Devereux RB. Prognostic implications of left ventricular hypertrophy. *Am Heart J.* 2001;141(3):334–341.
18. Staessen JA, Fagard R, Thijs L, et al. Randomised double-blind comparison of placebo and active treatment for older patients with isolated systolic hypertension. The systolic hypertension in Europe (Syst-Eur) trial investigators. *Lancet.* 1997;350(9080):757–764.
19. Lewington S, Clarke R, Qizilbash N, et al. Prospective Studies Collaboration. Age-specific relevance of usual blood pressure to vascular mortality: A meta-analysis of individual data for one million adults in 61 prospective studies. *Lancet.* 2002;360:1903–1913.
20. Wilson PW. Established risk factors and coronary artery disease: The Framingham Study. *Am J Hypertens.* 1994;7(7 Pt 2):7S–12S.
21. Coresh J, Wei GL, McQuillan G, et al. Prevalence of high blood pressure and elevated serum creatinine level in the United States: Findings from the Third National Health and Nutrition Examination Survey (1988–1994). *Arch Intern Med.* 2001;161(9):1207–1216.
22. Kaplan NM. Management of hypertensive emergencies. *Lancet.* 1994;344(8933):1335–1338.
23. Neal B, MacMahon S, Chapman N. Effects of ACE inhibitors, calcium antagonists, and other blood-pressure-lowering drugs: Results of prospectively designed overviews of randomised trials. Blood pressure lowering treatment Trialists' collaboration. *Lancet.* 2000;356(9246):1955–1964.
24. Wong ND, Thakral G, Franklin SS, et al. Preventing heart disease by controlling hypertension: Impact of hypertensive subtype, stage, age, and sex. *Am Heart J.* 2003;145(5):888–895.
25. He FJ, MacGregor GA. Fortnightly review: Beneficial effects of potassium. *BMJ.* 2001;323(7311):497–501.
26. Kotchen TA, McCarron DA. Dietary electrolytes and blood pressure. A statement for healthcare professionals from the American heart association nutrition committee. *Circulation.* 1998;98:613.
27. John JH, Ziebland S, Yudkin P, et al. Effects of fruit and vegetable consumption on plasma antioxidant concentrations and blood pressure: A randomised controlled trial. *Lancet.* 2002;359(9322):1969–1974.
28. Stamler J, Liu K, Ruth KJ, et al. Eight-year blood pressure change in middle-aged men: Relationship to multiple nutrients. *Hypertension.* 2002;39(5):1000–1006.
29. Klatsky AL, Friedman GD, Siegelaub AB, et al. Alcohol consumption and blood pressure Kaiser-permanent multiphasic health examination data. *N Engl J Med.* 1977;296(21):1194–2000.
30. Khot UN, Khot MB, Bajzer CT, et al. Prevalence of conventional risk factors in patients with coronary heart disease. *JAMA.* 2003;290(7):898–904.

31. Oliveria SA, Lapuerta P, McCarthy BD, et al. Physician-related barriers to the effective management of uncontrolled hypertension. *Arch Intern Med.* 2002;162:413.
32. Lindholm L, Ibsen H, Dahlof B, et al. Cardiovascular morbidity and mortality in patients with diabetes in the Losartan Intervention For Endpoint reduction in hypertension study (LIFE): A randomised trial against atenolol. *Lancet.* 2002;359(9311):1004–1010.
33. Dahlof B, Devereux RB, Kjeldsen SE, et al. Cardiovascular morbidity and mortality in the Losartan Intervention For Endpoint reduction in hypertension study (LIFE): A randomised trial against atenolol. *Lancet.* 2002;359(9311):995–1003.
34. Grundy SM, Cleeman JI, Rifkind BM, et al. Cholesterol lowering in the elderly population. Coordinating committee of the National Cholesterol Education Program. *Arch Intern Med.* 1999;159(15):1670–1678.
35. Third report of the National Cholesterol Education Program (NCEP) expert panel on detection, evaluation, and treatment of high blood cholesterol in adults (Adult Treatment Panel III). *Circulation.* 2002;106:3143.
36. ALLHAT Officers and Coordinators for the ALLHAT Collaborative Research Group. Major outcomes in high-risk hypertensive patients randomized to angiotensin-converting enzyme inhibitor or calcium channel blocker vs diuretic: The Antihypertensive and Lipid-Lowering treatment to Prevent Heart Attack Trial (ALLHAT). *JAMA.* 2002;288(23):2981–2997.
37. Kreisberg RA, Kasim S. Cholesterol metabolism and aging. *Am J Med.* 1987;82(1B):54–60.
38. Miettinen TA, Pyorala K, Olsson AG, et al. Cholesterol-lowering therapy in women and elderly patients with myocardial infarction or angina pectoris: Findings from the Scandinavian Simvastatin Survival Study (4S). *Circulation.* 1997;96(12):4211–4218.
39. Lewis SJ, Moye LA, Sacks FM, et al. Effect of pravastatin on cardiovascular events in older patients with myocardial infarction and cholesterol levels in the average range. Results of the Cholesterol and Recurrent Events (CARE) trial. *Ann Intern Med.* 1998;129(9):681–689.
40. Hunt D, Young P, Simes J, et al. Benefits of pravastatin on cardiovascular events and mortality in older patients with coronary heart disease are equal to or exceed those seen in younger patients: Results from the LIPID trial. *Ann Intern Med.* 2001;134(10):931–940.
41. Heart Protection Study Collaborative Group. MRC/BHF Heart Protection Study of cholesterol lowering with simvastatin in 20,536 high-risk individuals: A randomised placebo-controlled trial. *Lancet.* 2002;360(9326):7–22.
42. Shepherd J, Cobbe SM, Ford I, et al. West of Scotland Coronary Prevention Study Group. Prevention of coronary heart disease with pravastatin in men with hypercholesterolemia. *N Engl J Med.* 1995;333(20):1301–1307.
43. Downs JR, Clearfield M, Weis S, et al. Air Force/Texas Coronary Atherosclerosis Prevention Study. Primary prevention of acute coronary events with lovastatin in men and women with average cholesterol levels: Results of AFCAPS/TexCAPS. *JAMA.* 1998;279(20):1615–1622.
44. Grundy SM, Cleeman JI, Merz CN, et al. Implications of recent clinical trials for the National Cholesterol Education Program adult treatment Panel III guidelines. *Circulation.* 2004;110(2):227–239.
45. Grundy SM, Balady GJ, Criqui MH, et al. When to start cholesterol-lowering therapy in patients with coronary heart disease. A statement for healthcare professionals from the American heart association task force on risk reduction. *Circulation.* 1997;95(6):1683–1685.

25 Peripheral Arterial Disease

Gregory S. Cherr

CLINICAL PEARLS 321

SIGNIFICANCE OF PERIPHERAL ARTERIAL DISEASE FOR THE OLDER PATIENT 321

SYMPTOMS 321

DISEASE BACKGROUND 322
Pathophysiology of Peripheral Arterial Disease 322
Incidence and Prevalence of Peripheral Arterial Disease 323
Impact of Peripheral Arterial Disease on Survival 323
Impact of Peripheral Arterial Disease on Functional Status 323
Etiology of and Risk Factors for Peripheral Arterial Disease 323

EVALUATION OF THE PATIENT WITH PERIPHERAL ARTERIAL DISEASE 323
Differential Diagnosis of the Patient with Exercise-Induced Leg Pain 323
Differential Diagnosis of the Patient with Leg Pain at Rest 324
History 326
Physical Examination 327
Laboratory Examinations for Patients with Peripheral Arterial Disease 327
Radiologic Studies 327

MANAGEMENT OF THE PATIENT WITH PERIPHERAL ARTERIAL DISEASE 328
Lifestyle Recommendations 328
Medications 329

SURGICAL REVASCULARIZATION FOR THE PATIENT WITH PERIPHERAL ARTERIAL DISEASE 330
Indications 330
Results 330
Perioperative Risks 330
Preoperative Evaluation/Risk Reduction 330
Postoperative Care 331
Patient Monitoring/Secondary Prevention 331

AMPUTATION FOR THE PATIENT WITH PERIPHERAL ARTERIAL DISEASE 331
Indications 331
Results 331
Perioperative Risks 332
Preoperative Evaluation/Risk Reduction 332
Postoperative Care 332
Patient Monitoring/Secondary Prevention 332

ANGIOPLASTY/STENTING FOR THE PATIENT WITH PERIPHERAL ARTERIAL DISEASE 332
Indications 332
Results 332
Perioperative Risks 333
Preoperative Evaluation/Risk Reduction 333
Postoperative Care 333
Patient Monitoring/Secondary Prevention 333

CLINICAL PEARLS

- All patients with peripheral arterial disease (PAD) require atherosclerotic risk factor modification, antiplatelet therapy, and education regarding lifestyle modifications, including exercise therapy.
- Consider revascularization for disabling claudication, ischemic rest pain, gangrene, or ulcers.
- Below-knee amputation is recommended for ambulatory patients with adequate cognitive ability to participate in rehabilitation.
- Bedridden patients and those with severe dementia will have fewer complications with an above-knee amputation.
- Perioperative β-blockade is used to reduce the risk of coronary artery events.
- Surgery has better long-term results but higher perioperative risks.
- Technologic improvements in angioplasty/stenting have improved results and lowered the risk in patients.
- Percutaneous intervention is performed with local anesthesia and sedation; therefore, cardiac stress testing is rarely required.
- After surgery or angioplasty/stenting, surveillance vascular laboratory studies are used to monitor for progression of disease or graft/stent stenosis.

Peripheral arterial disease (PAD) is common among the elderly.[1,2] PAD may be asymptomatic or cause symptoms ranging from mild (claudication) to disabling (lower extremity gangrene). Furthermore, PAD is associated with a high risk of subsequent cardiovascular events such as stroke and myocardial infarction (MI).[2]

Recently, remarkable technologic and medical advances have been made in the care of patients with PAD. These developments have led to improvements in functional status, quality of life and survival.[2] Furthermore, these advances may benefit the most sick and frail patients with PAD. Medical treatment with 3-hydroxy-3-methylglutaryl coenzyme A (HMG-CoA) reductase inhibitors (statins) has improved survival, and cilostazol has been shown to significantly improve claudication symptoms.[3,4] Ongoing research is defining the role of medications such as clopidogrel and glycoprotein IIb-IIIa inhibitors. β-Blocker therapy has reduced the perioperative cardiac risk for surgical procedures.[5] Advances in radiologic equipment have allowed sophisticated combined open/endovascular procedures to be performed in the operating room. Finally, improved outcomes may be realized with new medical devices such as cuffed prosthetic bypass grafts and tissue-engineered bypass conduits.

Vascular surgery is undergoing rapid and profound changes involving minimally invasive endovascular procedures. Traditionally the purview of interventional radiologists, these procedures are increasingly being performed by both vascular surgeons and cardiologists. New therapies such as carotid angioplasty/stenting with distal protection devices and placement of covered stent grafts or drug-eluting stents will likely become the standard of care in the future.

Care of the patient with PAD is stimulating and demanding. Recent advances have only made this field more challenging and rewarding. This chapter will present a broad understanding of the issues relevant to the care of the patient with PAD.

SIGNIFICANCE OF PERIPHERAL ARTERIAL DISEASE FOR THE OLDER PATIENT

PAD is frequently underdiagnosed and undertreated in the elderly.[1,2] The incidence and prevalence of atherosclerotic occlusive disease (coronary, cerebrovascular, and PAD) increases with age. The survival of patients with atherosclerotic occlusive disease is increasing, although many patients live with significant (and possibly preventable) reductions in functional status and quality of life. The notion that atherosclerotic occlusive disease is a normal and untreatable part of aging is false. Quite the opposite, recognition and aggressive treatment of atherosclerotic occlusive disease and its associated risk factors have been shown to reduce the risk of primary or secondary ischemic events (such as MI, stroke, or PAD).[2,3] Therefore, appropriate therapy (both medical and surgical) plays a significant role in prolonging both the length and quality of life for our aging population.

SYMPTOMS

Patients with PAD may have no complaints or severe symptoms, including claudication or pain at rest. Patients with claudication typically describe exercise-induced calf or thigh/buttock pain that is reproducible and relieved by rest. However, a significant proportion of patients with PAD will not describe typical symptoms. Some patients avoid the pain by avoiding exercise altogether. Others describe milder pain that does not cause them to stop walking.[1,6] With increasing recognition of the spectrum of symptoms of milder PAD, greater vigilance is required to identify patients who may benefit from medical therapy and possibly arterial revascularization.

The symptoms of patients with more severe PAD are easier to recognize. Patients with ischemic rest pain describe a constant, throbbing pain often located in the toes or the ball of the foot. The pain is usually worse with leg elevation and improves with leg dependency. Frequently, narcotics reduce pain but do not completely alleviate it. These patients also note worsening pain with ambulation and sometimes foot ulceration or gangrene. Topics associated with PAD are listed in Table 25.1.

TABLE 25.1
TOPICS ASSOCIATED WITH PERIPHERAL ARTERIAL DISEASE

Diagnosis	ICD-9 Code
Atherosclerosis of the extremities with intermittent claudication	440.21
Atherosclerosis of the extremities with rest pain	440.22
Atherosclerosis of the extremities with ulceration	440.23
Atherosclerosis of the extremities with gangrene	440.24
Coronary artery disease	414.01
Remote myocardial infarction	412
Angina pectoris	413
Carotid artery disease without cerebral infarction	433.10
Carotid artery disease with cerebral infarction	433.11
Tobacco use disorder	305.1
History of tobacco use	V15.82
Diabetes mellitus with neurologic manifestations	250.6
Diabetes mellitus with peripheral circulatory disorders	250.7
Pure hypercholesterolemia	272.0
Hypertension	401.1
Peripheral embolism to legs	444.2
Atherothrombotic microembolism	445.02
Popliteal artery entrapment syndrome	443.9
Popliteal artery adventitial cystic disease	443.9
Thromboangiitis obliterans (Buerger disease)	443.1
Popliteal artery aneurysm	442.3
Polyneuropathy in diabetes	357.2
Chronic venous insufficiency with pain	459.39
Venous claudication	459.19
Deep venous thrombosis of common femoral vein	451.11
Deep venous thrombosis of superficial femoral, popliteal, or tibial veins	451.19
Spinal stenosis, lumbar region	724.02
Lumbar spondylosis with myelopathy	721.42
Lumbar region intervertebral disc disorder with myelopathy	722.73
Osteoarthritis of the hip	715.15
Osteoarthritis of the knee	715.16

DISEASE BACKGROUND

CASE ONE

A 68-year-old woman presents to her new primary care physician for an initial evaluation and describes left calf claudication at approximately half a mile. Past medical history is significant for diabetes, tobacco abuse, hypertension, and a left iliac angioplasty 2 years earlier. Medications include a β-blocker, angiotensin-converting enzyme inhibitor, and an oral hypoglycemic. Physical examination confirms the presence of reduced peripheral pulses. She is started on aspirin, a statin (after a fasting lipid profile reveals dyslipidemia), and bupropion (for tobacco cessation). After 6 months, her symptoms have progressed to claudication at two blocks. She is started on cilostazol and again encouraged to quit smoking. Six months later, her symptoms have become disabling, with pain at less than one block. She is referred to a vascular surgeon who confirms significant infrainguinal arterial disease with a lower extremity arterial study (ultrasound) and then arteriography. Angiography/stenting is unsuccessful and bypass surgery is advised. She has a moderate functional status, intermediate clinical predictors of a perioperative cardiac event and will undergo a high-risk procedure (bypass surgery). She has a cardiac stress test that reveals no evidence of ischemia. Perioperative β-blockade is maximized and she undergoes an uneventful femoral–popliteal bypass. To reduce the risk of graft thrombosis, ultrasound graft surveillance is performed in the postoperative period, at 6 months, and then annually.

Pathophysiology of Peripheral Arterial Disease

Atherosclerosis results from a chronic inflammatory state. The final common pathway for the many known risk factors for atherosclerosis is injury to the artery wall. This injury causes chronic inflammation and the subsequent development of atherosclerotic plaques. Persistent inflammation leads to plaque progression or rupture (with a subsequent acute ischemic event). Atherosclerotic risk factor reduction aims to reduce the triggers for chronic inflammation and the resulting plaque formation, progression, and eventual plaque instability.[7]

Incidence and Prevalence of Peripheral Arterial Disease

In community screening programs of older community-dwelling Americans, PAD has been found in 11% to 29% of subjects. In more than half of the subjects, PAD had not been previously diagnosed.[1,8] PAD was more prevalent in men than in women, but the ratio of men to women appears to be falling as more women develop cardiovascular diseases.[8] PAD was diagnosed in similar proportions of elderly white, black, Hispanic, and "other" subjects.[1]

Compared to coronary artery disease (CAD), patients with PAD receive less aggressive atherosclerotic risk factor modification and antiplatelet therapy.[1,8] Underdiagnosis and undertreatment of PAD likely represent a missed opportunity for treatment of claudication as well as secondary prevention of atherosclerotic events.[1,8]

Impact of Peripheral Arterial Disease on Survival

Patients with PAD have a significantly increased risk of death over time. The 5-year survival for patients with claudication is approximately 65% (and is consistent among many population-based studies).[2] Most patients die from CAD. The survival rate is worse for patients with ischemic rest pain or gangrene. Even when controlled for atherosclerotic risk factors (diabetes, hypertension, tobacco abuse, dyslipidemia) and prevalent cardiovascular disease (such as CAD or cerebrovascular disease), patients with PAD have a significantly worse survival compared to patients without PAD.[2]

Impact of Peripheral Arterial Disease on Functional Status

Approximately 25% of patients will have worsening symptoms over time, although only a small proportion (<5%) will require surgery. Amputation is a great fear for patients with PAD. These patients are reassured to know that only 1% to 2% of those with claudication will eventually require a major amputation.

The clinician should be alert to the impact of lifestyle adaptation on symptom reporting. Many patients with PAD report that their symptoms are stable when in fact they have progressively reduced their activity level to avoid symptoms.[9]

The long-term functional status for older patients undergoing amputation is poor. Compared to younger patients, older patients undergoing major amputation are less likely to achieve full mobility. The prognosis is even worse for older women and bilateral amputees. Patients undergoing below-knee amputation are two to three times more likely to regain full mobility than those with above-knee amputations.[2]

Etiology of and Risk Factors for Peripheral Arterial Disease

In the overwhelming proportion of patients, PAD is a manifestation of atherosclerotic occlusive disease. Other less common etiologies of PAD include arterial embolism, popliteal artery entrapment syndrome, popliteal artery adventitial cystic disease, arterial dissection, trauma, thromboangiitis obliterans (Buerger disease), and popliteal artery aneurysm.

The predominant risk factors for atherosclerotic PAD include increasing age, preexisting cardiovascular disease (CAD, cerebrovascular disease), hypertension, tobacco abuse, dyslipidemia, and diabetes mellitus.

EVALUATION OF THE PATIENT WITH PERIPHERAL ARTERIAL DISEASE

Differential Diagnosis of the Patient with Exercise-Induced Leg Pain

There are many causes of exercise-associated leg pain or weakness (Table 25.2). It is important to differentiate intermittent claudication from the other causes of exercise-induced leg pain.

Nerve Root Compression

Compression of a nerve root may cause peripheral nerve dysfunction and associated leg pain with exercise. Compression of a peripheral nerve root is typically caused by a herniated disc or osteophyte formation. Patients note leg pain that usually starts soon after walking and is often present upon standing. Typically, the pain is experienced along the back of the leg, although occasionally it is present in only the calf or lower leg. For some patients, the pain may be present at rest and exacerbated by exercise. Patients may also note leg weakness, numbness, or paresthesias. Stopping does not relieve symptoms unless the patient also sits or bends forward. The onset of symptoms is gradual and the patient may note a history of back problems. Surgical decompression of the nerve root may be indicated for patients with severe symptoms.

Osteoarthritis

Osteoarthritis of the hip or knee may produce exercise-induced leg pain. The pain is often worse in the morning and when beginning movement. The severity of pain is variable from day to day. Arthritis-associated pain is not promptly relieved by cessation of exercise. Finally, many patients note exacerbation of the symptoms of arthritis with changes in the weather. Exercise programs, nonsteroidal anti-inflammatory medications, and, occasionally, surgery are indicated for the treatment of symptomatic osteoarthritis.

TABLE 25.2
DIFFERENTIAL DIAGNOSIS OF EXERCISE-INDUCED LEG PAIN

Disease	Symptoms	Diagnosis
Claudication	Exercise-induced buttock, thigh or calf pain; reproducible	Atherosclerotic risk factors, prevalent cardiovascular disease, vascular laboratory study, arteriogram
Popliteal artery entrapment syndrome	Exercise-induced calf pain; reproducible	Arteriogram, MRI, CT scan, absence of traditional atherosclerotic risk factors
Popliteal artery adventitial cystic disease	Exercise-induced calf pain; reproducible	Arteriogram, MRI, CT scan, absence of traditional atherosclerotic risk factors
Thromboangiitis obliterans (Buerger disease)	Exercise-induced foot pain, pain at rest, ulcers, gangrene	Young patient with tobacco abuse and absence of other traditional atherosclerotic risk factors, arteriogram
Diabetic peripheral neuropathy	Pain (shooting, burning); unrelated to exercise	History, physical examination, nerve-conduction studies
Venous claudication	Exercise-induced leg pain with bursting, tight sensation	History of deep venous thrombosis and chronic venous disease, ultrasound
Osteoarthritis	Exercise-induced aching pain (knee, hip)	History, physical examination, x-rays
Spinal stenosis	Pain/numbness of back and/or legs; leg cramping or weakness; symptoms worse with exercise or standing	History, MRI

MRI, magnetic resonance imaging; CT, computed tomography.

Popliteal Artery Entrapment Syndrome

Popliteal artery entrapment syndrome is caused by obstruction of the popliteal artery by an abnormally located portion of the gastrocnemius muscle. Patients note exercise-induced calf or foot pain that is relieved by rest. Physical examination is normal with palpable pedal pulses. While those affected are often young, the diagnosis should be considered in any patient without atherosclerotic risk factors. Surgery is indicated to correct the anatomic abnormality and alleviate symptoms.

Popliteal Artery Adventitial Cystic Disease

Popliteal artery adventitial cystic disease is a rare cause of stenosis or occlusion of the popliteal artery. An idiopathic cystic lesion develops in the wall of the popliteal artery and encroaches on the lumen of the artery. Patients may present with typical symptoms of intermittent claudication with arterial stenosis but others may have ischemic rest pain if the popliteal artery is occluded. The diagnosis may be suspected in older patients without typical atherosclerotic risk factors. The location of the arterial pathology (isolated to the popliteal artery) should also alert the clinician to the possibility of popliteal artery adventitial cystic disease. Surgical repair is indicated to alleviate symptoms and prevent progression of the lesion. Emergency surgery is necessary for limb salvage in patients presenting with acute popliteal artery thrombosis.

Chronic Venous Insufficiency

Chronic venous insufficiency is caused by venous hypertension. Leg pain is typically mild and associated with leg heaviness or tiredness. The symptoms are usually worse at the end of the day and relieved by leg elevation or recumbency. Although primarily caused by venous valvular incompetence, a minority of patients will be symptomatic secondary to remote deep venous thrombosis and resulting venous obstruction. Physical examination reveals chronic skin changes of the calf (brawny edema or lipodermatosclerosis) and occasionally varicose veins. Treatment includes graded compression stockings, leg elevation, and skin care to prevent infection/ulcers. A minority of patients will benefit from surgical treatment of varicose veins or incompetent superficial veins (such as the greater saphenous vein).

Venous Claudication

Venous claudication is caused by severe venous hypertension. Patients with this rare disease note exercise-induced leg pain most often in the hip and thigh. The pain is described as a tight or "bursting" sensation. Rest relieves the pain and recovery may be aided by leg elevation. The patients have a history of severe venous obstructive disease from prior iliofemoral deep venous thrombosis. Physical examination usually reveals leg edema and lipodermatosclerosis. Treatment is supportive and includes graded compression stockings, leg elevation, and skin care. Some patients may benefit from surgical therapy with venous bypass or venous valve replacement, although the results of these procedures are generally disappointing.

Differential Diagnosis of the Patient with Leg Pain at Rest

There are many causes of leg pain at rest (Table 25.3). Chronic lower extremity ischemia is a common cause of

TABLE 25.3
DIFFERENTIAL DIAGNOSIS OF LEG PAIN AT REST

Disease	Symptoms	Diagnosis
Acute on chronic lower extremity ischemia	Previous claudication with progression to leg/foot pain at rest	History, physical examination, vascular laboratory study, arteriogram
Acute arterial occlusion	Abrupt onset of ischemia with leg pain, neuromuscular deficit	History, physical examination, electrocardiogram, cardiac echocardiogram, arteriogram, operation
Thromboangiitis obliterans (Buerger disease)	Foot pain, ulcers, gangrene	History, physical examination, arteriogram
Popliteal artery aneurysm	Abrupt onset of ischemia with leg pain, neuromuscular deficit	History, physical examination, ultrasound, arteriogram
Diabetic peripheral neuropathy	Pain (shooting, burning); unrelated to exercise	History, physical examination, nerve-conduction studies

leg pain at rest in the elderly. Patients note a gradual progression of symptoms from mild claudication to disabling claudication to pain at rest.

Peripheral Emboli

Peripheral emboli cause the abrupt onset of leg ischemia with severe pain and varying degrees of neuromuscular compromise. Most peripheral emboli originate in the heart and may be caused by a left ventricular aneurysm, acute MI, or arrhythmia. Other less common causes include valvular heart disease or paradoxical embolism. Most patients do not have a history of claudication. Urgent intervention is required to prevent limb loss and includes a bolus of unfractionated heparin (100 units per kg intravenously) and evaluation by a vascular surgeon.

Atherothrombotic Microembolism (Blue-toe Syndrome)

Atherothrombotic microembolism is an unusual cause of lower extremity pain at rest. Atheroembolism is the proximal to distal movement of microscopic debris such as cholesterol crystals, thrombus, or fibrinous platelet aggregates. The most common cause is aortoiliac arterial disease (aneurysm or occlusive disease), followed by infrainguinal occlusive arterial disease, degenerating arterial bypass grafts and diffuse "shaggy" atheromatous disease of the thoracic aorta. Patients complain of constant severe foot or toe pain. The symptoms are acute at onset and are unrelated to activity, foot position, and so on. Physical examination is remarkable for palpable foot pulses and violaceous discoloration of the toes or forefoot. Extremely small emboli may cause patchy ischemia, contiguous areas of ischemia and cyanosis, and the appearance of livido reticularis on physical examination. Treatment includes pain control, antiplatelet therapy, and prevention of recurrent atheroembolism (usually requiring arterial reconstruction). Early amputation is reserved for patients with superinfection, as many patients will have healing of lesions that initially appeared to be frankly gangrenous.

Peripheral Bypass Graft Occlusion

Leg pain at rest may be caused by occlusion of a bypass graft. Patients may note a gradual progression of claudication (more common with a vein graft) or acute ischemia with no antecedent symptoms (typical of a prosthetic bypass graft). Anticoagulation and recanalization of the bypass graft (thrombolytic therapy or surgery) should be considered to attempt limb salvage.

Arterial Dissection or Trauma

Arterial trauma may cause leg ischemia and pain at rest. Often overlooked is iatrogenic trauma that occurs during arteriography or femoral line placement. These procedures may also cause an arterial dissection that leads to leg ischemia. Finally, thoracic aortic dissection may progress to involve the iliac arteries and cause leg ischemia. Patients note severe interscapular or back pain and are typically hypertensive.

Thromboangiitis Obliterans (Buerger disease)

Thromboangiitis obliterans is an idiopathic disease resulting in severe inflammation of the medium and small arteries of the feet or hands. Patients may complain of calf or foot claudication, digital ulcers, or gangrene. Typically, patients affected are young (<50 years) tobacco abusers with arterial occlusive disease found only below the knee. Traditional atherosclerotic risk factors (beside tobacco abuse) are absent. Physical examination reveals cool extremities with diminished or absent distal pulses and often toe ulcers or gangrene. Treatment consists of pain control, assistance with tobacco cessation, and selective amputation. Revascularization is technically difficult as suitable distal target vessels are usually absent.

Thrombosed Popliteal Artery Aneurysm

Thrombosis of a popliteal artery aneurysm is an unusual cause of leg pain at rest. Patients note the acute onset of leg pain. A minority of patients will have claudication from chronic aneurysm occlusion with collateralization or distal embolization of aneurysm mural thrombus. Concomitant arterial aneurysms are common—a contralateral popliteal artery aneurysm is present in half of the patients, a femoral artery aneurysm in approximately 40%, and an abdominal aortic aneurysm in >50%. Physical examination may reveal the presence of another arterial aneurysm. The diagnosis of popliteal artery aneurysm can be confirmed by ultrasonography, computed tomography (CT) scan, or magnetic resonance imaging (MRI). For patients presenting with acute leg ischemia from a thrombosed popliteal aneurysm, thrombolytic therapy before revascularization increases the chances of limb salvage by allowing identification of outflow vessels.

Diabetic Neuropathy

Diabetic neuropathy is a frequent complication of diabetes in the elderly. Patients typically describe lower leg and foot pain that is unrelated to exercise. The pain is intermittent and is often described as "shooting," "burning," or "stabbing." Physical examination and, occasionally, nerve-conduction studies are used to confirm the diagnosis. Treatment with tricyclic antidepressants and gabapentin may provide some benefit.

Deep Venous Thrombosis

An extensive deep venous thrombosis may cause leg pain and associated leg edema. Although these patients usually have normal arterial circulation, peripheral pulses may be difficult to palpate due to leg edema. A warm foot with normal capillary refill helps to distinguish a patient with a deep venous thrombosis from one with ischemia, who typically will have a cool, cyanotic foot with sluggish or absent capillary refill.

History

A careful history is important to elicit the symptoms of PAD. Symptoms may include claudication and/or ischemic rest pain. Claudication is classically described as exercise-induced leg pain relieved promptly by rest. The symptoms are reproducible. The site of arterial disease dictates the location of leg symptoms. Patients with aortoiliac disease describe symptoms of the thigh and buttocks including aching pain associated with weakness or fatigue. Men may also have impotence. Patients with disease of the femoral, popliteal, or tibial arteries note a cramping pain of the calf with exercise.

Although many patients experience the "classic" symptoms described in the preceding text, a significant number may have atypical complaints.[1] Many patients complain of exercise-induced leg tiredness, heaviness, or weakness. Some patients may note exercise-induced pain that does not stop them from walking. Others may experience back pain. Finally, some patients may describe intermittent exercise-induced leg pain, likely due to variations in the pace of ambulation. As few as 10% to 15% of patients with PAD have typical symptoms of claudication.[1] Awareness of the association between atypical leg symptoms and PAD will allow the clinician to diagnose many more patients with PAD and therefore prescribe appropriate medical therapy for these patients at high risk for subsequent atherosclerotic events.

Patients with ischemic rest pain describe a constant, severe, throbbing pain. The symptoms are worst in the toes or foot. The pain is exacerbated by leg elevation (such as lying in bed) and relieved by dependency (which increases perfusion through the effects of gravity). Narcotics may provide partial relief, but rarely do they totally alleviate the symptoms. To reduce pain, many patients with chronic ischemic rest pain sleep in a chair. These patients often have significant associated leg edema because their feet are constantly dependent.

The following questions are important to help differentiate symptoms of PAD from other causes of leg pain with exercise or at rest:[2]

When you walk, where do you have pain?
When did you first have the symptoms?
Have the symptoms improved or worsened over time?
How far can you walk before experiencing symptoms?
How far can you walk before the pain causes you to stop?
How long does it take the pain to resolve when you stop walking?
Does the pain occur every time you walk a certain distance?
What actions help to alleviate the pain (standing, sitting, lying, bending forward)?

Along with a thorough physical examination, this information will help to determine the etiology of leg symptoms.[2]

A review of systems can establish the presence of atherosclerotic risk factors that may increase the index of suspicion for PAD. It is also important to elicit a history of current or remote symptoms of concomitant end-organ ischemia (MI, angina, stroke, or transient ischemic attack) or other comorbidities (such as chronic lung disease or renal insufficiency) that may affect arteriography or possible surgical intervention.

To help with perioperative risk assessment, functional status should be assessed. Because ambulation is limited in patients with symptomatic PAD, many activities are difficult to perform. The author has found stair climbing to be a good functional assessment in patients with symptomatic PAD. Because stair climbing is a short, intense activity, many patients are able to walk one or more flights of stairs before developing symptoms of PAD.

Physical Examination

The clinician needs to avoid the temptation to focus solely on the vascular examination of the extremity. A thorough physical examination is required and should include a complete assessment of the cardiovascular system. A careful examination may uncover the presence of significant pathology such as a carotid bruit, asymmetric arm blood pressures (indicating significant occlusive disease of the great vessels), cardiac arrhythmias, or an abdominal aortic aneurysm.

Assessment of peripheral pulses is an essential part of the physical examination for both symptomatic and asymptomatic elderly patients. For the asymptomatic patient, the absence of distal pulses indicates the presence of PAD and is an indication for aggressive atherosclerotic risk factor reduction. This will be discussed in detail in the section on "Medical Management."

For patients with symptomatic PAD, it is important to palpate the femoral, popliteal, dorsalis pedis, and the posterior tibial artery pulses. Distal pulses will be abnormal. Often, pulses are graded with a confusing array of numerical scales. A preferable approach is to describe the pulse as normal, diminished, or absent. A prominent femoral or popliteal pulse should raise the suspicion of an aneurysm.

The feet should also be inspected for the presence of ulcers, gangrene, or neuropathy. The presence of edema, muscle atrophy, or changes in the skin color or temperature should also be noted. Patients with chronic ischemia may have pallor with leg elevation, redness of the foot when lowering the leg (dependent rubor), or "trophic" changes of the legs and feet, including loss of hair, dry skin, and thickened toenails.

A handheld Doppler probe can provide a wealth of information at the bedside. The probe can be used to better assess patients with leg edema and nonpalpable pulses. The ankle–brachial index (ABI) may also be calculated, using a ratio of the highest ankle systolic pressure (from the dorsalis pedis artery or posterior tibial artery) divided by the highest arm pressure. A blood pressure cuff is placed just above the ankle with the Doppler probe over the dorsalis pedis or posterior tibial artery and slowly deflated. The systolic pressure is noted with return of the flow in the artery. An ABI >0.90 is considered normal. Patients with claudication usually have an ABI <0.70, while those with ischemic rest pain have a ratio <0.50. An ABI of <0.30 indicates severe, limb-threatening ischemia.

Laboratory Examinations for Patients with Peripheral Arterial Disease

A complete blood count with platelet count should be obtained for patients with claudication. The hemoglobin or hematocrit level is used to identify patients with anemia or polycythemia, both of which may exacerbate symptoms of claudication. A baseline platelet count is useful should a patient develop thrombocytopenia after exposure to heparin (raising the suspicion of heparin-induced thrombocytopenia). The serum creatinine and blood urea nitrogen levels should be obtained (if not previously done). Renal dysfunction is asymptomatic and is more common in diabetic and/or hypertensive patients (who are also at high risk for developing PAD). Patients with abnormal renal function are at increased risk for nephrotoxicity with administration of contrast media, and prior knowledge allows changes in therapy that may avoid this devastating complication. A fasting lipid profile should be obtained. For patients with PAD, aggressive treatment of dyslipidemia (elevated low density lipoprotein [LDL] or triglyceride, or reduced high density lipoprotein [HDL]) reduces the risk of subsequent atherosclerotic events.[3] If indicated by history, the presence of diabetes mellitus may be assessed with a fasting glucose, hemoglobin A_{Ic}, or oral glucose tolerance test. Evidence is accumulating regarding the importance of subtle elevations of the C-reactive protein for the prognosis of patients with cardiovascular diseases. However, further data are needed before recommending this test routinely for patients with PAD.

Radiologic Studies

Appropriate radiologic studies are crucial in the diagnosis and management of PAD.

A vascular laboratory test is essential for the diagnosis of PAD. Performance by an accredited vascular laboratory (Intersocietal Commission for Accreditation of Vascular Laboratories [ICAVL]) ensures that the studies are sensitive, specific, and subject to an ongoing quality assurance program. A "lower extremity arterial study" includes a combination of tests such as an ABI, segmental pressures/waveforms, and duplex ultrasound arterial imaging. These tests give an excellent appraisal of the blood flow to the ankle, foot, and toes. Performing a lower extremity arterial study with exercise (walking or toe-raises) may identify patients with mild reductions of leg perfusion at rest but severe ischemia with exercise. The lower extremity arterial study is quick, inexpensive, and risk free. It provides important screening information regarding leg perfusion, but further, more precise anatomic studies are required to plan possible intervention.

CT angiogram or magnetic resonance (MR) angiogram may provide further diagnostic information. Both studies require equipment and expertise that may not be available at all institutions. However, both studies may provide adequate anatomic detail to guide in planning further interventions for patients with PAD. CT angiogram requires administration of contrast media and may cause nephrotoxicity. The clinician should note that the MR angiogram might not accurately discriminate between severe stenosis and complete occlusion. In the future, improvements in technique will likely lead to MR angiogram being the diagnostic study of choice for patients with PAD.

For patients with symptomatic PAD, arteriography remains the gold standard for diagnosis and planning of therapeutic intervention. Angiography carries a risk of morbidity, including severe contrast reaction, nephrotoxicity (increased in patients with diabetes and those with preexisting renal dysfunction), hemorrhage, and atheroembolism (all <1%).[2] Arteriography is expensive and may be unpleasant or uncomfortable for the patient. When appropriate, angioplasty/stenting may be performed at the same time as the diagnostic study. Angioplasty/stenting should be performed by or in consultation with a vascular surgeon, as an inappropriate or poorly planned intervention may cause difficulty with subsequent attempts at limb salvage.

MANAGEMENT OF THE PATIENT WITH PERIPHERAL ARTERIAL DISEASE

Care of the patient with PAD includes antiplatelet therapy, aggressive atherosclerotic risk factor modification, and serial assessment of the severity of symptoms. A minority of patients will also require revascularization (either surgical or percutaneous).

The expectations of treatment include addressing the symptoms of PAD (prevention of progression of symptoms, reduction of pain, maintenance of functional status and improvement of quality of life) and secondary prevention of atherosclerotic events such as development of symptoms in the contralateral leg, stroke, or MI.

The most important issue for patients with PAD is the prevention of subsequent atherosclerotic events. The diagnosis of PAD conveys a risk for both worsening leg ischemia as well as for remote cardiovascular events such as MI or stroke. An aggressive medical plan should be formulated to target risk factors shown to increase the risk of future events (such as tobacco abuse) combined with antiplatelet therapy, exercise, and diet changes. Medications for patients with PAD are summarized in Table 25.4.

Lifestyle Recommendations

Aggressive atherosclerotic risk factor modification includes lifestyle recommendations. Patients should be encouraged to remain active and exercise regularly. Many frail elderly patients are hesitant to increase their activity for fear of exacerbating chronic medical conditions or causing injury to the legs by walking to the point of claudication. Patients with PAD are often reassured to learn that regular activity will often lead to a gradual increase in their pain-free walking distance. The mechanism of improvement in walking distance over time is likely multifactorial, with improvements in both leg function as well as cardiovascular performance.

Patients should also be counseled regarding a "heart-healthy" diet. Generally, this consists of a low-salt, low-fat diet. At present, inadequate data exist to fully understand the effect of low-carbohydrate, high-fat, and high-protein diets on atherosclerosis and cardiovascular events. Many patients benefit from frequent counseling (and positive feedback) regarding fundamental changes in eating habits, such as avoiding "fast food" or substituting fat-free milk for whole milk.

Obesity may be related to both claudication distance as well as risk of subsequent cardiovascular events for patients with PAD. Therefore, weight loss is a priority for these patients. Overweight and obese patients require honest advice regarding weight loss. Many strategies for weight loss complement the recommendations for exercise and diet. However, further guidance is often necessary for patients with significant weight problems. Changing these behaviors requires persistence from the health care provider.

Tobacco Abuse

Cigarette smoking is a risk factor for developing PAD and progression of the disease. Smokers are also at increased risk of amputation, MI, stroke, and death.[2] Therefore, tobacco cessation is a critical part of the medical management of PAD. The health care provider must give consistent counseling regarding the importance of tobacco cessation and possible strategies for quitting. A direct relationship exists between the amount of time the clinician spends counseling the patient and the

TABLE 25.4
MEDICATIONS FOR PATIENTS WITH PERIPHERAL ARTERIAL DISEASE

Medication	Indication	Quality of Evidence
Aspirin	PAD	Level A
Clopidogrel	PAD	Level A
Cilostazol	Nondisabling claudication	Level A
β-Blockade	Reduce perioperative risk of cardiovascular events for PAD surgery	Level A
Bupropion	Tobacco abuse	Level A
Nicotine replacement	Tobacco abuse	Level A
Statin	PAD and dyslipidemia	Level A

PAD, Peripheral arterial disease.

eventual tobacco cessation.[10] When available, support groups may be of benefit.[10] Medical therapy may double the success rate for tobacco cessation and includes nicotine replacement and/or bupropion (Evidence Level A).[10] Nicotine replacement is available as patches, gum, inhalers, and nasal sprays. The type of nicotine replacement therapy used should be individualized, as they are all equally effective.

Diabetes Mellitus

For patients with diabetes, intensive glycemic control reduces the risk of microvascular complications such as nephropathy and retinopathy. However, little evidence exists to prove that tight blood sugar control will prevent macrovascular events. Because patients with diabetes have such a high rate of cardiovascular events, aggressive modification of other atherosclerotic risk factors plays an even more important role for them.

Dyslipidemia

For patients with PAD, the National Cholesterol Education Program (NCEP)[3] guidelines recommend obtaining a fasting lipid profile. For patients with an elevated LDL despite dietary changes, statin therapy (HMG-CoA reductase drugs) should be considered (Evidence Level A). The NCEP guidelines recommend a treatment goal of an LDL <100 mg per dL (Evidence Level A).[3] Recent evidence suggests that therapy to lower the LDL even more is of benefit for patients with CAD. Further data are needed for patients with PAD. Finally, patients with low HDL or high triglyceride levels should be considered for alternative medications such as niacin or fibrate therapy.

Hypertension

Blood pressure control reduces the risk of subsequent MI, stroke, and cardiovascular death (Evidence Level A).[2] However, little data exist to evaluate the effect of treatment of hypertension on claudication and progression of PAD. Because PAD is considered equivalent in risk to CAD, treatment recommendations for patients with hypertension are similar for both sets of patients. In general, patients with PAD and hypertension should be treated using Joint National Committee (JNC) guidelines (Evidence Level B).[11] Occasionally, patients with symptomatic PAD may experience worsening symptoms when blood pressure is lowered precipitously. In general, β-blockade therapy is well tolerated by patients with claudication and may be prescribed as indicated by other cardiovascular conditions.

Foot Ulcer Prevention

For patients with diabetes, foot ulcers are the leading cause of hospitalization and often result in amputation.[2] Preventive therapy is critical to reduce the risk of foot ulceration. Besides a high prevalence of PAD, patients with diabetes are at increased risk for foot ulceration because of sensory and motor neuropathy. Abnormal foot sensation prevents the normal response to painful stimuli. Changes in foot shape are caused by motor neuropathy and lead to pressure points, often over the plantar portion of the metatarsal heads. Patients and families should be educated regarding the importance of regular foot examination, daily foot washing, and wearing clean socks and protective footwear at all times. When examining a patient with diabetes, the health care provider should regularly inspect the feet as well as reinforce the importance of diabetic foot care (Evidence Level C). Many patients with diabetes will also benefit from routine care from a podiatrist.

Patients with PAD and delirium or severe dementia are also at increased risk for foot ulceration. When incapacitated by an acute medical illness, a patient with PAD (even mild disease) may develop foot or leg pressure ulcers. Likewise, patients with severe dementia and PAD are prone to pressure ulcers. Prevention is important, as these ulcers can result in significant morbidity, limb loss, or even death. Strategies for prevention of pressure ulcers are based on pressure relief such as frequent turning and heel protectors.

Medications

Antiplatelet Therapy

All patients with PAD should be considered for antiplatelet therapy. Even for patients with asymptomatic PAD, antiplatelet therapy reduces the risk of subsequent cardiovascular events.[12] Aspirin (325 mg per day) or clopidogrel (75 mg per day) may be prescribed for patients with PAD (Evidence Level A).[12] Given its lower cost, aspirin would seem to be the best option for first-line therapy. Insufficient data exist to recommend routine use of both aspirin and clopidogrel.

Pentoxifylline

Pentoxifylline is a xanthine derivative with rheologic properties that cause increased red blood cell deformity and decreased blood viscosity. Although it is prescribed for patients with claudication, no convincing evidence exists to support the use of pentoxifylline for these patients.[2,4] Randomized, controlled trials have failed to prove the superiority of pentoxifylline over placebo for the treatment of claudication. A statistically significant number of patients can walk 25% farther on pentoxifylline, but a clinically insignificant number of patients can walk 100% farther before experiencing symptoms. The drug does not reduce the risk of subsequent cardiovascular events. Contraindications for pentoxifylline therapy include a history of allergic reaction to methylxanthines such as theophylline or caffeine. The drug is generally well tolerated with a low risk of side effects.

Cilostazol

Cilostazol is a phosphodiesterase inhibitor that inhibits platelet aggregation and causes direct artery wall dilation.[4] For patients with claudication, therapy with cilostazol (100 mg PO b.i.d.) results in a 50% increase in walking distance when compared to placebo[4] (Evidence Level A). No evaluation of the effect of cilostazol on health-related quality of life has been performed. Given its high cost and moderate benefits, its use should likely be restricted to patients with severe claudication who have failed conservative therapy (risk factor modification and exercise therapy) and are not candidates for revascularization (Evidence Level C). Because the antiplatelet effect of cilostazol is weak, aspirin or clopidogrel therapy should be continued. Congestive heart failure is a contraindication to cilostazol therapy. Side effects of cilostazol therapy include headache, dizziness, tachycardia, palpitations, and diarrhea.

SURGICAL REVASCULARIZATION FOR THE PATIENT WITH PERIPHERAL ARTERIAL DISEASE

The decision to proceed with surgery for patients with PAD requires an honest assessment of the benefits versus the risks of the proposed procedure. Patients with PAD and foot gangrene, nonhealing ulcers or ischemic rest pain are at high risk for subsequent limb loss, making the decision to proceed with surgery easier. The decision to intervene with patients who have claudication is more difficult, as a similar degree of claudication distance may result in widely varying degrees of disability for different patients. For example, claudication after walking 100 meters may be well tolerated in a frail patient with a poor functional status. The same degree of claudication in a mail carrier will result in unacceptable disability. Given the significant risk of morbidity or even death with vascular surgery, extensive counseling is required before the patient and surgeon decide to proceed with surgery. A summary of treatment options is given in Table 25.5.

Indications

The indications for bypass surgery include disabling claudication, ischemic rest pain, gangrene, or nonhealing ulcers (Evidence Level C).[2] The definition of "disabling claudication" is vague and varies from patient to patient. Baseline functional status seems to be the most important factor that influences the decision to intervene with a patient who has claudication.

Results

After bypass surgery, the risk of subsequent limb loss is low. The risk of amputation or further intervention on the ipsilateral leg is increased in noncompliant patients and those who continue to smoke cigarettes. The long-term mortality after bypass surgery is 40% to 50% at 10 years, with most deaths caused by cardiovascular disease. The risk of death is increased for patients with generalized atherosclerosis, diabetes, and critical limb ischemia (rather than claudication).[2]

The results for patients undergoing surgery vary among surgeons and hospitals. Most surgeons track their own perioperative results and can provide this information to the interested referring physician or patient.

Perioperative Risks

For patients undergoing open surgical revascularization for symptomatic PAD, perioperative risks include death (2% to 5%), MI (1% to 2%), early graft occlusion, bleeding, infection, wound complications, and leg swelling.

Preoperative Evaluation/Risk Reduction

Infrainguinal bypass surgery is a high-risk operation. Further information necessary to assess perioperative risk

TABLE 25.5
AVAILABLE TREATMENT FOR PERIPHERAL ARTERIAL DISEASE

Therapy	Indications	Quality of Evidence
Bypass surgery	Disabling claudication	Level C
	Gangrene	Level C
	Nonhealing foot ulcer	Level C
Atherosclerotic risk factor modification	PAD	Level A
Antiplatelet therapy	PAD	Level A
Angioplasty/stenting	Nondisabling claudication	Poor
	Disabling claudication	Level C
	Gangrene	Level C
	Nonhealing foot ulcer	Level C
Amputation	Prohibitive risk for surgery and unsuccessful angioplasty/stenting	Level C
	Nonreconstructible arteries	Level C

PAD, Peripheral arterial disease.

includes functional status, clinical predictors for cardiac events, and history of symptomatic CAD. With this information, the guidelines of the American College of Cardiology (ACC)/American Heart Association (AHA)[13] may be used to formulate a strategy for evaluation and management (such as proceeding with surgery, or obtaining a cardiac stress test or coronary angiogram [Evidence Level C]). Preoperative evaluation should result in an assessment of risk (high, moderate, or low risk for complications) that will help the surgeon to determine which operation (if any) to perform.

Aggressive perioperative β-blockade is used to reduce the risk of coronary artery events[5] (Evidence Level A). Antiplatelet therapy (aspirin, clopidogrel, or both) is continued at the discretion of the surgeon, as adequate data are lacking to guide the use of these medications in the perioperative period.

Postoperative Care

The recovery period after infrainguinal bypass surgery is variable. Patients with a good preoperative functional status undergoing surgery for disabling claudication are often discharged home within a few days. Patients with a poor functional status or those requiring toe amputation or open wound care often have a longer hospital stay. Evaluation by a physical therapist and occupational therapist early in the postoperative course facilitates return of normal functional status and identifies patients who may benefit from intensive rehabilitation.

Patient Monitoring/Secondary Prevention

After bypass surgery, all patients require continued atherosclerotic risk factor modification and antiplatelet therapy. After recovery, all patients should undergo surveillance lower extremity arterial studies in the vascular laboratory. Surveillance is performed to monitor for graft stenosis as well as progression of disease in the contralateral leg. Graft patency and limb salvage are improved when graft stenoses are identified and repaired before bypass graft thrombosis[2] (Evidence Level B). Ultrasound graft surveillance protocols vary among surgeons. Most surgeons obtain an initial study early in the postoperative course, with another study usually within 6 months of surgery and then annually.

AMPUTATION FOR THE PATIENT WITH PERIPHERAL ARTERIAL DISEASE

Major leg amputation presents many challenges for both the patient and the clinician. Most patients are reluctant to have an amputation and some refuse to consent to the operation (although many patients find relief after amputation, having suffered for long periods with pain, chronic wounds, and multiple prior procedures). Often, families must decide on surgery for elderly patients who are unable to give consent. Surgeons may see the amputation as evidence of the failure of previous interventions. Finally, elderly patients, families, and clinicians recognize that the procedure often leads to profound alterations in functional status, morbidity, or death. In this emotionally charged environment, a frank discussion of options (including palliative care) will help the patient and/or family to be satisfied with the decision to proceed with amputation. A team approach to care of the patient undergoing amputation will increase the potential for good outcomes. Included in this team are the primary care physician, surgeon, physiatrist, occupational and physical therapist, and prosthetist.

Indications

The indications for amputation include gangrene, ulceration, or ischemic rest pain with nonreconstructive vessels (usually occlusion of the distal target vessels in the calf and foot) or prohibitive risk from bypass surgery. Many patients with nonreconstructive vessels have had previous bypass surgery with subsequent bypass graft occlusion from progression of atherosclerosis. Prohibitive surgical risk is frequently based on poor functional status (bedridden patient) or severe dementia (and inability to cooperate with postoperative rehabilitation therapy).

Rarely, patients (usually with diabetes) present with foot infection resulting in sepsis and multisystem organ dysfunction. After resuscitation, emergency amputation is indicated to prevent progression of organ dysfunction and death.

Below-knee amputation is usually recommended for ambulatory patients with adequate cognitive ability to participate in rehabilitation. Walking with a below-knee prosthesis requires significantly less energy than an above-knee prosthesis, and a significant proportion of patients will eventually ambulate with a below-knee prosthesis. For bedridden patients and those with severe dementia, above-knee amputation is usually performed. In these patients, return to ambulatory status is not a realistic goal and the risk of wound complications is reduced with an above-knee amputation. After below-knee amputation, bedridden and severely demented patients usually develop a knee flexion contracture. Once a contracture develops, the stump is prone to pressure ulceration and chronic wound problems. This long-term complication is unusual with an above-knee amputation.

Results

After below-knee amputation, approximately 15% of patients will develop severe wound problems requiring conversion to above-knee amputation. Significantly, more patients with below-knee amputations will achieve full mobility with a prosthesis when compared to those with an above-knee amputation. Bilateral amputees, women, and elderly patients are less likely to have a good functional outcome.[2]

The long-term results after major leg amputation are dismal, reflecting the severe comorbidities present in these patients. After 5 years, approximately 50% of the patients undergoing below-knee amputation are alive, and another 30% will have a contralateral leg amputation. The outcomes are even more bleak for patients requiring an above-knee amputation.

Perioperative Risks

The perioperative mortality after below-knee amputation is 3% to 10% and rises to approximately 20% for patients submitted to above-knee amputation. The significant perioperative mortality reflects the severity of the comorbidities of these patients. Common perioperative complications include cardiac events (MI, congestive heart failure), infection (wound, pneumonia), deep venous thrombosis, and wound complications (more common with below-knee amputations).[2]

Preoperative Evaluation/Risk Reduction

The 3% to 20% perioperative mortality for patients undergoing major amputation illustrates the need for aggressive risk reduction. Patients often have a poor functional status and widespread atherosclerosis. However, little data exist that specifically address cardiac risk reduction before amputation. The severity of symptoms that would lead to a recommendation of major amputation (severe pain, foot gangrene, or infection) often preclude cardiac stress testing or the ability to intervene based on the results of these tests (such as delaying amputation until recovery from coronary artery angioplasty/stenting or bypass surgery). Most often, amputation proceeds under the assumption of significant CAD and medical therapy is maximized to reduce the risk of cardiac complications. Intervention commonly includes aggressive perioperative β-blockade and judicious use of intravenous fluid.

Postoperative Care

Evaluation by a physiatrist, physical therapist, and occupational therapist early in the postoperative period (or preoperatively, when possible) will facilitate attempts to maintain mobility. Deep venous thrombosis prophylaxis and adequate pain control are also important. After below-knee amputation, development of a knee flexion contracture will severely impair the ability to regain full mobility. Many different devices (such as splints or casts) are available to attempt prevention of contracture at the knee. These devices are used at the discretion of the surgeon or physiatrist.

After major amputation, the rehabilitation potential for severely demented or nonambulatory patients is poor. Instead, postoperative care should focus on adequate pain control and facilitating a prompt return to baseline functional status.

Patient Monitoring/Secondary Prevention

After amputation, all patients require atherosclerotic risk factor modification and antiplatelet therapy. Given the high risk of contralateral limb loss, frequent follow-up and aggressive treatment of leg symptoms are required to reduce the chances of subsequent amputation.

ANGIOPLASTY/STENTING FOR THE PATIENT WITH PERIPHERAL ARTERIAL DISEASE

Percutaneous revascularization of the lower extremity generally includes angioplasty and/or stenting. Compared to open surgical revascularization, the advantages of angioplasty/stenting include less morbidity and mortality, less pain, shorter hospital stays, and faster recovery. The disadvantages include an increased risk for restenosis, recurrent symptoms, and repeat interventions.

The field of percutaneous revascularization is changing quickly. Medications and technologies exist that, although attractive in concept, lack data to support their routine use in clinical practice. Some examples include glycoprotein IIb-IIIa inhibitors, covered stent grafts and laser atherectomy devices. These medications and technologies are also extraordinarily expensive. It is hoped that rigorous data will be forthcoming to guide in the use of these new therapies.

Indications

For patients with PAD, the indications for percutaneous intervention are the same as for open surgery. The indications for angioplasty/stenting include disabling claudication, ischemic rest pain, gangrene, or nonhealing ulcers[2] (Evidence Level C). The definition of "disabling claudication" is vague and varies from patient to patient. Baseline functional status seems to be the most important factor that influences the decision to intervene on a patient with claudication.

A small minority of clinicians has championed the use of angioplasty/stenting for patients with nondisabling claudication. Most, however, caution against the use of percutaneous interventions for these patients, citing the lack of proven benefit, high cost of intervention and subsequent reinterventions, and good results for patients compliant with atherosclerotic risk factor modification and lifestyle changes (including exercise therapy).[2]

Results

The results for percutaneous lower extremity revascularization are best for patients with the following characteristics: Disease of large vessels (aortoiliac disease), short segment lesions, stenotic lesions, and symptoms of claudication. The results are poorest for patients with the following characteristics: Disease of smaller vessels in the leg, long-segment lesions, occluded lesions, and symptoms of rest pain, gangrene, or nonhealing ulcers. Although no data exist to support the use of routine stent placement, stents are frequently deployed to treat lesions inadequately treated with angioplasty alone (immediate recoil) or with focal arterial dissection at the site of angioplasty.

Perioperative Risks

The risks of percutaneous revascularization are generally less than those of open bypass surgery. Mortality (<0.2%) and limb loss (<0.2%) are rare.[2] The advantages of reduced risks must be balanced with the inferior results after many types of percutaneous interventions.

Contrast nephrotoxicity is a major risk after angiography. The risk of contrast nephrotoxicity is increased with advanced age, preexisting renal dysfunction, and larger dye loads. The increased risk of nephrotoxicity found inpatients with diabetes is likely caused by associated renal dysfunction and not by the diabetes itself.

Patients undergoing percutaneous intervention may develop acute limb ischemia as a result of the procedure. Rarely, angioplasty/stenting is complicated by acute arterial occlusion. In this case, emergency bypass surgery is often required for limb salvage. Periprocedural plaque disruption may cause distal embolization and "blue-toe syndrome." Intervention may cause vessel perforation or bleeding, necessitating placement of a covered stent graft or open blood vessel repair.

Preoperative Evaluation/Risk Reduction

Percutaneous intervention is performed with local anesthesia and sedation. As it is a low-risk procedure, it rarely requires cardiac stress testing.

For patients taking metformin, contrast-induced renal dysfunction may cause profound metabolic acidosis. Metformin should be stopped on the day before angiography and restarted 48 hours postprocedure. Metformin therapy should only be resumed after blood chemistries have documented no evidence of renal dysfunction.

As contrast nephrotoxicity may cause permanent renal dysfunction, all efforts should be made to avoid this complication. Reducing the amount of contrast used will reduce the risk of nephrotoxicity. A number of strategies can be used to limit the dye exposure. MR angiography and duplex ultrasound arterial mapping are modalities that have proved helpful in selective cases. Alternative agents (carbon dioxide, gadolinium) may be used to limit the dose of contrast. Staggering procedures to administer smaller, serial doses of contrast will also reduce the risk of renal dysfunction. Periprocedural hydration reduces the risk of nephrotoxicity. Recent evidence indicates that sodium bicarbonate may further reduce the risk of renal dysfunction. Typically, sodium bicarbonate is administered in 5% dextrose solution (D5-W with 150 mEq/L of sodium bicarbonate [3 "amps" of sodium bicarbonate]).[14] *N*-acetylcysteine administration may also reduce the risk of nephrotoxicity (600 mg PO b.i.d.—two doses before and two doses after angiography).[15]

A number of interventions have not proven effective in reducing the risk of nephrotoxicity. Specifically, dopamine, fenoldopam, and furosemide do not prevent renal dysfunction after arteriogram.

Postoperative Care

Depending on the size of the sheaths used and the amount of heparin administered, patients may be required to remain supine for 3 to 6 hours after the procedure to reduce the risk of bleeding. A number of devices are available to close the arterial puncture site (with a percutaneously placed suture or collagen plug). Although more comfortable for the patient and more convenient for the provider, these devices may be associated with an increased risk of complications, including bleeding, pseudoaneurysm formation, arterial occlusion, embolization, and infection.[16] Aggressive antiplatelet therapy (aspirin and clopidogrel) after coronary intervention has been shown to improve patency and reduce recurrent ischemic coronary events. No data exist to support the use of combined antiplatelet therapy after peripheral intervention. However, many clinicians do prescribe a course of both aspirin and clopidogrel after percutaneous lower extremity revascularization.

Patient Monitoring/Secondary Prevention

All patients require atherosclerotic risk factor modification and antiplatelet therapy after lower extremity angioplasty/stenting. Given the high risk of restenosis and recurrent ischemia for most percutaneous interventions, frequent follow-up and serial duplex examinations are required to optimize results.

REFERENCES

1. Hirsch AT, Criqui MH, Treat-Jacobson D, et al. Peripheral arterial disease detection, awareness, and treatment in primary care. *JAMA*. 2001;286:1317–1324.
2. Dormandy JA, Rutherford RB. Management of peripheral arterial disease. TransAtlantic Inter-Society Concensus Working Group. *J Vasc Surg*. 2000;31:S1–S296.
3. Grundy SM, Becker D, Clark LT, et al. Executive summary of the third report of The National Cholesterol Education Program (NCEP) expert panel on detection, evaluation, and treatment of high blood cholesterol in adults (Adult treatment panel III). *JAMA*. 2001;285:2486–2497.
4. Beebe HG, Dawson DL, Cutler BS, et al. A new pharmacological treatment for intermittent claudication: Results of a randomized, multicenter trial. *Arch Int Med*. 1999;159:2041–2050.
5. Boersma E, Poldermans D, Bax JJ, et al. Predictors of cardiac events after major vascular surgery: Role of clinical characteristics, dobutamine echocardiography, and [beta]-blocker therapy. *JAMA*. 2001;285:1865–1873.
6. McDermott MM, Greenland P, Liu K, et al. Leg symptoms in peripheral arterial disease: Associated clinical characteristics and functional impairment. *JAMA*. 2001;286:1599–1606.
7. Libby P. Inflammation in atherosclerosis. *Nature*. 2002;420: 868–874.

8. http://www.vascularweb.org. Accessed on August 15, 2005.
9. McDermott MM, Liu K, Greenland P, et al. Functional decline in peripheral arterial disease: Associations with the ankle brachial index and leg symptoms. *JAMA*. 2004;292:453–461.
10. Anderson JE, Jorenby DE, Scott WJ, et al. Treating tobacco use and dependence: An evidence-based clinical practice guideline for tobacco cessation. *Chest*. 2002;121:932–941.
11. Chobanian AV, Bakris GL, Black HR, et al. The seventh report of the Joint National Committee on prevention, detection, evaluation, and treatment of high blood pressure. *JAMA*. 2003;289:2560–2572.
12. Tran H, Anand SS. Oral antiplatelet therapy in cerebrovascular disease, coronary artery disease, and peripheral arterial disease. *JAMA*. 2004;292:1867–1874.
13. Eagle KA, Berger PB, Calkins H, et al. American College of Cardiology/American Heart Association Task Force on Practice Guidelines. ACC/AHA guideline update for perioperative cardiovascular evaluation for noncardiac surgery—executive summary a report of the American College of Cardiology/American Heart Association Task Force on Practice Guidelines. *Circulation*. 2002;105:1257–1267.
14. Merten GJ, Burgess WP, Gray LV, et al. Prevention of contrast-induced nephropathy with sodium bicarbonate: A randomized controlled trial. *JAMA*. 2004;291:2328–2334.
15. Pannu N, Manns B, Lee H, et al. Systematic review of the impact of N-acetylcysteine on contrast nephropathy. *Kidney Int*. 2004;65:1366–1374.
16. Koreny M, Riedmuller E, Nikfardjam M, et al. Arterial puncture closing devices compared with standard manual compression after cardiac catheterization: Systematic review and meta-analysis. *JAMA*. 2004;291:350–357.

SUGGESTED READINGS AND RESOURCES

American Heart Association
http://www.americanheart.org/
Website, including information for clinicians and patients regarding PAD, heart disease, and cerebrovascular disease.

The 7th report of the Joint National Committee on Prevention, Detection, Evaluation, and Treatment of High Blood Pressure
http://www.nhlbi.nih.gov/guidelines/hypertension/express.pdf

Medical Articles, News, and Research Pertinent to the Care of the Patient with PAD
http://www.vascularweb.org

Cardiac Disease

26

Tarek Helmy *Amar D. Patel* *Nanette K. Wenger*

CLINICAL PEARLS 335

NORMAL AGE-RELATED CHANGES IN THE CARDIOVASCULAR SYSTEM 336

CORONARY HEART DISEASE 337
Signs and Symptoms 337
Differential Diagnosis 337

STABLE ANGINA 338
Definition 338
Pathophysiology 338
Incidence and Prevalence 339
Etiology 339
Risk Factors 339
Workup/Keys to Diagnosis 339
Management 340
Lifestyle Recommendations 340
Medications 340
Percutaneous/Surgical Interventions 342
Alternative Treatments 342

ACUTE CORONARY SYNDROMES 342

VALVULAR HEART DISEASE 344
Aortic Stenosis 344
Aortic Regurgitation 345
Mitral Regurgitation 345
Mitral Stenosis 346

ARRHYTHMIAS 347
Atrial Fibrillation 347
Ventricular Arrhythmias 350
Bradyarrhythmias 352

CLINICAL PEARLS

- Atypical symptoms of myocardial ischemia such as fatigue, dyspnea, worsening heart failure, syncope, and confusion are common in the elderly.
- The physical examination is usually unremarkable in patients with stable angina.
- Mnemonic for coronary heart disease (CHD) management: A, Aspirin and Antianginal therapy; B, β-Blockers and Blood Pressure; C, Cigarette smoking and Cholesterol; D, Diet and Diabetes; E, Education and Exercise.
- Bradycardia, conduction abnormalities, hypotension, hepatic or renal toxicity, and mental status changes are potential side effects of cardiovascular medications.
- High-risk characteristics of acute coronary syndrome (ACS): Worsening or prolonged chest pain, pulmonary edema, hemodynamic instability, mitral regurgitation (new or worsening), ventricular tachycardia, new bundle branch block, elevated cardiac biomarkers, or age >75 years.
- Symptoms of severe aortic stenosis include worsening dyspnea with exertion, heart failure symptoms, chest pain, or syncope.
- Symptomatic aortic stenosis requires prompt surgical evaluation, given the accelerated mortality once symptoms develop.
- Late peaking of the basal systolic murmur is the best indication of severe aortic stenosis in the elderly.
- Severe aortic regurgitation is oftentimes not associated with symptoms.
- Suppression of sinus tachycardia in critically ill patients with advanced aortic regurgitation should be avoided, as forward cardiac output is maintained by increasing the heart rate.
- Medical therapy for chronic mitral regurgitation consists of afterload reduction, diuretics, and maintaining an adequate volume status.
- Surgical intervention on regurgitant valvular lesions (both aortic and mitral) should be guided by echocardiographic parameters, and should not be delayed until symptoms develop.
- Mitral valve repair is better than mitral valve replacement given the preservation of the subvalvular apparatus, left

ventricular (LV) function, and the avoidance of oral anticoagulation.

- Patients with valvular disease or following valve replacement surgery should receive prophylaxis for infective endocarditis.
- There is an increased risk of conduction system disease in the elderly, given the age-related degradation and fibrosing of the system.
- Atrial fibrillation (AF) is the most common arrhythmia and accounts for one third of elderly patient hospitalizations for cardiac rhythm disturbances.
- A rate-control over rhythm-control strategy should be used in elderly patients with atrial fibrillation.
- Approximately 50% of AF-related strokes occur in elderly patients older than 75.
- An INR range of 1.6 to 2.5 is recommended in elderly patients older than the age of 75 with a history of gastrointestinal bleeding.
- Symptomatic bradycardia, high-grade AV block, bradycardia induced by medications used to treat arrhythmias, and postprocedural AV block that is not expected to resolve (catheter ablation of AV node or coronary artery bypass graft surgery [CABG]) are indications for pacemaker placement.

Cardiovascular diseases are prominent in the elderly population and account for a significant proportion of their morbidity and mortality.[1] Most deaths are due to the sequelae of coronary heart disease (CHD), whether in its acute presentation as myocardial infarction (MI) or from its long-term complications. Cardiovascular disease in the elderly also accounts for a large number of emergency department visits and hospitalizations, and a resultant increased need for ambulatory and custodial care. As the US population ages and medical therapy improves, the prevalence of cardiovascular conditions such as CHD, valvular heart disease, and arrhythmias will become increasingly prevalent at an elderly age.

CHD accounts for approximately 33% of all deaths in patients older than 65. Given the comorbidities in this population, noninvasive assessment for occult coronary disease becomes more difficult. The growing burden of CHD highlights the importance of secondary prevention measures. Percutaneous coronary interventional therapies have taken on an expanded role in the treatment of elderly patients, when medical management is ineffective or nonfeasible, and the surgical risk is high.

Valvular heart disease in the elderly is most often related to calcific and/or degenerative changes in the valve leaflets. Rheumatic heart disease has become less common. Management of calcific aortic stenosis (AS) is challenging given the dearth of clinical trial data in an elderly patient population. The expected benefits of pharmacologic management of valvular heart disease in the elderly are generally similar to the younger population. The decision to refer a patient for valvular surgery is difficult and must be tailored to each patient.

Cardiac dysrhythmias are very common at an elderly age, and occur even in clinically healthy persons. CHD, hypertension, and heart failure are important comorbidities that contribute to the development of rhythm disturbances in the elderly; these must be addressed when managing such patients. In recent years, significant advances in pharmacologic options and percutaneously implanted devices have aided in the treatment of atrial and ventricular arrhythmias. However, as in all aspects of medical care, the treatment of the total patient and not just the presenting disease should be at the forefront of a clinician's approach to managing elderly patients.

NORMAL AGE-RELATED CHANGES IN THE CARDIOVASCULAR SYSTEM

The cardiovascular system undergoes considerable change with aging. A decrease in the elasticity and compliance of the aorta results in a rapid increase in systolic blood pressure during left ventricular (LV) contraction and rapid decrease in diastolic blood pressure during ventricular relaxation. The increased pulse pressure accelerates the atherosclerotic process due to progressive damage of the endothelium. Additionally, the "stiffness" of the aorta also increases LV workload due to the higher pressures it must generate to overcome the aortic afterload. This leads to LV hypertrophy and fibrosis; impaired LV filling results because the myocardium is unable to relax appropriately during passive filling before the atrial systole (this is referred to as diastolic dysfunction). The contribution of the left atrial contraction to ventricular filling becomes more important; its loss (i.e., with atrial fibrillation [AF]) can lead to heart failure.

Aging is also associated with an increased incidence of sinus node dysfunction. Although the number of atrioventricular (AV) node cells remains relatively preserved, the number of sinus node cells can decrease by 50% to 75% in the aged heart. This leads to a decrease in the intrinsic and maximally obtainable sinus rate. As a result, sinus node dysfunction (sinus bradycardia, sinus arrhythmia, sinoatrial nodal block, sinoatrial arrest, and sick-sinus syndrome) is common. AV nodal disease is mainly manifest as a prolonged PR interval. Fibrosis of the conduction skeleton and pathways can lead to various types of heart block. These changes render elderly persons susceptible to developing symptomatic, age-related conduction system disease.

Cardiac valvular disease may occur with aging, but is not generally considered normal. In particular, thickening and calcification of the mitral annulus and the base of the aortic valve is not uncommon. Mild mitral regurgitation (MR) may be seen with age-related thickening of the valvular leaflets. Aortic valve sclerosis may develop from age-related changes and mild calcification of the basal portions of the valvular cusps.

Coronary atherosclerotic heart disease may develop as early as the first or second decade of life, with symptoms becoming evident as early as the third decade. The natural progression of atherosclerotic CHD becomes more severe as the patient ages. Aging may lead to more diffuse CHD, producing a state of overall low cardiac reserve and poor systemic function due to widespread ischemia. This makes elderly persons less tolerant to cardiovascular events. Elderly patients have a higher incidence of CHD extent and severity compared to younger patients. This places elderly patients at higher risk for cardiac events and poor outcomes.

CORONARY HEART DISEASE

Signs and Symptoms

A reduction in physical activity is common in the aged, especially those with CHD. Comorbidities such as chronic lung disease, peripheral vascular disease, and osteoarthritis make the performance of meaningful physical activity difficult. As a result, activity-related manifestations of CHD may not be apparent until the disease is significantly advanced. This may account for the relatively high number of acute ischemic presentations in this population.

Elderly patients commonly experience chest discomfort as a manifestation of CHD. It is usually described as a tightness or pressure, and may radiate to the neck, jaw, or arm. However, atypical symptoms of myocardial ischemia such as fatigue, dyspnea, or worsening heart failure may occur. These symptoms likely result from an ischemia-induced exaggerated increase in LV end-diastolic pressure in an already noncompliant LV, increasing pulmonary capillary wedge pressure that leads to pulmonary edema and symptoms of shortness of breath. Even neurologic symptoms such as syncope and confusion may be observed as manifestations of occult CHD. Atypical symptoms must be addressed as aggressively as typical angina; studies performed in large community settings have shown similar 3-year cardiac-related death rates.

Silent ischemia is at least twice as common as clinically evident CHD at an elderly age. The etiology is unclear but may be related to the development of a collateral circulation that would reduce the effective extent of ischemic burden with minimal physical activity. Other possibilities include mental status changes that may not allow proper memory or communication, autonomic dysfunction, or tolerance to pain due to endogenous endomorphins.

Differential Diagnosis

Manifestations of CHD in the elderly have a vast array of potential presentations. Given the later, and more often acute presentations of elderly patients with symptomatic CHD, early diagnosis allows for a wide assortment of therapeutic options. CHD in the elderly presents as several clinical syndromes (see Table 26.1). A heightened awareness should be maintained for atypical symptoms

TABLE 26.1
DIFFERENTIAL DIAGNOSIS OF CARDIOVASCULAR CONDITIONS IN THE ELDERLY

Ischemic (ICD-9)	Valvular (ICD-9)	Arrhythmia (ICD-9)
Angina pectoris (413.9)	**Mitral Valve Disease**	Atrioventricular block, complete (426.0)
Prinzmetals angina (413.1)	Stenosis—rheumatic (394.0)	First-degree atrioventricular block (426.11)
Coronary atherosclerosis (414.0)	Insufficiency—rheumatic (394.1)	Mobitz II atrioventricular block (426.12)
Unstable angina (411.1)	Stenosis and Insufficiency—rheumatic (394.2)	Other second degree atrioventricular block (426.13)
Acute coronary occlusion without myocardial infarction (411.81)	Mitral valve disorders—except rheumatic (424.0)	Left bundle branch (426.2)
Acute myocardial infarction (410)	**Aortic Valve Disease**	Other left bundle branch block (426.3)
Prior myocardial infarction (412)	Stenosis—rheumatic (395.0)	Right bundle branch block (426.4)
Postmyocardial infarction syndrome (411.0)	Insufficiency—rheumatic (395.1)	Bundle branch block, other (426.5)
Aneurysm and dissection of heart (414.1)	Stenosis and Insufficiency—rheumatic (395.2)	Anomalous atrioventricular excitation (426.7)
Ischemic heart disease NOS (414.9)	Aortic valve disorders—except rheumatic (424.1)	Paroxysmal supraventricular tachycardia (427.1)
	Tricuspid Valve Disease	Atrial fibrillation (427.31)
	Rheumatic—related (397.0)	Atrial flutter (427.32)
	Nonrheumatic (424.2)	Sinoatrial node dysfunction (427.81)
	Pulmonary Valve Disease	Paroxysmal ventricular tachcardia (427.2)
	Rheumatic—related (397.1)	Ventricular flutter (427.42)
	Nonrheumatic (424.3)	Ventricular fibrillation (427.41)
		Cardiac arrest (427.5)
		Premature beats, unspecified (427.60)
		Supraventricular premature beats (427.61)
		Other premature beats (427.69)

TABLE 26.2
DIFFERENTIAL DIAGNOSIS IN PATIENTS WITH CHEST PAIN

Head	Chest	Abdomen
Depression	Aortic dissection[a]	Perforated viscus[a]
Anxiety	Pulmonary embolus[a]	Esophageal rupture[a]
Panic attack	Pnuemothorax[a]	Esophagitis
Somatoform disorders	Recent chest trauma	Esophageal spasm
Delusional	Pericarditis	Esophageal reflux
	Pleurisy	Biliary colic
	Pulmonary hypertension	Cholecystitis
	Dysphagia	Choledocholithiasis
	Pneumonia	Cholangitis
	Muscle sprain/strain	Peptic ulcer disease
	Nerve impingement	Pancreatitis
	Costochondritis	
	Rib fracture	
	Sternoclavicular arthritis	
	Herpes zoster	

[a]Potentially life threatening conditions.

of myocardial ischemia. Alternate diagnoses of chest pain should be considered (see Table 26.2).

STABLE ANGINA

CASE ONE

Mr. A. is a 76-year-old who comes to the office, on the insistence of his wife, because of a 4-month history of increasing fatigue and shortness of breath. In addition to mild osteoarthritis, Mr. A. has a long history of hypertension and dyslipidemia, both of which are currently treated with medications. The patient has noticed a gradual decrease in his level of endurance to the point that he becomes extremely fatigued when maintaining his yard. Prior to the last 4 months, he was not limited in this activity. He has not experienced any chest discomfort when performing yard work, but notes that he develops an exertional shortness of breath that improves when he rests. The blood pressure is 155/90 mm Hg with an otherwise unremarkable physical examination. A 12-lead electrocardiogram (ECG) reveals normal sinus rhythm with poor R-wave progression and diffuse, nonspecific T-wave flattening. A nuclear myocardial perfusion study showed a moderate-sized, reversible anterior wall perfusion defect. Cardiac catheterization revealed three vessel coronary diseases with a left ventricular ejection fraction (LVEF) of 50%. The patient was sent for coronary artery bypass grafting. The procedure was successfully performed with some cognitive deficit as a postoperative event. Prior to discharge, the patient was started on metoprolol, lisinopril, atorvastatin, and aspirin. The patient was discharged with the intent of joining a cardiac rehabilitation program.

Definition

Angina is a syndrome typically characterized by chest discomfort that may be associated with jaw, neck, shoulder, back, or arm pain. This pain is typically brought on, or exacerbated by, exertion or emotional stress and is relieved by rest or nitroglycerin. Stable angina is said to be present if there is no substantial worsening of these symptoms, there is a predictable pattern of onset with exertion, and it lasts a short time (<10 to 15 minutes).

Pathophysiology

Angina results from significant narrowing of the coronary arteries, commonly the result of coronary atherosclerosis. Coronary disease is manifest by the development of atherosclerotic plaques. An injury to the endothelium by chemical, mechanical, or inflammatory events incites the process of atherosclerosis. Low-density lipoprotein cholesterol (LDL-C) diffuses into the area of the injured coronary endothelium and is then oxidized. This process initiates a cascade of events leading to a marked inflammatory reaction, which results in endothelial dysfunction. As a result of this inflammatory state, growth factors, cytokines, and chemotactic factors are released. This leads to the development of an atherosclerotic plaque, which is composed of a lipid core surrounded by smooth muscle cells and fibrous tissue. The plaque morphology that commonly causes stable angina consists of a small lipid core and is covered by a thick fibrous cap. Conversely, the plaque structure that typically leads to unstable angina is more vulnerable and dangerous, as it contains a large thrombogenic lipid core surrounded by a thin fibrous cap. Digestive enzymes, known as *matrix metalloproteinases,* are released around the plaque edge, leading to plaque rupture and the development of acute coronary syndromes.

Incidence and Prevalence

An estimated 3.6 million elderly patients have symptomatic CHD. The extent and severity of coronary disease increases with aging. The incidence of CHD is greater in younger middle-aged men than women; this disparity begins to diminish with aging, and after age 80, the incidence of CHD in men and women is comparable.

Etiology

The gradual progression of a stable coronary atherosclerotic lesion to approximately 70% of its luminal diameter (90% reduction in cross-sectional surface area) results in a significant decrease in coronary perfusion pressure across the stenotic area and commonly produces symptoms of myocardial ischemia. In the elderly, however, there is a greater likelihood of subcritical coronary artery stenoses ($\leq$70% stenosis) that span a significant length of the vessel. As a result of the dissipation of blood flow energy across a long stenotic segment, the poststenotic segment does not receive an adequate blood supply, causing symptoms.

Risk Factors

Risk factors for the development of CHD include age, sex, family history, dyslipidemia, hypertension, diabetes mellitus, cigarette smoking, renal insufficiency, obesity, and a sedentary lifestyle. The presence of peripheral vascular disease increases the likelihood of concomitant CHD.

Workup/Keys to Diagnosis

Physical Examination

The physical examination is usually unremarkable in patients with stable angina. A complete cardiovascular examination may lend clues to the presence of CHD. Elevated blood pressure, xanthomas, carotid bruits, abdominal bruits, and diminished pedal pulses increase the clinical suspicion for CHD. Examining a patient during an anginal episode may reveal signs of myocardial ischemia, such as a paradoxical splitting of S2, an S3 gallop, the presence or worsening of MR, bibasilar rales, and a chest wall heave. The resolution of these signs once the chest pain resolves is highly predictive of CHD. Conditions that may cause angina that are not necessarily associated with CHD may be identified (i.e., AS, hypertrophic cardiomyopathy).

Laboratory

Although there are no highly specific tests which suggest CHD, the history and physical examination may suggest the presence of other diseases which may cause or contribute to the development of functional angina (myocardial ischemia in the absence of significant hemodynamic coronary artery disease). Conditions that either substantially increase myocardial oxygen demand or decrease myocardial oxygen supply can lead to myocardial ischemia. The identification and treatment of these entities may result in a substantial reduction of symptoms (see Table 26.3).

Diagnostic Procedures

A 12-lead ECG should be obtained in all patients with symptoms suggestive of angina, although the normalcy rate will be at least 50% of patients presenting with stable angina. A normal ECG does not exclude severe CHD. ECG findings of left ventricular hypertrophy, bundle branch block, old Q-waves, AF, ventricular tachyarrhythmia, atrioventricular block, ST depression, ST elevation, and T-wave inversions may suggest CHD; however, these findings are not specific for the diagnosis of stable angina.

Stress testing is performed to establish the diagnosis of CHD and provide risk stratification and prognostic assessment. Given the high prevalence of CHD in the elderly, the sensitivity of stress testing is increased (84%) with a decrease in specificity (70%), thereby increasing the rates of false-positive results.[2]

TABLE 26.3
SYSTEMIC DISEASES THAT MAY POTENTIALLY EXACERBATE ISCHEMIA

Hematologic	Pulmonary	Cardiovascular	Other
Anemia	Hypoxemia as a result of	Aortic stenosis	Hyperthermia
Sickle cell disease	■ Pneumonia	Hypertrophic cardiomyopathy	Hyperthyroidism
Hyperviscosity syndromes	■ Asthma	Tachyarrhythmias	Hypertension
Leukemia	■ Chronic obstructive lung disease	Dilated cardiomyopathy	Anxiety
Thrombocytosis	■ Interstitial fibrosis	Arteriovenous fistulae	
Hypergammaglobulinemia	■ Obstructive sleep apnea		
	■ Pulmonary hypertension		

The adequate performance of an exercise test in the elderly poses concern, given the limited functional capacity of most patients. Although exercise testing is not contraindicated in this population, muscle weakness, deconditioning, improper gait, and coordination limit the usefulness of this test. The mechanical hazards of treadmill exercise testing in this population must be considered. Elderly patients are more likely to hold tightly on to the handrails, reducing the validity of metabolic equivalent (MET) assessment. Baseline ECG abnormalities such as left bundle branch block, pacemaker rhythm, or marked ST segment changes are contraindications to ECG-exercise testing. Patients with these baseline abnormalities must have adjunctive myocardial imaging (radionuclide or echocardiography). Although such indices as the Duke Treadmill score carry prognostic significance, their utility in risk assessment for patients older than 75 is largely irrelevant. If a patient is referred for exercise stress testing, more gradual exercise protocols should be considered. The ability to walk through the second stage of a Bruce protocol (>6 minutes) is a good prognostic factor and predicts low risk. In assessing risk, attention is paid to the chronotropic and ionotropic response to exercise and exercise-induced arrhythmias. When exercise testing cannot be performed, other options such as pharmacologic myocardial perfusion imaging or dobutamine stress echocardiography should be considered. These tests may be safer in the elderly and are more sensitive in identifying single- and two-vessel disease. The predictive value of these tests is greater than that of ECG-exercise testing alone.

Management

The initial management of elderly CHD patients should follow the mnemonic:[3]

A, Aspirin and antianginal therapy
B, β-Blockers and blood pressure
C, Cigarette smoking and cholesterol
D, Diet and diabetes
E, Education and exercise

These initial considerations should be included when treating patients with angina. As stated earlier, conditions that may exacerbate or provoke symptoms of angina should be managed. This may reduce the need for the intensification of medical treatment, if anginal symptoms resolve and the patient is not high-risk.

Lifestyle Recommendations

Lifestyle modifications include cigarette smoking cessation, dietary modification, education, and exercise.[4] The cessation of cigarette smoking should always be encouraged, as the elderly receive a similar benefit as younger individuals. Cigarette use declines with age, with 15% of men and 11.5% of women older than 65 years continuing to smoke cigarettes. Patients with symptoms of CHD are most likely to quit. The use of transdermal nicotine replacement patches (14 to 22 mg daily, then taper after 6 weeks) and bupropion (150 mg oral twice daily) should be considered as part of a smoking cessation strategy. For this to be successful, a structured approach should be implemented. Oftentimes, the utilization of allied health professionals to implement and carry out these measures with patients should be strongly considered.

Greater than one third of patients older than 65 years perform no leisure time physical activity. Patients must be counseled on the importance of weight control and exercise. Exercise has been associated with a reduction in blood pressure and insulin resistance in addition to an increase in high-density lipoprotein cholesterol (HDL-C). Moderate exercise has proven efficacious in reducing cardiovascular events. Studies have shown that the exercise trainability of elderly patients is similar to that of younger patients, and that the elderly derive significant benefit from exercise rehabilitation. A gradual and steady increase in physical activity is strongly suggested over short bursts of vigorous physical activity, which increases the likelihood of sudden cardiac death. Exercise-based cardiac rehabilitation should be recommended to all elderly patients with CHD. Walking 30 minutes most days of the week is reasonable.

The importance of patient education in the elderly cannot be overemphasized. Dietary education as it pertains to comorbid disease states (hyperlipidemia, diabetes, hypertension, heart failure) must be given during office visits. The maximal gain that patients receive from diagnostic and therapeutic technology is dependent on their understanding of their disease. Educating the patient about their disease, if necessary by health educators or the use of professionally prepared material, is of great importance. The presence of a spouse, significant other, or family member during the office visit is important in that they may help facilitate the interview and help better clarify matters to both the clinician and the patient.

Medications

The initiation of cardiovascular medications must be closely monitored, as elderly patients are more prone to side effects such as bradycardia, conduction abnormalities, hypotension, hepatic or renal toxicity, and possible mental status changes. Medications have to be started at lower doses and gradually titrated to prevent adverse effects. Aspirin is recommended in all elderly patients (75 to 325 mg daily) with CHD regardless of symptoms, provided that no contraindications exist (Evidence Level A).[5] Therapeutic classes of medications considered in this section focus on angiotensin-converting enzyme inhibitors (ACE-I), lipid-lowering agents, β-blockers, calcium-channel blockers, and nitrates.

ACE inhibitor therapy has been shown to reduce mortality in the secondary prevention of CHD (Evidence Level A).

The Heart Outcomes Prevention Evaluation (HOPE) trial ($n = 9{,}297$; mean age 66 ± 7 years; 55% $\geq$65 years) and the European Trial on Reduction of Cardiac Events with Perindopril in Stable Coronary Artery Disease (EUROPA) ($n = 12{,}218$; mean age 60 ± 9 years; 31% >65 years) showed a significant reduction in death, MI, and stroke in patients treated with ACE inhibitor therapy.[6,7] However, recent results from the Prevention of Events with Angiotensin Converting Enzyme Inhibition (PEACE) trial ($n = 8{,}290$; mean age 64 ± 8 years; 11% $\geq$75 years) demonstrated no additional reduction in the composite endpoint (cardiovascular death, MI, or coronary revascularization) in patients with preserved left ventricular function and intensive medical therapy who received trandolapril over placebo.[8] There is much controversy regarding the possible improved efficacy of "tissue-specific" ACE inhibitor (ramipril 2.5 to 20 mg PO daily or divided twice daily dosing; perindopril 4 to 8 mg PO daily; trandolapril 2 to 4 mg PO daily) over other ACE inhibitor preparations (lisinopril 20 to 40 mg PO daily; enalapril 10 to 40 mg PO daily; fosinopril 20 to 40 mg PO daily; benazepril 20 to 40 mg PO daily). There have been no studies specifically comparing ACE inhibitor types. Barring significant renal insufficiency, ACE inhibitor therapy should be considered in all patients with CHD, especially those with diabetes mellitus.

Lipid-lowering agents such as hydroxyl-methylglutaryl coenzyme A reductase inhibitors ("statins") are first-line agents in the treatment of dyslipidemia, even in those patients $\geq$65 years (Evidence Level A). In addition to a significant reduction in CHD mortality, treatment with statin therapy has demonstrated plaque stabilization, plaque regression, or the slowing of plaque progression. Randomized clinical trials, such as the PROspective Study of Pravastatin in the Elderly at Risk (PROSPER) demonstrated a 15% relative risk reduction in CHD death, nonfatal MI, and stroke over placebo (5,804 patients, aged 70 to 82, mean 75 ± 3 years).[9] Subset analysis from the elderly cohort (age range 65 to 69, $n = 4{,}891$; age range $\geq$70, $n = 5{,}806$) in the Heart Protection Study showed a significant reduction in the incidence of a first major coronary event, stroke, and revascularization when patients were randomized to simvastatin 40 mg over placebo over a 5-year follow-up period.[10] Benefits of statin therapy, even in patients with average cholesterol levels, have been well demonstrated. Statin therapy is recommended, even for CHD patients with mild elevations in LDL-C. The most recent update of the National Cholesterol Education Program has recommended that patients with high-risk CHD be treated to achieve a goal of LDL-C $\leq$70 mg per dL. This recommendation is supported by the results of the Treating to New Targets (TNT) Study ($n = 10{,}001$; mean age 61 ± 8.8 years) which demonstrated a 22% relative risk reduction in the composite primary endpoint (death, nonfatal MI, resuscitation after cardiac arrest, or stroke) of atorvastatin 80 mg compared to atorvastatin 10 mg over a 4.9-year follow-up period.[11] In patients with CHD and an LDL-C level >100 mg per dL despite maximal statin therapy, the consideration for newer agents such as ezetimibe (10 mg PO daily) may provide additional reduction. Ezetimibe inhibits both dietary and biliary cholesterol absorption at the intestinal brush border. Although this agent has not been specifically tested in the elderly population, a 10% to 15% decrease in LDL-C is expected. If these agents are not tolerated, agents such as bile acid sequestrants (cholestyramine) (Evidence Level A), fibric acid derivatives (gemfibrozil and clofibrozil) (Evidence Level A), and niacin (Evidence Level A) should be considered for low HDL-C and elevated triglycerides.

Antianginal agents, such as β-blockers, improve survival in patients after MI and are widely used for the first-line treatment of angina in the elderly (Evidence Level A). In the treatment of stable angina, β-blockers should be titrated to achieve a heart rate range of 55 to 60 beats per minute (atenolol 25 to 100 mg PO daily; metoprolol 25 to 100 mg PO twice daily; labetolol 100 to 400 mg PO twice daily). Exercise caution in the elderly to avoid the development of heart block. Diabetes mellitus is not a contraindication to the use of β-blockers. Contraindications to the use of β-blockers include marked bradycardia, sick-sinus syndrome, and high-grade AV block. Relative contraindications include reactive airway disease, severe depression, and peripheral vascular disease.

Although their mechanisms are different, both calcium channel blocker and nitrate preparations dilate epicardial coronary arteries and reduce myocardial oxygen demand. Calcium channel blockers are as effective as β-blockers in the treatment of angina. Although β-blockers should be considered as first-line therapy, initiation of calcium channel blockers may be considered if adequate reduction in symptoms is not achieved or if contraindications exist with β-blocker use (Evidence Level B). Recent study results suggest that amlodipine (OR 0.69, CI 0.54 to 0.088; $p = 0.003$) favors a reduction in cardiovascular events (cardiac death, nonfatal MI, revascularization, stroke, transient ischemic attacks, and hospitalization for heart failure or angina) over enalapril (OR 0.85, CI 0.67 to 1.07; $p = 0.16$) compared to placebo control, especially in those patients $\geq$65 years (49% relative risk reduction).[12] The reduction in cardiovascular events observed with the use of amlodipine was mainly driven by a significantly greater reduction in anginal symptoms requiring hospitalization. Long-acting nitrates are generally added to β-blocker or calcium channel blocker therapy if symptoms persist (Evidence Level B). There is no survival benefit with nitrate use, but symptom improvement occurs. The major contraindications to calcium channel blocker use include overt decompensated heart failure. Evidence of bradycardia, AV block, or sinus node dysfunction should discourage the use of nondihydropyridine calcium channel blockers (verapamil and diltiazem). Nitrates should be avoided in patients with severe AS or hypertrophic obstructive cardiomyopathy.

Percutaneous/Surgical Interventions

Percutaneous coronary intervention (PCI) and coronary artery bypass graft surgery (CABG) at an elderly age has significantly increased during the last 20 years. In large retrospective national registries of coronary revascularization, octogenarians compared to patients <80 years were more likely to have chronic lung disease, chronic kidney disease, cerebrovascular disease, peripheral vascular disease, three-vessel coronary artery disease, and left main coronary artery disease. The in-hospital mortality rates are higher in octogenarians undergoing PCI (3.8%) and CABG (4.2% to 8.1%) compared to patients <80 years (1.1% and 3.0%, respectively), most likely related to comorbid illnesses.[13,14] Randomized, multicenter clinical trials have demonstrated that invasive treatment (PCI or CABG) over medical therapy provided the most benefit in terms of improvement in quality of life and reducing angina, but few elderly patients were participants in these trials (Evidence Level A).[15] The decision to pursue revascularization in elderly patients must be made on an individual basis, and after careful consideration of the patient's overall condition. For example, those with severe functional or cognitive limitations at baseline would not be surgical candidates, given the high likelihood of overall poor postoperative recovery. Conversely, elderly patients who have a reasonable level of cognitive and functional ability with an acceptable degree of comorbidity should at least be considered for revascularization. Unfortunately, at this time, there are no prospective randomized studies that have been performed in the very elderly to make any substantive recommendations regarding the decision to pursue mechanical revascularization as it pertains to long-term outcomes.

Alternative Treatments

The use of antioxidant vitamins such as vitamin E, vitamin C, and β-carotene in population-based epidemiologic trials have not been shown to reduce the morbidity and mortality associated with cardiovascular disease, and are not recommended as they may actually increase risk (Evidence Level A).[16] Vitamins such as B_6, B_{12}, and folate are used to reduce homocysteine levels in patients with hyperhomocysteinemia, which is strongly associated with the development of CHD and peripheral vascular disease. Although these vitamins reduce homocysteine levels, clinical trials are needed to determine if a significant reduction in cardiovascular events occurs. ω-3 fatty acids (approximately 1 g per day) have shown benefit in atherosclerotic plaque regression in addition to a reduction in death, nonfatal MI and stroke. Randomized clinical trials are necessary to further define the health benefits of ω-3 fatty acids and their role in primary and secondary prevention. Garlic has not been shown to reduce blood pressure and cholesterol levels and is not recommended, as it may increase bleeding risk.

ACUTE CORONARY SYNDROMES

CASE TWO

Mrs. P. is a 75-year-old who comes to the office with complaints of feeling chest pressure over the past few months when she cleans around the house. During the past 1 to 2 days, she is beginning to feel more severe chest pressure; it is waking her up from sleep and lasts for 20 minutes. She notes more fatigue and has increasing shortness of breath, especially during these episodes of pain.

Acute coronary syndrome (ACS) describes a constellation of clinical symptoms that suggest acute myocardial ischemia. ACS encompasses unstable angina and acute MI (non–ST segment elevation and ST segment elevation).[17,18] Unstable angina is a clinical syndrome that results from the disruption of an atherosclerotic plaque. The ensuing cascade of events (platelet activation and thrombus formation) leads to a decrease in coronary blood flow, with possible subsequent MI and death. Patients usually present with chest discomfort; if these symptoms occur at rest or become progressively worse, prompt evaluation is strongly recommended. The clinician must decide if these signs and symptoms are suggestive of obstructive CHD (see Table 26.4) and determine patient risk for adverse cardiac events (see Table 26.5).

The history, physical examination, 12-lead ECG and cardiac biomarkers are all important for the initial ACS evaluation. Patients with low-risk clinical characteristics with subsequent normal ECGs and cardiac biomarkers can be sent for stress testing (exercise or pharmacologic) the same day or have the remainder of the evaluation performed as an outpatient in a timely fashion. Patients with high-risk clinical characteristics, ischemic ECG changes, or abnormal cardiac biomarkers should be hospitalized.

Unless a specific contraindication exists, initial medical therapy for ACS includes aspirin, heparin (fractionated or unfractionated), β-blockers, nitrates, and oxygen (all with Evidence Level A). The acute administration of statins and ACE inhibitor (Evidence Level B) has been proven to be of benefit as well. Additionally, clopidogrel (75 mg PO daily) has demonstrated a benefit in elderly patients with unstable angina and non–ST segment elevation MI in that it reduced the incidence of death, nonfatal MI, and stroke (Evidence Level A). Intravenous glycoprotein IIb/IIIa inhibitors (abciximab, eptifibitde, and tirofiban) given in the appropriate setting has decreased the occurrence of death, MI, and urgent revascularization (Evidence Level A). This benefit is extended to patients >65 years; however, dosing must be appropriately adjusted in the setting of diminished renal function. The treating clinician must be cautious with the initiation and titration of these medications given the potential for the exaggerated side effects that may occur.

TABLE 26.4
SIGNS AND SYMPTOMS THAT SUGGEST AN ACUTE CORONARY SYNDROME FROM OBSTRUCTIVE CORONARY HEART DISEASE

High Risk[a]	Intermediate Risk[a,b]	Low Risk[a,b]
Chest discomfort or left arm pain that reproduces documented anginal symptoms	Chest discomfort or left arm pain as chief symptom	Atypical history
Known CHD	Age >70 years	Normal ECG
New or worsening MR	Male gender	Normal cardiac biomarkers
Hemodynamic instability	Diabetes mellitus	Recent cocaine use
Pulmonary edema	Renal insufficiency	
Diaphoresis	Peripheral arterial disease	
New ST changes (≥0.05 mV) or T-wave inversion (≥0.02 mV)	Old Q waves or abnormal ST segments/T waves	
Elevated cardiac biomarkers	Normal cardiac biomarkers	

This table serves as an estimation of short-term risks and was developed as a guidance tool only.
[a]At least one finding must be present.
[b]High risk findings must not be present.
MR, mitral regurgitation; ECG, echocardiogram; CHD, coronary heart disease.
Adapted from Braunwald E, Mark DB, Jones RH, et al. *Unstable angina: diagnosis and management*. Rockville, MD: Agency for Health Care Policy and Research and the National Heart, Lung, and Blood Institute, US Public Health Service, US Department of Health and Human Services; 1994; AHCPR Publication No. 94-0602.

In patients with documented ACS, two main management strategies are considered: "Early invasive" or "early conservative." An early invasive approach, involving coronary angiography and revascularization, provides better outcomes (reduced incidence of death and MI) when compared to patients treated with a more conservative approach (Evidence Level A). This reduction in outcomes (death, MI, recurrent angina) was observed even at 6 months after the initial event. Elderly patients (65 to 80 years) in the high-risk group for adverse cardiac events should be strongly considered for an early invasive approach.[15] There is no conclusive clinical trial data suggesting the significant benefit of an early invasive or an early conservative approach in patients older than 80.

TABLE 26.5
RISK OF DEATH OR NONFATAL MYOCARDIAL INFARCTION IN PATIENTS WITH UNSTABLE ANGINA

High Risk[a]	Intermediate Risk[a,b]	Low Risk[a,b]
Increasing frequency of myocardial ischemia symptoms	Rest angina <20 min that resolves with rest or NTG	New-onset anginal symptoms with minimal exertion or at rest
Ongoing rest pain >20 min	Resolution of chest pain lasting longer than 20 min, now with high- or intermediate-risk characteristics for CAD	ECG is unchanged or normal during anginal episode
New or worsening MR	Peripheral arterial disease	Normal cardiac biomarkers
Pulmonary edema	Prior MI	
Presence of an S3	Cerebrovascular disease	
New or worsening rales	Prior aspirin use	
Hemodynamic instability	Age >70 years	
Elderly age (>75 years)	Inverted T waves >0.02 mV	
ST-segment changes (≥0.05 mV) with chest pain at rest	Significant Q waves	
Bundle-branch block (new)	Mildly elevated cardiac biomarkers	
Ventricular tachycardia—sustained		
Markedly elevated cardiac biomarkers		

This table serves as an estimation of short-term risks and was developed as a guidance tool only.
[a]At least one finding must be present.
[b]High risk findings must not be present.
NTG, nitroglycerin; ECG, echocardiogram; CAD, coronary artery disease; MR, mitral regurgitation.
Adapted from Braunwald E, Mark DB, Jones RH, et al. *Unstable angina: diagnosis and management*. Rockville, MD: Agency for Health Care Policy and Research and the National Heart, Lung, and Blood Institute, US Public Health Service, US Department of Health and Human Services; 1994; AHCPR Publication No. 94-0602. AHCPR Clinical Practice Guideline No. 10, Unstable Angina: Diagnosis and Management, May 1994.

VALVULAR HEART DISEASE

Aortic Stenosis

AS is a common valvular disease of the elderly.[19] The normal aortic valve area is 3 cm^2, and the hemodynamically significant effects of AS usually appear after 75% reduction of the valve area. Detection is crucial, because significant symptomatic AS is associated with increased mortality if untreated.

Etiology

Most cases are due to the calcification of a tricuspid aortic valve. Currently, aortic atherosclerosis is considered the underlying pathology. AS may develop prematurely in bicuspid aortic valves, whereas congenital AS is usually discovered early in life.

Pathophysiology

AS causes impairment to the forward cardiac output and imposes a pressure overload on the left ventricle. The decrease in cardiac output and in tissue perfusion, in particular with exercise, accounts for most of the symptoms in severe AS. With pressure overload, increased stress on the left ventricular wall leads to progressive LV hypertrophy. The result is a decrease in the compliance of the LV and the development of diastolic dysfunction. If the pressure overload is not relieved, a gradual decline in LV systolic function ensues.

The natural history of AS follows a certain timeline. There is usually a latent period when patients are asymptomatic, and morbidity and mortality are fairly low. Once symptoms develop, the disease takes on an accelerated course and survival is significantly decreased. Part of this high mortality rate is attributed to sudden cardiac death, which is common in these patients.

Signs and Symptoms

Symptoms associated with severe, hemodynamically significant AS include dyspnea that is worse with exertion, heart failure symptoms, chest pain, or angina. AS is one of the most important causes of syncope in the elderly patient. Syncope was initially thought to be due to decreased cardiac output with severe stenosis of the aortic valve, but recently a vasodepressor reflex (due to high left ventricular pressure) has been proposed as an alternative mechanism for syncope. Arrhythmias and sudden cardiac death are common in symptomatic patients with AS. Symptoms usually progress rapidly in elderly patients, and once symptomatic, only 50% of patients will survive for 5 years. The physical findings in severe AS include a slow rising carotid pulse with a small volume, usually associated with a thrill. In the elderly, this finding may be masked due to the decreased elasticity of the arterial wall. The apical impulse is prominent, sustained, and may be displaced laterally and inferiorly. A harsh systolic ejection murmur, heard at the base of the heart and radiating to the neck, and muffling of the second heart sound are also important signs of AS. The severity of the stenosis relates to the timing of peak murmur (peaks later in severe lesions) rather than to the harshness or loudness of the murmur. This murmur has to be differentiated from the more benign early peaking murmur of aortic sclerosis commonly heard in elderly patients. The lack of commissural fusion of the calcified aortic valve explains the absence of an ejection sound and muffling of the second heart sound. A fourth heart sound is usually heard with normal sinus rhythm. Onset of AF can precipitate heart failure in elderly patients due to a loss of the atrial contribution to ventricular filling in a poorly compliant ventricle with elevated pressures, in combination with the shorter ventricular filling period due to the rapid heart rate. Findings of other associated valvular lesions may be present. Dorsal kyphosis at an elderly age may be associated with decreased intensity of the murmur.

Diagnostic Testing

ECG findings are those typical for LV hypertrophy. Echocardiography with Doppler studies can evaluate the severity of AS noninvasively, with great accuracy. These parameters can be determined using planimetry as well as velocity across the LV outflow track. A direct measurement of the aortic valve gradient can be obtained at cardiac catheterization, which allows for calculating the valve area using the Gorlin equation (see Table 26.6). Cardiac catheterization should be performed in all elderly patients because of their high risk for CHD. Approximately 50% of patients undergoing aortic valve replacement surgery will have concomitant coronary disease warranting CABG, which significantly increases the operative risk.

Management

Surgical aortic valve replacement is the mainstay of therapy for severe AS. Surgical intervention should be guided by the onset and progression of symptoms in the presence of severe aortic valve stenosis. Asymptomatic patients can be managed conservatively with periodic monitoring, although sudden death may be the first symptom of critical AS. The onset of symptoms warrants surgical intervention. Aortic valve replacement surgery improves symptoms and long-term survival, even in patients with reduced left ventricular systolic function.

The valve replacement surgical mortality is higher for older patients, described in one series to be 12.4% for patients older than 75 years of age and 6.6% for patients younger than 75 years. Because bioprosthetic valves deteriorate more slowly in older patients, the choice between a mechanical and a bioprosthetic valve depends on the age of the patient and the risk of long-term anticoagulation. Aortic balloon valvotomy has no role in the long-term management of AS and is only considered as a bridge to

TABLE 26.6
ASSESSMENT OF AORTIC AND MITRAL VALVE STENOSIS SEVERITY

	Aortic Valve		Mitral Valve	
Severity	Mean Gradient (mm Hg)	Valve Area (cm^2)	Mean Gradient (mm Hg)	Valve Area (cm^2)
Normal	None	2.0–3.0	None	3.0–4.0
Mild	<25	1.5–2.0	<5.0	>1.5
Moderate	25–50	1.0–1.5	5.0–10	1.0–1.5
Severe	>50	<1.0	>10	<1.0
Critical	>80	<0.7	N/A	N/A

N/A, not applicable.

stabilize patients and improve the outcomes of subsequent valve surgery in critically ill patients.

Aortic Regurgitation

Etiology

Aortic regurgitation (AR) has many causes: Myxomatous degeneration, infective endocarditis, rheumatic heart disease, arterial hypertension, and congenital bicuspid valve being the most common. Other causes include trauma, aortic dissection, and syphilis.[19]

Pathophysiology

AR represents a left ventricular volume overload, which over time, and depending on the severity of the regurgitation, will cause the LV to dilate with progressive worsening in the systolic function.

Signs and Symptoms

In the early stages, AR is well tolerated, especially in younger patients, with preserved exercise tolerance. Exercise causes an increase in the heart rate, leading to a shortening of the diastolic phase of the cardiac cycle and the lessening of the regurgitant volume, as well as causing a decrease in the left ventricular afterload, leading to an increase in forward flow and diminished regurgitant volume. As the disease progresses and the ventricle continues to dilate, symptoms of heart failure become more pronounced. Typically, symptomatic AR suggests that the optimal time for surgery has passed.

Physical findings of severe AR include a wide pulse pressure, rapid carotid upstroke followed by abnormal collapse, nodding of the head, visible capillary pulsations in the nail beds, and "pistol shot" sound over the femoral artery. Cardiac examination reveals a diffuse hyperdynamic apical impulse and a long blowing diastolic murmur heard best at the left upper to midsternal border, and an apical diastolic rumble. With advanced heart failure, the typical findings of elevated jugular venous pressure, pulmonary edema, and peripheral edema are evident. Patients with advanced AR maintain forward cardiac output by increasing their heart rate; therefore sinus tachycardia should not be suppressed in critically ill patients.

Diagnostic Testing

Echocardiography is the gold standard test for evaluating the severity of AR. This is done by assessing the width of the regurgitant jet as well as measuring the pressure half time of the aortic flow. LV function and dimensions can also be accurately measured.

Management

Medical therapy consists of afterload reduction, diuretics, and sodium restriction. Nifedipine therapy in patients with severe AR and preserved systolic function may delay the need for surgery. Aortic valve replacement surgery should be considered in patients with severe AR and depressed LV function (<50% to 55%) or dilated LV (end systolic dimension >55 mm).

Acute AR is usually caused by trauma, aortic dissection, or infective endocarditis. The acute volume overload to a noncompliant ventricle results in acute pulmonary edema with normal left ventricular size. Of interest, the typical murmur of chronic AR is often absent in this setting; instead a soft first heart sound should raise suspicion of acute AR. The diagnosis of AR can be reliably made by echocardiography.

Mitral Regurgitation

Etiology

Common causes of MR in the elderly population include rheumatic heart disease, myxomatous degeneration of the leaflets, mitral valve prolapse, infective endocarditis and ischemic papillary muscle dysfunction or chordal rupture.[19]

Pathophysiology

MR is another form of volume overload on the LV, because the regurgitant fraction is added to the normal filling volume with every cardiac cycle. This leads to the progressive dilation of the LV with depression of systolic function in the advanced stage. The left atrium also dilates and may become more compliant, which protects against pulmonary vascular hypertension in the early stages of the disease; as the disease progresses, left atrial dimensions and pressure increase leading to pulmonary hypertension and congestion.

Signs and Symptoms

The clinical course of chronic MR is a gradual one; patients remain fairly compensated until deterioration of LV function occurs. Early symptoms are usually fatigue and weakness. The onset of an AF can precipitate heart failure due to the loss of the atrial contribution to ventricular filling. In the advanced stage, a clinical picture of congestive heart failure (CHF) with pulmonary congestion and poor cardiac output may be the presenting symptom. Physical findings include a diffuse displaced cardiac apical impulse, a holosystolic murmur at the apex radiating to the axilla, and signs of pulmonary hypertension and congestion. In severe MR, a diastolic rumbling murmur may be heard at the apex because of increased flow across the mitral valve. The presence of a loud second heart sound indicates pulmonary hypertension. This can also be associated with a right ventricular (RV) heave as the RV dilates.

Acute severe MR has a dramatic presentation of acute pulmonary edema and cardiogenic shock. This is usually due to papillary muscle dysfunction, a flail leaflet, or ruptured cordae in the setting of an acute MI, or infective endocarditis. Patients are severely ill and require immediate intervention. Intra-aortic balloon counterpulsation may be used as a temporary stabilizing measure to bridge the patient to surgery.

Diagnostic Testing

Echocardiography is very important in the diagnosis of MR. In addition to providing information about the severity of the MR, LV function, and dimensions, it can also define the leaflets involved, the probable etiology of MR, and the condition of the leaflets and the subvalvular apparatus. This information is crucial in assessing the feasibility of valve repair or reconstruction. The width of the regurgitant jet and the degree it fills the left atrium determine the severity of the MR. Other clues can be obtained from examining the flow pattern in the pulmonary veins.

Management

Medical therapy for chronic MR consists of afterload reduction, diuretics, and maintaining an adequate fluid balance. Mitral valve surgery is indicated when severe heart failure symptoms develop, or when there is an increase in the left ventricular dimensions (end diastolic dimension of >45 mm) or a decrease in the LVEF (<60%). Better results are achieved when surgery is performed before severe LV dysfunction occurs.

Mitral valve repair is superior to valve replacement because it preserves the subvalvular apparatus and tends to better preserve left ventricular function. It also avoids the issue of long-term anticoagulation. Mitral valve replacement is indicated when valve repair is technically not possible. The choice of a mechanical or a bioprosthetic valve depends on the age of the patient and their risk of anticoagulation. Mortality for mitral valve replacement surgery ranges between 10% and 14%. When combined with CABG, in cases of ischemic MR, the mortality increases toward 20% to 30%, especially in patients over the age of 80. Emergent surgery for acute severe MR carries a very high mortality, especially if combined with CABG in cases of ischemic MR in the setting of an acute MI.

Mitral Stenosis

Etiology

Mitral stenosis (MS) is less commonly seen in the elderly. It is usually rheumatic in etiology but is rarely due to progressive mitral annular calcification.[19]

Signs and Symptoms

The clinical picture is usually that of pulmonary congestion, and in the advanced stages right-sided heart failure. Symptoms are usually stable unless AF occurs. This is not uncommon, and may lead to clinical decompensation and the development of pulmonary edema.

Diagnostic Testing

Echocardiography is an excellent method to evaluate the thickness, mobility, and the calcification of the mitral valve leaflets. It is also useful in evaluating the subvalvular apparatus. A valve area can be measured using planimetry, or calculated using the pressure half time of the mitral valve flow. The pressure gradient across the mitral valve can also be determined. Left atrial dimensions and left ventricular function can also be assessed. Cardiac catheterization can directly measure the gradient across the mitral valve and calculate a valve area using the Gorlin equation (Table 26.6).

Management

The management of MS depends on the degree of the patient's symptoms as well as the presence of AF or pulmonary hypertension. Medical management is directed towards maintaining adequate fluid balance, and rate control in cases of AF, and is warranted as long as it provides symptomatic relief. As the symptoms progress, and AF develops, other strategies should be considered. Percutaneous balloon mitral valvuloplasty (commissurotomy) is now the first choice of intervention in suitable patients. It is far less invasive than surgical commissurotomy, yet the results are fairly comparable. The decision to proceed with valvuloplasty is based on an echocardiographic valve score, taking into account four variables: Leaflet thickness, mobility, calcification, and the subvalvular apparatus. Mitral valve replacement surgery is indicated in severely symptomatic patients who are not candidates for valvuloplasty. Patients with valvular disease or following valve replacement surgery should receive prophylaxis for infective endocarditis when indicated, as for dental or appropriate surgical procedures.

ARRHYTHMIAS

Upon initial presentation, patients may vary from having nonspecific symptoms, such as fatigue, that may not immediately direct the clinician to an arrhythmia diagnosis, to having quite specific symptoms, such as palpitations or syncope. A careful and specific history must be obtained in these instances, as patients typically have difficulty in fully describing their symptoms. Signs and symptoms such as palpitations, lightheadedness, dizziness, syncope, chest pain, shortness of breath, and diaphoresis should be addressed. Oftentimes, if a patient experiences palpitations, they (or the clinician) may be able to replicate their chest sensations by hand tapping the pattern and speed of the rhythm. This may help establish the rate and rhythm. For example, a rapid, but irregular rhythm suggests AF, whereas a fast regular rhythm may suggest ventricular tachycardia (VT) in the elderly. Additionally, the circumstances during which these arrhythmias are triggered are also important. Activities or circumstances such as exercise, gastrointestinal illnesses, assuming a recumbent position, alcohol consumption, cigarette smoking, emotional upset, and medication consumption that may be temporally associated with the arrhythmia should be identified.

Atrial Fibrillation

CASE THREE

Mrs. D. is an 82-year-old woman brought into the office from an assisted-living facility. It was at the assisted living facility that she was noted to have a fast irregular rhythm. In retrospect, she states that she has felt fatigued for the past few months and has felt light-headed at times when she is walking. She feels an occasional "fluttering" in her chest. On examination, her blood pressure is 169/74 mm Hg with a heart rate of 126 beats per minute. Auscultation reveals an irregular heart rhythm. An ECG reveals AF with a rapid ventricular rate.

Definition

AF is a supraventricular arrhythmia characterized by unsynchronized atrial activity resulting in the deterioration of mechanical atrial function.[20] The ventricular response to irregular atrial activity is dependent on the electrophysiological states of the AV node, vagal tone, sympathetic tone, and medications.

Pathophysiology

There are several mechanisms that contribute to the development and persistence of AF. Structural and morphologic changes within the atrial myocardium as a result of normal aging or progression of disease processes are explanations for the occurrence of AF. Morphologic changes lead to a patchy fibrosis, which prompts the development of changes in the electrophysiological mechanisms within the atrial myocardium. The nonhomogeneity of the atrial tissue causes an abnormal conduction and propagation of electrical activity, leading to the lack of synchrony of atrial contraction. Conduction abnormalities within the AV node (fatty or fibrotic infiltration) or autonomic innervation of the atrial myocardium may also cause AF. In many instances, it is not possible to determine the anatomic abnormality that is responsible for the development of AF.

Incidence and Prevalence

AF is the most common arrhythmia encountered in a clinical setting and accounts for approximately one third of elderly patient hospitalizations for cardiac rhythm abnormalities. The prevalence of AF is approximately 0.4% of the general population and increases with age. Cross-sectional studies have shown that more than 6% of patients older than 80 have AF. Age-adjusted incidence is higher in men (2% per year) compared to women (1.5% per year) older than 80. Furthermore, whites are twice as likely to develop AF compared to blacks.

Etiology

There are several etiologies of AF. The acute causes of AF that should be considered include pulmonary embolism, pericarditis, myocarditis, MI, hyperthyroidism, alcohol consumption ("holiday heart syndrome"), surgery, infection, and metabolic abnormalities. These episodes may be short-lived if the underlying condition is treated. Cardiovascular conditions associated with the development of AF include CHD, valvular disease (especially mitral valve disease), and hypertension, especially in the presence of left ventricular hypertrophy. Cardiomyopathies, such as hypertrophic cardiomyopathy, dilated cardiomyopathy, and restrictive cardiomyopathies (amyloidosis, hemachromatosis, endomyocardial fibrosis) may predispose the elderly to AF. Furthermore, genetic predisposition, diabetes mellitus, cardiac tumors, constrictive pericarditis, cor pulmonale, obstructive sleep apnea, idiopathic dilation of the right atrium, atrial septal defect, sinus node disease, ventricular pre-excitation, and supraventricular tachycardia increase the likelihood for the development of AF.

Workup/Keys to Diagnosis

Physical Examination

Physical examination of patients with AF includes an irregular pulse with corresponding irregular jugular venous pulsations. A variation in the loudness of the first heart sound may be appreciated. Proper auscultation to elicit valvular abnormalities should be performed. Additionally, in identifying potential etiologies for AF, attention should be directed toward the head, neck, and pulmonary examination.

Diagnostic Procedures

At least a single-lead ECG recorded during the arrhythmia is necessary to establish the diagnosis. In cases where paroxysmal AF is suspected, a 24-hour Holter monitor or event recorder may be used, depending on the presumed frequency of the arrhythmia.

Management

In evaluating and managing patients with AF, the clinician must consider the following:

1. Is the patient symptomatic when in AF? If so, what are the symptoms and how disabling are they?
2. Frequency, duration, and type of AF (paroxysmal, persistent, first episode).
3. The factors precipitating AF and maneuvers that may have been performed to terminate AF.
4. Have any medications helped in the past?
5. Are there any underlying cardiac conditions or treatable causes of AF?

A 12-lead ECG should be obtained, as findings such as left ventricular hypertrophy, prior MI and pre-excitation may be of help in establishing a cause for AF. If clinically indicated, a chest radiograph may be useful in examining the lung parenchyma and vasculature. A transthoracic echocardiogram is useful to assess the valvular apparatus, left ventricular size and function, atrial size, pulmonary artery pressures, and pericardial disease.

Medications

The three main strategies considered in treating AF in the elderly include rhythm control, rate control, and anticoagulation.[20] Recent clinical trial data have demonstrated the superiority of rate-control over rhythm-control strategies in elderly patients $\geq$65 years given the increased incidence of adverse events associated with antiarrhythmic use.[21,22] The decision to pursue direct current cardioversion in a patient must be made on an individual basis. If treatment of the underlying condition is possible (i.e., hyperthyroidism, infection or inflammatory states, myocardial ischemia, pulmonary embolus, alcohol use), every attempt must be made to identify and correct the causative factor(s). During this time, rate-controlling agents may be employed for rapid ventricular rates. Even after the treatment or the unsuccessful identification of the underlying condition, patients who continue to remain significantly symptomatic may be considered for cardioversion. However, if these patients have concurrent conditions such as sick-sinus syndrome, rheumatic heart disease with enlarged left atria ($\geq$6 cm), or chronic lung disease, they are not likely to benefit from cardioversion and are better served with rate-controlling therapy, given the low rate of successful cardioversion. At the current time, clinical trials are under way to evaluate the merits of rate control versus rhythm control in patients with AF and heart failure. Whichever strategy is to be considered, all patients must be placed on long-term anticoagulation, even if they appear to be in a restored and preserved sinus rhythm.

Medications for conversion to and the maintenance of sinus rhythm include amiodarone, dofetilide, and ibutilide (see Table 26.7, all with Evidence Level A). Amiodarone (intravenous or oral) can be used for the restoration of sinus rhythm and is equally effective in the conversion of AF and atrial flutter. Prior to initiation, serum samples should be obtained for baseline thyroid and liver function in addition to a chest radiograph and pulmonary function testing. Dofetilide has restricted use in the United States, requires 72 hours of inpatient observation, and must be dosed based on the patient's creatinine clearance. Due to the lack of negative ionotropic effects, dofetilide is useful in those with reduced left ventricular function, including those with CHF symptoms and CHD. Dofetilide seems more effective in converting atrial flutter than AF. Ibutilide is an intravenous preparation and is more effective in converting atrial flutter than AF. When all these agents are given in conjunction with electrical cardioversion, the success in the maintenance of sinus rhythm is increased. The common side effects of these agents include hypotension, rapidly conducting atrial flutter, torsades de pointes, and QT interval prolongation. There is a relative paucity of data regarding the initiation of antiarrhythmic therapy in the outpatient setting. The most worrisome occurrence is the development of proarrhythmia. Before such therapy is administered, the initiation of β-blockers or calcium channel blockers should be considered to avoid the development of rapid AV conduction. Other medications such as quinidine, procainamide, and disopyramide are not routinely used in elderly patients, given the higher incidence of cardiac and extra-cardiac side effects. Medications such as encainide, flecainide, and propafenone have limited utility in the elderly, given the significant limitations of use with concurrent comorbidities (CHF, obstructive lung disease, or CHD).

TABLE 26.7
COMMON MEDICATIONS USED TO TREAT ARRHYTHMIAS

	Oral	Intravenous	Arrhythmias Treated
Amiodarone	600–800 mg/d, divided dose until 10 g, then 200–400 mg/d as maintenance	5–7 mg/kg over 30–60 min, then 1.2–1.8 g/d (continuous) until 10 g total	Atrial fibrillation, atrial flutter, ventricular tachycardia
Dofetilide	CrCl (mL/min): Dose (μg b.i.d.) >60: 500 40–60: 250 20–40: 125 <20: Contraindicated	N/A	Atrial fibrillation, atrial flutter
Ibutilide	N/A	1 mg over 10 min, repeat 1 mg in 10 min if necessary	Atrial fibrillation, atrial flutter
Calcium Channel Blockers			
Verapamil	120–360 mg daily divided dose	0.075–0.15 mg/kg IV over 2 min	Atrial fibrillation
Diltiazem	120–360 daily divided dose	0.25 mg/kg over 2 min, then 5–15 mg/h	Atrial fibrillation
β-Blockers			
Atenolol	25–100 mg daily dose	N/A	Atrial fibrillation, ventricular tachycardia
Carvedilol	3.125–25 mg daily divided dose	N/A	Ventricular tachycardia
Esmolol	N/A	0.5 mg/kg over 1 min, then 0.05–0.2 mg/kg/min	Atrial fibrillation
Metoprolol	25–100 mg b.i.d.	2.5–5 mg over 2 min, up to three doses	Atrial fibrillation, ventricular tachycardia
Propanolol	80–240 mg daily divided dose	0.15 mg/kg	Atrial fibrillation
Digoxin	0.125 to 0.375 mg daily	0.25 mg every 2 h (maximum 1.5 mg)	Atrial fibrillation

CrCl, creatinine clearance; N/A, not applicable.

Direct current cardioversion may also be used to restore sinus rhythm. The success rate in the restoration of sinus rhythm varies from 70% to 90%, and is much higher than pharmacologic cardioversion. For elective cardioversion (Evidence Level C), patients must be adequately anticoagulated for 3 to 4 weeks prior to, and after cardioversion. If the duration of AF is clearly <48 hours, anticoagulation prior to, and after cardioversion is optional and is dependent on the risk to the patient. An alternative approach is to perform a transesophageal echocardiogram to exclude the presence of a left atrial or left atrial appendage clot or sluggish blood flow. If these findings are not present, direct current cardioversion may be performed while the patient is receiving intravenous heparin. Oral anticoagulation must be maintained for 4 weeks after successful cardioversion. In patients with concomitant AV nodal disease, electrical cardioversion may result in prolonged periods of asystole (secondary to prolonged sinoatrial recovery times) or severe bradycardia (secondary to transient complete AV node block).

Medications used to maintain rate control include digoxin (Evidence Level B), β-blockers (Evidence Level C), and nondihydropyridine calcium channel blockers (Evidence Level C) (Table 26.7). Digoxin in acute onset AF is of limited use and shows no difference in acutely reducing the heart rate. In persistent AF, digoxin is effective in rate control at rest, especially in those with CHF. Nondihydropyridine calcium channel blockers, such as verapamil and diltiazem are effective in acute rate control of AF, especially when administered intravenously. Persistent AF can be adequately treated with either of these calcium channel blockers, but caution must be exercised if they are to be administered in patients with heart failure, as they can cause further depression of left ventricular function. β-Blockers such as atenolol, metoprolol, or propanolol may be used in both acute and persistent AF. Combination therapy is often necessary and is effective in AF rate control. Digoxin in combination with atenolol or diltiazem has a synergistic effect on the AV node. This type of combination may be better in achieving adequate and consistent heart rate control. The major side effects of these medications include hypotension, heart block, bradycardia, and heart failure.

Multicenter randomized studies have demonstrated that long-term anticoagulation with warfarin decreases the stroke rate by 68% and mortality by 33% in patients with nonvalvular AF (Evidence Level A). Aspirin therapy, although less effective, affords a 20% to 25% reduction in stroke (Evidence Level A).[23] Approximately 50% of AF-related strokes are in elderly patients older than 75. The most frequent cause of disabling stroke in women is AF-associated. Independent risk factors for the development of AF-associated stroke are prior thromboembolism, heart failure with reduced LVEF <35%, hypertension, increasing age, and diabetes mellitus (see Table 26.8). A target international normalized ratio (INR) between 2 and 3 is

TABLE 26.8
RISK-STRATIFICATION FOR PRIMARY[a] PREVENTION OF THROMBOEMBOLISM IN PATIENTS WITH NONVALVULAR ATRIAL FIBRILLATION

High Risk	Intermediate Risk	Low Risk
Age >75 y Hypertension Reduced LVEF	Age 65–75 y Coronary artery disease Diabetes mellitus Thyrotoxicosis No high-risk features	Age <65 y No high-risk features Normotensive

[a]Patients with atrial fibrillation and prior thromboembolism are at high risk for stroke, and anticoagulation is recommended for secondary prevention in such instances.
LVEF, left ventricular ejection fraction.

recommended for patients with chronic or intermittent AF who are at high risk for thromboembolic events. In patients who are older than 75 years, and at a higher risk for bleeding, but with no clear contraindication to oral anticoagulation, the target is 2.0 (range 1.6 to 2.5). Aspirin, 325 mg, may be given to patients with contraindications to warfarin use, but the risk for stroke is high in the aged. In patients who have concurrent CHD and AF, the use of warfarin should be maintained with the use of clopidogrel 75 mg daily or aspirin 81 mg daily (Evidence Level C). Furthermore, in those with AF and recent coronary stent implantation, clopidogrel should be preferentially used over aspirin therapy in conjunction with warfarin. Oral anticoagulation, without heparin substitution, may be temporarily withheld in patients without mechanical heart valves for 1 week when diagnostic or surgical procedures need to be performed that carry an increased risk of bleeding (Evidence Level C). In patients with mechanical prosthetic heart valves, or those with increased risk for thromboembolic events, heparin (unfractionated or low-molecular weight) should be substituted for oral anticoagulation (Evidence Level C).

Percutaneous/Surgical Interventions

Many patients are unable to tolerate AV nodal blocking agents or antiarrhythmic agents, or have concomitant AV nodal disease, which becomes apparent after direct current cardioversion. In these patients, other percutaneous therapies such as AV node modification with a permanent pacemaker may be suitable. These patients must still be maintained on oral anticoagulation. Additionally, performing catheter ablation techniques to eliminate foci around the pulmonary veins, superior vena cava, right atrium, and the left atrium is a potentially curative approach, with success rates ranging from 70% to 85%. However, very limited data are available for elderly patients. Surgical therapies such as the maze operation create barriers between the atria to limit recurrent wavefront propagation, as is observed with sustained AF. The success rates for this procedure are approximately 90%.

Ventricular Arrhythmias

CASE FOUR

Mr. S. is a 70-year-old with a history of CABG who comes into the office with a reported episode of fainting. His family states that he was sitting in a local restaurant when he suddenly "blacked out," lost consciousness, and was slumped over for <5 seconds. He regained consciousness with no confusion after the episode. He did not have any seizure activity and had no prodromal symptoms. He did not go to the emergency room because he felt "all better" after the episode. He comes into the office with a report that it happened again 1 week later while he was walking on the driveway to get the newspaper. He is admitted directly from the office. An echocardiogram revealed an LVEF of 25%. Cardiac catheterization was performed and showed nonrevascularizable coronary disease. While in the hospital, several episodes of nonsustained ventricular tachycardia (NSVT) occur, despite electrolyte correction and maximal medical management. The patient is referred to cardiac electrophysiology for implantable cardiac defibrillator placement.

Definition

An ECG diagnosis of NSVT is suggested by the occurrence of three or more consecutive abnormally shaped premature ventricular complexes at a rate greater than 120 beats per minute with a QRS duration of 120 milliseconds and an ST-T vector in the opposite direction to the QRS deflection. The differentiating feature of NSVT and sustained VT is that the latter must last for at least 30 seconds or be associated with hemodynamic instability requiring intervention. If the ventricular activity is fragmented and chaotic without any evidence of organized deflections on ECG, the rhythm is ventricular fibrillation (VF).

Pathophysiology

Depending on the etiologies listed in the following text, the cause of VT or fibrillation (VT/VF) is different. As is commonly observed in elderly patients with CHD and a low LVEF, the presence of scar tissue formed in the area of damaged left ventricular myocardium acts as a nidus for the development of ventricular arrhythmias.

Incidence and Prevalence

The incidence of VT or ventricular fibrillation (VF) causing sudden cardiac death increases with age and accounts for approximately 300,000 deaths annually. In general, ventricular arrhythmias may be observed in up to 80% of the population older than 60. Premature ventricular contractions (PVCs) are common in the elderly, and are asymptomatic for the most part. VT is present in approximately 2% to 8% of elderly patients with heart disease and occasionally occurs in the absence of heart disease.

Signs and Symptoms

Although patients may present with similar signs and symptoms as observed with atrial arrhythmias, syncope and sudden cardiac death are more suggestive of VT/VF.

Etiology and Risk Factors

The etiologies for VT include CHD, left ventricular aneurysm, dilated cardiomyopathy, hypertrophic cardiomyopathy, arrhythmogenic RV dysplasia, prolonged QT interval, coronary artery spasm causing transient myocardial ischemia, R-on-T premature ventricular complexes, and depressed left ventricular function. With these underlying etiologies, VT may degenerate into VF, especially if prolonged VT occurs.

Workup/Keys to Diagnosis

Physical Examination

Generally, physical examination findings do not directly suggest a diagnosis of ventricular arrhythmias. Upon initial examination of the patient, ecchymoses, hematomas, or lacerations on the head, arms, or torso should be identified, as they are highly suggestive of a syncopal event. Physical examination findings that suggest CHF (increased jugular venous distention, rales, S3, ascites, and lower extremity edema) may be present.

Laboratory

Derangements in electrolyte levels, such as hypokalemia, hypomagnesemia, hypocalcemia, or hypophosphatemia, tend to make susceptible individuals develop ventricular arrhythmias. These levels should be checked and repleted, if necessary.

Diagnostic Procedures

An ECG should always be obtained on such patients as it may suggest concurrent CHD, prior MI, left ventricular aneurysm, or left ventricular hypertrophy. Abnormal QT interval prolongation may be noted. An echocardiogram revealing left ventricular dysfunction with significant wall motion abnormalities strongly suggests the presence of CHD. In select patients, the use of Holter monitoring to detect ventricular arrhythmias may be helpful.

In patients with NSVT, electrophysiological studies (EPS) and signal-averaged ECG (SAECG) have been used to further risk stratify patients.[24] Several studies have shown that sustained VT can be induced during EPS in up to 18% to 45% of cases with NSVT. The likelihood is increased in those with LV dysfunction. However, EPS cannot be recommended as a routine test, given the lower than needed sensitivity levels. For example, EPS performed in survivors of cardiac arrest with sustained VT failed to show inducibility of VT in up to 30% to 50% of cases. EPS is of benefit in select patients. SAECG is a computer-driven, noninvasive method that evaluates the terminal portion of the QRS. The presence of high-frequency, low-amplitude potentials at the terminal portion of the QRS has been shown to predict the occurrence of fatal arrhythmic events post-MI. In the post-MI setting, a normal SAECG has a high negative predictive value. The use, however, of SAECG is limited because of its low positive predictive value, low sensitivity, and sparse data for elderly patients.

Management

In assessing a patient with ventricular arrhythmias and the potential therapies available, the clinician must work with the family and the patient in deciding on the best management strategy for the patient, not just the dysrhythmia. For example, the presence of significant comorbidities may outweigh the utility and benefit of certain measures. In some instances, the life expectancy of the patient, notwithstanding the cardiac dysrhythmia, may be too limited to receive any potential benefit from invasive measures. Furthermore, the clinician must determine the extent of improvement in the overall quality of life that further therapy may provide. Potential reversible causes should be identified and corrected. If the etiology is presumed to be secondary to ischemia, patients should be referred for cardiac catheterization and cardiac surgery, if appropriate.

Medications

Medication choices for the treatment of ventricular arrhythmias in elderly patients are limited (Table 26.7). Several clinical trials have been prematurely terminated because of an increase in arrhythmogenic deaths in patients taking medications such as encainide, flecanide, moricizine, or sotalol. Medications that should be considered for ventricular arrhythmias are β-blockers and/or amiodarone. β-Blockers (Evidence Level A) reduce the occurrence of sudden cardiac death, especially in post-MI patients. The most common reasons for β-blocker intolerance are bronchospasm, depression, fatigue, and sexual dysfunction. β-Blockers used in conjunction with amiodarone (Evidence Level A) have a synergistic effect and are more effective in reducing fatal ventricular arrhythmias and sudden cardiac death. Even alone, amiodarone therapy has been shown to be useful in suppressing ventricular arrhythmias and sudden cardiac death in patients with ischemic or nonischemic cardiomyopathy with depressed LV function. Possible toxic effects include hypo- or hyperthyroidism (incidence 2% to 24%), persistent cough (i.e., chronic interstitial pneumonitis; 1% to 15%), transaminitis (15% to 50%), hepatitis (3%), corneal microdeposits (>90%), halo vision (<5%), photosensitivity (25% to 75%), gastrointestinal upset (4% to 30%), bradycardia, hypotension, and proarrhythmia (<1%).

Percutaneous/Surgical Interventions

Scar tissue surrounded by viable myocardium is a nidus for the development of sustained VT. In these instances, surgical resection of the scar tissue has been successful in eliminating VT. However, this procedure is reserved for certain types of monomorphic VT and carries a relatively high surgical mortality rate (>10%). In a percutaneous approach, EPS can be used to map and ablate VT pathways using radio-frequency energy. The types of VT that may be successfully ablated using radio frequency energy are RV outflow tract tachycardia, fascicular VT, bundle branch reentrant tachycardia, idiopathic VT, and appropriate but repeated shocks in those with implantable cardioverter defibrillators (ICD) on maximum medical therapy (Evidence Level A).

Several randomized clinical trials have demonstrated the superiority of ICD therapy over antiarrhythmic therapy in the prevention of cardiac arrest or death from arrhythmia (Evidence Level A).[25–28] Although the indications for ICD therapy are evolving, currently patients with a history of prior MI with LV systolic dysfunction (LVEF ≤35%) who demonstrate ventricular arrhythmias (spontaneous or inducible during EPS) are potential candidates. Furthermore, patients with a VT/VF arrest with no identifiable reversible cause or patients with syncope and EPS-inducible VT/VF that is refractory to medical therapy are candidates for ICD therapy. Several recent studies demonstrate the arrhythmic mortality benefit of ICD therapy in patients with nonischemic dilated cardiomyopathy and ischemic cardiomyopathy without documented ventricular arrhythmias (prophylactic ICD placement). These new data have moved the Centers for Medicare and Medicaid Services to modify its guidelines for ICD therapy to include patients with a diagnosis of nonischemic dilated cardiomyopathy for >9 months with an LVEF ≤30%. Furthermore, the previous requirement of a QRS duration ≥120 milliseconds has been withdrawn, given the improved survival benefit in patients with a QRS duration <120 milliseconds.

Bradyarrhythmias

> **CASE FIVE**
>
> Mr. J. is a 76-year-old with a past medical history of hypertension who comes to the office complaining of fatigue, dizziness, and feeling as though "my heart is going to jump out of my chest." He notes no temporal pattern or particular activities associated with his symptoms. He states that he has felt so dizzy and light-headed at times when walking in the house that he has had to grab onto furniture to keep from falling. He has never fallen and lost consciousness. An ECG shows marked sinus bradycardia of 30 beats per minute with junctional escape beats. The patient is referred for permanent pacemaker placement.

Bradycardias are common in the elderly and may be the result of conduction system aging or underlying cardiac disease. In particular, the progressive deterioration of the sinoatrial node, AV node, and/or bundle of His occurs over time, often leading to symptoms requiring pacemaker implantation.[26]

In assessing the patient for permanent pacemaker placement, potential reversible causes should be identified and corrected. Medications that have AV nodal blocking properties (e.g., β-blockers, nondihydropyridine calcium channel blockers, clonidine, digoxin) should be discontinued. Hypothyroidism should be ruled out as an etiology. In asymptomatic patients, those with a resting heart rate ≤40 beats per minute (junctional escape rhythm) or pauses of 3 seconds or more should be considered for pacemaker implantation. First degree AV block is usually of no consequence in the elderly patient, whereas the presence of second and third degree AV block suggests disease of an aging conduction system. Type II second degree AV block and third degree AV block are usually associated with a poor prognosis and warrant pacemaker placement (Evidence Level B). Type I second degree AV block is uncommonly associated with AV nodal disease and usually results from enhanced vagal tone, myocardial ischemia, or drug toxicity. This rhythm is transient and usually does not require pacemaker placement.

Other indications for pacemaker implantation include symptomatic bradycardia of any type (Evidence Level C), bradycardia induced by medications used to treat arrhythmias (Evidence Level C), after catheter ablation of the AV junction (Evidence Level C), postoperative AV block that is not expected to resolve (Evidence Level C), patients with concomitant neuromuscular disease and AV nodal disease (Evidence Level B), long QT syndrome (Evidence Level C), and bradycardia-induced VT (Evidence Level C).

One of the recent developments in heart failure therapy is the pacing of both ventricles (cardiac resynchronization therapy). Using a biventricular pacing system in patients with a prolonged QRS duration (≥120 milliseconds) or those with incomplete left bundle branch block (<120 milliseconds) with desynchronous contraction of both ventricles has resulted in a significant improvement in the 6-minute walk test, peak oxygen consumption, hospitalization rates, and quality of life. Ongoing studies of cardiac resynchronization therapy are being conducted to evaluate and validate methods to identify those patients who would benefit from biventricular pacing systems.

REFERENCES

1. Mittelmark MB, Psaty BM, Rautaharju PM, et al. Prevalence of cardiovascular diseases among older adults. The Cardiovascular Health Study. *Am J Epidemiol.* 1993;137:311–317.
2. Gibbons RJ, Balady GJ, Bricker JT, et al. ACC/AHA 2002 guideline update for exercise testing: Summary article: A report of the American College of Cardiology/American Heart Association Task Force on Practice Guidelines (Committee to Update the 1997 Exercise Testing Guidelines). *Circulation.* 2002;106:1883–1892.
3. Gibbons RJ, Abrams J, Chatterjee K, et al. ACC/AHA 2002 guideline update for the management of patients with chronic stable angina–summary article: A report of the American College of Cardiology/American Heart Association Task Force on practice guidelines (Committee on the management of patients with chronic stable angina). *J Am Coll Cardiol.* 2003;41:159–168.
4. Williams MA, Fleg JL, Ades PA, et al. Secondary prevention of coronary heart disease in the elderly (with emphasis on patients > or = 75 years of age): An American Heart Association scientific statement from the Council on Clinical Cardiology Subcommittee on Exercise, Cardiac Rehabilitation, and Prevention. *Circulation.* 2002;105:1735–1743.
5. A. T. Collaboration. Collaborative meta-analysis of randomised trials of antiplatelet therapy for prevention of death, myocardial infarction, and stroke in high risk patients. *BMJ.* 2002;324:71–86.
6. Yusuf S, Sleight P, Pogue J, et al. Effects of an angiotensin-converting-enzyme inhibitor, ramipril, on cardiovascular events in high-risk patients. The Heart Outcomes Prevention Evaluation Study Investigators. *N Engl J Med.* 2000;342:145–153.
7. Fox KM. Efficacy of perindopril in reduction of cardiovascular events among patients with stable coronary artery disease: Randomised, double-blind, placebo-controlled, multicentre trial (The EUROPA Study). *Lancet.* 2003;362:782–788.
8. Braunwald E, Domanski MJ, Fowler SE, et al. Angiotensin-converting-enzyme inhibition in stable coronary artery disease. *N Engl J Med.* 2004;351:2058–2068.
9. Shepherd J, Blauw GJ, Murphy MB, et al. Pravastatin in elderly individuals at risk of vascular disease (PROSPER): A randomised controlled trial. *Lancet.* 2002;360:1623–1630.
10. Heart Protection Study Collaborative Group. MRC/BHF Heart Protection Study of cholesterol lowering with simvastatin in 20,536 high-risk individuals: A randomised placebo-controlled trial. *Lancet.* 2002;360:7–22.
11. Larosa JC, Grundy SM, Waters DD, et al. Intensive lipid lowering with atorvastatin in patients with stable coronary disease. *N Engl J Med.* 2005;352:1425–1435.
12. Nissen SE, Tuzcu EM, Libby P, et al. Effect of antihypertensive agents on cardiovascular events in patients with coronary disease and normal blood pressure: The CAMELOT study: A randomized controlled trial. *JAMA.* 2004;292:2217–2225.
13. Alexander KP, Anstrom KJ, Muhlbaier LH, et al. Outcomes of cardiac surgery in patients > or = 80 years: Results from the National Cardiovascular Network. *J Am Coll Cardiol.* 2000;35:731–738.
14. Batchelor WB, Anstrom KJ, Muhlbaier LH, et al. Contemporary outcome trends in the elderly undergoing percutaneous coronary interventions: Results in 7,472 octogenarians. National Cardiovascular Network Collaboration. *J Am Coll Cardiol.* 2000;36:723–730.
15. TIME Investigators. Trial of invasive versus medical therapy in elderly patients with chronic symptomatic coronary-artery disease (TIME): A randomised trial. *Lancet.* 2001;358:951–957.
16. Tribble DL. AHA Science Advisory. Antioxidant consumption and risk of coronary heart disease: Emphasis on vitamin C, vitamin E, and beta-carotene: A statement for healthcare professionals from the American Heart Association. *Circulation.* 1999;99:591–595.
17. Braunwald E, Antman EM, Beasley JW, et al. ACC/AHA 2002 guideline update for the management of patients with unstable angina and non-ST-segment elevation myocardial infarction–summary article: A report of the American College of Cardiology/American Heart Association task force on practice guidelines (Committee on the Management of Patients With Unstable Angina). *J Am Coll Cardiol.* 2002;40:1366–1374.
18. Antman EM, Anbe DT, Armstrong PW, et al. ACC/AHA guidelines for the management of patients with ST-elevation myocardial infarction. *Circulation.* 2004;110:e82–e292.
19. Bonow RO, Carabello B, de Leon AC, et al. ACC/AHA guidelines for the management of patients with valvular heart disease. Executive summary. A report of the American College of Cardiology/American Heart Association Task Force on Practice Guidelines (Committee on Management of Patients With Valvular Heart Disease). *J Heart Valve Dis.* 1998;7:672–707.
20. Fuster V, Ryden LE, Asinger RW, et al. ACC/AHA/ESC guidelines for the management of patients with atrial fibrillation: Executive summary A report of the American College of Cardiology/American Heart Association Task Force on Practice Guidelines and the European Society of Cardiology Committee for Practice Guidelines and Policy Conferences (Committee to develop guidelines for the management of patients with atrial fibrillation) developed in collaboration with the North American Society of Pacing and Electrophysiology. *Circulation.* 2001;104:2118–2150.
21. Van Gelder IC, Hagens VE, Bosker HA, et al. A comparison of rate control and rhythm control in patients with recurrent persistent atrial fibrillation. *N Engl J Med.* 2002;347:1834–1840.
22. Wyse DG, Waldo AL, DiMarco JP, et al. A comparison of rate control and rhythm control in patients with atrial fibrillation. *N Engl J Med.* 2002;347:1825–1833.
23. The SPAF III Writing Committee for the Stroke Prevention in Atrial Fibrillation Investigators. Patients with nonvalvular atrial fibrillation at low risk of stroke during treatment with aspirin: Stroke prevention in atrial fibrillation III study. *JAMA.* 1998;279:1273–1277.
24. Iravanian S, Arshad A, Steinberg JS. Role of electrophysiologic studies, signal-averaged electrocardiography, heart rate variability, T-wave alternans, and loop recorders for risk stratification of ventricular arrhythmias. *Am J Geriatr Cardiol.* 2005;14:16–19.
25. The AVID Investigators. A comparison of antiarrhythmic-drug therapy with implantable defibrillators in patients resuscitated from near-fatal ventricular arrhythmias. The Antiarrhythmics Versus Implantable Defibrillators (AVID) Investigators. *N Engl J Med.* 1997;337:1576–1583.
26. Gregoratos G, Abrams J, Epstein AE, et al. ACC/AHA/NASPE 2002 guideline update for implantation of cardiac pacemakers and antiarrhythmia devices: Summary article: A report of the American College of Cardiology/American Heart Association Task Force on Practice Guidelines (ACC/AHA/NASPE Committee to Update the 1998 Pacemaker Guidelines). *Circulation.* 2002;106:2145–2161.
27. Connolly SJ, Gent M, Roberts RS, et al. Canadian Implantable Defibrillator Study (CIDS) : A randomized trial of the implantable cardioverter defibrillator against amiodarone. *Circulation.* 2000;101:1297–1302.
28. Ferrick KJ. Antiarrhythmic therapy in elderly persons: A device-based approach. *Am J Geriatr Cardiol.* 2005;14:10–15.

Heart Failure

27

Richard W. Pretorius

CLINICAL PEARLS 354

PATHOPHYSIOLOGY 355

ETIOLOGY 355

SYSTOLIC AND DIASTOLIC DYSFUNCTION 355

SYMPTOMS AND SIGNS OF HEART FAILURE 356
Electrocardiogram 356
Chest X-ray 356
Echocardiogram 356
Brain Natriuretic Peptide 357
Renal Insufficiency 357

TREATMENT 357
Diuretics 357
Angiotensin-Converting Enzyme Inhibitors 358
Angiotensin Receptor Blocking Agents 359
β-Blockers 359
Digoxin 359
Spironolactone 359
Hydralazine and Oral Nitrates 360
Other Modalities 360
Calcium Channel Blockers 360
Antiarrhythmics 360
Nonpharmaceutical Therapies 361

COMORBIDITY 361

HOSPICE 361

CLINICAL PEARLS

- Heart failure is the most common cause of hospitalization in the geriatric population.
- Fatigue and dyspnea on exertion are the most common symptoms, but they can be subtle and nonspecific.
- Survival has been increased by angiotensin-converting enzyme (ACE) inhibitors, β-blockers, and spironolactone.
- Recently, the combination of hydralazine and dinitrates has been shown to increase the survival of African Americans.
- No single test is diagnostic.
- Over 50% of patients with heart failure will have a normal ejection fraction.
- Treatment protocols provide direction, but treatment must be individualized and closely monitored.
- Early treatment of subtle findings such as mild hyponatremia can prevent hospitalizations.
- A gradual decline in cardiac function may go undetected for days or weeks resulting in an acute crisis that precipitates a hospitalization.
- Weighing a patient daily and using a sliding scale of a loop diuretic is often needed to maintain a patient at dry weight.

Heart failure occurs when the cardiac output is inadequate to meet the circulatory needs of the body. It is the most commonly coded diagnosis in Medicare patients, representing 1 million hospital admissions per year as a primary diagnosis and 3 million as one of the top three diagnoses.[1] It is the only cardiovascular disease that is increasing in both incidence and prevalence in the United States. It has an increased incidence with age that is exponential, exceeding 40% of the population by age 90. There are 5.5 million people in the United States with heart failure, including nearly 500,000 newly diagnosed each year and 300,000 who die annually. Because 90% of deaths and 80% of hospitalizations due to heart failure occur in patients older than 65 years, it is the quintessential geriatric ailment.[2,3] Heart failure consumes one fourth of all Medicare expenditures. Medicare paid an average of $16,514 for reimbursement for medical care for patients with heart failure in 1996, which was 431% of the average cost of $3,831 spent for other Medicare beneficiaries.[4] The annual cost of care of patients with heart failure is estimated to be nearly three times greater than that for patients with cancer and two times greater than that for patients with acute myocardial infarction.[4]

PATHOPHYSIOLOGY

The heart, which is primarily a pump, shows indications of failing when there is low cardiac output relative to the circulatory needs of the body. The resulting neurohormonal activation, with an elevation of natriuretic peptides and troponins, is a physiologic attempt to preserve cardiac output, although it occurs at the expense of further cardiac and vascular stress. In order to increase the effective circulatory volume, retention of sodium occurs—and continues to occur—even in the presence of established volume overload. Because sodium distributes equally between the plasma and the interstitial space (which together comprise the so-called sodium space), massive quantities of fluid can be retained over time if uncorrected. In the inadequately treated patient, the degree of fluid retention will exceed the degree of sodium retention as a consequence of the presence of other osmotically active molecules beside the sodium, and a relative hyponatremia will result.[5] Indeed, persistent hyponatremia in the geriatric patient most commonly indicates volume expansion, and every attempt should be made to treat the heart failure sufficiently to correct it. Morbidity increases from pneumonia in "wet lungs" or from hypoxia-induced (from the pulmonary edema and hypoperfusion) myocardial infarction.

> **CASE ONE**
>
> A woman in her late eighties who is not on medication and has not seen a physician in many years presents to the office with complaints of pronounced fatigue and dyspnea on walking across the room. She has been sitting in a chair for the past several nights. On examination, she has anasarca with large bilateral pleural effusions and massive peripheral edema. Her cardiac echocardiogram shows normal systolic function and no cardiomegaly. She is diagnosed with chronic diastolic heart failure. She is treated with a diuretic and eventually loses 50 pounds, 40% of her dry weight, over a period of 3 months and is ultimately maintained on a low-dose diuretic, an angiotensin-converting enzyme (ACE) inhibitor and a β-blocker. Despite presenting clinically with New York Heart Association (NYHA) class IV heart failure, she corrected to NYHA class I heart failure with appropriate treatment. Because of the gradual onset over a long period of time and the resulting compensatory physiologic changes, she presented with normal renal function and a chest x-ray that showed no vascular dilatation or congestion, although the increased oncotic pressure had produced large pleural effusions.

Although heart failure often presents as an acute event such as a myocardial infarction or an acute change in functional ability, as was the case here, the underlying disease process has frequently been present—and undetected—for a number of years. This particular patient, on additional questioning, not only had gradual onset of symptoms of heart failure over a 6-month period, but she also presented with mild untreated hypertension. Hypertension is the most common cause of diastolic heart failure. It is likely that the hypertension had been present for 10 to 20 years, causing chronic increased cardiac afterload that ultimately caused her heart failure.

ETIOLOGY

The etiology of heart failure is often multifactorial in the elderly although the final pathway of disease is one of two cardiac dysfunctions: Inadequate ventricular filling and/or inadequate ventricular emptying. Contributing factors to heart disease can be traced to the four basic structural components of the heart: Muscle, valves, coronary arteries, and electrical conduction system. Cardiac muscle disease includes cardiomyopathies (hypertrophic, restrictive, congestive, infiltrative, hypertensive). Valvular disease includes stenosis or regurgitation of any of the four valves (particularly stenosis of the aortic valve and regurgitation of the mitral valve). Coronary artery disease includes myocardial ischemia and myocardial infarction. Electrical disturbances include atrial fibrillation and other arrhythmias. Of these, coronary artery disease is the most common cause and accounts for nearly 70% of cases of heart failure.[6] Hypertension is the second most common cause and may account for up to 60% of cases in African Americans.[7] Valvular heart disease is the third most common cause. Consequently, treatment of ischemia is essential. It is the most important strategy to maximize myocardial function. Hypertension, insufficiently treated in two thirds of patients, should be treated proactively long before heart failure has the opportunity to develop. Finally, surgery for valvular heart disease can be considered regardless of age. Outcome is more dependent on general fitness than on age alone.[8]

SYSTOLIC AND DIASTOLIC DYSFUNCTION

Heart failure has traditionally been defined as decreased cardiac output associated with a left ventricular ejection fraction (LVEF) of <45%. This is the prototypical systolic dysfunction. In the past two decades, however, there has been increased recognition that the cardiac pump can fail due to one of two mechanisms: Inadequate filling (ventricular charge) or inadequate emptying (ventricular discharge). For many years, large double-blinded, randomized placebo-controlled trials of heart failure focused on patients with a decreased ejection fraction. More recent information has shown that most patients with heart failure have a normal ejection fraction.[9] Until large trials in diastolic dysfunction are published, treatment with diuretics, ACE inhibitors, and β-blockers is based on extrapolation from studies on systolic dysfunction, expert opinion, and empiric observation.

Systolic dysfunction accounts for approximately one third of the cases of heart failure; diastolic heart failure is present alone in another third of cases and combines with systolic heart failure in another third (see Table 27.1). Diastolic dysfunction increases with age, particularly in women. Men with heart failure have a normal LVEF 22% of the time when diagnosed at age 60. Prevalence with a normal LVEF increases to 33%, 41%, and 47% respectively when their age is in the seventies, eighties, and nineties. In women, heart failure with a normal LVEF occurs more frequently, at rates of 37%, 44%, 59%, and 73% when thier age is in the sixties, seventies, eighties, and nineties, respectively.[10] Seventy-three percent of hospitalized patients with heart failure and an LVEF of 50% or greater are women.[9]

SYMPTOMS AND SIGNS OF HEART FAILURE

The most common symptoms—fatigue, exercise intolerance, and weakness—are nonspecific and occur in well over 90% of heart failure cases. These symptoms are often incorrectly attributed to noncardiac causes including normal aging. Dyspnea on exertion occurs in 95% of patients with systolic heart failure and 85% of patients with diastolic heart failure. Orthopnea occurs in 60% to 70% of cases, and is slightly more common in systolic heart failure. Paroxysmal nocturnal dyspnea occurs approximately 50% of the time in both types.[11]

TABLE 27.1
DIFFERENTIAL DIAGNOSES WITH ICD-9 CODES

- Heart failure (428)
  - Congestive heart failure, unspecified (428.0)
  - Left heart failure (428.1)
  - Systolic heart failure (428.2)
    - Unspecified (428.20)
    - Acute (428.21)
    - Chronic (428.22)
    - Acute on chronic (428.23)
  - Diastolic heart failure (428.3)
    - Unspecified (428.20)
    - Acute (428.21)
    - Chronic (428.22)
    - Acute on chronic (428.23)
  - Combined systolic and diastolic heart failure
    - Unspecified (428.20)
    - Acute (428.21)
    - Chronic (428.22)
    - Acute on chronic (428.23)
  - Heart failure, unspecified (428.9)

Signs, like symptoms, may be nonspecific and require a high index of suspicion. Because an insidious onset permits the gradual development of compensatory physiologic processes, the physical examination may be essentially normal despite markedly reduced cardiac function. Rales, a displaced apical impulse and the presence of an S3 or S4 gallop occur approximately two thirds of the time in uncompensated heart failure. These signs occur almost twice as frequently as edema, which is present approximately one third of the time.[11]

The constellation of signs and symptoms is more sensitive for the diagnosis of heart failure than any individual test. Monitoring signs and symptoms is essential for determining the efficacy of therapeutic interventions. One highly useful clinical sign is dry weight. Unfortunately a patient's dry weight cannot be calculated from a formula. Dry weight is the weight at which the patient feels well and demonstrates optimized signs, symptoms, and laboratory parameters (particularly sodium, blood urea nitrogen, creatinine, and brain natriuretic protein).

Electrocardiogram

In most cases of heart failure the electrocardiogram (ECG) is abnormal. A normal ECG makes it unlikely that the patient has systolic heart failure because it has a high sensitivity (94%) for left ventricular systolic dysfunction, although it is less useful in the context of diastolic heart failure.[12] The ECG, including the left ventricular amplitude, is dynamic and subject to the variable forces acting upon the heart, particularly the degree of fluid overload.

Chest X-ray

Cardiomegaly occurs in 90% or more of patients with systolic heart failure but it is rarely present in patients with isolated diastolic heart failure.[13] Cardiomegaly is dependent upon the severity of the heart failure, the extent of myocardial hypertrophy and the degree of uncompensated vascular congestion. It may be absent in the setting of a "stunned myocardium" (due to sudden onset ischemia) or in the setting of diastolic heart failure with relatively compensated fluid balance. Similarly, signs of pulmonary congestion (pleural effusions, perihilar fullness, ground-glass opacities, peribronchovascular interstitial thickening, Kerley B lines) can be helpful but also depend on the acuity of the process. Patients who have a long-standing elevation in their pulmonary capillary wedge pressure may have little evidence of pulmonary edema.

Echocardiogram

The echocardiogram evaluates the function of the cardiac valves and distinguishes between patients with normal and decreased systolic ejection fractions. There are currently no universally accepted radiologic criteria for the diagnosis of diastolic heart failure, and objective evidence for diastolic dysfunction is often not definitive. Some would argue that the echocardiogram should at least demonstrate evidence of abnormal left ventricular relaxation, abnormal left ventricular filling, diminished diastolic distensibility, or diastolic stiffness. Others would argue that diastolic dysfunction is a diagnosis based on clinical evidence of heart failure in the setting of a normal ejection fraction. Because the echocardiogram is an indirect measure of cardiac function and not a direct measurement of the degree of tissue perfusion, one should be cautious about overinterpretation.

Brain Natriuretic Peptide

The brain natriuretic peptide (BNP) is released by ventricular myocytes when the ventricular wall is stretched or strained. BNP is elevated in patients with systolic dysfunction as well as in those with diastolic abnormalities on echocardiography. Although it is an expensive test, it is both sensitive and specific in the diagnosis of heart failure. Just as cardiac troponins have a central role in the workup of patients with chest pain, the BNP can be helpful in the patient with dyspnea. BNP values of <100 pg per mL in the emergency room indicate that heart failure is unlikely (sensitivity 90%, specificity 76%, negative predictive value 89%). Values of 100 to 400 pg per mL are intermediate and may indicate the need for other standard evaluation. Values >400 pg per mL are most likely from heart failure (positive predictive value 95%).[14] In the emergency room workup of dyspnea, BNP can decrease the emergency room stay by nearly 30 minutes, the hospital length of stay by 3 days, and the cost of hospitalization by $1,800.[15]

Renal Insufficiency

Renal insufficiency, one of the strongest predictors of mortality, is a common occurrence in heart failure, with at least one third of patients having moderate to severe impairment (an estimated glomerular filtration rate [GFR] <60 mL/minute/1.73 m^2). Nonsteroidal anti-inflammatory drugs (NSAIDs) should be used with caution in the setting of possible heart failure as they are associated with a doubling of the odds of a hospital admission for newly diagnosed heart failure and with a 10-fold increase in hospitalization for a patient with a history of heart disease. The use of NSAIDs in the presence of renal dysfunction and heart failure is a major contributing factor to decompensation. NSAIDs account for approximately 20% of hospital admissions with the diagnosis of heart failure.[16]

TREATMENT

Medications used in heart failure are reviewed in Table 27.2.

Diuretics

The retention of sodium and water is the hallmark feature of heart failure. Diuretics facilitate the excretion of sodium and water into the urine. They remain so essential in the treatment of heart failure that it is considered unethical to withhold loop or thiazide diuretics to conduct long-term trials. Frequent dosing adjustments are often required to prevent recurrences of either edema or dehydration even in stable patients. The most expedient way to maintain fluid balance is for the patient to obtain a daily weight and to adjust the dose of the diuretic accordingly (often by using a sliding scale that decreases the diuretic dose for a low weight and increases it for a high one). Because diuretics activate the renin-angiotensin-aldosterone system, they should usually be used in conjunction with ACE inhibitors when possible (Evidence Level A). Patients with diastolic dysfunction are highly sensitive to changes in volume and great care must be exerted to keep the weight from straying >1.0 to 1.5 kg above or below the patient's dry weight. Diuretics can improve symptoms within hours or days, unlike ACE inhibitors or β-blockers that take weeks or months for clinical benefit. Sudden fluid shifts, however, can trigger arrhythmias so weight loss should be limited to <0.5 to 1.0 kg per day or less. There is often no urgency in correcting the fluid balance in an elderly patient who may have had the gradual accumulation of excess fluid over many months. The electrolyte changes and the re-equilibration of osmotically active molecules across cellular membranes take time. Starting doses of furosemide can range from 20 mg every other day up to 40 mg daily and only occasionally need to be higher (Evidence Level B).

Metolazone, when used alone, is a mild diuretic and has a potency that is approximately equal to the thiazide diuretics. Unlike thiazide diuretics, however, it can produce diuresis in patients with severe renal insufficiency (GFR <20 mL per minute). Metolazone and furosemide administered either concurrently or sequentially have produced marked diuresis in some patients who were otherwise refractory to a maximal dose of furosemide alone. For instance, a patient who is taking high doses of furosemide and starts metolazone 2.5 mg (or sometimes 5 mg) 30 minutes before the furosemide may have a dramatic response and even risk contraction alkalosis from overdiuresis. Although the U.S. Food and Drug Administration has approved 600 mg per day as a maximal dose for furosemide, some patients who have renal insufficiency with persistent inadequate diuresis will respond to doses of 1,000 to 2,000 mg per day in divided doses. Patients with a decreased LVEF often tolerate high doses of diuretics. Patients with diastolic dysfunction and normal LVEF require higher left ventricular filling pressures and are less tolerant of intravascular depletion induced by diuretics. When the excess fluid has been adequately mobilized from both the intravascular and extravascular spaces,

TABLE 27.2
MEDICATIONS FOR HEART FAILURE

Medication	Initial (mg)	Target (mg)	Maximum (mg)
Loop diuretics			
Furosemide	20	Titrate	600–2,000 divided t.i.d.
Bumetanide	0.5	Titrate	5 b.i.d.
Ethacrynic acid	25	Titrate	200 b.i.d.
Torsemide	10	Titrate	100 b.i.d.
Other diuretics			
Hydrochlorothiazide	12.5	Titrate	50
Metolazone (half hour before loop diuretic)	1.25	Titrate	20
Spironolactone	25	50	200
ACE inhibitors			
Benazepril	5	20	40
Captopril	6.25 t.i.d.	50 t.i.d.	150 t.i.d.
Enalapril	2.5 b.i.d.	10 b.i.d.	20 b.i.d.
Fosinopril	5	20	40
Lisinopril	5	20	40
Quinapril	2.5 b.i.d.	10 b.i.d.	20 b.i.d.
Ramipril	1.25 b.i.d.	5 b.i.d.	10 b.i.d.
Trandolapril	0.5 b.i.d.	4 q.d.	4 q.d.
β-Blockers			
Bisoprolol	1.25	10	10
Carvedilol	3.125 b.i.d.	25 b.i.d.	50 b.i.d.
Metoprolol	6.25 b.i.d.	75 b.i.d.	75 b.i.d.
Metoprolol XL	12.5	200	200
Digoxin	0.125	Titrate	Titrate to avoid toxicity
Vasodilators			
Isosorbide dinitrate	10 t.i.d.	40 t.i.d.	40 t.i.d.
Hydralazine	10 t.i.d.	75 t.i.d.	100 t.i.d.

ACE, angiotensin-converting enzyme.

the dose of the diuretics can be reduced or occasionally stopped.

Diuretics may also cause electrolyte imbalance, particularly hypokalemia and hypomagnesemia, increasing the risk of sudden death from a ventricular arrhythmia. Diligent monitoring of electrolytes, renal function, weight, and fluid balance is essential in all patients with heart failure, but particularly those on diuretics. Electrolytes (sodium, potassium, and magnesium) and renal function (blood urea nitrogen and creatinine) should be obtained every 2 to 3 months in stable patients; weights should be obtained daily; fluid balance (as indicated by degree of edema and skin turgor) and any change in oral intake should be monitored weekly by caregivers and every 1 to 2 months by physicians. More frequent monitoring should be done in patients who are experiencing an exacerbation of their heart failure, particularly if a new dry weight needs to be determined (Evidence Level C).

Angiotensin-Converting Enzyme Inhibitors

The renin–angiotensin–aldosterone system begins with angiotensinogen, which is made in the liver. Renin converts it to angiotensin I in the kidney, which is then converted to angiotensin II by ACE. Angiotensin II, a potent vasoconstrictor, binds to receptor AT_1, which triggers detrimental cardiac effects, and receptor AT_2, which triggers beneficial cardiac effects. Angiotensin II also triggers the release of aldosterone, which causes sodium and fluid retention. An ACE inhibitor blocks both the formation of angiotensin II and the metabolism of bradykinin, a vasoconstrictor that causes sodium retention. An ACE inhibitor blocks three peptides—angiotensin II, aldosterone, bradykinin—whereas an angiotensin receptor blocker (ARB) blocks one peptide, angiotensin II, at the receptor AT_1.[17]

ACE inhibitors have been shown to be beneficial in patients with all degrees of heart failure severity and, along with diuretics, are considered a first-line therapy. They can improve the ejection fraction as well as reduce left ventricular hypertrophy by inhibiting ventricular remodeling. Because they decrease mortality in patients who have increased cardiovascular risk but still have normal left ventricular function, they have a role even in the preclinical stage of heart failure[18] (Evidence Level A). Their benefit comes from a decrease in cardiac afterload and blood pressure as well as an apparent direct effect on myocardial cells. Starting an ACE inhibitor can cause acute deterioration of renal function or more commonly a temporary diminution of renal function. In the Evaluation of Losartan in the Elderly study (ELITE) only 10.9% of patients had an increase in the serum creatinine concentration that was >0.3 mg per dL (26.5 mmol per L) and only 0.8% discontinued the ACE inhibitor due to the worsening of renal function.[19] Even in the Cooperative North Scandinavian Enalapril Survival Study (CONSENSUS), which compared 40 mg of enalapril with placebo in patients with advanced heart failure (NYHA IV), there was an additional increase in renal insufficiency of 17% in comparison with placebo and an additional discontinuation rate of 1.5%. The increase in renal creatinine is an initial finding that often reverses if the ACE inhibitor is continued. The mean initial increase in creatinine was 49% in the CONSENSUS study but recovered to 9% above baseline.[20]

Angiotensin Receptor Blocking Agents

ARBs have equal efficacy as ACE inhibitors and, according to guidelines from the American College of Cardiology and the American Heart Association, can be considered if an ACE inhibitor cannot be tolerated due to cough (5%) or angioedema.[3] They are not typically used as first-line agents because they have not been shown to decrease mortality in patients with heart failure.[17] ACE inhibitors and ARBs act on different enzymes in the renin-angiotensin-aldosterone system, raising hopes that their combined use could further decrease morbidity and mortality.[21] Unfortunately, early studies of combined ACE inhibitors and ARBs have failed to demonstrate improved exercise capacity, functional capacity, and quality of life.

β-Blockers

Heart failure activates the sympathetic nervous system and elevates the level of circulating catecholamines, with resultant tachycardia and peripheral vasoconstriction. While adrenergic activation is beneficial as an acute response, over time it has detrimental effects on exercise tolerance and mortality as the increased sympathetic drive increases arrhythmias. At the cellular level, increased norepinephrine causes myocyte hypertrophy, apoptosis, and myocardial ischemia. Clinical trials have shown that β-blockers reduce mortality by 35% in patients with asymptomatic left ventricular dysfunction (Evidence Level A). While some of the larger, earlier trials were done with bisoprolol, carvedilol, and metoprolol, current data do not support the preferential use of one β-blocker over another.[22] β-Blockers are usually well-tolerated but they should be started at low doses and then increased gradually, typically at 2-week intervals. Because β-blockers can initially worsen fluid retention, diuretics may need to be increased to maintain patients at their dry weight. Hypotension and dizziness, if a concern, can be minimized by administering the β-blockers at a different time of the day than the ACE inhibitors and diuretics. Fatigue and weakness, when they occur, usually resolve in a few weeks.

β-Blockers are contraindicated in patients with severe bronchospasm, systolic blood pressure <85 mm Hg, bradycardia that is symptomatic, or advanced heart block (in the absence of a pacemaker). β-Blockers should be started when the patient's heart failure is compensated. When the patient is decompensated, β-blockers may worsen symptoms and decrease LVEF. The previous recommendation to wait until 2 weeks after hospital discharge has been supplanted by a recommendation to start β-blockers once the patient is stable in the hospital. Clinically, improvement may take 3 to 6 months to be evident.

Digoxin

Digoxin is the only positive inotrope that has been shown to have benefit in heart failure (increased exercise capacity, decreased symptoms, decreased hospitalization), although it has not been shown to affect mortality. For patients who remain symptomatic despite appropriate doses of diuretics, ACE inhibitors, and β-blockers, digoxin is a reasonable choice. It can also be a good choice in the patient with atrial fibrillation and heart failure, due to its inotropic and rate-controlling properties, although it may not control heart rate as well as diltiazem. Because of its narrow therapeutic index and its propensity to increase toxicity in the presence of hypokalemia or hyperkalemia, potassium and digoxin levels should be carefully monitored. This is particularly true for the unstable patient who is not in fluid balance and in the patient who begins a new medication, such as amiodarone, that affects the digoxin level.

Spironolactone

Plasma levels of both renin and norepinephrine increase in correlation with the severity of the heart failure. The increased activity of the renin-angiotensin-aldosterone system is persistent and induces sustained sodium retention. When an aldosterone-blocking agent such as spironolactone binds to the mineralocorticoid receptors, substantial natriuresis and diuresis occur. This is in contrast to primary hyperaldosteronism where the action of aldosterone is less persistent and a steady state of sorts is achieved. Hyperaldosteronism increases renal sodium retention with the expansion of extracellular fluid by 1.5 to 2 L. At this point renal sodium retention ceases, fluid and sodium balance is restored and no detectable edema occurs. In heart failure the continued action of aldosterone can eventually result in the retention of 8 to 10 L or more of excess fluid.

Spironolactone is indicated in patients who have NYHA class IV heart failure and are symptomatic despite the use of the ACE inhibitor, β-blockers, digoxin, and diuretics (Evidence Level A). Baseline laboratory studies should include a serum potassium <5 mEq per L and creatinine <2.5 mg per dL. Potassium level should be monitored closely within 1 week of initiation, at least every 4 weeks for the first 3 months and every 3 months thereafter. The potassium level should also be monitored if there is a change in the dose of spironolactone, a change in any other medications that affects the potassium balance, a weight change of >2 kg, or an exacerbation of heart failure. In patients with severe heart failure (NYHA class IV) and abnormal LVEF who are already on diuretics and ACE inhibitors, even a low dose of spironolactone (25 to 50 mg) can decrease the risk of death by 30% and the risk of hospitalization by 35%.[23]

Hydralazine and Oral Nitrates

Hydralazine and isosorbide dinitrates have long been recognized as alternatives for patients who cannot use ACE inhibitors. In one large-scale study, the first Vasodilator Heart Failure trial, hydralazine, and oral nitrates decreased mortality by 25% to 30% compared to prazosin and placebo when each treatment was added to diuretic and digoxin therapy.[24] This compares favorably to enalapril, which decreased mortality by 28% when it was added to diuretic and digoxin therapy[25] (Evidence Level B). In a recent study designed exclusively for blacks, the African-American Heart Failure trial, the combination of isosorbide dinitrate and hydralazine reduced the annual death rate by 43% and the first hospitalizations by 33%. This was so impressive that the study was terminated early.[26] As there are 375,000 blacks with moderate to severe heart failure, approximately 15,000 lives could be saved yearly in the black population alone. Because these patients were already on standard therapy of neurohormonal-inhibitor drugs before the combination was added to their regimen, alternative mechanisms may be influencing the progression of heart failure.

The starting dose of isosorbide dinitrate is 10 mg three times per day, which can be titrated up to a maximum dose of 40 mg three times per day with an allowance for a 12-hour nitrate-free period to prevent the development of tolerance. The starting dose of hydralazine is 10 to 25 mg three times per day, which can be titrated up to a maximum dose of 100 mg three times per day.[26]

Other Modalities

Mobilizing fluid can sometimes be a challenge in elderly patients with refractory heart failure (NYHA class IV) who are on appropriate medications and are still unresponsive to high oral doses of furosemide. When diuretic resistance occurs, therapeutic options include higher doses of furosemide, constant furosemide infusion, concomitant low-dose dopamine infusion to increase renal blood flow, and potentiating diuretic activity by combining furosemide with metolazone. Another option may be to draw out fluid from the interstitial space into the intravascular space using small volumes of hypertonic saline. One protocol, studied in Italy, used 500 to 1,000 mg IV furosemide plus 150 mL of hypertonic saline (1.4% to 4.6%) over 30 minutes twice a day for 6 to 12 days, resulting in a long-term survival rate at 30 months of 55% versus 15% in a control group that received only the IV furosemide.[27]

Calcium Channel Blockers

Calcium channel blockers, in general, are contraindicated in heart failure. Although they have the benefits of anti-ischemic properties, increased coronary blood flow and systemic vasodilation, they have the disadvantages of a negative inotropic effect and reflex neurohormonal activation, with the risk of worsening of symptoms and increased mortality. Older agents such as diltiazem, nifedipine, and verapamil can exacerbate heart failure and increase mortality, particularly in patients after myocardial infarction and those with an ejection fraction <40%. The newer agents amlodipine and felodipine have less negative inotropic effects and appear to be safer in heart failure. While not indicated for heart failure, they have not been shown to increase mortality and may be considered for the management of hypertension in patients with systolic dysfunction. The role of calcium channel blockers in patients with diastolic dysfunction is not clear.[28]

Antiarrhythmics

Although there is a 40% to 50% mortality rate in heart failure from ventricular arrhythmias, class I antiarrhythmics are contraindicated because of the increased mortality associated with their proarrhythmic properties. Only amiodarone has shown either no significant effect on total mortality or a trend toward reduction in the risk of death. Amiodarone is not currently recommended for prophylaxis in heart failure due to its uncertain benefit and its toxicity to thyroid, eyes, lungs, and liver, although it can be used in the setting of ventricular fibrillation or sustained ventricular tachycardia. Patients on amiodarone should have a chest x-ray and thyroid and liver function testing done at baseline and every 6 months. Pulmonary function testing should be done at baseline and then repeated if abnormalities are noted on the chest x-ray.

Although half of the deaths from heart failure occur as a result of pump failure due to continued inotropic decline despite appropriate pharmacologic interventions, the other half are caused by sudden death due to an arrhythmia. The likelihood of arrhythmias can be decreased by vigilantly maintaining a favorable environment for inotropic function by optimizing oxygenation, carefully correcting electrolyte abnormalities and diligently keeping patients at their dry weights.

Nonpharmaceutical Therapies

Alcohol is a myocardial toxin and should be either avoided or restricted to one or two drinks per day because of its depressant effect on the myocardium. As obesity increases the volume of distribution and the necessary cardiac output, weight loss will decrease the required cardiac workload. High sodium intake is commonly discouraged, typically <2 g per day if fluid retention is present, although there are no good studies of salt restriction in the context of heart failure. Similarly, high fluid intake is discouraged as a way of avoiding fluid overload, although realistically a consistent fluid intake is probably the most practical approach, particularly in milder degrees of heart failure. In the setting of more severe heart failure where fluid overload is present despite appropriate therapy, a fluid restriction of 1.5 to 2 L daily may be considered.

COMORBIDITY

The prevalence of comorbid conditions in Medicare patients with heart failure is 1.77 times higher than among older patients without heart failure.[4] Of heart failure patients, 60% have two or more comorbid conditions, 20% have one and 20% have none. As the elderly heart is fragile, every effort should be made to treat comorbid conditions.[4] Any physiologic stress due to an uncontrolled disease process will, of necessity, put stress on the cardiovascular system, increasing the required cardiac output and worsening the heart failure. Self-monitoring for early symptoms of any disease process as well as preventive visits with one's physician every 1 to 2 months are critically important. In the nursing home setting, a talented charge nurse who knows the residents well and who is alert for subtle changes in behavior and functional level, usually the first indication of worsening cardiac output, can be invaluable. The influenza and pneumococcal vaccines decrease morbidity and mortality by reducing the cardiorespiratory stress caused by these infections (Evidence Level A). In the Group Health study, there was a 27% reduction in hospitalizations for congestive heart disease and a 50% reduction in all-cause mortality for vaccinated elderly patients over six seasons.[29]

HOSPICE

Heart failure is the most common noncancer diagnosis for hospice patients in the last year of life, representing one out of six of all hospice patients. Yet it is not easy to determine the length of the terminal stage, and only approximately 10% of patients with end-stage heart failure actually enroll in hospice programs.[30] Factors such as ejection fraction of <20% and severe heart failure at baseline (NYHA class III or IV) have limited predictive value.[31] Even for patients with 3 days or less to live, scoring criteria incorrectly estimate a 6-month survival in over 50% of patients. Furthermore, there is no significant decrement in quality of life for many patients as death approaches, and almost a third of nonhospitalized patients reported good-to-excellent quality of life less than a month before death.[32]

REFERENCES

1. Haldeman GA, Croft JB, Giles WH, et al. Hospitalization of patients with heart failure: National hospital discharge survey, 1985 to 1995. *Am Heart J.* 1999;137:352–360.
2. Friesinger GC, Butler J II. End-of-life care for elderly patients with heart failure. *Clin Geriatr Med.* 2000;16:663–675.
3. Hunt SA, Baker DW, Chin MH, et al. ACC/AHA guidelines for the evaluation and management of chronic heart failure in the adult: Executive summary. *J Am Coll Cardiol.* 2001;38:2101–2113.
4. Zhang JX, Rathouz PJ, Chin MH. Comorbidity and the concentration of healthcare expenditures in older patients with heart failure. *J Am Geriatr Soc.* 2003;51(4):476–482.
5. Andrew P. Hyponatremia: Terminology and more. *Can Med Assoc J.* 2004;170(13):1891–1892.
6. Gheorghiade M, Gattis WA, O' Connor CM. Treatment gaps in the pharmacological management of heart failure. *Rev Cardiovasc Med.* 2002;3:S11–S19.
7. Mathew J, Davidson S. Etiology and characteristics of heart failure in blacks. *Am J Cardiol.* 1996;78:1447–1450.
8. Freeman WK, Schaff HV, O' Brien PC, et al. Cardiac surgery in the octogenarian: Perioperative outcome and clinical follow up. *J Am Coll Cardiol.* 1991;18:29–35.
9. Klapholz M, Maurer M, Lowe AM, et al. Hospitalization for heart failure in the presence of a normal left ventricular ejection fraction: Results of the New York heart failure registry. *J Am Coll Cardiol.* 2004;43(8):1432–1438.
10. Aronow WE, Ahn C, Kronzon I. Association of diastolic heart failure with age and gender in 572 older patients with heart failure. *Chest.* 1998;113:867–869.
11. Zile MR, Brutsaert DL. New concepts in diastolic dysfunction and diastolic heart failure: Part 1: Diagnosis, prognosis, and measurements of diastolic function. *Circulation.* 1989;105:1389.
12. Davie AP, Francis CM, Love MP. Value of the electrocardiogram in identifying heart failure due to left ventricular systolic dysfunction. *BMJ.* 1996;312:222.
13. Gehlbach BK, Geppert E. The pulmonary manifestations of left heart failure. *Chest.* 2004;125(2):669–682.
14. Maisel AS, Krishnaswamy P, Nowak RM, et al. Rapid measurement of B-type natriuretic peptide in the emergency diagnosis of heart failure. *N Engl J Med.* 2002;347:161–167.
15. Mueller C, Scholer A, Laule-Kilian K, et al. Use of b-type natriuretic peptide in the evaluation and management of acute dyspnea. *N Engl J Med.* 2004;350:647–654.
16. Page J, Henry D. Consumption of NSAIDs and the development of congestive heart failure in elderly patients: An underrecognized public health problem. *Arch Intern Med.* 2000;160:777–784.
17. Scow DT, Smith EG, Shaughnessy AF. Combination therapy with ACE inhibitors and angiotensin-receptor blockers in heart failure. *Am Fam Physician.* 2003;68(9):1796–1798.
18. Dahlof B, Pennert K, Hansson L. Reversal of left ventricular hypertrophy in hypertensive patients: A metaanalysis of 109 treatment studies. *Am J Hypertens.* 1992;92:95–110.

19. Pitt B, Segal R, Martinez FA, et al. Randomized trial of losartan versus captopril in patients over 65 with heart failure. *Lancet.* 1997;340:747–752.
20. Yusuf S, Sleight P, Pogue J, et al. The Heart Outcomes Prevention Evaluation Study Investigators. Effects of an angiotensin-converting-enzyme inhibitor, ramipril, on cardiovascular events in high-risk patients. *N Engl J Med.* 2000;342(3):145–153.
21. Jong P, Demers C, McKelvie RS, et al. Angiotensin receptor blockers in heart failure: Meta-analysis of randomized controlled trials. *J Am Coll Cardiol.* 2002;39:463–470.
22. Kukin ML. [Beta]-blockers in chronic heart failure: Considerations for selecting an agent. *Mayo Clin Proc.* 2002;77(11):1199–1206.
23. Pitt B, Zannad F, et al. The effect of spironolactone on morbidity and mortality in patients with severe heart failure. *N Engl J Med.* 1999;341:709–717.
24. Cohn JN, Archibald DG, Ziesche S, et al. Effect of vasodilator therapy on mortality in chronic congestive heart failure: Results of a Veterans Administration Cooperative Study. *N Engl J Med.* 1986;314:1547–1552.
25. Cohn JN, Johnson G, Ziesche S, et al. A comparison of enalapril with hysdralazine-isosorbide dinitrate in the treatment of chronic congestive heart failure. *N Engl J Med.* 1991;325:303–310.
26. Taylor AL, Ziesche S, Yancy C et al. Combination of isosorbide dinitrate and hydralazine in blacks with heart failure. *N Engl J Med.* 2004;351:2049–2056.
27. Licata G, DiPasquale P, Parrinello G, et al. Effects of high-dose furosemide and small-volume hypertonic saline solution infusion in comparison with a high dose of furosemide as bolus in refractory congestive heart failure. *Am Heart J.* 2003;145:459–466.
28. Aronow WS. Epidemiology, pathophysiology, prognosis, and treatment of systolic and diastolic heart failure in elderly patients. *Heart Dis.* 2003;5:279–294.
29. Nichol KL, Wuorenma J. Benefits of influenza for low-, intermediate-, and high-risk senior citizens. *JAMA.* 1998;158: 1769–1776.
30. Zambroski CH. Hospice as an alternative model of care for older patients with end-stage heart failure. *J Cardiovasc Nurs.* 2004;19(1):76–85.
31. Fox E, Landrum-McNiff K, Zhong Z, et al. Evaluation of prognostic criteria for determining hospice eligibility in patients with advanced lung, heart, or liver disease. *JAMA.* 1999;282:1638–1645.
32. Levenson JW, McCarthy EP, Lynn J, et al. The last six months of life for patients with congestive heart failure. *J Am Geriatr Soc.* 2000;48:S101–S109.

28

Cerebrovascular Disease and Stroke

William D. Smucker

CLINICAL PEARLS 363

DIFFERENTIAL DIAGNOSIS OF STROKE SIGNS AND SYMPTOMS 364

DISEASE BACKGROUND 364
Description/Definition of Problem 364
Pathophysiology 364
Systems Impacted 365
Incidence and Prevalence 365
Impact on Function 365

WORKUP/KEYS TO DIAGNOSIS 366
Is the Patient Medically Stable? 366
Are the Signs and Symptoms Consistent with a Presumptive Diagnosis of a Stroke? 366
Did the Syndrome Develop Suddenly? 366
Is There Evidence of Focal Brain Dysfunction? 366
Do Diagnostic Studies Confirm a Stroke? 366
Is Cerebral Hemorrhage Present? 366
Does the Patient Fulfill Criteria for Thrombolysis? 368

MANAGEMENT 368
Prognosis 368
Determining Appropriate Location and Intensity of Stroke Management 368
Stroke Unit 369
General Medical Care of the Patient with Acute Ischemic Stroke 369
Assessing and Managing Risk of Complications Following Acute Stroke 370
Assessing and Managing Aspiration Pneumonia Risk 370
Assessing and Managing Deep Vein Thrombosis Risk 371
Assessing and Managing Risk of Urinary Tract Infection 371
Assessing and Managing Pressure Ulcer Risk 372
Assessing and Managing Poststroke Depression 372
Assessing Comorbid Coronary Heart Disease 372
Multidisciplinary Assessment of Function and Determination of Rehabilitation Needs 372
Lifestyle Recommendations 373
Medications 373
Surgical Interventions 374
Patient Monitoring/Secondary Prevention 374
Patient Education 376
Patient Monitoring 376

ACKNOWLEDGMENTS 376

CLINICAL PEARLS

- *Time is brain.*
- Thrombolytic therapy can improve survival and function if administered within 3 hours of stroke onset.
- Age alone is not a contraindication to thrombolytic therapy.
- Stroke unit care for patients with acute stroke is associated with improved survival, reduced complication rates and improved function.
- To prevent strokes, patients should control blood pressure, use antithrombotic therapy, lower lipids, control blood sugar, exercise regularly, and stop smoking.

- Benefits of warfarin outweigh the risks for most elderly patients with atrial fibrillation and a history of stroke or transient ischemic attack (TIA).
- Clinicians should routinely monitor elderly poststroke patients for cognitive decline, depression, and dependence in activities of daily living.

A clinician has several important opportunities to decrease the devastating physical, cognitive, and emotional effects of stroke. First, educating patients to seek emergent care for stroke symptoms may allow treatment to limit the extent of irreversible brain damage. Second, the identification and treatment of modifiable stroke risk factors can reduce the risk of first stroke and recurrent stroke. Third, once the stroke has occurred, preventive measures can decrease the risk of common stroke-related complications. Fourth, the treatment of stroke-related complications may reduce their impact on function, independence, and quality of life.

DIFFERENTIAL DIAGNOSIS OF STROKE SIGNS AND SYMPTOMS

A stroke or transient ischemic attack (TIA) causes focal brain ischemia, resulting in the sudden onset of focal neurologic symptoms such as unilateral weakness, numbness, or clumsiness, or it may cause global symptoms such as headache, nausea and vomiting, altered mental status, dizziness, or seizures. The differential diagnosis of conditions that can cause focal or global neurologic symptoms is exhaustive (see Table 28.1), but few conditions other than stroke cause a rapid onset of focal brain dysfunction.

Focal neurologic symptoms can also be caused by central nervous system conditions such as tumor, infection, seizures, demyelinating disease, or nutritional deficiencies. The focal symptoms may be due to conditions that affect the peripheral nerves, such as Bell palsy, optic neuritis, diabetic ophthalmoplegia, labyrinthitis, and mononeuropathies of the limbs. The causes of both global and focal neurologic symptoms include hypoxia, hypercarbia, hypotension, arrhythmia, hypoglycemia, hyperglycemia, electrolyte imbalance, systemic infection, hepatic or renal failure, adverse drug reaction, and seizures.

A stepwise approach to evaluation and treatment (see section Workup/Keys to Diagnosis) can help confirm the presence of a stroke and exclude competing diagnostic possibilities.

DISEASE BACKGROUND

Description/Definition of Problem

Over 700,000 Americans suffer a stroke each year. Age is the most important risk factor for stroke, with the peak incidence among those older than 80. With increasing age, strokes cause a greater degree of disability and result in a higher rate of mortality.

Pathophysiology

A stroke is caused by the sudden interruption of the cerebrovascular blood supply, causing focal brain ischemia and infarction. The signs and symptoms caused by focal ischemia are determined by the function of the damaged brain cells. A TIA is defined as the complete resolution (within 24 hours) of the signs and symptoms of brain ischemia.

Strokes are classified by pathophysiologic types because the acute treatment and subsequent preventive therapies

TABLE 28.1
CONDITIONS THAT MAY CAUSE STROKE-LIKE SYMPTOMS

Metabolic	Cardiovascular/ Pulmonary	Toxic	Infectious	Neurologic	Hematologic
Hypoglycemia (251.2) Hyperglycemia with hyperosmolar state (250.2) Dehydration (276.5) Hyponatremia (276.1) Hepatic encephalopathy (572.2)	Hypotension (458.8) Hypertensive encephalopathy (437.2) Syncope (780.2) Hypoxia (348.1) Pulmonary insufficiency, NOS (518.82)	Adverse drug effect (349.82) Intoxication (292.81)	Systemic infection (sepsis) (995.91) Encephalitis (323.9) Meningitis (322.9) Brain abscess (324.0)	Subdural hematoma (852.2) Bell palsy (351.0) Labyrinthitis (386.30) Postseizure paralysis (344.8) Petit mal status epilepticus (345.2) Brain neoplasm (191.9) Multiple sclerosis (340) Transient global amnesia (437.7) Mononeuritis of upper limb (354)	Hypercoagulable state (289.81)

NOS, not otherwise specified.

differ according to the pathophysiology. The two major types of stroke are ischemic and hemorrhagic.

In the elderly, most strokes are ischemic. An ischemic stroke occurs when a thrombus occludes a cerebral artery. The ischemic occlusion of a cerebral artery can be the result of a locally formed arterial thrombus (thrombotic stroke) or due to a thrombus that forms in the heart or larger arteries and embolizes distally (embolic stroke). One method of characterizing ischemic strokes according to anatomy and pathophysiology uses three ischemic stroke categories: Large artery atherosclerosis, small artery occlusion, and cardioembolism. Large artery atherosclerosis involves severe arterial narrowing or atherosclerotic plaque rupture leading to thrombus formation in the carotid, vertebral, basilar, middle cerebral, or anterior cerebral arteries. Small artery vascular occlusion of the penetrating cerebral arteries is due to arterial narrowing caused by vascular hypertrophy and thrombosis. Cardioembolic strokes occur when atrial fibrillation, prosthetic valves, diseased mitral and aortic valves, or areas of akinetic myocardium promote the formation of a cardiac thrombus within the heart that embolizes and occludes a cerebral artery.

A hemorrhagic stroke occurs when a cerebral artery ruptures due to conditions that make arteries stiff and fragile (e.g., atherosclerosis, hypertensive lipohyalinosis) or weak (e.g., arterial aneurysm, amyloid angiopathy). A bleeding disorder, brain tumor, arteritis, or trauma can also produce a cerebral hemorrhage.

Systems Impacted

A stroke can have deleterious effects on cognition, communication, mood, sensation, strength, stamina, independence in activities of daily living (ADL), and the ability to safely ingest adequate amounts of fluid and nutrients. Complications associated with a stroke include pneumonia, urinary tract infection (UTI), deep vein thrombosis (DVT), pulmonary embolus (PE), falls, fractures, pressure ulcers, and painful musculoskeletal conditions. Cognitive deficits and muscular weakness may increase falls and injuries. The occurrence of stroke signals not only the immediate risk of death due to the stroke or its acute complications, but also the future risk of acute illness and even death from ischemic cardiovascular events like myocardial infarction, claudication and critical limb ischemia, or recurrent stroke.

Incidence and Prevalence

The incidence of stroke varies according to an individual's risk factors for stroke. Table 28.2 lists common modifiable and nonmodifiable risk factors and conditions associated with stroke. Modifiable risk factors are conditions that may respond to lifestyle change, medication, or surgery, with a resultant decrease in the risk of first or recurrent stroke. Attention to all modifiable risk factors is important because multiple risk factors impart cumulative risk.

TABLE 28.2
STROKE RISK FACTORS

Modifiable risk factors

- High blood pressure
- Diabetes mellitus
- Hyperlipidemia
- Cigarette smoking
- Inactivity
- Obesity
- Heavy alcohol use
- Sleep apnea
- Estrogen use
- Atrial fibrillation
- Carotid artery stenosis

Nonmodifiable risk factors

- Increased age
- Male gender
- Family history
- Race (African American >Asian, Hispanic >white)
- Family history of stroke or heart attack before age 60

Impact on Function

Stroke is the leading cause of disability in the United States.[1] One survey of stroke survivors of age 65 and older found that 6 months after the stroke, 50% had hemiparesis, 35% experienced depressive symptoms, 30% required assistance with walking, 26% were dependent in some ADL, and 19% had aphasia.[1] Stroke frequently causes or exacerbates cognitive decline. Elderly stroke survivors often require prolonged rehabilitation, and approximately one fourth will need permanent care in a long-term care facility.[1]

CASE ONE

Mrs. M. is an 80-year-old widow, with a history of hypertension for 35 years, hypercholesterolemia for 15 years, and type 2 diabetes for 5 years. Her usual medications include hydrochlorothiazide 12.5 mg daily, lisinopril 20 mg daily, atorvastatin 40 mg daily, glipizide 10 mg twice daily, and aspirin 81 mg daily.

The emergency department calls you to tell you that 2 hours ago Mrs. M. called 911 after a fall. The fall was caused by the sudden onset of weakness in her right leg and arm that occurred while doing the dishes. The emergency squad reported that she was alert and conversant with right-sided weakness, but she had an otherwise normal neurologic examination. Her blood pressure was 180/100, heart rate 90 per minute and irregular, and blood glucose 125 mg per dL. The electrocardiogram monitor showed atrial fibrillation that lasted 15 minutes, converting to normal sinus rhythm spontaneously. Twenty minutes after the onset of her weakness, she recovered full strength.

WORKUP/KEYS TO DIAGNOSIS

The first hours of evaluating a patient with signs and symptoms of an acute stroke are critical. The three main objectives in this period are stabilization of the patient, confirmation of the diagnosis of stroke, and determination of eligibility for thrombolytic therapy. The clinical questions in the subsequent text can help guide this process.[2]

After stabilization, the clinician's tasks are to identify and reduce risk factors for early stroke-related complications, assess physical and cognitive status to determine the need for physical, occupational or speech therapy, characterize the type of stroke, and devise a comprehensive treatment plan that optimizes physical, cognitive, and emotional health and reduces the risk of recurrent stroke.

Is the Patient Medically Stable?

One must first confirm that the patient is medically stable and has optimum cerebral perfusion by assuring that the airway is adequate, oxygenation is normal, and that blood pressure and pulse are stable.

Are the Signs and Symptoms Consistent with a Presumptive Diagnosis of a Stroke?

Signs and Symptoms

Any abrupt decline in neurologic or cognitive function can be the sign of a stroke (see Table 28.3). Unlike other possible diagnoses, strokes occur suddenly, occur in a clinical context consistent with the pathology of the cerebral vessels, and produce signs and symptoms of focal brain dysfunction. Other elements that favor the diagnosis of a thrombotic or embolic stroke include a new neurologic deficit upon awakening, a prior history of transient cerebral ischemia, the presence of stroke risk factors, (Table 28.2) evidence of atherosclerotic cardiovascular disease, and the presence of valvular heart disease or cardiac arrhythmia.

TABLE 28.3
SIGNS AND SYMPTOMS SUGGESTIVE OF CEREBRAL ISCHEMIA

Major stroke syndromes

- Sudden confusion, difficulty speaking, or difficulty understanding speech
- Sudden difficulty seeing with one eye
- Sudden difficulty walking, severe dizziness, and/or loss of balance or coordination
- Sudden numbness or weakness of the face or in an arm or leg, especially if confined to one side of the body
- Sudden severe headache with no other known cause

Subtle syndromes that may be due to stroke

- Acute difficulty judging distance or depth
- Acute difficulty recognizing or paying attention to one side of the body or environment
- Acute difficulty with new learning
- Acute onset of impulsiveness or poor planning
- Acute onset of poor judgment
- Acute onset of poor safety awareness

Did the Syndrome Develop Suddenly?

Most stroke syndromes develop within seconds or minutes. Two important exceptions to this rule are the strokes that develop during sleep, creating a new neurologic deficit evident only upon awakening, and the thrombotic stroke that produces a progressive neurologic deficit that reaches maximum intensity over many hours. The gradual onset of neurologic deficits suggests diagnoses such as subdural hematoma (SDH), brain tumor, demyelinating disease, or nutritional deficiencies. Some causes of stroke-like neurologic symptoms can develop quickly (e.g., seizures, hypoxia, hypotension, arrhythmia, hypoglycemia, hyperglycemia) or more slowly (e.g., electrolyte imbalance, systemic infection, hepatic or renal failure, adverse drug reaction), but these causes tend to produce global, rather than focal, neurologic dysfunction.

Is There Evidence of Focal Brain Dysfunction?

Common signs and symptoms of brain ischemia are listed in Table 28.3. Most evaluations for acute stroke occur in emergency departments and will include the completion of a stroke severity assessment such as the National Institutes of Health Stroke Scale (NIHSS)[3] (see Table 28.4).

If a formal stroke scale has not been done, a focused physical examination to detect focal brain dysfunction should assess cognitive ability, speech abilities, visual fields, cranial nerve function, motor function, sensation, and gait. The physical examination should also assess cardiopulmonary status.

Do Diagnostic Studies Confirm a Stroke?

Diagnostic tests are used to confirm the presence of a stroke or of a condition masquerading as a stroke. The tests also evaluate comorbid illness that may contribute to stroke-like symptoms or influence subsequent management. Diagnostic protocols may vary and evolve according to new information and local custom. Table 28.5 lists essential and optional testing for the patient presenting with symptoms of acute stroke (Evidence Level C).[4]

Is Cerebral Hemorrhage Present?

Intracerebral hemorrhage is usually detected by the initial brain imaging study. Although computed tomography (CT) scan and magnetic resonance imaging have a 96% concordance for the diagnosis of hemorrhage, neither

TABLE 28.4
NATIONAL INSTITUTES OF HEALTH STROKE SCALE[3]

1.a. Level of consciousness:	0 Alert 1 Not alert, but arousable with minimal stimulation 2 Not alert, requires repeated stimulation to attend 3 Coma
1.b. Ask patient the month and their age:	0 Answers both correctly 1 Answers one correctly 2 Both incorrect
1.c. Ask patient to open and close eyes and then to grip and release the nonparetic hand:	0 Obeys both correctly 1 Obeys one correctly 2 Both incorrect
2. Best gaze (only horizontal eye movement):	0 Normal 1 Partial gaze palsy 2 Forced deviation
3. Visual field testing:	0 No visual field loss 1 Partial hemianopia 2 Complete hemianopia 3 Bilateral hemianopia (blind including cortical blindness)
4. Facial paresis (ask patient to show teeth or raise eyebrows and close eyes tightly):	0 Normal symmetrical movement 1 Minor paralysis (flattened nasolabial fold, asymmetry on smiling) 2 Partial paralysis (total or near total paralysis of lower face) 3 Complete paralysis of one or both sides (absence of facial movement in the upper and lower face)
5. Motor function—arm (right and left): Right arm______ Left arm______	0 Normal (extends arms 90 (or 45) degrees for 10 s without drift) 1 Drift 2 Some effort against gravity 3 No effort against gravity 4 No movement 9 Untestable (joint fused or limb amputated)
6. Motor function—leg (right and left): Right leg______ Left leg______	0 Normal (hold leg 30 degrees position for 5 s) 1 Drift 2 Some effort against gravity 3 No effort against gravity 4 No movement 9 Untestable (joint fused or limb amputated)
7. Limb ataxia:	0 No ataxia 1 Present in one limb 2 Present in two limbs
8. Sensory (use pinprick to test arms, legs, trunk and face—compare side to side):	0 Normal 1 Mild to moderate decrease in sensation 2 Severe to total sensory loss
9. Best language (describe picture, name items, read sentences):	0 No aphasia 1 Mild to moderate aphasia 2 Severe aphasia 3 Mute
10. Dysarthria (read several words):	0 Normal articulation 1 Mild to moderate slurring of words 2 Near unintelligible or unable to speak 9 Intubated or other physical barrier
11. Extinction and inattention:	0 Normal 1 Inattention or extinction to bilateral simultaneous stimulation in one of the sensory modalities 2 Severe hemi-inattention or hemi-inattention to more than one modality

Brott TG, Adams HP, Olinger CP, et al. Measurements of acute cerebral infarction: A clinical examination scale. *Stroke*. 1989;20:864–870.

TABLE 28.5

DIAGNOSTIC TESTS FOR THE INITIAL EVALUATION OF POSSIBLE STROKE[4]

Recommended:
Computed tomography scan of brain
Electrocardiogram
Blood glucose
Serum creatinine, urea, electrolytes
Complete blood count, including platelets
Prothrombin time and partial thromboplastin time
Oxygen saturation (pulse oximetry)
Optional (guided by history or physical findings)
Chest radiograph
Carotid duplex ultrasound examination
Magnetic resonance imaging of the brain
Magnetic resonance arteriography of the brain
Liver function tests
Serum ammonia level
Blood alcohol level
Toxicology screen
Electroencephalogram

Adapted from Adams HP. Guidelines for the early management of patients with ischemic stroke. *Stroke*. 2003;34:1056–1083.

imaging study can exclude the presence of hemorrhage with 100% accuracy.[5] The clinical suspicion of a hemorrhage may require further investigations, such as lumbar puncture or additional brain imaging. For example, compared to patients with ischemic stroke, patients with intracerebral hemorrhage are more likely to have a decreased level of consciousness, headache, vomiting, and very high blood pressures at initial presentation.

Does the Patient Fulfill Criteria for Thrombolysis?

The phrase "time is brain" highlights the importance of rapid assessment to determine the eligibility for thrombolytic therapy to diminish neuronal damage. Rapid assessment is essential because a patient may be a candidate for intravenous thrombolytic therapy if stroke symptoms have been present for <3 hours (Evidence Level A). Patients who awaken with stroke symptoms are not thrombolysis candidates. If intravenous thrombolysis is given beyond this 3-hour time limit, the likelihood of devastating intracerebral hemorrhage increases.

CASE ONE: PART TWO

Laboratory evaluation in the emergency department is unremarkable. Neurologic examination is completely normal (NIHSS score = 0). Blood pressure is 150/95; all other vital signs are normal. CT scan of the head reveals no intracerebral hemorrhage or acute infarction, but shows periventricular white matter changes and age-appropriate cerebral atrophy.

At this point, it is clear that Mrs. M. is medically stable, she had confirmed symptoms consistent with focal brain dysfunction, and diagnostic studies did not confirm an acute stroke or a cerebral hemorrhage. Mrs. M.'s evaluation was completed within 3 hours of symptom onset, but she was not a candidate for thrombolysis because her symptoms had resolved completely.

MANAGEMENT

Prognosis

Up to 25% of patients with an acute stroke will suffer either a worsening of neurologic deficit, a life-threatening complication, or death within the first 48 hours. Prediction of whether a complication will occur is imprecise. Some predictors of in-hospital death and poor functional recovery include advancing age, higher NIHSS at 6 hours[6] (see Table 28.6), an increasing number of neurologic deficits (i.e., weakness, aphasia, dysarthria, disturbed level of consciousness), atrial fibrillation, hyperglycemia (i.e., capillary glucose >108 mg per dL), relative decrease from admission systolic blood pressure in the first 24 hours of >20 mm Hg, need for mechanical ventilation, swallowing problems, and prior stroke.

Determining Appropriate Location and Intensity of Stroke Management

The appropriate management for acute stroke varies according to the type of stroke, the need for intensive monitoring and the need for aggressive support or control of vital organ functions. Patients with a thrombotic ischemic stroke who do not receive thrombolysis and are medically stable can be managed in a stroke unit rather than in an intensive care unit. In contrast, intracerebral hemorrhage is a true medical emergency because of the high incidence of neurologic deterioration and death.[7] It is prudent to consider early neurosurgical consultation and management in an intensive care unit for most patients with hemorrhage because rapid clinical deterioration and the development of increased intracranial pressure may require specialized medical management or surgical intervention. Patients with an acute TIA require a thorough diagnostic evaluation for stroke etiology because they have a high rate of recurrent stroke in the days and weeks following acute TIA. Therefore, it is prudent to admit patients with TIA to a stroke unit for observation, completion of diagnostic evaluations and institution of treatment to reduce stroke risk.[8]

CASE ONE: PART THREE

You make the provisional diagnoses of a TIA and new paroxysmal atrial fibrillation. You decide to admit her to

TABLE 28.6
PREDICTING PROGNOSIS IN ACUTE STROKE[6]

	Age				
NIHSS[a] at 6 h	60	65	70	75	80
	Risk of Death 100 d Poststroke				
5	0.03	0.04	0.05	0.07	0.09
10	0.07	0.09	0.11	0.14	0.17
15	0.14	0.18	0.22	0.26	0.31
20	0.27	0.32	0.38	0.43	0.50
25	0.44	0.50	0.57	0.62	0.68
30	0.63	0.69	0.74	0.78	0.82
	Risk of Incomplete Functional Recovery 100 d Poststroke				
5	0.19	0.22	0.27	0.32	0.37
10	0.47	0.53	0.59	0.65	0.70
15	0.78	0.82	0.85	0.88	0.90
20	0.93	0.94	0.96	0.97	0.97
25	0.98	0.99	0.99	0.99	0.99
30	0.99	0.99	0.99	0.99	0.99

[a]National Institutes of Health Stroke Scale (Table 28.4).
Table values derived from Weimar C, Konig IR, Kraywinkel K, et al. on behalf of the German Stroke Study Collaboration. Age and National Institutes of Health Stroke Scale score within 6 hours of onset are accurate predictors of outcome after cerebral ischemia. *Stroke*. 2004;35:158–162.

the stroke unit, with cardiac telemetry, to monitor for the early recurrence of symptoms, complete the diagnostic evaluation for TIA, and consider whether Mrs. M. should receive warfarin therapy.

Stroke Unit

Optimal care of hospitalized stroke patients occurs in specialized stroke units, if available[4] (Evidence Level A). Stroke unit care for patients with acute stroke decreases mortality and long-term morbidity. Stroke unit teams initially concentrate on stabilizing patients and monitoring for acute neurologic deterioration. The stroke unit's interdisciplinary team assesses the patient's risk factors for acute complications of stroke, measures physical and cognitive function, recommends pertinent rehabilitation to optimize physical and cognitive function, and addresses secondary stroke prevention measures.

General Medical Care of the Patient with Acute Ischemic Stroke

Once a patient is evaluated and stabilized, common medical concerns include monitoring, assessment and treatment of blood pressure, blood glucose, temperature elevations, and oxygenation (see Table 28.7).

Tissue plasminogen activator (tPA) administration protocols include measures to aggressively control blood pressure before and after thrombolysis. For most patients who do not receive thrombolysis, the normalization of elevated blood pressure during the first 24 to 48 hours is not necessary, and may be deleterious. Acutely elevated blood pressure is a common response to stroke. Blood pressure may decrease spontaneously over 8 to 12 hours. Elevated blood pressure should be treated only if the hypertension is associated with end-organ damage (i.e., myocardial infarction, congestive heart failure, aortic dissection, hypertensive encephalopathy) or if the systolic blood pressure is >220 mm Hg or the diastolic blood pressure is >120 mm Hg. During the first 24 to 48 hours following a stroke, the goal of blood pressure treatment is not normalization but a reduction of 10% to 15%. Caution is advised when actively lowering blood pressure, because an observational study of ischemic stroke showed that actively lowering systolic or diastolic blood pressure ≥20 mm Hg was associated with a higher frequency of infarct expansion, early deterioration of neurologic status and poor 3-month outcome.[10]

Hypoglycemia and hyperglycemia can adversely affect stroke outcomes, so capillary blood glucose should be monitored frequently during the initial hours following a stroke[4] (Evidence Level C). Hypoglycemia can damage neurons and should be corrected with glucose infusion[4] (Evidence Level B). Hyperglycemia can exacerbate ischemic damage and infarct progression, thereby increasing the risk of adverse clinical outcomes. Still, expert opinion varies on how aggressively one should control post-stroke hyperglycemia (capillary blood glucose >108 mg per dL) because few intervention studies exist and they

TABLE 28.7
GENERAL CARE FOLLOWING ACUTE STROKE

General Care Following Acute Stroke (Evidence Level)
BP control if not eligible for thrombolytic therapy (Evidence Level C[4])
1. Systolic BP <220 or diastolic BP <120
• Observe unless hypertensive encephalopathy, pulmonary edema, acute myocardial infarction, or aortic dissection present
2. Systolic BP >220 mm Hg or diastolic 121–140 mm Hg
• Goal is 10%–15% reduction of BP
• Labetalol 10–20 mg IV over 1–2 min, may repeat every 10 min to maximum of 300 mg, or
• Nicardipine 5 mg/h IV initially. Titrate by increasing by 2.5 mg/h every 5 min to maximum of 15 mg/h
3. Diastolic BP >140
• Goal is 10%–15% reduction of blood pressure
• Nitroprusside 0.5 μg/kg/min IV initially, titrate to goal BP with continuous BP monitoring
Monitor bedside capillary glucose
■ Hourly for 2 h, then every 2–4 h, unless unstable (Evidence Level C[4])
Correct hypoglycemia (Evidence Level B[4])
■ Infuse 10–20 mL of 50% glucose
For hyperglycemia (BG >108 mg/dL) in the first 24–48 h, options include
a. Infuse normal saline 100 mL/h and monitor glucose (Evidence Level B[10])
b. Infuse insulin to maintain glucose <126 mg/dL, >72 mg/dL (Evidence Level B[9])
Evaluate and treat fever (Evidence Level B[4])
Monitor oxygen saturation and maintain oxygen saturation ≥95% (Evidence Level C[4])

BG, blood glucose; BP, blood pressure.

have yet to confirm clinical improvements in stroke outcome. American Stroke Association guidelines recommend insulin treatment when blood glucose reaches 300 mg per dL[4] (Evidence Level C). A recent study demonstrated that insulin infusion to maintain capillary blood glucose within a range of 72 to 126 mg per dL is safe and effective. The same study showed that hyperglycemia tends to decline spontaneously, but incompletely, with saline infusion.[9]

Temperature elevation in the acute poststroke period adversely affects neuronal metabolism, and is associated with increased morbidity and mortality. Because fever may signal infection or phlebitis, patients should be evaluated, and temperature should be normalized with antipyretics[4] (Evidence Level B).

Tissue oxygenation is essential to limit neuronal damage and optimize organ function. Supplemental oxygen is not beneficial if oxygenation is normal. Oxygen saturation should be monitored regularly and oxygen administered as needed to maintain saturation ≥95% (Evidence Level C).[4]

Assessing and Managing Risk of Complications Following Acute Stroke

Common complications associated with acute stroke include aspiration pneumonia, DVT, PE, UTI, pressure ulcer, depression, and cognitive decline (see Table 28.8). Most complications associated with stroke occur within the first 14 days, but complications related to the initial stroke may continue to occur for many months after the acute event. Physical, occupational and speech therapists, nurses, and physicians comprise the core of a multidisciplinary stroke team that assesses functional status and risk factors for stroke complications and then creates a plan to reduce the risk of complications, optimize functional status, and reduce the risk of stroke recurrence.

Assessing and Managing Aspiration Pneumonia Risk

Swallowing disorders that may lead to aspiration and aspiration pneumonia occur in up to 65% of patients following an acute stroke. Patients at greatest aspiration risk are those with a depressed level of consciousness, high stroke severity score or orofacial weakness. Signs and symptoms suggestive of a swallowing problem include a "wet" or "gurgly" voice, a weak voice, or a weak cough. Because aspiration may be asymptomatic after a stroke, it is prudent to prevent patients from eating or drinking until a health professional has assessed their aspiration risk and performed either a screening or formal swallowing assessment (Evidence Level C).[13] Although some observational studies suggest that identifying and reducing aspiration risk factors can reduce the rates of aspiration pneumonia, no interventions have been conclusively proved to prevent aspiration pneumonia among stroke patients with dysphagia and aspiration. In fact, in one study of acute stroke patients followed up for 7 days, pneumonia developed in a high percentage of patients with dysphagia although they took nothing by mouth during that time.[16]

TABLE 28.8
ACUTE STROKE COMPLICATIONS: ASSESSING AND MANAGING RISKS

Acute Stroke Complications: Assessing and Managing Risks (Evidence Level)
Recurrent stroke
■ Aspirin 50–325 mg daily within 24–48 h of stroke (Evidence Level A[4])
■ Other antiplatelet agents not recommended in first 48 h (Evidence Level C[4])
Gastrointestinal bleeding risk due to aspirin use
■ Proton pump inhibitor or misoprostol for gastric cytoprotection (Evidence Level A[11])
■ Treat *Helicobacter pylori* infection if present (Evidence Level A[12])
Aspiration pneumonia
■ NPO until evaluated for aspiration risk (Evidence Level C[13])
■ Swallowing evaluation by trained health practitioner (Evidence Level B[13])
■ Modify diet to decrease aspiration risk (Evidence Level B[13])
Deep vein thrombosis
■ Anticoagulant prophylaxis (Evidence Level A[14])
• Prophylactic dose of unfractionated heparin
• Prophylactic dose of low-molecular-weight heparin
• Warfarin to achieve INR 2–3
■ Mechanical methods of prophylaxis if anticoagulants contraindicated (Evidence Level B[14])
• Intermittent pneumatic compression
• Graduated compression stockings
■ Do not use aspirin for DVT prophylaxis (Evidence Level A[14])
Urinary tract infection (Evidence Level C[4])
■ Avoid indwelling urinary catheter
■ Monitor urinary emptying and constipation
Pressure ulcer
■ Monitor skin daily (Evidence Level C[4])
■ Use pressure-reducing devices
■ Reposition frequently
■ Optimize nutrition and hydration
Shoulder pain and disability
■ Support limb if shoulder muscles are weak
■ Therapy for range of motion and strengthening
Depression
■ Monitor depressive symptoms and treat depression (Evidence Level A[15])
Falls
■ Assess physical, cognitive, and environmental risk factors
■ Treat osteoporosis

NPO, nothing by mouth; INR, international normalized ratio; DVT, deep vein thrombosis.

Assessing and Managing Deep Vein Thrombosis Risk

Twenty percent to 50% of patients develop DVT during the first 2 weeks after a stroke. DVT can lead to a PE, which causes up to 25% of deaths in the first month after an acute stroke. DVT is more likely in patients with lower-limb paresis, immobility, increasing age, congestive heart failure, chronic obstructive pulmonary disease, systemic illness, or a history of DVT.[14] Because DVT is frequently asymptomatic, prophylactic treatment is recommended for most acute stroke patients (Evidence Level A).[14] Preferred treatment options for DVT prophylaxis include low-dose unfractionated heparin (LDUH), low-molecular-weight heparin (LMWH), or vitamin K antagonists (e.g., warfarin), but not aspirin (Evidence Level A).[14] For patients with contraindications to anticoagulant treatment, the options for DVT prevention include intermittent pneumatic compression devices or graduated compression stockings (Evidence Level B).[14]

Assessing and Managing Risk of Urinary Tract Infection

Urinary incontinence and bladder dysfunction occurs in up to 80% of patients with acute stroke and persists in up to 25%. Urinary incontinence is more likely in those older than 75, and those with immobility, cognitive deficits, or communication disorders. Strategies to decrease UTI include avoiding indwelling bladder catheterization, optimizing bladder emptying by avoiding anticholinergic medications, and preventing constipation. The risk of constipation can be reduced by encouraging early ambulation, limiting narcotics, and anticholinergic medications, and optimizing nutrition and hydration.

Assessing and Managing Pressure Ulcer Risk

The clinician should participate in a comprehensive plan that includes assessment of modifiable and nonmodifiable risk factors for pressure ulcer (see Chapter 37). Stroke-related risk factors for skin breakdown include paralysis and immobility, decreased level of consciousness or comatose state, loss of limb sensation, muscle spasticity, and bowel or bladder incontinence. Additional pressure ulcer risk factors include prior skin ulcer, advanced atherosclerosis, poor nutrition, malignancy, diabetes, and advanced cardiac, pulmonary, or renal disease.

Early mobilization, pressure reducing mattresses, proper positioning with frequent turning, and attention to risk factor modification are reasonable strategies to try to reduce the risk of pressure ulcers.

Assessing and Managing Poststroke Depression

Depression affects up to 20% of patients following a stroke. Depression is more likely to occur among patients with greater stroke severity, greater functional impairment, and prior depression. Poststroke depression most often presents with emotional lability, anxiety, or vegetative symptoms (e.g., weight loss, lack of energy, poor sleep, loss of libido). Mortality is two to three times higher in patients with poststroke depression than in stroke patients who are not depressed.[15]

It is important to maintain a high index of suspicion for poststroke depression for at least a year after a stroke and to begin treatment as early as possible. For patients receiving antidepressants, those treated soon after acute stroke have a more rapid and more lasting recovery of ADL function[17] (Evidence Level A). Because clinical trials of antidepressants for poststroke depression have tested the efficacy of only a few medications, it is prudent to choose an antidepressant proved effective for these patients (i.e., citalopram, fluoxetine, nortriptyline)[15] (Evidence Level A).

Assessing Comorbid Coronary Heart Disease

Twenty percent to 30% of stroke patients have known or silent cardiovascular disease, and 2% to 5% suffer cardiac deaths in the weeks following acute stroke.[18] Cardiac disease prevalence is lowest in patients with small artery (lacunar) strokes, increases in the presence of carotid stenosis, and is highest in those with cardioembolic stroke. Noninvasive testing to detect asymptomatic coronary artery disease is reasonable after stroke or TIA for patients who have evidence of carotid or large vessel atherosclerosis, for those with a Framingham 10-year coronary heart disease risk of 20% or more, and for those who will be starting a program of aerobic exercise (Evidence Level C). This testing can generally be deferred until discharge from the stroke unit.[18]

Multidisciplinary Assessment of Function and Determination of Rehabilitation Needs

A comprehensive multidisciplinary assessment should characterize communication abilities, cognitive status, physical strength and sensation, and independence in ADL. Based on this assessment, the team should devise a plan to rehabilitate stroke-related deficits with the goal of optimizing functional independence. Because patients' functional status and rehabilitative needs continue to evolve over time, the clinician should regularly assess these domains as part of comprehensive outpatient management after stroke.

Communication problems occur in up to 30% of stroke patients and may affect auditory comprehension, verbal expression, or ability to read and write. The role of the speech therapist is to recommend a treatment plan that includes rehabilitation, environmental adaptations, and assistive devices as appropriate.

Following a stroke, up to 70% of patients older than 75 will manifest cognitive impairment and 30% will fulfill diagnostic criteria for dementia. In the months after a stroke, up to 50% of patients show gradual improvement in cognition, while others will show continued decline. Even if cognition is normal after a stroke, the incidence of subsequent dementia is 8% per year, highlighting the importance of the regular measurement of cognitive status.

Physical assessment should determine limb strength, muscle tone, range of motion, and sensation. Limb weakness affects up to 80% of patients with stroke and is associated with deconditioning, loss of function, spasticity, pain, and falls. Shoulder dysfunction and weakness are identified in up to 60% of patients with stroke. Care of the weak shoulder may include support to prevent subluxation, range of motion exercises to prevent a frozen shoulder, strengthening exercises, and occupational therapy for ADLs.

The combination of cognitive difficulties and muscular weakness increases the risk of falling and fracture. Fall injury prevention includes physical rehabilitation and assistive devices for ambulation when appropriate, attention to environmental hazards, and osteoporosis treatment.

CASE ONE: PART FOUR

Mrs. M.'s first 2 days of hospitalization were benign, with no recurrence of leg or arm weakness, maintenance of sinus rhythm, normalization of blood pressure without pharmacologic intervention, blood sugars under 130 mg per dL, normal swallowing evaluation, and continued independence in all ADLs. Low density lipoprotein (LDL) cholesterol was 115 mg per dL and hemoglobin A_{1c} 7.8%. The echocardiogram revealed normal ventricular function, mild left ventricular hypertrophy and trivial mitral insufficiency. Carotid ultrasonography showed 80% stenosis of the right carotid artery and <50% stenosis of the left carotid artery.

The consulting cardiologist recommended against warfarin for paroxysmal atrial fibrillation due to advanced age and fall risk. The neurologist recommended changing to a different antiplatelet agent. Mrs. M. is unsure about a consultation with a vascular surgeon for possible carotid endarterectomy. Mrs. M. understands that she is at high risk for a stroke and wants your advice about how to reduce her risk of a future stroke.

Lifestyle Recommendations

Patients who have suffered a stroke can reduce the chances of a future stroke or cardiovascular event by stopping smoking, reducing fat and cholesterol in their diet, limiting ethanol intake, increasing exercise, attaining a healthy weight, and complying with medication regimens to control blood pressure, hyperglycemia, and hypercholesterolemia, and reduce risk of thrombosis (Evidence Level B).[19]

Stroke survivors should be encouraged to engage in explicit regimens of aerobic and strength training following recovery from the acute illness. Stroke survivors benefit from a program of aerobic exercise for several reasons: They may be deconditioned due to hospitalization and stroke-related complications or premorbid inactivity; a return to optimum function requires strength and cardiovascular fitness; and most risk factors for stroke and cardiovascular disease are reduced by exercise.[20] Recommended exercise regimens include a daily total of 20 to 60 minutes of aerobic activities (e.g., walking, treadmill, stationary cycle) for 3 to 7 days of the week, weight training exercises that involve the major muscle groups 2 to 3 days a week, and stretching to improve flexibility before or after exercise sessions (Evidence Level C).[20] Because cardiovascular disease is so prevalent in stroke survivors, it is prudent to complete a pre-exercise evaluation, including a noninvasive cardiac stress test, prior to beginning active cardiorespiratory activities (Evidence Level C).

Medications

Thrombolytic Agents

Intravenous recombinant tPA given within 3 hours of acute ischemic stroke onset can reduce the rate of severe disability and death[4,19] (Evidence Level A). The absolute reduction in these outcomes is relatively small; this reduction translates into 14 fewer patients dead or dependent for every 100 receiving tPA rather than placebo. This benefit is offset by the occurrence of intracerebral hemorrhage. The rate of intracerebral hemorrhage seen in clinical trials ranged from 3% to 6% of patients, but in one community-based study it was 15%, probably due to tPA administration beyond 3 hours of symptom onset. Approximately 30% of all patients with ischemic stroke are potential tPA candidates, but only 8% or less of ischemic stroke patients arrive at the hospital and receive evaluation within 3 hours of symptom onset.

Advanced age alone should not be used as a criterion to withhold tPA. The use of tPA should be guided by a physician with expertise and experience using the medication according to established protocols. Patients whose acute ischemic stroke symptoms last longer than 3 hours, but less than 6 hours, may benefit from evaluation by clinicians experienced in interventional neurology and neurologic intensive care for consideration of intra-arterial tPA[21] (Evidence Level C). Experts recommend limiting intra-arterial thrombolysis to patients in clinical trials or those who give informed consent after careful evaluation by clinicians with expertise and experience with this intervention.[21]

Parenteral Anticoagulants

Parenteral anticoagulants include unfractionated heparin (UFH), LMWH, and pentasaccharides. Prophylactic doses of parenteral anticoagulants can effectively reduce DVT in patients with ischemic stroke who are bedridden, immobile, or have hemiparesis[4] (Evidence Level A). Parenteral anticoagulants should not be used for DVT prophylaxis for 24 to 48 hours after tPA administration, and should not be used following an acute intracerebral hemorrhage.

A treatment with full therapeutic doses of parenteral anticoagulants is not recommended for any subgroup of patients with acute stroke because therapeutic dose anticoagulation does not decrease the likelihood of subsequent stroke, but it does increase the chance of serious bleeding complications (Evidence Level A).[21]

Antiplatelet Agents

Most patients with acute ischemic stroke should receive 160 to 325 mg of aspirin daily within 24 to 48 hours of acute stroke (Evidence Level A).[4] Other antiplatelet agents are not recommended in the acute poststroke period (Evidence Level C).[4] Aspirin should not be given to patients with known contraindications, aspirin allergy, or within 24 hours of thrombolytic agents.

Long-term preventive therapy with an antiplatelet agent (aspirin, aspirin plus extended-release dipyridamole [ASA/ER-DP], clopidogrel) is recommended for patients after noncardioembolic ischemic stroke or TIA (Evidence Level A).[21] While the optimum dose of aspirin is debatable, doses >50 mg per day do not increase efficacy, but gastrointestinal toxicity increases with increasing dose (toxicity does not rise dramatically until one exceeds 325 mg daily). Therefore, expert guidelines recommend that aspirin doses ranging from 50 to 325 mg daily are appropriate.[21] ASA/ER-DP 25/200 mg twice daily offers some additional preventive benefit compared to aspirin alone (number needed to treat 15) (Evidence Level A).[22] Clopidogrel 75 mg daily is not superior to aspirin for patients whose initial cardiovascular event is a stroke or TIA (Evidence Level A).[23] Clopidogrel is reasonable for patients who are allergic or sensitive to aspirin (Evidence Level B).[21] Combining aspirin and clopidogrel is not appropriate for the prevention of ischemic stroke; the combination is not superior to clopidogrel alone for stroke prevention and it raises the incidence of serious gastrointestinal bleeding (Evidence Level A).[24]

Warfarin

Warfarin is indicated to prevent recurrent stroke for patients with atrial fibrillation (Evidence Level A).[25] Warfarin is not indicated for the prevention of noncardioembolic ischemic strokes (Evidence Level A),[21] but may be considered to prevent stroke recurrence in the clinical situations of cervical carotid or vertebral artery dissections, cerebral venous thrombosis, and known hypercoagulable states (Evidence Level C).[21]

Absolute contraindications to warfarin include bleeding diathesis (Evidence Level C), platelet count <50,000 (Evidence Level C), uncontrolled hypertension (>160/90) (Evidence Level B), and noncompliance with medications or monitoring (Evidence Level B).[12] Relative contraindications to warfarin include alcohol intake over 2 ounces daily (Evidence Level C)[12] and the regular use of a nonselective nonsteroidal anti-inflammatory drug (NSAID) without cytoprotection (Evidence Level B).[12] Falling is not a contraindication to warfarin therapy (Evidence Level B),[12] nor is the use of a cyclooxygenase-2 specific NSAID (Evidence Level A),[12] use of a nonselective NSAID plus misoprostol or a proton pump inhibitor (Evidence Level A),[12] or resolved peptic ulcer bleeding with *Helicobacter pylori* testing and treatment (Evidence Level A).[12]

Gastric Cytoprotection

It is prudent to consider coadministration of a proton pump inhibitor to decrease the risk of serious gastrointestinal bleeding for elderly patients on long-term aspirin therapy (Evidence Level A).[25] The risk of long-term aspirin therapy is further reduced by combining treatment of *H. pylori* infection, if present, with long-term proton pump inhibitor therapy. Misoprostol is an alternative to a proton pump inhibitor for cytoprotection.[12]

Surgical Interventions

A meta-analysis of randomized trials showed that carotid endarterectomy is beneficial, compared to medical therapy, for those patients with symptomatic stenosis of 70% or more (number needed to treat 6), but without subtotal occlusion. Endarterectomy is somewhat beneficial for those with symptomatic stenosis of 50% to 69% (number needed to treat 13), but is not better than medical therapy for stenosis <50% (Evidence Level A).[26] The benefits of endarterectomy persisted for 8 years of follow-up. In study populations, the operative risk of stroke or death associated with endarterectomy is 7% in the 30 days following surgery. Because no data exist to favor either the choice of performing endarterectomy 3 to 4 days after acute stroke symptoms have stabilized or deciding to wait up to 6 weeks, the timing of endarterectomy surgery is left to the discretion of the vascular surgeon.

The relatively new alternative to endarterectomy, carotid artery angioplasty and stenting, may be appropriate for select individuals as part of a research study.

> **CASE ONE: PART FIVE**
>
> Because Mrs. M. had symptoms that could be explained by either a large artery thrombus formed in her stenotic left carotid artery or a cardioembolism due to intermittent atrial fibrillation, you consult a vascular surgeon. The surgeon and neurologist recommend carotid endarterectomy. Mrs. M. agrees.

Patient Monitoring/Secondary Prevention

Assessing and Reducing Risk of Recurrent Stroke or Cardiovascular Events

A stroke or TIA should be considered a sentinel event signaling the presence of systemic atherosclerosis that places the patient at increased risk of morbidity and mortality from stroke, cardiovascular disease, and peripheral vascular disease. In the first 30 days following a stroke, most deaths are due to the initial stroke and its complications. In the year after a stroke, nearly half of the deaths will be due to cardiovascular events such as myocardial infarction, sudden death, aortic aneurysm, or critical limb ischemia, while 10% can be attributed to the initial stroke and 5% to a recurrent stroke.

The clinician should identify risk factors for recurrent stroke and cardiovascular disease and tailor treatment regimens to attain specific risk reduction goals for blood pressure and lipid levels. For instance, studies support a goal of systolic blood pressure <140 mm Hg (130 mm Hg if diabetes is present), diastolic blood pressure <90 mm Hg (80 mm Hg if diabetes is present), and a goal of LDL cholesterol <100 mg per dL (Evidence Level B).[19] Some experts suggest prescribing antihypertensive therapy with an angiotensin-converting enzyme inhibitor or angiotensin receptor blocker (ARB), and lipid-lowering therapy with a 3-hydroxy-3-methylglutaryl coenzyme A reductase inhibitor ("statin") regardless of baseline blood pressure or cholesterol level (Evidence Level B).[27] Strict control of blood sugar for those with diabetes is of unproven benefit for stroke prevention, but remains a reasonable goal because those with lower Hb A_{Ic} values have a lower risk of myocardial infarction.

Reducing the Risk of Thrombosis for Noncardioembolic Stroke

Patients with noncardioembolic ischemic stroke should receive an antiplatelet agent (Evidence Level A). Compared to placebo, antiplatelet therapy reduces the risk of recurrent stroke from 10.8% to 8.3%, which means that one would need to treat 40 patients for 1 year to prevent one stroke.[28] Antiplatelet therapy is also beneficial for the combined endpoint of stroke, myocardial infarction, or vascular death. Compared to placebo, antiplatelet therapy reduces the incidence of this combined endpoint from 21.4% to 17.8%, with a number needed to treat of 28 for this outcome.[28]

CASE ONE: PART SIX

Mrs. M. is near her ideal body weight, so you recommend targets for optimum cardiovascular health and stroke prevention of a diet low in cholesterol, LDL cholesterol <100 mg per dL, and Hb A_{lc}<7%. She is willing and able to increase the frequency and intensity of aerobic walking to improve blood pressure, lipids and blood sugar and to reduce the risk of recurrent stroke. Because she has not exercised regularly or vigorously for several years, you recommend outpatient stress testing prior to initiating an exercise program of walking for 30 minutes daily.

TABLE 28.9

CONGESTIVE HEART FAILURE, HYPERTENSION, AGE, DIABETES, AND STROKE ($CHADS_2$) SCORE AND STROKE RISK[30]

CHADS Score	Stroke Rate per 100 person-year
0	1.9
1	2.8
2	4
3	5.9
4	8.5
5	12.5
6	18.2

Scoring: 1 point each for recent congestive heart failure, history of hypertension, age ≥75, diabetes; 2 points for history of stroke or TIA $CHADS_2$, congestive heart failure, hypertension, age, diabetes, and stroke.

Adapted from gage BF, Waterman AD, Shannon W, et al. Validation of clinical classification schemes for predicting stroke: results from the National Registry of Atrial Fibrillation. *JAMA*. 2001;285:2864–2870.

Reducing the Risk of Thrombosis for Cardioembolic Stroke

Most elderly patients with sustained or paroxysmal atrial fibrillation should receive warfarin anticoagulation to achieve an international normalized ratio (INR) of 2.5 (range 2 to 3)[21] (Evidence Level A). Some patients with mechanical artificial cardiac valves should receive warfarin to achieve an INR of 3 (range 2.5 to 3.5)[29] (Evidence Level A).

Atrial fibrillation occurs in 5% of people older than 65. The rate of stroke in people with atrial fibrillation ranges from 4% to 18% per year. Stroke is more likely if atrial fibrillation occurs in those with the risk factors of increasing age, hypertension, prior stroke or TIA, diabetes, and left ventricular dysfunction. The stroke risk rises with increasing numbers of risk factors. Patients with valvular disease and atrial fibrillation have the highest risk of cardioembolic stroke.

Antithrombotic treatment with warfarin or aspirin reduces the relative risk of stroke due to atrial fibrillation by 65% and 20%, respectively. If a recurrent stroke occurs during warfarin therapy, it is less likely to result in severe disability or death.[25]

Clinicians are often hesitant to prescribe warfarin to patients with increasing age and frailty, despite multiple risk factors for stroke. Studies suggest that clinicians' decisions are influenced more by concerns about warfarin complications than by the stroke reduction benefits of warfarin. Interestingly, patients may reach a different decision about the risk-benefit ratio of warfarin than their physicians. For this reason, it is prudent to inform patients about the benefits and burdens of warfarin therapy and reach a shared decision about warfarin use. It is helpful to use a stepwise approach to determine the risks and benefits for individual patients.[12]

First, one must assess whether anticoagulation has the potential to improve the quality or length of life. If a person has advanced disease and a poor prognosis, warfarin may not provide a meaningful benefit.

The next step is to determine if the patient has a high or low risk for stroke due to atrial fibrillation. Generally, a person with atrial fibrillation is considered low risk for stroke if they are younger than 65 and their risk of stroke from all other factors is 1% or less per year. Low-risk patients with atrial fibrillation younger than 65 can be treated with aspirin rather than warfarin to reduce the risk of cardioembolic stroke.

Several methods exist for calculating stroke risk, but the simplest is the $CHADS_2$ score (see Table 28.9).[30] A high-risk patient with atrial fibrillation is one with a stroke risk >1%. Using the $CHADS_2$ score, a patient with atrial fibrillation who has experienced a TIA or stroke has a stroke risk of at least 4%, and experts would recommend warfarin prophylaxis. The expected relative benefit of warfarin therapy for such a patient is the difference between the estimated stroke rate (in this example, 4%) and the expected rate of stroke while taking warfarin (approximately 1% per year).

Next, determine the risk of bleeding complications due to warfarin. Among patients with atrial fibrillation, the rate of hemorrhage requiring hospitalization or transfusion is approximately 70 per 10,000 person-years for those on placebo and 130 per 10,000 person-years for those taking warfarin.[31] It is important to note that gastrointestinal or genitourinary bleeding during warfarin therapy may be due to occult malignancy in up to 30% of patients.[31]

Intracerebral bleeding and SDH cause a great degree of concern among clinicians and may negatively impact their decision to use warfarin. The rate of intracerebral bleeding among patients with atrial fibrillation receiving warfarin is approximately 30 per 10,000 patients per year, compared to 10 per 10,000 patients per year among those receiving placebo.[31] Most intracerebral bleeding episodes reported in clinical trials occurred when the INR was above 3. Intracranial bleeding is more likely if the systolic blood pressure is over 160 mm Hg or the diastolic blood pressure is above 90 mm Hg.[12]

Among community-dwelling elderly patients, SDHs occur at a rate of 4 per 10,000 patient-years. The risk of SDH for those taking aspirin is approximately 8 per 10,000 patient-years, compared to 12 per 10,000 patient-years for those taking warfarin. Seventy percent of SDH are related to head trauma, with 50% of head trauma incidents due to falls. Therefore, only 35% of SDHs in the elderly can be directly attributed to falls. One decision analysis estimated that falls increase the risk of SDH by only one to two additional cases per 10,000 patients. The analysis further estimates that, as the number of falls in the calculation was raised to 295 per year, warfarin was still expected to produce the best quality of life compared to aspirin or no therapy for atrial fibrillation. This decision analysis suggests that occasional falling should not be a major factor in the decision to withhold warfarin for elderly patients with atrial fibrillation.[32]

Next, create a plan based on the patient's medications and medical conditions to reduce the risk of bleeding. Some evidence suggests that it is possible to reduce the risks of bleeding while taking warfarin by limiting alcohol consumption, controlling blood pressure, treating *H. pylori* infection, and prescribing a proton pump inhibitor or misoprostol for those taking aspirin or an NSAID.[12] Similarly, a comprehensive evaluation for fall risk factors, with appropriate interventions, may reduce the risk of falls. Close monitoring to keep INR values within the range of 2 to 3 may reduce bleeding risk, because most bleeding events are associated with INR values over 3. Frequent INR monitoring is especially important when initiating warfarin, because bleeding risk varies over time. The risk of major bleeding is 3% per month in the first month of therapy, decreases to 0.8% per month in the subsequent 11 months and then stabilizes at 0.3% per month.[31]

Finally, discuss with the patient the relative values they place on reducing the risk of cardioembolic stroke with warfarin compared to the risk of bleeding complications, and reach a shared decision about warfarin use. The decision to use warfarin should also include a plan to reduce bleeding risk, monitor adequacy of anticoagulation, and monitor for complications.

CASE ONE: PART SEVEN

On the second postoperative day following carotid endarterectomy, Mrs. M. develops atrial fibrillation with a controlled ventricular rate. You review the benefits and adverse effects of warfarin for stroke prevention in paroxysmal atrial fibrillation. Mrs. M.'s risk factors of hypertension, age >75, diabetes, and TIA produce a $CHADS_2$ score of 5, which predicts 12.5 strokes per 100 person-years. She has no evidence of bleeding from the gastrointestinal, urinary, or genital tracts. Her bleeding risk is increased by current aspirin use. Options include discontinuing aspirin if warfarin were instituted for stroke prevention, or prescribing cytoprotection if aspirin were continued to reduce the risk of myocardial infarction. Her isolated fall due to TIA symptoms is not a contraindication to warfarin. She chooses to stop aspirin and start warfarin because she thinks that the benefit of reducing stroke risk with warfarin outweighs the possibility of a bleeding complication.

Patient Education

Ongoing care for a person who has had a stroke or TIA, and for their caregiver, should include education about stroke and cardiovascular disease that includes how to respond to acute signs and symptoms of a stroke or myocardial infarction, how to cope with functional impairments, how to access community resources that assist stroke survivors, how to control stroke risk factors, and how to monitor for important adverse medication effects. Such information may be provided by the inpatient multidisciplinary team, or accessed at the websites of the American Heart Association and the American Stroke Association.

Patient Monitoring

Subsequent outpatient visits should include a regular assessment of physical, cognitive, and psychological functioning, rehabilitation needs, a review of cardiovascular and cerebrovascular symptoms, an assessment of the completeness and adequacy of stroke risk factor reduction, and surveillance for potential adverse effects of medications. Caregivers of stroke survivors should be assessed periodically for stress and depressive symptoms related to caregiving.

ACKNOWLEDGMENTS

Maggie Reitenbach provided exceptional administrative and secretarial support. David Sperling provided valuable clinical and editorial insight.

REFERENCES

1. American Heart Association. *Heart Disease and Stroke Statistics*, 2004 Update. Dallas, TX: American Heart Association; http://www.americanheart.org/presenter.jhtml?identifier=3000090 accessed December 29, 2004.
2. Smucker WD, DiSabato JA, Krishen AE. Systematic approach to diagnosis and initial management of stroke. *Am Fam Physician*. 1995;52:225–234.
3. Brott TG, Adams HP, Olinger CP, et al. Measurements of acute cerebral infarction: A clinical examination scale. *Stroke*. 1989;20:864–870.
4. Adams HP. Guidelines for the early management of patients with ischemic stroke. *Stroke*. 2003;34:1056–1083.

5. Kidwell C, Chalela JA, Saver JL, et al. Comparison of MRI and CT for detection of acute intracerebral hemorrhage. *JAMA.* 2004;292(15):1823–1830.
6. Weimar C, Konig IR, Kraywinkel K, et al. German Stroke Study Collaboration. Age and national institutes of health stroke scale score within 6 hours after onset are accurate predictors of outcome after cerebral ischemia. *Stroke.* 2004;35:158–162.
7. Broderick JP, Adams HP, Barsan W, et al. Guidelines for the management of spontaneous intracerebral hemorrhage. *Stroke.* 1999;30:905–915.
8. Daffertshofer M, Mielke O, Pullwitt A, et al. Transient ischemic attacks are more than "ministrokes". *Stroke.* 2004;35:2453–2458.
9. Gray CS, Hildreth AJ, Alberti G, et al. GIST Collaboration. Poststroke hyperglycemia natural history and immediate management. *Stroke.* 2004; 35:122–126.
10. Castillo J, Leira R, Garcia M, et al. Blood pressure decrease during the acute phase of ischemic stroke is associated with brain injury and poor stroke outcome. *Stroke.* 2004;35:520–527.
11. Kimmey MB. Cardioprotective effects and gastrointestinal risks of aspirin: Maintaining the delicate balance. *Am J Med.* 2004;117(suppl 5A):72S–78S.
12. Man-Son-Hing M, Laupacis A. Anticoagulant bleeding in older persons with atrial fibrillation. Physicians fears often unfounded. *Arch Intern Med.* 2003;163:1580–1586.
13. Agency for Health Care Research and Quality. Diagnosis and treatment of swallowing disorders (dysphagia) in acute-care stroke patients. Summary, Evidence Report/Technology Assessment: Number 8, March 1999.Rockville, MD: http://www.ahrq.gov/clinic/epcsums/dysphsum.htm. Accessed December 29, 2004
14. Geerts WH, Pineo GF, Heit JA, et al. Prevention of venous thromboembolism. The seventh ACCP conference on antithrombotic and thrombolytic therapy. *Chest.* 2004;126:338S–400S.
15. Robinson RG. Poststroke depression: Prevalence, diagnosis, treatment and disease progression. *Biol Psychiatry.* 2003;54:376–387.
16. Kidd J. The natural history and clinical consequences of aspiration in acute stroke. *Q J Med.* 1995;88:409–413.
17. Narushima K, Robinson RG. The effect of early versus late antidepressant treatment on physical impairment associated with poststroke depression is there a time-related therapeutic window? *J Nerv Ment Dis.* 2003;191:645–652.
18. Adams RJ, Chimowitz MI, Alpert JS, et al. Coronary risk evaluation in patients with transient ischemic attack and ischemic stroke a scientific statement for healthcare professionals from the stroke council and the council on clinical cardiology of the American Heart Association/American Stroke Association. *Stroke.* 2003;34:2310–2322.
19. Akopov S, Cohen S. Preventing stroke: A review of current guidelines. *J Am Med Dir Assoc.* 2003;4(5):S127–S136.
20. Gordon NF, Gulanik M, Costa F, et al. Physical activity and exercise recommendation for stroke survivors. *Stroke.* 2004;35: 1230–1240.
21. Albers GW, Amarenco P, Easton JD, et al. Antithrombotic and thrombolytic therapy for ischemic stroke. The seventh ACCP conference on antithrombotic and thrombolytic therapy. *Chest.* 2004;126:483S–512S.
22. Diener HC, Cunha L, Forbes C, et al. European stroke prevention study 2. Dipyridamole and acetylsalicylic acid in the secondary prevention of stroke. *J Neurol Sci.*1996;143(1–2):1–13.
23. CAPRIE Steering Committee. A randomised, blinded trial of clopidogrel versus aspirin in patients at risk of ischaemic events (CAPRIE). *Lancet.* 1996;348:1329–1339.
24. Diener HC, Bogousslavsky J, Brass LM. MATCH Investigators. Aspirin and clopidogrel compared with clopidogrel alone after recent ischaemic stroke or transient ischaemic attack in high-risk patients (MATCH): A randomized, double-blind, placebo-controlled trial. *Lancet.* 2004; 364(9431):331–337.
25. Singer DE, Albers GW, Dalen JE, et al. Antithrombotic therapy in atrial fibrillation. The seventh ACCP conference on antithrombotic and thrombolytic therapy. *Chest.* 2004;126:429S–456S.
26. Rothwell PM, Eliasziw M, Gutnikov SA, et al. for the Carotid Endarterectomy Trialists' Collaboration. Analysis of pooled data from the randomised controlled trials of endarterectomy for symptomatic carotid stenosis. *Lancet* 2003;361:107–116.
27. Muir KW. Secondary prevention for stroke and transient ischaemic attacks. *BMJ.* 2004;328:297–298.
28. Antithrombotic Trialists' Collaboration. Collaborative meta-analysis of randomised trials of antiplatelet therapy for prevention of death, myocardial infarction, and stroke in high risk patients. *BMJ.* 2002;324:71–86.
29. Salem DM, Stein PD, Al-Ahmad A, et al. Antithrombotic therapy in valvular heart disease—native and prosthetic. The seventh ACCP conference on antithrombotic and thrombolytic therapy. *Chest.* 2004;126:457S–482S.
30. Gage BF, Waterman AD, Shannon W, et al. Validation of clinical classification schemes for predicting stroke: Results from the National registry of atrial fibrillation. *JAMA.* 2001;285:2864–2870.
31. Levine MN, Raskob G, Beyth RJ, et al. Hemorrhagic complications of anticoagulant treatment. The seventh ACCP conference on antithrombotic and thrombolytic therapy. *Chest.* 2004;126:287S–310S.
32. Man-Son-Hing M, Nichol G, Lau A, et al. Choosing antithrombotic therapy for elderly patients with atrial fibrillation who are at risk for falls. *Arch Intern Med.* 1999;159:677–685. 26:287S–310S.

29 Tremor

Lesley D. Wilkinson   Carol Stewart   Nancy Tyre

CLINICAL PEARLS 378

DIFFERENTIAL DIAGNOSIS 379
Description and Definition of Tremor 379
Incidence and Prevalence of Tremor 379
Signs and Symptoms of Tremor 380

TREMOR SYNDROMES 381
Parkinsonian Rest Tremors 381
Action and Postural Tremors 381
Toxic/Metabolic Tremor (Also Known as *"Enhanced Physiologic Tremor"*) 381
Essential Tremor 382

LESS COMMON ACTION AND POSTURAL TREMORS 383
Cerebellar Intention Tremor (or "terminal kinetic tremor") 383
Rubral Tremor 384
Orthostatic Tremor 384
Specific Task and Dystonic Tremors 384
Neuropathic Tremor 384
Palatal tremor (previously called *palatal myoclonus*) 384
Wilson Disease 384
Psychogenic Tremor 384

WORKUP AND DIAGNOSIS OF PATIENTS WITH TREMOR 384
A Focused History 384
Physical Examination 385
Laboratory Tests 385
Special Studies 386

MANAGEMENT 386
General Measures for Tremors 386
Lifestyle and Therapy 386
Medications 386
Surgery 393
Patient Resources 393

CONCLUSION 393

CLINICAL PEARLS

- Tremor is not part of normal aging.
- Tremor is common in the geriatric population. It can cause substantial disability and can severely diminish quality of life.
- Most geriatric patients with tremor will have one of three syndromes: Essential tremor (ET), toxic/metabolic tremor, or Parkinson disease (PD).
- Tremor at rest suggests PD; tremor with activity suggests essential or toxic/metabolic tremor.
- All patients with geriatric tremor should have medications and underlying disorders considered as etiologies for their tremor.
- Treatment for ET is initially β-blockers; second line is primidone.
- Physical therapy, weights for the arms, and surgery may be useful when pharmacologic treatment does not suffice.

Tremors are oscillating involuntary movements. Most older patients with tremor will ultimately prove to have one of the three major tremor syndromes—essential tremor (ET), Parkinson disease (PD), or toxic/metabolic tremor. However, there are many potential causes of tremor. Tremor in the older population is not unusual. It is the most common movement disorder. Up to 9% of people older than 80 have tremor, and >5 million people in the United States have tremors.

Normal aging does not include developing a tremor, but tremor is more likely to manifest with greater age. Although tremor may be associated with a variety of syndromes, many patients with tremor are otherwise healthy. Still, tremor itself can be a significant source of disability and diminished quality of life. Evaluation and treatment of tremor can significantly ameliorate chronic disabling symptoms and contribute to management of contributing diseases as well. This chapter will provide the practitioner with information to help confidently address this common and potentially disabling symptom.

DIFFERENTIAL DIAGNOSIS

Tremor is best differentiated by clinical examination.[1] There is a large differential, although most patients have one of three common entities: (i) ET, (ii) toxic/metabolic tremor, or (iii) PD. Table 29.1 provides an extensive list of causes for tremor, with an associated table, Table 29.2, listing drug-related causes.[2]

Description and Definition of Tremor

Tremor is an involuntary movement disorder with a regular and consistent movement. Other hyperkinetic movement disorders (such as choreas, tics, dystonias, and myoclonus, including asterixis, and spasms) involve irregular and/or variable movements. Tremor involves a rhythmic, oscillatory movement of part of the body. It is usually fairly consistent in frequency, but varies in amplitude. Movement is caused by contractions of reciprocally innervated antagonistic muscle groups firing either asynchronously or synchronously. Although there are some clear pathophysiologic pathways, overall tremor is poorly understood. Most tremors show positive positron emission tomography (PET) scan findings in the cerebellum but do not necessarily originate there. Much remains to be understood in all but a few unusual syndromes.

Incidence and Prevalence of Tremor

The incidence and prevalence of tremor in the general population is largely a factor of the prevalence and incidence of ET, which is the dominant tremor disorder. The next most common tremor is from PD. Other tremors are much less common. At least 7% to 8% of the entire geriatric population older than 60 suffers from tremor, and

TABLE 29.1
DIFFERENTIAL DIAGNOSIS OF TREMOR

Postural-action Tremors			
Essential tremor (333.1)	Also known as benign essential tremor or familial tremor	Variants can include primary writing tremor and orthostatic tremor that is limited to the legs and trunk while standing (ICD-9 Code Tremor NOS 781.0)	
Toxic/metabolic tremor or enhanced physiologic tremor Detected when increased sympathetic activity is present (ICD-9 codes based on underlying cause)	Toxin exposure: Bromides (967.3) Mercury (985.0) Lead (984) Arsenic (985.1) Toluene (982.0) Methyl ethyl ketone (982.0)	See separate drug table 29.2	Anxiety (300.00–300.02)/ excitement (298.1 or 309.29)/fright Muscle fatigue (780.79) Hypoglycemia (251.2) Thyrotoxicosis (242.9) Uremia (586) Liver failure (570) Fever (780.6) or hypothermia (991.6) Pheochromocytoma ■ malignant (194.0) ■ benign (227.0)
Combination and Other Tremors			
Parkinson disease—classically described as resting tremor (332.0) In rare cases, can be caused by exposure to toxins such as: Manganese (985.2) Carbon monoxide (986) Cyanide (989.0) Carbon disulfide (982.2)	**Intention tremor**—due to cerebellar outflow disease, potential causes include stroke (434), multiple sclerosis (340), midbrain trauma (851–854), heredodegenerative diseases of the cerebellum (334.0–334.9), severe essential tremor, Wilson disease, hepatocerebral degeneration (572.8), and mercury poisoning	**Rubral tremor**—potentially rest, action, postural and intention tremors, due to damage to midbrain including red nucleus, associated with ataxia and dysmetria (781.3) (If ataxia is a late effect due to a stroke, ICD-9 code is 438.84.)	**Wilson disease**—may be postural action alone or in combination with both rest and intention tremor (275.1)

TABLE 29.2
DRUGS THAT CAN CAUSE TREMOR

Drugs That Cause a Parkinsonian-like Tremor	Drugs That Cause a Toxic/Metabolic or Enhanced Physiologic Tremor
■ Neuroleptics (E939.3) including: • Haloperidol • Thioridazine • Aripiprazole (Abilify) ■ Metoclopramide HCl (E933.0) ■ Reserpine (E942.6) ■ Amiodarone (E942.9) ■ Valproic acid/sodium valproate (E936) ■ Methyldopa (E942.6) ■ Other dopamine-depleting medications	■ β-Agonists such as albuterol (E945.7), terbutaline, and isoproterenol (E941.2) ■ Pseudoephedrine and ephedrine (E941.2) ■ Epinephrine (E941.2) ■ Amphetamines (E939.7), including pemoline, methylphenidate, and dextroamphetamine ■ Antidepressants, tricyclics, or SSRIs (E939.0) ■ Lithium (E939.8) ■ Neuroleptics (E939.1–939.3) ■ Valproic acid/sodium valproate (E936) ■ Carbamazepine (E936.3) ■ Levodopa (E936.4) ■ Corticosteroids (E932.0) ■ Nicotine (305.1) ■ Caffeine (E939.7) or theophylline (E945.7) ■ Alcohol (291.8), benzodiazepine, or narcotic withdrawal (292.0) ■ Thyroid replacement medication (E932.7) ■ Tocainide (E942.9) ■ Amiodarone (E942.9) ■ Cyclosporine A (E933.1)

SSRIs, selective serotonin reuptake inhibitors.

it has been asserted that 9% of the population older than 80 suffers from a tremor.[3]

Signs and Symptoms of Tremor

The signs and symptoms of tremor (see Table 29.3) are the key to classifying, diagnosing, and treating these disorders.[1] This is an area of medicine where astute clinical diagnosis is still by far the most important factor in successful management.

There are three major tremor syndromes in the geriatric population, and multiple less common causes of tremors. While it can be impossible in some patients to precisely determine the classification of the tremor, even partial characterization is critical to adequately differentiate tremors and select management.

TABLE 29.3
SUMMARY OF THREE COMMON TREMOR DISORDERS

Symptom or Sign	Toxic/Metabolic	Essential Tremor	Parkinson Disease
Tremor type (when tremor occurs)	Action—i.e., actively using limb or holding against gravity	Action—i.e., actively using limb or holding against gravity	Rest
Most common location of tremor	Upper extremities	Upper extremities	Upper extremities
Other tremor locales	Not common	Often in neck (i.e., head or neck), voice; legs later and less common	Legs, lips, tongue, chin
Unilateral/bilateral	Mainly bilateral	Mainly bilateral	Unilateral or bilateral—often starts unilateral
Age	Any age, common in geriatrics due to drugs/illnesses	More common with elderly, but often presents in younger people	Much more common with elderly
Family history	Irrelevant	Present in at least 50% of patients	FHx not commonly present, but PD more likely with FHx
Associated signs	Signs of underlying illness, drug or toxin	Generally no associated signs	Parkinson signs (such as rigidity, masked facies, etc.)
Response to alcohol	None	Often temporary resolution	None

FHx, family history; PD, Parkinson disease.

The most crucial tremor distinction is between "resting" tremors and "action" tremors. Resting tremors occur when the patient is not using the affected body part and its muscles are entirely at rest. Action tremors arise when the patient is using the affected body part. Of course this includes situations when the patient is performing an activity with the limb/part, but it also includes when the patient is not moving the limb/part but is holding it against gravity. It is then referred to as a "postural" tremor. It is therefore particularly important to make sure a limb is truly at rest, and not being partially activated or held against gravity, when determining whether a tremor is an active or a resting tremor.

TREMOR SYNDROMES

Parkinsonian Rest Tremors

Tremors at (genuine) rest are virtually all parkinsonian. There is only a small subset of rest tremors that are not parkinsonian. Some patients with advanced/severe forms of action tremors, including ET, can show some rest component. When this occurs it usually represents a concordance of two common disorders: PD and ET. A minority may have a parkinsonian action tremor.[4,5] Wilson disease and rubral tremors can also have rest components. The site of the core pathology for PD and all Parkinson-type tremors is impairment of the substantia nigra pars compacta.

Incidence and Prevalence

Parkinson resting tremor is the second most common type of tremor. The prevalence of PD is in approximately 2% of the population older than 65.[6] Of patients with PD, 70% to 75% have the typical resting tremor, while 25% to 30% never develop tremor. The older the age of onset of PD, the less likely tremor will be the initial complaint and the more likely rigidity and paucity of motion will be the major expressions.

Signs and Symptoms of Parkinsonian Tremors

Classically, 50% to 80% of PD will begin insidiously with a tremor in one arm with a finger/hand "pill-rolling" motion, supination/pronation of the forearm, or flexion/extension at the elbow. The tremor worsens with stress and with the use of another limb or limbs, including walking, and improves with the use of the involved limb. There may be a concomitant action component, but the resting component is the key to determining the classification and diagnosis.

Typically as PD progresses, the tremor spreads to the other ipsilateral limb in 1 to 3 years, and to the contralateral limbs in 3 to 8 years.[6] Parkinsonian tremor can involve all four limbs plus the chin, lips, tongue, and neck. It essentially never involves the voice and does not cause head or neck tremor (yes/yes or no/no movements). PD can affect phonation (causing the voice to be too soft) but it does not cause a quavery voice. Tremors of the legs and feet, when present, are much more likely with PD than with ET.

Appropriately diagnosing a parkinsonian tremor is aided considerably by noting other PD features such as bradykinesia, stiffness or rigidity, micrographia, and reduced facial animation.

Etiologies of Parkinsonian Tremors

In addition to idiopathic PD, parkinsonian tremors can also be caused—far less commonly—by medications (Table 29.2),[2] and by vascular lesions, tumors, or infections that damage the substantia nigra. Manganese poisoning, carbon monoxide, cyanide, and carbon disulfide can also cause a parkinsonian syndrome. These causes are rare in actual practice but these exceptional situations must be kept in mind, as they may be reversible.[7,8]

Action and Postural Tremors

There are two common causes of action and postural tremors: (i) Toxic/metabolic tremor (or "enhanced physiologic tremor") and (ii) ET. It is difficult to differentiate these two types of tremor through symptoms or examination. Occasionally, symptoms from an underlying etiology may help to differentiate a toxic/metabolic tremor. There is generally no additional symptomatology in ET besides tremor. These tremors are primarily noted when holding the arms out against gravity or making goal-directed movements with the arms. The arms are generally involved in both of these etiologies.

Toxic/Metabolic Tremor (Also Known as *"Enhanced Physiologic Tremor"*)

CASE ONE

B.D. was a 65-year-old man who presented as a new patient due to an insurance change. He requested referral to oncology for treatment already under way for a recent diagnosis of lung cancer. At the time of presentation, he had no tremor. We discussed smoking cessation for this heavy smoker now diagnosed with lung cancer. He reported that he had virtually quit while taking bupropion. However, he had a significant tremor when he used bupropion, which had made it difficult for him to function and was intolerable. The tremor had resolved quickly upon cessation of bupropion. This is an example of a toxic/metabolic tremor. Since bupropion is not a direct enhancer of endogenous epinephrine, this particular medication's mechanism of action is unknown.

CASE TWO

M.G. was a 62-year-old woman without medical insurance who presented complaining of malaise, exercise intolerance, and anxiety. She reported that she had been anxious for years due to a kidnapping in the past that had left her with posttraumatic stress disorder. She felt that her tremor was due to this anxiety and had not changed recently. On examination she had a very noticeable postural tremor when holding out her hands. Her vital signs were unremarkable with normal pulse, temperature, and blood pressure. She had a loud heart murmur heard diffusely over the precordium. Laboratory tests were normal, with the exception of a thyroid-stimulating hormone (TSH) below the level of detection. She was treated with methimazole and had resolution of virtually all of her signs and symptoms, including 90% to 95% of her tremor. This illustrates an example of toxic/metabolic tremor successfully resolved by treating the underlying disorder.

Incidence and Prevalence

Toxic/metabolic tremor, also known as an *enhanced physiologic tremor*, does not have a well-defined incidence and prevalence because it is generally tied to an underlying disorder or medication, and it can resolve or improve when the condition ends. Toxic/metabolic tremor happens to most people at some point in their lives.

This type of tremor is so common in the geriatric population, particularly in the setting of polypharmacy or anxiety, that it should be considered in every patient with tremor.

Pathophysiology

The term *enhanced physiologic tremor* is based on the fact that all people have a normal, minimal physiologic tremor of about 4 to 12 Hz, which is virtually undetectable unless its amplitude is enhanced. It may be possible to appreciate a normal physiologic tremor when extending a hand holding a piece of paper or pointing a light.[9] Multiple etiologies can cause an increase in the amplitude of this tremor, making it clinically significant. Tremor is probably due to reflex oscillations produced by afferent muscle spindle pathways. Underlying causes are usually due to medication side effects or metabolic derangements; hence the term *toxic or metabolic* tremor.

Signs and Symptoms of Toxic/Metabolic Tremor

This is often difficult to differentiate from ET because it can present in a similar manner. Generally, patients show a tremor with the use of their hands. Tremor is not noticeable at rest. The tremor begins with either holding the arms up against gravity or using them for directed movements.

Etiologies of Toxic/Metabolic Tremor

Many of the disorders and/or medications that cause toxic/metabolic tremor are due to excess epinephrine, but there are a number of other medications which cause tremor without directly raising epinephrine. All patients with action/postural tremors should have these etiologies considered. Even in patients who also have ET, their tremor can be significantly worsened by contributions from an enhanced physiologic tremor.

Please see Table 29.1 for the large differential of toxic/metabolic tremor,[7,8,10] and Table 29.2[2] for medications known to contribute to tremor. Of note, bupropion is not even on the standard lists, so it is clear that additional medications can idiosyncratically cause tremor as well.

Essential Tremor

CASE THREE

A.T. was a 64-year-old woman. She reported a long-standing tremor, which had been getting worse recently to the point that she was having trouble eating soup or drinking water without making a mess and embarrassing herself. She had a history of hypertension and gastroesophageal reflux disease (GERD), and was on hydrochlorothiazide and ranitidine. She had no family history of tremor. On examination, her vital signs were stable and she was in no acute distress. Her tremor was not noticeable at rest. It became evident when she held her hands out, and worsened when she tried to pick up her pen and complete her new patient questionnaire. Her labs included a normal complete blood count (CBC), TSH, and chemistry panel. Her presentation was consistent with ET, so she was prescribed long-acting propranolol. This worked well for her hypertension, and minimized the tremor so that it no longer limited her activities.

Over the next 9 years, a head tremor and shaky voice became noticeable, although well tolerated. Her upper extremity tremor was somewhat more noticeable than it had been when she used her hands to get on the examination table. Even her gait seemed a little shaky by age 73.

A.T.'s case is illustrative of a fairly standard course for ET, though she was fortunate to respond so well to propranolol. She did not have a known family history, so it would not be labeled *familial*. At this point one might consider the addition of another pharmacologic agent, and perhaps physical therapy. The underlying mechanism of ET is not well understood despite multiple studies. There may be central oscillators in the thalamus and/or the inferior olive.

Incidence and Prevalence

The prevalence of ET in the geriatric population (age >60) is approximately 6%.[11] There are at least five million individuals in the United States living with it, and probably more. ET is the most common cause of chronic tremor in all ages. The greatest number of patients with ET is in the geriatric age-group, but there is an early demographic group as well, so quite a few older patients will have had their tremor for many years by the time they are encountered as geriatric patients. Little concrete information is available about the incidence of ET but it may be about 0.5% per year in those older than 65.[12]

ET is distributed equally between genders, but may be more likely in whites than in other ethnicities. The most important risk factor for developing ET is having a family history of ET.

Genetics

ET is frequently inherited as an autosomal dominant trait. At least half of ET patients have a family history of ET.[13,14] There are two loci that have been found to link with the manifestation of familial ET: 3q13 and 2p24.1. A rare variant has been found in a gene of indefinite function that maps in the 2p24.1 area and may be related to some familial ET.[15] There have also been families with hereditary ET in which they clearly do not link to any of the known chromosomal loci, or they do link to the 2p24.1 chromosomal locus but do not manifest the gene variant. There is apparently considerable genetic heterogeneity corresponding to its variable clinical presentations, time of onset, affected body part, and severity.

There have been two recent twin studies, which have shown 60% to 90% concordance rates for ET in monozygotic twins, and 30% to 60% concordance for dizygotic twins.[16,17]

Signs and Symptoms of Essential Tremor

ET usually begins in the upper extremities and affects the hands in 90% to 95% of cases. The frequency of the tremor is 4 to 12 Hz, usually closer to 4 to 6 Hz in the older population. It is a classic action and/or postural tremor. The patient is fine at rest, and then the tremor starts to show as they begin a motor movement with the affected part. It can begin unilaterally, but is usually bilateral. If it is persistently unilateral over years, it calls the diagnosis into question.[5]

ET is usually slowly progressive over time in a given patient. It commonly becomes more severe and spreads to other body parts, ultimately affecting the head (34% to 50%) with either yes–yes or no–no action, face (5%), voice (12% to 30%), trunk (5%) and lower limbs (15% to 20%).[18,19] It is unusual to affect only the head (1% to10% of patients)[20] or voice in isolation. In fact, if the voice is solely affected, dystonia needs to be considered. ET is associated with a quavering voice with normal phonation; dysphonia, even if subtle, suggests dystonia.

The tremor in ET either remains consistent as the patient holds out the arms against gravity and/or approaches a goal of movement, or there is a brief terminal increase as the goal is reached. When ET is more severe, this can cause significant disability due to interference with eating, drinking, writing, and other skilled motor activities. Many patients do ultimately have some disability, and patients with severe cases can be totally disabled. From 15% to 60% must alter their careers due to their tremor.[12]

In contrast, cerebellar tremors—which can also lead to severe disability—cause an increasing tremor amplitude as the patient performs the movement, not just as the goal is reached. So the amplitude grows to be quite large by the time the goal is reached. This variation may be hard to differentiate at times.

One feature of ET, which is not present in any other type of tremor, is that it is generally very sensitive to alcohol. Many patients will discover that a drink temporarily resolves, or at least significantly decreases, their tremor.

Until recently, ET has been believed to be an isolated problem, without associated symptoms. There is growing evidence that there can be associated findings, but they should not be those of PD (unless the patient suffers dual disease). Generally, patients are neurologically well. However, in keeping with the heterogeneity of ET, some patients can have subclinical cognitive abnormalities uncovered with careful testing. They can show postural instability and ataxic gait. They are more likely to have poor hearing, and they may show olfactory deficits.[12] Patients with severe ET may even have a resting tremor, though it is difficult to test for this carefully enough, because the limb must be at complete rest. ET-associated rest tremors will not be "pill-rolling" in nature. Some forms of ET may actually be a mild degenerative disease with associated symptoms and signs, but definitive characterization and delineation are not yet available. Formal inclusion/exclusion instruments for ET have been developed but are only useful as research tools. Ultimately the clinician must rely on symptoms and signs for diagnosis.

LESS COMMON ACTION AND POSTURAL TREMORS

All other tremor types are relatively uncommon in comparison to the three common ones: ET, PD, and toxic/metabolic. Nonetheless, they show distinct clinical pictures, and differing treatment modalities, so it is important to be aware of them even though they will present much less commonly in a standard practice.

Cerebellar Intention Tremor (or "terminal kinetic tremor")

These tremors are usually 5 Hz and are kinetic, or "intention" action tremors, so they show increasingly worse amplitudes as the motion progresses toward the goal. During physical examination, they are classically tested with "finger-to-nose" and "heel-to-shin" tests. Generally the patient will have additional cerebellar signs such as ataxia, dysmetria, and dysarthria. Titubation is a profound cerebellar tremor with a coarse postural tremor of the head and body when upright.

Cerebellar tremors are caused by cerebellar damage, particularly damage to the outflow tracts from the cerebellum to the thalamus. This damage is most commonly secondary to cerebral vascular accidents (CVAs), multiple sclerosis (MS), trauma, hereditary degenerative disorders, or even long-term alcohol use. Mercury poisoning can also cause a cerebellar tremor.[9,21]

MS is commonly associated with tremor. The details of the tremor are believed to be a direct consequence of the specific lesions developed by each patient. One study of 100 MS patients showed some detectable tremor in 58%, with moderate to severe tremor in 15%.[22] Another study showed a 25% prevalence of tremor, but only 3% severe tremor.[23]

Rubral Tremor

This tremor, also called *Holmes tremor*, is virtually always produced by midbrain damage, often near the red nucleus. It is slow, <5 Hz, may be slightly irregular, and can show a mixture of rest tremor, action tremor, and kinetic/intention tremor. It is virtually always accompanied by evidence of midbrain or cerebellar damage. There can be a delay of up to 2 years (or more) from the time of injury to the onset of tremor.[9]

Orthostatic Tremor

Although historically this tremor has been thought to be an atypical presentation of ET, it has a particular presentation, frequency, and treatment that suggests it is actually a distinct entity. Patients present with an unsteady feeling when standing because they experience uncontrollable shaking, with cramping calves and thighs in this position. An electromyography (EMG) demonstrates around 16 Hz in orthostatic tremor, and symptoms diminish when walking. The tremor is absent when the patient's feet are off the floor, and it is largely only postural and decreases with action. It does not respond to alcohol or the usual treatments for ET, and as we will discuss in the subsequent text, it is uniquely sensitive to clonazepam.[3,24]

Specific Task and Dystonic Tremors

Dystonic tremors occur when patients with dystonic spasms attempt to counteract the dystonic contractions. The symptoms can appear largely tremorous, concealing the underlying dystonia. Treatment and etiology are based on the underlying dystonia.[24]

Tremors specific to a skilled motor task also occur, and may be related to dystonia more than ET because they remain specific. Primary writing tremor is a common one. It is a coarse and slow tremor that causes the writing to be large and messy. Exact etiologies are unclear for this, but it does respond to using other muscle groups for the same task, so it may reside in the specific motor program used for the skilled task.[25,26]

Neuropathic Tremor

Patients with differing types of neuropathies may exhibit differing postural/action tremors. Weakness and/or loss of proprioception may underlie these tremors.

Palatal tremor (previously called *palatal myoclonus*)

Continuous tremors of the soft palate occur at 100 to 150 Hz due to degeneration of the olivary nucleus. This occurs when there is a lesion in a pathway from the contralateral dentate nucleus to the ipsilateral central tegmental tract. It is usually only bothersome if it causes eustachian tube opening and closing with concomitant clicking.[24]

Wilson Disease

Generally this rare (prevalence 1 per 40,000) hereditary disorder of copper metabolism presents before age 40 and most commonly by age 20. It would be an extremely uncommon diagnosis among the senior patient population. Wilson disease is an autosomal recessive disorder. It can present with parkinsonian and/or action tremors most classically. A postural tremor may appear to be "wing-beating." Common accompanying signs include parkinsonian features, dystonia, athetosis, and psychiatric symptoms, along with liver abnormalities.[24] The classic Kayser-Fleischer ring consisting of copper deposition on the cornea coincides with neurologic impairment.

Psychogenic Tremor

This is a tremor without evident organic etiology resulting from voluntary muscle activation. Signs and symptoms that suggest the diagnosis are (i) sudden onset and/or remission, (ii) unusual combinations of various tremor types, (iii) decreased frequency with distraction, (iv) frequency changes to coincide with that of voluntary movements with the contralateral extremity, (v) history of somatization, and (vi) tremor associated with vigorous muscle activation of opposing groups around a joint (this is appreciated as increased resistance and tremor resolves when resistance decreases).[21]

It is usually diagnosed by distracting the patient with competing tasks, either motor or cognitive, which make it difficult to maintain the voluntary tremor. It is almost impossible to maintain two different tremor frequencies voluntarily in two extremities.[10]

WORKUP AND DIAGNOSIS OF PATIENTS WITH TREMOR

As previously stated, the signs and symptoms of tremor are the key to classifying, diagnosing, and treating tremors. In addition to patients who present with the complaint of tremor, be alert to tremor in the geriatric patient that is not brought to your attention. Patients may be embarrassed or may not feel it is worthy of a physician's evaluation even when it is significant and symptomatic.

A Focused History

Be sure to obtain the following history elements:

- Patient and family description of the tremor
- Timeline, with onset, duration and development over time

- Affected body parts and severity
- Factors that improve and worsen the tremor, including response to alcohol
- Associated symptoms, such as gait problems, and neurologic symptoms
- General health, particularly symptoms of thyroid disease, diabetes and/or hypoglycemia, acute illness, or anxiety
- ALL MEDICATIONS
- Alcohol, benzodiazepine, smoking, and drug history
- Family history of tremor and other neurologic syndromes.

Physical Examination

For a fairly quick and reasonable assessment of tremor, the patient has to be examined by inspection at the beginning of the visit. Particularly note the affected areas, symmetry of the tremor, whether it is fast or slow, and whether it gets worse or better with each examination feature. The patient will then be asked to sit with the arms at true rest, holding the arms out against gravity, and then doing a goal-directed activity such as picking something up, writing words, or drawing a spiral, and doing finger-to-nose testing. The lower extremities should also be observed. Include sitting, standing, walking, and heel-to-shin testing. Abnormalities of the head and/or voice should be noted.

Look carefully for the physical examination features in Table 29.4 while narrowing down the diagnosis. These signs are key findings that can enable you to effectively diagnose tremor.

Laboratory Tests

Laboratory tests are primarily done to look for causes of toxic/metabolic tremor. Generally laboratory tests should include: (i) A chemistry panel with liver function tests (LFTs), electrolytes and glucose, (ii) thyroid function tests, and (iii) hemoglobin or hematocrit tests. It may be appropriate to screen for drugs of abuse or a pheochromocytoma if clinically suggested.

Tremors do not generally have other helpful laboratory tests except under unusual circumstances (Table 29.1). Testing for toxic levels of manganese, cyanide, toluene, methyl ethyl ketone, arsenic, bromides, mercury, or lead should be done with suspicion of excessive exposure. Carboxyhemoglobin testing can be done for CO exposure. (Testing for carbon disulfide requires a special lab.) Manganese, cyanide, carbon disulfide, and carbon monoxide toxicity can cause parkinsonian tremors, while arsenic, bromides, mercury, lead, and solvents cause action tremors (Table 29.1). Toxin-induced tremors will be highly unusual in an older population without occupational exposures but each of these toxicities can cause tremors, and rarely toxicity will be found, particularly in ethnic groups utilizing folk remedies.

In younger patients (<age 40), Wilson disease may need to be ruled out with serum ceruloplasmin. This is even less

TABLE 29.4
PHYSICAL EXAMINATION FEATURES OF VARIOUS TREMOR SYNDROMES

Physical Examination Features	Suggests or Helps Differentiate Tremor
■ Reduced movement ■ Masked facies ■ Worsening tremor with walking or use of contralateral extremities ■ Increased tone assessed at examination while trying to passively move upper extremities	Features of Parkinsonian syndrome
■ Tremor increases only at goal, vs. during the entire goal-directed movement	Likely to be essential tremor (More likely to be cerebellar tremor if it increases through entire movement and shows large amplitudes)
■ Cerebellar signs such as ataxia (wide gait), dysmetria (disorganized movement), nystagmus, and so on ■ Plus any additional general neurologic signs	Abnormalities suggest multiple sclerosis or CVA
■ Evidence of significant anxiety and/or sweating	Suggests either withdrawal or enhanced physiologic (toxic/metabolic) tremor due to endogenous epinephrine
■ Tremor stops, diminishes, or changes frequency when the patient is asked to do a voluntary rhythmic activity with other limbs ■ Tremor diminishes when using the affected limb in a way that interferes with coactivation of muscles	To assess suspicion for psychogenic tremor

Cogwheeling can be felt in any tremor if use of the extremity increases the tone with a superimposed sensation of the tremor; parkinsonian symptoms need to be appreciated with the extremity at true rest (e.g., not maintaining posture, weight against gravity).
CVA, cerebral vascular accident.

necessary in the geriatric population because it virtually never presents so late. We mention it even though it will be extremely rare to avoid missing the diagnosis in a patient with a classic tremor with additional dysarthria, dystonia, and PD.

Special Studies

Most tremor patients do not require any imaging or complex workup. The great majority will have a straightforward diagnosis. They will have a toxic/metabolic cause, will seem to have routine ET or will have a fairly classic Parkinson examination. Imaging is required only if there is a suspicion of an anatomic etiology, such as when there are cerebellar or rubral tremors with associated signs, especially if the tremor is unilateral. Palatal tremor also suggests an underlying lesion.

MS workup needs to be done if there is a clinical suspicion; however, tremor is not a common initial presenting symptom of MS.

Extremely rarely will there be a suspicion of rare causes of parkinsonian tremor and imaging may be appropriate to rule out tumors, CVA lesions, infections, or other causes of localized damage. Usually imaging is unnecessary with parkinsonian tremors, and the diagnosis of PD is confirmed by response to treatment.

MANAGEMENT

General Measures for Tremors

Diagnosis of the type of tremor is critical in the appropriate choice and success of therapy. Management measures are geared toward minimizing, and ideally alleviating, all tremors. The goal is to maintain the patient with the maximum function possible.

The primary management of toxic or metabolic tremor is, if at all possible, to remove the underlying cause (i.e., change medications if possible, treat any underlying disorders diagnosed during evaluation, etc.). Overall management for ET is outlined in Figure 29.1. Unusual causes of parkinsonian symptoms should be managed appropriately, particularly discontinuing or minimizing medications that can cause PD symptoms (Tables 29.1 and 29.2).

The first-line therapies for all irresolvable tremors are generally the least invasive, including medications, and physical and occupational therapies, as well as lifestyle modifications. Surgery is to be considered in patients who have not had adequate results with other approaches.

Lifestyle and Therapy

The first interventions to consider are changes related to patient habits. Even if the patient's tremor is not toxic/metabolic, caffeine, nicotine, and other stimulants—including over-the-counter medications such as pseudoephedrine—should be considered for elimination as they may temporarily exacerbate any type of tremor. While alcohol does generally decrease ETs temporarily, there can be a rebound exacerbation of tremor thereafter.[9]

Physical and rehabilitative therapy can provide exercises that may minimize tremors of the hands, arms, legs, and trunk through strength training. It is not proved, however, that this will improve function[27] (Evidence Level B, small randomized controlled trial [RCT]). Speech therapy may benefit those with speech tremors. Wrist weights can help decrease the amplitude of arm tremors during activity (Evidence Level B, small RCTs).

With PD in particular, the patient must be educated regarding the chronicity of the disease without overwhelming him/her. Family and caretakers should also be educated and their emotional needs as well as those of the patient should be addressed. Support groups are also available but may be overwhelming and unnecessary for the newly diagnosed PD patient with early stage disease.

Medications

The type of medication to be considered depends directly on the diagnosed tremor category. Underlying disorders should be appropriately addressed, such as thyrotoxicosis, MS, or drug toxicities. After any underlying etiologies are appropriately treated, medication is tailored to the patient's specific tremor problem.

Toxic/Metabolic Tremor

Sometimes the underlying etiology is not immediately reversible. Examples of this include patients being treated for thyrotoxicosis prior to thyroid medications beginning to work, patients on medications causing tremor where a therapy change is not an option, and patients with stage fright. Under these circumstances, β-blockers such as propranolol can often offer significant relief of symptoms (Evidence Level B, small RCTs). For situational anxiety, the propranolol dose is 20 to 60 mg immediate-acting 1 hour before the event. The dose for more chronic disorders starts at the same level daily and can be titrated up significantly, to dosing similar to ET (see Table 29.5).

Essential Tremor

Two types of drugs are the mainstay of treatment for this disorder,[1] β-blockers, especially nonselective β-blockers such as propranolol, and[2] primidone, an anticonvulsant medication. In both cases, the mechanism of action is unknown. Treatment is usually beneficial, but not generally adequate to wholly resolve tremor symptoms over time (see Fig. 29.1 for overall treatment of ET).

β-Blockers

These are the first-line treatment for ET. From 50% to 70% of patients respond to β-blockers with a 50% to 60%

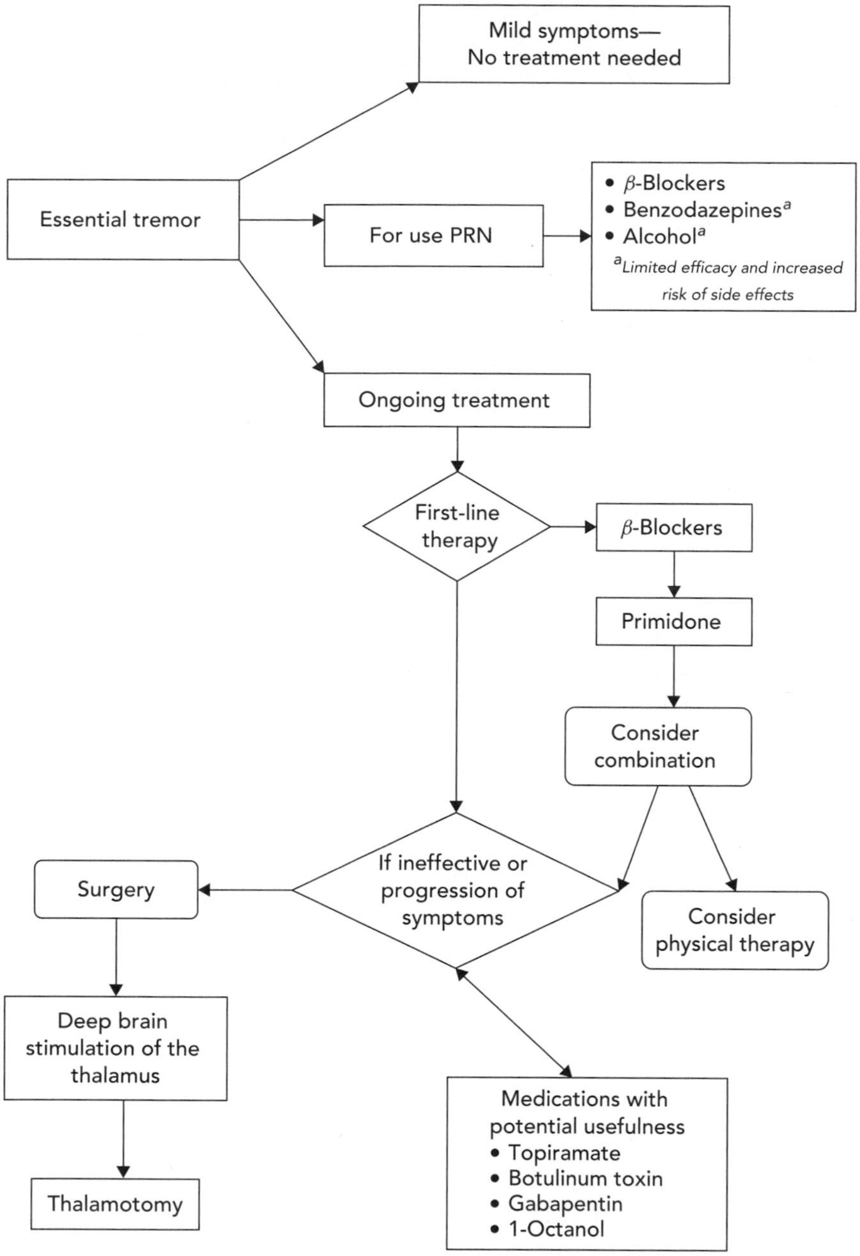

Figure 29.1 Treatment of essential tremor. PRN, treatments that a patient can receive on an "as needed" basis.

reduction in tremor amplitude[10] (Evidence Level B, smaller RCTs). The best-studied β-blocker has been propranolol; no other β-blockers have been shown to be more effective. In the geriatric population, doses should be started at low levels and titrated up; so beginning as low as 10 mg a day, or long-acting 60 mg per day, is reasonable. Ultimately, the usual doses with the greatest tremor control benefits are between 160 and 320 mg per day, whether in long-acting or divided preparations (see Table 29.5 for medication details).

Propranolol is usually most effective for upper extremity tremor, less so for head tremor, and even less so for voice tremor.

Other β-blockers that have been shown to be effective include metoprolol, timolol, sotalol, nadolol, and atenolol[10] (Evidence Level B, smaller, mostly short-duration RCTs). It is reasonable to use propranolol regularly and save the use of any other β-blockers for specific situations, such as patients who have relative contraindications to β-blocker use such as mild asthma, where metoprolol or atenolol may be the drug of choice, or patients who develop central symptoms such as depression or slowing, where nadolol (which is more peripherally acting) may be the drug of choice.[28] Side effects and relative contraindications for β-blockers are summarized in Table 29.5.

Primidone

The other drug that clearly demonstrates benefits in ET is primidone, which is an anticonvulsant. Studies on this

TABLE 29.5
PHARMACOLOGIC TREATMENT OF ESSENTIAL TREMOR

Dosing	Contraindications	Precautions	Adverse Reactions	Interactions
Propranolol[a] 10–320 mg/d Start low at 10 mg daily immediate-acting or 60 mg daily long-acting, increase gradually as needed to a maximum dose of 320 mg/d; do not stop abruptly	Unstable heart failure, asthma, diabetes mellitus, cardiogenic shock, sinus bradycardia, and greater than first-degree block	Impaired hepatic or renal function	Bradycardia, CHF, hypotension, lightheadedness, depression, agranulocytosis	Reserpine, calcium channel blockers, nonsteroidal anti-inflammatory drugs, haloperidol, aluminum hydroxide gel, ethanol, phenytoin, phenobarbitone, rifampin, chlorpromazine, antipyrine, lidocaine, thyroxine, cimetidine, theophylline
Primidone[a] 25–750 mg/d Start low at 25 mg q.h.s. (half of 50 mg tablet); increase gradually as needed to a maximum dose of 750 mg/d; Maximum benefit may be 250 mg or 500 mg but data not clear; do not stop abruptly	Porphyria, phenobarbital sensitivity	Monitor CBC and SMA-12 q6 mo	Ataxia, vertigo, nausea, vomiting, anorexia, fatigue, drowsiness, irritability, sexual impotence, diplopia, nystagmus, morbilliform rash, red cell hypo- or aplasia, agranulocytosis, granulocytopenia	Phenobarbital is a metabolite of primidone
Metoprolol[b] 100–400 mg/d in divided doses; Increase weekly as needed	Sinus bradycardia, second- or third-degree AV block, heart failure, cardiogenic shock	CHF, bronchospasm, COPD, hepatic dysfunction, diabetes, surgery, hyperthyroidism	Fatigue, dizziness, depression, diarrhea, rash, dyspnea, bradycardia, CHF, hypotension, bronchospasm, heart block	Bradycardia with catecholamine-depleting drugs, digitalis, felodipine, may increase effects of calcium channel blockers; may interfere with glaucoma screening tests
Atenolol[b] 25–100 mg/d, Increase weekly as needed	Sinus bradycardia, second- or third-degree AV block, heart failure, cardiogenic shock	Bronchospasm, renal dysfunction, diabetes, hyperthyroidism, pheochromocytoma, surgery, ischemic heart disease or failure	Heart failure, bronchospasm, Bradycardia, angina, MI, heart block dizziness fatigue, GI upset depression, orthostatic hypotension, cold extremities	Additive with catecholamine-depleting drugs, prazosin, digoxin; conduction abnormalities, bradycardia, heart block with calcium channel blockers

Nadolol[b]				
40–240 mg/d Increase at 3–7-d intervals as needed	Asthma, sinus bradycardia, second- or third-degree heart block, heart failure, cardiogenic shock	Ischemic heart disease, bronchospastic disease, COPD, renal or hepatic dysfunction, diabetes, hyperthyroidism, surgery, SLE	Bradycardia, dizziness, fatigue, cold extremities, heart failure, heart block, bronchospasm, GI upset, rash, pruritus	Hypotension, bradycardia with catecholamine-depleting drugs, general anesthetics, conduction abnormalities, bradycardia, heart block with calcium channel blockers, digitalis
Topiramate				
25–50 mg/d to 1.6 g/d in divided doses; titrate as needed, increasing by 25–50 mg at weekly intervals; tremor studied at migraine doses	Hypersensitivity	Discontinue if acute myopia or secondary angle glaucoma occur	Drowsiness, dizziness, ataxia, speech disorder, psychomotor slowing, nervousness, paresthesia, hypoesthesia, visual disorders, fatigue, weight loss, GI upset, anorexia, kidney stones, acidosis	Phenytoin, carbamazepine, valproic acid, digoxin, oral contraceptives, carbonic anhydrate inhibitors, anticholinergics
Gabapentin				
300 mg to 3.6 g/d in divided doses above 300 mg	Hypersensitivity	Avoid abrupt cessation, renal dysfunction, elderly	Somnolence, dizziness, ataxia, fatigue, nystagmus, visual disturbance, tremor, dyspepsia, dysarthria, amnesia, back pain, edema, dry mouth, constipation, twitching, pruritus	Alcohol, morphine and other CNS depressants

This chart does not include a complete listing in each category.
[a]The effect of propranolol and primidone together can be more than additive and are combined if the patient has not had an adequate response to either by itself.
[b]Patients who fail propranolol are unlikely to respond to another β-blocker. These are usually used to treat those who are unable to tolerate the side effects of propranolol.
CHF, congestive heart failure; CBC, complete blood count; COPD, chronic obstructive pulmonary disease; AV, atrioventricular; MI, myocardial infarction; SLE, systemic lupus erythematosus; GI, gastrointestinal; CNS, central nervous system.

drug have been small in number, but it seems to be similar in effectiveness to propranolol, or even slightly better[12,29] (Evidence Level B, small RCTs). It is considered second line due to its side effects. Dosing should start at 25 mg to 50 mg (one half to one whole 50 mg pill) at bedtime, and can be titrated up slowly as tolerated. Initial tolerability can be very poor, including an acute toxic reaction with the first dose that includes nausea, vomiting, and ataxia. Up to 20% or more of patients cannot tolerate primidone. It is used nonetheless, because it can work well for those who can tolerate it and longer-term side effects appear to be stable, possibly better than propranolol. After 50 mg is tolerated, patients may go up weekly to doses up to 750 mg. Doses above 250 mg may not further improve tremor control for most patients, however.[30]

Combination Propranolol and Primidone

A combination of the two treatments may provide benefits beyond either treatment by itself[31] (Evidence Level C, common opinion).

Additional Promising Drug Therapies for Essential Tremor

There are a number of other medications that have been tried for ET. None are routine standard of care at this point. All have small numbers of patients/studies to back up their efficacy. Quite a few additional medications have been tested and have failed to demonstrate efficacy when exposed to more rigorous trials.

1. Benzodiazepines, for example, are NOT a promising therapy. Their benefit is small (if any) and their side effects and addiction potential are well known. Among multiple other drugs that have failed to show efficacy, Levetiracetam, a new antiseizure medication, showed promise in early observations but has not been demonstrated to be effective (Evidence Level B, small RCTs).
2. Topiramate (Topamax) has one crossover study that showed a statistically significant benefit at 400 mg per day with side effects similar to use for seizures[32] (Evidence Level B, small RCT).
3. Gabapentin (Neurontin)—primarily used as an antiepileptic and pain medication—has had three small studies done (total 69 patients). It was well tolerated, and some patients responded well to it, but it was inconsistently statistically significant across the study population[10] (Evidence Level B, equivocal RCTs).
4. 1-Octanol is an 8-C alcohol currently used as a food-flavoring agent. In two very preliminary open-label studies it was successful in reducing ET without the intoxicating effects of ethanol. It is not available for clinical use at this time (Evidence Level B, preliminary data). An alcoholic drink may be effective for select patients for very short-term control when in socially appropriate situations.
5. Botulinum toxin A (Botox) can be helpful in head, neck, or voice tremors. It is not generally used in hand tremors because of weakness associated with tremor reduction. It is worth trying when significant head, neck, or voice tremors do not respond adequately to standard medication[31,33] (Evidence Level B, small RCTs).

Parkinson Disease

Treatment algorithms for PD are complex, and treatment of PD tremor is usually, but not always, incorporated under general treatment of PD. Treatment needs usually evolve over the course of the disease, and eventually combination regimens are required. PD disabilities due to bradykinesis and rigidity often overwhelm the symptoms of tremor as the disease progresses. The literature for PD management is extensive and evolving. At this point, there are no treatments proved to be disease-altering or neuroprotective, so for now all treatment is directed toward symptom minimization. Current possibilities for neuroprotective agents are listed in Table 29.6. Table 29.7 lists current PD treatments.

The most effective general PD treatment, levodopa, tends to develop complications with chronic therapy. About half of patients will suffer from fluctuations and/or dyskinesias after 5 years of therapy.[24] These may be cumulative medication side effects of carbidopa/levodopa or disease progression. Studies are unclear. Given that the length of therapy may be a limiting factor in carbidopa/levodopa use, it makes sense to begin PD therapy with other agents and change to carbidopa/levodopa only when necessary for symptom control.[18,24] However, geriatric patients also frequently suffer substantial side effects from nonlevodopa therapies, so it is challenging to determine the ideal therapy algorithm over time. PD care will usually involve neurology specialists or geriatricians with a special interest and expertise in PD.

TABLE 29.6
POSSIBLE NEUROPROTECTIVE AGENTS FOR PARKINSON DISEASE—(NONE PROVEN AS OF 2005)

Selegiline or rasagiline (selective MAO B inhibitors)
Glutamate-mediated toxicity blockers—riluzole
Mitochondrial mediators—coenzyme Q10, creatine, ginkgo biloba, nicotinamide, carnitine
Transplantation of human or porcine fetal nigral cells
Antioxidants—vitamin E, glutathione, iron chelators
Calcium channel blockers
Cyclosporine
Nonsteroidal anti-inflammatory agents
Estrogens

MAO B, monoamine oxidase type-B.

TABLE 29.7
CURRENT PARKINSON DISEASE TREATMENTS

Class	Medication and Dosage	Mechanism of Action	Precautions	Side Effects	Interactions
Antiviral	Amantadine 100 mg b.i.d.–t.i.d.	Unknown mechanism of action in PD; increases dopamine release, inhibits dopamine reuptake, stimulates dopamine receptors, anticholinergic effects	Benefit appears transient in some patients Best as short-term monotherapy in mild disease, can add L-dopa to this and increase benefit, adding this to L-dopa, however, of little benefit; may have a role in late PD for patients with dyskinesias and motor fluctuations	Livedo reticularis, nausea, ankle edema, orthostasis; infrequent—hallucinations, confusion, nightmares—more common if on other PD medications	Potentiates side effects of anticholinergic medications, including antihistamines, may require decreased dosage of those medications if used concurrently Caution with CNS stimulants, cotrimoxazole; can worsen tremor of PD in patients also on thioridazine, potential class effect with other phenothiazines
MAO B inhibitor	Selegiline 5 mg each morning Sometimes a second dose is added at noon, but with limited additional benefit	Symptomatic—treats early mild symptoms (and possibly) Neuroprotective—block free radical formation in dopamine metabolism	The whole theory of neuroprotection and its role in PD remains unproven	Nausea, headache, insomnia	Tricyclics, SSRIs, esp. fluoxetine, nonselective MAO inhibitors, meperidine, possibly other opiates Because of the selective nature of MAO B inhibitors, no hypertensive issues with tyramine foods
Anticholinergics	Benztropine 0.5 mg b.i.d. to 1–2 mg b.i.d.–t.i.d. Trihexyphenidyl 1 mg b.i.d. to 2 mg b.i.d.–t.i.d.	Shift the balance toward dopamine in the basal ganglia by blocking acetylcholine Benztropine may also inhibit presynaptic reuptake of dopamine	Alone—most useful in patients <70 with tremor, without akinesia or gait problems Adjunct therapy—may be useful in advanced PD with persistent tremor already on L-dopa or Dopamine agonist	Memory impairment, confusion, hallucinations, sedation, dysphoria, dry mouth, blurred vision, constipation, urinary retention—caution with BPH, impaired sweating, tachycardia	Class—Antipsychotics, tricyclic antidepressants
Dopamine agonists	Apomorphine 2 mg SC test dose, 2–10 mg SC t.i.d. Bromocriptine 2.5 mg to start, titrate to 5–10 mg q.i.d. Pramipexole 0.125 mg t.i.d. to 1.5 mg t.i.d. Ropinirole 0.25 mg t.i.d. to 1.0 mg t.i.d.	Directly stimulate dopamine receptors Can be considered for monotherapy in early PD, but no clear evidence that this is better than initial treatment with L-dopa	Ineffective in patients who have no therapeutic response to L-dopa Increased risk of side effects in the elderly, especially patients already suffering from dementia *Pergolide is another member of this class which has fallen into disuse due to increased risk of restrictive valvular heart disease*	Entire class—Nausea, vomiting, orthostatic hypotension, confusion, hallucinations, headaches Apomorphine—cutaneous reactions, rarely, chest pain, angina Pramipexole and ropinirole—sleep attacks	Class—Medications with dopamine antagonist activity, e.g., phenothiazines, butyrophenones Apomorphine—$5HT_3$ antagonist class (including, ondansetron, granisetron, dolasetron, palonosetron, and alosetron); effects on blood pressure may be increased by the concomitant use of alcohol, antihypertensive medications, and vasodilators (especially nitrates)

(continued)

TABLE 29.7
(continued)

Class	Medication and Dosage	Mechanism of Action	Precautions	Side Effects	Interactions
					Pramipexole—cimetidine Ropinirole—ciprofloxacin, estrogens
Dopamine precursor	Carbidopa/levodopa 25/100 mg start with half tab t.i.d. and increase to symptom control up to 25/250 mg q.i.d. Sustained-release formulations of this medication may be useful in some patients, but require higher total doses (up to 30% more)	Crosses blood–brain barrier where it is converted to dopamine to supplement the depleted supply in the corpus striatum	Appears to be effective for a limited time, 5–10 y, after which the dyskinesia and motor fluctuations associated with it limit its usefulness; many suggest delaying its use until absolutely necessary	Nausea, vomiting, somnolence, dizziness, headache, confusion, hallucinations, delusions, agitation, depression, potentially with suicidal tendencies, psychosis	Antipsychotics including phenothiazines, benzodiazepines, MAO inhibitors, phenytoin, pyridoxine, methionine, selegiline, iron therapy, and protein rich foods interfere with absorption
COMT inhibitors	Entacapone 200 mg with each dose of L-dopa, up to eight doses per day Tolcapone 100–200 mg t.i.d	Extend the duration of action of L-dopa, may allow reduction of L-dopa doses by 30%	Only useful in combination with L-dopa Taper either medication if decided to discontinue, can precipitate symptoms like neuroleptic malignant syndrome. Use of tolcapone requires monitoring of LFTs, recommended only if other treatments have failed	Dyskinesias, hallucinations, confusion, nausea, orthostatic hypotension, diarrhea, abdominal pain, orange urine Tolcapone—increased liver enzymes, very rare hepatotoxicity	Class—If used with caridopa/levodopa, potential interaction with desipramine, imipramine Entacapone—caution with drugs known to interfere with biliary excretion, glucuronidation, and intestinal β-glucuronidase including probenecid, cholestyramine, and some antibiotics (e.g., erythromycin, rifamipicin, ampicillin, and chloramphenicol) Tolcapone—caution with warfarin

PD, Parkinson disease; CNS, central nervous system; COMT, catechol-*O*-methyl transferase inhibitors; SSRIs, selective serotonin reuptake inhibitors; MAO, monoamine oxidase; BPH, benign prostatic hyperplasia; LFT, liver function tests.

Tremor in PD responds to most of the PD treatments.[18] Anticholinergics, selegiline, dopamine agonists, and carbidopa/levodopa all have been shown to have significant effects on PD tremor (Evidence Level B, small RCTs). No one agent is clearly superior, so treatment choices for tremor can be made on the basis of other PD considerations. In addition, long-acting propranolol (but not primidone) has been shown to have a significant effect on PD tremor; propranolol is not considered a general PD treatment but can be well tolerated and is worth considering for tremor symptoms (Evidence Level B, RCT).

Orthostatic Tremor

This tremor is rare, so studies on treatment are very small and not well controlled. It has been described as sensitive to clonazepam (begin clonazepam at 1 mg q.h.s and increase up to 2 to 6 mg daily) and gabapentin.[34] Medications that work for ET are often tried and can work for individual patients, but they do not work well in general. Some evidence suggests orthostatic tremor is not very responsive to medication of any kind[35] (Evidence Level B, small RCTs).

Dystonic Tremor

Treatment for this disorder involves treating the underlying dystonia, which is beyond the scope of this chapter. Botulinum toxin is often the most successful treatment.

Primary Writing Tremor

This may be a form of dystonic tremor, a form of ET, or a unique disorder.[9] Medications for both ET and dystonia may be tried, but often the most successful treatment is retraining and using a new type or size of pen or a typewriter to change the involved movements[26] (Evidence Level B, small RCTs).

Cerebellar Tremor and Rubral (Midbrain) Tremor

No medical therapies have been shown to be consistently effective to date. Multiple medications have worked on individual patients[9] (Evidence Level B, multiple preliminary trials and small RCTs). Of course, any underlying disorders should be treated as appropriate. Bracing the proximal portion of the limb and/or wrist weights may help to decrease the tremor amplitude and to increase functionality (Evidence Level B, at least one small RCT).

Surgery

Medically refractory, disabling tremors due to multiple etiologies may be ameliorated by surgery. With relatively recent developments in neurosurgical techniques, this can be an important and realistic alternative for patients with significant disability. The current state-of-the-art technique for a number of tremors is to implant electrodes in the ventral intermediate nucleus of the thalamus and perform continuous deep brain stimulation[36] (Evidence Level B, small RCTs).

Surgical treatment has been shown to provide significant tremor relief in ET, PD, and cerebellar tremors due to MS, with preliminary data for Holme (rubral) tremor as well (Evidence Level B, small RCTs). This type of surgery does not alter the course of disability due to anything other than tremor in PD or MS. A large fraction of patients—above 80%—achieve significant or even total relief of tremor symptoms, and most patients who have side effects are able to have them resolved with adjustment of the stimulation parameters. Side effects are almost entirely reversible if stimulation is turned off.[37]

Bilateral brain stimulation can be more helpful than unilateral, particularly for face or head tremors, though patients may be more likely to have side effects.[38]

Longer-term efficacy and side effects of surgery for tremor have been somewhat more variable but still very positive. Many PD patients become disabled by the spectrum of PD symptoms, so surgery has more overall benefit for PD. Deep brain stimulation in the subthalamic nucleus not only treats PD tremor but also improves all of the cardinal motor symptoms of PD.[37]

A number of ET patients become tolerant to the brain stimulation and there is the risk of device complications requiring repeated surgeries, including hardware replacements (up to 40%). However, at least half of ET patients derived long-term significant benefit from surgery even in the more pessimistic study. Other studies show even greater benefits for their patients with fewer complications[39,40] (Evidence Level B, small RCTs). Surgical care of severe refractory tremors can be a reasonable consideration.

Patient Resources

Despite all the treatment options listed in the preceding text, a number of patients will not have complete, ideal tremor control and will have to cope with their tremors over many years. The section "Suggested Readings and Resources" provides a listing of helpful patient resources.

CONCLUSION

Tremor is a common problem in the geriatric population. It can cause substantial disability. Identification and treatment of tremor are important to maintain patients' health and quality of life. There are a number of treatment options, though they often fall short of full amelioration of symptoms. Supportive relationships with tremor patients, including continuing tremor assessment and treatment adjustment, are therefore an important component of geriatric health care. Further developments are likely in the future care of tremors—both in our understanding of the etiology of tremors and in the ability to provide improved treatment options.

REFERENCES

1. Deuschl G, Bain P, Brin M. Consensus statement of the movement disorder society on tremor. Ad hoc scientific committee. *Mov Disord*. 1998;13(suppl 3):2–23.
2. Diederich NJ, Goetz CG. Drug-induced movement disorders. *Neurol Clin*. 1998;16(1):125–139.
3. Smith GN. Movement disorders. In: David AK, Johnson TAJ, Phillips DM, et al. eds. *Family medicine: Principles and practice*, 6th ed. New York, NY: Springer-Verlag; 2003: Chapter 66.
4. Elble RJ. Tremor and dopamine agonists. *Neurology*. 2002;58 (4 suppl 1):S57–S62.
5. Chaudhuri KR, Buxton-Thomas M, Dhawan V, et al. Long duration asymmetrical postural tremor is likely to predict development of Parkinson's disease and not essential tremor: Clinical follow up study of 13 cases. *J Neurol Neurosurg Psychiatry*. 2005; 76(1):115–117.
6. Christine CW, Aminoff MJ. Clinical differentiation of parkinsonian syndromes: Prognostic and therapeutic relevance. *Am J Med*. 2004;117(6):412–419.
7. Pappert EJ. Toxin-induced movement disorders. *Neurol Clin*. 2005;23(2):429–459.
8. Masdeu J, Rodriquez-Oroz MC, Chapter 78, abnormalities of posture and movement. In: Cassel Christine, ed. *Geriatric medicine: An evidence-based approach*, 4th ed. New York, NY: Springer-Verlag; 2003.
9. Zesiewicz TA, Hauser RA. Phenomenology and treatment of tremor disorders. *Neurol Clin*. 2001;19:651–680,vii.
10. Pahwa R, Lyons KE. Essential tremor: Differential diagnosis and current therapy. *Am J Med*. 2003;115(2):134–142.
11. Dogu O, Sevim S, Camdeviren H, et al. Prevalence of essential tremor: Door-to-door neurologic exams in Mersin province, Turkey. *Neurology*. 2003;61(12):1804–1806.
12. Louis ED. Essential tremor. *Lancet Neurol*. 2005;4(2):100–110.
13. Busenbark K, Barnes P, Lyons K, et al. Accuracy of reported family histories of essential tremor. *Neurology*. 1996;47(1): 264–265.
14. Lou JS, Jankovic J. Essential tremor: Clinical correlates in 350 patients. *Neurology*. 1991;41(2(Pt 1)):234–238.
15. Higgins JJ, Lombardi RQ, Pucilowska J, et al. A variant in the HS1-BP3 gene is associated with familial essential tremor. *Neurology*. 2005;64(3):417–421.
16. Tanner CM, Goldman SM, Lyons KE, et al. Essential tremor in twins: An assessment of genetic vs environmental determinants of etiology. *Neurology*. 2001;57(8):1389–1391.
17. Lorenz D, Frederiksen H, Moises H, et al. High concordance for essential tremor in monozygotic twins of old age. *Neurology*. 2004;62(2):208–211.
18. Elble RJ. Diagnostic criteria for essential tremor and differential diagnosis. *Neurology*. 2000;54(11 suppl 4):S2–S6.
19. Koller WC, Busenbark K, Miner K. Essential Tremor Study Group. The relationship of essential tremor to other movement disorders: Report on 678 patients. *Ann Neurol*. 1994;35(6):717–723.
20. Louis ED, Ford B, Frucht S. Factors associated with increased risk of head tremor in essential tremor: A community-based study in northern Manhattan. *Mov Disord*. 2003;18(4):432–436.
21. Cooper G, Rodnitzky R. The many forms of tremor: Precise classification guides selection of therapy. *Postgrad Med*. 2000; 108(1):57–70.
22. Alusi SH. A study of tremor in multiple sclerosis. *Brain*. 2001; 124(Pt 4):720–730.
23. Pittock SJ, McClelland RL, Mayr WT, et al. Prevalence of tremor in multiple sclerosis and associated disability in the Olmsted county population. *Mov Disord*. 2004;19(12):1482–1485.
24. Goetz CG. Hyperkinetic movement disorders. In: *Textbook of clinical neurology*, 2 nd ed. Philadelphia, PA: Elsevier Science; 2003:731.
25. Bain PG, Findley LJ, Britton TC, et al. Primary writing tremor. *Brain*. 1995;118(pt 6):1461–1472.
26. Espay A, Hung SW, Sanger TD, et al. A writing device improves writing in primary writing tremor. *Neurology*. 2005;64(9): 1648.
27. Bilodeau M, Keen DA, Sweeney PJ, et al. Strength training can improve steadiness in persons with essential tremor. *Muscle Nerve*. 2000;23(5):771–778.
28. Tarsy D. Tremor.UpToDate.http://www.utdol.com/application/topic.asp?file=move_dis/4697&type=A&selectedTitle=1~15, accessed 2/23/05.
29. Koller WC, Vetere-Overfield B. Acute and chronic effects of propanolol and primidone in essential tremor. *Neurology*. 1989; 39(12):1587–1588.
30. Serrano-Dueñas M. Use of primidone in low doses (250 mg/day) versus high doses (750 mg/day) in the management of essential tremor. Double-blind comparative study with one-year follow-up. *Parkinsonism Relat Disord*. 2003;10(1):29–33.
31. Lyons KE, Pahwa R, Comella CL, et al. Benefits and risks of pharmacological treatments for essential tremor. *Drug Saf*. 2003; 26(7):461–481.
32. Connor GS. A double-blind placebo-controlled trial of topiramate treatment for essential tremor. *Neurology*. 2002;59(1):132–134.
33. Brin MF, Lyons KE, Doucette J, et al. A randomized, double masked, controlled trial of botulinum toxin type A in essential hand tremor. *Neurology*. 2001;56(11):1523–1528.
34. Ondo W. Gait and balance disorders. In: *Medical clinics of North America*, Vol. 87 (4): WB Saunders; July 1, 2003:793–801,viii.
35. Gerschlager W, Munchau A, Kapzenschlager R, et al. Natural history and syndromic associations of orthostatic tremor: A review of 41 patients. *Mov Disord*. 2004;19(7):788–795.
36. Schuurman PR, Bruins J, Merkus MP, et al. A comparison of continuous thalamic stimulation and thalamotomy for suppression of severe tremor. *N Engl J Med*. 2000;342(7):461–468.
37. Walter BL, Vitek JL. Surgical treatment for Parkinson's disease. *Lancet Neurol*. 2004;3(12):719–728.
38. Ondo W, Almaguer M, Jankovic J, et al. Thalamic deep brain stimulation: Comparison between unilateral and bilateral placement. *Arch Neurol*. 2001;58(2):218–222.
39. Koller WC, Lyons KE, Wilkinson SB, et al. Long-term safety and efficacy of unilateral deep brain stimulation of the thalamus in essential tremor. *Mov Disord*. 2001;16(3):464–468.
40. Rehncrona S, Johnels B, Widner H. Long-term efficacy of thalamic deep brain stimulation for tremor: Double-blind assessments. *Mov Disord*. 2003;18(2):163–170.

SUGGESTED READINGS AND RESOURCES

International Essential Tremor Foundation
General information and research resource
P.O. Box 14005
Lenexa, KS 66285-4004
http://www.essentialtremor.org
(888) 387-3667
Support groups by area:
www.egroups.com/community/activa

Parkinson Disease
The up-to-date NIH resource
http://www.nlm.nih.gov/medlineplus/parkinsonsdisease.html
Tremor Action Network
P.O. Box 5013
Pleasanton, CA 94566-0513
tremor@tremoraction.org
http://www.tremoraction.org

We Move
Worldwide Education and Awareness for Movement Disorders
204 West 84th Street
New York, NY 10024
http://www.wemove.org

Youcan Toocan Inc.
Eating and drinking aids and other products
http://www.youcantoocan.com

Pulmonary Disease in the Elderly

30

Eleanor M. Summerhill

CLINICAL PEARLS 395

INTRODUCTION 396

PULMONARY SIGNS AND SYMPTOMS 396

NORMAL AGE-RELATED CHANGES IN THE RESPIRATORY SYSTEM 398
Changes in the Lung 398
Changes in the Chest Wall and Respiratory Muscles 399
Mechanics 399
Changes in Pulmonary Function 399
Arterial Oxygen Tension 400
Loss of Respiratory Reserve 400

ASTHMA IN THE ELDERLY 400
Epidemiology 400
Diagnosis 400
Treatment Considerations in the Elderly 402

CHRONIC OBSTRUCTIVE PULMONARY DISEASE 402
Epidemiology 403
Diagnosis 403
Treatment Considerations in the Elderly 403

PNEUMONIA 405
Pathophysiology and Clinical Presentation 405
Mortality 405
Diagnostic Evaluation 405
Causative Organisms in the Elderly 406
Treatment 407
Prophylaxis 407

TUBERCULOSIS 407
Tuberculin Skin Testing 409
Diagnosis and Treatment of Latent Tuberculosis Infection 409
Clinical Presentation, Diagnosis, and Treatment of Active Tuberculosis 410

SLEEP-DISORDERED BREATHING 410
Changes in Sleep Patterns with Aging 411
Obstructive Sleep Apnea 411
Diagnosis 411
Treatment 411

CONCLUSION 411

CLINICAL PEARLS

- Although the physiologic reserve of the respiratory system declines with age, dyspnea with usual activity is abnormal and should trigger an investigation for underlying disease.
- The perception of dyspnea appears to be blunted in the elderly and may delay seeking medical attention.
- An alveolar-to-arterial oxygen gradient of 20 to 25 mm Hg is the upper limit of normal in any population, and a higher gradient in the elderly patient warrants further evaluation.
- The most common causes of cough include postnasal drip, cough-variant asthma, chronic bronchitis, and gastroesophageal reflux disease. Therapy should be directed at the underlying mechanism following diagnostic evaluation.

- The differential diagnosis of asthma in the elderly is broad and often overlooked.
- Asthma may present at any age.
- The negative predictive value of methacholine challenge testing is higher than the positive predictive value, so that it is more useful in ruling out a diagnosis of asthma than establishing one.
- Special treatment considerations in the elderly with asthma and chronic obstructive pulmonary disease include a higher risk of adverse effects of medication and exacerbation of coexistent disease, medical noncompliance, and precipitation of bronchospasm by commonly used medications for comorbid illness.
- Although a number of medications are indicated for symptomatic relief in chronic obstructive pulmonary disease, smoking cessation and supplemental oxygen therapy are the only therapies shown to favorably impact outcome.
- Elderly patients with pneumonia often present with nonspecific symptoms and may not manifest the classic constellation of fever, dyspnea, and cough. This may lead to delayed diagnosis or misdiagnosis and a greater mortality risk.
- Initiation of appropriate antibiotic therapy for pneumonia within the first 8 hours of presentation has been shown to significantly reduce mortality.
- Prevention may be the best way to reduce the morbidity and mortality associated with pneumonia in the elderly. Recommended immunizations include the 23-valent pneumococcal polysaccharide and influenza vaccines.
- Because of the waning of cell-mediated immunity, the two-step purified protein derivative skin test is recommended in those elderly with an initial nonreactive test result.
- The risk of isoniazid-induced hepatitis is low. Therefore, isoniazid-based treatment regimens are recommended for the treatment of both latent and active tuberculosis in the elderly.
- Sleep patterns change with normative aging, and sleep disturbances such as insomnia, nocturnal awakening, and sleep-disordered breathing appear to be more common in the elderly population. Their clinical significance is unclear.

INTRODUCTION

With normal aging come changes in pulmonary function that reduce the physiologic reserve of the respiratory system. This progressive decline that occurs with advancing age in various organ systems is called *homeostenosis*. However, it is important to remember that despite this age-related decline, it is never normal for an individual to have the need to curtail normal activities because of pulmonary limitation. Dyspnea with usual activity is always abnormal and is indicative of underlying disease.[1]

As in many areas of medicine, there are few pulmonary diseases entirely unique to the geriatric population. However, the prevalence, presenting manifestations, diagnosis, and treatment may differ from those in younger adult populations. This chapter contains an overview of presenting signs and symptoms of pulmonary disease in the elderly, the normal physiology of the aging lung, and some specific disease processes particularly relevant to ambulatory geriatric clinical practice.

PULMONARY SIGNS AND SYMPTOMS

Pulmonary disease may be associated with a variety of signs and symptoms. The most common symptoms pointing to pulmonary pathology include dyspnea, cough, pleuritic chest pain, and hemoptysis.

Dyspnea is defined as an abnormally uncomfortable awareness of breathing[2] and is most often described as breathlessness or shortness of breath. Recently, dyspnea was defined by the American Thoracic Society (ATS) as "a subjective experience of breathing discomfort that consists of qualitatively distinct sensations that vary in intensity."[3] Dyspnea is a very common presenting symptom of pulmonary disease. However, as delineated in Table 30.1, dyspnea may also be indicative of cardiac disease, hematologic disease, neuromuscular disease, metabolic disease, deconditioning, and/or obesity, or it may be psychosomatic

TABLE 30.1
COMMON CAUSES OF DYSPNEA

Cardiovascular
Left ventricular failure
Valvular dysfunction
Pericardial effusion
Right-to-left shunt
Pulmonary
Obstructive airways disease
Parenchymal lung disease
Pulmonary vascular disease
Pleural disease
Respiratory muscle weakness
Neuromuscular disorders
Phrenic nerve paralysis
Metabolic and systemic illness
Mechanical
Upper airway obstruction
Chest wall and thoracic spine abnormalities
Exogenous obesity
Massive ascites
Hematologic
Anemia
Psychosomatic
Anxiety
Deconditioning

in origin. A thorough history including acuity of onset, exacerbating factors such as exertion and positional change, and associated symptoms are vital in determining the etiology of dyspnea. Abrupt onset points to relatively acute processes such as pulmonary infection, pulmonary embolism (PE), and congestive heart failure (CHF). Subacute or chronic presentations of dyspnea are more likely to be indicative of underlying chronic bronchitis, emphysema, interstitial lung disease (ILD), or chronic CHF. Dyspnea may occur at rest or may only be apparent on exertion. In making an assessment of the severity of chronic dyspnea, it is important that the practitioner ask the patient "what are your usual daily activities?" and "what activities have you had to discontinue recently?" because patients often reduce activities to minimize discomfort.[4]

Evidence suggests that the perception of dyspnea may be blunted in the elderly. This may be due to a number of complex processes involving the mechanical properties of the lung and chest wall, central and peripheral chemoreceptors, neural input and output, and deconditioning. For example, there is a lower response to hypercapnic hypoxemia in the elderly, largely because of a decrease in carbon dioxide sensitivity.[5] And, despite similar levels of decline in forced expiratory volume in 1 second (FEV_1), older subjects given methacholine bronchoprovocation testing noted less subjective discomfort compared to younger individuals. This may be due either to reduced number or activity of stretch receptors or to decreased perception of resistive respiratory loads.[6]

A history of positional change eliciting or exacerbating dyspnea may be helpful in elucidating the underlying etiology. Orthopnea, or dyspnea in the supine position, is characteristic of CHF. It is usually related to gravitational elevation of pulmonary and venous capillary pressures and a reduction of vital capacity (VC). However, it may also be indicative of bilateral diaphragmatic paralysis and may occur in obstructive lung disease. Paroxysmal nocturnal dyspnea, like orthopnea, is usually indicative of CHF. It may also be present in chronic bronchitis because of pooling of secretions or in asthma because of circadian changes in airway obstruction. Platypnea, which occurs in the upright position, is most often associated with orthodeoxia, or oxygen desaturation when upright. Platypnea and orthodeoxia may occur because of changes in ventilation–perfusion (V/Q) matching or may be indicative of intracardiac shunt.

The underlying etiology of dyspnea in the elderly may usually be elucidated by means of a thorough history (including tobacco and occupational exposures), physical examination, and simple diagnostic testing. Initial testing should include a chest radiograph (CXR), electrocardiogram (ECG), and complete blood count (CBC). If a pulmonary cause for dyspnea is suspected, further investigation is indicated. This should include pulse oximetry or arterial blood gas (ABG) analysis and pulmonary function tests (PFTs). PFTs include spirometry, inspiratory and expiratory flow loops, lung volumes, and diffusing capacity for carbon monoxide (D_{LCO}). If respiratory muscle weakness is suspected, maximal inspiratory and expiratory pressures should be obtained. If the cause of dyspnea remains unclear, echocardiography and, finally, cardiopulmonary exercise testing may help in differentiating between cardiac or pulmonary limitation and deconditioning.[1,4]

Cough is a common symptom referable to the respiratory system. It is a physiologic mechanism for clearing and protecting the airway. It may be stimulated by a number of different processes, including airway irritation or inflammation, parenchymal disease, CHF, or medications. Cough is generally categorized as either acute or chronic on the basis of a duration of $<$ or $>$3 weeks. In the overwhelming majority of cases, acute cough is related to either a viral or a bacterial upper respiratory tract infection. However, particularly in the elderly, acute cough may be a presenting manifestation of more serious illness such as pneumonia, aspiration, CHF, or PE.[7]

Studies have shown that chronic cough is usually due to one or a combination of four processes: Postnasal drip, cough-variant asthma, chronic bronchitis, or gastroesophageal reflux disease (GERD).[8,9] Other causes to consider in the elderly include bronchiectasis, CHF, ILD, bronchogenic lung cancer, postviral airway hyperreactivity, and recurrent aspiration.[7] An additional etiology that should be recognized in this population is angiotensin-converting enzyme (ACE) inhibitors. Approximately 5% to 20% of patients placed on ACE inhibitors will develop a dry cough. This is a class effect of these antihypertensive medications and is most likely related to the accumulation of the inflammatory mediators bradykinin or substance P, both of which are degraded by ACE. The development of cough is idiosyncratic and is not dose related. The time course may be quite variable, ranging from several hours to even months after initiation of ACE inhibitors. After discontinuing the medication, the cough generally resolves within 4 days.[10]

Evaluation of chronic cough should begin with a complete history and physical examination, as well as a CXR. If the CXR is normal, and nothing in the history and physical points to a diagnosis, the next most useful step is a methacholine challenge test to assess for bronchial hyperreactivity (BHR).[8] GERD may be silent. Therefore, if another cause of chronic cough cannot be found and treated, prolonged esophageal pH monitoring should be considered.[11] Some patients will be found to have more than one diagnosis. Therapy should be directed toward the underlying pathophysiologic mechanism of the cough. Specific therapy has been shown to be effective in patients compliant with the therapeutic regimen in 97% to 98% of cases.[8,9] Patients with chronic bronchitis, asthma, and postviral airway hyperreactivity respond to inhaled bronchodilators and corticosteroids; those with postnasal drip respond to decongestants and nasal steroid preparations and those with GERD to histamine-2 (H_2) blockers and proton pump inhibitors. Symptomatic treatment with antitussive agents such as dextromethorphan, and narcotics such as codeine is useful to supplement specific therapy, but is ineffective alone.

Pleuritic chest pain is most often sharp but may also be described as dull, achy, or a "catching" sensation. Characteristically, it worsens with deep inspiration, cough, or positional change. Pleuritic pain originates in the parietal pleura, which has extensive pain fiber innervation; the visceral pleura does not. Pain is usually relatively well localized over the area of involvement. However, if the diaphragmatic parietal pleura is affected, pain may be referred to the shoulder.[12] Inflammation in the peripheral lung parenchyma may spread to the visceral and then parietal pleura, causing pleuritic pain. Some of the most common causes of pleuritic chest pain include pneumonia, PE, pneumothorax, pleuritis due to acute viral infection or collagen vascular disease, pericarditis, and radiation pneumonitis.

Hemoptysis may be noted by the patient as ranging from blood-streaked sputum to the expectoration of gross blood. If massive (defined as >200 to 600 mL in a 24-hour period, depending on the author), it represents a medical emergency requiring hospitalization and immediate evaluation by a pulmonologist and/or thoracic surgeon.[13] Studies performed in the 1940s to 1960s found that the most frequent causes of hemoptysis included bronchiectasis, bronchogenic carcinoma, and tuberculosis (TB). More recently, bronchitis has become one of the most frequent etiologies of hemoptysis in developed countries. In contrast, TB is much less common.[14,15] Table 30.2 lists some of the more common etiologies of hemoptysis.

TABLE 30.2
MAJOR CAUSES OF HEMOPTYSIS

Airway diseases—most common
Bronchitis
Bronchogenic carcinoma
Bronchiectasis
Pulmonary parenchymal diseases
Lung abscess
Mycetoma
Necrotizing pneumonia
Parasitic infection
Fungal infection
Tuberculosis
Vascular
Pulmonary embolism
Pulmonary hypertension
Arterial–venous malformation
Systemic diseases
Goodpasture syndrome
Wegener granulomatosis
Systemic lupus erythematosus
Other systemic vasculitides
Cardiac
Mitral stenosis
Iatrogenic
Bronchoscopy
Swan-Ganz catheter–induced infarction
Pulmonary artery rupture
Transtracheal aspiration
Hematologic—rare
Coagulopathy

Evaluation should begin with a detailed history and physical, ruling out other sources of bleeding such as the upper respiratory or gastrointestinal tracts. Duration and amount of hemoptysis, smoking history, and features suggestive of the presence of bronchitis or a pulmonary parenchymal infection should be elicited. The most important diagnostic test is the CXR. Additional testing to consider includes a CBC, coagulation profile, renal function studies, and urinalysis. If the CXR is abnormal, it may be helpful in elucidating the underlying etiology. If normal or without localizing findings, studies have shown that independent risk factors for occult carcinoma include age >40 years, smoking history of >40 pack-years, and duration of hemoptysis of >1 week.[15–17]

If hemoptysis is not massive, <1 week in duration, occurs in the setting of acute bronchitis, and if CXR is normal, further workup is not usually necessary, provided there is resolution with appropriate antibiotic therapy. However, if there is an abnormal finding on CXR, hemoptysis is massive, persists for >1 week, occurs in a setting inconsistent with acute bronchitis, or two or more of the above patient risk factors for carcinoma are present, pulmonary or thoracic surgery consultation is advised for further evaluation.[15–17] Fiberoptic bronchoscopy and/or high-resolution computed tomography scanning are the next steps in evaluation, depending on the clinical setting, and may provide complementary information.[18,19] Further evaluation is particularly important in the geriatric population, which is at higher risk for carcinoma, especially those individuals with a significant history of smoking or second-hand exposure.

NORMAL AGE-RELATED CHANGES IN THE RESPIRATORY SYSTEM

Pulmonary function deteriorates with age, even in the healthy elderly population.[5,20] The anatomic and structural changes that occur with normal aging and result in diminished pulmonary function are discussed in the subsequent text.

Changes in the Lung

Changes in the lung associated with aging include smaller airway size, changes in the morphology of the alveolar ducts and sacs, and possibly, alterations in the composition and/or thickness of the alveolar basement membrane.[5,20]

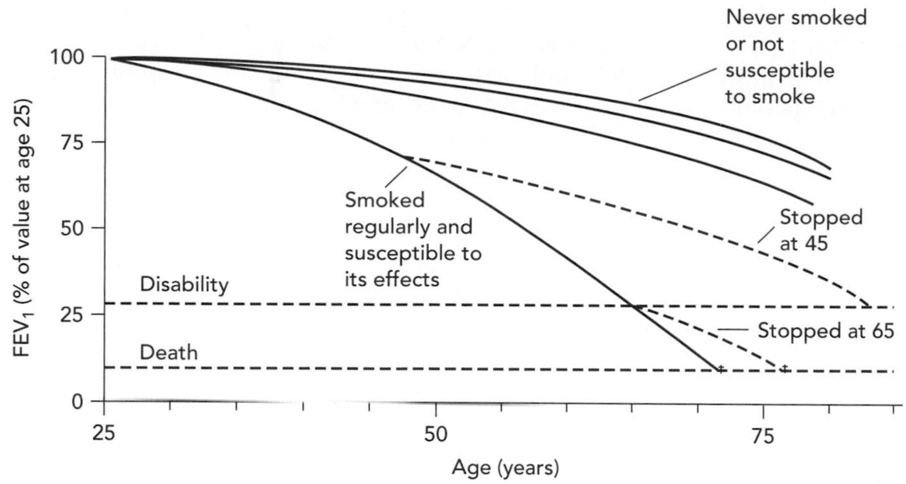

Figure 30.1 Decline in lung function with aging. As depicted in this graph, forced expiratory volume in 1 second (FEV_1) decreases over time with normative aging. In susceptible smokers, the rate of decline in FEV_1 has a much steeper slope. After smoking cessation, the rate of decline reverts to that of a nonsmoker. (From Fletcher C, Peto R. The natural history of airflow obstruction. *Br Med J.* 1977;1:1645–1648. Graph reproduced with permission from the BMJ Publishing Group).

Mean bronchiolar diameter, the main determinant of airways resistance, has been found to decrease significantly after age 40.[21] This change is thought to be the result of alterations in the collagenous matrix and elastic components of the underlying connective tissue, which support the airways, tethering them open.[20] With age, the alveolar ducts become enlarged, and the alveolar sacs shallower, resulting in a decrease in the airspace surface area–to–lung volume ratio.[22] In addition, there is some evidence that changes in the alveolar basement membrane composition and, thickness may also occur with aging.[5,20] Taken together, these changes contribute to a decline in the measured DLCO. This decline occurs later in women than in men, perhaps secondary to estrogen effects.[5,20]

Changes in the Chest Wall and Respiratory Muscles

The thoracic cage and respiratory muscles also undergo significant alterations. The chest wall becomes less compliant because of calcification of the intercostal cartilages, arthritis of the costovertebral joints, and in some individuals, osteoporosis and kyphoscoliosis of the spine. There is also an age-related decrease in diaphragm and intercostal muscle strength. The exact mechanism is unclear, and there is wide variability within the normal range.[5,20]

Mechanics

Taken together, the structural changes described in the preceding text are responsible for the changes in lung mechanics noted with normal aging. These include decreased elastic recoil, and therefore, increased lung compliance; increased airways resistance; premature airway closure; and decreased gas exchange capacity. These changes are similar to those encountered in emphysema, but without the same clinical consequences. In addition, there is increased chest wall stiffness leading to decreased compliance.

Changes in Pulmonary Function

Because of the loss of elastic recoil of the lung, increased chest wall stiffness, and decreased force generated by the respiratory muscles, there is a progressive decrease in VC. It has been estimated that forced vital capacity (FVC) declines about 14 to 30 mL per year in nonsmoking men, and 15 to 24 mL per year in nonsmoking women, starting at approximately 30 to 40 years of age. Rates for decline of FEV_1 are similar.[20] Of note, this rate of decline is markedly increased in susceptible tobacco smokers. Within a short period of smoking cessation, the rate of decline in FVC reverts to resemble a nonsmoker's decay curve, as shown in Figure 30.1.[23] With the reduction in FVC, there is a symmetric increase in residual volume (RV) so that total lung capacity (TLC) remains relatively constant (see Fig. 30.2). An exception is the patient with kyphoscoliosis.

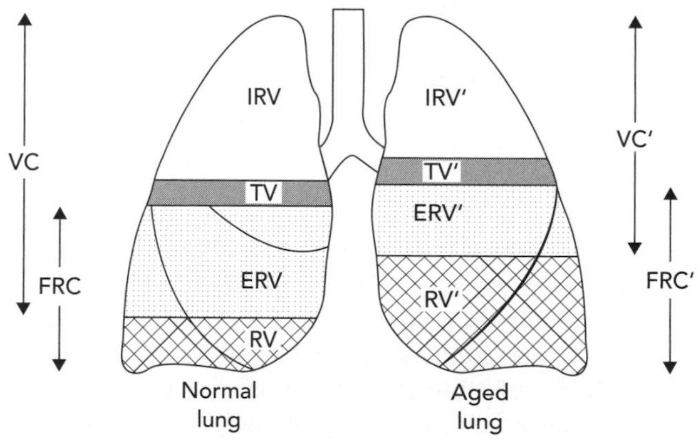

Figure 30.2 Changes in lung volume associated with aging. As depicted above, vital capacity (VC) decreases with aging. Correspondingly, residual volume (RV) and functional residual capacity (FRC) increase so that total lung capacity (TLC) does not significantly change. TV, tidal volume; IRV, inspiratory reserve volume; ERV, expiratory reserve volume. (From Chan ED, Welsh CH. Geriatric respiratory medicine. *Chest.* 1998;114:1704–1733. Reproduced with permission from Chest).

In these individuals, there is often a significant drop in TLC and a resultant restrictive defect. Just as RV increases with aging, so does functional residual capacity. Therefore, the small airways (terminal bronchioles) close early, especially in the dependent parts of the lung, leading to V/Q mismatching and increased dead space ventilation. These contribute to the increase in the alveolar-to-arterial oxygen gradient (A–a gradient).[5,20]

Arterial Oxygen Tension

In addition to increased dead space ventilation, there is also an increase in shunt fraction that occurs with aging. In combination with decreased gas exchange capacity, these processes result in a decrease in arterial oxygen tension (PaO_2) with aging. Recently, it was shown that this increase in alveolar to arterial (A–a) gradient is not linear after age 74. At sea level, PaO_2 in the healthy elderly patient remains approximately 83 mm Hg. Therefore, it must be emphasized that a maximum A–a gradient of 20 to 25 mm Hg is the upper limit of normal in any population. A gradient in excess of this is indicative of a pathologic process.[20,24]

Loss of Respiratory Reserve

The decrease in lung function associated with age results in diminished respiratory reserve. Although this loss of pulmonary reserve is not apparent during normal activities, it may be unmasked under conditions such as acute illness, surgery, or strenuous exercise. With aging, ventilatory performance becomes less efficient. This results in a greater utilization of oxygen ($\dot{V}O_2$) to achieve the same minute ventilation as in youth. In addition, the $\dot{V}O_{2\,max}$, a measure of pulmonary, cardiac, and metabolic performance, declines steadily after age 25 to 30, resulting in a decrement in maximum work capacity over time.[20]

ASTHMA IN THE ELDERLY

As defined by the National Asthma Education and Prevention Program (NAEPP) Expert Panel 1 in 1997, asthma is "a chronic inflammatory disease of the airways in which many cells, including mast cells, eosinophils, neutrophils, T-lymphocytes, and epithelial cells play a role. In susceptible individuals, this inflammation causes recurrent episodes of wheezing, breathlessness, chest tightness, and cough, especially at night or in the early morning. These symptoms are usually associated with widespread but variable airflow limitation that is at least partially reversible either spontaneously or with treatment. This inflammation also causes an associated increase in airway hyperresponsiveness to a variety of stimuli."[25]

Epidemiology

Asthma is considered a young person's disease, and therefore is a frequently overlooked diagnosis in the elderly. However, onset may be at any age. Given the presence of confounding factors such as tobacco smoking, secondhand smoke exposure, and occupational exposures, it is often impossible to distinguish asthma from chronic bronchitis in the older population. Asthma prevalence peaks in childhood at approximately 8% to 10% of the population and declines in young adulthood to a rate of 5% to 6%. Subsequently, there is another peak after age 70, with a prevalence rate of approximately 7% to 9%.[26] Elderly patients with asthma represent two distinct populations. One includes those with long-standing asthma or recrudescence of childhood or early adulthood asthma, and the other includes those with new- or recent-onset disease. Estimates of the incidence of new-onset asthma in the elderly have been highly variable. In one study, approximately 50% of asthmatics over the age of 70 had developed the disease after age 65. Those with early onset asthma had a greater likelihood of previous atopic disease and of chronic persistent airway obstruction, as occurs in chronic obstructive pulmonary disease (COPD).[27]

Diagnosis

The approach to making a diagnosis of asthma in the geriatric patient is similar to that in younger individuals. It is based on a compatible clinical history, physical examination, and objective assessment of reversible airflow limitation and/or bronchial hyperresponsiveness (BHR). The most common symptoms include episodic wheezing, dyspnea, and cough. Exertional dyspnea and paroxysmal nocturnal dyspnea are less frequently encountered. The differential diagnosis in this population is broad. Diseases that may present with similar symptoms include chronic bronchitis, emphysema, bronchiectasis, occupational asthma, recurrent aspiration, sarcoidosis, constrictive bronchiolitis, CHF, GERD, PE, laryngeal dysfunction, endobronchial tumors, and ACE inhibitor–induced cough.[20,25,26] The physical examination may be normal, or there may be evidence of hyperinflation and/or end-expiratory wheezing on examination of the chest. Other findings supporting the presence of atopic disease are helpful. These include nasal mucosal swelling and polyps, as well as eczema. Objective testing must show either a significantly reversible obstructive ventilatory defect or evidence of BHR. An obstructive ventilatory defect is demonstrated by spirometry showing a reduction in $FEV_1/FVC \leq 70\%$. Significant reversibility is defined as $\geq 15\%$ as well as ≥ 200 mL improvement in FEV_1 following administration of bronchodilator.[28] On occasion, full PFTs with a DLCO will be necessary to rule out emphysema or restrictive lung disease. If spirometry is normal, or there is an irreversible obstructive defect, methacholine challenge testing is helpful. BHR is present if there is a $\geq 20\%$ decrement in FEV_1. The negative predictive value of the methacholine challenge test is higher than the positive predictive value, making it more useful in excluding a diagnosis than establishing one. If the baseline FEV_1 is $\leq 65\%$ of the predicted value, methacholine

TABLE 30.3
STEPWISE APPROACH FOR MANAGING ASTHMA IN ADULTS

Classify Severity: Clinical Features Prior to Treatment or Achieving Adequate Control

Severity	Symptoms: Day / Nocturnal	Objective Testing: PEF or FEV_1 / PEF Variability	Medications Required to Maintain Long-Term Control
Step 4 **Severe persistent**	Continual	≤60% predicted	**Preferred treatment:** ■ High-dose inhaled corticosteroids *And* ■ Long-acting inhaled β_2-agonists *And*, if needed, ■ Corticosteroid tablets or syrup long term (2 mg/kg/day, generally do not exceed 60 mg/d; make repeat attempts to reduce systemic corticosteroids and maintain control with high-dose inhaled corticosteroids)
	Frequent	>30%	
Step 3 **Moderate persistent**	Daily	>60%–<80% predicted	**Preferred treatment:** ■ Low-to-medium–dose inhaled corticosteroids and long-acting inhaled β_2-agonists **Alternative treatment (listed alphabetically):** ■ Increase inhaled corticosteroids within medium-dose range *Or* ■ Low-to-medium–dose inhaled corticosteroids and either leukotriene modifier or theophylline
	>1 night/wk	>30%	If needed (particularly in patients with recurring severe exacerbations): **Preferred treatment:** ■ Increase inhaled corticosteroids within medium-dose range and add long-acting inhaled β_2-agonists **Alternative treatment:** ■ Increase inhaled corticosteroids within medium-dose range and add either leukotriene modifier or theophylline
Step 2 **Mild persistent**	>2 times/wk but less than once perday	80% predicted	**Preferred treatment:** ■ Low-dose inhaled corticosteroids **Alternative treatment (listed alphabetically):** ■ Cromolyn, leukotriene modifier, nedocromil, OR sustained release theophylline to a serum concentration of 5–15 hg/mL
	>2 nights/mo	20%–30%	
Step 1 **Mild intermittent**	≤2 d/wk	>80% predicted	■ No daily medication needed ■ Severe exacerbations may occur, separated by long periods of normal lung function and no symptoms; a course of systemic corticosteroids is recommended for exacerbations
	≤2 nights/mo	<20%	

Quick Relief **All patients**	■ Short-acting bronchodilator: 2–4 puffs of short-acting inhaled β_2-agonists as needed for symptoms ■ Intensity of treatment will depend on severity of exacerbation; up to three treatments at 20-min intervals or a single nebulizer treatment as needed; course of systemic corticosteroids may be needed ■ Use of short-acting β_2–agonist greater than two times a week in intermittent asthma (daily, or increasing use in persistent asthma) may indicate the need to initiate (increase) long-term control therapy

↓Step down
Review treatment every 1–6 mo; a gradual stepwise reduction in treatment may be possible

↑Step up
If control is not maintained, consider step-up. First, review patient medication technique, adherence, and environmental control.

Goals of Therapy: Asthma Control
- Minimal or no chronic symptoms day or night
- Minimal or no exacerbations
- No limitations on activities; no school/work missed
- Maintain (near) normal pulmonary function
- Minimal use of short-acting inhaled β_2-agonist
- Minimal or no adverse effects from medications

Reproduced from the NAEPP Expert Panel Report: Guidelines for the Diagnosis and Management of Asthma. Update on Selected Topics 2002. Bethesda, MD: NIH Publications 02-5074, 2003(25).

of the predicted value, methacholine challenge testing is potentially harmful and therefore not recommended.[25,29]

Treatment Considerations in the Elderly

Treatment is generally similar to that for younger individuals and should follow the stepped care approach outlined in Table 30.3 (Evidence Levels A and B), adapted from the NAEPP Expert Panel Report 2 update in 2002.[30] Using this approach, patients are assigned to the step that includes the most severe feature of their disease. The aim is to gain control as quickly as possible, with a short course of corticosteroids, if necessary, and then step down to the least medication needed to maintain control. Overreliance on short-acting β-agonists is one of the indicators of poor asthma control. In addition to pharmacotherapy, patients should be educated about environmental controls. Referral to an allergist or pulmonologist should be considered for patients who fit the criteria for steps 3 and 4.

Although treatment is similar in all age groups, there are a number of special considerations in the elderly. These include a higher risk for adverse drug effects, partially due to decreased metabolism and elimination of medications. Doses may therefore need to be adjusted, and multiple drug interactions may also be problematic. For example, theophylline clearance is reduced in the elderly patient, and age is an independent risk factor for developing life-threatening theophylline toxicity. In one study, individuals $\geq$75 years of age were shown to have a 16-fold greater risk of death from chronic theophylline intoxication than 25-year-olds.[31] In addition, it is metabolized in the liver by the cytochrome P-450 system, resulting in multiple drug interactions with many commonly used medications such as H_2-receptor antagonists and a number of antibiotics. The recommended initial starting dose in the elderly is 25% of the standard dose, and careful monitoring, maintaining levels in the therapeutic range of 8 to 15μg per L, is necessary.[25,26]

Asthma medications may also exacerbate coexisting medical conditions such as diabetes mellitus, cardiac disease, and osteoporosis. Older patients with ischemic heart disease and/or tachyarrythmias may be particularly susceptible to adverse effects from the administration of β_2-adrenergic receptor agonists (β-agonists) because of their chronotropic effects and dose-related hypokalemia. Concomitant use of inhaled anticholinergic agents may be a consideration in an effort to decrease β-agonist use, although the benefit of this regimen has not been proven. Oral corticosteroids and some inhaled corticosteroids, particularly when used at higher doses, increase the risk of osteoporosis and adrenal axis suppression. Therefore, as always, the lowest effective maintenance doses of these medications should be used. Bone densitometry is recommended at the beginning of treatment and again 6 months later, along with calcium and vitamin D supplementation, and if indicated, bisphosphonates (Evidence Level C).[25] Other side effects of systemic corticosteroids include hypertension, cataracts, impaired glucose metabolism, and confusion and agitation, particularly in the elderly with underlying cognitive impairment.

Medications used to treat common comorbid diseases in the elderly patient with asthma may precipitate bronchospasm. These include nonselective β_2-adrenergic receptor blockers (β-blockers), and to a lesser degree, selective β-blockers used to treat ischemic heart disease, arrythmias, and hypertension; β-blockers used in ophthalmologic preparations to treat glaucoma; and aspirin and other nonsteroidal anti-inflammatory agents used in aspirin-sensitive individuals.

The higher prevalence of underlying physical disabilities, neuropsychiatric disorders, and financial constraints put the elderly at high risk for medical noncompliance. Therefore, it is of utmost importance to teach the elderly to use mechanical devices such as spacers, turbohalers, or diskus inhalers to achieve optimal delivery of inhaled medications. Patients should be given detailed written instructions about dosage and timing of medications. In addition, cost should be considered when choosing a therapeutic regimen.

Because of the reduced awareness of bronchoconstriction in the elderly, there may be a delay in obtaining medical attention. The use of objective measures of airflow obstruction such as peak flow monitoring may therefore be especially important in this population. There are some concerns that there may be an increased risk of asthma mortality in the elderly. However, two recent studies that more stringently excluded patients with smoking-related COPD and emphysema suggest that mortality rates due to asthma itself are similar to those in younger populations.[20,26]

CHRONIC OBSTRUCTIVE PULMONARY DISEASE

COPD is the fourth leading cause of mortality and morbidity in the United States. Further increases in prevalence and mortality rates are predicted worldwide in the next decades.[32] *COPD* is a term that currently encompasses chronic bronchitis and emphysema. Asthma is no longer included in this nomenclature. Although some patients with asthma eventually develop irreversible airway obstruction clinically indistinguishable from COPD, the underlying inflammatory pathophysiology differs significantly. Recently, the Global Initiative for Chronic Obstructive Lung Disease (GOLD) expert panel defined COPD as "characterized by the finding of airflow limitation which is not fully reversible. The airflow limitation is usually both progressive and associated with an abnormal inflammatory response of the lungs to noxious particles or gases."[33]

Chronic bronchitis is defined as the presence of a productive cough for 3 months in each of 2 successive years for which other etiologies of chronic cough have been excluded. Emphysema is a histopathologic finding describing abnormal permanent enlargement and destruction of the airspaces distal to the terminal bronchioles.[33] Both these terms describe subsets of patients with COPD, and these two entities may coexist to variable degrees in the same patient. Neither term reflects the major impact of airflow limitation in COPD. Of note, airflow limitation in COPD may be partially, but never fully, reversible.

Epidemiology

Prevalence peaks in the sixth decade of life, reaching approximately 15% of all tobacco smokers.[32] It often presents insidiously, with patients and doctors alike attributing the symptoms of COPD to normal aging. In fact, it is not uncommon for patients to present with respiratory failure as their first manifestation of COPD. Tobacco smoking is by far the most important risk factor in the development of COPD, and evidence suggests that passive exposure may play a role as well. Nonetheless, not all smokers develop COPD. This suggests that other factors such as genetic susceptibility and environmental exposures act as disease modulators. At present, the only known genetic abnormality conferring susceptibility to COPD is α_1-antitrypsin deficiency. α_1-Antitrypsin is a circulating protease inhibitor that protects the lung from oxidative injury. Smokers with severe α_1-antitrypsin deficiency may develop premature, accelerated panacinar emphysema as early as the fourth or fifth decade of life. However, α_1-antitrypsin deficiency accounts for only a very small proportion of cases of emphysema. Other genetic risk factors for COPD are currently being investigated.

Occupational exposures to organic dusts, vapors, and other irritants can cause COPD independently of smoking and increase the risk in those who smoke concurrently. Indoor pollution due to the burning of fossil fuels has also been implicated. The role of outdoor pollution is less clear. Other associations include early childhood respiratory infections and lower socioeconomic status, but whether these act as independent variables is not well defined.[33]

Diagnosis

The diagnosis is made in the setting of a compatible history, physical examination, and PFTs. Cardinal symptoms include chronic cough, sputum production, and progressive dyspnea. Dyspnea presents initially on exertion, and then at rest as the disease becomes more severe. Wheezing is also commonly reported, particularly with upper respiratory infections. A history of significant smoking and occupational or environmental exposures is very helpful in making the diagnosis. Early in the disease process, physical findings may be absent. With progression of disease, decreased breath sounds, a prolonged expiratory phase, and possibly, wheezing may be noted on examination of the chest, along with an increased anteroposterior width. In addition, pursed-lip breathing, cyanosis, and cachexia may be observed. Findings consistent with cor pulmonale denote end-stage disease. These include elevated jugular venous pulsation, hepatojugular reflux, an enlarged liver that is tender to palpation and lower extremity edema.

PFTs are necessary to confirm the diagnosis and assess for severity of disease. Spirometry reveals an obstructive ventilatory defect that is not completely reversible after bronchodilator administration. RV is generally elevated because of air trapping. In patients with emphysema, TLC is usually increased because of a loss of elastic recoil of the lung and DLCO is diminished because of destruction of gas exchange units. CXR is not a sensitive method to make the diagnosis, but may be helpful in ruling out other disease processes. When present, the following findings support the diagnosis of COPD: Flattening of the diaphragms, elongation and narrowing of the cardiac silhouette, paucity of lung markings, bullous disease, and evidence of pulmonary artery hypertension. Additional testing should include an oxygen needs assessment at rest and with exercise, and nocturnal oximetry testing may also be considered. An ABG should be performed on all patients with an $FEV_1 \leq 40\%$ to assess for hypercarbia.[33] The differential diagnosis for COPD in this population is very similar to that listed in the preceding text for asthma.

Treatment Considerations in the Elderly

To prevent further lung injury, smoking cessation is the most important first step in the treatment of COPD. Once lost, lung function cannot be recovered. However, as discussed previously and depicted in Figure 30.1,[23] after smoking cessation the loss of lung function will revert to the rate seen in the nonsmoking elderly. The only other intervention with a proven impact on outcome in COPD is oxygen therapy (Evidence Level A). Supplemental oxygen is indicated in patients with $Pa_{O_2} < 55$ mm Hg or oxygen saturation $\leq$88%, as determined by oxygen needs assessment or nocturnal oxygen study. It is also indicated in patients with $Pa_{O_2} < 60$ mm Hg and either erythrocytosis or evidence of cor pulmonale.

A stepwise approach to the outpatient management of COPD is depicted in Table 30.4. Inhaled bronchodilators are the first-line agents. They have been shown to provide long-term symptomatic improvement, even without the demonstration of significant short-term effects on spirometry (Evidence Level A). Anticholinergic agents or long-acting β-agonists are generally the initial choice in patients with moderate COPD and daily symptoms. The onset and duration of action are longer than those of the short-acting β-agonists, and there is some evidence that they are slightly more effective in COPD.[32] Ipratropium bromide, which requires dosing four times daily, was until recently the only anticholinergic available in the United States. A once-daily medication, tiotropium bromide, was recently approved. In a double-blind randomized trial, tiotropium was found to be superior to ipratropium bromide in preventing exacerbations, improving FEV_1, and decreasing use of rescue β-agonists.[34] In another study, tiotropium was

TABLE 30.4
SEVERITY CLASSIFICATION AND THERAPY OF CHRONIC OBSTRUCTIVE PULMONARY DISEASE

Stage	Characteristics	Recommended Treatment	
0: At Risk	Chronic symptoms (cough, sputum) Exposure to risk factors Normal spirometry	■ Avoidance of risk factors ■ Influenza vaccination	
I: Mild COPD	FEV_1/FVC <70% $FEV_1 \geq 80\%$ predicted With or without symptoms	■ Short-acting bronchodilator when needed	
II: Moderate COPD	IIA FEV_1/FVC <70% $50\% < FEV_1 < 80\%$ predicted With or without symptoms	■ Regular treatment with one or more bronchodilators ■ Rehabilitation	■ Inhaled glucocorticosteroids if significant symptoms and lung function response
	IIB FEV_1/FVC <70% $30\% < FEV_1 > 50\%$ predicted With or without symptoms	■ Regular treatment with one or more bronchodilators ■ Rehabilitation	■ Inhaled glucocorticosteroids if significant symptoms and lung function response or if repeated exacerbations
III: Severe COPD	FEV_1/FVC <70% FEV_1 <30% predicted or presence of respiratory failure or right heart failure[a]	■ Regular treatment with one or more bronchodilators ■ Inhaled glucocorticosteroids if significant symptoms and lung function response or if repeated exacerbations ■ Treatment of complications ■ Rehabilitation ■ Long-term oxygen therapy if respiratory failure ■ Consider surgical treatments	

[a]$PaO_2 < 60$ mm Hg with or without $PaCO_2 > 50$ mm Hg while breathing air at sea level.
COPD, chronic obstructive pulmonary disease; FEV_1, forced expiratory volume in 1 second; FVC, forced vital capacity; PaO_2, arterial oxygen tension; $PaCO_2$, arterial carbon dioxide tension.
Adapted from Pauwels RA, Buist AS, Calverly PM, et al. Global strategy for the diagnosis, management, and prevention of chronic obstructive pulmonary disease. NHLBI/WHO Global Initiative for Chronic Obstructive Lung Disease (GOLD) workshop summary. *Am J Respir Crit Care Med.* 2001;163:1256–1276 with permission.

found to decrease dyspnea and the number of exacerbations and hospitalizations, and improve FEV_1 and quality-of-life scores compared to placebo. There was no statistically significant advantage over the use of the long-acting β-agonist salmeterol.[35] β-Agonists with a shorter onset and duration of action are more useful on an "as-needed" basis. They are the treatment of choice for patients with mild COPD without daily symptoms and for exacerbations. In addition, they may be used regularly in combination with an anticholinergic agent. This combination produces greater and more sustained improvements in FEV_1 than either alone.[33] In most stable COPD patients there is no evidence to support the use of bronchodilators through the nebulized route. However, this route may be preferable for individuals who are unable to correctly use various inhaler devices and spacers, even with appropriate education. Theophylline may be a useful therapeutic adjunct but is not a first-line agent because of potential toxicity. In addition to bronchodilating effects, theophylline also acts to improve respiratory muscle function, stimulate the respiratory center, reduce pulmonary vascular resistance, and potentiate diuresis. Glucocorticosteroids do not modify the course of COPD (Evidence Level A). Their use is recommended only in a limited number of patients. Inhaled glucocorticosteroids are indicated in patients who demonstrate a significant improvement of $\geq$15% in FEV_1 following a brief (6 to 12 week) therapeutic trial. They have also been shown to be beneficial in those with an FEV_1 $\leq$50% of the predicted value and frequent exacerbations (Evidence Level B).

Although there is no evidence to support long-term treatment with oral glucocorticosteroids, they have been shown to significantly improve symptoms and decrease length of hospital stay during exacerbations (Evidence Level A). The most common causes for exacerbations are tracheobronchial infections and air pollution. However, the cause is often never determined.[33] Recommended outpatient management of exacerbations includes a 10-day course of oral corticosteroids at a dose equivalent to 40 mg of prednisolone daily (Evidence Level C), nebulized bronchodilators, possibly theophylline (Evidence Level A), and antibiotics if there is evidence of bacterial tracheobronchitis (Evidence Level B). Indications for hospital admission include a marked increase in the intensity of symptoms over baseline, severe underlying COPD, worsening hypoxemia, new or worsening hypercarbia, altered mentation, new-onset arrhythmias, failure to respond adequately to initial outpatient management, the presence of high-risk comorbid conditions such as pneumonia or PE, new or worsening cor pulmonale, older age, and inadequate home support.[32,33] Because the medications used to treat asthma and COPD are similar, special treatment considerations in asthma in the elderly listed in the preceding text also apply to the treatment of COPD. The use of antitussive agents is felt to be contraindicated, and mucolytic agents are not recommended for routine use, although they may be of benefit in select circumstances (Evidence Level C).[33] Additional pharmacologic therapies such as leukotriene modifiers and antioxidant agents are presently under investigation.

Nonpharmacologic therapies include pulmonary rehabilitation, which has been shown to reduce symptoms and improve quality of life (Evidence Level A). Lung volume reduction surgery may be a consideration in a very small, select number of patients.[36] The use of noninvasive positive pressure ventilation in patients with stable hypercarbic respiratory failure is under investigation, but its use is not currently recommended. In general, patients older than 65 are not felt to be appropriate candidates for lung transplantation.

PNEUMONIA

Pneumonia is the leading infectious cause of death in the United States. In addition to being at increased risk of developing pneumonia, the elderly are at greater risk of dying from it, with 90% of mortality from this disease occurring in the elderly.[37] These increased risks in the older population may be explained by a number of factors. With aging, there is decreased respiratory reserve, a reduced ability to expectorate and clear pathogens, waning of humoral and cell-mediated immunity, and increased risk of aspiration. Other important factors linked to age include functional and nutritional status (which directly influence the immune response), comorbid disease, and a greater risk of oropharyngeal colonization with gram-negative and drug-resistant bacteria. In addition, the elderly often present with different clinical manifestations of illness compared to younger patients, leading to an increased risk of delayed diagnosis or misdiagnosis.[20,38]

Pathophysiology and Clinical Presentation

Most bacterial pneumonias are related to microaspiration of bacteria that colonize the oropharynx. According to one study, nocturnal microaspiration occurs at a rate of 45% in the elderly, and in 70% of those with impaired consciousness.[39] The risk of developing pneumonia is directly related to the size of the inoculum, the degree of virulence of the aspirated organism, and host defense mechanisms.

As in many other illnesses, the presentation of pneumonia in the elderly is often atypical. Rather than presenting with the classic constellation of fever, cough, and dyspnea, the elderly patient may come to medical attention with nonspecific symptoms. These may include overall functional decline, confusion, falls, or an exacerbation of an underlying disease such as diabetes or coronary artery disease. Often the elderly will present without respiratory complaints and will have no systemic signs of infection such as fever, tachycardia, or leukocytosis.[20,38] The absence of these systemic signs may be reflective of a poor host response to infection, leading to delayed diagnosis, misdiagnosis, and a greater mortality risk.[20,38,40]

Mortality

Most patients with pneumonia are treated on an outpatient basis. However, the elderly have a greater likelihood of being hospitalized because of the presence of significant comorbid disease. The two most commonly used mortality prognostic methods, the British Thoracic Society (BTS)[41,42] and the Pneumonia Outcomes Research Team (PORT)[43] rules, are helpful adjuncts in determining which patients may be safely treated on an outpatient basis and which patients should be hospitalized.[44,45] However, they have been shown to be significantly less sensitive and specific in populations aged $\geq$75 years.[38] Table 30.5 lists risk factors associated with a complicated course or mortality.[44] When multiple risk factors are present, hospitalization should be strongly considered.

Diagnostic Evaluation

Evaluation should always include a CXR and a measurement of arterial oxygen saturation by either pulse oximetry or, if hypercarbia is of concern, ABG analysis. An assessment of severity of illness may be made based on a combination of physical findings including vital signs, mental status, and evidence of volume depletion, along with the oxygen saturation measurement and radiographic findings. The number and severity of comorbidities also play a role in determining which patients require hospitalization. Sputum Gram stain and culture are not considered necessary for outpatient treatment unless there is a concern for drug-resistant pathogens or an organism not covered by the usual empiric therapies (Evidence Level B).[44,45]

Patients under consideration for hospitalization due to severity of illness, the presence of significant comorbidities, or lack of home social supports should also be evaluated with a CBC and differential, routine blood chemistries, liver function tests, and two sets of blood cultures. The first three tests help in risk stratification. Blood cultures within the first 24 hours of admission, preferably before initiation of antibiotic therapy, have been shown to improve mortality (Evidence Level A).[44] The recommendations of the ATS and Infectious Disease Society of America (IDSA) differ in regard to the utility of routine performance of sputum Gram stain and culture on admission. The argument made against

TABLE 30.5
MORBIDITY AND MORTALITY IN COMMUNITY-ACQUIRED PNEUMONIA

Factor	Characteristic
Age	>65 yr
Comorbidities	COPD Bronchiectasis Malignancy Diabetes mellitus Chronic renal failure CHF Chronic liver disease Chronic alcohol abuse Malnutrition Cerebrovascular accident Postsplenectomy History of hospitalization within the past year
Physical findings	RR >30 breaths/min Diastolic blood pressure <60 mm Hg Systolic blood pressure <90 mm Hg Pulse >125 beats/min
Laboratory data	WBC $<4 \times 10^9$/L or $>30 \times 10^9$/L, or absolute neutrophil count $<1 \times 10^9$/L Pa_{O_2} <60 mm Hg and/or Pa_{CO_2} >50 mm Hg on room air Serum creatinine >1.2 mg/dL, BUN >20 mg/dL Anemia (hematocrit <30%, hemoglobin <9 mg/dL) Coagulopathy Arterial pH <7.35
Radiologic data	Rapidly progressing infiltrate Multilobar involvement Pleural effusion Cavitary infiltrates

COPD, chronic obstructive pulmonary disease; CHF, congestive heart failure; RR, respiration rate; WBC, white blood cells; Pa_{O_2}, arterial oxygen tension; Pa_{CO_2}, arterial carbondioxide tension; BUN, blood urea nitrogen.
Data from Niederman MS, Mandell LA, Anzueto A, et al. Guidelines for the management of adults with community acquired pneumonia: Diagnosis, assessment of severity, antimicrobial therapy, and prevention. *Am J Respir Crit Care Med.* 2001;163:1730–1754 with permission.

this practice is that the yield is laboratory dependent, and the benefit of finding a specific etiologic agent in terms of cost or outcome has not been proven. However, the IDSA consensus panel supports this testing for the following reasons: An unexpected or resistant organism that may not respond to empiric therapy may be detected on a pretreatment specimen, empiric coverage may be narrowed later on the basis of these results, or the results may provide important epidemiologic data.[45]

Other testing that may be indicated in specific cases includes antigen testing for *Legionella* and influenza. *Legionella pneumophila* serogroup 1 accounts for approximately 70% of *Legionella* cases in the United States. *Legionella* urinary antigen level should be measured in all elderly patients with severe pneumonia or those with clinical features suggestive of Legionnaires disease (Evidence Level B). Urinary antigen testing has a sensitivity of 50% to 60% and a specificity of >95%. A nasopharyngeal washing should be sent for rapid influenza antigen testing in the appropriate clinical setting during the months of November through March. The sensitivities of the rapid tests range from 70% to 85%, with a specificity of >90%.[45] Lastly, if there is a pleural effusion present, diagnostic thoracentesis is imperative to identify the presence of complicated parapneumonic effusion or empyema.

Causative Organisms in the Elderly

The classification of pneumonia into "typical" and "atypical" forms is no longer of practical utility. Studies have shown that no radiologic or clinical pattern is sufficiently specific to reliably determine an etiologic diagnosis on the basis of these criteria alone. Organisms such as *Streptococcus pneumoniae* that tend to cause lobar consolidation and a productive cough were previously classified as typical. Organisms described as atypical include *Mycoplasma pneumoniae, L. pneumophila, Chlamydia pneumoniae,* and viruses. These organisms are more likely to be associated with a nonproductive cough and diffuse pulmonary infiltrates.

Pneumonia in all age-groups is currently categorized as either community-acquired pneumonia (CAP) or hospital-acquired pneumonia (HAP). CAP is defined as pneumonia that occurs in a patient with no history of hospitalization or residence in a long-term care facility for ≥14 days before the onset of symptoms.[44] HAP, or nosocomial pneumonia, is defined as occurring ≥48 hours following admission to a hospital or long-term care facility.[46]

The most common causative organism of CAP in the elderly is *S. pneumoniae*, followed by *Hemophilus influenzae*, and atypical organisms including *Legionella sp.*, influenza, and other viruses. Less commonly occurring pathogens, usually present only in patients with specific risk factors, include enteric bacteria, anaerobes, and *Staphylococcus aureus*.[38] An increasingly recognized pattern is that of mixed infections involving both typical and atypical pathogens. Although the importance of the atypical organisms in mixed infections remains unclear, outcome is improved if an antibiotic that covers atypical organisms, such as a macrolide or quinolone, is part of the therapeutic regimen (Evidence Level B).[44] Influenza predisposes to secondary bacterial infection with *S. pneumoniae, H. influenzae,* and *S. aureus*.

Of particular importance in patients coming from an institutional setting are lower respiratory tract infections caused by *S. aureus, S. pneumoniae*, gram-negative enterics, and anaerobes.[38] Drug-resistant *Streptococcus pneumoniae* (DRSP) is of particular concern in this population because risk factors include age ≥65 years, nursing home residence, and the presence of underlying cardiopulmonary disease. Pneumonia caused by DRSP increases the risk of empyema, and there is an increased mortality risk when the penicillin minimum inhibitory concentration values are ≥4 mg per dL.[38] These organisms are often also resistant to cephalosporins, macrolides, trimethoprim–sulfamethoxazole, and tetracyclines. At present, DRSP remains sensitive to vancomycin. Resistance to quinolones has been reported but remains rare. Further development of resistance is very much a concern.

Treatment

Initial choice of antibiotics is empiric and should be based on severity of illness, presence of comorbid disease, age, and whether the patient is living in the community or an institutional setting. Both ATS and IDSA have published guidelines for treatment of pneumonia. The current recommendations of the ATS are listed in Table 30.6. The importance of the administration of appropriate antibiotics within the first 8 hours of presentation cannot be stressed highly enough because this has been shown to significantly decrease mortality (Evidence Level B).[44,45]

Elderly patients who require broader antibiotic coverage include those at risk for aspiration, those living in a nursing home or institutional setting, and those who have recently been discharged from the hospital. Patients at risk for aspiration will require coverage for oral anaerobes. Oral agents with anaerobic coverage that may be used in the outpatient setting include ampicillin, clindamycin, metronidazole, and amoxicillin–clavulanate. In the hospital or nursing home setting ampicillin, clindamycin, metronidazole, ampicillin–sulbactam, and piperacillin–tazobactam may be used intravenously. For patients who develop pneumonia in the institutional setting or within a week of hospital discharge, the risk for *Pseudomonas sp.* and DRSP must be taken into consideration and coverage broadened appropriately.

Prophylaxis

The best way to reduce the morbidity and mortality associated with pneumonia in the elderly is through prevention. It is currently recommended that the elderly receive prophylactic vaccination against influenza (Evidence Level A) and *S. pneumoniae* (Evidence Level B). The influenza vaccine is given yearly, usually between mid-September and mid-November, before the start of the "flu season." The vaccine is a trivalent vaccine revised annually on the basis of worldwide surveillance to cover the two most highly anticipated strains of influenza A and influenza B. Efficacy is about 70% to 90% in healthy persons under age 65 when the match between the vaccine and the circulating strain is good. The vaccine is less efficacious in the elderly but has been shown to be cost-effective and reduce the occurrence of pneumonia, hospitalization, and all-cause mortality.[44,47] Nursing home and health care workers should also receive the vaccine to avoid transmission to at-risk patients.[44]

The 23-valent pneumococcal polysaccharide vaccine is active against the serotypes known to cause 85% to 90% of disease in the United States. The clinical efficacy in the elderly is somewhat controversial. It appears to be more effective in preventing pneumococcal bacteremia than pneumoccocal pneumonia in older adults.[48,49] It is on this basis that it is recommended for all adults >65 years of age.[44] Given the emergence of DRSP, vaccination may become increasingly important. A single dose is recommended at 65 years or older. A second immunization is not necessary unless the first vaccination was given before 65 years of age. If the first vaccination is given before 65 years of age, a second vaccination is recommended 5 years later because immunity wanes over 5 to 10 years.[44]

TUBERCULOSIS

After the development of effective treatment in the mid-20th century, the incidence of TB, caused by the *Mycobacterium tuberculosis* bacillus, declined steadily into the

TABLE 30.6
EMPIRIC MANAGEMENT OF COMMUNITY-ACQUIRED PNEUMONIA

Patient Characteristics	Empiric Therapy
Outpatients	
No cardiopulmonary disease or modifying factors	Advanced-generation macrolide (e.g., azithromycin or clarithromycin) ***or*** doxycycline
Cardiopulmonary disease and/or other modifying factors	β-Lactam (e.g., oral cefpodoxime, cefuroxime, high-dose amoxicillin, amoxicillin/clavulanate, or IV ceftriaxone) ***plus*** macrolide or doxycycline ***or*** Monotherapy with antipneumococcal fluoroquinolone (e.g., gatifloxacin, levofloxacin, moxifloxacin)
Inpatients	
Mild–moderate (non-ICU), no cardiopulmonary disease, no modifying factors	IV azithromycin alone ***or*** Doxycycline and β-lactam ***or*** Monotherapy with antipneumococcal fluoroquinolone
Mild–moderate (non-ICU) with cardiopulmonary disease and/or modifying factors, including institutional residence	IV β-lactam (e.g., ceftriaxone, cefotaxime, ampicillin/sulbactam, high-dose ampicillin) *plus* IV or oral macrolide or doxycycline ***or*** Monotherapy with IV antipneumococcal fluoroquinolone
Severe (ICU) with no *Pseudomonas* risks	IV β-lactam (ceftriaxone, cefotaxime) ***plus either*** IV azithromycin ***or*** IV fluoroquinolone
Severe (ICU) with *Pseudomonas* risks	IV antipseudomonal β-lactam (e.g., cefepime, imipenem, meropenem, piperacillin/tazobactam) ***plus*** antipseudomonal fluoroquinolone (e.g., ciprofloxacin) ***or*** IV antipseudomonal β-lactam plus IV aminoglycoside ***plus either*** IV macrolide (e.g., azithromycin) *or* IV nonpseudomonal fluoroquinolone

ICU, intensive care unit.
Adapted from Niederman MS, Mandell LA, Anzueto A, et al. Guidelines for the management of adults with community acquired pneumonia: Diagnosis, assessment of severity, antimicrobial therapy, and prevention. *Am J Respir Crit Care Med.* 2001;163:1730–1754 with permission.

mid-1980s. The incidence of TB then underwent a resurgence, peaking at 10.5 per 100,000 people in 1992. The reasons for this resurgence included human immunodeficiency virus (HIV) infection, immigration from endemic areas of the world, the emergence of multidrug resistant (MDR) TB strains, outbreaks in congregate living settings such as nursing homes and homeless shelters, and the deterioration of government-sponsored TB control programs. With reinvestment of public health resources into TB control, the incidence of TB has declined once more in recent years. In 2003, the case rate was 5.1 per 100,000, a 52% drop from 1992. Currently, the incidence of TB is highest in two populations: Immigrants from regions with a high prevalence of TB and the elderly. In 2003, approximately 20% of all cases of TB were in the 13% of people older than 65, for an incidence rate of 8.4 per 100,000.[50,51] This high rate is considered to be largely due to reactivation of latent TB following primary infection much earlier in life, when TB was far more prevalent in the US population.

Primary TB is acquired by inhalation of infected droplet nuclei. Although most cases are not clinically apparent, sometimes lymphadenopathy or an infiltrate may be present on CXR. In most hosts with intact cell-mediated immunity, the infection is walled off by activated T lymphocytes and macrophages that form granulomas. Tubercle bacilli may remain dormant for years within the granulomas. This is known as *latent tuberculosis infection* (LTBI). Before the host develops specific cell-mediated immunity, or in immunodeficient individuals, a bacillemia may occur at the time of primary infection, allowing widespread deposition of tubercle bacilli in a number of organs. If unchecked, this may lead to the development of miliary TB.

Individuals with LTBI are not infectious, and the only sign that an infection has taken place may be a positive result for a tuberculin skin test. As many as 10% of patients with a positive result for a tuberculin skin test will reactivate. The risk is greatest in the first 2 years after conversion.[51] Rates of reactivation are relatively high in the elderly because of the waning of cell-mediated immunity that comes with aging along with the presence of comorbid diseases. However, reactivation TB is not the only reason for the increased incidence of disease in this population. The importance of institutional epidemics, particularly in nursing homes, has become well recognized.[52] Therefore, all nursing home residents and employees without a known previously positive result for a purified protein derivative (PPD) test should be tested at the time of initial admission or employment and periodically thereafter.

Tuberculin Skin Testing

Tuberculin skin testing is performed using the PPD test. The test is neither 100% sensitive nor specific. False-positives may occur in individuals previously infected with other, usually opportunistic, mycobacteria or following immunization with the bacille Calmette-Guérin (BCG) vaccine. False-negative results for PPD tests are common in the elderly. A two-step PPD is therefore recommended. An elderly patient with distant exposure may have a negative result for an initial test, but may be positive for PPD when tested again 1 to 3 weeks later. In this case, the first exposure to PPD activates immune memory, and the later positive result should not be construed as a new conversion. An individual with a negative result for a second test should be classified as uninfected.[53] The test should be read 48 to 72 hours after the PPD is placed intradermally on the volar aspect of the forearm. The amount of induration, not erythema, is measured. Three cut points have been determined for defining a positive result for a tuberculin skin reaction on the basis of the sensitivity and specificity of the test along with the degree of risk of disease in specific groups. These cut points are delineated in Table 30.7, taken from the ATS and Centers for Disease Control and Prevention (CDC) guidelines.[54] Because of the poor positive predictive value of PPD testing in low-prevalence groups, targeted TB testing is currently recommended only in high-risk groups.

Diagnosis and Treatment of Latent Tuberculosis Infection

All patients with a positive PPD require a CXR to exclude active pulmonary disease. Testing for HIV is also advisable. Patients with a positive PPD and no evidence of active disease are considered to have LTBI. Treatment of documented recent converters is indicated, regardless of age. Treatment of patients with long-standing LTBI is less clear-cut, and the potential risks and benefits must be weighed on an individual basis. The preferred regimen is a 9-month course of isoniazid (INH) daily in both HIV-positive and HIV-negative individuals (Evidence Level A), unless there is a specific contraindication. This regimen has been shown to be 70% to 90% effective in preventing reactivation.[54]

Recently, the risk of INH-induced hepatitis in the elderly has been shown to be much less than previously supposed. In fact, the risk in select elderly patients with no history of underlying liver disease or alcohol abuse may be

TABLE 30.7
CRITERIA FOR TUBERCULIN POSITIVITY

Reaction >5 mm of Induration	Reaction >10 mm of Induration	Reaction >15 mm of Induration
HIV positive persons	Recent immigrants (i.e., within the last 5 y) from high-prevalence countries	Persons with no risk factors for TB, including those tested at the start of employment or residence in a high-risk congregate setting
Recent contact with patients with TB	Injection drug users	
Fibrotic changes on chest radiograph consistent with prior TB	Residents and employees of the following high-risk congregate settings: Prisons and jails, nursing homes and other long-term facilities for the elderly, hospitals and other health care facilities, residential facilities for patients with AIDS, and homeless shelters	
Patients receiving organ transplants and other immunosuppressed patients (receiving the equivalent of >15 mg/d of prednisone for ≥1 mo)	Mycobacteriology laboratory personnel	
	Patients with silicosis, diabetes mellitus, chronic renal failure, some hematologic disorders (e.g., leukemias and lymphomas), other specific malignancies (e.g., carcinoma of the head, neck, or lung), weight loss of >10% of ideal body weight, gastrectomy, and jejunoileal bypass	
	Children younger than 4 y or infants, children, and adolescents exposed to adults at high risk	

TB, tuberculosis; HIV, human immunodeficiency virus; AIDS, acquired immunodeficiency syndrome.
Adapted from the American Thoracic Society and the Centers for Disease Control. Targeted tuberculin testing and treatment of latent tuberculosis infection. *Am J Respir Crit Care Med.* 2000;161:S221–S247 with permission.

as low as that in younger populations.[55,56] Baseline liver function tests are no longer routinely recommended for patients without an increased risk of hepatotoxicity such as chronic liver disease, regular alcohol use, HIV infection, or pregnancy. Recent studies have shown that clinical monitoring, which includes patient education about symptoms of hepatotoxicity, is very effective in preventing fulminant hepatic failure and death (Evidence Level B). Patients are instructed to immediately discontinue their medications and seek medical attention for symptoms of hepatotoxicity including anorexia, nausea, vomiting, and jaundice.

Alternative regimens for the treatment of LTBI include combination therapy with rifampin and pyrazinamide (PZA) for 2 months or rifampin alone for 4 months (Evidence Level B). Although combination therapy with rifampin and PZA has been shown to be as effective as INH for 9 months, recently there have been reports of severe and fatal hepatotoxicity.[57] Therefore, this regimen is now recommended only in patients without underlying liver disease or a history of significant alcohol use. It is not recommended for patients taking other potentially hepatotoxic medications. This regimen should be considered only when patient compliance with a longer regimen appears unlikely, and close medical follow-up is feasible. Liver enzymes must be measured at baseline and at 2, 4, and 6 weeks, and patients must be closely monitored for hepatotoxicity. When any of these regimens are given as intermittent therapy (i.e., twice weekly), they must be given as directly observed therapy (DOT), preferably by the local department of health. Concurrent administration of vitamin B_6 along with INH is necessary to protect against peripheral neuropathy.

Clinical Presentation, Diagnosis, and Treatment of Active Tuberculosis

As with many diseases in the elderly, TB often presents atypically. Patients aged >65 are significantly less likely to present with the classic constellation of cough, fever, night sweats, hemoptysis, and weight loss. In addition, radiographic patterns may differ. The CXR may reveal typical upper lobe infiltrates with cavitation, or unresolving infiltrates in the lower or middle lobes. TB should always be considered if pneumonia fails to improve with conventional therapy. Evaluation should include a complete history and physical along with a PPD test and CXR. Although the most common presentation of reactivation TB in the elderly is pulmonary, extrapulmonary and disseminated TB must also be considered in the appropriate clinical settings. Extrapulmonary sites may be involved in approximately 20% of cases. These may include the lymph nodes, pleura, meninges, genitourinary systems, weight-bearing bones such as the vertebral bodies (Pott disease), bone marrow, and joints. Because the diagnosis of TB may be difficult in the elderly, maintaining a high index of suspicion is very important. In one study, only 26% of TB cases found at autopsy in patients aged >65 years were diagnosed before death.[58]

Evaluation should include a complete history and physical examination, PPD test, and examination of appropriate specimens for acid-fast bacilli (AFB). It is important to recognize that the PPD test is best used to screen individuals at risk for LTBI. It is not as helpful in the diagnosis of active TB because it may be negative in up to 25% of these patients.[51] If the burden of the organism is low, the bacilli may not be detected on the specimen before culture. The sensitivity of sputum AFB smears improves to 96% if three specimens are obtained. If the clinical picture and CXR suggest active TB but no sputum is available, diagnostic bronchoscopy with washings should be performed. Although culture for mycobacteria remains the diagnostic gold standard, it may take up to 6 weeks to grow and identify the organism. More rapid tests involving amplification and detection of ribosomal ribonucleic acid have recently been developed. Although specificity approaches 100% and sensitivity is >95% in smear-positive individuals, the sensitivity is much lower in smear-negative individuals (40% to 77%).[51]

Because active TB in the elderly most often represents a recrudescence of old disease, MDR is usually not an issue. However, the initial therapy should include INH, rifampin, PZA, and ethambutol daily for 8 weeks, or until the susceptibility pattern is known. Ethambutol may be discontinued if the organism is found to be susceptible to INH. This is followed by INH and rifampin daily or twice weekly by DOT for an additional 16 weeks (Evidence Level A). Alternative regimens may be found in the published joint ATS, IDSA, and CDC 2003 guidelines.[57] All patients must have baseline measurements of liver enzymes and clinical monitoring for adverse reactions during the treatment period. Those with increased risk of hepatoxicity and/or baseline liver enzyme abnormalities should have monthly testing of liver enzymes as well. In addition, clinical monitoring and visual testing is recommended when the treatment regimen includes ethambutol at higher doses or for >2 months.

SLEEP-DISORDERED BREATHING

Sleep patterns change with normal aging, and sleep disturbances such as insomnia and nocturnal awakening are more common in the elderly. There is some evidence to suggest that the incidence of snoring and obstructive sleep apnea (OSA) also increase with age. However, the clinical significance of these findings is unclear. Perhaps the definition of normal sleep needs to be adjusted in the elderly population because the currently used indices do not appear to accurately predict clinically significant disease.

Changes in Sleep Patterns with Aging

With advancing age, there appears to be a decrease in the amount of sleep obtained per day, and a concurrent decline in sleep efficiency. In general, nocturnal awakenings become far more frequent and prolonged. At the same time, there is more of a propensity to nap during the day, as measured by the multiple sleep latency test (MSLT). Sleep architecture also changes with age. Although the amount of rapid eye movement (REM) sleep remains relatively constant, REM latency is shorter. This finding is also present in depressed individuals, which may therefore act as a confounding factor. Evidence suggests that there is also a reduction in slow, or delta wave activity, which is characteristic of the deeper stages of nonrapid eye movement sleep.[59]

Insomnia and poor sleep quality are frequent complaints in the elderly. This may often be due to normative changes in sleep patterns. Other common causes to consider in the elderly include sleep-disordered breathing, comorbid medical illnesses, depression, medications, and poor sleep hygiene. Evaluation should begin with a detailed history and physical, a review of medications, depression screening, and a discussion about sleep hygiene.

Obstructive Sleep Apnea

Sleep-disordered breathing includes a number of clinical syndromes, the most common of which is OSA. Signs and symptoms of OSA include snoring, choking, witnessed apneic episodes, and frequent nocturnal awakening. Daytime complaints include hypersomnolence, frequent morning headaches, intellectual impairment, and falling asleep while driving. OSA is caused by episodic, repetitive, upper airway obstruction by the soft tissue structures of the nasopharynx and hypopharynx. Sleep fragmentation results from repetitive arousals in response to apneic episodes, causing daytime somnolence. Factors that increase the risk for OSA include obesity, a large neck size (>16.5 cm in men, and >16.0 cm in women), a crowded oropharynx with large tonsils, low palate and large tongue, retrognathia, micrognathia, hypothyroidism, cardiopulmonary disease, and neuromuscular disease. The influence of gender is less pronounced in the elderly because women in this age-group are postmenopausal and the effects of estrogen are no longer an issue.[60]

Diagnosis

OSA is diagnosed by polysomnogram or sleep study. During the study, electroencephalograpy (EEG), electrooculography (EOG), chin and leg electromyography (EMG), pulse oximetry, airflow, and chest and abdominal muscle movements are recorded. An obstructive apnea is defined as cessation of airflow for at least 10 seconds, with continued ventilatory effort noted through rib cage EMG monitoring. Apneas are generally associated with significant oxygen desaturations and arousals from sleep. Hypopneas may also be present. They are defined as a reduction in airflow or a respiratory effort of 30% or greater, associated with a 4% oxygen desaturation.[61] Central hypopneas and apneas, associated with lack of both airflow and ventilatory effort, may also be found. These may be idiopathic or associated with central nervous system or cardiac disease.[59] The severity of sleep apnea is usually expressed as the apnea–hypopnea index (AHI), or respiratory disturbance index (RDI), which is the number of apneas and hypopneas per hour of sleep.

OSA is estimated to occur at a rate of 2% to 4% in the general population.[60] The prevalence of OSA in the elderly appears higher, but estimates of prevalence have varied widely depending on the criteria used. On the basis of an AHI of ≥ 5, one group found that sleep apnea was present in 2.9% of 60-year-olds, 33.3% of 70-year-olds, and 39.5% of 80-year-olds.[62] However, the threshold AHI was low and the relationship of the AHI to clinical findings unclear.

Untreated OSA has been found to be associated with systemic hypertension, coronary artery disease, CHF, stroke, arrythmias, and not surprisingly, an increased incidence of auto accidents. In younger patients, increased mortality has also been demonstrated. However, studies in the elderly have failed to clearly demonstrate OSA as an independent risk factor for mortality.[59,60]

Treatment

Treatment does not differ from that recommended for younger patients. It should include identification and management of reversible contributing factors such as obesity, hypothyroidism, and nasal or posterior pharyngeal obstruction. The treatment of choice for OSA is continuous positive airway pressure (CPAP). This may be administered by nasal prongs, mask, or full-face mask. Patient tolerance is a major problem with this form of treatment. Compliance is increased in those patients for whom CPAP achieves significant symptomatic relief. Current Medicare criteria for coverage for treatment with CPAP include an AHI of ≥ 15 events per hour or an AHI of ≥ 5 but ≤ 14 events per hour associated with documented excessive daytime sleepiness, cognitive impairment, mood disorder, insomnia, systemic hypertension, coronary artery disease, or stroke.[63] In select cases, oral appliances, adenotonsillectomy, or uvulopalatopharyngoplasity may be helpful. Tracheostomy is occasionally necessary. Sedatives and alcohol should be avoided in these patients.

CONCLUSION

When caring for the elderly, it is useful for clinicians to be cognizant of the normative physiologic changes associated with the aging respiratory system. Treatment may differ in the elderly because of a greater propensity for adverse reactions to medications, the increased risk of pharmaceutical interactions, and underlying comorbid disease. In addition, it is important to remember that the presenting signs and symptoms of pulmonary disease are often subtle and nonspecific in the geriatric patient. This may lead to delayed diagnosis or misdiagnosis, contributing to increased morbidity and mortality in the elderly patient.

REFERENCES

1. Silvestri GA, Mahler DA. Evaluation of dyspnea in the elderly patient. *Clin Chest Med.* 1993;14(3):393–404.
2. Manning HL, Schwartzstein RM. Pathophysiology of dyspnea. *N Engl J Med.* 1995;333:1547–1552.
3. American Thoracic Society. Dyspnea mechanisms, assessment, and management: A consensus statement. *Am J Respir Crit Care Med.* 1999;159:321–340.
4. Mahler DA, Fierro-Carrion G, Baird JC. Evaluation of dyspnea in the elderly. *Clin Geriatr Med.* 2003;19:19–33.
5. Zeleznik J. Normative aging of the respiratory system. *Clin Geriatr Med.* 2003;19:1–18.
6. Connolly MJ, Crowley JJ, Charan NB, et al. Reduced subjective awareness of bronchoconstriction provoked by methacholine in elderly asthmatic and normal subjects as measured on a simple awareness scale. *Thorax.* 1992;47(6):410–413.
7. Irwin RS, Widdicombe J. Cough. In: Murray JF, Nadel JA, eds. *Text book of respiratory medicine,* 2nd ed. Philadelphia, PA: WB Saunders; 1994:529–544.
8. Irwin RS, Corrao WM, Pratter MR. Chronic persistent cough in the adult: The spectrum and frequency of causes and successful outcome of specific therapy. *Am Rev Respir Dis.* 1981; 123:413–417.
9. Irwin RS, Curley FJ, French CL. Chronic cough: The spectrum and frequency of causes, key components of the diagnostic evaluation, and outcome of specific therapy. *Am Rev Respir Dis.* 1990; 141:640–647.
10. Israili ZH, Hall WD. Cough and angioneurotic edema associated with angiotensin-converting enzyme inhibitor therapy. *Ann Intern Med.* 1992;117:234–242.
11. Irwin RS, Zawahu JK, Curley FJ, et al. Chronic cough as the sole presenting manifestation of gastroesophageal reflux. *Am Rev Respir Dis.* 1989;140:1294–1300.
12. Moore KL. *Clinically oriented anatomy,* 2nd ed. Baltimore, MD: Williams & Wilkins; 1985:146–147.
13. Thompson AB, Teschler H, Rennard SI. Pathogenesis, evaluation, and therapy for massive hemoptysis. *Clin Chest Med.* 1992; 13:69–82.
14. Johnston H, Reisz G. Changing spectrum of hemoptysis: Underlying causes in 148 patients undergoing diagnostic flexible fiberoptic bronchoscopy. *Arch Intern Med.* 1989;149:1666–1668.
15. Hirshberg B, Biran I, Glazer M, et al. Hemoptysis: Etiology, evaluation, and outcome in a tertiary referral hospital. *Chest.* 1997; 112:440–444.
16. Jackson CV, Savage PJ, Quinn DL. Role of fiberoptic bronchoscopy in patients with hemoptysis and a normal chest roentgenogram. *Chest.* 1985;87:142–144.
17. Poe RH, Israel RH, Marin MG, et al. Utility of fiberoptic bronchoscopy in patients with hemoptysis and a nonlocalizing chest roentgenogram. *Chest.* 1988;92:70–75.
18. Set PAK, Flower CDR, Smith IE, et al. Hemoptysis: Comparative study of the role of CT and fiberoptic bronchoscopy. *Radiology.* 1993;189:677–680.
19. McGuinness G, Beacher JR, Harkin TJ, et al. Hemoptysis: Prospective high-resolution CT/bronchoscopic correlation. *Chest.* 1994;105:1155–1162.
20. Chan ED, Welsh CH. Geriatric respiratory medicine. *Chest.* 1998;114:1704–1733.
21. Niewoehner DE, Kleinerman J. Morphologic basis of pulmonary resistance in the human lung and effects of aging. *J Appl Physiol.* 1974;36:412–418.
22. Gillooly M, Lamb D. Airspace size in lifelong non-smokers: Effect of age and sex. *Thorax.* 1993;48:39–43.
23. Fletcher C, Peto R. The natural history of chronic airflow obstruction. *Br Med J.* 1977;1:645–648.
24. Cerveri I, Zoia MC, Fanfulla F, et al. Reference values of arterial oxygen tension in the middle-aged and elderly. *Am J Respir Crit Care Med.* 1995;152:934–941.
25. National Asthma Education and Prevention Program. *Expert panel report 2: Guidelines for the diagnosis and management of asthma.* Bethesda, MD: NIH Publication 19–4051; 1997.
26. Braman SS. Asthma in the elderly. *Clin Geriatr Med.* 2003;19: 57–75.
27. Braman SS, Kaemmerlen JT, Davis SM. Asthma in the elderly. A comparison between patients with recently acquired and long-standing disease. *Am Rev Respir Dis.* 1991;143(2): 336–340.
28. American Thoracic Society. Lung function testing: Selection of reference values and interpretive strategies. *Am Rev Resp Dis.* 1991;144:1202–1218.
29. American Thoracic Society. Guidelines for methacholine and exercise challenge testing—1999. *Am J Respir Crit Care Med.* 2000; 161:309v329.
30. National Asthma Education and Prevention Program. *Expert panel report: Guidelines for the diagnosis and management of asthma.* Update in Selected Topics 2002. Bethesda, MD: NIH Publication 02–5074; 2003.
31. Shannon M, Lovejoy FH. The influence of age vs. peak serum concentration on life-threatening events after chronic theophylline intoxication. *Arch Intern Med.* 1990;150:2045–2048.
32. ATS Statement. Standards for the diagnosis and care of patients with chronic obstructive pulmonary disease. *Am J Respir Crit Care Med.* 1995;152:S77–S121.
33. Pauwels RA, Buist AS, Calverly PM, et al. Global strategy for the diagnosis, management, and prevention of chronic obstructive pulmonary disease. NHLBI/WHO Global Initiative for Chronic Obstructive Lung Disease (GOLD) workshop summary. *Am J Respir Crit Care Med.* 2001;163:1256–1276.
34. Vincken W, Van Noord JA, Greefhorst AP, et al. for the Dutch/Belgian Tiotropium Study Group. Improved health outcomes in patients with COPD during 1 yr's treatment with tiotropium. *Eur Respir J.* 2002; 19:209–216.
35. Brusasco V, Hodder R, Miravitlles M, et al. Health outcomes following treatment for six months with once daily tiotropium as compared to twice daily salmeterol in patients with COPD. *Thorax.* 2003;585:399–404.
36. National Emphysema Treatment Trial Research Group. Patients at high risk of death after lung volume reduction surgery. *N Engl J Med.* 2001; 345:1075–1083.
37. Granton JT, Grossman RF. Community-acquired pneumonia in the elderly patient: Clinical features, epidemiology, and treatment. *Clin Chest Med.* 1993;14:537–553.
38. Niederman MS, Ahmed QAA. Community-acquired pneumonia in elderly patients. *Clin Geriatr Med.* 2003;19:107–120.
39. Huxley E, Viroslav J, Gray W, et al. Pharyngeal aspiration in normal adults and patients with depressed consciousness. *Am J Med.* 1978;64:564–567.
40. Starczewski AR, Allen SC, Vargas E, et al. Clinical prognostic indices of fatality in elderly patients admitted to the hospital with acute pneumonia. *Age Ageing.* 1988;17:181–186.
41. Farr BM, Sloman AJ, Fisch MJ. Predicting death in patients hospitalized for community-acquired pneumonia. *Ann Intern Med.* 1991;115:428–436.
42. Neill AM, Martin IR, Weir R, et al. Community-acquired pneumonia: Aetiology and usefulness of severity criteria on admission. *Thorax.* 1996;51:1010–1016.
43. Fine MJ, Auble TE, Yealy DM, et al. A prediction rule to identify low-risk patients with community-acquired pneumonia. *N Engl J Med.* 1997;336:243–250.
44. Niederman MS, Mandell LA, Anzueto A, et al. Guidelines for the management of adults with community acquired pneumonia: Diagnosis, assessment of severity, antimicrobial

therapy, and prevention. *Am J Respir Crit Care Med.* 2001;163: 1730–1754.
45. Bartlett JG, Dowell S, Mandell LA, et al. Practice guidelines for the management of community-acquired pneumonia in adults. *Clin Infect Dis.* 2000;31:347–382.
46. Campbell GD, Neiderman MS, Broughton WA, et al. Hospital-acquired pneumonia in adults: Diagnosis, assessment of severity, initial antimicrobial therapy and preventative strategies. *Am J Respir Crit Care Med.* 1995;153:1711–1725.
47. Nichol KL, Nordin J, Mullooly J, et al. Influenza vaccination and reduction in hospitalizations for cardiac disease and stroke among the elderly. *N Engl J Med.* 2003;348:1322–1332.
48. Shapiro ED, Berg AT, Austria R, et al. The protective efficacy of polyvalent pneumococcal polysaccharide vaccine. *N Engl J Med.* 1991;325:1453–1460.
49. Jackson LA, Neuzil KM, Yu O, et al. Effectiveness of pneumococcal polysaccharide vaccine in older adults. *N Engl J Med.* 2003;348:1747–1755.
50. Centers for Disease Control and Prevention. *Reported tuberculosis in the United States.* Atlanta, GA: Centers for Disease Control and Prevention; 2003.
51. American Thoracic Society and the Centers for Disease Control. Diagnostic standards and classification of tuberculosis in adults and children. *Am J Respir Crit Care Med.* 2000; 161:1376–1395.
52. Centers for Disease Control and Prevention. Prevention and control of tuberculosis in facilities providing long-term care to the elderly: Recommendations of the advisory committee for elimination of tuberculosis. *Morb Mortal Wkly Rep.* 1990; 39(RR-10):7–20.
53. Zevallos M, Justman JE. Tuberculosis in the elderly. *Clin Geriatr Med.* 2003;19:121–128.
54. American Thoracic Society and the Centers for Disease Control. Targeted tuberculin testing and treatment of latent tuberculosis infection. *Am J Respir Crit Care Med.* 2000;161:S221–S247.
55. Stead WW, To T, Harrison RW, et al. Benefit risk considerations in preventative treatment for tuberculosis in elderly persons. *Ann Intern Med.* 1987;107:843–845.
56. Salpeter SR. Fatal INH-induced hepatitis: Its risk during chemoprophylaxis. *West J Med.* 1993;159:560–564.
57. American Thoracic Society, Centers for Disease Control, and Infectious Diseases Society of America. Treatment of tuberculosis. *Morb Mortal Wkly Rep.* 2003;52(RR-11):1–77.
58. Reider HL, Kelly GD, Block AB, et al. Tuberculosis diagnosed at death in the US. *Chest.* 1991;100:678–671.
59. Feinsilver SH. Sleep in the elderly: What is normal? *Clin Geriatr Med.* 2003;19:177–188.
60. Redline S, Strohl KP. Recognition and consequences of obstructive sleep apnea hypopnea syndrome. *Clin Chest Med.* 1998; 19(1):1–19.
61. Meoli AL, Casey KR, Clark RW. Hypopnea in sleep-disordered breathing in adults. *Sleep.* 2001;24(4):469–470.
62. Hoch CC. Comparison of sleep-disordered breathing among healthy elderly in the seventh, eighth, and ninth decades of life. *Sleep.* 1990;13(6):502–511.
63. Centers for Medicare and Medicaid Services. Continuous positive airway pressure (CPAP). In: *Medicare Coverage Issues Manual, Revision 150.* Baltimore, MD:US Department of Health and Human Services; 2001:16–17.

31 Renal Function and Failure

Robert D. Lindeman

CLINICAL PEARLS 414

RENAL FUNCTION WITH NORMAL AGING 415

CLINICAL PRESENTATIONS OF RENAL DISEASE 415
Commentary 417
Urinary Abnormalities 417
Azotemia 419

LABORATORY TESTS AND DIAGNOSTIC PROCEDURES 419
Laboratory Tests 419
Imaging Techniques 419
Renal Biopsy 420

ACUTE RENAL INSUFFICIENCY OR FAILURE 420
Prerenal Acute Renal Insufficiency 420
Intrarenal Etiologies of Acute Renal Failure 420
Other Intrarenal Causes of Acute Renal Insufficiency 420
Postrenal Acute Renal Failure (Obstruction) 421

RENAL VASCULAR DISEASE 421
Renal Artery Stenosis 421

CHRONIC KIDNEY DISEASE 421
Control of Hypertension 422
Nutritional Modifications 422

END-STAGE RENAL DISEASE 423
Dialysis 423
Transplantation 423

DISORDERS OF SODIUM AND WATER BALANCE 423
Commentary 424
Dehydration and Volume Depletion 424
Hyponatremia 424
Hyponatremia in the Elderly 426
Hypernatremia 426

DISORDERS OF POTASSIUM BALANCE 427
Commentary 427
Hypokalemia 428
Hyperkalemia 428

DISORDERS OF ACID–BASE BALANCE 430
Metabolic Acidosis 430
Metabolic alkalosis 430

CLINICAL PEARLS

- When hematuria is found on dipstick examination of the urine and no red cells are seen on microscopic examination, one needs to test for urinary myoglobin to rule out rhabdomyolysis.
- Hematuria in patients on Coumadin is not normal. Further studies are warranted to find the source of the bleeding.
- If one encounters persistent pyuria with negative urine cultures, consider tuberculosis as a possible diagnosis.
- The serum urea nitrogen (SUN) to creatinine ratio is useful in distinguishing prerenal azotemia (e.g., dehydration, congestive heart failure) and postrenal azotemia (e.g., obstruction) from azotemia due to primary renal disease. A ratio >20 to 1 suggests one of the two former etiologies.

- A rapid rise in SUN and serum creatinine concentrations after starting a patient with hypertension on an ACE (ACE) inhibitor or angiotensin II receptor blocker (ARB) should suggest the possibility of bilateral renal artery stenosis.
- Nonsteroidal anti-inflammatory drugs (NSAIDs) can cause acute onset of nephrotic syndrome and/or deterioration of renal function (acute interstitial nephritis) months after starting these agents.
- When a previously healthy older person comes in with acute onset of hypertension/heart failure, consider acute postinfectious glomerulonephritis, even if protein and cellular elements are scant or absent in the urine.
- Multiple myeloma/light chain cast nephropathy should be ruled out in any elderly patient with unexplained renal insufficiency.
- An important clue in distinguishing hyponatremia associated with primary salt depletion from the syndrome of inappropriate antidiuretic hormone (SIADH) is the SUN level. The SUN is elevated in the former and tends to be normal or subnormal in the latter, unless preexisting renal disease was present.
- If an elderly patient is found to have unexplained hypokalemia, question him about the heavy use (abuse) of cathartics and enemas. Patients usually will not tell you unless you ask specifically.
- Be aware of the potential for life-threatening hyperkalemia in elderly patients with cardiovascular disease (CVD) (especially those with preexisting renal disease) when started on any of a number of CVD medications that compromise the renin–angiotensin–aldosterone system, specifically ACE inhibitors, ARB, β-adrenergic antagonists (blockers), and the potassium-sparing diuretics. Potassium supplements given along with thiazide or loop diuretics are usually not necessary in the treatment of hypertension, and they can be dangerous unless closely monitored.

RENAL FUNCTION WITH NORMAL AGING

Renal function, as measured by the glomerular filtration rate (GFR), declines after the age of 40 years at a mean rate of approximately 1% per year, accelerating in later years. This observation was first reported in cross-sectional studies. In the Baltimore Longitudinal Study of Aging,[1] however, one third of the participating volunteers followed serially, many for periods >20 years, showed no decline in renal function over time, although the whole study population showed a mean decrease similar to that observed in cross-sectional studies. This would appear to indicate that a decline in renal function with age is not inevitable (i.e., there is no involutional senescence), but rather the decrease in mean values is related to intervening pathology (e.g., atherosclerosis) in only part of the population. Renal mass also is lost with age.

Despite significant anatomic changes and loss of kidney function with age, the older kidney is capable of maintaining body fluid, electrolyte, and acid–base balance within the normal range under most circumstances. However, when challenged by environmental and disease-related stressors, such as large volume changes or acid loads, it takes the older kidney longer to correct abnormalities that develop.

CLINICAL PRESENTATIONS OF RENAL DISEASE

The clinical presentations of renal disease are not significantly different in old compared to young adults. Early recognition of a decline in renal function is important to permit early diagnosis and treatment of treatable causes. Even if no specific curative treatment is available, there are usually interventions (e.g., aggressive control of hypertension and nutritional measures) that can at least slow the progression of the disease process.

The first indication of renal disease may be picked up on a routine screening urinalysis (proteinuria, hematuria, pyuria, casts) without associated signs or symptoms. Loss of large amounts of protein in the urine can lead to hypoalbuminemia (nephrotic syndrome) and edema formation. Renal disease is often asymptomatic until more than two thirds of normal renal function is lost. The first symptoms associated with azotemia (increased serum urea nitrogen [SUN]) are fatigue, anorexia, nausea, somnolence, and confusion. By the time the patient develops these symptoms, unless a reversible cause can be found, they are at a point where dialysis is generally necessary.

Table 31.1 lists the most common disease entities (i.e., the diseases that should come to mind first in your differential diagnosis) by presenting manifestations. Hematuria (red cells) and pyuria (white cells) may present with or without red cell or white cell casts in the urine. Casts tell you that the cells are coming from the level of the glomerulus or tubule. Proteinuria may be either acute or chronic in onset, and may vary in quantity from nonnephrotic to nephrotic in quantity. Azotemia also may be acute or chronic at onset, and protein and cellular elements (red and white cells, casts) may or may not be present. An attempt has been made to list disease entities in the order of decreasing probability under each of the subcategories. This list would become too unwieldy if made all-inclusive, so it has been limited to the most common entities. Your nephrologist and/or urologist can help you sort out the more complex and puzzling cases.

CASE ONE

A 65-year-old man comes into your office noting the insidious onset of ankle edema during the day and waking up with swelling around the eyes in the mornings over the last month. His blood pressure is 150/86 mm Hg after 5 minutes of quiet lying, and he has 2+ edema of

TABLE 31.1
DIFFERENTIAL DIAGNOSIS OF KIDNEY DISEASES BY PRESENTING MANIFESTATIONS

1. **Proteinuria**
   a. Nonnephrotic
      Hypertensive glomerulosclerosis (403.9)
      Diabetic glomerulopathy, early (250.4)
      Focal/segmental glomerulosclerosis (582.1)
      Tubulointerstitial nephritis, chronic (582.89)
   b. Nephrotic (>3 g/d)
      Membranous glomerulopathy (581.1)
      Other GN (see Table 31.2)
      Interstitial nephritis, acute (580.89)
      Renal amyloidosis (277.3/581.81)
2. **Hematuria**
   a. With red cell casts
      Rapidly progressing GN (580.4)
      Other GN (Table 31.2) Acute postinfectious GN (580.0)
   b. Without red cell casts
      Urinary tract infection
         Cystitis (595.), prostatitis (601.)
         Pyelonephritis (590.)
      Malignancy
         Bladder (188.9)
         Kidney (Hypernephroma) (189.0)
      Anticoagulant therapy (964.2)
      Kidney stones (592.)
      Trauma (866.)
      Vascular occlusion/infarction (593.81)
      Polycystic kidney disease (753.1)
3. **Pyuria**
   a. With white cell casts
      Pyelonephritis (590.)
      Tubulointerstitial nephritis (582.)
   b. Without white cell casts
      Urinary tract infection
         Cystitis (595.), prostatitis (601.), urethritis (597.)
      Urinary tract tuberculosis (016.)
4. **Azotemia**
   a. Acute (with cellular elements)
      ATN (584.5)
         Ischemic, e.g., endotoxin shock
         Toxic, e.g., rhabdomyolysis
      Rapidly progressive GN (580.4)
      Acute interstitial nephritis (580.89)
      Other GN (Table 31.2)
      Acute postinfectious GN (580.0)
   b. Acute (without cellular elements)
      Prerenal acute renal failure (584.9)
         Dehydration, congestive heart failure, hypotension
      Nonoliguric ATN (584.5)
      Obstructive uropathy (599.6)
      Renal vein thrombosis (453.4)
      Bilateral renal artery thrombosis or embolism (593.81)
      Cholesterol embolization (593.89)
   c. Azotemia, chronic onset
      Diabetic glomerulosclerosis (250.4/583.81)
      Hypertensive nephrosclerosis (403.9)
      Focal/segmental glomerulosclerosis (582.1)
      Other GN (Table 31.2)
      Tubulointerstitial nephritis, chronic (582.89)
         Analgesic nephropathy (583.89)
      Urinary tract obstruction (599.6)
         Benign prostatic hypertrophy (600.01)
         Vesicoureteral reflux (593.7)
      Renal artery stenosis, bilateral
      Multiple myeloma/light chain nephropathy (203.0)
      Polycystic kidney disease (753.13)
      Renal amyloidosis (250.4/583.81)

The list is not all-inclusive but gives the most common causes in the elderly in approximate order of frequency.
ICD-9 codes are shown after each diagnosis.
ICD-9 codes for diseases of the kidney and urinary tract (excluding diseases of the male and female genital organs) will fall between 580 and 600. Specific disease entities, for example, glomerular diseases, will have different codes, depending on whether they are acute (580) or chronic (582). They can also be classified on the basis of whether they have nephrotic proteinuria (581) or whether proteinuria is unspecified, presumably nonnephrotic (583). Following this code number, there is a period and further qualifying code numbers that define the lesion better (0.0 to 0.7). Where renal involvement is secondary to some systemic disease, the systemic disease is first identified, followed by a code for the renal involvement. This ends with 0.81 if there is a specified pathologic renal lesion from a list provided, with 0.89 if there is a specific renal lesion identified but not on this list, and with 0.9 if the renal lesion is not identified by pathology.
GN, glomerulonephritis; ATN, acute tubular necrosis.

the lower extremities. The rest of the physical examination is unremarkable. A dipstick urine check reveals 3+ proteinuria with a few red cells and white cells per HPF on examination of the sediment.

His SUN is 18 mg per dL, his serum creatinine concentration is 1.5 mg per dL, and his electrolytes are all normal. His serum albumin is 2.8 g per dL and serum total cholesterol is 320 mg per dL. A 24-hour urine sample contains 8 g of protein.

He is referred to a nephrologist who is unable to determine the cause of his nephrotic syndrome after a battery of additional blood tests (antinuclear antibody [ANA], anti-DNA, antineutrophil cytoplasmic antibody [ANCA], etc.) are all negative. A renal biopsy is performed, which shows evidence on microscopic examination of a membranous glomerulopathy with diffuse thickening of the basement membrane, but no hypercellularity.

Commentary

Patients with nephrotic syndrome generally sleep lying flat so that eye puffiness is often noted on arising in the morning. In contrast, the patient with congestive failure and edema sleeps in a more upright position favoring development of lower extremity edema instead.

The most common primary renal lesion causing nephrotic syndrome in the older adult is membranous glomerulopathy. In one biopsy series, the incidence was 35% followed by minimal change disease (16%) and primary amyloidosis (12%).[2]

There exists considerable disagreement among nephrologists whether membranous glomerulopathy should be treated with immunosuppressive agents and/or corticosteroids. Although these patients will sometimes appear to respond to these agents, some patients will also improve spontaneously. The complications associated with the therapy must be weighed against the potential benefits. This decision is probably best left to the consulting nephrologist.

Urinary Abnormalities

Proteinuria

The normal urine protein (albumin) excretion is <30 mg per day (<2 mg per dL on spot urine check) and is not different in the old compared to the young. Macroproteinuria (albuminuria) by definition is a urinary protein excretion of >300 mg per day (or >20 mg per dL). Urinary protein excretions between 30 and 300 mg per day represent microproteinuria (albuminuria). The urine dipstick is not very sensitive and is adequate only for screening purposes, because a 1+ reading will be obtained at a protein concentration of roughly 30 mg per dL and a 2+ reading at roughly 100 mg per dL. Anything more than a trace of urinary protein should warrant quantitation with a timed urine specimen. The dipstick does not detect low-molecular-weight proteins. If one suspects that Bence-Jones proteinuria (light chain immunoglobulins seen with multiple myeloma [MM] that are responsible for tubular toxicity/obstruction) or tubular proteins are present, a sulfosalicylic acid test of the urine is needed.

Early damage to kidneys from diabetes and/or hypertension can be detected by testing the urine for microalbuminuria using semiquantitative dipsticks (Chemstick Micral, Boehringer Mannheim Corporation, Indianapolis, Indiana 46256; Micral, Roche Laboratories; Hemacue Urine Albumin, Bayer DCA 2000).

When quantitative studies are performed, the ratio of urine protein (albumin) to urine creatinine in a random urine sample (normally <30 mg protein per g of creatinine) corrects for variations in urine concentration due to hydration and is far more convenient than timed urine collections. Recent studies[3,4] have convincingly shown not only that microalbuminuria is a marker for risk of cardiovascular and renal disease, especially in patients with diabetes, but that treatment of those developing significant microalbuminuria with ACE inhibitors or angiotensin II receptor blockers (ARBs) reduces subsequent microalbuminuria and risk of cardiovascular and renal disease (Evidence Level A).

Definition

Nephrotic syndrome by definition is loss of >3 g of protein in the urine per day. Anything less than this is considered nonnephrotic proteinuria. The nephrotic syndrome is generally accompanied by hypoproteinemia, hyperlipidemia, and edema. There may also be evidence of hypercoaguability and increased susceptibility to infections due to loss of select proteins. Hypertension and impairment in renal function (increased SUN and serum creatinine concentrations) are part of the nephritic syndrome, but are also often present.

Table 31.2 lists the causes of nephrotic syndrome. For further descriptions as to the diagnosis, pathology, and treatment of these different entities, one may consult any of the following references: Cameron,[2] Couser,[5] Lindeman,[6] or Burkhart.[7] A number of serologic tests are important adjuncts to the differential diagnosis of glomerular and vascular (vasculitis) lesions responsible for the nephrotic syndrome. Serologic testing refers to the use of immunoassays to detect the presence of disease-relevant antibodies in serum or to determine the serum level of a specific antigen such as complement. Table 31.3 lists some of the more commonly used tests and the renal diseases they are designed to detect. Additional tests are described elsewhere in more detail.[8]

Hematuria

Hematuria exceeding 3 to 5 RBC/HPF deserves further evaluation. Red cell casts, best seen on an unspun urine specimen because they are so fragile, are indicative of a

TABLE 31.2
CAUSES OF NEPHROTIC SYNDROME DUE TO GLOMERULAR DISEASE

I. Primary glomerular diseases
   A. Membranous glomerulopathy (581.1)
   B. Membranoproliferative GN (581.2)
   C. Mesangial proliferative GN (IgA nephropathy) (581.2)
   D. Focal and/or segmental glomerulosclerosis (581.1)
   E. Minimal change disease (581.3)
   F. Crescentic or rapidly progressive GN (anti-GBM, immune complex, pauci-immune) (580.4)

II. Glomerular diseases associated with systemic illnesses
   A. Metabolic (diabetes mellitus, amyloidosis) (250.4/581.81)
   B. Immune systemic lupus erythematosis (710.0/581.81), polyarteritis nodosa (446.0/581.81), Henoch-Schonlein purpura (287.0/581.89), cryoglobulinemia (273.2/581.89), Wegener granulomatosis (446.4/581.89), Goodpasture (446.21/581.89)
   C. Neoplastic (leukemia, lymphoma, MM [203.0], carcinoma)
   D. Nephrotoxic (gold, penicillamine, nonsteroidal antiinflammatory drugs, lithium, heroin) (581.89)
   E. Allergic (insect stings [989.5/581.89], poison ivy and oak [692.6/581.89])
   F. Infectious
      1. Bacterial (acute postinfectious GN [580.0], infective endocarditis [421.0/581.89], syphilis [095.4/581.89])
      2. Viral (human immunodeficiency virus [042/581.89], hepatitis B and C [070.9/581.89])
      3. Protozoal (malaria) (084.9/581.89)
      4. Helminthic (schistosomiasis [120/581.89]), filariasis (125.9/581.89)
   G. Heredofamilial (Alport syndrome) (759.89)
   H. Miscellaneous (malignant hypertension) (403)

Anti-GBM, antiglomerular basement membrane antibody; GN, glomerulonephritis; MM, multiple myeloma.

TABLE 31.3
SEROLOGIC TESTS AVAILABLE FOR THE EVALUATION OF THE PATIENT WITH EVIDENCE OF GLOMERULAR AND/OR VASCULAR DISEASE (NEPHROTIC SYNDROME/RENAL INSUFFICIENCY), INDICATIONS FOR THEIR USE (TO RULE OUT SPECIFIC DISEASE ENTITIES), AND ESTIMATED FREQUENCY OF POSITIVE TESTS FOR THESE INDICATIONS

Serologic Test	Indications	Percent Positive (%)
Antistreptolysin antibody	Recent β-hemolytic streptococcal infection	>80
Streptozyme (rapid test kit)	APSGN	
Anti-DNase B antibody	Pyoderma-associated APSGN	80–90
Complement (C3, C4, CH50)	Acute GN—Low in APSGN	90
	Diffuse SLE	90
	Focal SLE	75
	Membranoproliferative GN	50–90
Antinuclear antibody	SLE	95–99
Anti-dsDNA	Same (more conclusive when positive)	40–70
(Anti-dsDNA)	Used to monitor response to therapy	
ANCA	Rapidly progressive GN	80–90
(p-ANCA/c-ANCA)	Wegener granulomatosis (pauci-immune crescentic and necrotizing GN/vasculitis)	
Anti-GBM	Goodpasture syndrome (pulmonary-renal syndromes)	90–100
IgA	IgA nephropathy	40–50
HBV and HCV serologies	HBV and HCV–associated glomerular diseases	
HIV serology	HIV-associated glomerular diseases	
Serum protein electrophoresis	MM amyloidosis, macroglobulinemia, etc.	80
Urine protein electrophoresis	Bence-Jones proteinuria (MM)	20
Serum immunoelectrophoresis	MM, amyloidosis, macroglobulinemia, etc.	
Cryoglobulin	Cryoglobulinemia-associated GN	

APSGN, acute poststreptococcal glomerulonephritis; Anti-dsDNA, anti-double-stranded DNA antibody; ANCA, antineutrophil cytoplasmic antibody; SLE, systemic lupus erythematosis; Anti-GBM, antiglomerular basement membrane antibody; IgA, immunoglobulin A; HBV, hepatitis B virus; HCV, hepatitis C virus; MM, multiple myeloma.

glomerular source (glomerulonephritis [GN]). Red cells that have lost their biconcave shape also suggest a glomerular origin, whereas biconcave red cells suggest that the bleeding is coming from the lower part of the urinary tract. Associated proteinuria and/or an elevated serum creatinine concentration also suggest renal parenchymal (glomerular) disease.

Work-up for isolated hematuria should include a urine culture, a platelet count, prothrombin time (PT), and partial thromboplastin time (PTT) to rule out a coagulopathy, and imaging studies of the kidney and urinary tract (renal ultrasound or intravenous pyelography). If these are nondiagnostic, a urologic consult for cystoscopy is warranted. In approximately 80% of older adults, the source of bleeding is the bladder, prostate, or urethra. Malignancies account for one third of all cases of hematuria in adults, most commonly involving the bladder, but the kidney (hypernephroma) and prostate may also be sources. After a comprehensive evaluation, no cause for bleeding will be found in approximately 10% of cases. In the absence of significant proteinuria, <10% of the cases of hematuria will be glomerular in origin.

Pyuria and casts

White cells and white cell casts result from infectious or inflammatory reactions in the kidney and urinary tract. White cell and granular casts indicate a renal origin that can be either glomerular (GN) or tubular (interstitial nephritis) in origin. Sterile pyuria should suggest the possibility of tuberculosis.

Azotemia

The primary clinical function of the kidney that requires monitoring is the GFR. The most practical and reproducible clinical measure of the GFR is the creatinine clearance. Participants in the Baltimore Longitudinal Study of Aging showed a 30% decline in mean clearances between the age of 30 and 80 years, yet the mean serum creatinine concentrations rose insignificantly (from 0.81 to 0.84 mg per dL).[9] As creatinine clearance rates decrease with age, the production of creatinine added to the circulation from muscle metabolism also falls at nearly the same rate. The practical implication of this observation is that the serum creatinine concentration of the older person must be interpreted with this in mind when used to determine or modify dosages of drugs cleared totally, such as aminoglycoside antibiotics (gentamycin), or partially, such as digoxin, by the kidney. Additionally, some drugs, for example, trimethoprim, cimetidine, and cephoxitin, compete with creatinine for tubular secretion, resulting in an increase in serum creatinine concentration without any change in creatinine clearance.

The SUN and urea clearance similarly make use of endogenously produced urea as the test substance. Because much of the filtered urea can be reabsorbed in the tubules at low flow rates, vigorous hydration is necessary to make the clearance results interpretable. SUNs are also affected by the rate of urea production (that is, protein intake and tissue catabolism) and hence serum creatinine concentrations are generally more useful in estimating GFR. As discussed in the following text, however, the SUN to serum creatinine ratio can be useful in separating pre- and postrenal causes of azotemia from azotemia due to primary renal disease.

A formula derived by Cockroft and Gault has been widely used to predict creatinine clearances using serum creatinine concentration, age, and weight for men as follows:

$$\text{Creatinine clearance (milliliters per minute)} = \frac{(140 - \text{Age in years}) \times \text{Weight (in kilograms)}}{72 \times \text{Serum creatinine (milligrams per deciliter)}}$$

For women, this value is multiplied by 0.85. Investigators from the Multicenter Diet in Renal Disease study (MDRD)[10] have developed a series of new predictors of creatinine clearance using serum creatinine concentration and additional confounders that they feel produce a more accurate estimate.

LABORATORY TESTS AND DIAGNOSTIC PROCEDURES

Laboratory Tests

Table 31.2 lists laboratory (serologic) tests that are available to help distinguish between the different pathologic entities responsible for nephrotic syndrome and/or acute and chronic renal insufficiency. The indications for each of these tests are also shown. Additional tests can be found elsewhere in more detail.[8] Interpretation of serum and urine osmolality and electrolytes (sodium, potassium) will be discussed later.

Imaging Techniques

A variety of imaging techniques are available to evaluate the genitourinary system.

Ultrasonography is noninvasive and safe, and it can provide many diagnostic clues, showing kidney size, hydronephrosis of the collecting system, and solid and cystic renal masses. An intravenous pyelogram (IVP) shows more detail of the collecting system, including sites of obstruction and other pathology, (for example, papillary necrosis). However, it is best to avoid use of intravenous contrast in older patients with diabetes mellitus, renal insufficiency, hypertension, and especially MM, as these patients are prone to develop acute renal failure (ARF). If it becomes necessary to use contrast agents, it is important to ensure that the patient is well hydrated. Computed tomography (CT) scans, magnetic resonance imaging (MRI), isotopic renography, and angiography are additional procedures available to further evaluate selected renal disorders.

Renal Biopsy

For patients with suspected primary glomerular disease or unexplained renal failure, a renal biopsy may be indicated after all other available means for establishing a diagnosis have been exhausted. Renal biopsy should not be withheld because of age alone. At least half of all primary glomerular lesions responsible for the nephrotic syndrome are potentially treatable (e.g., membranous glomerulopathy, minimal change disease, vasculitis), and so trials of immunosuppressive and/or corticosteroid therapy may be warranted. However, when a lesion known to be unresponsive to these agents is diagnosed, for example, primary amyloidosis, it is important to not subject older patients to the potentially serious side effects of these drugs.

ACUTE RENAL INSUFFICIENCY OR FAILURE

The primary care clinician is in a unique position to impact care in patients with acute renal insufficiency (ARI), both in terms of prevention and early detection. With a careful medical history, physical examination, and laboratory values (urinalysis, SUN, and creatinine concentrations), one can usually determine whether the cause is prerenal, intrarenal, or postrenal in origin.

Prerenal Acute Renal Insufficiency

Prerenal ARI occurs when poor perfusion of the kidney causes a failure in renal function. Loss of sodium and body fluids (intravascular volume depletion), decreased cardiac output (congestive heart failure), sepsis, internal redistribution of fluid volume, and certain drugs (diuretics, ACE inhibitors, ARBs) contribute in different combinations in most cases. In several reports, intravascular volume depletion accounted for over half of the cases of ARF. The decreased ability of the older patient to retain sodium and concentrate urine and, most importantly, the impairment of the thirst mechanism all contribute to their susceptibility. With acute hypotension from any cause, the decrease in renal perfusion stimulates sympathetic activity and release of vasoconstrictor substances that further reduce GFR. If the hemodynamic disturbances are promptly corrected, the patient usually, but not always, recovers. Older patients are generally slower to respond.

It is important to distinguish between prerenal ARI due to dehydration, hypotension, and congestive heart failure, and the ischemic acute tubular necrosis (ATN) or renal cortical necrosis that can develop in more severe cases. In prerenal azotemia, the SUN to serum creatinine ratio is usually >20 to 1. In patients with oliguria, a urine osmolality >500 mOsm per L and/or a urine sodium concentration <20 mEq per L suggests prerenal azotemia. When ATN develops, the damaged tubules lose their ability to concentrate urine and dilute sodium. However, these guidelines are not always reliable in differentiating prerenal ARI from ATN. If still in doubt, the response to volume repletion with salt and water may help, but it is important to recognize that older persons often have a delayed response to volume expansion, and aggressive replacement can result in volume overload and pulmonary edema.

Intrarenal Etiologies of Acute Renal Failure

ATN can be ischemic or nephrotoxic in origin. The causes of ischemic ATN are the same as those described under prerenal ARI, only more severe. Major surgical procedures under general anesthesia with or without associated hypotension account for most of the remaining cases.

Nephrotoxic ATN can be caused by some of the antibiotics used in treating serious infections, most notably the aminoglycoside class (e.g., gentamycin). These antibiotics are now rarely used outside the hospital because other effective antibiotics are available, and monitoring blood levels of the antibiotic is essential, especially in older persons. Other drugs that may be responsible are penicillins, cephalosporins, ciprofloxacin, NSAIDs, and the thiazide and furosemide diuretics. Older persons are also at increased risk of developing radiocontrast dye–induced ARF. Although newer agents are safer, it is still best to avoid the use of intravenous contrast dyes in persons with preexisting impairment of renal function, MM, vascular disease, diabetes, or intravascular volume depletion. Hydration before and after procedures employing contrast agents is effective in reducing the incidence and severity of ARF in older adults.

Rhabdomyolysis and ARF can be seen with the use of certain drugs, such as HMG-CoA reductase inhibitors (statins), with hypokalemia, and with acute immobilization resulting in muscle damage (e.g., acute alcohol intoxication or stroke). The myoglobin in urine turns the color brown. Myoglobin should be suspected when the urine dipstick test for blood is positive, but no red cells are seen on microscopic examination. Laboratory procedures are available to confirm the presence of myoglobin in the urine.

Other Intrarenal Causes of Acute Renal Insufficiency

Postinfectious acute glomerulonephritis (AGN) often presents in adults with circulatory congestion, suggesting heart failure. In contrast, AGN presents in younger persons with edema and hypertension. The urinalysis may fail to show significant proteinuria and/or hematuria that would suggest an intrarenal cause. These observations (lack of protein and cellular elements in the urine), together with low urinary sodium concentrations and high SUN to serum creatinine ratios, suggest prerenal ARF. Whereas streptococcal infection is the most common cause in younger persons, a wide array of other infectious agents can cause AGN in older persons. Drug users and alcoholics are especially at increased risk.

Acute or subacute GN may also be an immunologic consequence of a systemic disease, for example, lupus erythematosis, vasculitis, cryoglobulinemia, and Wegener granulomatosis. Other forms of primary renal disease (e.g., crescentic GN with or without glomerular immune deposits, membranoproliferative GN, and mesangioproliferative GN [IgA nephropathy]) may also present with an acute deterioration in renal function.

Acute interstitial nephritis (AIN) is an entity caused by a variety of medications, the most important being the nonsteroidal anti-inflammatory drugs (NSAIDs). A typical picture might be the onset of nephrotic syndrome and worsening ARF in a patient who has been on NSAIDs for close to a year. An increase in eosinophils in blood and urine is not as common in these patients as it is in penicillin-induced AIN. The renal abnormalities may improve after discontinuing the medication but permanent damage may persist, resulting in either chronic kidney disease (CKD) or even progressing to end-stage renal disease (ESRD) requiring dialysis or transplantation. The AIN results from a delayed hypersensitivity response to the NSAID; the nephrotic syndrome results from changes in glomerular permeability mediated by prostaglandins and other cytokines.

In a review[11] of 259 renal biopsies done for ARF in adults aged 60 and older (remembering that when the cause of ARF has been established by history and laboratory examination, a renal biopsy is not done), the following diagnoses were made: Pauci-immune crescentic GN 31%, AIN 19%, ATN with nephrotic syndrome 8%, ATN without nephrotic syndrome 7%, atheroemboli 7%, light chain cast nephropathy (MM) 6%, postinfectious GN 5.5%, antiglomerular basement membrane antibody nephritis 4%, and IgA nephropathy or Henoch-Schönlein syndrome 4%.

Postrenal Acute Renal Failure (Obstruction)

It is important to recognize postrenal causes of ARF because they are common and are usually treatable. Prostatic hyperplasia is the most frequent cause, but tumors and urethral strictures can also cause obstruction. Diabetes mellitus and other causes of peripheral neuropathy can result in bladder distension and overflow incontinence with ureteral reflux and increased hydrostatic pressure at the renal tubular level. The latter results in decreased urine flow rates and enhanced urea reabsorption, and so the SUN to serum creatinine ratio may exceed 20. The diagnosis can be made by ultrasound evaluation of the urinary tract or bladder postvoiding or by catheterization of the bladder. If a large residual is found, an indwelling catheter can be left in place for several weeks and a trial given to see if the residual remains. By this time, a referral to an urologist is indicated.

RENAL VASCULAR DISEASE

Renal Artery Stenosis

Nearly half of all normotensive and hypertensive persons aged 60 years and older with evidence of lower body atherosclerosis show some obstruction (>50% narrowing) of a renal artery or arteries. In most instances, the obstruction is not clinically important. In some, however, severe hypertension and/or renal insufficiency may develop that is potentially correctable with angioplasty or surgery. Therefore, any patient with suspected renal artery stenosis (RAS) warrants a diagnostic workup, and if a significant stenosis is found, the patient should be referred for further evaluation.

Findings suggestive of hemodynamically significant RAS include the onset of severe hypertension or significant worsening of existing hypertension, a persistent hypokalemia, a failure to control hypertension on previously effective medications, the onset of azotemia without a recognizable cause and without abnormalities on urinalysis, and/or a significant worsening of azotemia when started on ACE inhibitors or ARBs. Diagnostic procedures to screen for RAS include a flat plate of the abdomen (looking for differences in kidney size), a hypertensive IVP, a captopril renogram (the ACE inhibitor causes an acute fall in blood flow through the affected kidney), a serum renin concentration, and a serum concentration or urinary excretion of aldosterone.

Occlusive Disease of the Renal Arteries

Embolization or thrombosis of the renal arteries can result in either acute or chronic renal failure with or without changes in the urinalysis and urine sediment. Symptoms vary from a slowly progressive silent event to severe, acute flank pain and tenderness, hematuria, hypertension, fever, nausea, and vomiting (renal infarction).

Renal Cholesterol Embolization

Renal cholesterol embolization most commonly occurs after either aortic surgery or angiography in patients with diffuse atherosclerosis (dislodging atheromatous material), but it may also occur spontaneously. The usual course is a progressive renal insufficiency and worsening hypertension, but oliguria or even anuria, fever, eosinophilia, embolization to other organs and extremities (digital infarcts), and livido reticularis may be seen. Cholesterol emboli can be observed on fundoscopic examination, and cholesterol crystals can be seen in skin and kidney biopsies.

CHRONIC KIDNEY DISEASE

The most common causes of CKD in older adults are hypertensive nephrosclerosis, diabetic glomerulosclerosis, focal/segmental glomerulosclerosis, interstitial nephritis, and amyloidosis. Although a chronic elevation of serum creatinine concentration represents a loss of renal function that likely will not be recovered, defining the underlying pathology may help prevent a further decline in function. The best example of this is the relentless decline in kidney function in diabetic glomerulopathy that can be attenuated with ACE inhibitors or ARBs. These agents act not only by lowering the systemic blood pressure but also by reducing the glomerular hyperperfusion and hyperfiltration responsible for the mesangial proliferation and sclerosis by vasodilating the glomerular efferent arterioles.

Factors influencing morbidity and mortality in patients on dialysis are operative for an extended period before ESRD is present and need for dialysis is imminent. Only a minority of patients (20 to 25%), however, are referred to a nephrologist prior to the initiation of dialysis.[12] Conditions related to renal failure present before the onset of dialysis include hypertension, anemia, lipid abnormalities, renal osteodystrophy, and metabolic acidosis.

As CKD progresses, older patients should have a consultation with someone knowledgeable regarding renal care and nutrition. An NIH Consensus Development Conference in 1993[12] recommended early referral to a renal team (nephrologist, dietitian, nurse, social worker, and mental health professional), for example, when the serum creatinine concentration reaches 2.0 mg per dL in men and 1.5 mg per dL in women. This will allow time to establish a working relationship, to acquaint the patient with the various modes of renal replacement therapy, and to provide information on dialysis access, nutritional modifications, avoidance of potentially nephrotoxic drugs, and potential financial support for services. Quality of life is an important concern in the predialysis period; maintenance of physical strength, appetite, and sense of well-being, as well as physiologic function warrant strong consideration in the decision to initiate dialysis. Late referral is associated with an increased incidence of complications, the need for emergency placement of vascular access and dialysis, and long-term access problems.

Control of Hypertension

Control of hypertension in all kinds of CKD, especially diabetic nephropathy, has repeatedly been shown to slow the progression of the disease and to decrease morbidity and mortality in cardiovascular disease. In patients with established azotemia, the initial lowering of blood pressure may increase the azotemia, but if one can carry a patient past this initial period, there will often be a return to pretreatment levels of SUN and serum creatinine concentrations, regardless of the agents used. A recent report from the Modification of Diet in Renal Disease Study suggests that lowering the mean arterial blood pressure (MABP) below the usual target blood pressure—to MABP 92 mm Hg (equivalent to 125/75 mm Hg) as opposed to 107 mm Hg (equivalent to 140/90 mm Hg)—is even more effective in slowing the progression of renal failure[13] (Evidence Level A).

Nutritional Modifications

The Modification of Diet in Renal Disease Study has also shown that restriction of protein intake to 0.7 g per kg of body weight in patients with creatinine clearances <55 mL per min will marginally slow the progression of the renal disease process[14] (Evidence Level A) and, thereby, very likely delay the onset of symptoms of uremia. This level of protein intake can maintain nutritional status in noncatabolic patients without placing undue burden on the capacity to eliminate potentially toxic metabolites including acid, potassium, sulfate, phosphate, and unidentified uremic toxins. If there is evidence of excessive catabolism, that is, malnutrition or muscle wasting, or if urinary protein losses are high, one may have to increase protein intake to as much as 1.0 to 1.2 g per kg of body weight per day.

A dietitian should design a dietary prescription, not only for protein but also for energy, fat, carbohydrate, sodium, phosphate, and micronutrient intake. Restriction of fat intake and lowering of serum cholesterol and triglyceride concentrations with statins also appear to have a renoprotective effect. Sodium restriction and/or diuretic therapy may become necessary to prevent edema and circulatory overload. A metabolic acidosis should be vigorously treated to maintain serum bicarbonate concentrations in the normal range (with alkalinizing agents if necessary) because acidosis increases bone dissolution and inhibits osteoblastic activity. Multivitamin supplements (pyridoxine, folic acid, vitamin B_{12}, and others) are indicated because these patients often become vitamin deficient, especially after starting hemodialysis whereby vitamins are removed from the circulation.

Anemia resulting from CKD often requires more aggressive treatment in elderly patients than in younger patients because of coexisting heart disease. Red blood cell indices do not provide a reliable estimate of iron deficiency in uremia. Iron deficiency should be excluded by the evaluation of serum iron and ferritin levels and iron should be given only if indicated. A depletion of renal erythropoietin stores begins early in the course of CKD. The management of non-iron-deficiency anemia has been changed radically by the availability of erythropoietin (epoetin α). Correction of hematocrits to levels in the 30% to 35% volume range results in improved cardiac function, exercise tolerance, central nervous system (CNS) function, appetite, and sexual function. Epoetin α is started at a dose of 50 to 100 U per kg subcutaneously three times a week (it can be given intravenously once dialysis is started).

Hyperphosphatemia, hypocalcemia, and hyperparathyroidism become problematic early in the course of CKD. Phosphate (phosphorus) retention stimulates parathyroid

(PTH) hypersecretion in an attempt to increase urinary phosphate excretions and lower serum phosphate levels back to normal. Therefore, maintenance of serum phosphate levels in the normal range is essential for the prevention of secondary hyperparathyroidism. Antacids are given with meals to bind intestinal phosphate in ingested foods and prevent absorption. Calcium carbonate antacids (two 500-mg tablets with each meal) are the phosphate binders of choice. Toxicity may result from aluminum-containing (bone demineralization, dementia, anemia) and magnesium-containing (respiratory depression) antacids in patients with renal failure.

Hypocalcemia results from inadequate vitamin D activity, necessary for calcium absorption from the intestines. The kidney manufactures the 1α-hydroxylase enzyme, which is necessary for converting the carrier form of vitamin D_3 (25-OH cholecalciferol) to the active form of vitamin D_3 (1,25-$(OH)_2$ cholecalciferol). Lack of the 1α-hydroxylase enzyme results in hypocalcemia, which is the primary stimulus for PTH activity. This, in turn, leeches calcium from the bone, producing osteopenia. Hypocalcemia can be prevented by giving vitamin D in its active form (calcitriol 0.25 to 0.50 μg daily) along with adequate amounts of calcium in the diet (1,000 to 2,000 mg per day). Aggressive attempts to raise the serum calcium levels without adequate lowering of serum phosphate can result in the development of metastatic calcifications. If the hyperparathyroidism has existed for a long time, the gland may have hypertrophied to the extent that lowering the serum phosphate and raising the serum calcium will not shut off the continuing overactivity. In this case, parathyroidectomy may be necessary.

END-STAGE RENAL DISEASE

In 1997, more than half of all patients on chronic dialysis were aged 65 years and older. Diabetes mellitus and hypertension were the most common causes of ESRD, and there were disproportionately high rates in minorities (Hispanics, blacks). There are at least two reasons why an increasing number of older adults are on dialysis. First, there is increased referral and acceptance of older adults onto dialysis, especially those with significant comorbidity. Secondly, there are increased survival rates in these individuals primarily related to better management (prevention) of the atherosclerotic diseases and their complications.

Dialysis

Dialysis becomes necessary when azotemia reaches a point where the earliest symptoms appear (fatigue, nausea, vomiting, loss of appetite, confusion). Some nephrologists like to start dialysis before symptoms appear, especially in patients with diabetes, as they feel that these patients do better in the long run. The method of dialysis, that is, hemodialysis versus peritoneal dialysis (usually chronic ambulatory peritoneal dialysis [CAPD]), depends on the patient's wishes and comorbidities, the physician's expertise, and available resources. Neither method offers any advantage in terms of survival rates when patients with similar risk factors are compared. The functional status and quality of life are no less satisfactory in old dialysis patients when compared with younger patients. Physical and occupational therapies are important components of care in patients on dialysis as they generally undergo an accelerated loss of physical function that can be slowed by exercise programs. For many older adults, the time spent on dialysis in a dialysis unit is a time to socially interact with other patients on dialysis and with nursing staff. It is important for the nephrologist and primary care clinician to be in frequent communication to reach agreement on the aspects of the patient's care for which each will be responsible.

Transplantation

Transplantation in older persons remains uncommon and controversial, primarily because of the reluctance to allocate a scarce resource (the donor kidney) to an older person with a limited life expectancy. However, older adults with a renal transplant have better survival rates compared to those on dialysis. One report[15] showed a 5-year survival rate of 81% for patients with a transplant compared to 51% for patients on dialysis. The results in older patients continue to improve because of better patient selection, improved perioperative care, and the use of safer, more effective immunosuppression. Older adults develop a senescence of their immune system and hence require less aggressive immunosuppression therapy.

DISORDERS OF SODIUM AND WATER BALANCE

Sodium is the primary extracellular cation and is responsible for maintaining the state of hydration outside the cell. The serum sodium concentration can be accurately and precisely measured in the clinical laboratory, allowing one to classify states of sodium balance as normal (serum sodium concentration 135 to 145 mEq per L), hyponatremic, or hypernatremic. Water balance is determined by the clinical assessment of extracellular fluid volume (ECFV), which is much more subjective. Excessive water retention eventually results in the formation of edema. Water deficiency can develop either from a primary loss of water (dehydration), in which case hypernatremia develops, or from a primary loss of sodium with its osmotically obligated water (volume depletion). Patients with the latter maintain normal serum sodium concentrations until the volume depletion becomes sufficient to stimulate antidiuretic hormone release. If fluid losses are then replaced without salt, the water is retained and hyponatremia develops.

CASE TWO

An 86-year-old man was seen in the office because of the insidious onset of "confusion" (memory loss) over the preceding year. He had not been eating well and had to be encouraged (reminded) to drink fluids. His blood pressure was 130/70 mm Hg and his pulse was 88. On standing, his blood pressure dropped to 120/66 mm Hg and his pulse increased to 100. He had poor skin turgor with "tenting" of the forearm skin and dry mucous membranes. The rest of the history and physical examination was unremarkable (no edema). His serum sodium was 122 mEq per L. Other pertinent laboratory findings were a hematocrit of 40%, a serum potassium of 4.3 mEq per L, a serum chloride of 84 mEq per L, and a serum bicarbonate of 26 mmol per L. His SUN was 7 mg per dL, and serum creatinine was 1.0 mg per dL. His chest x-ray was unremarkable.

Commentary

One must decide whether this patient's hyponatremia is due to primary salt depletion or syndrome of inappropriate antidiuretic hormone (SIADH). In very elderly patients, the poor skin turgor can be explained by subcutaneous loss of fat, and dry oral mucous membranes can be explained by mouth breathing. He did not have an appreciable fall in blood pressure or increase in pulse rate on standing, which is against a primary salt depletion. The subnormal SUN and low SUN to serum creatinine ratio favor SIADH. If the SUN and serum creatinine concentrations had both been high, this would have been problematic, because both a primary salt depletion and SIADH with preexisting renal disease could then explain the findings.

It is important to make the distinction between these two entities as the former is treated by replacement with isotonic or hypertonic solutions of salt and the latter is treated with fluid restriction. A misdiagnosis could result in increased dehydration in the first instance and overhydration with pulmonary edema in the second.

Dehydration and Volume Depletion

The presenting signs and symptoms of dehydration/volume depletion in the elderly include altered mental status (confusion, delirium, stupor, coma), lethargy, reduced skin turgor, dry mucous membranes, tachycardia, and orthostatic hypotension. What is sometimes confusing is that all of these may occur in the elderly with a normal ECFV. Often there is a history to suggest dehydration/volume depletion (e.g., decreased food and fluid intake, febrile illness, polyuria, diabetes mellitus, chronic renal disease, use of diuretics, or a history of vomiting, diarrhea, or nasogastric suction). There may also be a history of impaired ability to get to a water source. Increased hematocrit, SUN, and serum creatinine concentrations are common, and the SUN to serum creatinine ratio is generally >20. The urine sodium concentration is usually low (<20 mEq per L) but can be above that if renal or adrenal disease is present. Hypokalemia, hypercalcemia, and hyperglycemia with glycosuria (osmotic diuresis) can cause polyuria and decreased concentrating ability that could lead to dehydration.

Mild dehydration (fluid loss <5% of body weight) can be treated with increased oral water or clear fluid intake unless a gastrointestinal (GI) disorder or impaired mental state precludes this. For more severe dehydration, replacement of fluid losses with normal saline (0.9% sodium chloride), even if the serum sodium concentration is slightly elevated, is necessary. Generally, it is better to replace the sodium deficit (intravascular volume deficit) before being concerned about the replacement of free water. More details on treatment are included in the sections on hypo- and hypernatremia.

Hyponatremia

The causes of hyponatremia are listed in Table 31.4. A low serum sodium concentration may result from[1] a loss of sodium in excess of osmotically obligated water (primary salt depletion),[2] a retention of water in excess of sodium (dilutional hyponatremia), or a combination of both as one sees in the SIADH. The initial pathology of SIADH is retention of water, resulting in an expanded ECFV. This then stimulates increased urinary sodium excretion, resulting in loss of osmotically obligated water so that ECFV returns to or toward the normal range.

A reduction in serum sodium concentration to <120 mEq per L, regardless of etiology, may produce symptoms ranging from mild, nonspecific complaints, such as malaise, irritability, muscle weakness, and change in personality, to marked CNS impairment. Serious CNS impairment results from a shift of fluid along osmotic gradients from the hypotonic ECFV into the isotonic brain cells, thereby increasing brain volume and intracranial pressure. Depending on the severity of the hyponatremia and the state of hydration, a spectrum of alterations in consciousness ranging from confusion to coma may appear. Seizures are often the manifestations that prompt immediate attention.

Hyponatremia with Contracted Extracellular Fluid Volume (Primary Salt Depletion)

In conditions where primary salt depletion with dehydration is suspected, a measure of urinary sodium concentration may be helpful in the differential diagnosis. If it is <10 mEq per L, suspected etiologies would include inadequate salt intake, excessive sweating, or gastrointestinal losses. If it is greater than this value, inappropriate renal losses of salt and water could be due to excessive use of diuretics, adrenal or pituitary insufficiency, or intrinsic renal

TABLE 31.4
HYPONATREMIC SYNDROMES

I. Hyponatremia with contracted extracellular volume (ECFV)
  A. Urinary sodium $<$10 mEq/L
    1. Inadequate intake
    2. Excessive sweating
    3. Excessive gastrointestinal loss (diarrhea, bowel, and biliary fistulas)
  B. Urinary sodium $>$10 mEq/L
    1. Severe metabolic alkalosis due to vomiting
    2. Excessive urinary losses (salt wasting)
      a. Adrenal insufficiency (Addison disease, hypoaldosteronism)
      b. Renal disease (renal tubular acidosis, interstitial nephritis)
      c. Diuretic induced
II. Hyponatremia with normal ECFV
  A. Displacement syndromes (hyperglycemia, hyperlipidemia, hyperproteinemia)
  B. Syndrome of inappropriate antidiuretic hormone
    1. Malignancies, especially small cell carcinoma of lung
    2. Pulmonary diseases, including positive pressure breathing
    3. Cerebral conditions (trauma, infection, tumor, stroke)
    4. Drugs (sulfonylureas, thiazides, antitumor agents, psychotropics, antidepressants)
    5. Other (myxedema, porphyria, idiopathic)
  C. Water intoxication (schizophrenia)
III. Hyponatremia with expanded ECFV (dilutional hyponatremia)
  A. Congestive heart failure
  B. Cirrhosis
  C. Nephrotic syndrome (hypoalbuminemia)
  D. Renal failure

ECFV, extracellular fluid volume.

disease (e.g., renal tubular acidosis, salt-losing nephritis, or renal insufficiency). In severe vomiting with a metabolic alkalosis and bicarbonaturia, urinary sodium along with the bicarbonate may be increased despite hypovolemia and hyponatremia. Epstein and Hollenberg[16] have shown that there is a reduction in the ability of the older person to conserve sodium when placed on a salt-restricted diet. This may make the elderly more susceptible to the development of salt-depletion hyponatremia during episodes of acute illness.

Treatment is generally best accomplished using isotonic saline (0.9%) as replacement; however, in patients with severe, symptomatic conditions, small amounts of hypertonic saline (3% or 5%) can be used initially. Often it remains unclear whether one is dealing with a primary salt loss syndrome or SIADH because urinary sodium excretions may be high in both situations. In the elderly, ECFV is hard to assess. An important clue in making the differential diagnosis may be the SUN because this becomes elevated in primary salt depletion and is normal to subnormal in SIADH, that is, assuming that there was no preexisting renal impairment.

Hyponatremia with Expanded Extracellular Fluid Volume (Dilutional Hyponatremia)

Impairment in water excretion occurs commonly in conditions in which salt excretion is also severely impaired. Patients with advanced cardiac, hepatic, or renal disease and generalized edema are often placed on diets that sharply restrict salt intake without placing limitations on fluid intake. Once hyponatremia begins to develop, restriction of water intake may become necessary.

Although total ECFV in these patients is increased, the blood volume returning to the heart and in the arterial vascular system tends to be decreased, stimulating baroreceptors in the right atrium and arterial system to retain sodium and baroreceptors in the left atrium and arterial system to stimulate ADH release and retain water. A decrease in GFR and/or an increase in sodium reabsorption in the proximal tubule limits water excretion by decreasing delivery of sodium and water to the distal nephron where dilution of urine below isotonic levels takes place. Under these conditions, while urine concentration is maintained near isotonic levels, the intake of fluids generally greatly exceeds the intake of sodium (i.e., the individual is ingesting hypotonic solutions, resulting in the generation of the hyponatremia). Treatment initially consists of salt and fluid restriction; if the use of loop diuretics and hypertonic saline becomes necessary, this requires hospitalization.

It is very difficult for a normal person to ingest sufficient water to develop symptomatic hyponatremia (water intoxication). Some patients with schizophrenic illnesses, however, have been reported to be capable of ingesting sufficient fluid to lower their serum sodium concentrations into the symptomatic range.

Hyponatremia with Normal Extracellular Fluid Volume (Syndrome of Inappropriate Antidiuretic Hormone)

A diagnosis of SIADH is made after other causes of hyponatremia have been excluded. The following criteria must be met: (i) The extracellular fluid osmolality and sodium concentration must be decreased; (ii) the urine must be hypertonic to serum; (iii) urinary sodium excretion exceeds 10 mEq per L; (iv) adrenal, renal, cardiac, and hepatic functions are normal; and (v) hyponatremia can be corrected by water restriction. Persistence of circulating ADH is considered inappropriate when neither hyperosmolality nor volume depletion is present. The inability to excrete water because of high ADH levels leads to volume expansion that, in turn, promotes urinary salt loss. SIADH is seen in patients with a number of neoplasms, most commonly oat cell carcinoma of the lung. Any condition impairing blood flow through the pulmonary circulation, such as positive pressure breathing, creates a decreased filling of the left atrium that stimulates ADH release. The reported causes of this syndrome, especially those related to drug therapy, continue to grow as seen in Table 31.4. Recent reports have raised concerns about the association between the selective serotonin reuptake inhibitor (SSRI) antidepressants and hyponatremia, with the elderly again at highest risk.[17]

Normovolemic hyponatremia may also result from the addition of an uncharged solute, such as glucose, which increases the serum osmotic pressure and draws water from inside the cell to expand and dilute the ECFV. This promotes an increased loss of sodium in the urine, reducing total body stores of this cation. Normovolemic hyponatremia (pseudohyponatremia) can also result from a displacement of water in a serum sample with abnormal amounts of large-molecular-weight solute (e.g., protein or lipids), so that one has a false perception of the amount of serum water originally present when it is further diluted in the process of quantifying serum sodium concentration.

Hyponatremia in the Elderly

Surveys of older persons in both acute and chronic care facilities show a high prevalence of hyponatremia. Kleinfeld et al.[18] reported that 36 of 160 patients (23%) in a nursing home had serum sodium concentrations chronically below 132 mEq per L (mean 120 mEq per L). In most patients, the low serum sodium concentration was not explained except by the presence of chronic debilitating disease and old age. Miller et al.[19] also found that 11% of an ambulatory geriatric clinic population had hyponatremia (serum sodium concentration <135 mEq per L). SIADH appeared to be the cause in approximately 60% of the cases of hyponatremia, with a quarter of these (seven cases) having no apparent underlying etiology other than age. Others[20] have found a similar high incidence of "idiopathic" SIADH (60%) in hospitalized elderly patients, but they were asymptomatic unless the sodium concentration fell below 110 mEq per L, and the subsequent course was benign, not requiring treatment. Anderson et al.[21] prospectively evaluated the prevalence, cause, and outcome of patients with hyponatremia in an acute care facility. The prevalence was 2.5% with the mean age being 60 years. Two thirds were iatrogenic. The most frequent cause was SIADH (normovolemic hyponatremia), accounting for 34% of cases; hypovolemia (dehydration), hypervolemia (dilutional hyponatremia), and hyperglycemia each accounted for another 16% to 19% of cases; and renal failure (overhydration) and error each accounted for 8% to 10%. Nonosmotic (baroreceptor) stimulation of ADH release was a major factor in all cases. Elderly persons appear to be more susceptible to the development of SIADH-like hyponatremia. The antidiuresis and hyponatremia observed postoperatively has been observed primarily in elders, as has been the hyponatremia observed with drugs such as the sulfonylureas, the SSRI antidepressants, and the thiazide diuretics. Further discussions on the possible causes of SIADH in the elderly are found elsewhere.[6] One recent additional finding to be added to these possible explanations is provided by Ishikawa et al,[22] who reported that urinary aquaporin-2 (AQP-2) excretions were increased in elderly patients with hyponatremia due to SIADH. The urinary excretion of AQP-2 reflects the activity of arginine vasopressin (AVP) on the collecting ducts in producing channels through which water can be absorbed back into the medullary portions of the kidney. This could explain why patients with SIADH might be retaining more water with resultant hyponatremia.

The first step in the management of fluid retention associated with either SIADH or dilutional hyponatremia is stepwise fluid restriction to levels as low as 500 mL per day. In the hospital, furosemide, a diuretic that will reduce urine concentration to near isotonic levels, can be given followed by an infusion of hypertonic salt solution. Other drugs that interfere with the concentrating ability of the kidney and thereby increase urine outputs are lithium and the antibiotic democlocycline. Vasopressin inhibitors are in the clinical trial stage and may be available for clinical use shortly.

Hypernatremia

An increase in serum sodium concentration is generally a result of a loss of body water in excess of salt (dehydration), although it also can result from ingestion or administration of large amounts of salt without sufficient water or from excessive amounts of adrenal steroids (cortisone). Elderly persons have a diminished thirst sensation that is further impaired by CNS dysfunction, such as stroke.[23] Hypernatremia often occurs in elderly who are bedfast or physically handicapped and hence do not receive adequate replacement fluids. A net deficit of water can also be associated with vomiting and/or diarrhea, pituitary or nephrogenic diabetes insipidus, an osmotic diuresis (e.g., hyperosmolar nonketotic diabetic acidosis), and hyperpyrexia (excessive sweating).

Hypernatremia reflects an increase in serum osmolality, which results in a shift of water from intracellular to extracellular spaces. One consequence of this shift is a shrinkage of brain cells, causing intracranial injury to blood vessels with venous thrombosis, infarction, and/or hemorrhage. The earliest manifestation of hypernatremia is thirst, followed by confusion and lethargy, and, ultimately, delirium, stupor, and coma. Because intravascular volume is preserved at the expense of cell water, changes in blood pressure and pulse rate are not prominent features of hypernatremic dehydration.

Once hypernatremia has occurred, restoration of fluids becomes necessary. The amount of water (or dextrose and water if given parenterally) needed can be estimated using the formula:

$$\text{Water deficit (milliliters)} = \frac{\text{Patient's serum Na}^{+} - 140 \text{ mEq per L}}{140 \text{ mEq per L (Normal Na}^{+})} \times 60\% \text{ of body weight (Body water in kilograms or liters)}$$

Example: A 70-kg man with a serum sodium concentration of 154 mEq per L

$$= \frac{154 - 140}{140} \times 70 \times 0.60 = 4.2 \text{ L fluid deficit}$$

The total body water is used rather than ECFV (20% of body weight) because as water is given, the osmolality in the ECFV falls, resulting in a shift of water along osmotic gradients back into the cell.

To avoid a recurrence in individuals with demonstrated impaired thirst, a fluid prescription establishing the quantity of fluid to be ingested daily may become an important part of preventative management.

DISORDERS OF POTASSIUM BALANCE

Potassium is the primary intracellular cation, with <2% of the total body potassium contained in the extracellular fluid compartment. Therefore, the serum concentration of potassium may not accurately reflect total body potassium stores. Flux of potassium into cells occurs with cell growth, intracellular nitrogen and potassium deposition, and increases in extracellular pH; potassium leaves the cell with cell destruction, glucose utilization, and decreases in extracellular pH. When one is interpreting serum potassium concentrations, factors that affect the ratio of intracellular to extracellular concentration must be kept in mind, because normally a steep concentration gradient is maintained. For example, the patient with diabetic ketoacidosis has a high serum potassium concentration, but rehydration, correction of the acidosis with sodium bicarbonate, and treatment of the hyperglycemia with insulin combine to produce a dramatic decrease in serum potassium concentration. Age alone does not appear to affect the ability to maintain this concentration gradient. Isotopic dilution studies and muscle biopsies, however, have been used to demonstrate that intracellular potassium stores can be depleted in a variety of clinical conditions commonly seen in elderly patients, such as metabolic and respiratory acidosis, congestive heart failure, cirrhosis, and uremia, with serum potassium concentrations remaining within normal limits.

CASE THREE

A 74-year-old man with long-standing, mild, type 2 diabetes mellitus well controlled on glyburide comes in for follow-up 1 month after being started on 25 mg of hydrochlorothiazide per day as additional treatment for mild systolic hypertension (156/84 mm Hg) and 1+ lower extremity edema that was felt possibly to be early evidence of congestive heart failure. He had previously been placed on an ACE inhibitor (lisinopril 10 mg daily). He was also started on an oral potassium chloride supplement 20 mEq twice daily. Baseline renal function and electrolytes were unremarkable. He now notes some apprehension (anxiety) and generalized weakness that has come on since his prior visit. An electrocardiogram is done which shows peaking of the T waves. Repeat laboratory values show a SUN of 22 mg per dL, serum creatinine of 1.5 mg per dL, serum sodium of 138 mEq per L, serum potassium of 6.2 mEq per L, serum chloride of 106 mEq per L, and serum bicarbonate of 22 mmol per L. The primary care clinician now has to decide whether to just stop the potassium chloride supplement or employ further means to lower the serum potassium concentration. He elects the former.

Commentary

This patient has multiple reasons for developing what could become a potentially lethal hyperkalemia. In one study of patients receiving potassium supplements along with thiazide diuretics,[24] two significant risk factors for hyperkalemia were identified. The first was a decrease in renal function. This patient had a normal SUN and serum creatinine until placed on a thiazide diuretic. Then it became slightly elevated, indicating that renal function (GFR) was less than half of the normal. Soon after starting treatment with a thiazide diuretic, there is often an increase in SUN and serum creatinine concentration as ECFV and renal perfusion fall, but over time these values tend to return to normal as ECFV increases. The second factor in this study[24] is age. In patients under the age of 50 years, the frequency of incident hyperkalemia was 0.8% compared to 4.2% to 6.0% with advancing age in age-groups older than 50 years. Older individuals under all conditions (normal and restricted salt intakes, supine vs. upright positions) have much lower plasma renin activities and urinary aldosterone excretions, explaining this observation at least partially.[25] This failure of the renin–aldosterone system in older patients, most notably seen in patients with interstitial nephritis and diabetes, may produce a type IV renal tubular acidosis with hyperkalemia (hyporeninemic hypoaldosteronism). The lack of renin and aldosterone decreases the amount of sodium reabsorbed in the distal nephron in exchange for both potassium and hydrogen, leading to the hyperkalemic acidosis. Other drugs used to treat hypertension and cardiovascular disorders (β-adrenergic blocking agents, ACE inhibitors, ARBs, potassium-sparing diuretics) act similarly in compromising the renin–angiotensin–aldosterone system, thereby decreasing potassium secretion in the distal nephron. Similarly, the inability to excrete hydrogen ion leads to a metabolic acidosis that increases the flux of potassium from inside the cells into the extracellular spaces.

The serum potassium concentration was reaching a level where a lethal cardiac arrhythmia was a real possibility in this patient. This is probably more true in any elderly person with preexisting cardiovascular disease. By just electing to stop the potassium supplement and doing nothing further to lower the potassium level, the primary care clinician was taking a calculated risk that this was adequate. To be safe, it might have been better to use one of the measures mentioned in the following text to lower the serum potassium concentration.

Hypokalemia

Table 31.5 lists the causes of hypokalemia. The most frequent cause of hypokalemia is the use of loop and/or thiazide diuretics to treat hypertension and/or edema. A frequently overlooked cause of hypokalemia in the elderly is the excessive use of enemas and purgatives, a behavior that should be suspected whenever unexplained hypokalemic alkalosis is observed.

Although the normal kidney is not as efficient in conserving potassium as it is for sodium, when intake is restricted or losses are excessive, it can reduce urinary excretions below 20 mEq per day. Because little potassium is normally lost through the gastrointestinal tract, it takes 2 to 3 weeks on a virtually potassium-free diet for a normal person to reduce his/her serum potassium concentration to 3.0 mEq per L. A reasonable criterion for establishing a diagnosis of urinary potassium wasting when the serum potassium concentration falls below 3.5 mEq per L would be the daily excretion of >20 mEq. The etiologies of excessive urinary potassium loss can be divided into four categories: (i) Pituitary-adrenal disturbances, (ii) renal defects, (iii) drug-induced losses, and (iv) idiopathic/miscellaneous.

Multiple pathophysiologic mechanisms occur in many, if not most, cases to explain the development of hypokalemia. As an example, the patient with vomiting not only has a reduction in potassium intake and some loss of potassium in the vomitus but is also losing hydrogen ions, producing a metabolic alkalosis. This, in turn, shifts potassium intracellularly and augments urinary potassium losses. The contracted extracellular volume then increases proximal tubular sodium and bicarbonate reabsorption that further enhances the metabolic alkalosis and induces a secondary hyperaldosteronism that increases urinary potassium losses.

The structural and functional defects associated with potassium deficiency are listed in Table 31.6. These involve the kidney, the myocardium and the cardiovascular system, the neuromuscular and the CNS, and the gastrointestinal tract. The characteristic electrocardiographic changes are ST segment depression, T-wave flattening, and prominent U waves. The cardiac function can be affected, resulting in atrial and ventricular ectopic beats, ventricular tachycardia, and even sudden death from ventricular fibrillation. Potassium deficiency can also contribute to impairments in carbohydrate metabolism and protein synthesis.

Because an alkalosis (chloride depletion) usually accompanies hypokalemia, replacement therapy should be instituted with potassium chloride rather than with the alkaline salts of potassium (the exception would be the patient with renal tubular acidosis). Foods rich in potassium (citrus and tomato juices, bananas, meats, and vegetables) provide the safest way to administer potassium. When additional oral replacement therapy is needed, commercial preparations come in liquid, tablet, and powder forms, usually in 20 mEq doses.

Routine replacement potassium therapy, at least in patients with hypertension placed on diuretic therapy with normal serum potassium levels, is not necessary. Rather, it is better to monitor serum potassium levels because an occasional patient will develop hypokalemia that does potentiate the possibility of ventricular arrhythmias.[26] A significant incidence of life-threatening hyperkalemia in patients receiving supplements means that the potential for benefit must be weighed against the risks.[23]

Hyperkalemia

Hyperkalemia is most commonly observed in patients with impaired renal function. However, patients with chronic renal failure who maintain good urine flow rates do not develop significant hyperkalemia until the azotemia becomes life threatening. Because the distal nephron has such a large capacity for secretion of potassium, hyperkalemia develops only when there is some associated factor present, such as (i) oliguria (ARF), (ii) excessive endogenous or exogenous potassium load (supplements, medication, catabolism), (iii) metabolic or respiratory acidosis, (iv) spironolactone, triamterene, or amiloride therapy, (v) a deficiency of endogenous steroid (aldosterone, cortisol), or (vi) administration of a drug that inhibits potassium secretion in the distal nephron (e.g., an ACE inhibitor or angiotensin II receptor blocker [ARB], a β-adrenergic antagonist [blocker], or an NSAID). Other drugs that can interfere with potassium secretion and

TABLE 31.5
CAUSES OF HYPOKALEMIA

I. Inadequate intake
II. Excessive sweating
III. Dilution of extracellular fluid volume
IV. Shift of potassium intracellularly
  A. Increase in blood pH (alkalosis)
  B. Glucose and insulin
  C. Familial hypokalemic periodic paralysis
V. Excessive gastrointestinal losses
  A. Vomiting
  B. Biliary, pancreatic, and intestinal drainage from fistulas and ostomies
  C. Chronic diarrhea (chronic infections and inflammatory lesions, malabsorption, villous adenomas of colon and rectum, catechol-secreting neural tumors, abdominal lymphomas, islet cell tumors of pancreas, excessive use of enemas and purgatives)
VI. Increased urinary losses (potassium wasting)
  A. Pituitary-adrenal disturbances (primary and secondary aldosteronisms due to renal artery stenosis, Cushing syndrome due to adrenal adenomas, carcinomas and/or hyperplasia, pituitary corticotropin hypersecretion, ectopic corticotropin secretion secondary to tumor, 11β-hydroxysteroid dehydrogenase deficiency due to Barter syndrome or licorice ingestion [glycyrrhizic acid inhibits the enzyme responsible for the conversion of cortisol to cortisone])
  B. Renal disorders (distal or proximal renal tubular acidosis, renin-secreting renal tumor, salt-losing nephritis, diuretic phase of acute tubular necrosis, postobstructive diuresis)
  C. Drug induced (thiazide and loop diuretics, large nonabsorbable anions, e.g., carbenicillin, cistplatin, aminoglycosides, amphotericin B, respiratory alkalosis due to acetylsalicylic acid, adrenergic agonists used to treat bronchospasm)
  D. Idiopathic, familial, and other pathologies (Liddle and Gitelman syndromes, hypomagnesemia, lysozymuria due to leukemia)

produce hyperkalemia include some of the bronchodilators (β_2 agonists), heparin, and trimethoprim.

The clinical manifestations of hyperkalemia are often subtle and may occur only shortly before death occurs from cardiac arrhythmia. Anxiety, restlessness, apprehension, weakness, stupor, and hyporeflexia should alert the clinician to the potential existence of this imbalance in patients at risk. Characteristic electrocardiographic changes are the peaking of T waves followed by the widening and loss of P waves and ultimately the widening of the QRS complex.

Therapy should be started when the serum potassium concentration exceeds 5.5 mEq per L; a true medical emergency exists when it exceeds 7.0 mEq per L. Acute treatment is with glucose, insulin, and sodium bicarbonate to shift potassium intracellularly and with calcium and sodium salts that act as physiologic antagonists. Sodium

TABLE 31.6
MANIFESTATIONS OF HYPOKALEMIA

I. Myocardial and cardiovascular
  A. Focal myocardial necrosis
  B. Electrocardiographic changes (depressed ST segments, inversion of T waves, accentuated U waves, arrhythmias)
  C. Other (potentiation of digitalis toxicity, salt retention, hypotension)
II. Neuromuscular and psychiatric
  A. Muscle weakness to flaccid paralysis
  B. Muscle pain and tenderness (rhabdomyolysis)
  C. Depressive reaction (anorexia, constipation, weakness, lethargy, apathy, fatigue, depressed mood)
  D. Acute brain syndrome (memory impairment, disorientation, confusion)
III. Renal
  A. Defect in urine-concentrating ability (polyuria)
  B. Paradoxical aciduria
  C. Sodium retention
IV. Gastrointestinal
  A. Decreased motility and propulsive activity of intestine
  B. Paralytic ileus
V. Metabolic
  A. Carbohydrate intolerance–delayed insulin release
  B. Growth failure due to impaired protein synthesis

polystyrene sulfonate (Kayexalate) resins are used to remove excess potassium from the body and can be given orally or in enema form (orally 15 mg one to four times daily and rectally 25 to 100 mg in a retention enema). To avoid constipation and fecal impaction with oral administration of these resins, lactulose solution (15 to 30 mL) can be given three times daily, titrating the dose. When hyperkalemia is due to a mineralocorticoid deficiency, 0.1 mg. of 9-fluorohydrocortisone (Florinef) can be given daily. Dialysis is used rarely as a last resort.

DISORDERS OF ACID–BASE BALANCE

Alterations in acid–base balance are generally described in terms of changes in the carbon dioxide–bicarbonate system because these changes reflect shifts in all other buffer systems in the blood and tissues and they can be easily quantified. An acidosis results from the introduction of excess acid into body fluids and an alkalosis results from an excess loss of acid. The body must cope with two types of acid, specifically carbonic acid derived from the hydration of carbon dioxide, and fixed hydrogen ions. The lungs remove the volatile carbon dioxide generated during metabolism. Retention of carbon dioxide (hypoventilation) results in a respiratory acidosis; excessive loss of carbon dioxide (hyperventilation) results in a respiratory alkalosis. The hydrogen ions and associated organic (lactate, β-hydroxybutyrate) and inorganic (phosphate, sulfate) anions are buffered in body fluids and can be excreted only by the kidney or lost through other fluids (e.g., the GI tract). On a normal diet, the body generates hydrogen ions from the metabolism of protein and fats and must excrete approximately 1 mEq of hydrogen ion per kg of body weight per day to stay in balance. Although acid–base parameters remain normal in the elderly under basal conditions, the ability of the older person to correct imbalances after an acute event is impaired.

Acid–base imbalances can be separated into a metabolic acidosis (low pH, pCO_2, bicarbonate), metabolic alkalosis (high pH, pCO_2, bicarbonate), respiratory acidosis (low pH, high pCO_2), and respiratory alkalosis (high pH, low pCO_2). Measurement of serum bicarbonate in venous blood alone may not be adequate to characterize an imbalance, in which case, an arterial sample is necessary to measure pH and pCO_2 and to calculate bicarbonate. Most primary disturbances are accompanied by a compensatory correction to maintain pH as close to normal as possible. This is the reason a person with a metabolic acidosis, for example, develops hyperventilation (compensatory respiratory alkalosis).

Metabolic Acidosis

In a patient with a metabolic acidosis, it is useful to determine if an anion gap exists. Normally, the difference between the sodium concentration and the sum of the chloride and bicarbonate concentrations is <12 mEq per L. When the difference is larger, an anion gap exists, indicating that some unmeasured anion is present, which is either organic (lactate, β-hydroxybutyrate, salicylate, formate) or inorganic (phosphate, sulfate). If no anion gap exists, the serum chloride concentration increases as the serum bicarbonate decreases (hyperchloremic acidosis). The causes of a metabolic acidosis are shown in Table 31.7.

TABLE 31.7
CAUSES OF METABOLIC ACIDOSIS

With anion gap
A. Azotemic renal failure
B. Diabetic and starvation ketoacidosis
C. Methyl alcohol intoxication
D. Paraldehyde intoxication
E. Ethylene glycol intoxication
F. Salicylate intoxication
G. Lactic acidosis
  1. Circulatory insufficiency and shock
  2. Metformin therapy
  3. Primary

Without anion gap
A. Diarrhea and fistula drainage (bicarbonate loss)
B. NH_4Cl ingestion
C. Renal tubular acidosis
D. Ureterosigmoidostomy

Treatment of a metabolic acidosis first depends on the identification of the cause and correcting it (e.g., treatment of diabetic ketoacidosis). Sodium bicarbonate or sodium citrate/citric acid solutions (Shohl solution) can be given orally (the latter avoids the buildup of gas in the intestinal tract). In some cases, rehydration with normal saline will suffice to correct the imbalance, as the replacement of sodium chloride allows one to increase the urinary excretion of ammonium chloride. If a more severe acidosis is present, one to two ampoules of sodium bicarbonate (44 mEq per 50 mL) can be given by infusion generally added to other solutions of normal saline or dextrose and water.

Metabolic alkalosis

A metabolic alkalosis results from an excess intake of alkali (e.g., sodium bicarbonate) or abnormal losses of acid (e.g., pernicious vomiting). Volume contraction (dehydration) produces a metabolic alkalosis by increasing the sodium and bicarbonate reabsorption in the proximal tubules and is often seen in patients who are on aggressive diuretic therapy. A metabolic alkalosis also occurs with potassium depletion owing to a shift of acid from the extracellular to intracellular spaces, and an increase in the exchange of hydrogen ion secretion for sodium ion reabsorption in the distal nephron.

A metabolic alkalosis can be subdivided on the basis of the amount of chloride in the urine and on whether it can be corrected with chloride administration. Chloride-responsive alkalosis (urine chloride <20 mEq per L) is generally due to excessive vomiting or administration of diuretics. Chloride-unresponsive alkalosis is usually accompanied by hypokalemia and is due to cortisone or aldosterone excess.

Treatment can again be accomplished by giving isotonic normal saline. With repletion of the chloride, the excess sodium will be excreted in the urine as sodium bicarbonate. In cases of mineralocorticoid excess, the underlying cause must be treated before saline replacement will be effective.

REFERENCES

1. Lindeman RD, Tobin JD, Shock NW. Longitudinal studies on the rate of decline in renal function with age. *J Am Geriatr Soc.* 1985;33:278–285.
2. Cameron JS. Nephrotic syndrome in the elderly. *Semin Nephrol.* 1996;16:319–329.
3. De Zeeuw D. Albuminuria, not only a cardiovascular/renal risk marker, but also a target for treatment. *Kidney Int.* 2004;66(Suppl 92):2–4.
4. Levey AS, Coresh J, Balk E, et al. National Kidney Foundation practice guidelines for chronic kidney disease: Evaluation, classification, and stratification. *Ann Intern Med.* 2003;139:137–147.
5. Couser WG. Section 3. Glomerular and vascular diseases. In: Jacobson HR, Striker GE, Klahr S, eds. *The principles and practice of nephrology*, 2nd ed. St. Louis: Mosby;1995:102–200.
6. Lindeman RD. Chapter 49. Renal and electrolyte disorders. In: Duthie EH Jr, Katz PR, eds. *Practice of geriatrics*, 3rd ed, Philadelphia, PA: WB Saunders;1998:546–561.
7. Burkhart JM, Canzanello VJ. Chapter 56. Renal disease. In: Hazzard WR, Bierman EL, Blass JP, et al. eds, *Principles of geriatric medicine and gerontology*, 3rd ed, New York, NY: McGraw-Hill;1994:637–655.
8. Foster MH. Chapter 10. Serologic evaluation of the renal patient. In: Jacobson HR, Striker GE, Klahr S, eds. *The principles and practice of nephrology*, 2nd ed. St. Louis: Mosby;1995:71–85.
9. Rowe JW, Andres R, Tobin JD, et al. The effect of age on creatinine clearance in men: Cross-sectional and longitudinal study. *J Gerontol.* 1976;31:155–163.
10. Levey AS, Bosch JP, Lewis JB, et al. A more accurate method to estimate glomerular filtration rate from serum creatinine: A new prediction equation. Modification of Diet in Renal Disease Study Group. *Ann Intern Med.* 1999;130:461–470.
11. Haas M, Spargo BH, Wit EC, et al. Etiologies and outcomes of acute renal insufficiency in older adults. A renal biopsy study of 259 cases. *Am J Kidney Dis.* 2000;35:433–447.
12. National Library of Medicine. *NIH Consensus Development Program. 93. Morbidity and mortality of dialysis. How does early medical intervention in pre-dialysis patients influence morbidity and mortality. Health Services/Technology Assessment Text (HSTAT)*, Bethesda, MD: National Library of Medicine;2003, (http://consensus.nih.gov).
13. Sarnak MJ, Greene T, Wang X, et al. The effect of a lower target blood pressure on the progression of kidney disease: Long-term follow-up of the Modification of Diet in Renal Disease Study. *Ann Intern Med.* 2005;142:342–351.
14. Levey AS, Greene T, Beck GJ, et al. Dietary protein restriction and the progression of chronic renal disease: What have all the results of the result of the MDRD study shown? *J Am Soc Nephrol.* 1999;10:2426–2439.
15. Schaubel D, Desmentes M, Mao Y, et al. Survival experience among elderly end-stage renal disease patients. A controlled comparison of transplantation and dialysis. *Transplantation.* 1995;60:1389–1394.
16. Epstein M, Hollenberg N. Age as a determinant of renal sodium conservation in normal man. *J Lab Clin Med.* 1976;87:411–417.
17. Kirchner V, Silver LE, Kelly CA. Selective serotonin reuptake inhibitors and hyponatremia: Review and proposed mechanisms in the elderly. *J Psychopharmacol.* 1998;12:396–400.
18. Kleinfeld M, Casimir M, Borra S. Hyponatremia as observed in a chronic disease facility. *J Am Geriatr Soc.* 1979;27:156–161.
19. Miller M, Hecker MS, Friedlander DA, et al. Apparent idiopathic hyponatremia in an ambulatory geriatric population. *J Am Geriatr Soc.* 1996;44:404–408.
20. Hirshberg R, Ben-Yehuda A. The syndrome of inappropriate antidiuretic hormone secretion in the elderly. *Am J Med.* 1997;103:270–273.
21. Anderson RJ, Chung HM, Kluge R. Hyponatremia: A prospective analysis of its epidemiology and the pathogenetic role of vasopressin. *Ann Intern Med.* 1978;102:164–168.
22. Ishikawa SE, Saito T, Fukagawa A, et al. Close association of urinary excretion of aquaporin-2 with appropriate and inappropriate arginine vasopressin-dependent antidiuresis in hyponatremia in elderly subjects. *J Clin Endocrinol Metab.* 2001;86:1665–1671.
23. Phillips PA, Rolls BJ, Ledingham JG, et al. Reduced thirst after water deprivation in healthy elderly men. *N Engl J Med.* 1984;311:753–759.
24. Lawson DH. Adverse reactions to potassium chloride. *Q J Med.* 1974;171:433–440.
25. Weideman P, DeMyttenaeu-Bursztein S, Maxwell MH, et al. Effect of aging on plasma renin and aldosterone in normal man. *Kidney Int.* 1975;8:325–333.
26. Siegal D, Hulley SB, Black DM, et al. Diuretics, serum and intracellular electrolyte levels, and ventricular arrhythmias in hypertensive men. *JAMA.* 1992;267:1083–1089.

Gynecology and Breast Disease

32

Barbara A. Majeroni

CLINICAL PEARLS 432

THE GYNECOLOGIC EXAMINATION IN THE ELDERLY PATIENT 432

CANCER SCREENING IN THE ELDERLY 433

DISORDERS OF THE VULVA AND VAGINA 434
Physiologic Changes 434
Skin Disorders 435
Infections and Infestations 436
Cancers 437

DISORDERS OF THE UPPER GENITAL TRACT 438
Physiologic Changes 438
Prolapse 438
Postmenopausal Bleeding 438
Malignancies of the Upper Genital Tract 439

HORMONE REPLACEMENT THERAPY 440
Risks and Benefits 441
Alternative Treatments for Vasomotor Symptoms 441

BREAST DISEASE 442
Lumps 442
Nipple Discharge 442
Breast Infections 442
Paget Disease of the Breast 443
Inflammatory Carcinoma 443
Evaluating a Breast Mass in a Patient at the End of Life 443

CLINICAL PEARLS

- The most common presenting complaint in carcinoma of the vulva is itching.
- Vaginal Candidiasis is less common in post menopausal women than in younger women.
- The most common benign affliction of the female genitalia is contact dermatitis.
- The incidence of breast cancer increases with age. Most women in whom breast cancer is diagnosed have no identifiable risk factors.
- Any vaginal bleeding in an elderly woman requires a diagnosis. Malignancy must be considered because of its life-threatening consequences.

Gynecologic care in the geriatric population presents some challenges not found in younger women. Performing an examination may be more difficult in women who have arthritis or have lost joint mobility or control because of strokes. Recommendations for screening change as women age, and the differential diagnosis for common complaints, such as vaginal itching, change after menopause because estrogen effects are lost. Many gynecologic cancers occur at higher rates in the elderly, and these diagnoses can be easily missed if they are not considered.

THE GYNECOLOGIC EXAMINATION IN THE ELDERLY PATIENT

Although many older women who have had regular pelvic examinations throughout their lives continue to do so without difficulty, some women are fearful of such examinations. The reasons are many and include embarrassment, fear that they may be unclean or smell, that the examination will be painful, that some pathology may be found, and physical limitations to positioning themselves on the table.

It is especially important for physicians working with older women to be aware of these fears and the intimate nature of the gynecologic examination. In the outpatient setting, it is helpful to talk to the patient while she is still dressed and then leave the room while she disrobes. This will give her a chance to bring up questions and concerns in a more dignified setting and may help reduce her embarrassment. The breast examination should not be overlooked because it may be forgotten at other visits. Drapes should be carefully positioned so that the examiner can see the patient's face, to determine whether she is in pain or frightened.

In many elderly women the introitus is narrowed, but the length of the vagina is usually not shortened, so if an alternate-sized speculum is needed, a medium Pederson speculum, which has a narrow blade, may be better than a small Graves speculum, which has a broader, shorter blade.

In patients with physical limitations, alternate positions can be used. A woman with osteoarthritis of the knees or hips will often be unable to flex adequately to move to the bottom of the table to allow room for the speculum handle. Placing her feet in the stirrups helps spread her legs as far as she is able to tolerate. The speculum can then be inserted upside down, so the handle is away from the table and an adequate view of the vagina and cervix can be obtained (see Fig. 32.1). This works best with a plastic speculum with an integrated light source but can also be done with other light sources. Women who are paraplegic or hemiplegic may not be able to position themselves into the stirrups at all. In such cases, the women can be positioned on their side with hips flexed, while an assistant supports the legs. This places the woman's perineum at the end of the table. With the assistant lifting up on the buttocks, the examiner can view the vulva and insert the speculum from behind the patient (see Fig. 32.2).

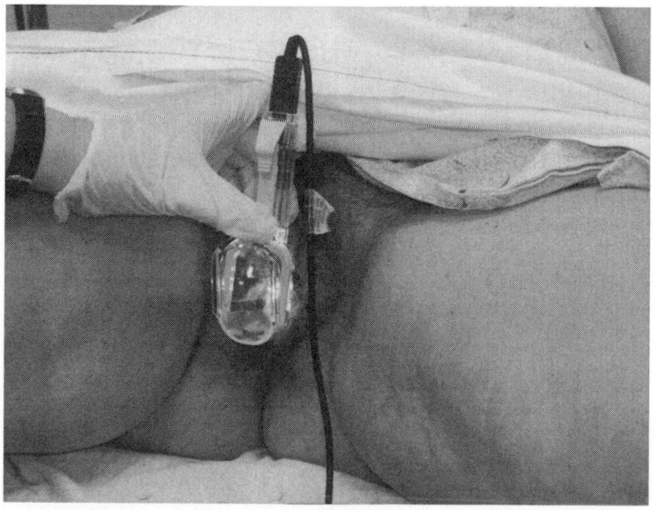

Figure 32.1 When a patient is unable to flex her knees or hips far enough to move to the end of the table, the speculum can be inserted upside down. This works particularly well with a plastic speculum with an internal light source. (Photo by Channa Kolb.)

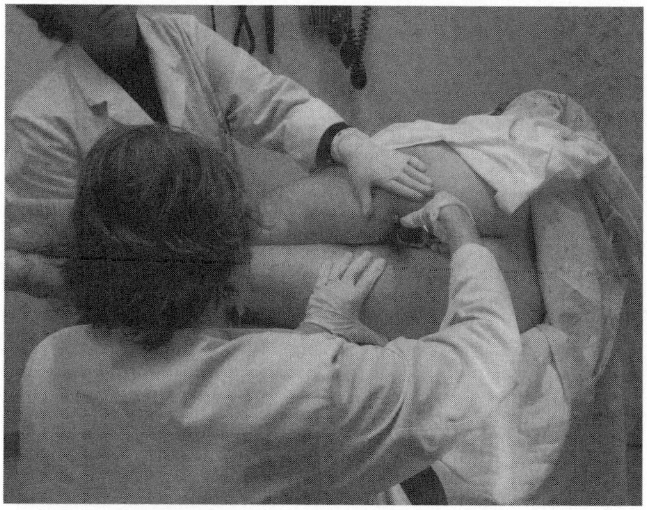

Figure 32.2 Patients unable to use the stirrups because of paraplegia or hemiplegia can be adequately examined in the lateral position from behind with the help of an assistant to support the legs and raise the buttocks. (Photo by Channa Kolb.)

Probably the most difficult patients to examine are those with advanced dementia. These women become confused about who the examiner is and what they are doing. These women are generally examined only when there is a clear indication, and the examination may have to be done under anesthesia.

CANCER SCREENING IN THE ELDERLY

Determining whether a screening intervention is warranted depends, in part, on the effect it will have on the life of the individual. Will intervention during an asymptomatic period reduce morbidity and extend the meaningful quality of life more than waiting until the disease reveals itself by symptoms? Is effective treatment available? Will this particular patient be able to tolerate treatment for disease if it is detected? Preventive medicine in the elderly has been described as a means of maintaining normal aging and preserving the potential for successful aging. Consensus on guidelines for screening have been elusive.

Most guidelines, including those of the American Cancer Society, agree that women older than 70 do not require Papanicolaou (Pap) smears provided they have had three technically satisfactory normal Pap smears within the last 10 years.[1] The U.S. Preventive Services Task Force sets the age at 65. The mortality rate for cervical cancer is more than sixfold higher in women 50 years old and older compared to that in younger women. Because most deaths from cervical cancer occur in women who have not had a Pap smear in the last 5 years, a woman who has not had Pap smears is a candidate for the procedure. Although women whose life expectancy is <5 years are unlikely to benefit from screening Pap smears, a recent study reported high rates of this screening procedure in women older than 75 (79%), and even in those older than 80 (72%).[2] The authors point out that the median life expectancy for women in the United States exceeds 5 years until age 90.

Breast cancer is the most common malignancy among women in the United States (excluding skin cancer). It is the second leading cause of death from cancer in this group (lung cancer is the first). Both incidence and mortality from breast cancer increase with age through age 84. The American Cancer Society recommends clinical breast examination yearly for women after the age of 40. Mammograms are recommended every 1 to 2 years from age 40 to 49, and annually thereafter. An upper age limit has not been defined. Most clinical trials that looked at screening mammography had upper age limit criteria ranging from 64 to 74 years. It has been suggested that medical comorbidity and life expectancy should be considered for women aged 75 or older because the benefit-to-risk ratio of screening mammography continues to shift adversely with advancing age.[3] A meta-analysis concluded that screening mammography in women aged 70 to 79 is moderately cost-effective and yields a small increase in life expectancy. However, there is no consensus recommendation.

DISORDERS OF THE VULVA AND VAGINA

CASE ONE

Mrs. M., who is 70 and married, is being seen for a routine follow-up of her hypertension. Near the end of the visit, she mentions that she has been having some itching "down there" and wonders whether she might have a yeast infection. On further questioning, her physician learns that she has no discharge, and the itching has been present for about 6 months and seems to be getting worse. On physical examination, the skin of the labia minora has a thin, white wrinkled appearance, with some extension onto the labia majora. There are a few excoriated areas. No vaginal discharge is present. A scraping of the involved area for potassium hydroxide (KOH) preparation reveals no fungal elements. Her physician elects to do a punch biopsy to confirm the diagnosis, and starts her on a high-potency steroid ointment. The biopsy confirms lichen sclerosus. The physician explains to Mrs. M. that this is not a yeast infection but a chronic skin condition that will get worse if it is not treated. Because there is an increased risk of vulvar carcinoma in patients with lichen sclerosus of the vulva, the physician makes sure that she knows that it is important for her to come in for regular checkups so the area can be examined and any suspicious lesions biopsied.

As the ovaries age, reduced secretion of estradiol after menopause results in inevitable physical changes in the vulva and vagina of older women. Vaginal atrophy results in a pale, narrow structure. The squamous epithelium is thinner, with less glycogen to interact with lactobacilli. This results in decreased vaginal secretions and a more alkaline pH, which lowers defense mechanisms. The collagen support of the pelvic floor diminishes, which can result in cystocele, rectocele, or vaginal or uterine prolapse.

Symptoms, such as vaginal soreness or vaginal or vulvar itching, occur in this age-group, but the differential is not the same as that in younger women (see Table 32.1).

Physiologic Changes

Atrophic Vaginitis

Decreased estrogen levels after menopause result in many changes in vaginal tissue. There is reduced blood flow, decreased collagen content, and mucosal thinning. The pH is also increased. Many women experience symptoms of vaginal dryness, pruritis, dyspareunia, and soreness. Although oral hormone replacement is effective in treating these symptoms, many women and their physicians are choosing to avoid this option in light of reports of increased risks of breast cancer. Topical estrogen preparations provide effective treatment for women who are symptomatic[4] (Evidence Level A). Several products are available, including conjugated equine estrogen vaginal creams and estradiol vaginal creams, tablets, and rings. Side effects are rare. These products should not be used in women with current breast cancer, undiagnosed vaginal bleeding, or a history of endometrial cancer or thromboembolic disease. They are indicated for short-term treatment. Studies have not been performed to confirm the safety of prolonged use (over 6 months.) In women for whom estrogen is contraindicated, options are limited. For dyspareunia, the use of a water-soluble lubricant should be encouraged. Some women find that topical application of vitamin A and D ointment helps the dryness. Caution should be used when applying lotions to the vulva because some hand lotions contain alcohol or other chemicals that can act as irritants.

Vulvodynia

Vulvodynia is a condition of chronic pain or burning of the vulva with no clear underlying cause. It is often exacerbated by sitting and relieved by lying down. Occult infections should be ruled out. Many women are treated repeatedly for presumed yeast infections with no definitive diagnosis. Bacterial vaginosis does not cause pain, so if a patient reports ongoing pain from repeated episodes of bacterial vaginosis, vulvodynia should be considered. Tricyclic antidepressants are sometimes helpful[5] (Evidence Level C), as well as topical steroid ointments and topical anesthetic creams. Gabapentin has been reported to be effective[6] (Evidence Level B). Sitting on a rubber ring may

TABLE 32.1
SOME CAUSES OF VULVAR OR VAGINAL PRURITIS IN POSTMENOPAUSAL WOMEN

Condition (ICD-9)	Diagnosis	Treatment
Atrophic vaginitis (627.3)	Examination	Topical estrogen
Contact dermatitis (692.9)	Examination, trial of elimination	Remove irritant
Lichen sclerosus (701.0)	Examination, biopsy	Topical steroids
Lichen simplex chronicus (698.3)	Examination, biopsy	Topical steroids
Seborrheic keratosis (702.19)	Examination	Cryotherapy or curettage only if symptomatic
Vulvar carcinoma (184.4)	Examination, biopsy	Surgery
Psoriasis (696.1)	Examination (±biopsy)	Various topical treatments
Bullous pemphigoid (694.5)	Examination, biopsy	Topical steroids, tetracycline, dapsone
Trichomonas (131.01)	Wet mount	Oral metronidazole
Candidiasis (112.1)	KOH preparation	Oral fluconazole (Diflucan) or topical imidazoles
Condyloma accuminata (078.11)	Examination	Destruction by cytotoxic agents or ablation
Pubic lice (132.2)	Examination	Topical 1% permethrin
Scabies (133.0)	Examination, history, ID mite	Topical 5% permethrin
Vulvodynia (625.8)	History	Tricyclic antidepressants, topical anesthetics, gabapentin

KOH, potasium hydroxide; ID, identify.

relieve some of the discomfort. Pelvic floor exercises have been helpful to some women. Referral to a pain clinic may be indicated.

Skin Disorders

Contact Dermatitis

The most common benign affliction of the female genitalia is contact dermatitis, also called *eczematoid* or *irritant dermatitis*. In the geriatric population, common causes include incontinence pads, over-the-counter creams and lotions used to alleviate dryness, detergents, soaps, feminine hygiene sprays, and moisture due to stress or urge incontinence. Also, cleansing the vulva vigorously with a rough washcloth can cause an irritant dermatitis. Women who do self-care should be encouraged to use a mild soap and cleanse the area with their fingers, rinsing it thoroughly and patting dry. If there is some incontinence, pads or undergarments should be changed frequently. The main treatment of contact dermatitis involves identification of the irritant and its removal.

Lichen Sclerosus

Lichen sclerosus is a benign, chronic, progressive dermatologic condition characterized by marked inflammation, epithelial thinning, and distinctive dermal changes (see Fig. 32.3). Although it can develop on any skin surface, more than 85% of cases occur in the anogenital region where it causes pain and itching. Lichen sclerosus usually occurs in postmenopausal women and is one of the most common conditions treated in vulvar clinics. Vulvar pruritis, which is the hallmark of the disease, may be intense. The classical appearance is thin, white wrinkled skin localized to the labia minora and/or labia majora, although the whitening may extend over the perineum and around the anus in a keyhole manner. The vaginal mucosa is not affected. Diagnosis should be confirmed histologically with a biopsy using immunofluorescent staining. There is an increased risk of vulvar malignancy in patients with lichen sclerosus, so the skin of the vulva should be examined at least

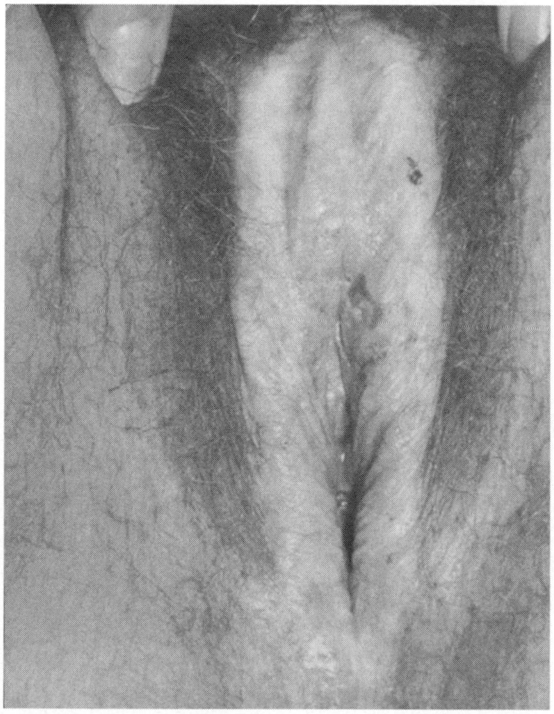

Figure 32.3 Lichen sclerosus of the vulva. (Photo by Flora L Williams, provided courtesy of Dr Wilma F. Bergfeld, Department of Dermatology, Cleveland Clinic.)

yearly. Treatment is recommended for all patients, even if asymptomatic, to prevent the progression of the disease. Untreated, it can lead to shrinkage of the vulvar skin and introital stenosis. Superpotent topical corticosteroids, such as clobetasol[7] (Evidence Level A, randomized controlled trial) or halobetasol propionate 0.05% ointment daily for 6 to 12 weeks and then one to three times per week for maintenance, have been shown to be efficacious. Steroid ointments are preferred over creams because creams may contain irritants not found in ointments. For severe lesions, intralesionsal injections of triamcinolone seem to be effective[8] (Evidence Level B).

Psoriasis

Psoriasis on the vulva may appear as an erythematous patch without scales. Because psoriasis is usually multifocal, the diagnosis is usually made by finding more typical areas on other skin surfaces.

Vulvar Lichen Planus

Lichen planus may be isolated to the vulva or may be part of a generalized skin eruption. It is uncommon but may present with complaints of vaginal or vulvar soreness, pruritis, burning, or dyspareunia. Papulosquamous lichen planus consists of small, intensely pruritic violaceous papules that arise on keratinized and perianal skin. Hypertrophic lichen planus resembles other hypertrophic lesions and may appear similar to squamous cell carcinoma. A biopsy may be needed to make the distinction. Erosive lichen planus presents with bright red erosions with white striae or a white border (Wickham striae) often visible along the margins. Common locations are the labia minora and the vestibule. Vaginal involvement has been reported in up to 70% of patients with erosive lichen planus. These lesions are persistent and resistant to treatment. Lichen planus has been treated with high-dose corticosteroid ointments. Hydrocortisone suppositories are effective for vaginal lichen planus[9] (Evidence Level B). Topical tacrolimus has recently been shown to be safe and effective[10] (Evidence Level B) for lichen planus of the vulva.

Bullous Pemphigoid

Bullous pemphigoid is an uncommon rash and is more likely to be seen in the crural folds than actually on the vulva, but it does present with moderate to severe itching. It may begin with erythematous patches that look like hives. After 1 to 3 weeks, the lesions become dark red as vesicles and bullae appear on their surfaces. Peripheral blood eosinophilia occurs in 50% of patients. Diagnosis is by biopsy. Treatment includes controlling itching with an antihistamine, such as hydroxyzine. Topical steroids and oral antibiotics such as tetracycline, erythromycin, or dapsone are used. Unresponsive cases may require oral steroids.

Infections and Infestations

Candida

The most common symptom of candidiasis is vulvar or vaginal itching. External soreness and dysuria can also occur. Women with diabetes are more susceptible to *Candida* infections, especially if their glucose level is uncontrolled. The loss of estrogen after menopause reduces the glycogen layer in the vaginal mucosa and increases the vaginal pH, making the vagina less hospitable to *Candida*. *Candida* vaginitis is much less common in the geriatric population than it is in younger women. In obese women with moist areas in the crural folds or beneath the pannus, *Candida* can cause an intertrigo that is difficult to eradicate. *Candida* is diagnosed by the finding of branching hyphae on a KOH preparation or by fungal culture. Topical azoles such as butoconazole, clotrimazole, miconazole, terconazole, or tioconazole are the most commonly recommended medications.[11] A single oral dose of fluconazole is recommended by the Centers for Disease Control and Prevention (CDC) for *Candida* vaginitis.[12] Severe cases may require a second dose 3 days later[13] (Evidence Level A).

Trichomonas

The physiologic changes in the genital tract of postmenopausal women make it inhospitable to some sexually transmitted diseases. *Chlamydia* infection and gonorrhea are extremely rare in the geriatric population. *Trichomonas*, on the other hand, tolerates the increased vaginal pH and can be found in older women. This organism may continue to be present in an asymptomatic state for months to years, so it is occasionally seen in women who have recently not been sexually active. When the infestation is heavy, symptoms include irritation, itching, and a profuse, thin vaginal discharge, which may have an odor. In 30% to 60% of women with *Trichomonas* infection, there is a foamy or frothy discharge in the upper vagina. Diagnosis is most commonly made by the visualization of motile trichomonads in a saline wet mount of the vaginal secretions, which is reported as being 60% to 80% sensitive. Culture has high sensitivity (>95%) and specificity (>95%) and should be considered in the presence of elevated numbers of leukocytes and the absence of motile trichomonads or clue cells on the wet mount or when microscopy is unavailable. A deoxyribonucleic acid (DNA) probe is also available and accurate.[14] Trichomonads may be reported on Pap smears, but this is insensitive, and false-positives are common.[15] Liquid-based Pap smears appear to have fewer false-positives.[16] *Trichomonas* infection should be treated even if asymptomatic because it causes a chronic inflammatory state, which may predispose to other infections. Treatment is oral metronidazole. The CDC recommends a single 2-g dose.[12] For recurrent cases, longer courses, such as 500 mg twice a day for 7 days, can be used. The sexual partner should be treated. Topical treatments are ineffective. Tinidazole is an alternative treatment for resistant *Trichomonas*,[11] which is also given orally in a single 2-g dose. Both drugs interact with alcohol, so the patient should be cautioned to avoid any alcohol-containing products while taking the medication, and for 72 hours afterward in the case of tinidazole, which has a longer half-life.

Bacterial Vaginosis

Bacterial vaginosis generally does not cause pain or itching, but it may cause an irritating vaginal discharge and/or an odor. Some women present complaining of a urinary tract infection because they notice the odor when they sit down to void. This condition is not an infection, but a change in the vaginal flora, with an overgrowth of anaerobes, which release aromatic amines, causing the odor in response to an elevated pH. The normal lactobacilli that maintain the vaginal pH disappear. In older women, there are fewer lactobacilli, and the normal vaginal pH is higher than that in women during the child-bearing years. Clinical diagnosis of bacterial vaginosis is made by identifying three of Amsel's criteria, which are (i) a homogeneous or milky discharge, (ii) an increased vaginal pH (>4.5), (iii) a positive whiff test (which is the release of an amine or fishy odor when a few drops of 10% KOH are added to the vaginal secretions), and (iv) >20% of the vaginal epithelial cells on wet mount are clue cells[17] (Evidence Level B). Clue cells are vaginal epithelial cells with edges that appear fuzzy because they are studded with coccobacilli. The elevated vaginal pH criteria is unreliable in the elderly. The gold standard is a Gram stain of vaginal secretions, but this is generally used only in research settings. The recommended treatment for bacterial vaginosis is oral metronidazole 500 mg b.i.d. for 1 week.[12] Alternatives are intravaginal metronidazole gel or clindamycin cream. Oral clindamycin has also been used but may be less effective. A single 2-g dose of metronidazole has been used but has a high recurrence rate.

Pubic Lice (Phthirus Pubis)

Infestations with pubic lice are extremely pruritic. There is an incubation period of approximately 4 weeks. Diagnosis is by the observation of the lice, which are 1 to 2 mm long gray-brown organisms, or nits, which are 0.5-mm brown or white ovoid structures attached to the hair shafts. Excreta may be seen as tiny red dots on the skin among the hair. Recommended treatment is topical, 1% permethrin (Nix) or 4% piperonyl butoxide—0.33% pyrethrins (Rid, Pronto)[18] applied to the affected areas and washed off after 10 minutes. Clothing and bed linens should be washed before reuse. Because of some resistance, the CDC currently recommends a second treatment after 1 week.

Scabies

Scabies is caused by an infestation with *Sarcoptes scabiei*, sometimes called the *itch mite*. After a 4-week incubation period, most patients develop severe pruritis in affected areas, which may be worse at night or after bathing. Scattered red papules may be seen. In the elderly, scabies may present with bullous lesions. If the lesions are misdiagnosed and treated with topical steroids, they become diffusely erythematous and crusted. The diagnosis can be confirmed by demonstrating the presence of the mite from a skin scraping of a papule or burrow or from beneath the fingernails. This is frequently difficult. The female mite has a rounded body with four pairs of legs and is <0.5 mm long. A history of exposure to others with scabies can be helpful in identifying this as the cause of itching. Recommended treatment is permethrin 5% cream (Elimite),[18] applied to all areas of the body from the neck down and washed off after 8 to 14 hours. One percent lindane lotion (Kwell) is an alternative treatment, but there is some resistance against this drug and a danger of neurotoxicity if used inappropriately. Lindane treatment requires a second application a week later. Crotamiton 10% cream (Eurax) has also been used but appears to be less effective. A single oral dose of ivermectin 3 mg (Stromectol) has also been used successfully. The itching may persist for as long as 4 weeks after successful eradication of the mites. Antihistamines may be helpful for symptomatic control of the itching.

Cancers

Carcinomas of the Vulva

More than half of all carcinomas of the vulva occur in women aged 60 to 79 years.[19] Whereas human papilloma virus (HPV) is found in approximately 50% of vulvar carcinomas, HPV-negative tumors are frequently found in older women. Ninety percent of primary vulvar malignancies are squamous cell carcinomas. They usually appear as ulcerated areas or polypoid masses on the vulva. The most common presenting complaint is itching. Carcinoma *in situ* has varying appearances. The classic lesion is scaly with a red background dotted with white, hyperkeratotic islands. Other lesions may be entirely red or white. Diagnosis can only be made by biopsy of suspicious lesions.

Malignant Melanoma

Malignant melanoma is the most common nonsquamous cancer of the vulva. The average age of presentation is 60 years, but it varies widely from 10 to 96 years. The most common locations are on the labia minora and the clitoris. Suspicious lesions should be biopsied early because survival is directly related to the depth of invasion.

Paget Disease

Paget disease of the vulva is an intraepithelial neoplasia. The appearance may vary from moist, oozing ulcerations to exzematoid lesions with scaling and crusting. It may resemble carcinoma *in situ*. Most patients are in their sixties or seventies. The most common presenting complaint is vulvar pruritis or soreness. Unlike mammary disease, which is frequently associated with underlying malignancy, vulvar disease is solely intraepithelial in >90% of cases.[20] However, there is a tendency for local recurrence and rare cases of local malignancy have been reported to follow the initial intraepithelial lesion. Treatment is wide and deep local excision. An association with mammary disease has been reported, so the finding of Paget disease of the vulva should prompt a careful breast examination.

Invasive Epidermoid Carcinoma

The most common invasive neoplasm of the vagina is invasive epidermoid carcinoma. Approximately two thirds of all patients are older than 50. A bloody vaginal discharge is the most common presenting symptom. In some series, vaginal prolapse has been an associated finding.

Bartholin Gland Carcinoma

Enlargement of the Bartholin gland in a postmenopausal woman should raise suspicion of malignancy.

Verrucous Carcinoma

As the name implies, verrucous carcinoma may have a warty appearance. Treatment is wide excision, but recurrences are common. Verrucous carcinoma may be found concurrently with squamous cell carcinoma.

Other Cancers

Many other cancers can occur on the vulva but are rare. These include basal cell carcinoma, neurofibrosarcoma, leiomyosarcoma, fibrosarcoma, lymphoma, and rhabdomyosarcoma. Primary cancers of the vagina are uncommon. Fibrosarcomas and leiomyosarcomas have been reported. The vagina may be involved in malignancies arising from adjacent areas, such as the cervix, rectum, or ovary. Metastases from cancers of the endometrium, uterus, and less commonly, the kidney, breast, or colon may involve the vagina. Postmenopausal bleeding or vaginal discharge may be the presenting complaint.

DISORDERS OF THE UPPER GENITAL TRACT

Physiologic Changes

Without estrogen stimulation, the organs of the female reproductive tract become senescent. The average weight of the ovary declines from 14 g in the fourth decade to approximately 5 g postmenopausally. On bimanual examination, the ovaries are generally not palpable in women older than 60. The uterus becomes smaller. Endocervical glandular tissue becomes less active, and the squamocolumnar junction and transition zone migrate high into the endocervical canal. Cervical erosions and ulcerations become more common, and the incidence of many gynecologic cancers increases.

Prolapse

Pelvic organ prolapse is frequently a result of collagen loss and ligament atrophy in women with postmenopausal estrogen deficiency. Risk factors include multiparity, operative vaginal delivery, obesity, advanced age, estrogen deficiency, neurogenic deficiency of the pelvic floor, connective tissue disorders, prior pelvic surgery with disruption of natural support, and chronically increased abdominal pressure.[21] Cystocele results from the downward displacement of the bladder and anterior vaginal wall. The presence of a cystocele does not predict incontinence. A cystourethrocele is a cystocele combined with distal prolapse of the urethra with or without urethral hypermobility. A rectocele results from the downward displacement of the posterior vaginal wall and the rectum. Uterine prolapse is the descent of the uterus into the lower vagina, or in severe cases, through the vaginal introitus. Enterocele occurs after hysterectomy, with symptoms of bulging in the vagina and low back pain. Symptoms related to prolapse may be relieved by lying down.

Diagnosis of prolapse is by physical examination, which must be done both in the supine (dorsal lithotomy) and standing positions. When evaluating for prolapse, the traditional examination should be supplemented with a site-specific examination of the vagina using either a single-bladed speculum (e.g. Sims speculum) or a Graves speculum taken apart so the blades can be used separately as single-sided retractors. Mild prolapse can be managed with pelvic floor exercises or physical therapy. Women with moderate prolapse and those who are not good surgical candidates are often treated with a pessary, which should be changed monthly to avoid erosions. In addition to preventing progression of prolapse, some women have shown improvement in the stage of prolapse after using a pessary[22] (Evidence Level B). Women with severe prolapse should be referred for surgery.

Postmenopausal Bleeding

The incidence of vaginal bleeding has been reported as 42 per 1,000 person-years >3 years after menopause.

Any vaginal bleeding in an elderly woman requires a diagnosis. Although there are many causes of bleeding other than cancer, malignancy must be ruled out because of its life-threatening consequences. The initial evaluation should include a complete pelvic examination, with Pap smear (if the patient has a cervix) and a pelvic ultrasound. Urinalysis and rectal examination with stool testing for occult blood are helpful in evaluating for bleeding from adjacent structures. Further testing may be suggested by the

TABLE 32.2
CAUSES OF VAGINAL BLEEDING IN ELDERLY WOMEN

Benign causes (ICD-9)
Atrophic vaginitis (627.3), atrophic cervicitis (622.8)
Hormone replacement therapy (962.2)
Polyps (622.7, 219.0)
Trauma (922.4)
Cervicitis, cervical ulcers (616.0)
Endometrial hyperplasia (621.30)
Genital prolapse (618.9)
Leiomyomata uteri (fibroids) (218.9)
Malignant Causes
Endometrial carcinoma (182.0)
Cervical carcinoma (180.9)
Thecal cell tumors of ovary (183.0)
Ovarian cancer (183.0)
Invasive epidermal carcinoma of vagina (184.0)
Adenocarcinoma of the uterus (182.0)
Uterine sarcoma (182.0)
Metastases to vagina from other cancers (198.82)
Nongynecologic Causes
Disease in adjacent organs, hepatic, postradiation

results of the initial screen. Table 32.2 lists some reasons for vaginal bleeding in the elderly woman.

Important elements of the history include duration of the bleeding. Were there any precipitating factors, such as trauma? Are there any associated symptoms, such as pain, fever, weight loss, and change in bowel or bladder habits? What medical problems does the patient have—hepatic, renal, or thyroid disease, or bleeding disorder? On the initial pelvic examination, careful assessment of the vaginal mucosa will rule out injuries due to thinning of the skin from atrophy or trauma. Vaginal carcinoma or metastatic disease to the vagina may be observed. Examination of the cervix for ulcerations or friable lesions is important. A Pap smear should be done, and any visible lesion needs to be biopsied, even if the Pap smear is normal. Palpation of the uterus and ovaries should be included. In addition, a general examination should be done to assess for signs of systemic illness.

Any woman with postmenopausal bleeding in the absence of estrogen replacement therapy must be evaluated for endometrial cancer because age is a significant risk factor for this disorder. Outpatient endometrial biopsy has a high overall accuracy in diagnosing endometrial cancer when the specimen contains enough endometrial tissue for a diagnosis. A positive test result is more accurate for ruling in disease than a negative test result is for ruling it out[23] (Evidence Level A). The Pipelle endometrial biopsy device is more accurate in postmenopausal women than in younger women, with detection rates of 99.6% in this group[24] (Evidence Level A). In women with cervical or vaginal stenosis, an endometrial biopsy may be difficult or impossible. The alternative evaluation is using ultrasound. A recent meta-analysis concluded that using a cut-off of 5 mm for endometrial thickness, a negative result for an ultrasound can reliably rule out endometrial pathology.[25] The ultrasound also evaluates for uterine and ovarian tumors. Management of bleeding depends on the cause that is identified.

CASE TWO

Mrs. S. had not been feeling well for a few months. She was tired and lacked energy and was losing weight, but she said, "What can you expect at 74 years?" What brought her to the office today was that she had been finding blood on her underwear. The bleeding was occurring frequently enough that she had started wearing sanitary napkins. This concerned her. Her history revealed vaginal bleeding intermittently for the past 3 weeks; some vague abdominal discomfort, not really pain; no change in bowel or bladder habits or appetite; and a 10-lb weight loss since her last visit 3 months ago. On physical examination, she is alert and thin. General examination is unremarkable. There are no lesions of the vulva, vagina, cervix, or rectum. The uterus is normal sized and nontender. The left ovary is palpable, the right is not. After obtaining consent, an endometrial biopsy is obtained using a Pipelle. Because the ovary is palpable (they usually are not at this age), her doctor schedules her for a pelvic and transvaginal ultrasound. A few days later, the pathology from the endometrial biopsy is reported as endometrial hyperplasia. The ultrasound shows enlargement of the left ovary, and her family doctor refers her to a gynecologist for further evaluation and treatment. She is taken to surgery and her postoperative diagnosis is thecal cell tumor (thecoma) of the ovary. Disease was confined to the ovary, giving her a good prognosis. Because the tumor produced estrogen, causing endometrial hyperplasia and bleeding, it was found at an earlier stage than many ovarian cancers.

Malignancies of the Upper Genital Tract

Many cancers are more common in women after menopause. The following are some gynecologic cancers that are seen in elderly women.

Endometrial Cancer

Endometrial cancer is the most common gynecologic cancer in the elderly, mostly affecting women in the postmenopausal age-group. It ranks fourth in terms of incident cancers and eighth in terms of age-adjusted mortality. In the United States, rates are higher in whites and Asian women than black women, but black women have higher mortality rates because of presenting more often with regional or distant disease.[26] Risk factors include use of unopposed estrogen, obesity, diabetes, nulliparity, and hypertension. Risk is reduced by combination oral contraceptive pills, smoking, low fat diets, and physical exercise.

Postmenopausal bleeding is the presenting complaint in 75% of patients. At the time of diagnosis, 75% of women have disease confined to the uterus, which has a favorable prognosis. Treatment is surgical for localized disease, followed by radiation if disease is outside the uterus. Women who have been diagnosed with endometrial cancer have an increased risk of developing other cancers including intestinal malignancies, renal cell carcinoma, bladder carcinoma, squamous cell skin carcinoma, connective tissue malignancies, and leukemia.[27]

Cervical Cancer

Worldwide, cervical cancer is the most common gynecologic malignancy. In less-developed areas of the world, this is the cancer that causes the most deaths among women. Incidence rates are three times higher in women aged 50 and older (15.8 per 100,000) than those among younger women, and mortality rates are more than sixfold higher among women older than 50. In elderly women who have never been screened, it may present as an advanced lesion. Highest rates are seen in Vietnamese, Hispanic, Native Alaskan, Korean, and black women. Lowest rates are seen among Japanese and non-Hispanic whites. More than 80% are squamous cell carcinomas. Risk factors include early age at first intercourse, multiple sexual partners, history of sexually transmitted diseases, and cigarette smoking. With advanced disease, symptoms may include an offensive vaginal discharge or post coital or postmenopausal bleeding. Pain is a late sign and is often related to diffuse pelvic infiltration or bone metastases. The presenting sign may be obstructive renal failure. Although high-risk types of HPV, 16 and 18, are frequently associated with cervical cancer, the high prevalence of HPV compared to the incidence of cervical cancer suggests that other cofactors are involved.[28] Treatment is usually radical hysterectomy with pelvic node dissection or radiation therapy.

Ovarian Cancer

Cancer of the ovary is frequently seen in the elderly. The peak incidence is in the fifth and sixth decades. It is the most common fatal gynecologic malignancy. More women die from ovarian cancer than from cervical and uterine cancer combined. The principal reason for the high death rate is the advanced stage of disease at diagnosis in 70% to 75% of cases, with an overall 5-year survival rate of only 20% to 30%. Symptoms tend to be very nonspecific, such as abdominal discomfort, malaise, bloating, fatigue, back pain, weight loss, or weight gain due to ascites. The highest incidence is among white women in northern and western Europe and North America. More than 50% of patients are aged 60 to 79. Ninety percent of ovarian cancers in older women are epithelial adenocarcinomas. Granulosa cell tumors are less common, but up to 60% of these occur after menopause. They may present with vaginal bleeding due to endometrial hyperplasia. Risk for ovarian cancer is increased by exposure to ionizing radiation and a high fat diet. The risk is reduced by a history of oral contraceptive use, the number of live births, and long-term breastfeeding.[29] Women using estrogen-only replacement therapy, particularly for 10 or more years, have been shown to be at significantly increased risk of ovarian cancer[30] (Evidence Level B).

No effective screening for ovarian cancer has been identified. The American College of Obstetrics and Gynecology recommends an annual pelvic examination for preventive health care.[31] CA125 is a tumor-associated antigen that is expressed by approximately 80% of epithelial cell ovarian cancers, but it may also be increased in the presence of other cancers (e.g., pancreatic, breast, bladder, and lung) and in benign disease (e.g., diverticulitis, leiomyoma, endometriosis, benign ovarian cyst, and renal disease). Transvaginal ultrasound has been suggested but has low specificity for ovarian cancer screening, which could result in many women undergoing potentially unnecessary surgery. Further studies are under way to assess the impact of screening on ovarian cancer mortality.[32] A high index of suspicion should be maintained in any postmenopausal woman with ovarian enlargement. Diagnosis is usually confirmed at laparotomy. Treatment is surgical with postoperative chemotherapy. Radiation therapy is usually limited to unresectable, symptomatic recurrence for palliation.

Fallopian Tube Cancer

Fallopian tube cancer is the rarest of the gynecologic cancers, with an incidence of 3.6 cases per million women. The peak incidence is between the age of 60 and 64. Usually a papillary adenocarcinoma, fallopian tube cancer may present as vaginal bleeding, unexplained vaginal discharge, or pelvic pain. A pelvic mass is found in approximately 65% of patients and ascites in 15%. Ultrasound may be helpful in making the diagnosis. Treatment is surgical.

HORMONE REPLACEMENT THERAPY

CASE THREE

Mrs. C., aged 70, came to the office to discuss whether she ought to stop her estrogen therapy, conjugated estrogen (Premarin) 0.625 mg daily, which had been started when she was 58 years old because of severe hot flashes. She had a hysterectomy at age 40 because of heavy bleeding from fibroids. She read an article in the newspaper about an increased risk of breast cancer in women who were taking hormones. A second cousin was recently diagnosed with breast cancer at age 80, and this raised her concern. She had tried to stop the estrogen once in the past, but her hot flashes had returned, and she was concerned that it might happen again. Her physician reviewed the evidence with her, explaining that the use of unopposed estrogen did not seem to significantly increase the risk of breast cancer but that there was an increased risk of stroke. This patient was a slender woman with osteoporosis, and estrogen does have some benefit in reducing the rate of fractures in women with osteoporosis. After their discussion, the patient and her doctor together decided to continue the estrogen for now, but to lower the dose to 0.3 mg a day and consider discontinuing it if her hot flashes did not return.

Risks and Benefits

For many years, hormone replacement therapy has been widely used on the basis of evidence from observational and animal studies suggesting that estrogen replacement was associated with increased survival in women with coronary artery disease and decreased risk of death from breast and colon cancer, as well as reduction in osteoporotic fracture risk. With reports of the prospective randomized studies of the Women's Health Initiative (WHI), recommendations have changed. The WHI studied women aged 50 to 79 years (average age 63 years). The combined estrogen and progesterone arm of the study was stopped after 5.2 years because of an increased breast cancer risk (relative risk 1.24, confidence interval 1.01 to 1.54) and increased rate of cardiovascular events, including stroke, coronary heart disease, and venous thromboembolic events. There was a significant decrease in fractures and a nonsignificant decrease in colon cancer[33] (Evidence Level A).

The estrogen-alone trial, which studied women who had previous hysterectomies, was projected for 9 years and was stopped after 6.8 years because of increased risk of stroke and the finding of no significant cardiovascular protection. The researchers did not identify any increased risk of breast cancer in this group. There was a significant increase in venous thromboembolism in the treated group, and total fracture rate was significantly decreased[34] (Evidence Level A).

In the WHI memory study, which looked at women aged 65 and older, there was an increased probability of dementia in the hormone-treated group, indicating that hormone replacement therapy did not confer the expected cognitive benefit[35] (Evidence Level A).

Hormone replacement therapy reduces hot flashes and other vasomotor symptoms and is the only U.S. Food and Drug Administration (FDA)—approved treatment for this indication. Some authors have recommended using estrogen and progestin treatment for this indication in women with a uterus, but stopping it within 5 years, if possible, because of the increased risks. In women without a uterus, estrogen alone can be used, but the patients should be aware that they are at increased risk for stroke. They point out that although both regimens confer fracture protection, this benefit does not outweigh the risk for most women.[36]

Not everyone agrees with the conclusions drawn from the WHI data. It has been pointed out that the increased risk of breast cancer did not reach statistical significance and that the absolute risk of breast cancer remains small.[37] The Medical Association of Clinical Endocrinologists has issued a statement that menopausal hormone therapy considerations must be individualized and that, in the absence of contraindications, hormone therapy remains appropriate for moderate to severe vasomotor symptoms associated with estrogen deficiency.

Alternative Treatments for Vasomotor Symptoms

The average age at menopause is 51 years (range 45 to 55). Given an increasing life expectancy, many women can be expected to spend one third to one half of their lives in the postmenopausal years. Hot flashes are the most debilitating symptom. More than 75% of women experience hot flashes during menopause and >25% remain symptomatic for >5 years. Hormone replacement therapy is the most effective treatment, but for women who have contraindications or have decided against estrogen therapy, other options are available.

Progestins alone can provide relief from menopausal symptoms. Megestrol acetate, depomedroxyprogesterone acetate, and transdermal estrogen cream have all been studied and result in an 80% to 90% reduction in hot flashes. Side effects include vaginal bleeding, weight gain, mood changes, and breast discomfort.[38] Some antidepressants may be useful. Venlafaxine (Effexor) produced 37% to 61% reduction in hot flashes in a randomized controlled trial[39] (Evidence Level A). Another randomized controlled trial showed a 50% reduction in hot flashes with fluoxetine (Prozac)[40] (Evidence Level A). An almost 65% reduction was reported with controlled-release paroxetine (Paxil-CR), but some women experienced gastrointestinal (GI) upset, headache, or sexual dysfunction[41] (Evidence Level A). Also, there is a potential drug interaction with tamoxifen that should be kept in mind. Paroxetine inhibits the CYP2D6 enzyme system, which is necessary to convert tamoxifen to an active metabolite, endoxifen. Use of the two together results in reduced levels of endoxifen, which may reduce the effectiveness of tamoxifen in preventing the recurrence of breast cancers[42] (Evidence Level B). Some other selective serotonin reuptake inhibitors, fluoxetine, sertraline, and fluvoxamine, have also been shown to inhibit CYP2D6, but not as potently as paroxetine. Gabapentin (Neurontin) at a dose of 900 mg was associated with a 45% reduction in hot flashes.[43] (Evidence Level A). Clonidine and methyldopa have been used, but have high rates of side effects. Selective estrogen receptor modulators, such as raloxifene, have no beneficial effect and may make the hot flashes worse.

There is limited safety and efficacy data on the use of dietary supplements for vasomotor symptoms. Phytoestrogens, especially isoflavones, have been thought to have potential because of their estrogenic activity, but little data are available. The clinical data on soy isoflavones are conflicting. Only three studies went beyond 16 weeks, and all three failed to show benefit. In addition, long-term use of soy supplements has been reported to induce endometrial hyperplasia[44] (Evidence Level A). Black cohosh is one of the most popular supplements used for menopausal symptoms. Published studies have yielded mixed results. Mild GI side effects may be self-limiting. Overdose can cause dizziness, tremors, headache, nausea, and vomiting. There have been case reports of hepatic failure with black cohosh, but causality has not been established. Dietary supplements derived from red clover have not been studied extensively. There are no data on safety or efficacy beyond 3 months. Vitamin E may be of some benefit, but data are lacking. It appears to be safe.

BREAST DISEASE

Lumps

More than 25% of breast abnormalities in women aged 50 to 70 are described as a breast mass. In the general population, only 10% of women presenting with breast masses are found to have cancer, but this risk increases in the older population. After age 30, there is a steep increase in the incidence of breast cancer. Except for a plateau between the age of 45 and 55, the incidence continues to increase with age. The risk of a woman aged 30 to 40 being diagnosed with breast cancer is 1 in 257. At age 70 to 80, this risk is 1 in 24. Most women in whom breast cancer is diagnosed have no identifiable risk factors. A thorough breast examination should be included in every woman's annual physical. Most breast tumors, particularly cancerous ones, are asymptomatic and are discovered only by physical examination or screening mammography. Any mass within the breast of a patient older than 65 years has a high likelihood of being malignant.

There are many potential causes of breast masses that are not cancers. Some of these include cysts (less common in older women), fibroadenomas, infections, benign nonproliferative lesions, and fat necrosis following trauma. However, every palpable mass must be evaluated to rule out invasive carcinoma. When a mass is identified on examination, the patient should be sent for a diagnostic mammogram. This differs from a screening mammogram in that it is interpreted individually and may include extra views of the involved area. This can help characterize the mass and document the extent of the lesion and any associated lesions. If a suspicious mass is palpable on examination but does not show up on a mammogram, it should still be biopsied.[45] Ultrasound can sometimes be helpful in distinguishing solid from cystic lesions. If the lesion is a simple cyst, aspiration may be all that is necessary. In the case of a solid lesion, when there is any question of malignancy, it is best to proceed to biopsy. Depending on the size, location, and nature of the lesion, this could be done by fine needle aspiration, core biopsy, or excision.

Nipple Discharge

Advancing age is associated with an increased risk of cancer in patients presenting with nipple discharge. In women younger than 40 years with a nonphysiologic discharge, <3% have malignancies; in women from 40 to 60 years old, the number rises to 10%; and in women older than 60 years, 37% presenting with a nonphysiologic nipple discharge have a malignancy. Physiologic nipple discharge, which is usually bilateral, milky, from multiple ducts, and not spontaneous, is uncommon in older women. Causes may be endocrine abnormalities, hyperprolactinemia, or drug side effects. Nonphysiologic discharge is usually unilateral, may be from a single duct, may be spontaneous, and serous, serosanguinous, sanguinous, multicolored, or purulent. The differential in postmenopausal women includes papillomas, duct ectasias, nonlactational infection, ductal carcinoma *in situ*, and invasive cancer. A careful physical examination should be done, searching for underlying breast masses and eliciting the discharge to determine whether it is from a single duct or multiple ducts and observe the nature of the discharge. The discharge can be tested for occult blood. Some clinicians send the discharge for cytology by moving a glass slide across a drop of the discharge on the nipple then spraying it with Pap smear fixative. This is not used much because of the low sensitivity (35% to 67%). The patient is generally referred to a breast surgeon for a duct excision, which is both diagnostic and therapeutic.

Breast Infections

Breast infections most commonly present as cellulitis or abscesses, with tenderness, fluctuance, erythema, induration, and less frequently, breast swelling. In some cases there may be fever and leukocytosis, lymphadenopathy, and a mass. Infections are commonly mixed, involving aerobes and anaerobes. Common organisms reported are *Staphylococcus aureus, Staphylococcus epidermidis, Proteus mirabilis, Peptostreptococcus* species, *Bacteroides* species, and *Pseudomonas aeruginosa*.

Large abscesses (>3 cm) benefit from prompt surgical drainage. Patients with smaller abscesses can often be aspirated and treated as an outpatient with oral antibiotics, such as amoxicillin/clavulanate or clindamycin. If a mass or induration persists, the patient should be evaluated for the possibility of an inflammatory carcinoma with an incisional biopsy of indurated tissue.

Candida infection is common on the underside of the breast, where it rests against the chest wall. It is usually bilateral and presents as red, weeping tissue in the inframammary fold. Diagnosis can be confirmed with a KOH smear of a skin scraping examined for fungal elements or by fungal culture. Treatment is with topical antifungals and the emphasis is on keeping the area clean and dry.

Other causes of breast infection are rare and are more likely to be seen in patients who are immunocompromised. These include *Mycobacterium tuberculosis*, which can present with recurrent abscesses with sinus formation or an ill-defined mass. Fungal infections such as actinomycosis, blastomycosis, histoplasmosis, sporotrichosis, and coccidiomycosis can affect the breast. Most fungal infections present as ill-defined masses with associated lymphadenopathy, although actinomycosis has been reported to mimic inflammatory breast disease. Parasitic diseases, leprosy, and syphilis can also affect the breast, the latter presenting as chancres or gummas.

Paget Disease of the Breast

The peak age of onset of Paget disease of the breast is between 50 and 60, but cases have been reported in patients from 26 to 88 years old. It presents as a lesion that appears similar to eczema on the nipple and areola. It is associated with underlying breast cancer in 97% of cases, which present with or without a palpable mass or mammographic abnormality. Because of this, treatment has traditionally been mastectomy. Studies are under way evaluating breast-conserving therapy with radiation as an alternative treatment.

Inflammatory Carcinoma

Inflammatory carcinoma has the appearance of acute inflammation with redness and edema. There may be no distinct palpable mass because the tumor infiltrates through the breast with no distinct margins, or there may be a dominant mass. This cancer is usually treated with chemotherapy and radiation. The peak age of onset is 50; it then plateaus.

Evaluating a Breast Mass in a Patient at the End of Life

When a woman is terminally ill, or has a limited life expectancy, she may choose to refuse diagnostic or therapeutic surgical procedures, chemotherapy, or radiation. Although as physicians, we are trained to try to prolong life, there may be times when it is appropriate to allow the patient to choose quality of life over prolonging it with procedures or treatments that will make her uncomfortable or weaker than she already is. Tamoxifen has been used for palliative treatment in women with a short life expectancy. A comparison of surgery plus tamoxifen versus tamoxifen alone found that morbidity and mortality were significantly higher in the tamoxifen-alone group, but the curves did not diverge for the first 3 years[46] (Evidence Level A). In a woman with a short life expectancy or who is unable to tolerate surgery, tamoxifen may be a reasonable choice. If the patient has capacity to decide, or if she has clearly made her wishes known to a health care proxy, the physician should respect her right to refuse treatment and support her with comfort care during the time that she has left.

REFERENCES

1. Saaslow D, Runowicz CD, Solomon D, et al. American Cancer Society Guidelines for the early detection of cervical neoplasia and cancer. *CA Cancer J Clin*. 2002;52:342–362.
2. Walter LC, Lindquist K, Covinsky KE. Relationship between health status and use of screening mammography and Papanicolaou smears among women older than 70 years of age. *Ann Intern Med*. 2004;140:681–688.
3. ACOG. ACOG practice bulletin: Breast cancer screening. *Obstet Gynecol*. 2003;101:821–831.
4. Nothnagle M, Taylor JS. Vaginal estrogens for relief of atrophic vaginitis. *Am Fam Physician*. 2004;69:2111–2112.
5. Davis GD, Hitchison CV. Clinical management of vulvodynia. *Clin Obstet Gynecol*. 1999;42:221–233.
6. Ben-David B, Friedman M. Gabapentin therapy for vulvodynia. *Anesth Analg*. 1999;89:1459–1460.
7. Bracco GL, Carli P, Sonni L, et al. Clinical and histologic effects of topical treatments of vulvar lichen sclerosus. A critical evaluation. *J Reprod Med*. 1993;38:37–40.
8. Mazdisnian F, Degregorio F, Palmieri A. Intralesional injection of triamcinolone in the treatment of lichen sclerosus. *J Reprod Med*. 1999;44:332–334.
9. Anderson M, Kutzner S, Kaufman RH. Treatment of vulvovaginal lichen planus with vaginal hydrocortisone suppositories. *Obstet Gynecol*. 2002;100:359–362.
10. Byrd JA, Davis MD, Rogers RS 3rd. Recalcitrant symptomatic vulvar lichen planus: Response to topical tacrolimus. *Arch Dermatol*. 2004;140:715–720.
11. Drugs for sexually transmitted infections. *Treat Guidel Med Lett*. 2004;2:67–74.
12. Centers for Disease Control and Prevention. Sexually transmitted diseases treatment guidelines 2002. *MMWR*. 2002;51:RR6.
13. Sobel JD, Kapernick PS, Zervos M, et al. Treatment of complicated Candida vaginitis: Comparison of single and sequential doses of fluconazole. *Am J Obstet Gynecol*. 2001;185:363–369.
14. DeMeo LR, Draper DL, McGregor JA, et al. Evaluation of a deoxyribonucleic acid probe for the detection of *Trichomonas vaginalis* in vaginal secretions. *Am J Obstet Gynecol*. 1996;174:1339–1342.
15. Krieger JN, Tam MR, Stevens CE, et al. Diagnosis of Trichomoniasis, comparison of conventional wet mount examination with cytologic studies, cultures, and monoclonal antibody staining of direct specimens. *JAMA*. 1988;259:1223–1227.
16. Lara-Torre E, Pinkerton JS. Accuracy of detection of *Trichomonas vaginalis* organisms on a liquid-based Papanicolaou smear. *Am J Obstet Gynecol*. 2003;188:354–356.
17. Amsel R, Totten PA, Speigel CA, et al. Nonspecific vaginitis. Diagnostic criteria and microbial and epidemiologic associations. *Am J Med*. 1983;74:14–22.
18. Flinders DC, DeSchweinitz P. Pediculosis and scabies. *Am Fam Physician*. 2004;69:341–348.
19. Rotmensch J, Yamada SD. Neoplasms of the vulva and vagina. In: Kulfe DW, Pollock RE, Weichselbaum RK, et al. eds. *Cancer Medicine 6*. Hamilton, Ont: BC Decker; 2003:1769–1777.
20. Di Saia P. Vulvar and vaginal disease. In: Scott JR, Di Saia PJ, Hammond CB, et al. eds. *Danforth's obstetrics and gynecology*, 8th ed. Philadelphia, PA: Lippincott Williams & Wilkins; 1999:779–804.
21. Kohli N, Goldstein DP. *Overview of the clinical manifestations, diagnosis, and classification of pelvic organ prolapse*. www.UptoDate.com, accessed 12/4/2004, 2004.
22. Handa VL, Jones M. Do pessaries prevent the progression of pelvic organ prolapse? *Int Urogynecol J*. 2002;13:349–351.
23. Clark TJ, Mann CH, Shah N, et al. Accuracy of outpatient endometrial biopsy in the diagnosis of endometrial cancer: A systematic quantitative review. *Brit J Obstet Gynaec*. 2002;109:313–321.
24. Dijkhuizen FP, Mol BW, Brolmann HA, et al. The accuracy of endometrial sampling in the diagnosis of patients with endometrial carcinoma and hyperplasia: A meta analysis. *Cancer*. 2000;89:1765–1772.
25. Gupta JK, Chien PF, Voit D, et al. Ultrasonographic endometrial thickness for diagnosing endometrial pathology in women with postmenopausal bleeding: A meta analysis. *Acta Obstet Gyn Scand*. 2002;81:799–816.

26. Purdie DM, Green AC. Epidemiology of endometrial cancer. *Best Pract Res Clin Obstet Gynecol.* 2001;15:341–354.
27. Hemminki K, Aaltonen L, Li X. Subsequent primary malignancies after endometrial carcinoma and ovarian carcinoma. *Cancer.* 2003;97:2432–2439.
28. Jhringran A, Eifal PJ, Wharton JT, et al. Neoplasms of the cervix. In: Kufe DW, Pollack RE, Weichselbaum RK, et al. eds. *Cancer Medicine 6.* Hamilton, Ont: BC Becker; 2003:1779–1809.
29. Goodman MT, Howe HL. Descriptive epidemiology of ovarian cancer in the United States, 1992–1997. *Cancer.* 2003;97(Suppl 10):2615–2630.
30. Lacey JV Jr, Mink PJ, Lubin JH, et al. Menopausal hormone replacement therapy and risk of ovarian cancer. *JAMA.* 2002; 288:334–341.
31. ACOG Committee on Gynecologic Practice. The role of the generalist obstetrician-gynecologist in the early detection of ovarian cancer. *Obstet Gynecol.* 2002;100:1413–1416.
32. Menon U. Ovarian cancer screening. *CMAJ.* 2004;171: 323–324.
33. Rossouw JE, Anderson GL, Prentice RL, et al. Risks and benefits of estrogen plus progestin in healthy postmenopausal women: Principle results from the Women's Health Initiative randomized controlled trial. *JAMA.* 2002;288:321–333.
34. Anderson GL, Limacher M, Assaf AR, et al. Effects of conjugated equine estrogen in postmenopausal women with hysterectomy: The Women's Health Initiative randomized controlled trial. *JAMA.* 2004;291:1701–1712.
35. Shumaker SA, Legault C, Rapp JR, et al. Estrogen plus progestin and the incidence of dementia and mild cognitive impairment in post menopausal women: The Women's Health Initiative Memory Study: A randomized controlled trial. *JAMA.* 2003; 289:2651–2662.
36. Aubuchon M, Santoro N. Lessons learned from the WHI: HRT requires a cautious and individual approach. *Geriatrics.* 2004; 59:22–26.
37. Bluming AZ. Hormone replacement therapy: The debate should continue. *Geriatrics.* 2004;59:30–37.
38. Miller RG, Ashar BH. Managing menopause: Current therapeutic options for vasomotor symptoms. *Adv Stud Med.* 2004;4:484–492.
39. Loprinzi CI, Kugler JW, Maillard JA, et al. Venlafaxine in the management of hot flashes in survivors of breast cancer: A randomized, controlled trial. *Lancet.* 2000;356:2059–2063.
40. Loprinzi CI, Sloan JA, Perez EA, et al. Phase III evaluation of fluoxetine for treatment of hot flashes. *J Clin Oncol.* 2002;20:1578–1583.
41. Stearns V, Beebe KI, Iyengar M, et al. Paroxetine controlled release in the treatment of menopausal hot flashes. *JAMA.* 2003; 289:2827–2834.
42. Stearns V, Johnson MD, Rae JM, et al. Active tamoxifen metabolite concentrations after coadministration of tamoxifen and the selective serotonin reuptake inhibitor paroxetine. *J Natl Cancer Inst.* 2003;95:1758–1764.
43. Guttso T Jr, Kurlan R, McDermott MP, et al. Gabapentin's effects on hot flashes in postmenopausal women: A randomized, controlled trial. *Obstet Gynecol.* 2003;101:337–345.
44. Unfer V, Casini MI, Constable I, et al. Endometrial effects of long term treatment with phytoestrogens: A randomized, double blind, placebo controlled study. *Fertil Steril.* 2004;82:145–148.
45. Smith-Bindman R. Diagnostic imaging in the differential diagnosis of vaginal bleeding and breast mass. *Adv Stu Med.* 2004; 4:476–482.
46. Fennessy M, Bates T, MacRae K. Late follow-up of a randomized trial of surgery plus tamoxifen versus tamoxifen alone in women aged over 70 years with operable breast cancer. *Brit J Surg.* 2004; 91:699–704.

33

Diabetes and Thyroid Disorders in the Elderly

Sara E. Young   *Richelle J. Koopman*   *Arch G. Mainous III*

CLINICAL PEARLS 445

DIFFERENTIAL DIAGNOSIS 446

TYPE 2 DIABETES MELLITUS 446
Description/Definition of Problem 446
Pathophysiology 446
Systems Impacted 447
Prevalence 447
Genetics 447
Signs and Symptoms 447
Course/Timeline 447
Risk Factors 447
Workup/Keys to Diagnosis 448
Management 448
Cardiovascular Disease 449
Peripheral Arterial Disease 449
Retinopathy 450
Nephropathy 450
Foot Care/Neuropathy 450
Diabetes Education 451
Influenza and Pneumococcal Immunization 451
Lifestyle Recommendations 451
Medications 452
Alternative or Integrative Medicine 454
Comorbidity Concerns 455
Hypertension 455
Dyslipidemia 456

THYROID DISEASE 456
Hypothyroidism 457
Hyperthyroidism 459

CLINICAL PEARLS

- Healthy elderly patients with diabetes should be encouraged to achieve the same glycemic, lipid, and blood pressure goals as younger patients.
- Elderly patients with diabetes mellitus are at increased risk for cardiovascular disease.
- Diet, exercise, and pharmacologic therapy recommendations for elderly patients with diabetes must be made in the context of decreased functional status, comorbidity, and polypharmacy.
- Use of angiotensin-converting enzyme (ACE) inhibitors or angiotensin II receptor blockers (ARBs) should be considered for individuals with diabetes with evidence of microalbuminuria and/or hypertension.
- Depression is a common comorbid condition of diabetes and unrecognized depression can interfere with diabetes care in older patients.
- With normal aging, the thyroid gland becomes more nodular, with 90% of women over age 80 having nodules.
- Subclinical hypothyroidism becomes increasingly common in older women.
- Amiodarone can precipitate hyperthyroidism, although hypothyroidism is more common.
- Cardiac disease is an important consideration in the treatment of older patients with hypo- or hyperthyroidism.
- Symptoms of thyroid disease are subtle and may mimic other diseases in older populations with multiple medical problems.

Endocrine disease is common in the elderly. Recent estimates suggest that at least 20% of patients over the age of 65 have diabetes. Elderly patients with diabetes have higher rates of premature death, functional disability, and comorbid illnesses such as hypertension, congestive heart disease, and stroke compared to those without diabetes. Similarly, thyroid disease in the elderly is approximately twice that in younger individuals. Because of the morbidity associated with thyroid disease, the U.S. Preventive Services Task Force suggests that clinicians should be aware of subtle signs of thyroid dysfunction in the elderly.

Some characteristics of aging complicate diagnosis and management. Elderly patients with hypothyroidism are more likely than younger patients to present with cardiovascular symptoms or neurologic findings, thereby contributing to difficulties in diagnosis. With aging, lean body mass decreases and body fat increases, whereas decreased physical activity is common, all of which play a role in insulin resistance. Because elderly patients often have multiple diseases and take many medications that often mimic or mask the usual presentation of endocrine disease, diagnosis and management become more complex. Moreover, the care of older adults with diabetes and thyroid disease is complicated by their clinical and functional heterogeneity.

DIFFERENTIAL DIAGNOSIS

The differential diagnosis of endocrine disorders is discussed in Table 33.1.

CASE ONE

Mrs. M. is a 68-year-old who comes to your office for follow-up of hypertension. She is obese and has not lost weight despite your advice on diet and exercise at her last visit. She complains of fatigue over the last 2 months. On further questioning, she has noted blurring of vision and vaginal itching without polyuria. She has a blood pressure of 142/93 mm Hg and a normal examination except for vaginal candidiasis. You order a fasting plasma glucose, which is 148 mg per dL. A second fasting plasma glucose of 164 mg per dL confirms your suspicions that Mrs. M. has developed diabetes mellitus.

TABLE 33.1
PARTIAL LIST OF ENDOCRINE DISORDERS (ICD-9)

Pituitary and Neurohypophyseal Disorders

Acromegaly (253.0)
Panhypopituitarism (253.2)
Pituitary dwarfism (253.3)
Hyperprolactinemia (253.1)
Diabetes insipidus (253.5)
Syndrome of inappropriate antidiuretic hormone (253.6)

Thyroid Disorders

Simple Goiter, unspecified (240.0)[a]
Nontoxic uninodular goiter (241.0)
Nontoxic multinodular goiter (241.1)
Toxic diffuse goiter (242.00)
Toxic uninodular goiter (242.1)[a]
Toxic multinodular goiter (242.2)[a]
Hyperthyroidism (242.90)[a]
Hypothyroidism, postablative (244.1)[a]
Hypothyroidism, postsurgical (244.0)[a]
Hypothyroidism, unspecified (244.9)[a]
Thyroid cyst (246.2)
Thyroiditis, acute (245.0)[a]
Thyroiditis, chronic, Hashimoto (245.2)[a]
Thyroiditis, subacute (245.1)[a]
Euthyroid sick syndrome (790.94)

Adrenal Disorders

Cushing syndrome (255.0)
Hyperaldosteronism (255.1)
Adrenogenital disorders (255.2)
Corticoadrenal insufficiency (255.4)
Pheochromocytoma (255.6)

Disorders of Carbohydrate Metabolism

Diabetes 1, uncomplicated (250.01)
Diabetes 1, uncontrolled (250.03)
Diabetes 2, without complications, controlled (250.00)
Diabetes 2, without complications, uncontrolled (250.02)
Diabetes 2, with unspecified complications (250.90)
Hypoglycemia, diabetes 1 (250.81)
Hypoglycemia, diabetes 2 (250.80)

Other Endocrine Disorders

Multiple endocrine neoplasia syndromes (258.0)
Carcinoid syndrome (259.3)

[a]Topics covered in this chapter.

TYPE 2 DIABETES MELLITUS

Description/Definition of Problem

Type 2 diabetes mellitus is a common, potentially debilitating condition characterized by hyperglycemia and insulin resistance. The discussion is limited to type 2 diabetes because type 1 diabetes, although important, is not commonly seen in the geriatric population.

Pathophysiology

Type 2 diabetes is largely a defect of the action of insulin at the level of the cell. The disease is characterized by high levels of circulating insulin and relative resistance to the action of insulin. Obesity plays an important role in the development of type 2 diabetes; obesity itself, and especially obesity in the abdominal region, leads to some degree of insulin resistance. β-Cell destruction and ketoacidosis are not prominent features of type 2 diabetes. Ketoacidosis in the elderly patient with hyperglycemia should initiate a search for other causes of acidosis, such as lactic acidosis when used with metformin.

Prior to the onset of clinical diabetes, patients may be diagnosed with one of the two defined prediabetes conditions: Impaired fasting glucose (IFG) and impaired glucose tolerance (IGT). IFG is defined as a fasting plasma glucose from 100 mg per dL (5.6 mmol per L) to 125 mg per dL (6.9 mmol per L). IGT is defined as a 2-hour plasma glucose from 140 mg per dL (7.8 mmol per L) to 199 mg per dL (11.0 mmol per L) in the course of a glucose tolerance test.[1] People with insulin resistance are at approximately a fivefold risk for diabetes, but this risk can be modified by modest weight loss and lifestyle modifications.

Systems Impacted

Elderly patients are at risk for many of the long-term complications of type 2 diabetes including cardiovascular disease (CVD), nephropathy and end-stage renal disease, peripheral vascular disease, neuropathy, and retinopathy and blindness. CVD is the primary cause of morbidity and mortality for patients with type 2 diabetes. In addition to being an independent risk factor for CVD, diabetes also tends to coexist with other risk factors for CVD, specifically hypertension and hyperlipidemia. When combined with the decreased sensation of diabetic neuropathy, the poor healing associated with peripheral vascular disease puts the elderly person with diabetes at a 10-fold risk for amputation.

These complications of type 2 diabetes have important consequences for the geriatric patient. Activities of daily living can be severely impacted by decreased exercise tolerance associated with heart disease. Joint deformity and amputation associated with peripheral neuropathy and peripheral vascular disease can further limit mobility as well as stability of gait. Additionally, the decreased visual sensation of retinopathy and decreased peripheral sensation of neuropathy may isolate the elderly patient and pose important safety risks, including falls. Poor vision, the result of diabetic retinopathy, may also complicate the ability to read medication bottles, read blood glucose meters, or correctly use insulin injections.

Type 2 diabetes has also been linked to cognitive decline in older persons. The changes in functional and cognitive status of the older patient must be assessed and integrated into the management plan. Urinary incontinence is also an important consequence of diabetes in older persons. Urinary incontinence may be multifactorial in its origin and the clinician should consider the contributions of polyuria associated with poor glycemic control, neurogenic bladder, cystocele and atrophic vaginitis in women, urinary tract infections, and vaginal candidiasis associated with poor glycemic control.

Older persons are at greater risk than younger persons with type 2 diabetes for nonketotic hyperglycemic–hyperosmolar coma. This dangerous and potentially life-threatening complication is largely the result of uncontrolled hyperglycemia in combination with inadequate fluid intake. Neglected or undiagnosed diabetes may be an important factor in the development of this complication, but infection or newly prescribed drugs that affect glucose tolerance can also be predisposing factors, especially for elders who live alone or in institutional settings.

Prevalence

Type 2 diabetes is equally prevalent in men and women. The risk for type 2 diabetes increases with age. The combined prevalence of diagnosed type 1 and type 2 diabetes among those aged 60 and older increased from 12.7% (1988 to 1994) to 15.2% (1999 to 2000).[2] Undiagnosed diabetes was estimated to affect an additional 4.2% of Americans aged 60 and older during 1999 to 2000; an additional 14.6% had IFG.[3]

Genetics

A family history of type 2 diabetes is a risk factor for the development of diabetes. Currently it is thought that there are many different causes of type 2 diabetes, and its genetic basis is likely also multifactorial.

Signs and Symptoms

Type 2 diabetes tends to progress from an asymptomatic stage to overt symptoms. However, when symptoms do begin to occur, they may be vague and nonspecific and, therefore, may not trigger recognition in either the patient or their physician. Hyperglycemia results in a catabolic state that may cause weight loss and fatigue. Patients may also experience the classic "polys" of polydipsia, polyuria, and polyphagia, although these symptoms also may be subtle. Prolonged hyperglycemia may also result in increased susceptibility to infection, including both bacterial and monilial skin infections, and vaginal candidiasis in women.

Course/Timeline

Type 2 diabetes typically has an insidious onset, with a prolonged preclinical period before the disease is detected. The time from onset of type 2 diabetes to clinical diagnosis has been estimated to last an average of 9 to 12 years. Additionally, patients likely pass from normal glucose tolerance through several years in the prediabetic states of IGT and IFG and on to type 2 diabetes.

Complications of type 2 diabetes accrue with the duration of the disease, although their development can have quite a variable course. In general, diabetes needs to be present for approximately 10 years before patients begin to have its complications. However, because there may be a delay of diagnosis for many years, in certain cases, complications may begin to appear soon after diagnosis.

Risk Factors

There are a variety of risk factors for type 2 diabetes. The major risk factors for type 2 diabetes that have been suggested for clinicians by the American Diabetes Association (ADA) are the following:[1]

Age ≥45 years
Overweight (BMI ≥25 kg per m^2)

Family history of diabetes in a parent or sibling
Habitual physical inactivity
Race/ethnicity (nonwhite)
Previously identified IFG or IGT
History of gestational diabetes mellitus of delivery of a baby weighing >9 lbs
Hypertension ($\geq$140/90 mm Hg)
High-density lipoprotein (HDL) cholesterol $\leq$35 mg per dL (0.90 mmol per L)
Triglyceride level $\geq$250 mg per dL
Polycystic ovary syndrome
History of vascular disease

Workup/Keys to Diagnosis

Physical Examination

The physical examination for diagnosing diabetes and ongoing management should include the following:[1]

Height and weight measurement
Blood pressure determination and orthostatic measurements, when indicated
Funduscopic examination
Oral examination
Thyroid palpation
Cardiac examination
Abdominal examination (e.g., for hepatomegaly)
Evaluation of pulses by palpation and with auscultation
Hand and finger examination
Foot examination
Skin examination (for acanthosis nigricans and insulin-injection sites)
Neurologic examination
Signs of diseases that can cause secondary diabetes (e.g., hemochromatosis, pancreatic disease).

Laboratory Studies

Biochemical criteria for the diagnosis of diabetes are discussed in Table 33.2.

TABLE 33.2
BIOCHEMICAL CRITERIA (VENOUS PLASMA) FOR THE DIAGNOSIS OF DIABETES, IMPAIRED GLUCOSE TOLERANCE, AND IMPAIRED FASTING GLUCOSE

	Glucose Concentration mg/dL (mmol/L)
Diabetes mellitus:	
Fasting and/or	$\geq$126 ($\geq$7.0)
2-h post glucose load	$\geq$200 ($\geq$11.1)
Impaired glucose tolerance	
Fasting (if measured)	<126 (<7.0)
And 2-h post glucose load	$\geq$140 and <200 ($\geq$7.8 and <11.1)
Impaired fasting glucose	
Fasting	$\geq$100 and <126 ($\geq$5.6 and <7.0)
And 2-h post glucose load (if measured)	<140 (<7.8)

Management

Ongoing Management

For established elderly patients with type 2 diabetes, the management plan should be formulated as an individualized therapeutic alliance among the patient and family, the physician, and other members of the health care team. Any plan should recognize diabetes self-management education as an integral component of care. Treatment goals are to prevent metabolic decompensation and control factors that contribute to the high risk of cardiovascular complications in the elderly patient with diabetes. Control of hyperglycemia and identifying and controlling hypertension, lipid disorders, and smoking are all important goals in a diabetes care plan for the elderly patient. Long-term treatment plans must consider the individual patient's remaining life expectancy, existing diabetes complications, coexisting medical and neuropsychiatric disorders, and the ability and commitment of the patient and the caregiver to adhere to the proposed, often complex, treatment plan. Elderly persons are at increased risk for adverse effects related to all aspects of treatment including diet, exercise, and medication (see Table 33.3).[4,5]

Glycemic control is critical to managing patients with type 2 diabetes. The UK Prospective Diabetes Study (UKPDS) showed the benefits of intensive glycemic control for preventing or delaying the development and progression of long-term complications. The UKPDS, the largest and longest interventional trial conducted in patients with type 2 diabetes, conclusively showed the significant benefits of improving glycemic control with intensive treatment using insulin, sulfonylurea, or metformin.[6] Epidemiologic analysis of 10-year UKPDS data showed a continuous relationship between the risk of microvascular complications and glycemia, such that for every 1 percentage point reduction in HbA_{Ic} there was a 37% reduction in the risk of microvascular complications.[7] The major barrier for the implementation of intensive glycemic control, from both the physician's and the patient's perspectives, is the increased incidence of hypoglycemia.

Severe hyperglycemia produces excessive fatty acid mobilization and oxidation, muscle wasting by excessive protein catabolism, excessive glucose production, and loss of glucose in the urine. Precipitating factors include infection, pancreatitis, myocardial infarction (MI), dehydration, cerebrovascular accident, and alcohol abuse. Commonly used medications that can cause hyperglycemia include corticosteroids, β-blockers, β-agonists, thiazides, furosemide, antipsychotic agents, phenothiazines, thyroid hormone preparations, calcium channel blockers, estrogen, phenytoin, gemesterol acetate, opiates, and nicotinic acid.

TABLE 33.3
ONGOING MANAGEMENT GOALS AND RECOMMENDED FREQUENCY OF TESTING AMONG PATIENTS WITH TYPE 2 DIABETES

	Management Goals
Glycemic control	
HbA_{1c}	<7.0%
Preprandial plasma glucose	90–130 mg/dL (5.0–7.2 mmol/L)
Postprandial plasma glucose	<180 mg/dL (<10.0 mmol/L)
Blood pressure	<130/80 mm Hg
Lipids	
LDL	<100 mg/dL (<2.6 mmol/L)
Triglycerides	<150 mg/dL (<1.7 mmol/L)
HDL	>40 mg/dL (>1.1 mmol/L)
	Recommended Frequency of Tests
Glycemic control (HbA_{1c})	Two times per year in individuals at goal; quarterly in those who have changed therapy or have not achieved goal
Blood pressure	Should be measured at every routine visit
Lipids	Should be measured annually
Smoking cessation	Should be part of ongoing treatment plan
Nephropathy (microalbuminuria)	Should be measured annually
Neuropathy	Should have comprehensive foot examination performed annually
Retinopathy	Should be performed annually by an ophthalmologist or optometrist

LDL, low-density lipoprotein; HDL, high-density lipoprotein.

Risk factors for developing hypoglycemia include advanced age, inconsistent caloric intake, high doses of insulin, delay in eating meal after administration of rapid-acting insulin, and hypoglycemia unawareness.[8]

Recommendations

Elderly patients with diabetes who are otherwise healthy should be treated to achieve the same glycemic, blood pressure and lipid targets as younger people[1,4,5] (Evidence Level C).

In elderly patients with multiple comorbidities, a high level of functional dependency, or limited life expectancy, more conservative goals should be used[1,4] (Evidence Level C).

Cardiovascular Disease

CVD is the leading cause of mortality in individuals with diabetes. Studies have shown the efficacy of reducing cardiovascular risk factors in preventing or slowing CVD. Emphasis should be placed on reducing cardiovascular risk factors, when possible, and clinicians should be alert for signs and symptoms of atherosclerosis. A risk factor—based approach should be used in the initial diagnostic evaluation and follow-up to identify coronary heart disease (CHD) in asymptomatic diabetic patients. At least annually, cardiovascular risk factors (dyslipidemia, hypertension, smoking, family history of premature coronary disease, and presence of micro- or macroalbuminuria) should be assessed. Diagnostic cardiac stress testing is indicated in patients with typical or atypical cardiac symptoms and an abnormal resting electrocardiogram (ECG). Screening cardiac stress testing should be considered in those with a history of peripheral or carotid occlusive disease, those with a sedentary lifestyle who plan to begin a vigorous exercise program, and those with two or more of the risk factors noted in the preceding text.

Recommendations

In patients with congestive heart failure (CHF), metformin is contraindicated. The thiazolidinediones are associated with fluid retention and can complicate management of CHF[1] (Evidence Level C).

An angiotensin-converting enzyme (ACE) inhibitor should be considered in patients older than 55 years with another cardiovascular risk factor to reduce the risk of cardiovascular events[1] (Evidence Level A).

β-Blockers should be considered in patients with a prior MI or in patients undergoing major surgery to reduce mortality[1] (Evidence Level A).

Peripheral Arterial Disease

Signs and symptoms suggestive of peripheral arterial disease include cold feet, atrophy of subcutaneous tissues, hair loss, intermittent claudication, and decreased or absent dorsalis pedis and posterior tibial pulses. Ankle-brachial index (ABI)/Doppler pressures at the ankle and toes should be obtained when concern for ischemic change in the forefoot arises on the basis of history and physical examination. Refer patients with significant claudication or a positive ABI for further vascular assessment.

Recommendation

Initial treatment recommendations involve behavior changes that include stopping smoking and a monitored program of physical activity; other management considerations include medications and surgical options[1] (Evidence Level C).

Retinopathy

Up to 21% of patients with type 2 diabetes have retinopathy at the time of first diagnosis of diabetes, and most develop some degree of retinopathy over time. Other common age-related eye disorders, such as glaucoma, cataract, and macular degeneration, are also more common among individuals with diabetes. The duration of diabetes is probably the strongest predictor for development and progression of retinopathy, an important cause of blindness. Diabetic retinopathy has few visual or ophthalmic symptoms until visual loss develops. The protective effects of glycemic control and blood pressure control on development and progression of retinopathy has been confirmed for patients with type 2 diabetes. Epidemiologic analysis of 10-year UKPDS data showed a continuous relationship between the risk of microvascular complications and glycemia, such that for every 1% reduction in HbA_{1c} there was a 37% reduction in the risk of microvascular complications.[7] Aspirin therapy does not prevent retinopathy or increase the risk of hemorrhage. Laser photocoagulation can reduce the risk of vision loss in patients with proliferative changes.

Recommendations

Patients should have an initial dilated and comprehensive eye examination by an ophthalmologist experienced in diagnosis and management of diabetic retinopathy shortly after diabetes diagnosis[1] (Evidence Level B).

Ophthalmic examinations for retinopathy should be repeated annually. If the patient has ophthalmic symptoms, established retinopathy, glaucoma, cataracts, A_{1c} >8.0%, type 1 diabetes, or blood pressure >140/80 mm Hg with abnormal findings, more frequent follow-up may be needed. Persons who are at lower risk may be examined every 2 years[1] (Evidence Level B).

Nephropathy

Diabetic nephropathy occurs in 20% to 40% of patients with diabetes and is the leading cause of end-stage renal disease. Persistent microalbuminuria is a marker for development of nephropathy in type 2 diabetes. Random spot urine collection, measuring the albumin-to-creatinine ratio, is the preferred screening method for microalbuminuria. Microalbuminuria is diagnosed when at least two out of three tests measured within a 6-month period show levels of 30 to 299 μg per mg creatinine. Urinary albumin excretion over baseline values may occur with: Exercise within 24 hours, infection, fever, CHF, marked hyperglycemia, or marked hypertension. Glomerular filtration rate (GFR) is already affected by aging, and various calculation methods appear to be more accurate than creatinine clearance measured from 24-hour urine samples at predicting GFR. Standard formulas include the Cockcroft-Gault equation and the Levey equation. ACE inhibitors and angiotensin II receptor blockers (ARBs) have been shown to delay the progression to macroalbuminuria and delay the progression to nephropathy in patients with type 2 diabetes, hypertension, and microalbuminuria. Nutrition deficiency may occur in some individuals and lead to muscle weakness. Protein-restricted meal plans should be designed by a registered dietitian. Radiocontrast media are particularly nephrotoxic in patients with diabetic nephropathy, and azotemic patients should be carefully hydrated before receiving any contrast.

Recommendations

All patients with type 2 diabetes should be screened for microalbuminuria at diagnosis and annually thereafter[1] (Evidence Level C).

ACE inhibitors or ARBs should be used in the treatment of both micro- and macroalbuminuria (Evidence Level A); if one class is not tolerated then the other should be given a trial[1] (Evidence Level C).

If ACE inhibitors, ARBs, or diuretics are used, monitor serum potassium levels for the development of hyperkalemia[1] (Evidence Level B).

Consider referral to a physician experienced in the care of diabetic renal disease when the GFR has fallen to <60 mL/minute/1.73 m^2, or if difficulties occur in the management of hypertension or hyperkalemia[1] (Evidence Level B).

Optimize glucose and blood pressure control to reduce the risk and slow the progression of nephropathy[1] (Evidence Level A).

Protein restriction to approximately 10% of daily calories, <0.8 g/kg body wt/day, is routinely prescribed when nephropathy is diagnosed[1] (Evidence Level B).

Foot Care/Neuropathy

Amputation and foot ulceration are the most common sequelae of diabetic neuropathy and are major causes of morbidity and disability. Diabetes is responsible for the largest number of nontraumatic amputations in the United States. For many, amputation is the eventual result of a nonhealing ulcer. Ulcers are caused by diabetic neuropathy and vascular insufficiency. Early recognition and management of risk factors can prevent or delay adverse outcomes. The risk of ulcers or amputations is increased in people who have had diabetes for more than 10 years, are male, have poor glucose control, poor vision, or have evidence of macrovascular or microvascular complications. Gait and balance should be assessed. Patients with diabetes and high-risk foot conditions should be educated about the risk factors and appropriate management, including the implications of loss of protective sensation, importance of daily foot monitoring (using other senses such as visualization or palpation), and proper care of the nails and skin of the feet.

Diabetic peripheral neuropathy has a prevalence of 20% to 50% in select patient populations with diabetes. The prevalence of peripheral neuropathy increases with length of time with diabetes, making it of special concern for older populations. The presence of peripheral neuropathy in older individuals is an important occurrence, as it is associated with an increased risk for falls and for diabetic foot ulcerations that can ultimately lead to amputations. People with neuropathy should have well-fitted walking shoes or athletic shoes.

In-office screening for peripheral neuropathy can be accomplished with the use of monofilament testing. To perform monofilament testing, assess insensitivity to slight pressure with the monofilament applied to three areas of the foot: The hallux, and the first and fifth metatarsal heads.

Recommendations

All older adults with diabetes should receive an annual foot examination to identify high-risk foot conditions such as peripheral neuropathy with loss of protective sensation, altered biomechanics, evidence of increased pressure or decreased skin integrity, bony deformity, peripheral vascular disease, vascular status, history of ulcers or amputation, or severe nail pathology[1] (Evidence Level C).

Perform a visual inspection of diabetic patients' feet at all routine visits[1] (Evidence Level C).

The foot examination in a primary care setting should include the use of a Semmes-Weinstein 5.07 (10 g) monofilament, tuning fork, palpation, and visual examination[1] (Evidence Level B).

Diabetes Education

Self-monitoring of blood glucose allows patients to monitor their response to therapy or while adjusting medications, nutrition therapy, and physical activity. Self-monitoring can be useful in avoiding hypoglycemia. Daily monitoring is particularly important in patients using insulin to evaluate for asymptomatic hypoglycemia. The optimal frequency and timing of monitoring is unknown but should be individualized to the needs and goals of each patient. Physicians should evaluate the patient's monitoring technique and ability to use data to guide treatment, as the accuracy and utility of self-monitoring is dependent on both the instrument and the user. Barriers to self-monitoring in elderly patients may include visual deficits, decreased dexterity with equipment and cognitive deficits. "Home orders" suggesting what action to take given a particular self-monitored blood glucose (SMBG) value can help guide patients or their caregivers.

Recommendation

Patients or their caregivers should be instructed on self-monitoring techniques and taught how to use the information obtained from self-monitoring to adjust therapies such as food intake, activity, and medications to achieve glycemic goals[1] (Evidence Level C).

Influenza and Pneumococcal Immunization

Influenza and pneumonia are common preventable infectious diseases associated with significant morbidity and mortality in the elderly and in people with chronic diseases. Systematic strategies to target those who are 65 years or older, nursing home or assisted-living residents, hospitalized patients, or those having additional chronic cardiopulmonary disorders should be implemented to vaccinate those particularly at risk. Family members of patients with diabetes, caregivers, and health care workers should consider vaccination because influenza is spread by person-to-person transmission. Anaphylactic hypersensitivity to chicken eggs or other vaccine components is a contraindication to influenza vaccination. Immunization is not recommended in patients with a history of Guillain-Barré syndrome within 6 weeks of a previous influenza vaccination. Chemoprophylaxis should be considered in patients with contraindications to vaccination and taken for the duration of the influenza season.

Recommendations

The injectible trivalent influenza vaccine should be recommended for all elderly patients with diabetes yearly beginning each fall/September[1] (Evidence Level C).

The injectible pneumococcal vaccine is indicated in people older than 64, patients with diabetes, and those with chronic cardiopulmonary or renal disease because these individuals are at high risk for invasive pneumococcal infections[1] (Evidence Level C).

Pneumococcal revaccination one additional time is recommended in patients who were younger than 60 when initially vaccinated; consider revaccination in patients with compromised immune systems, chronic renal disease, or nephrotic syndrome[1] (Evidence Level C).

Lifestyle Recommendations

Changes in lifestyle, including diet and exercise, are important interventions to limiting morbidity from diabetes in elderly patients.

Nutrition education programs can improve metabolic control among older people with diabetes. The glycemic index evaluates the source and amount of carbohydrate ingested and can be used as a way of controlling nutrition. The ADA recommends a diet of 50% to 60% of calories as carbohydrates, 10% to 20% of calories as monosaturated fats, 10% to 20% of calories as protein, and <30% of calories from fat, with saturated fat accounting for <7% and polyunsaturated fat calories <10% total. Caution should be taken with weight loss diets in older people with diabetes, particularly in long-term care settings, as these patients tend to be undernourished and underweight rather than overweight.

Decrease in physical activity can contribute to the decrease in muscle mass and decrease in insulin sensitivity seen in patients who are diabetic or obese, and this can develop with aging. The physician needs first to assess the older patient's ability to safely increase physical activity, then tailor the types of activities to the individual's functional status and environmental limitations while providing exercise goals. Evaluation of the patient before giving an exercise prescription should include a detailed medical evaluation screening for existing micro- and macrovascular complications. Elderly diabetic patients are at high risk for underlying CVD; graded exercise testing or its alternatives may help determine the suitability of a moderate to high-intensity exercise (>60% of maximal heart rate) program for elderly patients. Patients with a known history of coronary artery disease should be evaluated for risk of ischemia and arrhythmias during exercise. Activities should have minimal potential for trauma, such as walking, stationary bicycling, gardening, or yard work. Exercise programs at senior centers and health clubs, or walking in the mall are often easily accessible and can provide social interaction (and supervision) as well.

All patients with diabetes should have their smoking history and smoking status assessed. CVD risks decrease within 2 to 3 years of stopping smoking to those of people who have never smoked. Counseling for smoking cessation should be a routine element in caring for patients with diabetes. If the patient with diabetes who smokes is not willing to quit, then continue to provide brief motivational counseling to encourage cessation of tobacco use. If the patient who smokes is motivated to quit, physicians can assist them by helping to set a quit date and prepare to quit, offering medication, and suggesting behavioral interventions. Pharmacologic agents can increase rates of smoking cessation when partnered with behavioral interventions.

Lifestyle interventions focusing on nutrition therapy should be considered as therapeutic interventions to prevent and control type 2 diabetes in the elderly[1] (Evidence Level A).

A regular physical activity program, adapted to the presence of complications, is recommended for all patients with diabetes who are capable of participating[1] (Evidence Level B).

Assessing smoking status and implementing smoking cessation programs among elderly patients with diabetes should be done[1] (Evidence Level B).

Medications

Oral Medications

Unique challenges to management of diabetes in older patients involve their overall health status, coexisting illnesses, psychologic well-being, cognitive functioning, and their social environment. Treatment goals must be explicit, practical, and realistic. Preventing hypoglycemia should be a treatment goal because of the risks of physical injury and fractures during an acute episode, as well as the risks of MI and stroke. Signs of hypoglycemia include confusion, drowsiness, shakiness, cold sweats, headache, tachycardia, extreme hunger, diarrhea, or gas. On the other hand, fear of hypoglycemia can lead to suboptimal glycemic control. When individualized treatment goals and glycemic targets as close to normal as possible are not being met by use of diet and exercise within three to 6 months of diagnosis it is appropriate to consider the addition of oral agents. The potential for polypharmacy and drug interactions is high in the elderly patient, who may also be taking medications for coexisting medical problems.

Five classes of oral agents target hyperglycemia by different mechanisms: Sulfonylureas and meglitinides increase insulin secretion, biguanidines decrease hepatic gluconeogenesis and enhance insulin sensitivity in muscle, thiazolidinediones enhance insulin sensitivity, and α-glucosidase inhibitors delay carbohydrate absorption. No particular agents have been shown to be more efficacious. Beyond assuring that patients have no contraindications to particular agents, such as hepatic or renal impairment or CHF, these agents have no major pharmacologic differences in the elderly. Starting at a relatively low dose and titrating slowly based on the individual's response would be a prudent approach when initiating any of these antidiabetic agents.

Second generation sulfonylurea agents are favored in elderly patients because of potency greater than first generation agents and because they have a nonionic bond to plasma proteins that may reduce drug–drug interaction.[9,10] Glipizide is metabolized in the liver to inactive metabolites, reducing the risk of hypoglycemia. The availability of long-acting glipizide may allow for daily or twice-daily dosing and perhaps enhance compliance. Glyburide's metabolized by-products have hypoglycemic activity until eliminated in the urine and bile; therefore glyburide should be used with caution in elderly patients. Chlorpropamide, having a prolonged half-life and being renally excreted, increases the risk for hypoglycemia and this risk increases with age. This agent also may cause the syndrome of inappropriate secretion of antidiuretic hormone and has an antabuse-like alcohol sensitivity reaction. Chlorpropamide should not be used in older patients because of these risks.[9,10] Suflonylurea therapy can cause weight gain and hypoglycemia. Patients treated with sulfonylureas can exhibit β cell "exhaustion" at a rate of approximately 10% of patients per year; after 10 years of therapy approximately 50% of patients will become nonresponders to sulfonylureas.

Meglitinides such as repaglinide and nateglinide target postprandial hyperglycemia as they stimulate immediate postprandial insulin release. Rapid return to baseline may lower late hypoglycemic events. Frequent premeal dosing may make it difficult for compliance. Repaglinide is metabolized by the liver and has mostly biliary elimination although the half-life varies considerably in elderly patients. Nateglinide should be used cautiously in patients with renal or hepatic impairment.[9,10]

Metformin acts principally to reduce hepatic gluconeogenesis. Metformin is the most commonly prescribed biguanide and is considered safer than the earlier biguanides, which were withdrawn from the market because they caused lactic acidosis. Metformin is preferred in obese patients with insulin resistance because of its ability to increase insulin-mediated glucose uptake and utilization in peripheral tissues such as muscle. Metformin should be avoided in elderly patients with heart failure, with renal or hepatic insufficiency, or during acute illness because of increased risk of lactic acidosis.[9,10] Gastrointestinal side effects such as diarrhea, nausea, vomiting, flatulence, and abdominal discomfort may limit patient acceptability. Monitor serum creatinine at least annually and with dose changes in older patients on metformin. A timed urine collection for measurement of creatinine clearance is recommended for patients 80 years or older or those with reduced muscle mass who are taking metformin.[9,10] Metformin should be withheld before radiologic studies requiring contrast and renal function should be assessed prior to reinstituting metformin.

Thiazolidinediones such as rosiglitazone and pioglitazone are some of the newest and most expensive antidiabetic agents. They enhance glucose uptake and utilization in peripheral tissues. When used as monotherapy these agents do not cause hypoglycemia and they may be used in combination with other agents such as insulin, sulfonylureas, or metformin. The thiazolidinediones can cause fluid retention and worsen CHF; therefore they should not be used in elderly patients with heart failure. Thiazolidinediones should not be used in patients with hepatic impairment. These agents are hepatically metabolized and it is recommended that liver enzymes should be monitored at baseline and then periodically.[9,10]

α-Glucosidase inhibitors such as acarbose and miglitol target postprandial hyperglycemia by working on the reversibly inhibiting brush border enzymes of the proximal intestinal epithelium. These agents work at the intestine with little systemic action and have low risk for hypoglycemia. They should be avoided in patients with renal failure. They can be used as monotherapy or in combination with insulin or sulfonylureas. Common gastrointestinal side effects such as diarrhea and flatulence, the need for dosing before each meal, and cost may limit patient acceptability (see Table 33.4).

Insulin Therapy

When lifestyle therapies and oral agents have not met the individualized treatment goals of the patient, then insulin therapy should be instituted. Insulin therapy and its adjustments should be highly individualized in the elderly patient. Insulin has few contraindications and few drug interactions. Insulin is renally metabolized. Its use does require that the patient or caregiver have proper education and skills in monitoring of blood glucose, administration of insulin, and treatment of hypoglycemia. Potential challenges limiting the feasibility of insulin therapy in elderly patients include cognitive impairment, impaired vision, or impaired manual dexterity.

Difficulties with mixing insulin preparations and drawing up the correct amount of insulin can be addressed in a number of ways. Prefilled syringes of insulin can be prepared by a visiting nurse, caregiver, or relative. Prefilled syringes may be stored in a refrigerator for 3 to 4 weeks, and mixtures of regular insulin and NPH insulin are stable when refrigerated. Premixed insulins, such as 70/30 insulin or 75/25 lispro insulin, are an alternative in patients who have difficulty mixing insulins. Visually impaired older patients may find scale magnifiers useful to enlarge syringe numbers and markings, and a talking glucometer or large number glucometer may aid self-monitoring of blood glucose. Difficulties with manual dexterity can be addressed with vial holders and needle guides.

To enhance compliance and prevent errors in administration, the prescribed insulin regimen should be as simple as possible. Monitoring of blood glucose should vary in frequency depending on the individualized treatment goals and insulin regimen, but self-monitoring and recording of values in a logbook should be encouraged because it is necessary for the physician to assess the appropriateness of an insulin regimen. Most elderly patients with diabetes need finger stick blood glucose monitoring once a day, although more frequent monitoring up to four times a day may be necessary when adjusting or initiating insulin therapy.

An initial insulin daily dose is typically 0.2 to 0.5 units per kg of weight.[9,10] A single daily dose of intermediate-acting insulin may be sufficient in elderly patients with type 2 diabetes mellitus who have retained insulin secretory capacity; morning administration may allow for more feasible monitoring for hypoglycemia in the daytime. If daily insulin requirement exceeds 50 units or glycemic goals are not being met, then multiple daily dosing regimens should be initiated. Twice-daily dosing regimens

TABLE 33.4
CHARACTERISTICS OF SELECTED ORAL AGENTS FOR GLYCEMIC CONTROL

Oral Agent for Glycemic Control	Expected HbA_{Ic} Reduction as Monotherapy (%)	Initial Dose	Doses/d	Daily Dose Range (mg/d)	Side Effects and Disadvantages
Second-generation sulfonylureas	1–2				Weight gain Gastrointestinal upset Hypoglycemia
Glipizide		2.5 mg q.d.	1–2	2.5–40	
Glipizide XL		5 mg q.d.	1	5–20	
Glyburide		1.25 mg q.d.	1	1.25–20	
Meglitinides	0.5–2				Hypoglycemia Weight gain Complex premeal dosing
Repaglinide		0.5 mg t.i.d.	3–4	1.5–16	
Nateglinide		60–120 mg t.i.d.	3	180–360	
Biguanides	0.5–3				Contraindicated in patients with hepatic dysfunction, renal dysfunction, or heart failure Gastrointestinal upset Concern for lactic acidosis
Metformin		500 mg q.d.	1–3	500–2550	
Thiazolidinediones	1–1.5				Weight gain Contraindicated in patients with hepatic dysfunction or heart failure Edema
Pioglitazone		15–30 mg q.d.	1	15–45	
Rosiglitazone		2 mg b.i.d. or 4 mg q.d.	1–2	4–8	
α-Glucosidase inhibitors	0.5–1				Gastrointestinal upset Liver function test elevations Complex premeal dosing
Acarbose		25 mg q.d.	1–3	25–300	
Miglitol		25 mg q.d.	1–3	25–300	

commonly divide the dose into two-thirds before breakfast and one third before the evening meal. If postprandial hyperglycemia is noted, then addition of short-acting insulin to the intermediate-acting insulin regimen may be warranted. If a twice-daily dosing regimen includes both intermediate-acting and short-acting insulins, each dose will typically contain two-thirds of the dose as the intermediate-acting insulin and one third of the dose as the short-acting insulin (see Table 33.5).

Aspirin Therapy

Aspirin is recommended for secondary prevention of CVD in men and women with diabetes because it has been shown to reduce subsequent vascular events and reduce cardiovascular mortality in multiple randomized clinical trials (RCTs) and meta-analyses. Use of aspirin for primary prevention of vascular events in patients with diabetes older than 40 or with additional risk factors (family history of CVD, hypertension, smoking, dyslipidemia, albuminuria) likewise has provided risk reduction.

Recommendations

Aspirin once a day in doses ranging from 75 to 162 mg is recommended in all patients with diabetes without contraindications to use[1] (Evidence Level A). Contraindications include allergy to aspirin, increased bleeding tendency, recent gastrointestinal bleeding, active liver disease, and other anticoagulation therapy.

Other antiplatelet agents may be considered in patients at high risk of CVD who are not candidates for aspirin due to allergy (Evidence Level C).

Alternative or Integrative Medicine

Use of alternative therapies, some of which may impact blood glucose, is increasingly widespread in the United States. There is insufficient evidence to draw definitive conclusions about the efficacy of individual herbs and supplements for glucose control in patients with diabetes. Use of herbal remedies, reported in 20% of individuals with diabetes, has not been shown to improve glucose control and may even be harmful in individuals with

TABLE 33.5
CHARACTERISTICS OF INSULINS

Category	Preparations Available	Onset (h)	Peak (h)	Duration (h)
Short-acting	Regular	0.5–1	2–3	3–6
	Lispro	0.1–0.25	0.25–0.5	3–4
Intermediate-acting	NPH	2–4	4–10	10–18
	Lente	3–4	4–10	16–24
Long-acting	Ultralente	6–10	8–24	18–30
	Insulin glargine	—	none	24

diabetes.[11] Potential interactions between supplements and conventional therapy should be assessed. A prevalence study showed that individuals with diabetes were 1.6 times more likely to use alternative therapies than individuals without diabetes.[12] Most patients do not openly share use of alternative therapies with their health care provider. It is recommended that patients be specifically asked about their alternative therapy practices.

Comorbidity Concerns

Management guidelines for older patients with diabetes that advocate screening for the geriatric syndromes of polypharmacy, depression, cognitive impairment, urinary incontinence, persistent pain, and injurious falls cite studies showing increased prevalence of these syndromes in diabetic patients or are based on expert opinion.[4]

Polypharmacy, with its potential health and financial burdens, can be a major problem for older adults with diabetes who require multiple medications to manage glycemia, hypertension, hyperlipidemia, and other conditions. Careful review of medications, how the patient uses them, and evaluation for potential side effects is important at all visits. Consider asking the patient to maintain an updated list of all current medications, including nonprescription drugs. Patients or their caregivers should be educated on the expected benefits, risks, and potential side effects of medications. Each drug should have a clearly documented indication for its use. Drug-disease or drug–drug interactions should be considered, particularly before starting a new medication or if the patient presents with depression, falls, cognitive impairment, or urinary incontinence.

Depression is more common in adults with diabetes, and older adults are underdiagnosed and undertreated for depression. Unrecognized depression can interfere with diabetes care in older patients. The American Geriatrics Society recommends screening for depression during the initial evaluation of diabetes and if there is an unexpected clinical decline. Older patients with diabetes with new-onset or recurrent depression should be treated or referred for pharmacologic and psychologic treatment of depression.

Diabetes in older adults is associated with decreased cognitive function. Physicians should evaluate older patients' cognitive function when considering particular treatments and ability to perform diabetes self-care. Evaluation for delirium and other reversible causes of cognitive impairment should be performed if a clinical decline is noted; evaluations may include a review of the medication list, screening for depression, vitamin B_{12} deficiency, hypothyroidism, and neuroimaging. A recent Cochrane Review found no convincing evidence that treatment of diabetes influenced prevention or management of cognitive impairment.[13]

Risk factors for urinary incontinence that are more common in the diabetic elderly include polyuria from hyperglycemia, medication side effects, urinary tract infections, monilial vaginitis, neurogenic bladder, and autonomic insufficiency leading to fecal impaction. Urinary incontinence significantly affects quality of life but is often unrecognized by physicians unless symptoms are routinely assessed. Reversible causes of urinary incontinence should be sought and treated.

Older persons with diabetes have significant risk factors that may lead to injurious falls, including frailty, visual impairment, peripheral neuropathy and neuropathic pain, polypharmacy, and hypoglycemia. Geriatric syndromes including falls are often underreported, underdetected, associated with significant functional decline, and may have reversible contributing factors that could be addressed if found on routine screening with a comprehensive geriatric assessment.

Hypertension

Hypertension is a common comorbidity among elderly patients with diabetes and can lead to considerable morbidity and mortality. Control of hypertension is markedly effective in reducing risk for microvascular and macrovascular events in middle-aged patients. Antihypertensive medications are effective preventing stroke and heart attack/CHD and cerebrovascular morbidity and mortality in elderly people, based on meta-analyses of elders mainly in their 60s and 70s and chiefly using thiazides and β-blockers.[14] It is unclear what the effects of treatment are in the very old (older than 85) or frail elders with many severe competing comorbidities. Individual evaluation of the benefit-to-risk ratios are necessary. Risks may exceed the benefits, as when an elderly patient has orthostasis and recurring falls related to hypertensive medications.

Recommendations

Elderly patients should have blood pressure lowered gradually to avoid complications and side effects[4] (Evidence Level C).

All routine diabetes visits should include blood pressure measurement[1] (Evidence Level C).

Goals for blood pressure in patients with diabetes are systolic <130 mm Hg and diastolic <80 mm Hg if it can be safely achieved[1] (Evidence Level B).

Patients with systolic blood pressure ≥130 mm Hg or diastolic blood pressure ≥80 mm Hg should have measurement repeated on a separate day. Patients with blood pressure repeatedly between 130 and 139 mm Hg systolic or 80 to 89 mm Hg diastolic should be given lifestyle modification therapy alone for at most 3 months. If target blood pressures are not reached then pharmacologic therapy should be started[1] (Evidence Level C).

Patients who are hypertensive, having systolic blood pressure ≥140 mm Hg or diastolic blood pressure ≥90, should have lifestyle modification and pharmacologic therapy with antihypertensives to achieve goal blood pressure[1] (Evidence Level A).

Autonomic neuropathy may be assessed with orthostatic blood pressure measurements[1] (Evidence Level C).

ACE inhibitors, ARBs, β-blockers, diuretics, and calcium channel blockers have all demonstrated reduction in CVD events in persons with diabetes[1] (Evidence Level A).

It is recommended that all patients with diabetes and hypertension be treated with a regimen including either an ACE inhibitor or ARB[1] (Evidence Level C).

Dyslipidemia

There is a high incidence of CVD in older patients with diabetes and higher mortality once they have CVD. Over 65% of deaths in older diabetics are due to CVD. Treatment with lipid-lowering agents reduces cardiovascular risk. Priority is given to LDL cholesterol lowering, HDL cholesterol raising, and then triglyceride lowering. Overall health status can guide decisions on the feasibility of correcting dyslipidemias in older patients with diabetes. For patients with known coronary arterial disease (CAD), diabetes, and LDL >100 mg per dL, pharmacologic therapy should be instituted at the same time as lifestyle interventions are initiated. For patients with diabetes without known CVD pharmacologic therapy to achieve lipid level goals is recommended for LDL cholesterol level ≥130 mg per dL. In patients with LDL between 100 and 129 mg per dL treatment strategies include medical nutrition therapy and pharmacologic treatment with a statin. Pharmacologic therapy is recommended in patients who do not reach lipid goals with lifestyle modifications. Use of statins (HMG-CoA reductase inhibitors) has strong evidence for use, whereas less evidence supports using fibrates in the elderly.[15] Severe hypertriglyceridemia (triglyceride levels ≥1,000 mg per dL) carries a risk for acute pancreatitis, necessitating severe dietary fat restriction to <10% of calories and pharmacologic therapy.

Some studies have raised concerns about an association between low cholesterol and increased risk of cancer or hemorrhagic strokes, and low cholesterol as a predictor of early death in nursing home residents. The PROspective Study of Pravastatin in the Elderly at Risk (PROSPER) clinical trial showed potential benefits of lipid lowering, through lifestyle modifications and pharmacologic agents, outweighed potential risks in patients younger than 82 years old.[16] Patients who have a life expectancy of at least 10 years and who are active, cognitively intact, and willing to undertake the responsibility of self-management should be encouraged to do so and be treated using the stated goals for younger adults with diabetes.

Recommendations

Test for lipid disorders annually and more often if needed to achieve goals; patients with low-risk lipid levels should be reassessed every 2 years[1] (Evidence Level C).

Target lipid levels for adults with diabetes are LDL cholesterol <100 mg per dL, HDL cholesterol levels >40 mg per dL (in women the goal may be 10 mg per dL higher), and triglyceride levels <150 mg per dL[1] (Evidence Level B).

Lifestyle modifications such as reduction of saturated fat and cholesterol intake, weight loss, increased physical activity and smoking cessation have been shown to improve lipid profiles in patients with diabetes and should be considered[1] (Evidence Level A).

THYROID DISEASE

CASE TWO

Mrs. J. is a 72-year-old who presents complaining of fatigue and swelling of her legs. Upon further questioning, you learn she has a history of several years of constipation and also has noted that she frequently feels cold while others are comfortable with the temperature. Physical examination findings include coarse hair and diminished deep tendon reflexes with a slow return phase. You suspect hypothyroidism and order a thyroid-stimulating hormone (TSH), which is 168 μu per mL. Following this you order a free T_4, which is 1.2 μg per dL. Your diagnosis of primary hypothyroidism is confirmed.

Hypothyroidism

Description/Definition of Problem

Hypothyroidism is relatively common in the elder population, secondary only to diabetes as the most common endocrine disorder in the geriatric population. Primary hypothyroidism is the most common form of hypothyroidism and results from a failure of the thyroid gland itself, with insufficient secretion of thyroid hormone. This is often the result of Hashimoto autoimmune thyroiditis, although thyroid autoantibodies are often not detectable at the time of diagnosis. Hypothyroidism can also be secondary to radioablation or surgical removal of the thyroid gland for the treatment of hyperthyroidism, tumor, and drugs such as lithium, interferon, and amiodarone. Secondary hypothyroidism occurs when there is failure of the hypothalamic–pituitary axis due to disease of the hypothalamus or pituitary. Hypothyroidism associated with goiter due to iodine deficiency remains uncommon in the United States since the iodination of table salt.

Pathophysiology and Genetics

The most common cause of primary hypothyroidism, Hashimoto thyroiditis (also called *autoimmune thyroiditis* or *chronic lymphocytic thyroiditis*) is an autoimmune condition characterized by antibodies to thyroid peroxidase and thyroglobulin. Autoimmune destruction and progressive fibrosis of the thyroid gland result in dimunitions of the two principal thyroid hormones that circulate in the blood, T_3 and T_4, which exist largely bound to plasma proteins.

A predisposition to Hashimoto thyroiditis can be inherited in an autosomal dominant fashion and is also linked to other autoimmune diseases, such as pernicious anemia and systemic lupus erythematosis. A family history of thyroid or other endocrine diseases such as diabetes is also a risk factor for primary hypothyroidism.

Systems Impacted

Almost all systems of the body appear to require optimal levels of thyroid hormones. Oxidative metabolism and the basal metabolic rate are very sensitive to the level of circulating thyroid hormones. Therefore, the effects of thyroid hormone deficiency, as seen in clinical hypothyroidism, are multiple. Notable systems affected by hypothyroidism include the central and peripheral nervous system, carbohydrate and lipid metabolism, temperature regulation, the cardiovascular system, and the digestive system.

Prevalence/Gender

Clinical hypothyroidism has a prevalence of 1% to 2% in the general US population, but rises with age to a prevalence of 5% to 8% in those older than 55 years. Women have a greater prevalence than men, and the disease is also more prevalent in whites than blacks. There is a continued rise in prevalence with age, with a further increase in those older than 75 years.[17] The U.S. Preventive Services Task Force concluded in 2004 that there was insufficient evidence to recommend routine screening for asymptomatic individuals, but that clinicians should be alert for symptoms of thyroid disease and must test appropriately.

Signs and Symptoms

Because deficiency of thyroid hormone affects almost every system in the body, the signs and symptoms of hypothyroidism are multiple. However, they can be subtle, especially in older patients and in mild or early disease, and, therefore, may be confused with other disease states. Common signs and symptoms include weakness and fatigue, cold intolerance, dry coarse skin and hair, sallow complexion, weight gain, edema (pedal and periorbital), slowed speech and cognition, thickening of the tongue, hoarse voice, and constipation. Deep tendon reflexes are diminished, with slowing in the relaxation phase of the reflex. Edema in the tissues of the wrist in combination with effects on the peripheral nervous system may cause symptoms consistent with carpal tunnel syndrome. Similarly, paresthesias of the feet may signal tarsal tunnel syndrome because of a similar mechanism. Often in hypothyroidism, a cluster of symptoms is present whereas others are absent.

Myxedema coma is a severe complication of hypothyroidism, which is almost exclusively limited to people aged 60 years and older, with over 80% of cases occurring in women and a preponderance occurring in the winter months.[18] Myxedema coma often follows a precipitating stress such as infection, new medication, stroke, trauma, surgery, or exposure to cold. This severe complication consists of marked edema, severe slowing or alteration of cognitive processes with possible psychosis, bradycardia, hypothermia, hypoventilation, ileus, and alopecia. Overt coma and seizures can also occur, but are not necessary for diagnosis.

Impact on Function

Patients with appropriately treated hypothyroidism generally experience little impact on function. However, those with undetected hypothyroidism or lapses in treatment will have fatigue, as well as other effects consistent with the earlier-mentioned signs and symptoms. One of the most important considerations in the geriatric patient with untreated or undertreated hypothyroidism is its effect on cognition. Slowing of the mental processes and adverse effects on memory and cognition may be confused with depression or dementia.

Etiology and Course/Timeline

In primary hypothyroidism, the precipitating disease process is often autoimmune thyroiditis. In the acute stage of thyroiditis, during which patients may be asymptomatic or have minimal symptoms such as sore throat or neck fullness, patients may be hyperthyroid, euthyroid, or hypothyroid. Patients may progress to primary hypothyroidism over the course of several months. Antithyroid antibodies are initially present during acute thyroiditis, but are usually absent by the time hypothyroidism is clinically detected.

Risk Factors

In addition to the risk factors of female gender, older age, family history of thyroid disease, and family or personal history of other endocrine or autoimmune disease, medications can be a precipitating factor for hypothyroidism (in particular, use of the antiarrhythmic drug amiodarone, commonly used in the management of atrial fibrillation). Amiodarone contains iodine and has structural similarities to thyroxine. Amiodarone can precipitate hyperthyroidism, although hypothyroidism is more common. In the course of long-term therapy with amiodarone, approximately 10% of patients will develop thyroid abnormalities. Amiodarone can be withdrawn if it is safe to do so, or the patient can be started on appropriate therapy for hypothyroidism or hyperthyroidism.[19] Other medications that can cause hypothyroidism, largely through effecting a decrease in TSH secretion, are dopamine, glucocorticoids, and phenytoin.

Recommendations

Patients receiving amiodarone should be screened for thyroid disease at baseline and every 6 months during treatment[19] (Evidence Level C).

Workup/Keys to Diagnosis

Physical Examination

Signs of hypothyroidism that can be found on physical examination are numerous, but they may not all be present in any single patient. There may be modest weight gain. Bradycardia and/or hypothermia may be present. The appearance of the face is often described as "doughy," likely due to sallow complexion, dull facial expression, lip and periorbital edema, thickening of the tongue, drooping of the eyelids (because of decreased adrenergic stimulation), and myxedematous changes of the tissues. Hair is sparse and coarse. Skin is dry and cool to the touch. Response time is increased and changes in memory or cognition may be observed. Abdominal distention may be present, most often because of constipation. Deep tendon reflexes are diminished and are often characterized by a slow return phase. Examination of the neck most often reveals no abnormalities of the thyroid gland itself.

Laboratory

The thyroid is regulated by the hypothalamic–pituitary axis. The hypothalamus secretes thyrotropin-releasing hormone (TRH), which stimulates the pituitary to release TSH. This in turn stimulates the thyroid to secrete two hormones, T_3 and T_4, which are metabolically active in the body. In turn, T_3 and T_4 have a negative feedback on the pituitary gland, inhibiting further secretion of TSH.

For the laboratory diagnosis of hypothyroidism, measurement of serum TSH and free T_4, along with clinical examination, will usually indicate the diagnosis. A high TSH and low free T_4 indicate primary hypothyroidism. Secondary hypothyroidism, a failure of the hypothalamic–pituitary axis, will necessarily yield a low TSH. Subclinical hypothyroidism is present when TSH is mildly elevated, but free T_4 is normal. Subclinical hypothyroidism becomes increasingly common in older women.

Recommendations

The evidence is insufficient to recommend for or against routine screening for thyroid disease in adults (Evidence Level C).

Imaging and Diagnostic Procedures

Thyroid imaging such as ultrasonography and radionuclear scanning are unnecessary for the diagnosis of hypothyroidism in the absence of a structural abnormality of the thyroid on physical examination. If a thyroid nodule, goiter, or thyroid enlargement is detected on physical exam, imaging as well as fine needle aspirate or biopsy may be indicated.

Management

General Measures, Medications, and Patient Monitoring

The mainstay of treatment for clinical hypothyroidism is the replacement of thyroid hormone with a levothyroxine preparation. Levothyroxine is a synthetic hormone preparation. Most brand and generic forms of levothyroxine have minimal differences in bioequivalence. Using the same brand or generic form consistently in a patient will likely yield the best therapeutic results. Most healthy young adults require approximately 1.6 μg of levothyroxine/kg of body weight/day; however, the elderly require only 1.0 μg/kg/day.[21] Initiation of therapy in the elderly should be slower than that commonly used in healthy young adults to minimize the possibility of cardiovascular adverse effects because of rapid increase in pulse or blood pressure. Therefore, elder persons should be initiated at a dose of 0.025 mg of levothyroxine per day. The dosage can then be increased every 6 weeks by 0.025 to 0.050 mg per day, with monitoring by TSH.[22,23] The dosage is increased until TSH becomes normal. It is important that TSH be measured no sooner than 6 weeks after a change in medication dosage. Additionally, the clinical exam should help inform decisions about raising or lowering the dose of levothyroxine. Once a stable dose of levothyroxine is reached, TSH can be monitored every 6 to 12 months.[23]

With age, thyroid hormone requirements tend to decrease. Treatment of subclinical hypothyroidism in older adults is controversial, but is probably not warranted and may lead to excessive bone loss. However, patients with subclinical hypothyroidism should be monitored periodically for progression of disease.[22]

Lifestyle Recommendations

It is important to emphasize to the patient with primary hypothyroidism that the disease is always going to require thyroid hormone replacement. Therefore, patients should be cautioned to avoid lapses in therapy and advised to take their medication every day. Normal exercise and diet should be advocated, consistent with the patient's overall state of health and other medical conditions.

Alternative or Integrative Medicine

The synthetic hormone preparation of levothyroxine has largely replaced previous methods of thyroid hormone replacement, which involved ground thyroid glands from animals. These preparations had highly variable concentrations of thyroid hormones. However, ground, dessicated thyroid hormone preparations are still commercially available but are not recommended.[23]

Hyperthyroidism

Description/Definition of Problem

The term "hyperthyroidism" encompasses several heterogeneous disorders which are all characterized by elevated circulating thyroid hormone. Although Graves disease is the most common disease causing hyperthyroidism in young people, toxic multinodular goiter (MNG) becomes more common in the elderly. Therefore, we will focus our discussion on toxic MNG, a common cause of hyperthyroidism in this age-group. Other causes of hyperthyroidism include Graves disease, excessive administration of thyroid hormone, cancer of the thyroid, the hyperthyroid phase of thyroiditis (see hypothyroidism in the preceding text), and secondary hyperthyroidism due to medications such as amiodarone or to the elaboration of thyroid hormone—like substances from tumors such as those of the ovary.

Pathophysiology

With normal aging, the thyroid gland becomes more nodular, especially in women. In fact, thyroid nodules can be found in 90% of women aged 80 and older.[24] Most of these nodules remain benign and are also euthyroid. In some patients, however, the nodules are quite active and result in a hyperthyroid state, toxic MNG. These hyperfunctioning nodules secrete excess thyroid hormone and inhibit TSH production through the negative feedback loop of the hypothalamic–pituitary axis. However, the toxic thyroid nodule is not responsive to TSH and, therefore, continues to secrete high levels of thyroid hormone, despite the absence of stimulation from the pituitary in the form of TSH. The rest of the thyroid gland, in the absence of TSH, remains quiescent.

Systems Impacted

As was previously discussed for hypothyroidism, almost all systems of the body are affected by circulating levels of thyroid hormones. Therefore, the effects of thyroid hormone excess are multiple, especially among the central and peripheral nervous system, carbohydrate and lipid metabolism, temperature regulation, the cardiovascular system, and the digestive system.

Prevalence/Gender

The prevalence of hyperthyroidism in the elderly due to all causes varies between 0.5% and 2.5%, depending on the criteria used, and is more common in elderly women and in whites as opposed to blacks.[17,22] However, hyperthyroidism in patients older than 60 contributes to 10% to 15% of all cases of thyrotoxicosis.[25]

Signs and Symptoms

Typical symptoms of hyperthyroidism are heat intolerance, diaphoresis, anxiety, weakness and fatigue, diarrhea, palpitations, and weight loss despite increased appetite. However, symptoms may be more atypical in the elderly or may be mistakenly attributed to normal aging or to other comorbid medical conditions. Typical signs of hyperthyroidism are tachycardia, tremor, goiter, warm moist skin, hyperreflexia, proximal muscle weakness, and atrial fibrillation. Patients with toxic MNG, unlike those with hyperthyroidism due to Graves disease, usually do not have pretibial edema or exopthalmos.

Thyroid storm is a life-threatening emergency with abrupt onset of severe thyrotoxicosis and is proportionately more common in elder populations. Patients with thyroid storm may present with fever, tachycardia, marked weakness, psychosis, jaundice, atrial fibrillation, cardiovascular collapse, and shock. Thyroid storm usually results from unsuspected or untreated disease and may be precipitated by stresses such as infection, surgery, or trauma.

Impact on Function

Hyperthyroidism can have a variety of effects on many systems. However, in elderly patients with concomitant medical conditions, the effects will often be most pronounced in systems where there is already some deficit. For example, patients with underlying cardiac disease will be likely to manifest atrial fibrillation and CHF. Those with underlying dementia will exhibit more marked cognitive decline.

Risk Factors

In addition to hypothyroidism, the antiarrhythmic medication amiodarone can also cause overt hyperthyroidism. Lithium can also cause increased secretion of TSH.

Recommendations

Patients receiving amiodarone should be screened for thyroid disease at baseline and every 6 months during treatment[19] (Evidence Level C).

Subclinical Hyperthyroidism

Subclinical hyperthyroidism is defined in those patients with normal levels of circulating thyroid hormone but a low TSH. In one study of patients aged 60 and older with subclinical hyperthyroidism, only 2% progressed to overt hyperthyroidism over a period of 4 years.[26] Therefore, it is recommended that the patient with an isolated low TSH be managed with periodic monitoring of clinical status and repeated laboratory studies. In a minority of patients, isolated low TSH may be associated with the development of atrial fibrillation in the absence of other laboratory abnormality. These patients should probably be treated for both atrial fibrillation and hyperthyroidism. The management of subclinical hyperthyroidism continues to evolve.

Workup/Keys to Diagnosis

Physical Examination

On physical examination, patients with toxic MNG will likely have thyroid enlargement and may demonstrate weight loss, tremor, anxious affect, hyperreflexia, and tachycardia. More serious cardiovascular findings may include atrial fibrillation and signs of ischemia or heart failure.

Laboratory, Diagnostic Procedures

A highly sensitive TSH assay showing a low TSH value will accurately and easily diagnose hyperthyroidism. Serum thyroxine T_4 may also assist in diagnosis in those who are suspected to have a sudden onset of disease.

Although hyperfunctioning thyroid ("hot") nodules are less likely than hypofunctioning ("cold") nodules to represent thyroid carcinoma, fine needle aspiration should generally be performed to rule out thyroid malignancy.[24] As opposed to the uniform follicular appearance of Graves disease, the histology of toxic MNG demonstrates follicles of varying size, shape, and intensity of iodine metabolism.

Imaging

Nuclear thyroid scanning with radioactive iodine (RAI) is particularly useful in determining the functional status of thyroid nodules in the patient presenting with single or multiple thyroid nodules.[24] In toxic MNG, RAI uptake is increased in the nodule(s) and decreased in the rest of the gland. For large goiters, tracheal deviation may be present on chest x-ray. Chest x-ray may also reveal CHF in cases where there is cardiac decompensation.

Management

General Measures

The treatment of hyperthyroidism depends on its etiology. However, in all patients, and especially in older patients with CVD, the use of a β-blocker to control tachycardia and other symptoms is warranted. Antithyroid medications and therapies usually take some time to have their effect, and so the use of a β-blocker in the interim is protective for the older patient. β-Blockers may have effects on exercise tolerance and mood, and therefore should be monitored carefully in the older patient.

Medications

The transient hyperthyroidism of subacute thyroiditis is unlikely to need treatment. Nonsteroidal antiinflammatory medications may be used for neck pain. For other hyperthyroid states, antithyroid therapy is usually indicated and may involve antithyroid medications, RAI therapy, or surgical intervention. The antithyroid medications methimazole and propylthiouracil (PTU) work quickly by decreasing thyroid hormone secretion but require long-term use. Discontinuation of the medication or inconsistent adherence will lead to relapse of the disease, which may be especially hazardous in the older patient where discontinuation may precipitate or exacerbate existing cardiac problems. Also, these medications require frequent monitoring and dosage adjustments and may cause allergic reactions, hepatitis, and agranulocytosis.

For the elderly patient with Graves disease, thyroid ablation using RAI is the treatment of choice.[21] RAI ablation works by slowly destroying thyroid tissue over several weeks, and therefore the concomitant use of a β-blocker to control symptoms is important. A common effect of radioactive thyroid ablation is hypothyroidism, although this may take years to develop.

The treatment of toxic MNG with RAI ablation is somewhat more complex because, unlike in Graves disease, the uptake of the thyroid tissue is nonuniform, with more uptake in the hyperfunctioning nodule and less in the rest of the gland. Hypofunctioning nodules have relatively little iodine uptake and therefore are unlikely to be affected by RAI ablative therapy. The necessary RAI dose for toxic MNG is often greater than that required for Graves disease, and the nonnodular normal thyroid tissue may often be unaffected by the treatment. Although this may lead to less posttreatment hypothyroidism, this functioning thyroid tissue may develop new nodules over time. Therefore, surgical treatment for toxic MNG is a good treatment option.[24]

Recommendations. Antithyroid medications are useful in the management of Graves disease in children and in pregnant women, but they are not the treatment of choice in the older patient[21] (Evidence Level C).

Patients need to be monitored post–thyroid ablation therapy with TSH determinations to detect hypothyroidism, at which time replacement therapy with levothyroxine can be initiated[21] (Evidence Level C).

Surgical Interventions

Total thyroidectomy is a preferred choice for the management of hyperthyroidism from toxic MNG. It eliminates both the hyperthyroid state and the potential for future nodule formation. Patients need to be treated with β-blockers and antithyroid medications in the perioperative period to control the hyperthyroid state. Postoperatively, patients will necessarily become hypothyroid, and replacement therapy with levothyroxine will need to be initiated[24] (Evidence Level C).

REFERENCES

1. American Diabetes Association. Clinical practice recommendations. *Diabetes Care*.2005;28(suppl 1): http://www.diabetes.org/for-health-professionals-and-scientists/cpr.jsp.
2. Harris MI, Goldstein DE, Flegal KM, et al. Prevalence of diabetes, impaired fasting glucose, and impaired glucose tolerance in U.S. adults. *Diabetes Care*.1998;21:518–524.
3. Cowie CC, Rust KF, Byrd-Holt D, et al. Prevalence of diabetes and impaired fasting glucose in adults—United States, 1999–2000. *Morb Mortal Wkly Rep*.2003;52:833–837.
4. California Healthcare Foundation/American Geriatrics Society Panel on Improving Care for Elders with Diabetes. Guidelines for Improving the care of the older person with diabetes mellitus. *J Am Geriatr Soc*.2003;51:S265–S280.
5. Canadian Diabetes Association. Clinical practice guidelines for the prevention and management of diabetes in Canada. *Can J Diabetes*.2003;27(suppl 2):http://www.diabetes.ca/cpg2003/.
6. United Kingdom Prospective Diabetes Study (UKPDS) Group. Intensive blood-glucose control with sulphonylureas or insulin compared with conventional treatment and risk of complications in patients with type 2 diabetes (UKPDS 33). *Lancet*.1998;352: 837–853.
7. Stratton IM, Adler AI, Neil HA, et al. Association of glycaemia with macrovascular and microvascular complications of type 2 diabetes (UKPDS 35): Prospective observational study. *BMJ*.2000;321:405–412.
8. Davis S, Alonso M. Hypoglycemia as a barrier to glycemic control. *J Diabetes Complications*.2004;18:60–68.
9. Mooradian AD, McLaughlin S, Boyer CC, et al. Diabetes care for older adults. *Diabetes Spectr*.1999;12:70.
10. Oiknine R, Mooradian AD. Drug therapy of diabetes in the elderly. *Biomed Pharmacother*.2003;57:231–239.
11. Egede LE, Zheng D, Ye X, et al. The prevalence and pattern of complementary and alternative medicine use in individuals with diabetes. *Diabetes Care*.2002;25:324–329.
12. Yeh GY, Kaptchuck TJ, Eisenberg DM, et al. Systematic review of herbs and dietary supplements for glycemic control in diabetes. *Diabetes Care*.2003;26:1277–1294.
13. Areosa Sastra A, Grimley Evans J. Effect of the treatment of Type II diabetes mellitus on the development of cognitive impairment and dementia. (Cochrane Review). In: *The cochrane library*, Issue 3, Chichester, UK: John Wiley and Sons;2004.
14. Snow V, Weiss KB, Mottur-Pilson C. The evidence for tight blood pressure control in the management of type 2 diabetes mellitus. *Ann Intern Med*.2003;138:587–592.
15. Snow V, Aronson MD, Hornbake ER, et al. Lipid control in the management of type 2 diabetes mellitus: A clinical practice guideline from the American College of Physicians. *Ann Intern Med*.2004;140:644–649.
16. Shepherd J, Blauw GJ, Murphy MB, et al. Pravastatin in elderly individuals at risk of vascular disease (PROSPER): A randomized controlled trial. *Lancet*.2002;360(9346):1623–1630.
17. Bagchi N, Brown TR, Parish RF. Thyroid dysfunction in adults over age 55 years. A study in an urban US community. *Arch Intern Med*.1990;150:785–787.
18. Wall CR. Myxedema coma: Diagnosis and treatment. *Am Fam Physician*.2000;62:2485–2490.
19. Siddoway LA. Amiodarone: Guidelines for use and monitoring. *Am Fam Physician*.2003;68:2189–2196.
20. U.S. Preventive Services Task Force. Screening for thyroid disease. http://www.ahrq.gov/clinic/uspstf/uspsthyr.htm. Accessed March, 2006.
21. AACE Thyroid Task Force. American Association of Clinical Endocrinologists medical guidelines for clinical practice for the evaluation and treatment of hyperthyroidism and hypothyroidism. *Endocr Pract*.2002;8:457–469.
22. Wallace K, Hofmann MT. Thyroid dysfunction: How to manage overt and subclinical disease in older patients. *Geriatrics*.1998;53:32–38.
23. Hueston WJ. Treatment of hypothyroidism. *Am Fam Physician*.2001;64:1717–1724.
24. Hurley DL, Gharib H. Thyroid nodular disease: Is it toxic or nontoxic, malignant or benign? *Geriatrics*.1995;50:24–31.
25. Davis PJ, Davis FB. Hyperthyroidism in patients over the age of 60 years: Clinical features in 85 patients. *Medicine*.1974;53: 161–181.
26. Sawin CT, Geller A, Kaplan MM, et al. Low serum thyrotropin (thyroid-stimulating hormone) in older persons without hyperthyroidism. *Archives of Internal Medicine*.1991;151:165–168.

34 Immune and Inflammatory Disease in Older Adults

David R. Thomas

CLINICAL PEARLS 462

AGING OF THE IMMUNE SYSTEM 464

RHEUMATOID ARTHRITIS 464
- Systemic Lupus Erythematosus 465
- Sjögren Syndrome 466
- Scleroderma 467
- Psoriatic Arthritis 468

NONRHEUMATOID DISEASES WITH IMMUNE ETIOLOGY 468
- Vasculitis 468
- Polymyalgia Rheumatica and Giant Cell Arteritis 468
- Amyloid Disease 469
- Multiple Sclerosis 470
- Type 1 and 2 Diabetes 471
- Hashimoto Thyroiditis 471
- Soft Tissue Rheumatism 471
- Gout 471

CLINICAL PEARLS

- Musculoskeletal system disorders are among the most frequent complaints of older persons and account for a large portion of the care of older persons by primary care physicians.
- Aging is characterized by progressively increased concentrations of glucocorticoids and catecholamines and the decreased production of growth and sex hormones, a pattern reminiscent of that seen in chronic stress.
- The manifestations of immune disease are clearly related to the proinflammatory nature of cytokines, although the trigger for the initiation of the cytokine cascade is usually not known.

The classification of immune and inflammatory diseases is undergoing a considerable change. Traditional schemes have focused primarily on musculoskeletal conditions. Rheumatoid arthritis has served as a "prototype" disease in inflammatory arthritis research. However, most of the inflammatory mechanisms occurring in the rheumatoid synovium may also occur in tissues affected by other disorders, such as progressive systemic sclerosis, systemic lupus erythematosus, or the salivary glands of Sjögren syndrome patients. Improved understanding of the inflammatory cascade and immune complex diseases has increased the number of conditions attributed to inflammatory and immune complex disease.

Autoimmune diseases present as clinical syndromes caused by the activation of T cells or B cells, or both, in the absence of an ongoing infection or other discernible cause. While the trigger that initiates the cytokine cascade is not always known, the manifestations of disease are clearly related to the proinflammatory effect of cytokines. Tissue damage from trauma or infection, or some as yet unknown trigger of the immune system, activates the inflammatory cells and the subsequent release of the cell-associated proteins called *cytokines*.

TABLE 34.1
EXAMPLES OF PRO-AND ANTI-INFLAMMATORY CYTOKINES

Major Anti-inflammatory Cytokines	Major Proinflammatory Cytokines
Interleukin-1Ra	Interleukin-1r
Interleukin-4	Tumor necrosis factor-α r
Interleukin-6	Interleukin-18r
Interleukin-10	
Interleukin-11	
Interleukin-13	
Tumor necrosis factor-β	

Ra, receptor antagonist; r, receptor.

Cytokines act principally in a paracrine fashion. In other words, their activity is local, at the site of release. Their concentrations in tissues are therefore several times higher than those found in the peripheral circulation. These cytokines act through specific cell receptors locally and systemically. Cytokines both initiate and regulate acute-phase reactants. Locally, these are expressed as inflammation, and systemically hepatic acute phase proteins are produced with resulting fever and granulocytosis.[1]

This cascade is designed to isolate and destroy microbial pathogens and to activate tissue repair processes to facilitate a return to the physiologic homeostasis. The cascade is regulated by a complex interactive balance of soluble serum factors (s), receptors for cytokine (r), and receptor antagonists (Ra).

Interleukin (IL)-1s and tumor necrosis factor (TNF-α) are the cytokines responsible for the earliest acute phase reaction. Both cytokines induce a second wave of cytokines, including IL-6 and chemokines. IL-6 is an anti-inflammatory and immunoregulatory cytokine required for moderating the local and systemic inflammatory responses. Chemokines regulate the influx of leukocytes to the site of inflammation. The bioactivity of TNF-α and IL-1β is inhibited by naturally occurring antagonists such as IL-1 receptor antagonist (Ra) and soluble TNF receptors (sTNFR), as well as the anti-inflammatory cytokine IL-10. Examples of pro- and anti-inflammatory cytokines are given in Table 34.1.

A large number of conditions associated with the activated cytokine cascade produce musculoskeletal symptoms and illness.[2] Rheumatoid disorders are classical diseases of the cytokine cascade. Other cytokine cascade disorders, such as osteoporosis and Paget disease, primarily affect the musculoskeletal system. Others, such as metastatic carcinoma and multiple myeloma, cause secondary effects in the musculoskeletal system. Still others reflect immune disorders of the endocrine system, such as type 1 diabetes mellitus or thyroid disorders. Therefore, an increasing number of conditions are being recognized as primary immune complex disease.

Many autoimmune mechanisms can be confused with primary musculoskeletal disorders. For example, hyperthyroidism can be associated with manifestations resembling rheumatoid arthritis, in addition to producing radiologic findings due to the loss of skeletal calcium. Similarly, hypothyroidism in a person with long-standing rheumatoid arthritis may produce symptoms which may be attributed to the rheumatoid process. These crossover symptoms create diagnostic challenges.

Disorders in the musculoskeletal system are among the most frequent complaints of older persons, and account for a large portion of their care by primary care physicians (see Table 34.2). These disorders fall into three categories: (i) The classic rheumatoid diseases, (ii) conditions not generally regarded as rheumatoid in nature whose clinical manifestations are expressed in the musculoskeletal system, and (iii) a wide range of localized musculoskeletal disorders that fall under the general category of "soft tissue rheumatism."

TABLE 34.2
COMMON INFLAMMATORY CONDITIONS OF AGING (ICD-9 CODE)

Primary Joint Disease	Joints Often Involved	Joints Minor Presentation
Ankylosing spondylitis (720.0)	Crohn disease (555.9)	Amyloidosis (277.3)
Gout (274.0)	Giant cell arteritis (446.5)	CREST syndrome (710.1)
Polymyalgia rheumatica (725.0)	Psoriasis (696.0)	Hashimoto thyroiditis (245.0)
Rheumatoid arthritis (714.0)	Scleroderma (710.1)	Immune thrombocytic purpura (287.3)
Soft tissue rheumatism (727.3)	Sjögren syndrome (710.2)	Multiple sclerosis (340.0)
	Systemic lupus erythematosus (710.0)	Primary Raynaud (443.0)
		Vasculitis (287.0)

CREST, Calcinosis, Raynaud phenomenon, Esophageal dysmotility, Sclerodactyly, and Telangiectasia.

AGING OF THE IMMUNE SYSTEM

Aging is characterized by progressively increased concentrations of glucocorticoids and catecholamines and decreased production of growth and sex hormones, a pattern suggestive of that seen in chronic stress. Aging has also been associated with increased levels of circulating inflammatory components including elevated concentrations of TNF-α, IL-6, IL-1Ra, and sTNFR, acute phase proteins such as C-reactive protein (CRP) and serum amyloid A, and high neutrophil counts. Plasma levels of TNF-α have been positively correlated with IL-6, sTNFR-II, and CRP in centenarians, suggesting an activation of the entire inflammatory cascade. However, the increase in circulating inflammatory factors in healthy elderly humans is limited, and far less than levels seen during acute infections at any age.[3,4]

There remains uncertainty as to whether changes in cytokine levels are due to age itself or to underlying disease.[5] The increase in plasma levels of IL-6 with age may occur because of catecholamine hypersecretion and sex-steroid hyposecretion[6]—or acquired physiologic insults (visceral obesity, smoking, stress, etc.),[7] subclinical infections such as *Chlamydia pneumoniae* or *Helicobacter pylori*, or, finally, dental infections and asymptomatic bacteriuria.[8]

Proinflammatory cytokines are thought to play a pathogenetic role in age-associated diseases such as Alzheimer disease, Parkinson disease, atherosclerosis, type 2 diabetes, sarcopenia, and osteoporosis.[9] Low-grade inflammatory activity in older populations is related to dysregulated cytokine production, which is further exacerbated by age-associated pathology. Cause–effect or effect–cause awaits further study for many conditions attributed to aging that may have a basis in immune function.

RHEUMATOID ARTHRITIS

Rheumatoid arthritis occurs worldwide and is estimated to occur in 1% to 2% of the population, with a female to male ratio of 3:1. High levels of TNF-α and IL-1β have been demonstrated in synovial fluid and in the circulation of patients with rheumatoid arthritis.[10,11] The role of these proinflammatory cytokines has been bolstered by recent interventions involving TNF-α and IL-1 inhibitors.[12] An antigen, yet unknown, appears to initiate the autoimmune response. Suspect triggers such as the Epstein-Barr virus, the influenza virus, or the hepatitis C virus, are associated with joint symptoms that are exactly like rheumatoid arthritis; however, unlike true rheumatoid arthritis symptoms, these last only a few weeks.

Rheumatoid arthritis is diagnosed by the presence of five of seven diagnostic criteria, as shown in Table 34.3. The rheumatoid factor is present in 80% of patients. However, 5% of the elderly may have a false-positive rheumatoid factor. Citrullinated peptides are present in 90% of patients with rheumatoid arthritis, but due to their cyclic pattern may not be detected in half the patients tested. Radiologic changes on magnetic resonance imaging (MRI) are useful in diagnosing classic joint erosions.

The treatment of rheumatoid arthritis has been markedly improved by the recognition that bone erosions occur early in the disease; therefore therapy should be instituted promptly. Because rheumatoid arthritis is both most

TABLE 34.3
REVISED DIAGNOSTIC CRITERIA FOR RHEUMATOID ARTHRITIS CLASSIFICATION

Criteria	Description
Arthritis of three or more joint areas	Morning stiffness in and around the joints, lasting at least one hour before maximal improvement
Arthritis of three or more joint areas	At least three joint areas (out of 14 possible areas; right or left PIP, MCP, wrist, elbow, knee, ankle, MTP joints) simultaneously have had soft tissue swelling or fluid (not bony overgrowth alone) as observed by a physician
Arthritis of hand joints	At least one area swollen (as defined in the preceding text) in a wrist, MCP, or PIP joint
Symmetric arthritis	Simultaneous involvement of the same joint areas (as defined in the preceding text) on both sides of the body (bilateral involvement of PIPs, MCPs, or MTPs, without absolute symmetry is acceptable)
Rheumatoid nodules	Subcutaneous nodules over bony prominences or extensor surfaces, or in juxta-articular regions as observed by a physician
Serum rheumatoid factor	Demonstration of abnormal amounts of serum rheumatoid factor by any method for which the result has been positive in $<$5% of normal control subjects
Radiographic changes	Radiographic changes typical of RA on posterior or anterior hand or wrist radiographs, which must include erosions or unequivocal bony decalcification localized in, or most marked adjacent to, the involved joints (osteoarthritis changes alone do not qualify)

For classification purposes, a patient has rheumatoid arthritis if at least four of these criteria are satisfied (the first four must have been present for at least 6 weeks).
MCP, metacarpophalangeal; PIP, proximal interphalangeal; MTP, metatarsophalangeal; RA, rheumatoid arthritis.
Arnett FC, Edworthy SM, Bloch DA, et al. The American Rheumatism Association 1987 revised criteria for the classification of rheumatoid arthritis. *Arthritis Rheum.* 1988;31:315–324.

aggressive and most responsive to treatment in the first 2 years, it is now recommended that drug therapy begins within months of diagnosis.

Treatment options for rheumatoid arthritis can be divided into disease-modifying treatments and non–disease-modifying treatments. Non–disease-modifying treatments such as anti-inflammatory agents can be used to control symptoms and pain, but do not affect the progression of the disease.

Disease-modifying drugs modify the progression of the disease. A meta-analysis of clinical trials has suggested that the efficacy of methotrexate, sulfasalazine, intramuscular gold, and penicillamine is similar. Antimalarial drugs (e.g., chloroquine and hydroxychloroquine) are less effective. Penicillamine, because of concern about its toxicity, and oral gold, because of its marginal efficacy, are rarely used today.

Corticosteroids are potent suppressors of the inflammatory response in rheumatoid arthritis but have significant dose-dependent side effects. Controversy exists for when, if, and how corticosteroids should be used to treat rheumatoid arthritis. Corticosteroids clearly decrease the radiographic evidence of disease progression of rheumatoid arthritis. As a result, 30% to 60% of patients receive corticosteroids in low doses (e.g., $\leq$10 mg of prednisone per day) (Evidence Level B).

Methotrexate is considered the first-line disease-modifying agent and is generally used to compare other therapies. Side effects often limit the use of methotrexate but concomitant administration of folic acid (1 to 3 mg per day) significantly decreases many toxic effects without a measurable decrease in efficacy.

Newer treatment options are based on the observation that synovial inflammation in rheumatoid arthritis is produced by macrophage-derived cytokines. Several products that inhibit the actions of TNF-α (infliximab, etanercept, and adalimumab) and one that inhibits the action of IL-1 (anakinra) are available to treat rheumatoid arthritis. Blockade of TNF-α by etanercept or a monoclonal antibody (infliximab) is highly effective in preventing erosions when used in combination with methotrexate. Leflunomide, a pyrimidine antagonist that blocks deoxyribonucleic acid synthesis by the enzyme dihydroorotate dehydrogenase, has an efficacy similar to that of methotrexate and can be used either alone or in combination with methotrexate.

Blockade of IL-1r with a recombinant IL-1Ra antagonist is less effective than blockade of TNF-α in patients with rheumatoid arthritis, but it may retard the development of bone erosions.[13] The long-term safety of these new agents, particularly with respect to the risk of infections, cancer, and other autoimmune diseases, is still of some concern.[14]

Improvement in rheumatoid symptoms can be documented by the American College of Rheumatology (ACR) scale.[15] An ACR 20 is defined as a reduction by 20% or more in the number of tender and swollen joints, plus similar improvement in at least three of the following five measures: Pain, global assessments by the patient and the physician, self-assessed physical disability, and levels of acute phase reactant. Improvements of ACR 50 to 70 should be the aim of treatment. Failure to achieve this much improvement should trigger a referral or a change in therapy.

Blockade of TNF-α by anticytokine drugs is also effective in Crohn disease, refractory psoriatic arthritis, and ankylosing spondylitis.

Systemic Lupus Erythematosus

Systemic lupus erythematosus (SLE or lupus) is a multisystem, chronic autoimmune disorder involving a number of self-antigens. The annual incidence of lupus is about 5 per 100,000 persons. The incidence peaks for women in late middle age, and somewhat later for men. Lupus occurs within families, but there is no identified gene or genes that have been linked to the disorder. Environmental factors have also been implicated in the development of lupus, including infections, antibiotics in the sulfonamide and penicillin groups, exposure to excessive stress, and ultraviolet light.

Lupus can occur at any age and in either sex, but it occurs more frequently in women than men, with a ratio of 9:1. In persons older than 60, the sex ratio declines to 4:1. Estrogen may play a role in lupus. The symptoms often increase before menstruation and during pregnancy, but the link remains speculative.

Lupus occurs when antibodies are produced against the components within the nucleus of cells. These autoantibodies then react with body tissues as if the tissue were an antigen, and immune complexes are formed. These immune complexes accumulate in the joints, kidneys, skin, blood, and other tissues, activating the complement cascade, inflammation, pain, and organ damage.

Although the tissue inflammation is widespread, most patients present with isolated manifestations, leading to confusion with other diseases such as immune thrombocytic purpura, primary Raynaud, or rheumatoid arthritis. Polyarthritis and skin manifestations are the presenting features in about 75% of patients. Glomerulonephritis, lymphadenopathy, anemia, leucopenia, pleurisy, mouth ulcers, and central nervous system symptoms are other clinical features. Most patients have constitutional symptoms. The diagnosis of lupus can be made by finding four or more symptoms over time of a list of 11 clinical criteria developed by the American Rheumatism Association, shown in Table 34.4.

The management of SLE is complicated by the range of disease manifestations, the relapsing nature of the disease, and the lack of standardized criteria for remission. For example, whether an abnormal serologic result should be treated in the absence of clinical signs of the disease is not clear. There is no evidence that prophylactic treatment with a low dose of a glucocorticoid is beneficial.

TABLE 34.4
CRITERIA FOR DIAGNOSIS OF SYSTEMIC LUPUS ERYTHEMATOSIS

Symptom Or Criteria	Description
Malar rash	Red rash over cheeks and the bridge of the nose
Discoid rash	Red, scaly rash on the face, scalp, ears, arms, or chest
Photosensitivity	Unusual reaction to the sun
Oral ulcers	Small sores on the moist lining of the nose or mouth
Arthritis	Pain in the joints of the hands, arms, shoulders, feet, legs, hips, or jaws which may move from joint to joint and be accompanied by heat, redness, and swelling
Serositis	Pleurisy—chest pain or abnormal sounds heard by physician. Inflammation of the lining of the heart. Documented by ECG or heard by physician
Renal	Excessive protein and/or cellular casts in the urine
Neurologic	Seizures and/or psychosis
Hematologic (blood)	Disorder which can include a decrease in the number of red and white blood cells or platelets
Immunologic	Immunologic positive anti-DNA test
ANA	ANA positive

ECG, electrocardiogram; DNA, deoxyribonucleic acid; ANA, antinuclear antibody.
Tan EM, Cohen AS, Fries JF, et al. The 1982 revised criteria for the classification of systemic lupus erythematosus. *Arthritis Rheum.* 1982;25:1271–1277.

Arthritis and serositis can often be controlled by aspirin or other nonsteroidal anti-inflammatory drugs. Glucocorticoid therapy has not been shown to prevent progression of lupus nephritis, a major cause of morbidity in lupus. A regimen that includes cyclophosphamide is more effective in preserving renal function than is treatment with a glucocorticoid alone.[16] Clinical trials of monoclonal antibodies have shown high toxicity and poor efficacy. Antibodies against IL-10 may prove effective.

Sjögren Syndrome

Sjögren syndrome is a relatively common autoimmune disorder characterized by manifestations of keratoconjunctivitis sicca (90%) and xerostomia (80%), as shown in Table 34.5. In sharp contrast to the low frequency of lupus in older people, primary Sjögren syndrome has a frequency approximating that of rheumatoid arthritis. Arthralgia is reported in as many as 53% of patients and myalgia in as many as 22% of patients.

Primary Sjögren syndrome is often confused with rheumatoid arthritis both clinically and serologically. A secondary Sjögren syndrome is present in 10% to 20% of patients with rheumatoid arthritis and 38% of patients with late-onset lupus. It also occurs in patients with systemic sclerosis and mixed connective tissue disease. In the absence of other connective tissue disease, primary Sjögren syndrome is diagnosed. About a third of all cases of Sjögren syndrome are primary.

The diagnosis is complicated by the fact that xerostomia and xerophthalmia occur in 15% to 25% of otherwise normal older people. These symptoms should be differentiated from those associated with true Sjögren syndrome by the absence of systemic manifestations.

A Schirmer test can provide an effective and inexpensive diagnostic test. To perform the test, a piece of filter paper 0.25 cm wide and 3 cm long is folded, and one end is placed on the lower eyelid. In the presence of normal tears, at least 1.5 cm of the paper will be saturated in five minutes. In patients with keratoconjunctivitis sicca, the moistening covers 0.5 cm or less of the paper. Another procedure for confirming the presence of keratoconjunctivitis sicca involves slit lamp examination following intraocular instillation of rose bengal dye.

Anti-SS-A/Ro and anti-SS-B/La antibodies, if present, are also helpful in supporting the clinical diagnosis. Although the disorder can usually be diagnosed on the basis of its clinical manifestations and immunologic reactions, confirmation requires biopsy, usually obtained from the lip. Demonstration of diffuse lymphocytic infiltration of the mucosal glands confirms the presence of Sjögren syndrome.

The diagnostic criteria for Sjörgren syndrome requires four or more of the following criteria, one of which must be a biopsy: Symptoms of dry eye, signs of dry eye (Schirmer test or rose bengal test), symptoms of dry mouth, tests of salivary function (abnormal flow rate, scintigram, or sialogram), presence of anti-SS-A/Ro or anti-SS-B/La antibodies, and positive minor salivary gland biopsy.

Treatment of Sjögren syndrome is predominantly symptomatic. Artificial tears without preservatives and lemon-and-glycerine mouth rinses are the backbone of therapy. Corticosteroid eye medications should not be used because they may cause further damage to the cornea. Systemic corticosteroids in low doses may be helpful in patients with enlarged tender salivary glands and severe extra glandular symptoms. Immunosuppressive therapy for Sjörgren syndrome with oral cyclosporine, methotrexate, or hydroxychloroquine has not shown benefit.

TABLE 34.5
MANIFESTATIONS OF SJÖGREN SYNDROME

	Glandular Manifestations
Keratoconjunctivitis sicca	Diminished tear production due to destruction of the active secretory apparatus Tears are quantitatively and qualitatively altered, with increased osmolarity, diminished IgA, lysozyme, and lactoferrin content Patients may report dry eyes, grittiness, burning, photophobia, or reduced visual acuity
Xerostomia	Diminished saliva production manifested as a dry mouth, odynophagia, halitosis, excessive oral pathology and infections, and dysgeusia
	Extraglandular Manifestations
Respiratory disease	Dryness of the upper and lower respiratory tract may lead to inspissated secretions, chronic cough, and recurrent infection. Interstitial infiltrates also occur Serositis with pleural effusions may predominate
Renal disease	Interstitial nephritis and tubular dysfunction, most commonly manifesting as renal tubular acidosis, but may progress to complete Fanconi syndrome
Neurologic	Peripheral and cranial neuropathy, central nervous system involvement in a small minority of patients with multifocal lesions throughout the white matter resembling multiple sclerosis both clinically and radiologically
Arthritis	Arthralgia and/or nonerosive arthritis characterized by tenderness, swelling, or effusion involving two or more peripheral joints
Raynaud phenomenon	Intermittent attacks of digital pallor followed by cyanosis and/or rubor of the fingers, toes, ears, nose, tongue, induced by exposure to cold, stress, or both, in the absence of any other associated disease or anatomical abnormality
Cutaneous vasculitis	Cutaneous purpura and/or rash
Non-Hodgkin lymphoma	Occurs with increased frequency, often in the mucosa-associated lymphoid tissue

Garcia–Carrasco M, Ramos-Casals M, Rosas J, et al. Primary Sjögren syndrome: Clinical and immunologic disease patterns in a cohort of 400 patients. *Medicine.* 2002;81:270–280.

Untreated keratoconjunctivitis sicca can lead to loss of vision, and decreased saliva is associated with dental problems. Five percent to 10% of patients with long-standing Sjögren syndrome develop B-cell lymphoma. Others develop renal tubular dysfunction. Most patients, however, have good survival rates but decreased quality of life due to symptoms.

Scleroderma

In scleroderma, fibroblasts behave autonomously and produce excess elements of the extracellular matrix, particularly type I collagen. The fibroblasts are activated by T-cell–derived cytokines, suggesting that immune activation initiates the pathology of scleroderma. Scleroderma can be localized or diffuse (see Table 34.6). Systemic effects target the skin and gastrointestinal tract, causing profoundly debilitating symptoms. Mortality (approximately 40% over 5 years) is due to pulmonary fibrosis and renal involvement. Approximately 20% develop erosive arthritis. Scleroderma can also coexist with erosive rheumatoid arthritis, lupus, multiple sclerosis, and perinuclear antineutrophil cytoplasmic antibody–associated vasculitis.

Antinuclear antibody is positive in 70% of patients with scleroderma. Anti-RNP, found in mixed connective tissue disorder, is positive in 20% to 30% of patients with scleroderma, lupus, and Sjögren syndrome. Rheumatoid factors are present in up to one-third of patients. Scl-70 antibody has been noted in approximately one-third of scleroderma cases. There is variability in the presence of anti-Ro in scleroderma (12%), SLE (35%), and Sjögren syndrome (40%

TABLE 34.6
CLASSIFICATION OF SCLERODERMA

I. Limited (CREST syndrome)	Long-standing Raynaud Skin changes limited to hands, face, feet, and forearms Skin calcification and telangiectasia GIT involvement Late pulmonary hypertension Dilated nailfold capillary loops without dropout
II. Diffuse (Systemic sclerosis)	Truncal and acral involvement Skin changes within 1 year of Raynaud onset Tendon friction rubs Early interstitial lung disease Diffuse gastrointestinal tract involvement Nailfold capillary dilation and dropout

CREST, Calcinosis, Raynaud phenomenon, Esophageal dysmotility, Sclerodactyly, and Telangiectasia; GIT, gastrointestinal tract.

to 70%). Anticytoplasmic antibody is very common in limited scleroderma but rare in diffuse scleroderma. From 60% to 70% of patients with CREST (Calcinosis, Raynaud phenomenon, Esophageal dysmotility, Sclerodactyly, and Telangiectasia) syndrome have anticentromere antibodies.

CREST syndrome is characterized by limited cutaneous involvement, but severe Raynaud and calcinosis lead to profound functional limitations. Renal involvement does not usually occur in the limited form, but respiratory involvement with pulmonary hypertension may be a significant problem.

Corticosteroids have not been shown to be useful in delaying the progression of skin involvement in scleroderma. However, they may be helpful in controlling pain caused by arthralgia or myalgia. Similar benefits may be achieved with nonsteroidal anti-inflammatory agents. Nifedipine and angiotensin-converting enzyme inhibitors have shown to be effective in reducing symptoms in Raynaud phenomenon. Pentoxifylline may have an additive effect. Methotrexate, cyclosporine, cyclophosphamide, and extra corporeal photopheresis have been successful in decreasing skin symptoms but have not so far shown good effect in modifying systemic symptoms.

Angiotensin-converting enzyme inhibitors, including captopril and enalapril maleate are effective in controlling high blood pressure in systemic sclerosis, and may protect renal function. Cyclophosphamide alone, or in combination with low-dose prednisone has been found effective in the treatment of severe interstitial lung disease. Etanercept has improved skin symptoms but did not improve pulmonary symptoms.[17]

Psoriatic Arthritis

Psoriatic arthritis is a chronic inflammatory arthritis associated with psoriasis. It is often accompanied by bony proliferation and osteolysis at tendon, ligament, and capsular insertions. In epidemiologic studies, the incidence of psoriatic arthritis was estimated to be 6.59 per 100,000.[18] Psoriatic arthritis has been reported in about 6% of patients with psoriasis.

Clinical manifestations include dactylitis, enthesitis, osteoperiostitis, large joint oligoarthritis, arthritis mutilans, sacroiliitis, spondylitis, and distal interphalangeal arthritis. Psoriatic arthritis can be confused with rheumatoid arthritis or ankylosing spondylitis. However, spondyloarthropathies, such as psoriatic arthritis, are characterized by primary tendon or ligament inflammation rather than synovial inflammation. There is no consensus on the etiology or diagnostic criteria. A combination of negative rheumatoid factor, dactylitis, any typical radiographic feature, and involvement of less than four metacarpal phalangeal joints has a sensitivity of 90% and specificity of 89% for the diagnosis of psoriatic arthritis.

Management of psoriatic arthritis includes pain control, steroidal and nonsteroidal anti-inflammatory drugs, and disease-modifying agents. Methotrexate is a disease-modifying drug with demonstrated effectiveness in psoriasis and can improve nail lesions (Evidence Level A). Sulphasalazine, which has antibacterial, anti-inflammatory and immunomodulatory effects, is effective in treating persistent peripheral arthritis. Drugs such as lithium, β-adrenergic blocking agents and antimalarials can aggravate psoriasis and may therefore worsen psoriatic arthritis.

Blockade of TNF α with etanercept and intermittent infusion of infliximab, with or without methotrexate, has been effective in refractory psoriasis, but little is known about the effect on psoriatic arthritis. Psoriasis responded to treatment with IL-10 in several small and short-term clinical trials. A number of other biologic agents have also been successfully used to treat psoriasis in small pilot studies. These include antibodies against CD4, antibodies against the high-affinity IL-2r CD25 (daclizumab), and antibodies against the CD11, a component of the adhesion molecule leukocyte function-associated antigen type 1.

NONRHEUMATOID DISEASES WITH IMMUNE ETIOLOGY

Vasculitis

Vasculitis is an inflammation of blood vessel walls, which can cause tissue infarction or impair the function of the tissues supplied by the particular blood vessels. Different vasculitides have a predilection for different combinations of organs, for reasons that are still not entirely clear. A restricted or differential molecular expression in the endothelium of these organs may explain this phenomenon. A number of distinct syndromes have been described. A useful classification is in terms of the size of the vessel affected. A classification of vasculitis and a brief description of clinical features is given in Table 34.7.

Polymyalgia Rheumatica and Giant Cell Arteritis

The frequency of polymyalgia rheumatica in older patients approximates that of rheumatoid arthritis. Giant cell arteritis (also known as temporal or cranial arteritis) is an inflammatory vasculitis which often involves the short posterior ciliary vessels, resulting in an ischemic optic neuropathy. If not recognized and treated appropriately, preventable blindness may result. Temporal arteritis occurs in approximately 8% to 10% of patients with polymyalgia rheumatica.

Clinical features of polymyalgia rheumatica include severe aching and stiffness, absence of objective inflammation of the large joints, and in most cases a strikingly elevated erythrocyte sedimentation rate and elevated CRP. Visual difficulties, such as zigzag lines in a visual field or a general dimness of vision, soreness or claudication of the masseter muscles, and tenderness over the temporal artery are important clues to the presence of this disorder.

TABLE 34.7
CLASSIFICATION OF VASCULITIS

Large Vessel Vasculitis	
Giant cell arteritis	Unilateral headache, facial pain, and jaw claudication Sudden or painless visual loss, affecting part or all of the visual field Diplopia may occur Most common type of primary systemic vasculitis
Takayasu arteritis	Vasculitis of arteries leading to claudication of the arm, loss of arm pulses, variation in blood pressure of >10 mm Hg between the arms, arterial bruits, angina, aortic regurgitation, syncope, stroke, and visual disturbance May cause bowel ischemia or infarction, renovascular hypertension, and renal impairment
Medium Vessel Vasculitis	
Polyarteritis nodosa	Vasculitis leading to gut ischemia or infarction, angina or myocardial infarction, cortical kidney infarcts leading to hypertension and renal failure, and peripheral neuropathy May be associated with hepatitis B virus
Wegener granulomatosis	Upper respiratory tract disease or sinusitis in 90% of cases; bleeding, obstruction, and collapse of the nasal bridge; serous otitis media with conductive deafness; and tracheal stenosis Pulmonary symptoms of cough, hemoptysis, and dyspnea, or life-threatening hemorrhage Kidneys affected in up to 80% of cases with blood, protein, and casts in the urine Ocular manifestations including conjunctival hemorrhages, scleritis, uveitis, keratitis, proptosis, or ocular muscle paralysis Gastrointestinal hemorrhage, coronary artery ischemia, and neurological system symptoms may occur
Churg-Strauss syndrome	Atopic tendency, usually asthma May affect coronary, pulmonary, cerebral, and splanchnic circulations Rashes with purpura, urticaria, and subcutaneous nodules common Glomerulonephritis may develop, but renal failure uncommon
Small Vessel Vasculitis	
Henoch-Schönlein purpura	Purpura over the lower limbs and buttocks, hematuria, abdominal pain, bloody diarrhea, and arthralgia
Cryoglobulinemic vasculitis	Purpura, arthralgia, distal necroses, peripheral neuropathy, abdominal pain, and glomerulonephritis Because of hepatitis C virus infection in >80% of cases
Isolated cutaneous leukocytoclastic vasculitis	Associated with drug hypersensitivity (e.g., hydralazine, propylthiouracil)
Goodpasture disease	Rapidly progressive glomerulonephritis or presence of pulmonary hemorrhage, or both
Thromboangiitis Obliterans	
SLE	See text
Rheumatoid arthritis	See text

SLE, systemic lupus erythematosus.
Table developed from Savage COS, Harper L, Cockwell P, et al. Vasculitis. *BMJ.* 2000;320:1325–1328.

Rapid response to a test dose of prednisone, 15 mg per day for 2 or 3 days, supports the diagnosis. Once the condition is suspected, prednisone in a dose of 60 to 80 mg per day should be started (Evidence Level A). Biopsy of the temporal arteries is usually undertaken in suspected cases to rule out temporal artery arteritis. Obtaining a biopsy should not delay the initiation of prednisone therapy because of the very real hazard that the patient will develop blindness while the results of the biopsy are pending. The biopsy can be falsely positive, since the histologic change in the artery can be uneven, despite active disease. Prednisone therapy does not change the histology in the artery for several days, so the biopsy can be performed even after prednisone has been started.

Serial determinations of the erythrocyte sedimentation rate or CRP may be helpful in following the clinical course but are not infallible. Gradual lowering of the dose is guided by symptoms. The corticosteroid dose may be reduced to 10 mg per day over 6 months and then more slowly to a maintenance of 5 to 10 mg per day. Maintenance treatment may be required for as long as 2 years. While the condition often subsides during the course of 1 or 2 years, the symptoms may continue in some patients indefinitely, flaring up as the dose of prednisone is gradually decreased.

Amyloid Disease

Amyloidosis is a heterogeneous group of disorders characterized by extracellular deposition of fibrillar protein. Amyloidosis can be classified as primary amyloidosis, secondary amyloidosis, familial amyloidosis, senile systemic amyloidosis, or localized amyloidosis. Three different types of amyloid proteins have been described. The first type (AL) occurs in primary amyloidosis and in amyloidosis associated with multiple myeloma. The second type (AA) occurs in secondary amyloidosis. The third type (often a transthyretin) is associated with familial amyloid polyneuropathy.

Amyloid has also been associated with chronic hemodialysis (a β_2-microglobulin), with the histopathologic lesions of Alzheimer disease (β/A4 amyloid protein), and with non–insulin-dependent diabetes mellitus. Amyloid associated with aging in skin and endocrine organs may represent another biochemical form of amyloidosis.

A unique protein (a pentraxin) called *AP* (or serum AP) is associated with all forms of amyloid. Isotopically labeled serum AP has been used in a scintigraphic test to confirm the diagnosis of amyloidosis. The gold standard for the diagnosis of amyloidosis is a biopsy, showing a characteristic green birefringence with a Congo red stain.

In primary amyloidosis, the heart, lung, skin, tongue, thyroid gland, liver, spleen, kidney, intestinal tract, and vascular system may be involved. Amyloid fibrils infiltrate the myocardium, impairing ventricular contraction and relaxation. The most common clinical cardiac manifestations are congestive heart failure and arrhythmia, accounting for death in 40% of persons with primary amyloidosis.[19] The median survival in primary systemic amyloidosis is <18 months. Actuarial survival for patients in one study was 51% at 1 year, 16% at 5 years, and 4.7% at 10 years.[20]

Secondary (AA) amyloidosis involves the spleen, liver, kidney, adrenal, and lymph nodes. Vascular involvement may be widespread, though clinically significant involvement of the heart is rare. Secondary amyloidosis occurs in patients with chronic infectious or inflammatory processes. Nephrotic syndrome, congestive heart failure, orthostatic hypotension, carpal tunnel syndrome, and peripheral neuropathy are frequent findings. Secondary amyloidosis may complicate psoriasis. Electrophoresis of the serum reveals a protein spike in only 40% of patients, but immunoelectrophoresis shows a monoclonal protein in 68% of patients. Treatment for amyloidosis is unsatisfactory but includes melphalan, prednisone, colchicine, and dimethyl sulfoxide.[21]

Dialysis-related amyloidosis is a complication in patients on long-term hemodialysis. It is characterized by chronic arthralgia, periarticular soft tissue swelling, carpal tunnel syndrome, diffuse destructive arthropathy and spondylarthropathy, lytic bone lesions, and occasional pathologic fractures. The histologic prevalence of dialysis-related amyloidosis is much greater than suspected on clinical grounds. Thirty percent of patients are affected after <4 years on hemodialysis, and 90% are affected after 7 years on hemodialysis. Renal transplantation is the best treatment of dialysis-related amyloidosis. In patients unsuitable for transplantation, high flux membranes should be used from the start of dialysis. Palliative treatment includes analgesics, low-dose prednisone in severe cases, and surgical treatment of complications.[22]

Age-related amyloidosis may be systemic or localized. The systemic forms include associated-myeloma (AL) amyloidosis and senile systemic amyloidosis. Amyloid derived from transthyretin is the only clear-cut systemic form related to age. In localized amyloidosis, the fibril protein precursors are synthesized in the tissue involved by the amyloid. This localized age-related amyloidosis does not appear to cause clinical disease in most cases. The significance of aortic amyloidosis, amyloidosis of seminal vesicles, amyloid of the endocrine glands, and articular amyloidosis remains unknown.[23]

Multiple Sclerosis

Multiple sclerosis is an immune-related disease and the most common primary disease of the central nervous system. In multiple sclerosis, the myelin sheath that surrounds the axon is destroyed and is replaced by hard, plaque-like lesions. The loss of myelin leads to the impairment of nerve conduction through the damaged axons. Multiple sclerosis results from the interaction of an unknown environmental factor with the immune system of susceptible individuals. Once activated, the immune system causes the destruction of the myelin sheath. Multiple sclerosis is characterized by periods of remission and relapse over many years, which suggests that the immune response is variable.

Multiple sclerosis is more common in women and usually presents in early adulthood. Approximately half of all multiple sclerosis patients require the use of a walking aid within 10 years after clinical onset. Frequent relapse and poor recovery in the first years of clinical disease predict a more rapid deterioration. These patients frequently present to geriatricians when they require nursing home care.

Multiple sclerosis can be clinically categorized as either relapsing-remitting, observed in 85% to 90% of patients, or primary progressive multiple sclerosis. Relapses typically present subacutely, with symptoms developing over hours to several days, persisting for several days or weeks, and then gradually dissipating. The attacks are likely caused by activated, myelin-reactive T cells, causing acute inflammation with associated edema.

Approximately 40% of relapsing-remitting patients stop having attacks and develop a progressive neurodegenerative secondary disorder known as secondary progressive multiple sclerosis. The primary progressive form of multiple sclerosis is characterized by a persistent gradual clinical decline without remissions. Progressive patterns of multiple sclerosis have a poor response to any form of immunotherapy.

The diagnosis of multiple sclerosis is made by clinical history, neurologic examination, and MRI. Multiple central nervous system lesions separated in time are the hallmark of diagnosis. MRI permits an early and a more precise diagnosis of the disease. In patients experiencing their first episode suggestive of central nervous system demyelination with MRI evidence of at least three typical lesions, more than half of those developing multiple sclerosis experience an additional relapse within 1 year of their first episode. If there are no lesions seen on MRI, the probability of developing multiple sclerosis is substantially less.

Several immunomodulating therapies have been used in treating multiple sclerosis. These include immunosuppressive drugs such as prednisone, mitoxantrone, and cyclophosphamide, interferon β-1a, and glatiramer acetate (a major histocompatibility complex [MHC]-binding protein that engages the T-cell receptor).

Type 1 and 2 Diabetes

Evidence of an autoimmune reaction to the B cells occurs in approximately 90% of persons with type 1 diabetes mellitus. It is likely that environmental factors trigger the onset of diabetes in those with a genetic predisposition. Attempts at preventing type 1 diabetes have included inducing immune tolerance through the intravenous or subcutaneous administration of insulin in persons at risk. Results with oral insulin have been disappointing, but systemic insulin may be more promising. Cyclophosphamide has ameliorated type 1 diabetes if started early.

Type 2 diabetes mellitus is not usually thought of as an immune disease, but evidence suggests that a proportion of individuals with the metabolic syndrome have preexisting elevations in inflammatory cytokines. Type 2 diabetes mellitus may be induced by inflammatory disease in a subset of individuals.

Hashimoto Thyroiditis

Hashimoto thyroiditis is the most common type of thyroiditis and the most common cause of hypothyroidism. In Hashimoto thyroiditis, there is a gradual loss of thyroid epithelial cells, associated with activation of T cells. Antithyroid antibodies can be detected in the blood of patients with Hashimoto thyroiditis. The autoimmune response might be initiated either by a viral or bacterial infection that triggers T-cell activity, which cross reacts and then targets thyroid cells.

Soft Tissue Rheumatism

The largest number of musculoskeletal complaints among older people results from localized conditions involving tendons, bursa, muscle sheets, and muscles themselves. These conditions can be grouped into "soft tissue rheumatism." The symptoms produced by these conditions are due to the triggering of the inflammatory cascade by trauma, although the effect remains localized. Almost any part of the musculoskeletal systems can be affected, ranging from "pulled muscles" to plantar fascitis.

The pain may be perceived in a wide region due to the shared enervation of many connective tissues with specific areas of the skin (dermatomes). Thus, pain due to inflammation of a shoulder joint may be manifested by aching in the upper arms. Pain due to inflammation of the hip is often perceived as pain in the knee. Referred pain may also occur because of the irritation of a nerve root at its point of exit from the vertebral canal or to irritation as the nerve trunk passes by an inflamed structure such as a sacroiliac joint. Thus, pain in the shoulder may result from osteoarthritis in the neck, or arthritis of the lumbosacral spine may be perceived as pain or numbness in the foot.

The diagnosis of these disorders rests primarily on a careful history and a deliberate physical examination. For example, inflammation of the shoulder joint itself is only one cause of shoulder pain. Shoulder pain may also be referred from the cervical roots, from intrathoracic conditions such as an apical lung tumor or pleural disease, from the heart as a result of myocardial ischemia, or from subdiaphragmatic irritation due to gallbladder disease, abscess, or tumor. Even when the symptoms are due to structures in the shoulder region, they may reflect inflammation of or damage to the tendon sheaths or bursa surrounding the shoulder, or inflammation of any of the three joints comprising the shoulder. An examination for shoulder pain should address not only the extent and location of swelling, weakness, tenderness, and crepitus on the motion of the shoulder structures themselves and their surrounding tissues, but also the status of the neck, cervical and axillary lymph nodes, and the abdomen.

Treatment of localized soft tissue rheumatism involves local applications of heat, limitation of activity, gentle exercises to maintain range of motion, and judicious use of steroidal or nonsteroidal anti-inflammatory drugs. The gastrointestinal effects of these drugs limit the usefulness of these agents over time. Localized injections into the joint, tendon sheaths, or bursa often result in symptomatic improvement that can last for many months. Two or three injections may be performed at intervals of 4 to 8 weeks. More than three injections during a year are seldom indicated.

If localized soft tissue rheumatism pain continues for several months, it may lead to a chronic pain syndrome. Although this syndrome is resistant to therapy, use of acupuncture, relaxation therapy, or psychological therapy may be of benefit. In some cases, actual nerve block may be necessary.

Gout

Gout is found exclusively in humans. The incidence of gout varies in populations from 0.20 to 0.35 per 1,000, with an overall prevalence of 1.6 to 13.6 per 1,000. The clinical manifestations of gout increase with age and increasing serum urate concentration. The annual incidence rate of gout is 4.9% for urate levels >9 mg per dL, 0.5% for values between 7 and 8.9 mg per dL, and 0.1% for values <7 mg per dL. The cumulative incidence of gout reaches 22% after 5 years for serum urate values >9 mg per dL. In addition to

TABLE 34.8
CLINICAL DIAGNOSTIC CRITERIA FOR GOUT

An elevated serum urate concentration (hyperuricemia)
Recurrent attacks of acute arthritis where monosodium urate monohydrate crystals are demonstrable in synovial fluid leukocytes
Aggregates of sodium urate monohydrate crystals (tophi) deposited chiefly in and around joints, which sometimes lead to deformity and crippling
Renal disease involving glomerular, tubular, and interstitial tissues and blood vessels
Uric acid urolithiasis

These manifestations can occur in various combinations.

pain, gout produces limitation of activity in about 9.2% of male patients with the disorder.

Plasma monosodium urate remains in solution to approximately 7 mg per dL at body temperature. A serum urate value in excess of 7 mg per dL carries an increased risk of gouty arthritis or renal stones. For these reasons, hyperuricemia is defined as a true serum urate concentration >7 mg per dL. A variety of factors may cause higher serum urate concentrations. Serum urate levels correlate strongly with serum creatinine and urea nitrogen levels, body weight, height, age, blood pressure, and alcohol intake. Criteria for the diagnosis of gout are shown in Table 34.8.

Management of gout is aimed at lowering the serum urate and controlling the acute flare of disease. Control of pain for an acute episode can be obtained with steroidal and nonsteroidal anti-inflammatory agents. The dose of steroids should be relatively high, in the range of 40 to 60 mg of prednisone. No differences in response among the types of nonsteroidal anti-inflammatory drugs have been shown (Evidence Level B).

Approximately, two thirds of patients with acute gout respond to colchicine within hours when the drug is initiated within 24 hours of the onset of pain. A common dosing regimen is one 0.6-mg tablet every hour for up to three hours, for a maximum of three tablets. The use of colchicine on a long-term basis is common, but not supported by good evidence. Low-dose daily colchicine may be associated with severe adverse effects, including myopathy and myelosuppression. Concurrent treatment with erythromycin, simvastatin, and cyclosporine predisposes patients to adverse effects by altering the elimination of colchicine. Nonetheless, using colchicine for the first few months of urate-lowering therapy may be helpful.

The principal indications for long-term uric acid–lowering therapy in patients with gout are macroscopic subcutaneous tophi, more than three acute attacks of gout per year, or documented hyperuricemia. Asymptomatic hyperuricemia alone is not an indication for treatment. Treatment decisions should be based on the underlying cause of the hyperuricemia. Approximately 75% of patients with primary gout have substantially decreased renal urate excretion. Uricosuric drugs such as probenecid increase renal urate clearance and are considered first-line agents for such patients. A 24-hour urinary urate excretion <800 to 1,000 mg will identify patients who underexcrete urate. Alternatively, allopurinol, which inhibits uric acid synthesis through xanthine oxidase, can be used.

In patients with intact renal function, the dose of antihyperuricemic agents can be increased every 3 to 4 weeks for the first few months of therapy to decrease serum urate levels to between 4.6 and 6.6 mg per dL. Treatment is associated with a 30% reduction in recurrences of gouty arthritis, compared with patients whose serum urate levels remained above or below this range.

REFERENCES

1. Suffredini AF, Fantuzzi G, Badolato R, et al. New insights into the biology of the acute phase response. *J Clin Immunol.* 1999;19:203–214.
2. Thomas DR. The relationship between functional status and inflammatory disease in older adults. *J Gerontol A Biol Sci Med Sci.* 2003;58:995–998.
3. Baggio G, Donazzan S, Monti D, et al. Lipoprotein(a) and lipoprotein profile in healthy centenarians: A reappraisal of vascular risk factors. *Faseb J.* 1998;12:433–437.
4. Cohen HJ, Pieper CF, Harris T, et al. The association of plasma IL-6 levels with functional disability in community dwelling elderly. *J Gerontol.* 1997;52:M201–M208.
5. Gardner EM, Murasko DM. Age-related changes in Type 1 and Type 2 cytokine production in humans. *Biogerontology.* 2002;3:271–290.
6. Straub RH, Miller LE, Scholmerich J, et al. Cytokines and hormones as possible links between endocrinosenescence and immunosenescence. *J Neuroimmunol.* 2000;109:10–15.
7. Yudkin JS, Kumari M, Humphries SE, et al. Inflammation, obesity, stress and coronary heart disease: Is interleukin-6 the link? *Atherosclerosis.* 2000;148:209–214.
8. Crossley KB, Peterson PK. Infections in the elderly. *Clin Infect Dis.* 1996;22:209–215.
9. Miller RA. The aging immune system: Primer and prospectus. *Science.* 1996;273:70–74.
10. Eastgate JA, Wood NC, DiGiovine FS, et al. Correlation of plasma interleukin-1 levels with disease activity in rheumatoid arthritis. *Lancet.* 1988;2:706–709.
11. Saxne T, Palladino MA, Heinegard D, et al. Detection of tumor necrosis factor-alpha but not tumor necrosis factor-beta in rheumatoid arthritis synovial fluid and serum. *Arthritis Rheum.* 1988;31:1041–1044.
12. Firestein GS. Evolving concepts of rheumatoid arthritis. *Nature.* 2003;423:356–361.
13. Maini RN, Taylor PC. Anti-cytokine therapy for rheumatoid arthritis. *Annu Rev Med.* 2000;51:207–229.

14. Olsen NJ, Stein CM. Drug therapy: New drugs for rheumatoid arthritis. *N Engl J Med.* 2004;350:2167–2179.
15. Felson DT, Anderson JJ, Boers M, et al. Preliminary definition of improvement in rheumatoid arthritis. *Arthritis Rheum.* 1995; 38:727–735.
16. Mills JA. Medical progress: Systemic lupus erythematosus. *N Engl J Med.* 1994;330:1871–1879.
17. Sapadin AN, Fleischmajer R. Treatment of scleroderma. *Arch Dermatol.* 2002;138:99–105.
18. Shbeeb M, Uramoto KM, Gibson LE, et al. Epidemiology of psoriatic arthritis in Olmsted County, Minnesota, USA, 1982–1991. *J Rheumatol.* 2000;27:1247–1250.
19. McCarthy RE 3rd, Kasper EK. A review of the amyloidoses that infiltrate the heart. *Clin Cardiol.* 1998;21(8):547–552.
20. Kyle RA, Gertz MA, Greipp PR, et al. Long-term survival (10 years or more) in 30 patients with primary amyloidosis. *Blood.* 1999; 93:1062–1066.
21. Kyle RA, Greipp PR. Amyloidosis (AL). Clinical and laboratory features in 229 cases. *Mayo Clin Proc.* 1983;58:665–683.
22. Jadoul M. Dialysis-related amyloidosis: Importance of biocompatibility and age. *Nephrol Dial Transp.* 1998;13(Suppl 7): 61–64.
23. Mimassi N, Youinou P, Pennec YL. Amyloidosis and aging. *Ann Med Interne.* 2002;153:383–388.

Oral Conditions

35

Jude A. Fabiano

- CLINICAL PEARLS 474
- EVALUATION OF THE ORAL CAVITY 475
- DENTAL DECAY (CARIES) 477
- PERIODONTAL DISEASE 479
- DIET AND NUTRITION 481
- XEROSTOMIA 481
- OROFACIAL PAIN 482
- ORAL MEDICINE AND THE ELDERLY 483
- ORAL CANCER 483
- ORAL MUCOSITIS 485
- ORAL CANDIDIASIS 485
- TRAUMATIC LESIONS 486
- BURNING MOUTH SYNDROME (STOMATOPYROSIS) 487
- ORAL CONDITIONS AND SYSTEMIC DISEASE 487
- PERIOPERATIVE CONSIDERATIONS 487
- ATHEROSCLEROSIS, CARDIOVASCULAR DISEASE, AND STROKE 488
- DIABETES 488
- ASPIRATION PNEUMONIA/CHRONIC OBSTRUCTIVE PULMONARY DISEASE 488
- DEMENTIA 489
- CONCLUSION 489

CLINICAL PEARLS

- Oral health is intimately associated with general health and well-being.
- Poor oral health negatively affects nutrition and systemic health.
- Dental caries and periodontal disease are preventable.
- Xerostomia can have devastating effects on the health of the hard and soft tissues of the oral cavity.
- Root surface dental decay, often a secondary effect of xerostomia, has an increased incidence in older adults.
- Medications with xerostomic side effects should be avoided when possible.
- Diagnosis of orofacial conditions in elderly persons may be confounded by coincident medical and dental conditions, multiple medications, and vague histories.
- The 5-year survival rate of oral cancer has not improved over the past 30 years. Early diagnosis is crucial.
- Proper oral hygiene in older adults prevents several life-threatening systemic conditions.
- Follow current recommendations regarding antibiotic prophylaxis and anticoagulant therapy as they relate to dental procedures.

Good oral health has emerged as a critical factor in maintaining general health in geriatric individuals. The oral cavity provides an entrance to the body for every nutrient necessary for life except oxygen. Over the past several decades, the number of older adults who have retained some or all of their natural teeth has dramatically increased. While this has resulted in improved masticatory function and self-image, the risk for acute and chronic oral disease persists later in life. Periodontal disease, dental caries, root surface caries, infections, oral cancer, malocclusion, missing teeth, and weakness of the orofacial musculature can all inhibit the intake of nutrients and impact the general health of an individual. Compromised oral health has been linked to cardiovascular and cerebrovascular disease, pneumonia, and diabetes. In addition, feelings of social well-being and self-image, quality of life, life satisfaction, and psychological well-being are directly related to an individual's oral health.

Oral health problems are among the most common chronic conditions found in older people. While only 35% of patients 75 years and older visit a dentist annually, almost 90% of this group see physicians. It is critical, therefore, that physicians be familiar with oral pathology, perform thorough intraoral examinations on their elderly patients and be prepared to manage and/or refer patients for definitive treatment.

This chapter provides basic knowledge of the oral conditions that affect the systemic health and quality of life of older people, and of oral findings related to systemic conditions found in these individuals.

EVALUATION OF THE ORAL CAVITY

Key to identifying and assessing oral conditions is the ability to perform a comprehensive hard and soft tissue oral examination. A complete head and neck examination should precede the intraoral examination, including physical inspection of the head, facial form, skin, eyes, ears, nose, temporomandibular joint, neck, thyroid gland, and cranial nerves. Intraoral physical examination should then proceed as follows:

- *Lips.* Pale pink, homogeneous in color, well-defined border with skin. Bidigital palpation performed to identify uniform submucosal consistency and thickness (see Figs. 35.1 and 35.2).

  Common Abnormalities: Ulcerations, irregular surface, white thickenings, recurrent herpetic lesions.

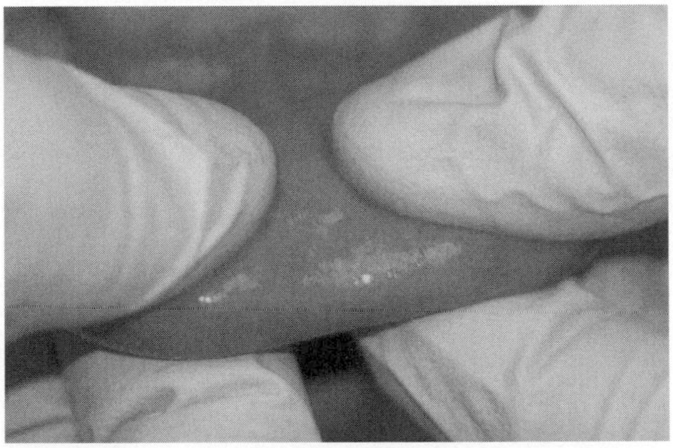

Figure 35.2 Bidigital palpation on lower lip. (See color insert.)

- *Buccal Mucosae.* Uniformly pink/red in color; visualize Stensen duct and check for normal salivary flow. Bidigital palpation to rule out submucosal thickenings or tumors (see Fig. 35.3).

  Common Abnormalities: Biteline hyperkeratosis, fibromas, candidiasis.

- *Buccal Vestibule.* Located at the junction of buccal mucosae and alveolar process. Examine for elevations or depressions. Palpate at height/depth of vestibule to identify tenderness or swelling (see Figs. 35.4 and 35.5).

  Common Abnormalities: Inflammatory lesions associated with dental abscesses.

- *Hard Palate.* Utilize direct visual inspection. Uniform pink color. Evaluate rugae, palatal raphe, palatine papilla, and maxillary tuberosities (see Fig. 35.6).

  Common Abnormalities: Maxillary torus, candidiasis, papillary hyperplasia.

- *Soft Palate:.* Utilize direct vision/mouth mirror; depress tongue if necessary. "Ah" for elevation, which should be

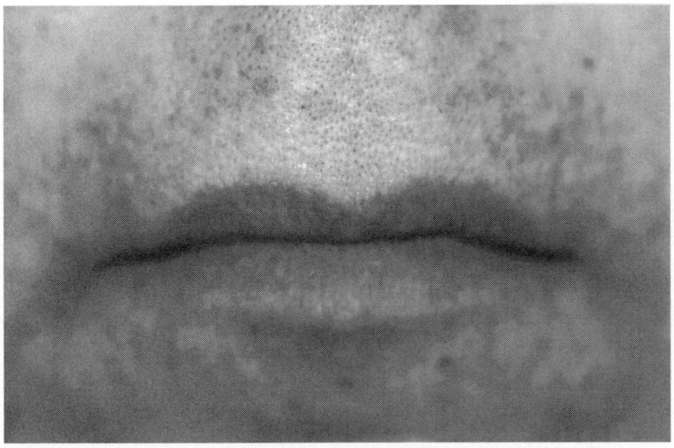

Figure 35.1 Normal appearance of lips. (See color insert.)

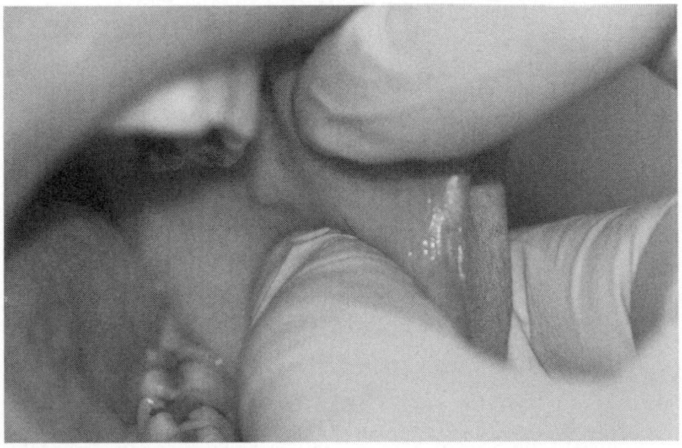

Figure 35.3 Bidigital palpation of buccal mucosa. (See color insert.)

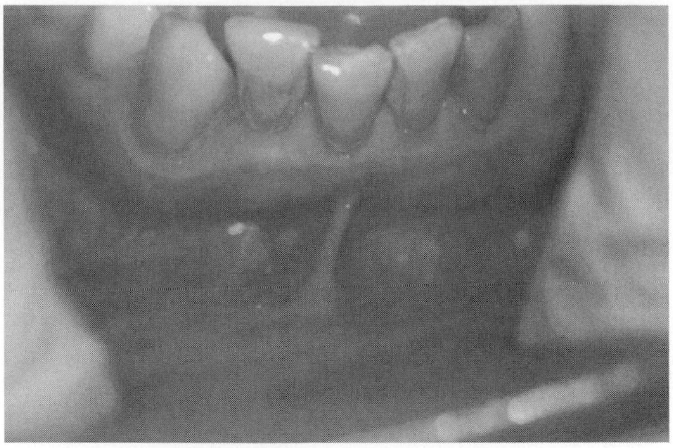

Figure 35.4 Visual examination of anterior buccal vestibule, mandibular arch. (See color insert.)

bilaterally uniform. Evaluate uvula for size, color, and texture (see Fig. 35.7).

Common Abnormalities: Candidiasis, swelling, ulcerations, nicotine stomatitis.

- *Oropharynx.* Depress tongue and have patient say "ah." Evaluate tonsils (usually atrophic in elders) and posterior wall of pharynx (see Fig. 35.8).

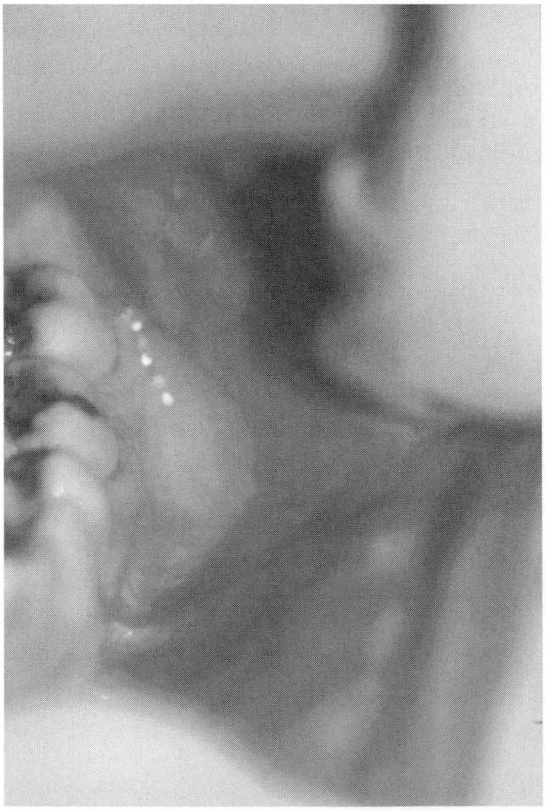

Figure 35.5 Visual examination of posterior buccal vestibule, mandibular arch. (See color insert.)

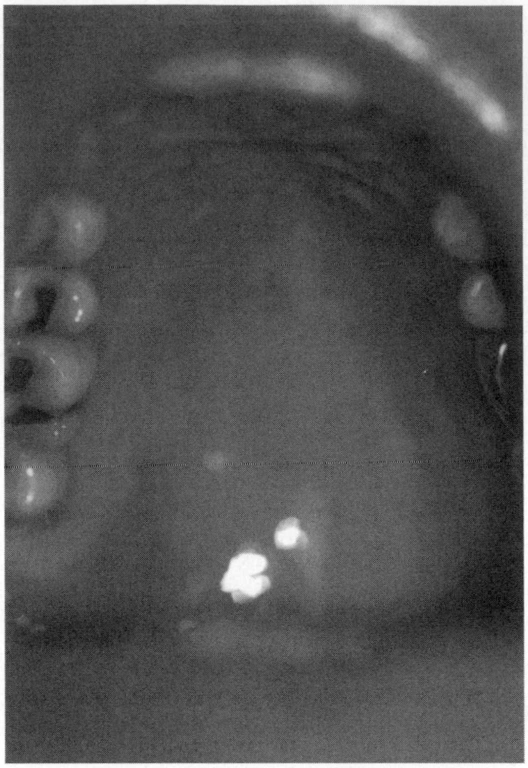

Figure 35.6 Visual examination of hard palate. (See color insert.)

Common Abnormalities: Erythema, exudate, asymmetry.

- *Tongue.* Have patient extrude tongue and wrap tip with gauze to properly visualize lateral borders. Assess ventral, lateral, and dorsal surfaces, including papillae, lingual frenum, and vasculature (see Figs. 35.9 and 35.10).

Common Abnormalities: Ulcerations, fibromas, "brown/black hairy tongue" (especially in smokers), geographic tongue. Posterior one third of lateral border is most frequent site of oral cancer.

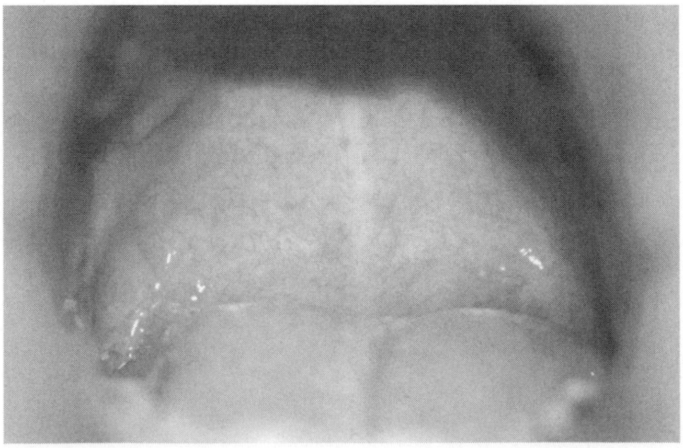

Figure 35.7 Visual examination of soft palate. (See color insert.)

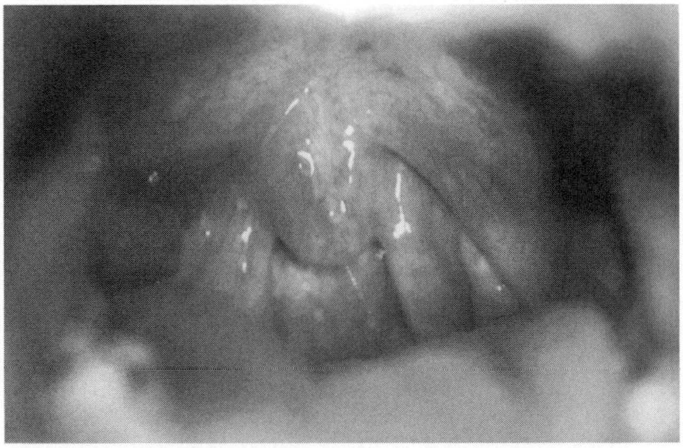

Figure 35.8 Visual examination of oropharynx. (See color insert.)

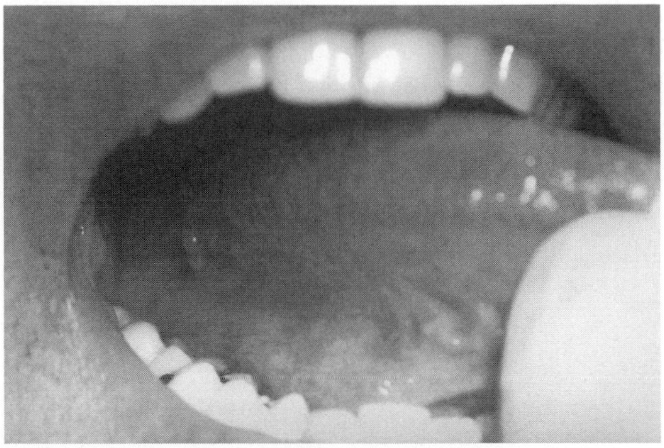

Figure 35.10 Visual examination of lateral surface of tongue, including lingual tonsil. (See color insert.)

- *Floor of Mouth.* Visualize as tongue is elevated. Uniform red color. Evaluate Wharton ducts for salivary flow. Bidigital palpation to evaluate submandibular salivary glands, lymph nodes, symmetry (see Fig. 35.11).

  Common Abnormalities: Ulcerations, varicosities, mucocele.

- *Gingivae.* Observe color (pink), frenal attachments, and recession.

  Common Abnormalities: Inflammation secondary to periodontal disease, recession, hyperplasia, fistulae (see Fig. 35.12).

- *Teeth.* Number present/absent, gross decay, plaque/calculus, mobility, discoloration, and occlusion (Fig. 35.12).

  Common Abnormalities: Decay, mobility, gingival abrasion, fractures, lost/fractured restorations, ill-fitting prosthesis.

DENTAL DECAY (CARIES)

CASE ONE

Mr. K., a 68-year-old in good general health and taking no medications, has been visiting his dentist every 6 months for an oral examination and prophylaxis (cleaning). Mr. K. historically had a very low caries rate and had not been diagnosed with a carious lesion in over 15 years. Four months prior to his most recent dental visit, Mr. K. was placed on nifedipine for the management of mild hypertension. Shortly after the initiation of the drug, Mr. K. experienced a feeling of dryness in his mouth that affected his ability to properly chew food, swallow, and speak. To counteract these difficulties, he began to suck on lemon drops and to drink soda frequently during the day and during the night as well. Four months after the initiation of the nifedipine therapy, dental examination revealed multiple root surface carious lesions, some moderate in size. Mr. K.'s physician was consulted, an alternative antihypertensive agent without xerostomic side effects was identified and the nifedipine was replaced. The carious lesions were restored and the

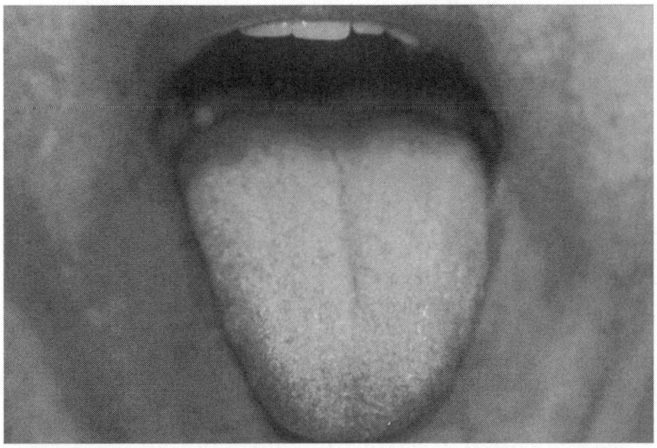

Figure 35.9 Visual examination of dorsal surface of tongue. (See color insert.)

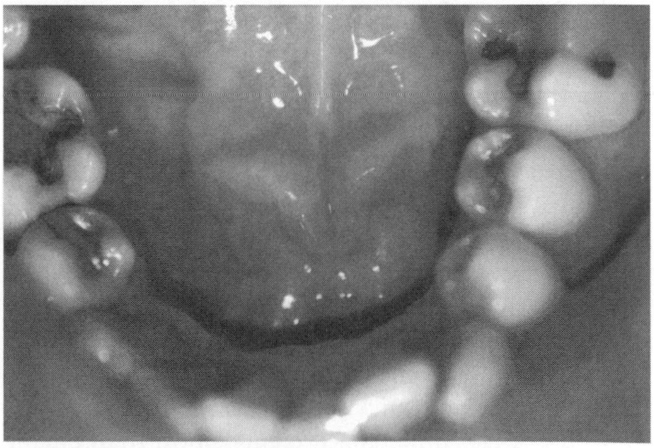

Figure 35.11 Visual examination of floor of the mouth, including Wharton ducts. (See color insert.)

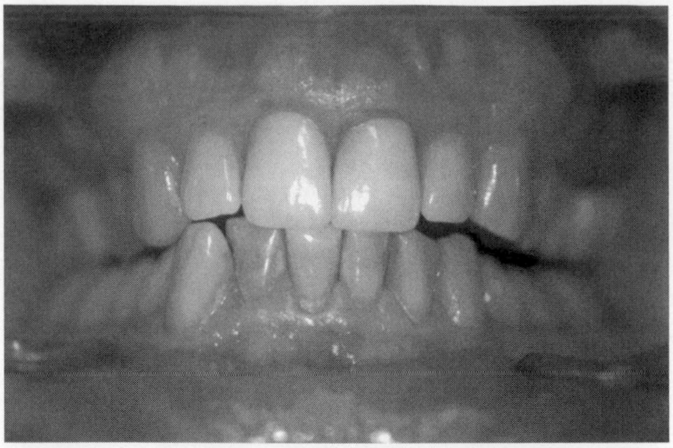

Figure 35.12 Visual examination of anterior gingival and teeth. (See color insert.)

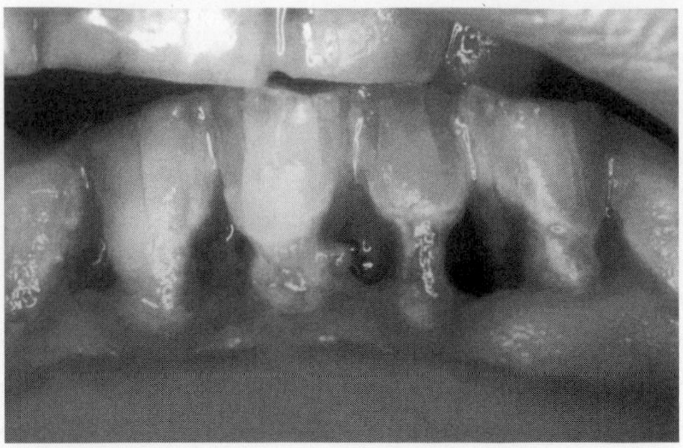

Figure 35.13 Root surface caries. (See color insert.)

patient was placed on daily topical fluoride treatments and instructed to use sugarless lemon drops and frequent sips of water, not sugar-containing beverages, to reduce the feeling of dry mouth. Mr. K. was subsequently placed on a 3-month examination interval. No additional carious lesions have formed and Mr. K. no longer has the feeling of dryness in his oral cavity.

Dental caries is the demineralization of the calcified structures of the tooth caused by *Streptococcus* species and other intraoral bacteria. Caries may occur on the smooth, pit and fissure and root surfaces of the tooth. Smooth and pit and fissure caries occur on the enamel surface and have a higher incidence in children and young adults. Root surface caries typically affect older adults and develop on the dentin surface of the root in areas where gingival recession has occurred. As an increased number of older people maintain their natural teeth, they are predisposed to root surface caries. Other local factors, such as xerostomia, increased sugar intake, acidic foods and drinks, and medications, increase the likelihood that root surface caries will develop.

Dental decay is preventable, with the removal of bacteria-harboring dental plaque. Dental caries occur when three components are present:

- A tooth surface (enamel and/or dentin)
- A fermentable substrate (i.e., sugar)
- Bacteria that metabolize fermentable substrates into acids.

The acids produce a result in the demineralization of the tooth surface and cavitation. Removal of one of the three components will interrupt the decay process and prevent caries from developing. Pit and fissure and smooth surface caries occur on enamel, the hardest substance in the body, and may take months to develop. However, root surfaces are not covered with enamel. Their surface has a thin layer of cementum, which quickly dissolves and exposes dentin. Dentin has a less mineralized composition than enamel, and the decay process on this surface will develop much more rapidly.

Root surface caries is a particularly difficult management issue in the older adult (see Fig. 35.13). Approximately half of all adults 75 years and older have at least one tooth with root surface decay. Individuals who have been caries-free for decades may develop a number of root surface carious lesions in a matter of weeks. Usually this type of episode follows a major change in the oral environment. Medications that cause dry mouth as a side effect are often a contributor. This, coupled with the attempts to counter the dry mouth by frequent use of high-sugar, acidic drinks, and/or candy lozenges, results in the rapid demineralization of the dentin on the root surface and may result in irreparable cavitation and the subsequent loss of the tooth. Care should be taken to avoid medications with a xerostomic effect, and to advise patients to see a dentist for frequent, regular evaluations when their use is unavoidable. Other factors contributing to caries in older adults include history of previous caries, number of existing dental restorations, dietary habits, lack of fluoride exposure, and presence of partial dentures, which often cause food retention and subsequent plaque formation, diminished oral and/or manual motor control, being dependent on others for oral hygiene, systemic disease(s), and infrequent dental visits.

Unless properly treated, dental caries can lead to abscess formation of the hard and soft tissues of the oral cavity, cellulitis (including Ludwig angina), infection of proximal structures (cavernous sinus thrombosis), septicemia, and systemic seeding (subacute bacterial endocarditis). Extraction of the infected tooth may be necessary, affecting dental occlusion, mastication, and nutritional intake.

Prevention of dental caries is focused on:

- The mechanical removal of dental plaque through proper brushing and flossing;
- The reinforcement of the composition of enamel through fluoride treatments;
- Diet modification;
- The use of antimicrobial rinses;
- Early attention to salivary dysfunction; and
- Professional prophylaxis and intervention at appropriate intervals.

Management of dental caries is through removal of the carious lesion and repair of the tooth with the appropriate dental material. Management of dental infections is primarily mechanical, either through root canal therapy, incision, and drainage or extraction. Use of antibiotics should be reserved for the treatment of established abscess formation, and inappropriate prescription of antibiotics should be avoided. Referral to the appropriate dental professional should be the first course of action.

Table 35.1 highlights medications that are useful in the management of oral conditions often found in elderly people.

PERIODONTAL DISEASE

CASE TWO

Ms. H. is an 84-year-old with a medical history significant for Parkinson disease. She has been a resident in a long-term care facility for 8 years and is currently confined to bed for most of the day. She has severe tremor of her extremities and head and neck, making oral hygiene difficult at best. The gross amounts of bacteria-harboring dental plaque and calculus that have formed on her teeth and gingival tissues have contributed to the development of a severe case of periodontitis. Ms. H. has dysphagia associated with Parkinson disease and frequently aspirates particles of food during swallowing. Following a case of pneumonia due to cultivable oral flora in her sputum, Ms. H. was placed on a vigorous daily regimen of oral hygiene and frequent oral prophylaxis to reduce the development of dental plaque and calculus, which directly reduced the severity of her periodontitis and her risk of subsequent aspiration pneumonia events.

Periodontal disease (gingivitis and periodontitis) is a host-mediated response to bacteria found in dental plaque resulting in the destruction of the supporting structures of the teeth, namely the gingiva and associated soft tissues, periodontal ligament, and alveolar bone. It is a chronic, progressive condition affecting >80% of people older than 65 and is the most common reason for tooth loss in individuals older than 40. Evidence exists indicating that periodontal disease can increase the risk for cardiovascular disease and respiratory diseases, and accelerate the progression of diabetes (see section "Oral Conditions and Systemic Disease").

Signs and symptoms of periodontal disease include erythema and inflammation of the gingival tissue, bleeding of the gingival tissue during brushing, and tooth mobility (see Fig. 35.14). Gingival recession is found in most older adults, although it is not always due to a disease process ("long in the tooth"). It is significant because it exposes root surfaces, which leave the tooth susceptible to root surface caries (see section "Dental Decay"). In advanced stages

TABLE 35.1
MEDICAL MANAGEMENT OF ORAL CONDITIONS

Indication	Medication/Directions	Strength of Evidence of Effectiveness
Caries prevention	■ 0.2% neutral NaF rinse Disp: 480 mL bottle Sig: Rinse 10 mL for 1 min and expectorate; do not swallow Repeat weekly	A
	■ 1.1% neutral NaF dental cream (PreviDent 5,000) Disp: 2 oz tube Sig: Place 1/2 inch ribbon on toothbrush, then brush for 2–3 min and expectorate; do not swallow; do not rinse or eat for 30 min following treatment Perform twice daily	A
Periodontal disease	■ Chlorhexidine gluconate 0.12% (Peridex, PerioGard) Disp: 16 oz bottle Sig: After brushing and flossing teeth, rinse 1/2 oz for 30 s twice daily and expectorate	A
Xerostomia	Saliva substitutes ■ Sodium carboxymethylcellulose 0.5% aqueous solution (Saliva Substitute, Salivart) Disp: 8 fl oz Sig: Rinse as frequently as needed	C
	Salivary stimulants ■ Pilocarpine HCl (Salagen) tablets 5 mg Disp: 21 tablets Sig: Take 1–2 tablet(s) 1/2 h prior to meals	B

(continued)

TABLE 35.1
(continued)

Oral mucositis	Topical analgesic rinses	C
	■ Diphenhydramine (Benadryl) elixir 12.5 mg/5 mL and attapulgite (Kaopectate) Disp: Mix equal parts of both liquids (4 oz each) to obtain 8 oz Sig: Rinse one teaspoon every 2 h for 1 min and expectorate	C
	■ Aminacrine (Kamillosan liquid) 30 mL Disp: Mix 30 drops in 100 mL of warm water Sig: Rinse 5–10 mL four times daily for 1 min and expectorate	C
	■ Dyclonine HCl (Dyclone) 0.5% or 1% Disp: 1 oz bottle Sig: Rinse one teaspoon for 2 min and expectorate	B
	Intravenous therapy ■ Palifermin (60 μg/kg/d) intravenously for 3 d immediately before starting high-dose chemotherapy and total-body irradiation (conditioning therapy) and then again for 3 d after stem-cell transplantation.	
Oral candidiasis	Candidiasis	
	■ Nystatin (Mycostatin, Nilstat) oral suspension 100,000 U/mL Disp: 240 mL Sig: Rinse 5 mL four times daily for 2 min and swallow until finished	A
	■ Nystatin lozenge (Mycostatin pastilles) 200,000 U Disp: 70 pastilles Sig: Dissolve one pastille in mouth five times daily for 14 d; do not chew or swallow whole	A
	■ Clotrimazole (Mycelex) troches 10 mg Disp: 70 troches Sig: Dissolve one troche in mouth five times daily for 14 d; do not chew or swallow whole	A
	Angular cheilitis	A
	■ Nystatin-triamcinolone acetonide (Mycolog II, Mytrex) ointment Disp: 15 mg tube Sig: Apply to affected areas four times daily for 10–14 d	
	■ Clotrimazole-betamethasone dipropionate (Lotrisone) cream Disp: 15 mg tube Sig: Apply to affected areas four times daily for 10–14 d	

NaF, sodium fluoride.

of periodontal disease, pain, swelling, and acute abscess formation may occur.

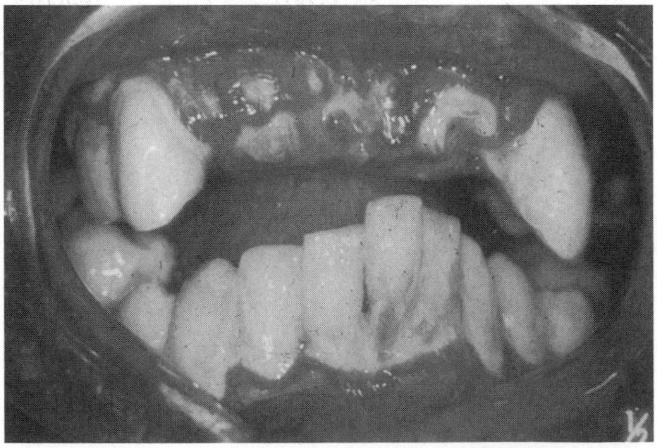

Figure 35.14 Severe periodontal disease. (See color insert.)

Management is based on prevention, and early recognition of periodontal disease is by far the best management approach. Removal of dental plaque through proper oral hygiene practices is key and includes:

- Brushing with a soft, polished tipped bristle toothbrush, including those that are battery-operated or have modified handles, at least twice per day;
- Flossing between all teeth every day;
- Proper use of antimicrobial rinses, such as chlorhexidine; and
- Frequent professional oral prophylaxis and/or periodontal therapy.

Recent developments in surgical and bone-grafting procedures have increased the success of periodontal treatments. Gingival hyperplasia may develop in older individuals associated with the use of phenytoin, cyclosporine, and calcium channel blockers. Selection of an appropriate alternative medication in most cases will reverse the condition. However, in selective cases surgical removal of the hyperplastic tissue may be necessary.

DIET AND NUTRITION

CASE THREE

Mr. J., a 78-year-old with a medical history significant for well-controlled insulin-dependent diabetes, was diagnosed with severe periodontal disease that necessitated removal of all of his remaining maxillary (upper) natural teeth. Immediately following the dental extractions, a maxillary interim (temporary) denture was placed to restore minimal masticatory function, postoperative instructions were given, and the patient was dismissed in satisfactory condition. Mr. J. returned the following day for reevaluation. On his way to the dental operatory he became light-headed, lost his balance and collapsed into the arms of the dental auxiliary. He was placed in a supine position and upon questioning stated that while he administered his normal dose of insulin this morning, he had not eaten due to the "strange feeling of the denture" in his mouth. Glucometer testing indicated a blood glucose of 48 mg per dL. Following a sugar-containing beverage, a blood glucose level of 136 mg per dL was recorded. Proper insulin administration and food ingestion instructions were again reviewed and he was discharged in satisfactory condition in the company of a responsible adult. He reported no subsequent events on follow-up appointments.

Satisfactory oral health in older people also involves masticatory ability that allows consumption of foods of all types and consistencies. Impaired chewing ability often restricts food choices to predominately soft, easy-to-chew items, therefore limiting many foods essential for proper nutrition. Adequate mastication is not only dependent on the absence of caries and periodontal disease, but on the number of remaining natural teeth, the number of occlusal (grinding) contacts existing regarding posterior teeth, the amount and type of saliva, and the proper function of the orofacial musculature. Inability to properly chew food and xerostomia also alter taste perception and may further limit food selection.

Compromised masticatory ability places the patient at risk of consuming below-optimum amounts of specific nutritional components, including vitamins A, B_6, and C, folic acid, carotene, calcium, niacin, and dietary fiber. Without healthy teeth, they consume less protein and more carbohydrates. Maintenance and restoration of natural teeth and/or clinically acceptable prosthetic replacement of missing posterior teeth are associated with a more varied food item selection and a better nutritional intake.

The ability to masticate properly is also dependent on the quality and quantity of saliva to allow proper bolus formation, initiate the digestive process, and provide adequate lubrication for swallowing. Conditions that negatively affect the orofacial musculature, particularly the muscles of mastication, certainly contribute to older people's limited food choices. Attention must therefore be given to all of the multiple components of the masticatory system and to optimizing the effects of each component to maximize a varied food intake, chewing efficiency, and nutritional status.

XEROSTOMIA

CASE FOUR

Ms. N., a 74-year-old with a medical history significant for Parkinson disease, presented with the chief complaint of a "loose upper denture." Clinical examination revealed a well-fitting maxillary complete denture with inadequate retention secondary to the lack of sufficient saliva to create a proper denture/tissue seal. Ms. K. stated that the denture, which had been fabricated 4 years ago, "fit fine" until she noticed a dryness in her mouth approximately 6 months ago. Further questioning revealed the addition to her anti-parkinsonism medications of trihexyphenidyl (Artane) at approximately the same time the denture retention issue developed. She was unable to eat her normal diet and lost 16 pounds over that same period. Following consultation with Ms. K.'s physician the trihexyphenidyl was discontinued, which did not have a negative effect on her symptoms and resulted in increased salivary flow, improved denture retention and the return of her normal eating habits.

Saliva is formed by the major salivary glands and numerous minor salivary glands, with most saliva produced by the major salivary glands. Two types of saliva are produced: Mucous and serous. Saliva acts to lubricate the oral cavity, increases the pH of the oral cavity, which protects against caries formation and promotes remineralization of tooth surfaces, aids in digestion and taste sensation, maintains mucosal integrity, is critical for proper denture stability and retention and functions as an antimicrobial agent.

Xerostomia is the subjective feeling on the part of an individual of decreased saliva and a dry mouth. It is a common complaint in older people; however, it is not always associated with objective findings of diminished salivary flow. The aging process itself is not the cause of xerostomia. Mouth breathing, obstruction of major salivary ducts, side effects of medications, metabolic changes, and many local and systemic disease processes and/or treatments contribute to this condition. Over 500 medications have been identified as causing xerostomia, and most drug-induced xerostomia is reversible. Patients often experience a decreased salivary flow with neoplasms of the head and neck and with surgical intervention and/or radiotherapy of these tumors. Radiation therapy may affect both the quality and quantity of saliva produced, often resulting in thick, mucous saliva. Xerostomia has been associated with increased and often rampant caries formation, compromised chewing and swallowing ability, inability to wear dentures, breakdown of mucosal tissues, and microbial overgrowth, including *Candida* sp of the oral cavity and bacterial sialadenitis.

Treatments for xerostomia are based on removing the cause or on replacement therapies. Alternate medications should be substituted whenever possible for agents that cause xerostomia. Drug families identified as causing xerostomia include anticholinergics, antihistamines, antihypertensives, anti-parkinsonians, antidepressants, bronchodilators, diuretics, and sedatives. Proper shielding and tissue preservation techniques should be utilized in patients receiving radiotherapy for tumors of the head and neck. Early diagnosis and treatment of conditions causing xerostomia, such as Sjögren syndrome, are essential in maintaining salivary function.

While the ideal salivary substitute has yet to be developed, several methods are recommended to aid in the lubrication of the oral cavity and reduce discomfort in those patients with xerostomia:

- Frequent sips of cool water and/or allowing ice chips to melt in the mouth
- Drinking milk, which has lubricating and moisturizing properties, with meals
- Use of a cool mist air humidifier, especially while sleeping
- Decreased use of alcoholic drinks and alcohol-containing mouthwashes
- Decreased intake of caffeine
- Use of sugar-free gum (Xylitol), candies (Koolerz, Smint Mints), and beverages to stimulate salivary flow
- Application of a lubricant (Vaseline) on lips
- Sleeping on one's side to avoid/reduce mouth breathing
- Use of saliva substitutes
  - Liquids (Saliva Substitute, Salivart, Xero-Lube)
  - Tablets (Salix)
  - Sprays (Optimoist)
  - Gels (Oralbalance)
  - Toothpaste (Biotene toothpaste).
- Use of cholinergic agonists, when appropriate
  - Pilocarpine, 5 to 7.5 mg t.i.d.
  - Cevimeline, 30 mg t.i.d.
- Immaculate oral and prosthesis hygiene
- Daily application of fluoride to teeth
- Frequent, regular professional oral evaluation and prophylaxis.

OROFACIAL PAIN

CASE FIVE

Mr. F., an 80-year-old with a medical history significant for rheumatoid arthritis, presented to his dentist with the chief complaint of difficulty in chewing and pain on the right side of his head. Clinical examination revealed swelling of and tenderness to palpation associated with the right temporal artery. Additional questioning of the patient revealed recent visual disturbances of the right eye. A preliminary diagnosis of giant cell (temporal) arteritis was substantiated by an elevated erythrocyte sedimentation rate of 140 mm per hour. The patient was immediately placed on prednisone 60 mg per day to reverse the ophthalmic effects and prevent permanent loss of vision.

While giant cell arteritis and polymyalgia rheumatica may occur separately, they often occur in the same individual, especially in those older than 60. Jaw claudication secondary to diminished blood flow to the muscles of mastication, which results in pain during chewing, swallowing, and/or talking, is a common complaint and may be the presenting symptom.

Older people often develop pathologic conditions of the head and neck that produce painful symptoms of differing character, duration, and intensity. Determining the etiology of orofacial pain is hampered by other coincident medical and dental conditions, multiple medications, and vague histories. It is important to remember that symptoms, including pain, from systemic conditions may radiate to the head and neck and mimic pain with an odontogenic cause. Assessment of pain in older adults may be facilitated by the use of the Visual Analog Scale and FACES Scale (e.g., see "Wong-Baker FACES Pain Rating Scale" citation in the Selected Reading), both of which have high reliability and validity, and by thorough cranial and autonomic nerve examinations. They are easy to use and aid in the assessment of pain and evaluation of the effectiveness of treatment.

The source of pain in older people can be from conditions that have an inflammatory/infectious, neoplastic, traumatic, developmental, and/or psychological origin. It is not uncommon for the painful area to be distant from the location of the cause of the pain. An intracranial tumor exerting pressure on a cranial nerve may result in pain being felt on the distal distribution of the nerve. If the tumor causing the pain is metastatic, the primary lesion may be quite distant indeed.

Diagnosis should be approached in a systematic manner. Locating the distribution of pain may point to a specific dermatome(s), unilateral/bilateral nature, and recruitment of additional pain pathways. Determination of the origin of the tissue involved as well as examining the character and duration of the pain will narrow the differential diagnosis.

Pain-producing conditions that characteristically occur in older individuals:

- Arthritis of the cervical vertebrae may limit mobility of the head and neck and produce pain. Diagnosis should be confirmed by imaging techniques to rule out other causes. Physical therapy and analgesics are of benefit.
- Carotidynia, tenderness of the carotid bulb, may cause neck pain related to head movement. Treatment with

nonsteroidal anti-inflammatory drugs is recommended and usually effective.

- Eagle syndrome, the mineralization of the stylohyoid ligament that essentially elongates the styloid process, may produce short bursts of sharp pain when the head is turned from side to side and/or on swallowing. Surgical resection of the mineralized ligament will eliminate the painful symptoms.

Table 35.2 outlines the varying sources, characteristics, and duration of orofacial pain found in older adults.

ORAL MEDICINE AND THE ELDERLY

Oral medicine, the study of oral disease caused by local or systemic conditions, has become an important branch of medicine and dentistry, particularly in older adults. These individuals present with a greater frequency of medically compromising conditions, many with oral findings, oral mucocutaneous disease, and/or orofacial pain. The net result is often compromised nutrition, communication disorders, poor self-image, and reduced quality of life. Oral conditions, such as periodontal disease, may play a role in the development of life-threatening conditions, such as cardiovascular disease and aspiration pneumonia. The health of oral tissues, therefore, is critical to the overall health of older people.

ORAL CANCER

CASE SIX

Mr. M., a 62-year-old with a 45-year history of heavy cigarette smoking, presented for a periodic oral examination and oral prophylaxis. Intraoral examination revealed a 4 × 5 mm white papule on the left lateral posterior one third of his tongue. No history or clinical signs of trauma were present. Palpation of the floor of the mouth and cervical triangles did not reveal enlarged lymph nodes. It was agreed that an excisional biopsy of the area be performed, and the lesion was removed in toto. Histologic examination revealed a well-differentiated carcinoma *in situ*. The area healed without incident and the patient was placed on a 2-month recall.

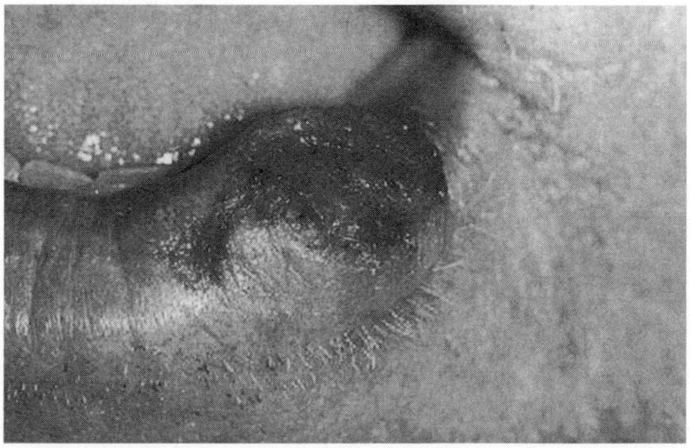

Figure 35.15 Advanced oral cancer of lower lip. (See color insert.)

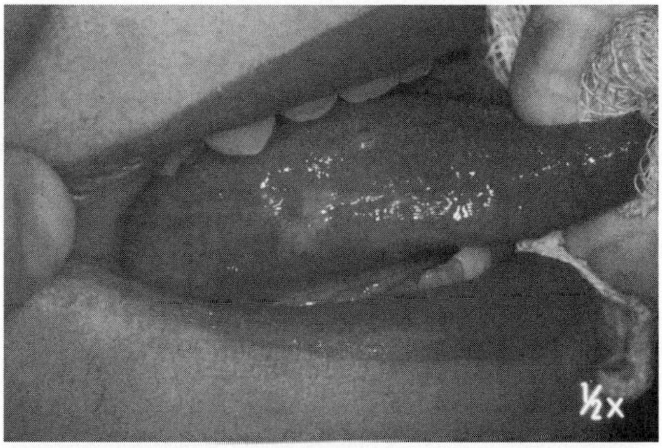

Figure 35.16 Oral cancer of lateral border of tongue. Note red and white areas of lesion. (See color insert.)

The median age of diagnosis of oral cancer is 64 years. It comprises approximately 3% of all cancers (31,000 cases per year). Of note is the fact that the 5-year survival rate of 50% has not improved to any extent over the past 30 years. The highest incidence is in African American men, followed in order by white men, African American women, and white women. Early detection, diagnosis, and treatment of stage I and II lesions are associated with improved recovery and survival. Over 90% of head and neck cancers are squamous cell carcinomas. Tobacco and alcohol use are the major risk factors. Smokers have a

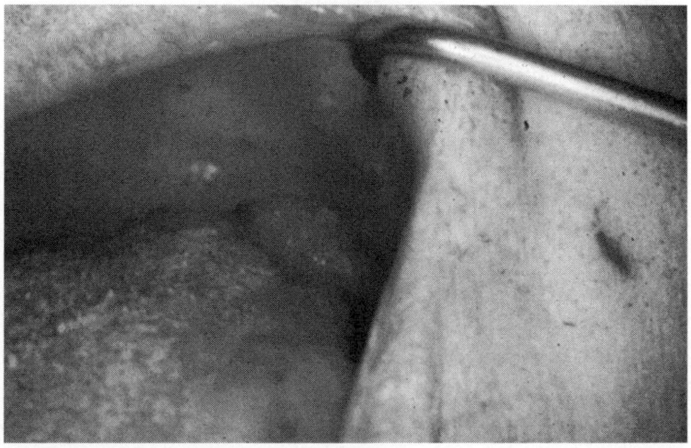

Figure 35.17 Oral cancer of posterior tongue/lingual tonsil. (See color insert.)

TABLE 35.2
DIFFERENTIAL DIAGNOSIS OF OROFACIAL PAIN IN OLDER ADULTS

	Eliciting/Accompanying Factors	Character of Pain	Duration of Pain
Odontogenic (Dental) Pain	May be intermittent or continuous Spontaneous in nature May be affected by temperature or pressure on offending tooth	Dull, aching, throbbing, lancinating Mild/moderate/severe	Brief—minutes/hours
Fractures	Associated with atrophic bone, usually mandibular	Sharp, ache, deep	Short—hours/days
Eagle Syndrome	Mineralization of stylohyoid ligament Surgical correction necessary	Sharp pain related to head movement Mild/moderate/severe	Long—weeks/months
Sinusitis	Change in head position Valsalva maneuver Pain involving the posterior maxillary dentition	Nonpulsating, aching, pressure Mild/moderate/severe	Short—days
Migraine	Usually unilateral Spontaneous onset Nausea and vomiting Sensoriphobia	Throbbing Severe	Short—hour/days
Cluster Headache	High prevalence in men Spontaneous, repetitive Tearing, ptosis, nasal obstruction Occurs at same time of day, often during sleep	Boring, sharp, burning, excruciating Severe	Brief—minutes/hours
Temporomandibular Disorder	History of trauma and/or bruxism Trismus Deviation TMJ sounds/pain on palpation Dental occlusal discrepancies	Dull ache Mild/moderate/severe	Long—weeks/months
Temporal Arteritis	Pain in the scalp (when combing hair) Orbital pain Claudication of the masticatory muscles Sudden onset	Deep, aching, throbbing, burning Moderate/severe	Short—hours/days
Neuralgias **Trigeminal** **Glossopharyngea**	Sudden onset Trigger point in dermatome of affected nerve	Sharp, knife-like, sudden, excruciating, lancinating Severe	Very brief—seconds (may be recurrent)
Postherpetic Neuralgia	Previous herpes zoster infection May be scarring	Mild/moderate/severe	Long—weeks/months
Tension-Type Headache	Usually bilateral Nausea and vomiting are rare May be related to stress, anxiety and depression	Dull, nonpulsating, pressure, tightness Mild/moderate	Short—hours/days
Atypical Facial Pain	"Wastebasket" term Usually unilateral and continuous May spread to a large area of the face Relationship between the pain source and site may be absent	Constant, pulling, deep, aching Mild/moderate/severe	Long—weeks/months
Neoplastic Pain	Caused by pressure on a cranial nerve, ulceration, and/or infection May be accompanied by paresthesia	Sharp, knife-like Moderate/severe	Long—weeks/months
Cervical Arthritis	Chronic neck pain Confirm diagnosis with imaging	Ache, sharp Mild/moderate/severe	Long—weeks/months
Carotidynia	Inflammation of the carotid bulb Anti-inflammatory medications are effective	Tenderness on palpation, pain on affective side of neck Mild/moderate/severe	Long—weeks/months
Cardiac Pain (Angina)	Pain on exertion radiating to lower and rarely upper jaw May also occur at rest	Sharp, deep, pressure Moderate/severe	Short—minutes
Gastrointestinal Pain	Epigastric in location May be similar to cardiac pain in distribution	Burning, dull Moderate/severe	Short—minutes/hours
Psychological Pain	Often associated with depression Distribution may not follow known pathways	Vague, dull, ache Mild/moderate/severe	Long—weeks/months/years

TMJ, temporomandibular joint.

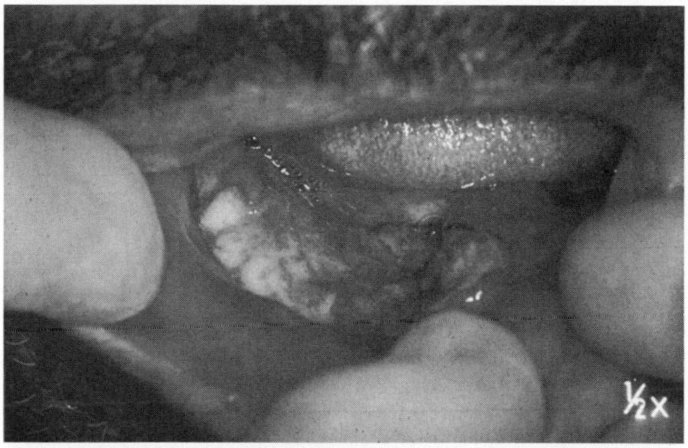

Figure 35.18 Advanced oral cancer of floor of the mouth. (See color insert.)

five to nine times greater risk than nonsmokers, and snuff users have a four times greater risk. Moderate-to-heavy alcohol users have been shown to have a three to nine times greater risk of developing oral cancer in studies controlled for tobacco use. Recent findings have found an association between the human papilloma virus and some oral cancers.

Signs and symptoms can be variable. Lesions can be ulcerative, erythematous, and/or leukoplakic and are found on the tongue, especially the posterior one third of the lateral border, floor of the mouth, buccal mucosa, gingiva, lips, oropharynx, retromolar pad, and palate (see Figs. 35.15 through 35.18). Pain may not be associated with early lesions but is usually present in advanced cases. Paresthesia may be a sign of neural involvement. Untreated lesions often spread to the lymphatic system of the head and neck, clinically producing enlarged lymph nodes. Verrucous carcinoma (comprising approximately 3% of all oral cancers) is a slow growing, diffuse, white thickening of the buccal mucosa, buccal vestibule, edentulous alveolar ridge, and/or gingival. It is often associated with smokeless tobacco use, is well differentiated and has a much better prognosis than typical squamous cell carcinoma.

Surgical management is most often the primary treatment, followed by radiation, chemotherapy, or any combination of the three. If a lesion is discovered, a conventional biopsy with histologic examination of the tissues is the most reliable means of diagnosis. Superficial lesions can be managed with local excision and regular follow-up. Invasive lesions should be managed through a multidisciplinary approach. Imaging studies will aid in the diagnosis and determination of treatment methods. Five-year survival rates are improved in patients with clear surgical margins, well-differentiated cell type, early staging, and negative nodes. The high risk of second primary lesions mandates close monitoring for a minimum of 5 years following initial tumor resolution.

ORAL MUCOSITIS

CASE SEVEN

A dental consult was requested for Mr. G., a 58-year-old with a diagnosis of stage IV non-Hodgkin lymphoma who was admitted for chemotherapy and bone marrow transplant. His chief oral complaint was of pain and burning of the oral tissues. Oral examination revealed diffuse ulcerative lesions, primarily of the buccal and labial mucosae. A diagnosis of mucositis secondary to cancer chemotherapy was made. Treatment with aminacrine (Kamillosan) liquid has been shown clinically to resolve ulcerated areas within 24 to 36 hours, so this was ordered for Mr. G.

Tissue destruction and altered functional abilities of the oral cavity following radiation therapy and/or chemotherapy results in oral mucositis. Oral mucositis is characterized by inflammation and ulceration of the oral mucosa secondary to destruction of the squamous epithelium, vasculature, connective tissue, salivary glands, muscle, and bone. It occurs in 60% to 92% of patients undergoing these therapies. The severity of the mucositis is related to the cumulative dose and type of fraction schedule for radiation therapy, timing and type of chemotherapy, type of tissue irradiated, location of radiation field, and local factors, including preexisting dental conditions, presence of irritating substances (i.e., alcohol, tobacco), and age.

Signs and symptoms of oral mucositis are pain, difficulty in mastication, dysphagia, malnutrition, dehydration, infection (especially candidiasis), and taste alteration.

Management of this condition is preventive and symptomatic. Dental treatment prior to the initiation of radiation and/or chemotherapy to eliminate infection and restore good oral health will markedly reduce the risk of oral complications. Regular dental evaluations during and following cancer treatment will help prevent severe complications. Proper oral hygiene and use of topical fluorides will help minimize dental caries and periodontal disease. Use of aminacrine (Kamillosan) liquid or analgesic and anesthetic oral rinses will help reduce the pain associated with oral mucositis and aid in nutritional intake. Palifermin (Kepivance), a recombinant human keratinocyte growth factor, has been shown to decrease the incidence and duration of severe oral mucositis in patients with hematologic cancers undergoing chemotherapy, with or without radiation, followed by a bone marrow transplant.

ORAL CANDIDIASIS

CASE EIGHT

Miss H. is a 77-year-old with a medical history significant for moderately well-controlled type 2 diabetes mellitus,

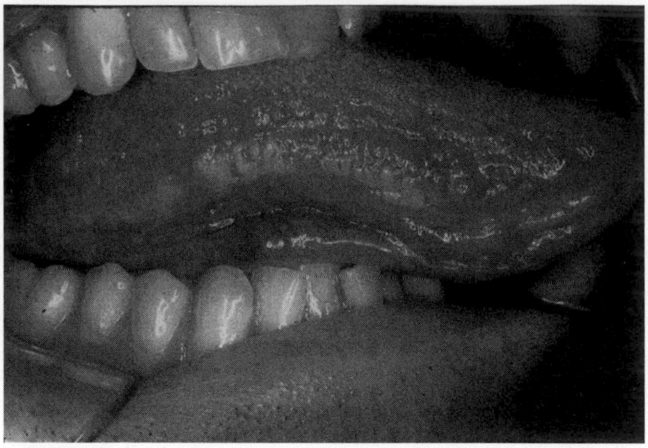

Figure 35.19 Candidiasis of lateral border of the tongue. (See color insert.)

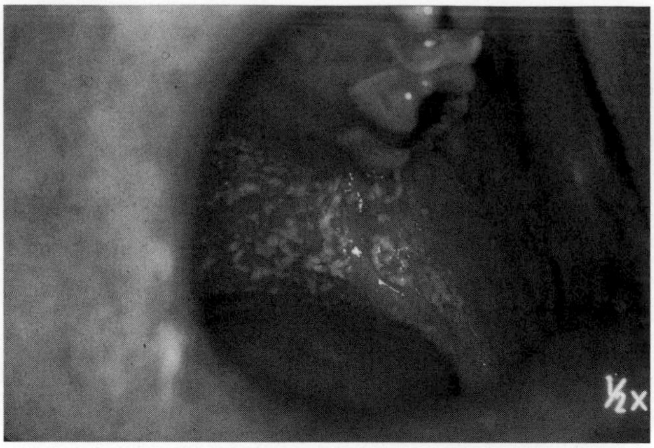

Figure 35.20 Candidiasis of soft palate. (See color insert.)

moderate obesity, and moderate asthma. Her medications included glyburide 15 mg per day and albuterol inhaler one to two puffs q4–6h. Miss H. presented with a 2-day history of moderate pain and mild swelling of the mandibular right buccal vestibule associated with a periodontally involved mandibular right second molar. After the affected area was incised and drained under local anesthesia, the patient was placed on amoxicillin 250 mg. t.i.d. for 10 days. Three days later, Miss H. presented with a chief complaint of a sore mouth with white patches on her tongue and the inside of her cheeks. Examination of the mouth revealed diffuse white papular areas that were easily removed with a tongue blade, leaving a bleeding mucosal surface. A clinical diagnosis of candidiasis was made and the patient was prescribed a 14-day course of nystatin oral suspension (400,000 units q.i.d.) to be rinsed for 1 minute and swallowed. Resolution of the mandibular swelling and the candidiasis was evident at the reexamination of the patient 1 week later.

Candidiasis is the most common fungal infection to affect the oral cavity. *Candida* sp is a normal component of the oral flora, and most infections caused by these organisms are opportunistic. It is common in patients who wear dentures, have poor oral hygiene, have nutritional deficiencies, and are xerostomic, immunocompromised, debilitated, or receiving prolonged antibiotics and/or oral inhalants. Oral candidiasis may be the result of the compromised medical condition of the individual, from the therapeutic management of the patient or a combination of both.

Signs and symptoms may vary from being totally asymptomatic to having a burning or painful complaint with no overt signs, to having a white coating on the oral mucosa that when wiped away reveals raw, bleeding areas (see Figs. 35.19 and 35.20). Systemic candidiasis may affect the mucosal lining of the esophagus and pulmonary tract. *Candida* sp, is often the cause of angular cheilitis (inflammation and tissue breakdown at the corners of the mouth). Diagnosis is by history, clinical signs and symptoms, and a positive cytologic smear, culture, or biopsy.

Management of uncomplicated candidiasis is with any number of topical antifungal medications, including nystatin oral suspension (200,000 to 400,000 units q.i.d.) rinsed and swallowed. Other antifungal medications include clotrimazole and fluconazole. Patients with dentures should be instructed to remove the dentures before the antifungal treatment is administered. The dentures are then to be thoroughly cleaned and soaked in an effective disinfectant or antifungal medication, as the prosthesis will harbor the organism and may result in reinfection of the oral tissues if inserted into the mouth untreated. In patients with systemic infections or compromised immunity, administration of amphotericin B, which requires intravenous administration, may be necessary. Angular cheilitis may be treated with nystatin ointment or clotrimazole cream.

TRAUMATIC LESIONS

CASE NINE

Mrs. T., a 61-year-old with a 35-year history of multiple sclerosis, was referred by her neurologist for evaluation of self-inflicted oral trauma caused by uncontrolled movements of the head and neck resulting in constant biting of her buccal mucosae and tongue. This activity caused painful ulcerations of the oral tissues preventing normal eating and speaking. Physical examination confirmed the presence of uncontrollable, irregular movements of her head and mandible that caused the oral structures to be trapped between her teeth and form the traumatic lesions. Intraoral examination revealed several macerated ulcerations and hyperkeratotic areas on the lateral borders of the tongue and buccal mucosae. Reduction of the movements and subsequent

> self-inflicted oral trauma were obtained by applying a cervical collar, which reduced the head movements, and a flat occlusal splint, which prevented the soft tissues from becoming trapped between the teeth. Healing of the lesions occurred over the 3 weeks following intervention. Reexamination of the patient 7 months later demonstrated a significant decrease in traumatic injury to the oral tissues and a corresponding improvement in eating and speech.

Traumatic injury to the oral mucosa in the elderly patient may be due to any number of causes, including cheek, lip, or tongue biting, ill-fitting dentures, fractured teeth or dental restorations, improper brushing of teeth and/or flossing, or dysfunctional motor activity.

Signs and symptoms are typically painful, ulcerated areas with erythematous borders and/or hyperkeratotic areas. Often these lesions present in a similar manner as do more serious conditions, including squamous cell carcinoma, and the transient nature of traumatic lesions must be recognized to avoid misdiagnosis and unnecessary treatment.

Management of traumatic lesions includes the identification and elimination of the cause and subsequent evaluation of the healing of the area. If no or limited resolution of the traumatic lesion occurs after an adequate healing period (2 to 4 weeks in an elderly patient), then further testing, including biopsy, is recommended.

BURNING MOUTH SYNDROME (STOMATOPYROSIS)

> **CASE TEN**
>
> Mrs. W., a 67-year-old, presented with a 2-month history of burning pain of the mouth, primarily of the tongue, that was absent on waking but presented and increased in intensity over the course of the day. She identified the intensity of her oral pain at four on the Visual Analog Scale. Intraoral examination was within normal limits. Medical history was remarkable for anxiety and depression. Laboratory findings were normal. No definitive cause was identified. Treatment was palliative and consisted of a rinse comprised of equal parts of diphenhydramine (Benadryl) elixir and attapulgite (Kaopectate), which resulted in mild relief. Reports on subsequent follow-up examinations demonstrated variable intensity in symptoms, with no evident cause and effect.

While burning mouth syndrome (BMS) has no identifiable etiology, it has been associated with various nutritional deficiencies, anxiety, depression, type 2 diabetes mellitus, salivary flow changes, allergic reactions, candidiasis, dentures, and/or parafunctional behavior. BMS is often diagnosed in postmenopausal women. However, no condition has been definitely linked to BMS. Detailed oral and systemic clinical, radiographic, and laboratory evaluation of the patient may not often specify a cause.

Signs and symptoms are generally the occurrence of burning pain localized to the tongue and, infrequently, other oral soft tissues with normal mucosal findings. There are reports that BMS patients demonstrate the same personality characteristics seen in other chronic pain patients.

Management should be tailored to each patient and may be multidisciplinary in nature. Palliative treatment includes topical analgesic rinses (see section "Oral Mucositis") and/or chronic pain protocols.

ORAL CONDITIONS AND SYSTEMIC DISEASE

Millions of older people have complex medical conditions that have an adverse effect on oral health. The incidence of compromised oral health is increasing due to advancing age, medical health, complications of medical treatment, and lack of oral health care, particularly in the institutional setting. As the current population continues to age, these problems will place a significant strain on health care providers and systems. An association between oral conditions and systemic disease has been demonstrated in a large number of epidemiologic studies regarding older individuals. Periodontal disease in particular has been linked to aspiration pneumonia, atherosclerosis, cardiovascular diseases, stroke, diabetes mellitus, and arthritis.

PERIOPERATIVE CONSIDERATIONS

Physicians are often consulted by dentists regarding antibiotic prophylaxis and anticoagulation considerations. Current American Heart Association/American Dental Association recommendations call for antibiotic prophylaxis in high-risk cardiac conditions when selective invasive dental procedures are performed. Prevention of infection of prosthetic joints is recommended by the American Academy of Orthopedic Surgeons/American Dental Association when:

1. An invasive dental procedure is to be performed;
2. The prosthetic joint is within 2 years of placement;
3. The patient has had previous prosthetic joint infections; and/or
4. The patient is immunocompromised.

Many dental procedures may be safely performed on patients receiving anticoagulant therapy within therapeutic INR levels. Interruption of anticoagulant therapy should be on the basis of the invasiveness of the dental procedure, the risk of abnormal bleeding, and the risk of thromboembolism in the absence of anticoagulant therapy. It is recommended that a current INR level be available prior to any invasive procedure.

Recommendations regarding these clinical concerns are reviewed periodically and the reader is advised to refer to the most current literature on the subject (please refer to American Dental Association citations in "Selected Reading").

ATHEROSCLEROSIS, CARDIOVASCULAR DISEASE, AND STROKE

CASE ELEVEN

Mr. S., a 75-year-old, presented for fabrication of maxillary and mandibular complete dentures following the removal of his remaining natural teeth due to severe periodontal disease. Medical history included a long-term history of smoking, myocardial infarction following unstable angina, for which quadruple coronary bypass surgery was performed, and light-headedness on standing, which was being managed with meclizine. A screening panoramic radiograph revealed bilateral radiopacities inferior to the mandible at the level of C3 and C4 vertebral bodies, consistent with calcification affecting the carotid arteries. Subsequent referral and sonographic evaluation revealed extensive arthrosclerotic changes and severe bilateral carotid stenosis, 90% of the right external and internal carotid arteries, 70% of the left internal carotid artery, and 55% of the left external carotid artery. Carotid digital subtraction angiography demonstrated a stenosis >95% at the origin of the right internal carotid artery for a 2.5 cm. segment. The left internal carotid showed a 65% stenosis. The patient underwent right carotid endarterectomy with a satisfactory outcome.

Several recent studies have implicated chronic inflammatory conditions, including periodontitis, with atherosclerosis after adjusting for other common risk factors. Poor oral health, especially when in combination with smoking, is a risk factor for death due to cardiovascular disease and cerebrovascular accidents. Periodontitis has been shown to elevate levels of C-reactive protein and fibrinogen, reliable markers for atherosclerosis. Specific oral bacteria associated with periodontitis have been demonstrated in atheromas in coronary vessels. Signs of carotid calcifications on panoramic radiographs are highly associated with positive ultrasound readings, and the extent of carotid calcifications and the severity of periodontal disease have been shown to be related. In fact, successful treatment of periodontitis has been shown to reduce the levels of inflammatory markers associated with increased risk of cardiovascular and peripheral arterial disease. While the effects of periodontitis may have occurred over many years and are often most severe in elderly patients, it is important to treat existing periodontal disease, eliminate chronic inflammation, and minimize additional local and systemic damage.

DIABETES

CASE TWELVE

Ms. H., a 73-year-old, presented for comprehensive dental care. Medical history was significant for long-term (39 years) poorly controlled insulin-dependent diabetes, congestive heart failure, myocardial infarction (age 64), and peripheral artery disease. Oral evaluation revealed multiple missing teeth and severe periodontitis and alveolar bone loss associated with the remaining natural teeth. Removal of hopelessly involved teeth and initiation of proper oral hygiene, including frequent professional oral prophylaxis, and partial denture fabrication improved the patient's oral health, allowing for improved food selection, enhanced nutritional intake, and normal glucose levels.

Diabetes and periodontitis have a mutually deleterious effect on one another. Poorly controlled diabetes has been associated with a three times greater incidence of periodontal disease, and the duration of diabetes is related to the severity of periodontitis. Degenerative vascular changes, impairment of the immune system, and altered metabolism caused by diabetes contribute to impaired synthesis of collagen and impaired wound healing, predisposing factors to periodontitis.

Periodontitis, because of the release of inflammatory proteins into the circulation, can result in altered insulin function and increased glucose levels. The highly inflamed gingival tissues associated with periodontitis may allow bacteria and inflammatory mediators to readily enter the blood stream and negatively affect normal insulin activity. Good oral health allows proper mastication, selection of healthy foods, and improved nutrition. It appears that proper management of periodontal disease and the subsequent elimination of chronic inflammation has a positive effect on the control of glucose levels in the patient with diabetes.

ASPIRATION PNEUMONIA/CHRONIC OBSTRUCTIVE PULMONARY DISEASE

CASE THIRTEEN

Mr. F., an 80-year-old with a 42-year history of hereditary spastic paraparesis and periodontitis associated with poor oral hygiene, progressively developed significant dysphagia over the past 10 years. He has been tube fed for 2 years. Over the past 10 months, he has had three episodes of pneumonia, the last two resulting in admission to the intensive care unit. Bacterial isolates from sputum samples identified several oral pathogens, including *Actinobacillus actinomycetemcomitans*, a bacterium commonly associated with periodontal disease. Recovery from each episode was prolonged and had residual effects on the patient's swallowing ability.

Proper oral hygiene was instituted to reduce the bacteria-harboring plaque associated with his remaining teeth. However, his dysphagia progressed to the point that a gastrostomy tube was placed to allow proper nutrition and prevent aspiration.

Dental plaque may serve as a reservoir for oral and respiratory bacteria and may be the cause of aspiration pneumonia in elderly individuals, particularly those with dysphagia. Patients with significant dental plaque accumulations in nursing home facilities and hospitals are at greater risk for nosocomial infection, as it has been shown that the dental plaque of these patients becomes colonized with respiratory organisms. Recurrent aspiration may introduce these pathogens into the respiratory tract and cause pneumonia. Poor oral health has been identified as a risk factor for aspiration pneumonia. Institution of proper oral hygiene, including the use of a daily rinse containing 0.12% chlorhexidine gluconate, has been shown to reduce the rate of pneumonia by 40% to 50%.

Some evidence exists that associates periodontal disease with chronic obstructive pulmonary disease (COPD). Aspiration of saliva containing respiratory pathogens, enzymes, and host-derived mediators may cause lung inflammation and infection in the lower airway, leading to exacerbation of COPD and diminished respiratory function and disease progression. Reduction of bacteria-harboring dental plaque by improvement of oral hygiene may prevent the aspiration of significant numbers of these pathogens, reducing the incidence of pneumonia, and subsequent worsening of COPD.

DEMENTIA

CASE FOURTEEN

Ms. K., a 71-year-old with a 4-year history of rapidly progressing Alzheimer disease (AD), was evaluated at the request of her caregiver. With mild restraint of the patient's head, visual oral examination of her dentition was possible. Significant accumulations of dental plaque covered her teeth; however, multiple carious lesions were visible involving the coronal and root surfaces of the teeth. Prior to the onset of AD, the patient had meticulous oral hygiene and was caries-free for 20 years. Management of the patient was not possible in the conscious state. After consultation with her caregiver, who was her health care proxy, it was decided to treat Ms. K. in the operating suite utilizing general anesthesia. Multiple dental restorations were performed to maintain several reasonably healthy teeth, preserve some masticatory function, and prevent making the patient completely edentulous. Most of her teeth, however, required extraction due to extensive dental decay. The patient tolerated the procedure without incident. Proper oral hygiene and topical fluoride programs were started by her caregiver, reducing the accumulation of dental plaque and the rate of dental caries.

Individuals with dementia have been shown to have a higher incidence of oral diseases. Several longitudinal studies conclude that the rate of oral conditions appears to be related to dementia severity, not the specific dementia diagnosis. Heavy dental plaque accumulation, directly related to poor or absent oral hygiene, is associated with the development of dental caries. As noted in the preceding text, dental plaque also predisposes the patient to aspiration pneumonia and cardiovascular disease. Patients with dementia also have decreased use of dentures and increased denture-related oral conditions, and they visit a dentist less frequently than those without dementia.

Dental management is difficult in those with severe dementia. Attention should be given to oral hygiene, avoiding medications with a xerostomic effect, removal of unrestorable teeth, frequent oral examination, and aggressive topical fluoride programs. Oral or intravenous sedation or general anesthesia may be necessary to provide adequate dental care.

CONCLUSION

The health of the hard and soft tissues of the oral cavity directly affects the systemic health of an individual. This is particularly true in elderly people, who have limited functional capacity and a compromised response to challenges affecting general health. Oral health is essential for proper nutrition, positive self-image, and favorable quality of life. Prevention of several fatal systemic conditions is directly related to proper oral hygiene and the maintenance of oral health. Physicians are encouraged to routinely examine the oral cavity and take steps to promptly intervene when abnormal findings are identified.

SELECTED READING

Abdollahi M, Radfar M. A review of drug-induced oral reactions. *J Contemp Dent Pract*. 2003;3(4)1:010–031.

American Academy of Oral Medicine. *Clinician's guide to oral health in geriatric patients*. Baltimore, MD: American Academy of Oral Medicine; 1999a.

American Academy of Oral Medicine. *Diagnosis and treatment of chronic orofacial pain*. Baltimore, MD: American Academy of Oral Medicine; 1999b.

American Dental Association; American Academy of Orthopedic Surgeons. Antibiotic prophylaxis for dental patients with total joint replacements. *J Am Dent Assoc*. 2003;134(7):895–899.

American Dental Association; American Heart Association. Prevention of bacterial endocarditis: Recommendations by the American Heart Association by the committee on rheumatic fever, endocarditis and kawasaki disease. *JAMA*. 1997;277:1794–1801.

Beers MH, Berkow R, eds. *The merck manual of geriatrics*, 3rd ed. Whitehouse, NJ: Merck Research Laboratories; 2000.

Chiappelli F, Bauer J, Spackman S, et al. Dental needs of the elderly in the 21st century. *Gen Dent*. 2002;50(4):358–363.

Ciancio SG, ed. *American Dental Association to Dental Theraputics*, 3rd ed. Chicago, IL: ADA Publishing; 2004.
Helgeson MJ, Smith BJ, Johnsen M, et al. Dental care considerations for the frail elderly. *Spec Care Dentist*. 2002;22(3 suppl):40S–53S.
Holm-Pedersen P, Loe H, eds. *Textbook of geriatric dentistry*, 2nd ed. Munksgaard: Munksgaard Publishing; 1996.
Jakobsson U. Pain management among older people in need of help with activities of daily living. *Pain Manag Nurs*. 2004;5(4):137–143.
Lamster IB. Oral health care services for older adults: A looming crisis. *Am J Public Health*. 2004;70(9):14–17.
Navazesh M. Dry mouth: Aging and oral health. *Compend Contin Educ Dent*. 2002;23(10 suppl):41–48.
Neville BW, Day TA. Oral and precancerous lesions. *CA Cancer J Clin*. 2002;52(4):195–215.
Rankin KV, Jones DL, Redding SW, eds. *Oral health in cancer therapy: A guide for health care professionals*, 2nd ed. Dallas, TX: Dental Oncology Education Program; 2003.
Scannapieco FA, Bush RB, Paju S. Associations between periodontal disease and risk for atherosclerosis, cardiovascular disease and stroke. A systemic review. *Ann Periodontol*. 2003a;8(1):38–53.
Scannapieco FA, Bush RB, Paju S. Associations between periodontal disease and risk for nosocomial bacterial pneumonia and chronic obstructive pulmonary disease. A systematic review. *Ann Periodontol*. 2003b;8(1):54–69.
Spielberger R, Stiff P, Bensinger W, et al. Palifermin for oral mucositis after intensive therapy for hematologic cancers. *N Engl J Med*. 2004;351(25):2590–2598.
Vernillo AT. Dental considerations for the treatment of patients with diabetes mellitus. *J Am Dent Assoc*. 2003;134(10 suppl):24S–33S.
Wayne DB, Trajtenberg CP, Hyman DJ. Tooth and periodontal disease: A review for the primary-care physician. *South Med J*. 2001;94(9):925–932.
Williams RC. A century of progress in understanding periodontal disease. *Compend Contin Educ Dent*. 2002;23(5 suppl):3–10.
Wisconsin Geriatric Education Center. *Geriatric oral health: The missing link to comprehensive care*. http://www.cuph.org/wgec/index.jsp (Accessed August 23–28, 2004).
Wong-Baker FACES Pain Rating Scale. http://www.ndhcri.org/pain/Tools/Wong-Baker_Faces_Pain_Rating_Scale.pdf (Accessed February 24, 2005).

36

Common Dermatologic Conditions in Aging

Charles A. Cefalu   Lee Nesbitt

- CLINICAL PEARLS 491
- INTRINSIC VERSUS EXTRINSIC CHANGES OF AGING 492
- PHOTOAGING 492
- BENIGN LESIONS 494
- DERMATITIS 496
- BULLOUS LESIONS 498
- COMMON DERMATOLOGIC BACTERIAL/PARASITIC/FUNGAL INFECTIONS 499
- PREMALIGNANT AND MALIGNANT LESIONS 503
- SKIN MANIFESTATIONS OF VASCULAR DISEASE 508
- MISCELLANEOUS SKIN CONDITIONS 509

CLINICAL PEARLS

- Intrinsic skin aging or physiologic changes are structural, clinical, and immunologic. Secondary changes (wrinkling, coarseness, and roughness) are due to extrinsic factors, such as exposure to ultraviolet rays of the sun.
- Terbinafine and itraconazole are safe, have high cure rates in onychomycosis, and require only 3 months of treatment.
- Early treatment of herpes zoster with oral antiviral agents halts the progression of the disease, decreases incidence of visceral and cutaneous dissemination, promotes healing, reduces the duration and intensity of acute pain, and reduces the duration and frequency of postherpetic neuralgia.
- Treatment of squamous and basal cell carcinoma depends on the size of the lesion and extent or numbers of lesions, morphology, location, and patient's compliance.
- Risk factors for melanoma include very fair skin, family history, dysplastic or numerous nevi, blue eyes, blond or red hair, freckling, frequent sunburn, inability to tan, and immunosuppression.
- Seborrheic keratoses have a "stuck-on" appearance, are brown black in color, and occur most commonly on the back, chest, and face. Indications for removal are cosmetic.
- Melanoma are infiltrative lesions with diverse coloring—ranging from brown, black, gray to red—with irregular margins.
- The best treatment for seborrheic dermatitis of the scalp (dandruff) is prevention using regular shampoos containing tar or selenium sulfide.
- Allergic contact dermatitis typically presents as a vesicular or bullous eruption in the area of contact with an allergen around the waist, cap or hat line (rubber lining), or the finger, neck, or wrist (ring, necklace, or watch).

- Xerosis occurs more commonly with aging because of a reduction in water contact and barrier function and is best managed by avoidance of frequent bathing or showering with hot water and harsh soaps.
- Severe fungal infections of the feet, scalp, and nails are best treated with a course of oral antifungal therapy.
- Scabies in the nursing home setting may be epidemic and may present as a seborrheic dermatitis-like rash. Diagnosis is made by the finding of mite excreta or eggs on the hair shaft.
- Ulceration of the skin of the lower extremities may result from chronic vascular insufficiency of either arterial or venous origin.

This chapter discusses the common dermatologic conditions of aging. Topics discussed include histologic changes with normal aging (intrinsic) and premature aging (external photoaging). There will be a brief discussion of common benign and malignant lesions, common infections, common papulosquamous disease processes, and a miscellaneous category. No amount of text can fully describe the common dermatologic conditions of aging. Therefore, the chapter text is accompanied in most cases by color plates that characterize most of these skin diseases (also see Table 36.1 for differential diagnosis).

INTRINSIC VERSUS EXTRINSIC CHANGES OF AGING

Skin changes with aging can be categorized as either intrinsic (related to physiologic changes secondary to longevity) or extrinsic (environmentally induced changes). Intrinsic changes can be further subdivided into structural changes, clinical manifestations of these changes, and physiologic and immunologic changes.

Structural changes in the epidermis include flattening of the dermoepidermal interface, generalized loss of melanocytes, focal melanocyte clustering, basal cell heterogeneity, and loss of Langerhans cells. Dermal changes include decreased density, increased size and cross-linking of collagen bundles, elastic fiber loss, decreased vascularity, and reduced ground substance. There is also a decrease in the number of sweat glands, thinning and ridging of the nails, a generalized decrease in the number and thickness of terminal hairs, loss of melanocytes from hair bulbs, focal conversion of vellus to terminal hairs, and decreased innervation and generalized atrophy of tissue.

Clinical changes related to these structural changes include an increased frequency of benign and malignant epidermal neoplasms, irregular pigmentation, a propensity to blister formation, development of lentigo senilis, development of superficial skin laxity, decreased insulating capacity and surface markings, a predisposition to tear-type injury, thermoregulatory disturbances, the development of pallor, xerosis, hypothermia and hyperthermia, brittle nails, diffuse hair loss, coarse hair, hair graying, loss of manual dexterity, propensity to injury, and diffuse thinning of the scalp hair leading to baldness.[1,2]

Owing to a reduction in dermal clearance of chemical agents with normal aging, older patients have a propensity to persistence of contact dermatitis with slower healing. In addition, the topical administration of potentially noxious medications or chemicals to the skin surface may result in the sudden onset of a severe inflammatory dermatitis because the inflammatory response with aging is delayed at onset. The immune response is also depressed with normal aging such that both the percentage of T cells and its absolute number are decreased. This is directly related to the reduced ability to respond to specific antigens. Clinically, this may manifest as a decline in skin hypersensitivity to specific antigens and the ability to determine immune status. Skin testing with specific agents such as tuberculin, mumps, or *Candida* may result in a false-negative or weaker hypersensitivity reaction.

An increase in B-cell dysfunction also occurs, resulting in a raised incidence of autoantibodies and increased immunoglobulin-A (IgA) and IgG levels. This may manifest itself clinically as false-positive antigen–antibody reactions between foreign antigens (laboratory reagents to detect clinical disease) and autoantibodies including rheumatoid factor and initial testing for syphilis.

Lastly, the quantity of epidermal 7-dehydro-cholesterol per unit area decreases linearly with aging and can result in diminished vitamin D production, development of osteomalacia, and clinical fracture.[2]

PHOTOAGING

Extrinsic aging of the skin refers to the effects of environmental exposure, principally chronic ultraviolet light exposure. The extent of ultraviolet damage over time depends on the depth of penetration of ultraviolet light in the skin as determined by the wavelength. Ultraviolet radiation involving a wavelength of 290 to 320 nm causes most of the acute and chronic exposure. Wavelengths of sunlight involving 320 to 400 nm are also important in causing damage because they have greater depths of penetration. Ultraviolet light causes damage to skin by effecting DNA injury, decreased DNA repair, or both, as well as oxidation, lysosomal damage, and altered collagen structure.

Clinical correlates of this damage include wrinkling, coarseness, and roughness of skin, with mottled pigmentation. The mottled pigmentation is due to the development of solar lentigos, seborrheic keratoses, ephelides or freckles, hypopigmentation, and telangiectasias. Skin malignancies are also more common in photodamaged areas of the skin.

The role of oxidative stress and the use of antioxidants to prevent extrinsic aging have received much attention in the last several years. Although various *in vitro* and animal studies have shown that low–molecular-weight antioxidants exert protective effects against oxidative stress (particularly vitamins C and E, ascorbate, tocopherol, and

TABLE 36.1
DIFFERENTIAL DIAGNOSIS OF COMMON DERMATOSES IN THE ELDERLY

Benign	Premalignant	Malignant
Solar lentignes (liver or brown spots) (692.70)[a]		Lentignes maligna melanoma (172)[a]
Sebaceous hyperplasia (706.9)[a]		Nodular basal cell carcinoma (173)[a]
Milia (epidermal cysts) (706.2)[a]		Malignant melanoma (172.9)[a]
Acrochordons		
Seborrheic keratoses (702.19)[a]		
Dermatosis papulosa nigra (709.8)[a]		
Erythema ab igne (692.82)		
Favre-Racouchot syndrome		
Vascular Lesions		
Senile purpura (287.2)[a]		
Cherry hemangioma (228.01)[a]		
Venous lakes (benign venous angiomas) (228.01)[a]		
Nodular Lesions		
Keratoacanthoma (238.2)[a]		
Dermatoses		
Seborrheic dermatitis (690.10)[a]		
Allergic contact dermatitis (692.9)[a]		
Xerosis (dry skin) (708.6)[a]		
Stasis dermatitis (459.81)[a]		
Neurodermatitis (698.3)[a]		
Dermatitis medicamentosa (693)[a]		
Bullous Lesions		
Bullous pemphigoid (694.5)[a]		
Erythema multiforme Bullosum (695.1)[a]		
Staphylococcal scalded skin syndrome		
Bullous impetigo (684)[a]		
Insect bites		
Second-degree burns		
Epidermolysis bullosa Acquisita (757.39)		
Linear immunoglobulin-α bullous disease		
Dermatitis herpetiformis (694.0)		
Viral, Fungal, and Parasitic Dermatoses		
Herpes zoster (shingles) (053.9)[a]		
Tinea cruris (110.3)[a]		
Tinea pedis (110.4)[a]		
Erythrasma (039.0)[a]		
Onychomycosis (110.1)[a]		
Psoriasis (696.1)[a]		
Pediculosis (132.9)[a]		
Scabies (133.0)[a]		
Dysplastic nevi[a]	Actinic keratosis (702.0)[a]	Squamous cell carcinoma (173)[a]
		Basal cell carcinoma (173)[a]
		Malignant melanoma (172.9)[a]
Vascular Ulcers		
Arterial (707.9)[a]		
Venous (454)[a]		
Pressure ulcers (707)		
Miscellaneous Dermatoses		
Rosacea (695.3)[a]		
Acne vulgaris (706.1)		
Lupus erythematosus (695.4)		
Bromoderma		
Iododerma		
Papular syphilid		
Seborrhea (706.3)		
Hyperkeratotic Dermatoses		
Corn (700)[a]		
Callus (700)[a]		

[a]Topics covered in this chapter.

lipoic acid [LA]), controlled long-term studies evaluating the efficacy of low–molecular-weight antioxidants in the prevention or treatment of extrinsic aging are lacking.[3]

Treatment of photodamage involves prevention of cumulated exposure through the use of broad-spectrum sunscreens that shield the skin from the effects of ultraviolet light. Tretinoin has been used in high concentrations to reverse some of the cosmetic changes of aging. Tretinoin increases the thickness of the superficial skin layers, reduces pigmentary changes and roughness, and increases collagen synthesis, but only when used for long periods of time. Concentrations of between 0.02% and 0.05% cream have been shown to be an effective treatment option. A recent study demonstrated the effectiveness of a 0.25% solution. This concentration proved tolerable and achieved clinical response in as little as 1 month[4] (Evidence Level B). Another study showed that 0.1% cream is superior to 0.05% emollient cream with respect to speed of improvement over a 24-month period[5] (Evidence Level B).

α-LA is a potent scavenger with anti-inflammatory properties. It has been shown to be effective in significantly reducing skin roughness when used in a 5% cream and combined with laser profilometry over a 12-week period[6] (Evidence Level B). Pyruvic acid, an α-keto acid, when applied in a 50% preparation to achieve a peel, was shown to produce a smoother texture, less-evident fine wrinkles, lightening of hyperpigmentations (freckles and lentigines), thinning of the epidermis, and thickening of the dermis, with limited or no discomfort in the postpeel period[7] (Evidence Level B).

Surgical options for the treatment of photodamage include the use of chemical peeling agents, dermabrasion, and laser resurfacing. All of these procedures essentially work by destroying the surface populations of keratinocytes, followed by repopulation of the surface with keratinocytes deep from within the sun-protected follicular structures. Few clinical trials, however, have proved their effectiveness[8] (Evidence Level C). One-pass short-pulse erbium: YAG laser has also been shown to be safe and effective, with minimal side effects and rapid healing within 3 to 5 days[9] (Evidence Level B). Lastly, the use of 40% urea cream combined with δ-aminolevulinic acid (δ-ALA) with exposure to activating light (photodynamic therapy [PDT]) for 7 days has been compared with the use of δ-ALA and light therapy alone and followed up for 1 and 5 months respectively. Both treatments were found to be safe and effective in significantly reducing the severity of photodamage[10] (Evidence Level B).

Although wrinkling may be a sign of photodamage and extrinsic aging, wrinkling in a site with limited sun exposure may be a marker of general health status or intrinsic aging, particularly in women[11] (Evidence Level C).

The use of botulinum toxin for treatment of wrinkles has increased greatly in recent years. It is generally used in the following locations: Glabella, brow, crow's feet, upper lip wrinkling lines, depressor anguli oris, nasolabial folds, mentalis, and neck. Although the treatment is considered to be safe and well tolerated, the injecting surgeon should be familiar with the potential complications of therapy[12] (Evidence Level C). Hormone replacement therapy may also slow the progress of intrinsic aging of the skin. However, it does not limit the number and depth of wrinkles[13,14] (Evidence Level B).

BENIGN LESIONS

Solar lentigines are circumscribed, pigmented, nonmalignant macular lesions referred to as *brown* or *liver spots*. They typically have a diameter of approximately 0.5 cm and are induced by ultraviolet radiation. In rare cases, they may progress into a lentigo maligna melanoma with characteristic diameters in the 3 to 6 cm range and with irregular pigmentation and shape with irregular borders. A change in size or color of the lesion should prompt investigation and resection. Without adequate resection, solar lentigines have a 50% risk of developing into a malignant melanoma and a 10% risk of metastatic spread[15] (Evidence Level C).

Sebaceous hyperplasia is a sebaceous gland that has the appearance of a yellow nodule with a central pore. Although the number of sebaceous glands remains stable with age, their size may increase, and sebum production decreases. This results in increased visibility, especially in sun-exposed areas. These lesions should be differentiated from nodular basal cell cancer. Cancerous lesions are differentiated from hyperplasia by the presence of telangiectatic blood vessels and a translucent appearance. Suspicion of malignancy should be followed by biopsy[15] (see Fig. 36.1) (Evidence Level C). Treatment options include laser therapy, electrodesiccation, and topical bichloracetic acid. Curettage is a less optimal form of therapy because of scarring. For diffuse multiple lesions, oral isotretinoin has been shown to be effective[16] (Evidence Level B).

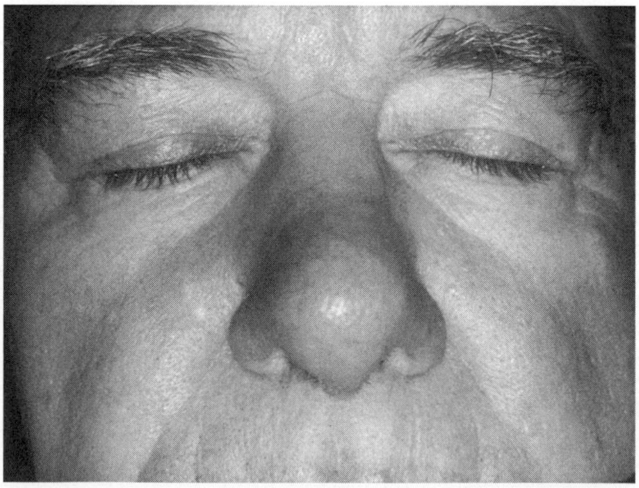

Figure 36.1 Lesions of sebaceous hyperplasia. (See color insert.)

Milia are epidermal cysts that frequently occur on sun-damaged facial or periorbital skin and measure approximately 1 mm in diameter. Although they may be of concern to the patient for cosmetic reasons, they have no malignant potential. They may be removed with a comedone or needle extractor[15] (Evidence Level C).

Acrochordons are skin tags with a flesh-colored appearance and typically occur on the neck and axillae, especially in the obese elderly. They are benign. Indications for removal include cosmetic problems or irritation[15] (Evidence Level C). Treatment options include electrocautery or scissor excision at the base of the stalk or cryotherapy. Local anesthesia is usually not necessary.[16]

Seborrheic keratoses are common in the elderly and typically have a "stuck-on" appearance, are brown black in color, and may occur on any part of the body, but more frequently in seborrheic areas such as the back, chest, and face. The lesions typically range in size from 2 to 10 mm in diameter. Melanomas tend to have more diverse colors ranging from brown, blue, black, and gray to red. In addition, the surface of keratoses is rough as opposed to melanomas in which the surface is smooth. Dermatosis papulosa nigra is a variant that occurs more commonly on the face of dark-skinned individuals, and in multiple ways. Patients have a hereditary predisposition for development and there is no relationship between its occurrence and exposure to sunlight[15] (see Fig. 36.2) (Evidence Level C). Excisional biopsy may be required if the diagnosis is in question. Otherwise, because of their cosmetically unappealing appearance, especially with multiple ones, patients will often request removal. Cryosurgery, curettage, and excision are the most common methods of treatment. Except for extremely thick lesions, cryotherapy with liquid nitrogen is effective, but repeat treatments may be necessary. Shaving the lesion or use of curettage with electrocautery after administration of local anesthesia provides an additional option. Although these lesions are typically asymptomatic, keratoses may become irritated or inflamed by chafing with clothing. Topical steroids may be useful for symptomatic relief[16] (Evidence Level B).

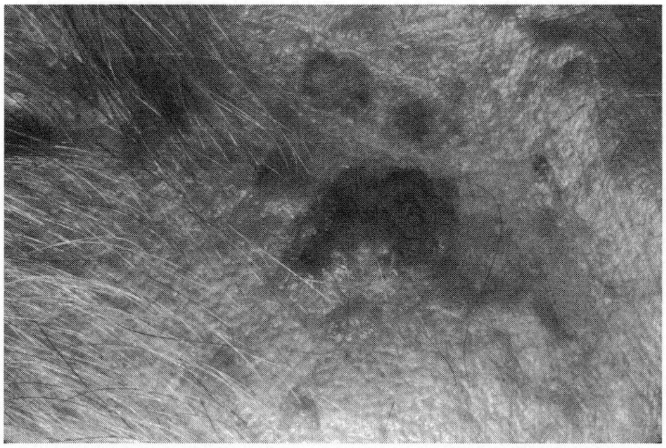

Figure 36.2 Lesions of seborrheic keratoses. (See color insert.)

Senile purpura or ecchymosis involves the development of purplish discolorations in the dermis. They are a result of increased fragility and rupture of the dermal capillaries and blood vessels, with resultant extravasation of blood into the surrounding tissue. Senile purpura is commonly seen on the dorsal forearm and hands. Prevention includes wearing long-sleeved shirts to reduce shear and friction. Caregivers should be cautioned to handle frail patients gently to prevent bruising and skin tears. Patients may need reassurance that the development of senile purpura is not a sign of a bleeding disorder.

Cherry hemangiomas are bright red papules that range from 1 to 5 mm in diameter, increase with advancing age, and appear commonly on the trunk. Although their etiology and pathogenesis are unknown, there appears to be no association with exposure to the sun. Treatment has traditionally involved hyfrecation[15] (Evidence Level C). The use of potassium titanyl phosphate (KTP) vascular laser has been shown to be superior to hyfrecation because only one treatment, rather than two, is necessary. There were also fewer side effects with laser therapy[17] (Evidence Level B).

Venous lakes, also referred to as *benign venous angiomas*, are flat, compressible, and soft and range from 4 to 6 mm in diameter. They appear as bluish red lesions most commonly on the lower lips or the ears of older patients. Excision may be indicated for cosmetic reasons or if it cannot be distinguished from melanoma[15] (see Fig. 36.3) (Evidence Level C). The use of carbon dioxide vaporization is also associated with excellent cosmetic results that can

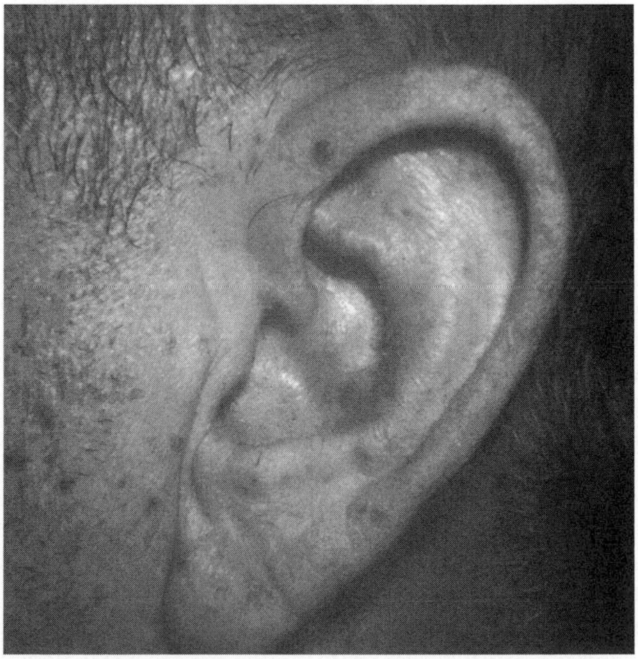

Figure 36.3 Appearance of the lesions of venous lakes, or benign venous angiomas, in the ear. (See color insert.)

be achieved in one session[18] (Evidence Level B). Infrared coagulation is another option but requires several treatment sessions and is associated with minimal scarring.[19]

Keratoacanthoma is a rapidly growing lesion that typically occurs on the sun-exposed areas of the face and upper extremities with aging. Although usually a solitary lesion, it may present in multiple ways. It may also occur less commonly on the lower extremities in older women. The lesion begins as a papular one, enlarging over a 4-week period to 2 cm or more. An umbilicated, keratinous core develops, and after 4 to 6 months the core is expelled with involution of the lesion, resulting in a hypopigmented scar. Although the exact cause is unknown, ultraviolet light, human papillomavirus, and prolonged exposure to coal tar derivatives are thought to be the risk factors. It is not known whether the lesion is truly benign or has potential for malignancy. However, because of its histologic similarity to squamous cell carcinoma, and potential for scarring, total removal is the preferred treatment for solitary lesions. Small lesions can be treated with electrodesiccation and curettage or through blunt dissection. For lesions occurring around the nose or ears, Mohs surgery (described in detail later in this chapter) provides an alternative. Other alternatives include intralesional fluorouracil, intralesional methotrexate, intralesional 5-interferon-α-2a, or radiotherapy for patients with recurrent or larger lesions[16] (Evidence Level B).

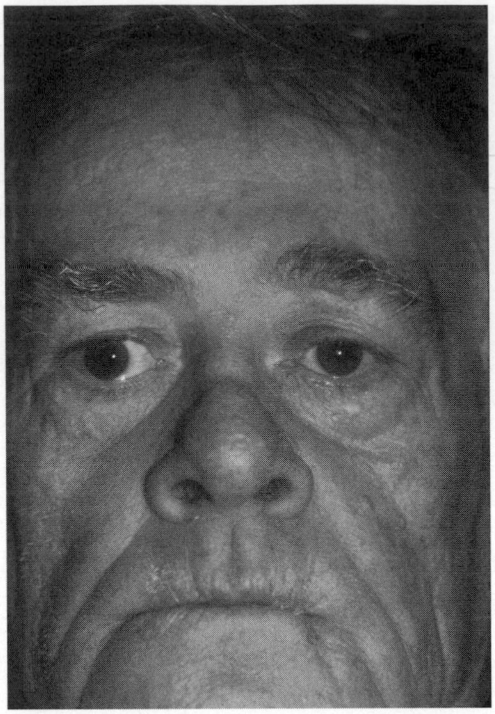

Figure 36.4 Seborrheic dermatitis—appearing as a greasy scaling and erythema of the scalp and skin areas. (See color insert.)

DERMATITIS

Seborrheic dermatitis principally affects the central part of the face, around the ears and nose, the eyebrows and eyelashes. It can be severe in patients with Parkinson disease and other central nervous system (CNS) disorders, including acquired immunodeficiency syndrome (AIDS). Clinically, it appears as a greasy scaling and erythema of the scalp and skin areas. Pityrosporon orbiculare (Malassezia furfur), saprophytic fungi, have been associated with seborrheic dermatitis but the exact cause is unknown. Treatment of scalp areas involves the use of antiseborrheic shampoos containing tar or selenium sulfide or 2% chloroxine. Treatment of other affected areas includes the use of ketoconazole cream or a mild to moderate potency topical corticosteroid for acute cases. Maintenance therapy, especially for the scalp area, is usually successful in preventing a flare[8,15] (see Fig. 36.4) (Evidence Level A). Tacrolimus 0.1% ointment applied for 28 days has been shown to be 70% to 99% effective, with only local burning and irritation as side effects[20] (Evidence Level B). Ciclopirox shampoo, which has an active antifungal ingredient, has been shown to be an effective and safe treatment for seborrheic dermatitis of the scalp[21] (Evidence Level B). A 4-week treatment of ketoconazole 2% has been shown to be significantly more effective than 1% zinc pyrithione for seborrheic dermatitis of the scalp[22] (Evidence Level B). However, lithium gluconate (8%) has been shown to be even more effective than ketoconazole 2% in achieving complete remission at 2 months with comparable safety[23] (Evidence Level B).

Allergic contact dermatitis typically presents as vesicles or bullae in the area of contact with an allergen. A clinical cue to the diagnosis is the characteristic location of the lesions around the waist line (belt or rubber lining), cap or hat line, or the finger or neck (ring or necklace). In other instances, a history of recent contact exposure to chemicals or allergens may be helpful in elucidating the cause (e.g., gardening). Mild to moderate symptomatology related to itching and localized distribution may be treated with typical corticosteroids and lubrication, whereas severe symptoms of itching and involvement may require systemic steroids in a dose of 40 to 60 mg per day for 5 to 10 days. With recurrent episodes of dermatitis in which the causative agent is unknown, patch skin testing may be useful[15] (see Fig. 36.5) (Evidence Level C).

Xerosis, or dryness of the skin, is common in the elderly and may present simply as rough, itchy skin, or more severely as a scaly, dry, cracked appearance (eczema craquelé). Chronic rubbing and scratching result in thickening or lichenification of the skin. It is the most common cause of itching or pruritus in the elderly. It is due to a reduction in water content and barrier function with aging of the epidermis. Environmental factors such as drying from exposure to hot water, too frequent bathing or showering with harsh soaps, decreased humidity from cold and windy weather ("winter itch"), or

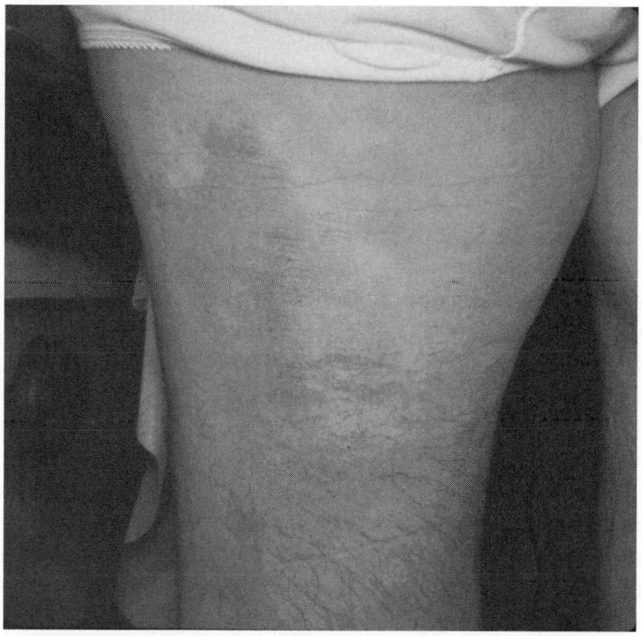

Figure 36.5 Allergic contact dermatitis, presenting as vesicles or bullae in the area in contact with an allergen. (See color insert.)

dry heat from central heating may exacerbate the process. Common areas of involvement include the anterior legs, extensor aspects of the arms and forearms, and dorsum of the hands. Severe cases can result in cellulitis. Prior to initiating treatment, it is very important to rule out other causes of pruritus such as contact allergens, medications (including vitamins) or foods, metabolic diseases (renal, liver, or thyroid disease), parasitic infections (scabies), anemia, paraproteinemia, papillary duct disease, neoplasia (lymphoma), or psychogenic causes (neurosis). Treatment may require the use of a humidifier, the use of moisturizing agents containing lactic acid or α-hydroxy acids to reduce roughness and scaling, and mild soaps such as Basis or Aveeno. The addition of mild topical steroids may be necessary on an episodic basis when irritation or inflammation is prominent[8,15,24] (Evidence Level C). The use of sedating antihistamines such as hydroxyzine and diphenhydramine should be avoided in the elderly because of their anticholinergic properties and risk of precipitating delirium, cognitive dysfunction, functional decline, and other side effects (blurred vision, constipation, urinary retention).[25,26] Prevention of exacerbations involves taking tepid and less frequent baths and the regular use of emollients after showering to "seal in" moisture. Older patients should be discouraged from using bath oil because it may make the tub or shower slippery, predisposing the patient to falls[8,15] (Evidence Level C). In general, cleansing of the skin with mild synthetic surfactants and/or emollients is ideal for managing xerosis because these agents cause minimal barrier disturbance, allowing the skin to better absorb topically applied agents[27] (Evidence Level B). Comprehensive management of xerosis in nursing home residents can prevent stasis dermatitis and ulcer formation, which is discussed in the subsequent text[28] (Evidence Level B).

Stasis dermatitis can occur from any clinical condition that results in dependent edema and venous insufficiency, and it can be acute or chronic in nature. It is characterized as being red, edematous, eczematous fluent areas of skin. It should be distinguished from tinea infection by the performance of potassium hydroxide scrapings and fungal cultures when necessary.[29] When secondary bacterial infection occurs, heralded by warmth, redness, swelling and pain, systemic antibiotics, warm compresses, and leg elevation may be necessary until resolution occurs. Repeated infection may result in damage to lymphatic drainage, lymphedema, and pigmentation. In the chronic state of stasis dermatitis, lichenification, fibrosis, and atrophy of pigmented skin and scarring may occur over a healed ulceration.

It may be necessary to use leg elevation and moist dressings for the acute exudative phase of stasis dermatitis, systemic antibiotics if there is evidence of infection or cellulitis, and subsequently use moderate to potent glucocorticoid ointment for a limited period. Definitive therapy for stasis dermatitis and ulcer prevention involves control of hypertension, correction of anemia and malnutrition, weight reduction in obese patients, exercise, mobilization, and control of dependent edema. Una boot dressings replaced weekly or intermittent pneumatic compression devices can limit edema and create an opportunity for healing. Corrective surgery of varicosities and/or elastic stockings worn daily also provides long-term benefits[29,30] (see Fig. 36.6) (Evidence Level C).

Neurodermatitis or lichen simplex chronicus refers to a nonspecific group of chronic, pruritic conditions of unknown cause. Owing to the urge to scratch, which leads to relief and a vicious repetitive cycle of more pruritus and scratching, hyperpigmentation, lichenification (leathery thickness), redness, and scaliness develop over time. Treatment involves the use of potent corticosteroids with

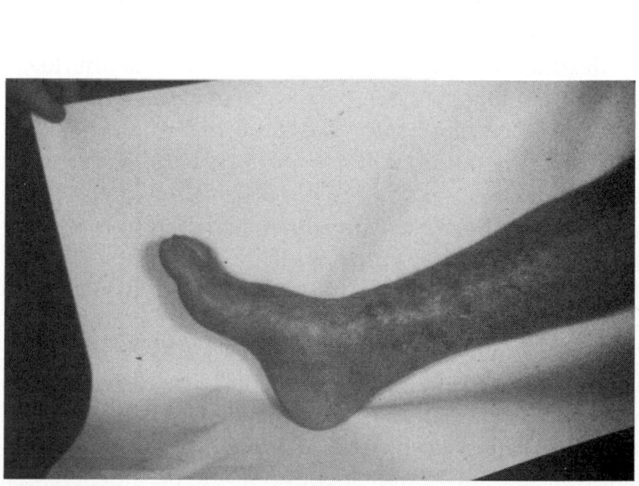

Figure 36.6 Stasis dermatitis, characterized by red, edematous areas of the skin. (See color insert.)

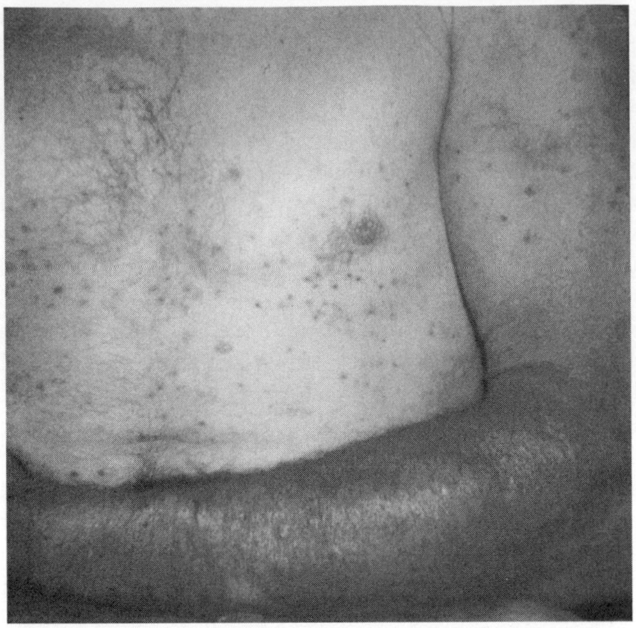

Figure 36.7 Neurodermatitis or lichen simplex chronicus. (See color insert.)

an occlusive dressing of emollients and behavior modification or stress management. Differential diagnosis includes the exclusion of irritant or allergic contact dermatitis[8] (see Fig. 36.7). Triggering factors such as irritants, allergens, and cutaneous bacterial, viral, or fungal infections should be identified and eliminated when possible[31] (Evidence Level C).

BULLOUS LESIONS

Bullous pemphigoid usually occurs in patients between the age of 60 and 80 and primarily in women over the age of 50. It is characterized by the presence of tense bullae filled with straw-colored fluid on erythematous or normal skin most commonly of the distal extremities, followed by the lower abdomen, groin, and axilla (intertriginous) in flexural areas. It may also be localized to the lower extremities. In some cases, papules or urticarial plaques may be as prominent as frank blisters. Pruritus is a cardinal and initial manifestation lasting for weeks or months, followed by blister development. Bullous lesions may evolve into erosions and crusting, with subsequent postinflammatory pigmentation without scarring. The acute process may last for several months to years but is typically self-limited, with alternating episodes of remissions and exacerbations.

Histopathologic examination reveals the etiology of the disease because the pemphigoid blister is subepidermal with a normal epidermis. It also includes the presence of an inflammatory eosinophilic dermal infiltrate with deposition of IgG and complement C3 at the dermoepidermal junction. Circulating autoantibodies may also be present in 60% to 70% of patients. The titer of autoantibodies does not correlate with disease activity. Bullous pemphigoid is not related to the development of internal malignancy, as previously thought. Therefore, workup is indicated only if other signs and symptoms are present. Skin biopsy may be necessary for diagnostic purposes. Drugs such as captopril, furosemide, phenacetin, penicillins, antipsychotics, and aldosterone antagonists, as well as ultraviolet light, are also associated with the disease.

Treatment depends on severity. Localized involvement can be treated with topical corticosteroids and tetracycline or dapsone, nicotinamide, azathioprine, methotrexate, cyclosporine, or chlorambucil. Most cases require systemic doses of corticosteroids in a regimen of 1 mg/kg/day (40 to 60 mg) of prednisone given until no new blisters develop, with gradual tapering thereafter. For the most severe cases, intravenous pulse corticosteroids, plasmapheresis, immunoglobins, or intravenous pulse cyclophosphamide are the options. Although mortality is low, the disease can be very uncomfortable because itching may be severe. The differential diagnosis includes other less common blistering diseases such as epidermolysis bullosa acquisita, linear IgA bullous disease, and dermatitis herpetiformis. Management should include dermatologic consultation[11,15,25,32] (see Fig. 36.8) (Evidence Level A).

Erythema multiforme bullosum appears as large hemorrhagic bullae on an erythematous base without scaling, and in the severe form it is referred to as *Stevens-Johnson syndrome*. The bullae occur on the palms and soles and less commonly on the buccal mucosa, conjunctiva, and

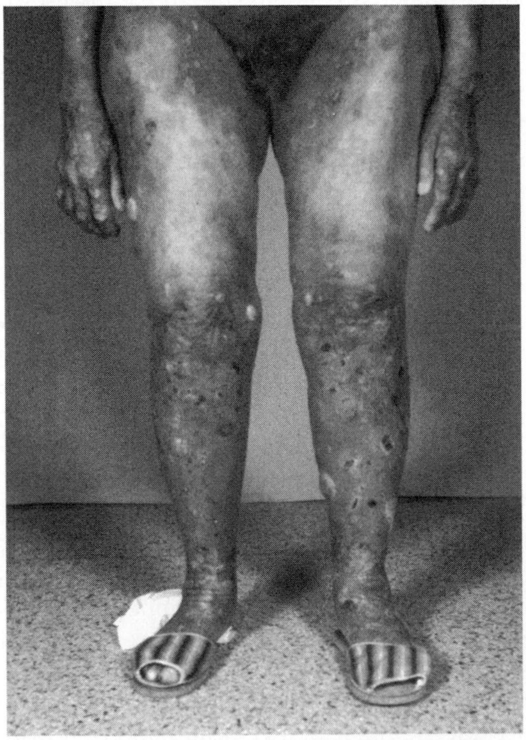

Figure 36.8 Bullous pemphigoid localized to the lower extremities. (See color insert.)

glans penis. There is usually sparing of the trunk area. Itching is not a common manifestation. When the presentation involves large and expanding bullae, the lesions may appear flaccid and a desquamating process develops, which is referred to as *toxic epidermal necrolysis* (TEN). The disease process may also present with internal manifestations such as Loeffler syndrome with eosinophilia, albuminuria, hematuria, and elevated blood urea nitrogen and sedimentation rate. Differential diagnosis primarily involves ruling out staphylococcal infection and, in severe forms, staphylococcal scalded skin syndrome (discussed later). Histologic examination typically reveals sparing of the stratum corneum and stratum granulosum with staphylococcal infection, as opposed to TEN in which the entire epidermis is involved. Causative agents include a long list such as bacterial, viral, and mycotic infections, collagen diseases, drugs, vaccines, allergenic contact agents, hormonal changes, and internal malignancy. Treatment involves symptomatic treatment of itching and burning and treatment of the suspected cause. Topical antibiotics for secondary infection and systemic corticosteroids may also be necessary for severe cases. Untreated cases are often very symptomatic and may last 2 to 3 weeks. Severe cases should be referred to a dermatologist for aggressive treatment[15,33] (see Fig. 36.9) (Evidence Level A).

Bullous impetigo may be caused by *Staphylococcus aureus* or *Streptococcus* (group A-B-hemolytic) species, with the majority caused by the former. These two organisms are the common causes of skin infections in the elderly. Although they may be part of the normal skin flora, alteration in skin architecture due to trauma, disease, malnutrition, or other processes may result in skin infections. Insect bites and various other types of dermatitis may also cause alteration in skin architecture. Bullous impetigo is characterized by thin-walled bullae (with a very fragile roof consisting only of stratum corneum) filled with clear to cloudy fluid that ultimately ruptures, resulting in an erythematous rim around the periphery of the lesion with a honey-colored, crusty exudate. Although impetigo tends to be self-limiting, in the presence of altered immune states associated with aging and disease, systemic manifestations may develop as a complication, as occurs with poststreptococcal glomerulonephritis. Treatment involves a 5- to 10-day course of an oral broad-spectrum antibiotic such as cloxacillin, dicloxacillin, or cephalexin, or a 2- to 5-day course of azithromycin and topical mupirocin ointment applied to the lesions until they heal[32] (Evidence Level A).

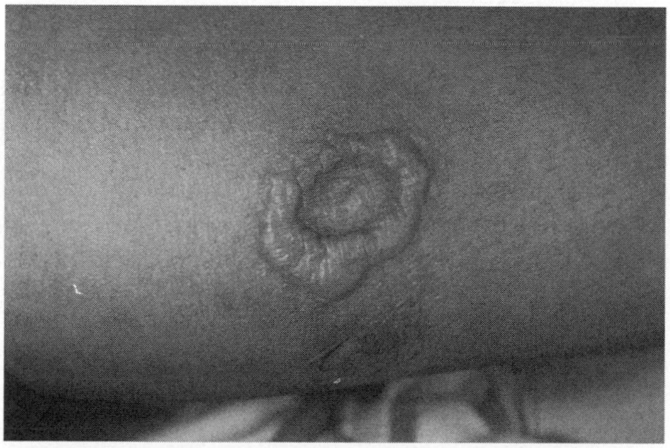

Figure 36.9 Erythema multiforme bullosum appearing as large hemorrhagic bullae on an erythematous base without scaling. (See color insert.)

COMMON DERMATOLOGIC BACTERIAL/PARASITIC/FUNGAL INFECTIONS

Herpes zoster (shingles) is the most common viral infection of the skin in the elderly. It is a reactivation of latent varicella-zoster virus (VZV) or chickenpox. The presentation is that of a grouped band of inflammatory vesicles and bullae following the pattern of a dermatome distribution. Malaise, skin tenderness, paresthesias, itching, tingling, or pain over the involved dermatome occur days to weeks before the outbreak of the rash. The rash may begin as erythematous macules and papules, progressing rapidly to vesicles. Pain can be severe in the elderly. Vesicles become pustules and eventually crust over in 7 to 10 days. Full resolution of the rash can take 2 to 3 weeks.

This reactivation occurs within the sensory neurons of the dorsal root ganglion. A risk factor for development and morbidity is advanced age. The decline in cell-mediated immunity with aging is thought to be a major factor responsible for the prevalence of shingles with aging. Other risk factors include recent surgery, trauma, immunosuppression (human immunodeficiency virus [HIV], malignancy, or use of corticosteroids). Shingles, and its complications, occurs 20 to 100 times more frequently in immunosuppressed patients. It occurs equally in men and women, and typically only once in life.

The infection is contagious to patients who have not had varicella infection. It is spread by direct contact with the lesions but can also be caused by the aerosol from patients with disseminated herpes zoster. According to a recent study, the incidence rate of herpes zoster is 215 per 100,000 person years. More than two thirds of reported cases occur in persons 50 years of age or older.

From 10% to 15% of herpes zoster cases involve the trigeminal nerve distribution. In such cases, an ophthalmologic examination is warranted. Involvement of the nasociliary branch of the trigeminal nerve can lead to lesions in the eye and development of neurotrophic keratitis and ulceration, scleritis, or uveitis. Less commonly the facial or auditory nerves can be involved. This pattern is referred to as *Ramsay-Hunt Syndrome* (external ear or tympanic members resulting in facial palsy with or without tinnitus, vertigo, or deafness). Secondary bacterial infection as well as postherpetic neuralgia (associated with advanced age and characterized as pain that persists or appears after the rash has healed or 30 days after onset of rash) can occur.

Differential diagnosis includes other conditions causing localized pain such as pleurisy, myocardial infarction, renal colic, cholecystitis, and glaucoma. Contact dermatitis, burns, and insect bites may also be considered. However, characteristic lesions and pattern make the diagnosis simple in most cases. A Tzanck smear taken from the base of the vesicle (stained with either hematoxylin-eosin, Giemsa, or Papanicolaou) will show multinucleated giant cells and epithelial cells containing intranuclear inclusion bodies. Differentiation from herpes simplex can be confirmed by direct fluorescent antibody staining. A viral culture may also be helpful in making the definitive diagnosis, but isolation of the virus may be difficult. Herpes simplex does not occur in a true dermatome pattern and tends to be recurrent.

Treatment of the uncomplicated case involves intervention within 72 hours of onset of rash, if possible, with oral antiviral agents such as acyclovir (800 mg five times per day for 7 to 10 days), valacyclovir (1 g three times per day for 7 days), or famciclovir (500 mg three times per day for 7 days). Early intervention is associated with halting the progression of disease, an increase in the rate of clearing of virus from vesicles, decreased incidence of visceral and cutaneous dissemination, decrease in ocular complications when eye involvement is present, a reduction in the duration and intensity of acute pain, and duration and frequency of postherpetic neuralgia. Oral corticosteroids have not been shown to be beneficial in preventing postherpetic neuralgia. Wet compresses and topical antibiotics such as bacitracin or mupirocin are useful for treating secondary bacterial infection (see Fig. 36.10) (Evidence Level A).

Postherpetic neuralgia is more common in patients with ophthalmic zoster, very severe initial pain, severe skin lesions, or very high viral antibody titers. Although the pathophysiology is unknown, it resolves in approximately 1 to 3 months in 50% of patients, but in others it can be persistent and disabling. Options for the management of pain include narcotics, nonsteroidal anti-inflammatory drugs, epidural injection of local anesthetics, corticosteroids, antidepressants, capsaicin, and acupuncture. The only approved agent for postherpetic neuralgia is capsaicin, but many patients may not be able to tolerate the burning sensation associated with topical administration[8,15,34,35] (Evidence Level A).

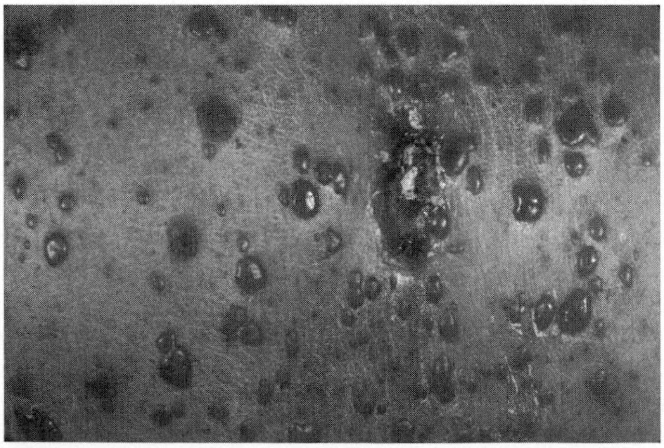

Figure 36.10 Herpes zoster (shingles), presenting as a grouped band of inflammatory vesicles and bullae following the pattern of a dermatome distribution. (See color insert.)

Tinea cruris, tinea pedis, candidiasis, and onychomycosis are common in the elderly. Candidiasis is a yeast infection that is more common in the elderly because of the decreased elasticity of the skin with aging and increased skin folds. Factors that promote candidiasis include decreased mobility, moisture, friction, and poor hygiene. It also occurs more commonly in the obese and patients with diabetes. A common denominator is usually skin-to-skin contact. Antibiotic therapy may also be a precipitant. Common intertriginous areas include the inframammary abdominal folds, groin, anogenital folds, flexural areas, submammary areas, perioral area, and axilla. The clinical presentation is that of an erythematous or beefy red, macerated, mildly malodorous, and moist area with weeping pustules when associated with secondary infection. In the bedridden patient, it may present on the back where moisture and occlusion of the skin occurs, or in the oral cavity (oral thrush) in those taking corticosteroids (orally or by inhaler), antibiotics, or immunosuppressives, or in those with systemic illnesses. In cases in which the diagnosis is in question, a potassium hydroxide (KOH) preparation of the scrapings of the area will typically show the presence of spores and pseudohyphae consistent with yeast infection. Management of candidiasis or intertrigo involves the practice of good hygiene and the use of cool compresses using Burow solution (a drying agent) three times per day to promote dryness. The use of topical anticandidal agents such as miconazole, nystatin, ketoconazole, econazole, or other antifungal creams applied several times per day is effective in clearing the rash when used for 10 to 14 days or more. The areas should also be kept dry, with skin exposure to air to promote drying. Recurrent attacks may require preventive treatment in the form of absorbent (drying) powders[8,32] (see Fig. 36.11) (Evidence Level B).

Tinea pedis, commonly referred to as *athlete's foot*, is a common fungal infection (trichophyton species) of the foot in older patients. It typically presents as an erythematous dermatitis with itching, scaling, and maceration, and sometimes fissuring and ulcerations, most commonly in the interdigital areas. Secondary bacterial infection may occur. The infection may also present with vesicle formation, particularly in the instep, toe webs, and soles of the feet (vesicular tinea pedis). Diagnosis may be confirmed by KOH preparation but the test may not be diagnostic by itself. Management includes the use of topical antifungal agents such as clotrimazole, ketoconazole, econazole, terbinafine, tolnaftate, or ciclopiroxolamine in mild to moderate cases. Systemic treatment involving the use of

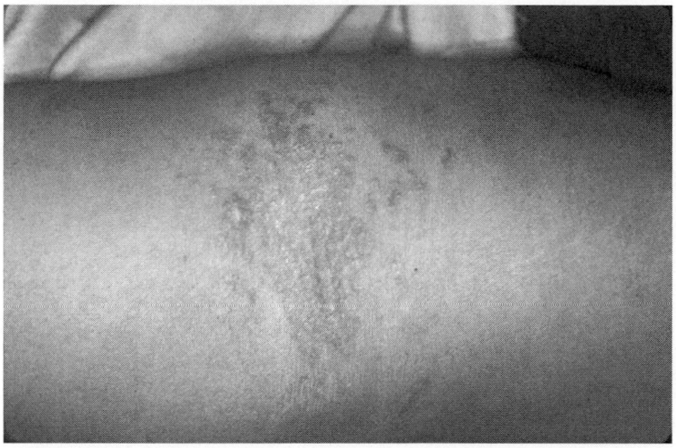

Figure 36.11 Candidiasis. (See color insert.)

oral terbinafine, itraconazole, or fluconazole may be necessary for severe, extensive, or persistent infections. Once the infection is clear, recurrent infections associated with occupational factors (regular exposure to moisture) may require the use of drying agents such as benzoyl peroxide and/or waterproof shoe wear. The vesicular form requires the use of oral griseofulvin 500 mg twice a day or ketoconazole 200 mg daily. The duration of therapy depends on the response to treatment, which typically takes longer in the older patient, but should generally be continued for 8 to 12 weeks[8,15,29,32,36,37] (see Fig. 36.12) (Evidence Level A).

Tinea cruris, commonly referred to as *jock itch* or *crotch itch,* is the counterpart of tinea pedis, occurring in the groin area (intertriginous). It is typically associated with itching and presents as an erythematous scaling dermatitis. Moisture and lack of ventilation is a key factor contributing to its development. It is more common in men. Differential diagnosis includes erythrasma, which clinically appears very similar. As opposed to tinea, direct microscopy is negative for fungal forms but the Wood lamp typically demonstrates characteristic coral-red fluorescence. Treatment for mild to moderate cases

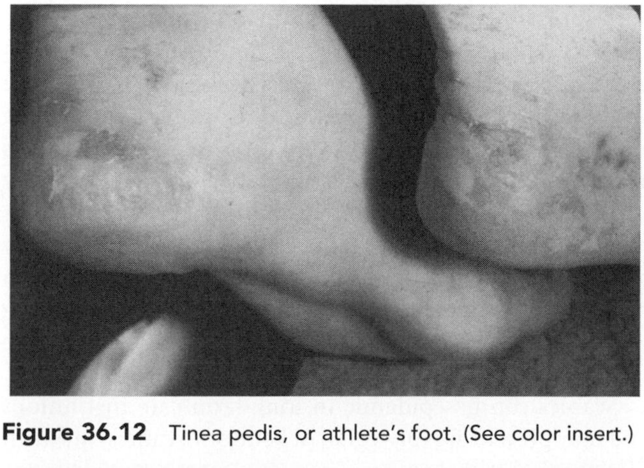

Figure 36.12 Tinea pedis, or athlete's foot. (See color insert.)

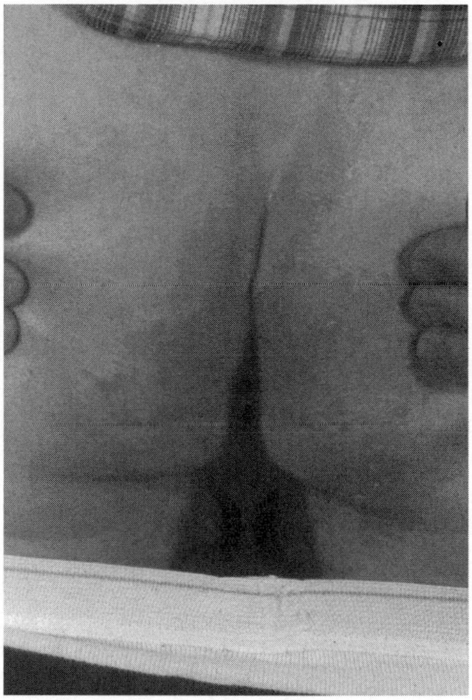

Figure 36.13 Tinea cruris, or jock itch or crotch itch, presenting as erythematous scaling dermatitis. (See color insert.)

of tinea cruris involves the use of topical antifungal creams, as indicated in the preceding text, for several weeks. For severe cases, oral antifungal therapy with griseofulvin, itraconazole, terbinafine, or fluconazole is effective. Duration of therapy depends on response. For cases with associated inflammation, the initial use of a combination topical corticosteroid and antifungal agent may be necessary for 7 to 10 days. Treatment of erythrasma involves topical application of benzoyl peroxide wash and erythromycin or tetracycline 250 mg four times per day orally for 14 days[32,36,37] (see Fig. 36.13) (Evidence Level A).

Onychomycosis (fungal nail infection) has traditionally been considered a recalcitrant problem (especially in the elderly) often caused by the dermatophyte tinea unguium. Rarer causes are yeasts and molds. It is present in 20% of patients aged 40 to 60 and 50% of those older than 70. It is caused by the dermatophyte trichophyton species. Other than being a cosmetic issue, cases are asymptomatic except when associated with secondary bacterial infection, ulcerations of the nail bed, and discomfort related to tight fitting foot wear. Morbidity includes pain with walking, compromised tactile function of the nails, and secondary infection. A complication is the difficulty with routine nail care. The most common form involves distal and lateral subungual onychomycosis, in which the initial presentation is a white patch on the nail that darkens over time, with the nail becoming opaque and thick, followed by cracking. There may also be associated yellowing of the nail and accumulation of subungual debris. Older patients are at greater risk for onychomycosis because of age-associated reduction in immune function and circulation to the distal foot (peripheral vascular disease), the presence of tinea pedis, using tight-fitting or occlusive footwear, slower growth of the nails with age, and increased frequency of trauma to the feet and toes.

Other causes of thickened yellow nails should be ruled out before making a diagnosis, including psoriasis or previous trauma. This is especially important because treatment involves several months of expensive systemic antifungal therapy. Diagnosis can be made by identification of hyphae on KOH preparation or by pathologic examination of the nail stained with periodic acid Schiff (PAS), which is confirmatory. Fungal culture may also be performed, which has the advantage of identification of the specific pathogen, but may take weeks for identification.

Older, less expensive oral antifungal agents include griseofulvin and ketoconazole, which require at least a year of therapy and are associated with high relapse rates, drug interactions, and side effects. Itraconazole, terbinafine, and fluconazole are newer, more expensive agents but have the advantages of 3 months of therapy, safer profile, higher cure rates (65% to 85%), higher affinity (and therefore concentration in the nails), and efficacy against most dermatophytes that cause the disease. Only terbinafine and itraconazole in doses of 200 to 250 mg daily are approved by the U.S. Food and Drug Administration for use. Itraconazole should not be used in combination with terfenadine, astemizole, or cisapride because fatal ventricular arrhythmias, prolonged QT intervals, and *torsades de pointes* have been reported, resulting in death. Its use with digoxin, warfarin, and oral hypoglycemics may alter the doses of these agents because it is an inhibitor of the P-450 cytochrome oxidase system. Topical treatment with amorolfine or ciclopirox (Penlac) may be beneficial. It may also be necessary to initially perform debridement of the affected nails in severe cases. Prevention includes the avoidance of moisture (or tight-fitting dark shoes), use of clean socks (white preferable), good hygiene practices, regular benzoyl peroxide washings, and topical application of antifungal creams[25,32,37] (see Figs 36.14 and 36.15) (Evidence Level A).

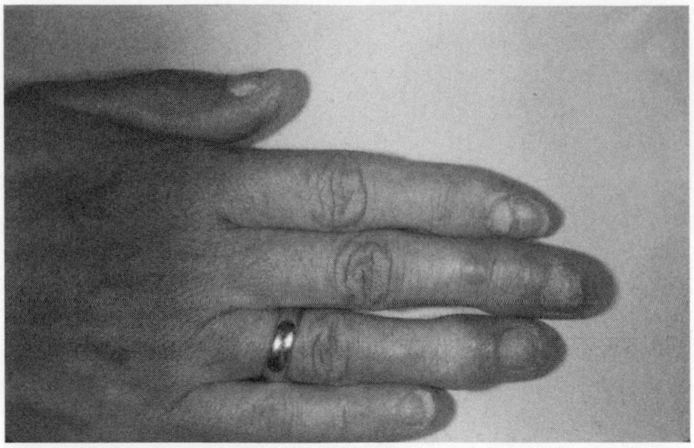

Figure 36.15 Onychomycosis of fingernails. (See color insert.)

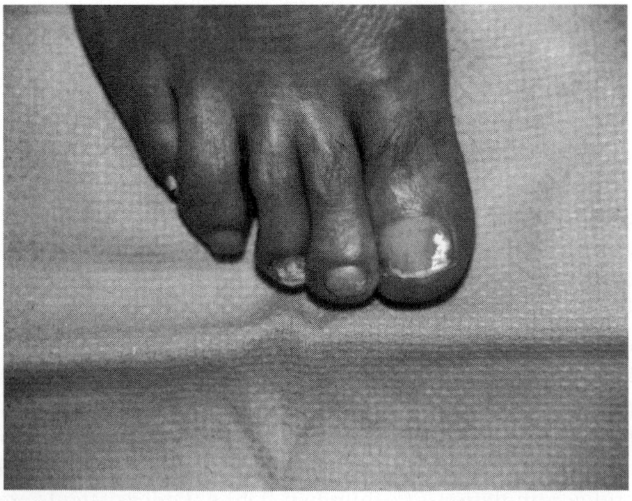

Figure 36.14 Onychomycosis of toenails. (See color insert.)

Pediculosis and scabies constitute common parasitic infections in the elderly. The infection is transmitted by direct contact with infected individuals, clothes, or bedding. During infestation with scabies, the female mite (typically 3 to 50) becomes fertilized on the skin surface and "burrows" through superficial layers of skin, laying eggs that produce linear burrows or "crooked" or " raised lines" on the skin surface. The burrow is the most diagnostic lesion. This causes the development of severe pruritus associated with erythematous papules and, occasionally, nodules days to weeks later, when a hypersensitivity reaction to the mite saliva and secretions occurs. Typical locations include the hands, axilla, the areola in women, and periumbilical areas in men (pediculosis corporis). Scratching may be so intense that it causes bleeding or weeping eczematous areas. Excoriations may develop as a result, which should raise suspicion of scabies. Diagnosis can be confirmed by finding mite excreta or eggs on the hair shaft, and more rarely the mite on a scraping of a lesion. When suspected by its location and characteristic lesions, even in the absence of definitive scraping, scabies should be treated with topical permethrin 5% applied from the neck line to the toes, rinsed off after 8 to 12 hours, and repeated in 1 week. In patients who have only been exposed, a single treatment is sufficient. In addition, clothing and bedding should be washed in hot water. When the entire family is affected, all family members should be treated at the same time to prevent reinfection. Use of topical corticosteroids may also be necessary to reduce the initial inflammatory response. If it appears that the rash has not responded to permethrin, treatment with lindane or malathion lotion should be considered because resistant strains develop (see Figs 36.16, 36.17) (Evidence Level B).

Scabies can be epidemic in long-term care institutions and may present as Norwegian or keratotic scabies, in which

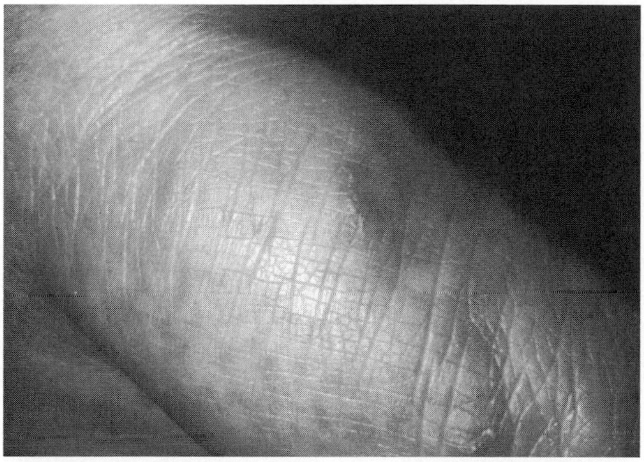

Figure 36.16 Scabies, characterized by linear burrows or crooked or raised lines. (See color insert.)

thousands of mites cause infestation and the development of a seborrheic dermatitis-like rash. It is treated with oral ivermectin, in two 12-mg doses taken a week apart, accompanied by cleansing of the clothes and bedding.

Pediculosis capitis (scalp) and pediculosis pubic (pubic region) are diagnosed by finding nits, eggs, or lice stuck to the hair shafts. In the scalp, the lice can commonly be found on the nape of the neck. Treatment involves destruction of the eggs and nits. Permethrin shampooing of the scalp performed twice, 1 week apart, and combing out of the nits with a special comb is effective. Shaving the affected area is also as effective as combing the scalp (pediculosis capitis)[8,32] (Evidence Level B).

PREMALIGNANT AND MALIGNANT LESIONS

Keratoacanthoma is a bud-shaped, skin-colored, rapidly growing, slightly reddish lesion arising from a hair follicle that occurs in people older than 60 years. It typically occurs on sun-exposed hair-bearing areas of the skin. The natural progression of the lesion is rapid growth to approximately 10 to 25 mm in diameter followed by slow involution over 2 to 6 months, and rarely over a 12-month period. Because the lesion typically looks like a carcinoma, and because of cosmetic issues, complete resection is often performed[15] (Evidence Level B).

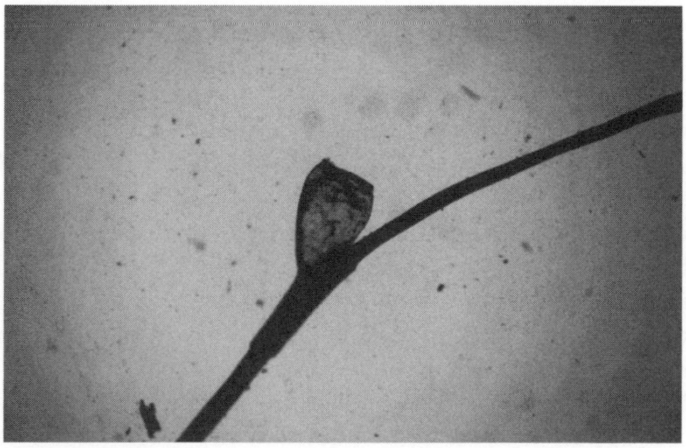

Figure 36.17 Pediculosis—presence of eggs on the hair shaft. (See color insert.)

Actinic keratoses, also called *solar keratoses*, are the most common premalignant skin lesion with aging. The lesion of actinic keratosis appears as a single pinhead-sized area of white scale or multiple flat, rough, or slightly elevated scaly macules or papules on a hyperemic base measuring 0.2 to 1.5 cm. A key characteristic of the lesion is its propensity to recur after being picked or scratched off by the patient. The skin surrounding the lesion may also show signs of damage such as wrinkling, dryness, and yellow discoloration. The lesions are a precursor of invasive squamous cell carcinoma and a risk factor for the development of basal cell carcinoma and melanoma. They affect 60% of light-complexioned persons older than 40 with a genetic predisposition and typically occur in chronically sun-exposed areas such as the face, scalp (in bald-headed people), dorsum of the hands and arms, trunk, neck, and forearms. Male gender and chronic sun exposure may predispose an individual to the development of a large number of these lesions. However, there is an increased prevalence in the white population with age, regardless of gender or sun exposure. In the 65- to 74-year-old age-group, 55% of men and 37% of women with high sun exposure develop actinic keratoses, compared to 19% of men and 12% of women with low sun exposure. They are extremely rare in the African American population.[25,32]

The lesion of actinic keratosis is composed of a clone of anaplastic keratinocytes confined to the lower layers of the epidermis. Over time, without treatment, the lesion may develop into squamous cell carcinoma *in situ* (with invasion of atypical cells within the epidermis). This may progress to invasive squamous cell carcinoma when the abnormal cells invade the epidermal–dermal junction. The pigmented variety of actinic keratoses may result in a brown color and present difficulty in recognition. The natural history of actinic keratoses, according to one study, includes spontaneous resolution of some of the lesions. There is a 22% increase in the total number at 1-year follow-up and a 1% conversion rate to invasive squamous carcinoma, or 10% to 20% conversion over 10 years. Other studies have shown a conversion rate of between 12% and 25%. The rate of metastatic spread is much lower with squamous cell carcinomas that develop from actinic keratoses than it is with those that develop from burns or chronic wounds.[25,32,38]

Treatment of actinic keratosis typically involves a variety of modalities including liquid nitrogen cryotherapy, curettage, laser resurfacing, electrodessication, chemical cauterization with phenol or trichloroacetic acid, excisional biopsy, dermabrasion, or chemical peel with topical 5-fluorouracil. The choice of these options depends on the extent of lesions, the extent of involvement, and the general health of the patient. Use of liquid nitrogen is associated with blistering or crusting at the site of the treatment in a week. For extensive involvement, the use of topical 5-fluorouracil or dermabrasion is recommended. The benefit of using topical 5-fluorouracil is that it can uncover patients with moderate actinic damage and subclinical lesions. The cream is applied twice daily to the entire sun-damaged area or region of affected skin rather than only to lesions. After 2 to 3 weeks of therapy, the damaged skin containing keratoses becomes red, tender, and even eroded. The treatment is then stopped and a cortisone topical cream may be used to control uncomfortable symptoms of the inflammatory process (Evidence Level A).

Dermabrasion is another option for eradicating large numbers of actinic keratoses, especially on the face or scalp, because the symptomatic period is typically of less duration. Dermabrasion may be associated with a better cosmetic result as well because this process destroys the skin uniformly, whereas topical 5-fluorouracil destroys damaged skin but not surrounding aging skin. Dermabrasion also appears to be effective in the prevention of long-term recurrence of dyskeratotic or malignant cutaneous lesions. Ultrapulse CO_2 laser resurfacing is a more recent advance in treatment and appears to be superior to dermabrasion, especially for lesions of the periorbital, nasal alae, perioral, and vermillion border areas.

Other promising topical agents include tretinoin, imiquimod, and diclofenac sodium (COX-2 inhibitor). Imiquimod is an immunomodulator that enhances the immune response by activating one of the interleukin receptors in the skin. Diclofenac sodium topical gel has been shown to clear 30% of the actinic keratosis with 90 days of therapy, according to one study. PDT is an investigational therapy that involves the application of topical 5-ALA to lesions, followed by light exposure for 20 minutes, 16 hours later. It has been shown to have a 50% to 88% response rate in the eradication of lesions. Dermatologic consultation should be performed in the case of multiple lesions or when the diagnosis is in question[25,38] (see Fig. 36.18).

Basal cell carcinoma is the most common skin malignancy and carcinoma in the United States. It typically arises on chronically sun-exposed skin. The lesion may present in three distinct clinical patterns: Nodular, morpheaform, and superficial. The nodular (noduloulcerative) presentation is the most common variety. It appears as a waxy, translucent, or pearly appearing papule. It commonly also has a raised, pale, rolled border and central ulceration and crusting. This may give the classical appearance of the so-called rodent ulcer. The border may be indistinct but is best delineated by the application of pressure to the skin around the papule. The presence of telangiectasias overlying the papule is also characteristic, which may result in an increased risk of bleeding, friability, and poor healing. Although metastasis is rare, the lesion slowly enlarges, with resulting destruction of the underlying tissue secondary to local invasion.

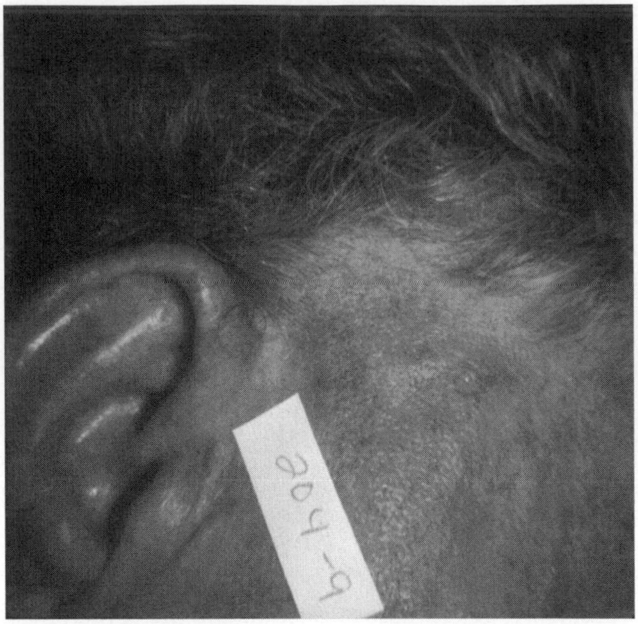

Figure 36.18 Lesions of actinic keratoses, or solar keratoses, appearing as a single pinhead-sized area of white scale or multiple flat, rough, or slightly elevated scaly macules or papules on a hyperemic base measuring 0.2 to 1.5 cm. (See color insert.)

Other less common presentations of basal cell carcinoma include the morpheaform (fibrosing) type, which appears as a scar with atrophy or an indurated yellowish plaque with an ill-defined border. Ulceration may occur at a later date. These are also referred to as *basosquamous carcinomas* because they have microscopic features of both types of skin cancer. They tend to be more aggressive than the modular type. The superficial, multifocal type appears as one or several erythematous papules, macules, or patches with fine scaling, and sometimes as superficial erosion. The patches become surrounded by a pearly border that appears to be fine and threadlike, with small areas of ulceration and crusting. The pigmented variety of basal cell carcinoma is less common but is easily confused with a melanoma (discussed in the subsequent text)[8,24,25,38] (see Fig. 36.19).

Squamous cell carcinoma appears as chronic erythematous papules, plaques, or nodules with scaling, crusting, or ulceration of the center and irregular borders. The edges of the lesion appear to be discrete or "heaped-up" and fleshy in appearance, as opposed to basal cell carcinoma, which has a clear appearance. When a squamous cell carcinoma *in situ* originates from an actinic keratosis it grows thicker, with the pink macular or papular area developing into an erythematous raised base. It may even develop an overlying keratin horn. Squamous cell carcinoma *in situ* may also appear as tan to red, or actually be the same color as the skin. In such cases, palpation rather than visual inspection is likely to be more successful in locating the lesion.

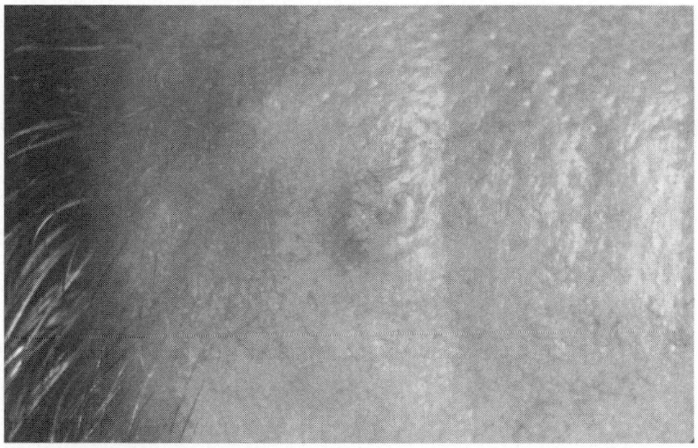

Figure 36.19 Basal cell carcinoma of the nodular type. (See color insert.)

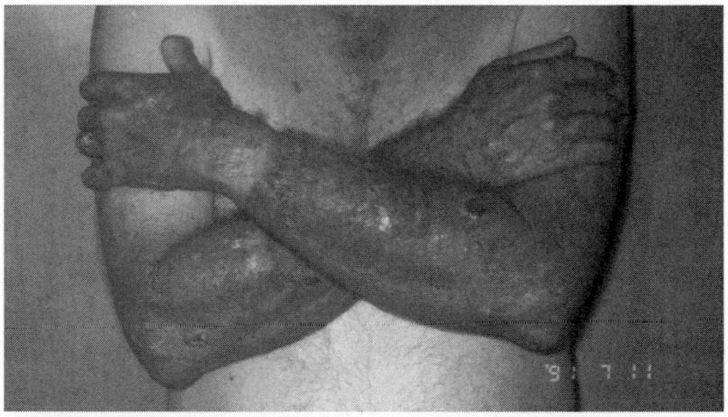

Figure 36.21 Squamous cell carcinoma—in the arms. (See color insert.)

Lesions that develop from actinic keratoses are less likely to metastasize than others. Their size ranges from an initial several millimeters to, ultimately, as large as 2 cm. With invasion, the borders of the lesion become more indurated and with distinct borders. A shallow ulceration may develop. If left untreated or improperly treated, and with continued growth and time, the lesion thickens, invading subcutaneous tissue, nerve, muscle, and bone. The lesion of squamous cell carcinoma typically develops in chronically sun-exposed or damaged skin, at sites of chronic inflammatory or chemical injury, long-standing nonhealing wounds (chronic leg ulcer), and in burn and radiation scars. Other risk factors include viral oncogenesis, immunosuppression, psoralen ultraviolet A (PUVA) therapy, arsenic exposure, and hydrocarbon exposure (see Figs 36.20–36.22).

A special type of squamous cell carcinoma, Bowen disease, may occur anywhere on the skin but is more common on covered areas, especially on the glans penis, vulva, and oral mucosa (and sometimes referred to as *erythroplasia of Queyrat*). It appears as a slow-growing patch of scaling skin with a sharp irregular border and areas of crusting. Lesions tend to be multiple in 55% of cases. Risk factors for Bowen disease include chronic exposure to arsenic (from an old remedy for asthma, exposure to insecticides, or well water), papovaviruses, and oncornaviruses. A typical presentation of Bowen disease secondary to chronic arsenic exposure involves the palms and soles, occurring in 40% of such exposures. Bowen disease is associated with a 15% to 30% risk for the development of internal malignancy[8,24,38] (see Fig. 36.23).

Treatment of squamous and basal cell carcinoma depends on the diagnosis, lesion size and extent or numbers of lesions, morphology, location, and compliance of the patient (see Fig. 36.24). When the presentation is characteristic, an excisional biopsy can be performed with confirmation by tissue diagnosis. When in question, an incisional biopsy can be performed by shaving the lesion or by punch biopsy to further determine definitive

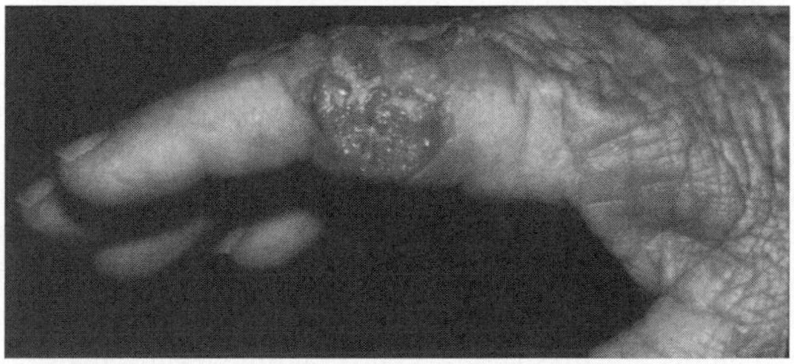

Figure 36.20 Squamous cell carcinoma—in the fingers. (See color insert.)

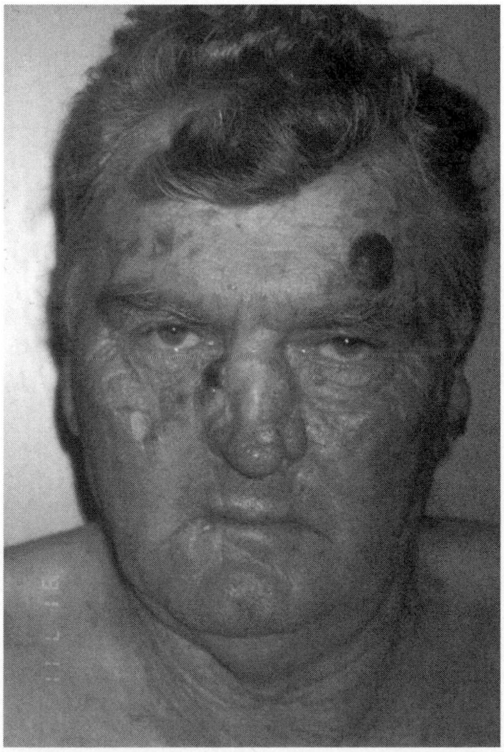

Figure 36.22 Squamous cell carcinoma—on the face. (See color insert.)

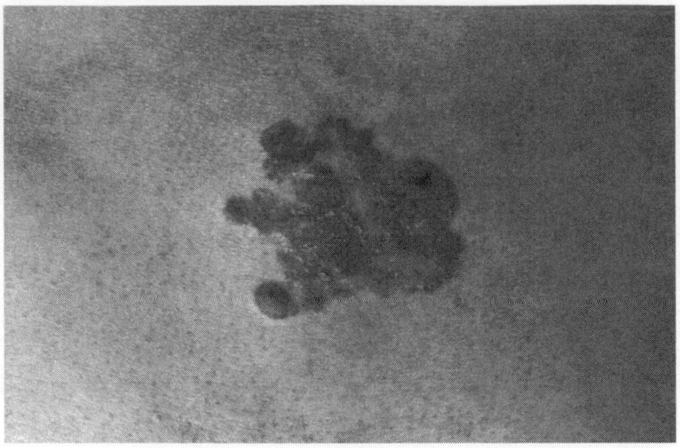

Figure 36.23 Bowen disease, characterized by a slow-growing patch of scaling skin with a sharp irregular border and areas of crusting. (See color insert.)

treatment. Standard techniques for eradication of the lesion include electrodessication and curettage (burning), cryosurgery (freezing), radiation therapy (x-ray), surgical excision, application of 5-fluorouracil applied topically or interlesionally, PDT, laser therapy, and excision by Mohs micrographic surgery. Although not approved yet, imiquimod (application of 5-ALA activated by visible light treatment) has shown success in areas in which loss of tissue is cosmetically or functionally unacceptable.[8,24,37,39]

Burning of the lesion may be performed by electrodessication, cautery, or laser. The advantage of this process is that it is quick and simple, requiring little operative skill. Disadvantages of the process are that normal skin may be destroyed or there may be incomplete destruction of the lesion, with recurrence in 7.7% to 13.2% of cases. A black scab results with healing that may take several months to heal and leave a scar with a sunken appearance. Electrodessication or cautery typically involves three scraping and burning cycles performed during a single sitting. Freezing of the lesion through cryosurgery is also quick and simple. As is the case for burning, disadvantages include incomplete removal followed by recurrence or destruction of normal skin, resulting in a depressed scar with healing in 1 to 2 months.

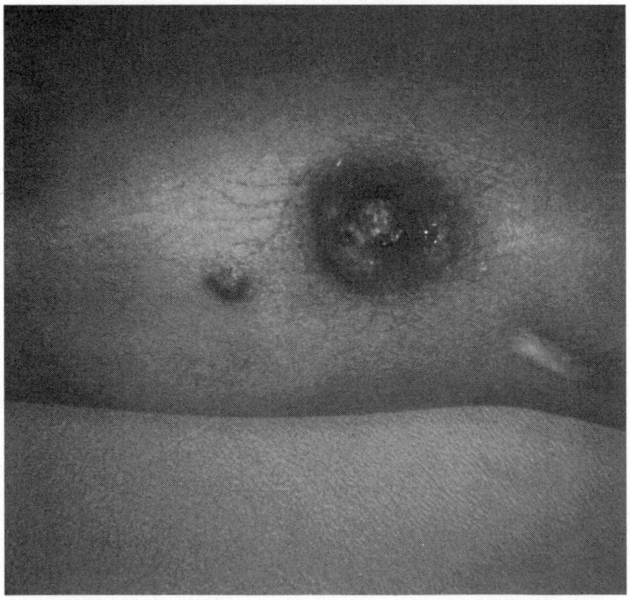

Figure 36.24 Dysplastic nevus. (See color insert.)

If cryotherapy is used, the freezing process may need to be repeated several times over several visits because the freezing process may not initially kill cancer cells. Two 30-second freeze–thaw cycles should be used at each treatment. This method is associated with a 95% cure rate for facial lesions. The advantage of this method is that it is quick and easy to perform, without the need for anesthetic injection.

A disadvantage of electrodessication and cautery, cryotherapy, 5-fluorouracil, or imiquimod therapies is that complete removal of the lesion cannot be confirmed. 5-Fluorouracil and imiquimod therapy are preferred therapies for mild early disease that is superficial and in which surgical therapy might result in a cosmetically poor result.

X-ray radiation therapy is another option but has the disadvantage of causing a recurrence of 7.5% at 5 years secondary to the radiation process itself. However, in specific situations in which radiation therapy ablation is appropriate, such therapy is typically delivered in fractional treatments or in small increments over many visits to reduce the risk of recurrence from overexposure. Basosquamous carcinomas should be excised completely because of their more aggressive nature.

Standard surgical excision is the fourth option for removing skin cancers. The advantage of this process is that the surgeon can usually see the borders of the lesion and resect normal skin outside the borders of the lesion. The disadvantage is that this method requires multiple cross-sectional microscopic cuts and subsequent slide preparations to examine the borders of the lesion to ensure that the entire tumor and any roots are removed. In rare cases, residual cancer may be left behind in the periphery, where the resection occurs. The cure rate is slightly better than that achieved with electrodessication and curettage or cryosurgery.

Lastly, Mohs micrographic surgery provides the most definitive form of surgery for skin cancers, with the highest cure rates of approximately 99%. It is most appropriate for large squamous or basal cell carcinoma >1 cm in size, for tumors with indistinct borders, tumors in close proximity to cosmetic or functional structures (nerves or muscles), or for recurrent lesions in which other forms of therapy have failed. In this procedure, surgical excision and curettage of the lesion is performed. Then the edges of the remaining skin borders are serially examined pathologically at the time of surgery. Additional sections of tissue are removed depending on the presence of residual tumor.

The process is continued until no residual tumor is found microscopically.[38,39]

Dysplastic nevi are atypically appearing nevi, so-called atypical nevi. They are markers of risk for and potential precursors of melanoma. The lifetime risk of melanoma with dysplastic nevi is 18%, whereas the lesions themselves have a 7- to 70-fold increased risk of becoming melanoma. In patients with a history of or a family member with melanoma, the risk is 100%. The lesion has an irregular border and varies in color.[38]

Melanoma is the most serious of all skin cancers. It poses the greatest health risk, with an incidence that has tripled in the last half century. However, it is curable if diagnosed and treated in the early stages. Risk factors for melanoma include fair skin, positive family history, numerous or dysplastic nevi, blue eyes, blond or red hair, and sunlight exposure (especially blistering intermittent sunburns in childhood). Because these lesions are asymptomatic, regular skin examinations and early recognition in high-risk patients is key to a favorable prognosis. Freckling, frequent sunburn, and inability to tan increase the risk by two to three times, and immunosuppression increases the risk by 10-fold. Patients with a family history have a 400-fold risk. A new pigmented lesion or change in the size, surface, color, or borders of a preexisting nevus should raise suspicion for melanoma and prompt the clinician to perform biopsy on the lesion.

The main clinical features of melanoma include variation in color and pigmentation pattern, notching, and irregularity of the border of the lesion. The "A, B, C, D, E" criteria for evaluation of pigmented lesions is useful in this regard. "A" stands for asymmetry, as opposed to an oval or round shape typical of benign lesions. "B" stands for border irregularity, as opposed to the even and symmetric borders consistent with a benign lesion. "C" stands for color variegation, in that a single lesion has many shades of brown, black, blue black, red, or white (amelanotic melanoma). "D" stands for diameter of the lesion, with malignant lesions 6 mm or larger in diameter and benign lesions typically smaller than 6 mm. "E" stands for elevation. In general, the most frequent sites for melanoma in men are the back, head, neck, and chest, whereas in women, the most common areas are the arms, head, neck, lower legs, and back.[7,8,25,32,38]

There are four clinical types of melanoma: Lentigo maligna, superficial spreading type, modular type, and acral lentiginous. Lentigo maligna appears as an irregularly shaped brown or tan macule. It occurs almost exclusively in elderly white men. It may have a very long *in situ* phase, lasting years and appearing as a freckle (Hutchinson freckle or lentigo maligna). In this phase, it may not have an irregular border, a pigmented mottled appearance, or variegated colors. With time, one or more papules or nodules develop within the macule or patch, which may herald the presence of invasion. It is then termed *lentigo maligna melanoma*. It is most commonly seen on sun-damaged, atrophic skin.

Superficial spreading melanoma usually presents as an irregularly shaped papule, plaque, or macule, with great variation in color, that spreads laterally and may appear anywhere on the body. Over time, nodules appear within the lesion, which is usually >6 mm in diameter. This is the most common type, involving 70% to 80% of cases.

The nodular type appears as a black or gray papular nodule that grows rapidly and extends vertically into the skin, rather than laterally. Acral lentiginous maligna usually presents as a black or dark brown patch or macule that expands slowly over years and is usually found on the soles, nail beds, or palms, with highest incidence in those aged 65 years or older. It is also more common in darker-pigmented people and is diagnosed later than other melanomas, and therefore, usually has an unfavorable prognosis.

When in doubt as to the etiology of the lesion, the patient should be referred for evaluation promptly. Treatment consists of surgical excision and lymph node dissection or adjuvant therapy, depending on depth, which is the critical factor that determines prognosis. Patients with lesions <0.76 cm in depth have 5-year survival rates of >95%. However, patients with lesions of >4 mm have 5-year survival rates of <50%. Other factors associated with a poor prognosis include advanced age, anatomic sites of the scalp, hands and feet, male sex, and ulceration.

Two systems are commonly used to stage melanomas. The traditional system uses three stages: Skin involvement only, nodal involvement, and lastly distant metastasis. Stage I is further classified according to the thickness of the lesion. The Clark anatomic level of invasion or the Breslow tumor thickness indices are used to estimate survival prognosis. Clark level I indicates confinement to the epidermis. Clark level II indicates that tumor cells have invaded into the papillary dermis (99% 5-year survival). Clark level III indicates that tumor cells are filling the papillary dermis (95% 5-year survival). Clark level IV indicates that tumor cells have invaded the reticular dermis (75% 5-year survival). Clark level V indicates that tumor cells have invaded the subcutaneous tissue (39% 5-year survival). For the Breslow index, prognosis is based on thickness: <0.85 mm thickness (99% survival at 5 years), 0.85 to 1.69 mm thickness (95% 5-year survival), 1.7 to 3.64 mm thickness (78% 5-year survival), and >3.65 mm thickness (42% 5-year survival).

Another system involves the American Joint Committee on Cancer staging system, which divides patients into four stages by the classic tumor, node, metastasis (TNM) system classification.

Excisional biopsy into the fat tissue is the recommended method of removal. Current recommendations for resection include the following: For lesions <1 mm deep, excise with 1-cm margins; for lesions with intermediate thickness,

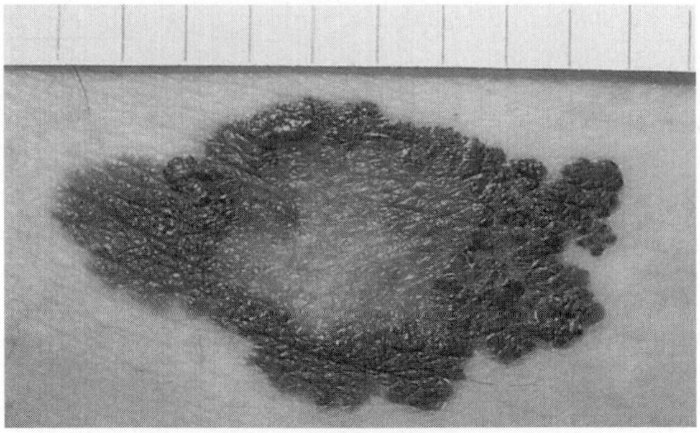

Figure 36.25 Melanoma—"A, B, C, D, E" (asymmetry, *b*order irregularity, color variegation, *d*iameter of the lesion, elevation) criteria for evaluation of pigmented lesions. (See color insert.)

excise with 2- to 4-cm margins; and for lesions with tumors deeper than 4 mm, excise with 3-cm margins. Elective lymph node dissection, to search for occult nodal disease, and selective nodal dissection have not been proved to be effective. However, node sampling may aid in the staging of the disease in patients with melanomas >1 mm thickness. Most recently, Mohs micrographic surgery has been employed as the treatment of choice. This technique allows examination of the entire periphery of the excised tissue. It allows a narrower 1 cm margin of excision in most cases.

Metastasis occurs most commonly to the skin, subcutaneous tissue, and lymph nodes. Visceral metastasis occurs more frequently in the lungs, liver, brain, bone, and intestine. For metastatic disease, various chemotherapeutic and immune therapies are in use. More recently, use of interferon-α-2b has been shown to increase survival in a cohort of patients with metastatic disease. Regular screening for melanoma should be performed on all patients with a history of first-degree relatives with melanoma[7,8,25,32,38,40] (see Fig. 36.25) (Evidence Level A).

SKIN MANIFESTATIONS OF VASCULAR DISEASE

Chronic arterial insufficiency of a severe nature or chronic venous insufficiency of the lower extremities can cause chronic skin ulcers. Historical factors, associated symptoms, physical findings, and location are important clues as to the differentiation of these ulcers, including characteristics of the ulcer.

Ischemic arterial ulcers are well demarcated and circular or "punched out" in appearance. They are typically gray with a pale area of skin surrounding the borders. They are painful and do not bleed when touched. A history of other vascular disease (e.g., hypertension, coronary artery disease, hypercholesterolemia, long-standing diabetes, and stroke); claudication associated with pain of the hip, buttock, or legs when ambulating; and numbness, tingling, or weakness of the lower extremity are characteristic. Lack of pulse, pallor, loss of hair, thinning and shininess of the skin, and change in temperature of the anterior legs and dorsum of the feet (colder) are characteristic physical findings. Ischemic arterial ulcers are typically located on bony prominences and in patients with diabetes are typically found on the heels, dorsa of the toes, and medial and lateral malleoli.

Treatment for mild to moderate distal disease involves good control of diabetes; antiplatelet therapy with aspirin, pentoxifylline, and cilostazol; and local care with cleaning agents to prevent infection. Severe arterial disease may require surgical vascular reconstruction, depending on the preoperative risk of the patient[41,42] (Evidence Level C).

Venous insufficiency ulcers occur after chronic thickening of the skin associated with hyperpigmentation and have a more irregular border than arterial ulcers. A key ingredient in their development is chronic edema. Risk factors for venous insufficiency include genetic predisposition, prolonged standing in one position for long periods, prolonged intra-abdominal pressure against the iliac veins (e.g., during pregnancy), a history of thrombophlebitis, or any condition that causes chronic edema formation (e.g., congestive heart failure, hypoproteinemia, and chronic anemia). Ulcers are typically found on the anterior/medial lower leg. The ulcer is typically preceded by minor trauma producing a red or blue-red patch. Venous ulcers have irregular shaggy brown to brown-red borders, which are hard because of scarring. They are painful when the patient is standing. The pain is typically relieved with elevation. When severe, the ulcers may be associated with the production of a transudate. Exudates indicate infection.[41,43] A cycle of chronic ulcer development with healing results in lichenification, fibrosis, and atrophic pigmentation of the skin with scarring over the healed ulcers.

Treatment of a venous insufficiency ulcer may require debridement of necrotic tissue and application of moist saline dressings with frequent change, as well as the use of systemic antibiotics when associated with lymphangitis or cellulitis. When clear of systemic infection, the ulcer may be treated with aluminum acetate solution soaks, zinc oxide or benzoyl peroxide antibiotic ointments, and topical antibiotics and autolytic agents. Further trauma must be avoided.

Oral zinc sulfate, 200 mg three times per day, has been shown to be useful adjunctive therapy. Stanozolol, 2 to 4 mg daily for 3 to 6 months, may be useful for recurrent ulcerations. A form of compression therapy such as an Unna paste boot and/or physiologic or biosynthetic wound dressing can be used for final healing. Lastly, grafting may be necessary in cases involving large ulcers with healthy granulation tissue in the base. Once edema has been treated, vascular reconstruction may also be an option[29,43] (Evidence Level A).

In the absence of edema or stasis, when in an unusual location, or when the ulcer does not respond to therapy in 6 weeks, a biopsy of the lesion should be performed to exclude diseases such as syphilis, diabetes, rheumatoid arthritis, immunodeficiency, carcinoma, or systemic lupus erythematosus.

MISCELLANEOUS SKIN CONDITIONS

Rosacea is a chronic inflammatory condition that usually starts in middle age. It presents as erythema associated with telangiectasia, pustules, papules, and often, hypertrophy of the sebaceous glands. It usually presents in the central facial (flushing) region (cheeks) but may also present in the nasal area and in the eye (e.g., conjunctivitis, iritis, and blepharitis). Severe cases can result in scarring and papularity, referred to as *rhinophyma* (more common in men). The chin and brow are occasionally involved.

Mild disease appears as a slight flushing of the nose and cheeks, forehead, and chin. With severe disease, the skin becomes deeper red or purplish red, with chronic dilatation of the superficial capillaries and inflammation of acneiform pustules and deep-seated pustules, furuncles, or cystic nodules causing abscesses, sinuses, and scarring. It is more common in women, but the most severe form is more common in elderly men. The etiology is poorly understood but may be secondary to a host of factors that cause vasomotor lability, including alcohol and caffeine use, fluorinated steroids, heat, increased vascularity, increased production of sebum, reaction to the follicular mite *Demodex folliculorum*, and even menopause. Differential diagnosis includes acne vulgaris, lupus erythematosus, bromoderma, iododerma, and papular syphilid. Rosacea and seborrhea may appear together.

Mild cases can be treated with 1% hydrocortisone cream and elimination of suspected precipitants. A 5% precipitated sulfur preparation or benzoyl peroxide lotion applied twice daily may also be helpful if *Demodex folliculorum* is suspected. The treatment of choice for moderate to severe cases is long-term oral administration of tetracycline used at minimal doses of 250 mg daily. Metronidazole 200 mg twice daily may also be used as an alternative but is less safe when used chronically. Both agents provide suppressive relief but no cure. Topical metronidazole provides a safe alternative when used in combination with tetracycline. For acute flares or inflammation with pustule formation, ice-cold boric acid compresses or Vleminckx compresses, as well as the use of nonfluorinated steroid lotions or creams, may be effective. For treatment-resistant cases, isotretinoin can produce dramatic improvement, but relapses over a period of weeks or months are common. Finally, the use of oral estrogen in a low dose may be effective in women with severe rosacea[29,44] (see Fig. 36.26) (Evidence Level A).

Corns and calluses are hyperkeratotic lesions that develop over bony prominences or in areas of friction or increased pressure. They tend to develop where the plantar fat pad has become atrophied. There may be associated bursae formation and edema and erythema formation when associated with pain and when the lesions extend deep. Treatment involves surgical debridement of the lesion for symptom relief. Debridement will reveal whether soft tissue breakdown or ulceration has occurred and will confirm that the lesion is not a wart. Preventive management involves weight dispersion and the use of a shock-absorbing material in the form of a cushion or pad in the insole of the shoe. Custom-molded shoes are expensive and often unnecessary. Extensive surgical management should only be used as a last resort[45] (Evidence Level C).

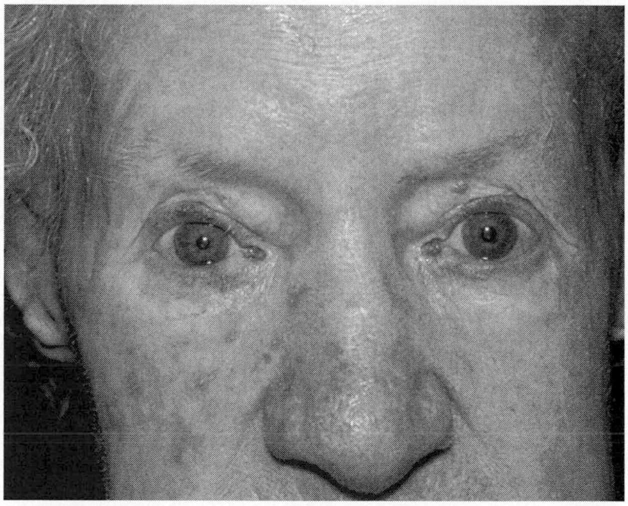

Figure 36.26 Rosacea, presenting in the central facial region and the nasal area. (See color insert.)

Dermatitis medicamentosa is a term used to describe dermatitis secondary to a drug eruption. This condition may be erythematous, lichenoid, eczematous, acneiform, urticarial, bullous, fixed drug, exfoliative, nodular, photosensitive, or purpuric. Corticosteroids, bromides, and iodides can cause an acneiform-type eruption on the skin. Penicillins and other antibiotics are more likely to cause a urticarial eruption. Bismuth, barbiturates, sulfonamides, antihistamines, and penicillins may cause an erythematous drug eruption. Iodides, penicillamine, and bleomycin may cause a bullous eruption. Phenothiazines, chlorothiazide, demeclocycline, griseofulvin, and oral hypoglycemic agents may cause a photodermatitis. Gold may cause an exfoliative drug eruption. Gold, quinidine, methyldopa, or antituberculous, antiarrhythmic, or anticonvulsant agents may cause a lichenoid or eczematous drug eruption. Finally, sulfathiazole or salicylates may cause a nodular drug eruption.[29]

REFERENCES

1. Turner ML. Skin changes after forty. *Am Fam Physician.* 1984;29(6):173–181.
2. Fenske NA, Conard CB. Aging skin. *Am Fam Physician.* 1988;37(2):219–230.
3. Podda M, Grundmann-Kollmann M. Low molecular weight antioxidants and their role in skin aging. *Clin Exp Dermatol.* 2001;26(7):578–582.

4. Kligman DE, Draelos ZD. High-strength tretinoin for rapid retinization of photoaged facial skin. *Dermatol Surg*. 2004;30(6): 864–866.
5. Lowe N, Gifford M, Tanghetti E, et al. Tazarotene. 1% cream versus tretinoin 0.25% emollient cream in the treatment of photodamaged facial skin: A multicenter, double-blind, randomized, parallel-group study. *J Cosmet Laser Ther*. 2004;6(2):79–85.
6. Beitner H. Randomized, placebo-controlled, double blind study on the clinical efficacy of a cream containing 5% alpha-lipoic acid related to photoageing of facial skin. *Br J Dermatol*. 2003;149(4):841–849.
7. Ghersetich I, Brazzini B, Peris K, et al. Pyruvic acid peels for the treatment of photoaging. *Dermatol Surg*. 2004;30(1):32–36.
8. Sumaira Z, Aasi MD. Dermatological diseases and disorders. *Geriatric review syllabus*, 5th ed. New York, NY: Blackwell Publishing; 2002–2004:390–399.
9. Avram DK, Goldman MP. The safety and effectiveness of a single-pass erbium:YAG laser in the treatment of mild to moderate photodamage. *Dermatol Surg*. 2004;30(8):1073–1076.
10. Touma D, Yaar M, Whitehead S, et al. A trial of short incubation, broad-area photodynamic therapy for facial keratoses and diffuse photodamage. *Arch Dermatol*. 2004;140(1):33–40.
11. Purba MB, Kouris-Blazo A, Wattanapenpaiboon N, et al. Can skin wrinkling in a site that has received limited sun exposure be used as a marker of health status and biological age? *Age Ageing*. 2001;30(3):227–234.
12. Klein AW. Contraindications and complications with the use of botulinum toxin. *Clin Dermatol*. 2004;22(1):66–75.
13. Henry F, Pierard-Franchimont C, Cauwenbergh G, et al. Age-related changes in facial skin contours and rheology. *J Am Geriatr Soc*. 1997;45:220–222.
14. Pierard GE, Letawe C, Dowlati A, et al. Effect of hormone replacement therapy at menopause on the mechanical properties of skin. *J Am Geriatr Soc*. 1995;43:662–665.
15. Mash MJ, Fedor M, Bonnington L. Skin. *Primary care geriatrics-A case-based approach*, 4th ed. St. Louis, MO: Mosby; 2002:468.
16. Luba MC, Bangs SA, Mohler AM, et al. Common benign skin tumors. *Am Fam Physician*. 2003;67(4):729–738.
17. Dawn G, Gupta G. Comparison of potassium titanyl phosphate vascular laser and hyfrecator in the treatment of vascular spiders and cherry angiomas. *Clin Exp Dermatol*. 2003;28(6):581–583.
18. del Pozo J, Pena C, Garcia Silva J, et al. Venous lakes: A report of 32 cases treated by carbon dioxide laser vaporization. *Dermatol Surg*. 2003;29(3):308–310.
19. Ah-Weng A, Natarajan S, Velangi S, et al. Venous lakes of the vermillion lip treated by infrared coagulation. *Br J Oral Maxillofac Surg*. 2004;42(3):251–253.
20. Meshkinpour A, Sun J, Weinstein G. An open pilot study using tacrolimus ointment in the treatment of seborrheic dermatitis. *J Am Acad Dermatol*. 2003;49(1):145–147.
21. Gupta AK, Bluhm R. Ciclopirox shampoo for treating seborrheic dermatitis. *Skin Therapy Lett*. 2004;9(6):4–5.
22. Pierard-Franchimont C, Goffin V, Decroix J, et al. A multicenter randomized trial of ketoconazole 2% and zinc pyrithione 1% shampoos in severe dandruff and seborrheic dermatitis. *Skin Pharmacol Appl Skin Physiol*. 2002;15(6):434–441.
23. Dreno B, Chosidow O, Revuz J, et al. The Study Investigator Group. Lithium gluconate 8% versus ketoconazole 2% in the treatment of seborrheic dermatitis: A multicenter, randomized study. *Br J Dermatol*. 2003;148(6):1230–1236.
24. Kurban RS, Kurban AL. Common skin disorders of aging: Diagnosis and treatment. *Geriatrics*. 1993;52(8):56–69.
25. Danahy JF, Gilchrest BA. Geriatric dermatology. *Reichel's care of the elderly-clinical aspects of aging*, 5th ed. Philadelphia, PA: Lippincott Williams & Wilkins; 1999:513–524.
26. Willcox SM, Himmelstein DU, Woolhandler S. Inappropriate drug prescribing for the community-dwelling elderly. *JAMA*. 1994;272(4):292–295.
27. Subramanyan K. Role of mild cleansing in the management of patient skin. *Dermatol Ther*. 2004;17(suppl 1):26–34.
28. Norman RA. Xerosis and pruritus in the elderly: Recognition and management. *Dermatol Ther*. 2003;16(3):254–259.
29. Beacham BE. Common dermatoses in the elderly. *Am Fam Physician*. 1993;47(6):1445–1450.
30. Fitzpatrick TB, Johnson RA, Wolff K, et al. *Color atlas & synopsis of clinical dermatology-common & serious diseases*. New York, NY: McGraw-Hill; 2001:468–473.
31. Senti G, Wuthrich B. Therapy of neurodermatitis (atopic dermatitis). *Ther Umsch*. 2001;58(8):304–308.
32. Norman RA. Geriatric dermatology. *Clinical geriatrics*. Boca Raton, FL: The Parthenon Publishing Group; 2003:367–377.
33. Arnold HL, Odom RB, James WD. Erythema and urticaria. *Andrews' diseases of the skin-clinical dermatology*. 8th ed. Philadelphia, PA: WB Saunders; 1990:131–136.
34. Twersky JI, Schmader K. Zoster. *Principles of geriatric medicine and gerontology*, 5th ed. New York, NY: McGraw-Hill; 2003:1133–1137.
35. Pilot F, Alper BS, Vanderhoff BT. Management of herpes zoster and postherpetic neuralgia. *Am Fam Physician Monogr*. 2004: 3–20.
36. Arnold HL, Odom RB, James WD. Diseases due to fungi and yeasts. *Andrews' diseases of the skin-clinical dermatology*, 8th ed. Philadelphia, PA: WB Saunders; 1990:331–335.
37. Goldstein AO, Smith KM, Ives TJ, et al. Mycotic infections-effective management of conditions involving the skin, hair, and nails. *Geriatrics*. 2000;55(5):40–52.
38. Balin AK. Skin cancer. *Principles of geriatric medicine and gerontology*. 5th ed. New York, NY: McGraw-Hill; 2003:747–750.
39. Stulberg DL, Crandell B, Fawcett R. Diagnosis and treatment of basal cell and squamous cell carcinomas. *Am Fam Physician*. 2004;70(8):1481–1481.
40. Gordon ML, Hecker MS. Care of the skin at midlife: Diagnosis of pigmented lesions. *Geriatrics*. 1997;52(8):56–69.
41. Cefalu CA. Peripheral vascular disease in the elderly. *Reichel's care of the elderly-clinical aspects of aging*, 5th ed. Philadelphia, PA: Lippincott Williams & Wilkins; 1999:167–177.
42. Peripheral Arterial Disease (PAD)-Peripheral Vasodilators, Hemorrheologic Agents and Anti-Platelet Agents. *Geriatric pharmaceutical care guidelines*. Covington, KY: Omnicare, Inc.; 2004:469.
43. Arnold HL, Odom RB, James WD. Cutaneous vascular diseases. *Andrews' diseases of the skin-clinical dermatology*, 8th ed. Philadelphia, PA: WB Saunders; 1990:982–984.
44. Arnold HL, Odom RB, James WD. Acne. *Andrews' diseases of the skin-clinical dermatology*, 8th ed. Philadelphia, PA: WB Saunders; 1990:263–264.
45. Kosinski M, Ramcharitar S. In-office management of common geriatric foot problems. *Geriatrics*. 1994;49(5):43–47.

37

Prevention and Treatment of Pressure Ulcers: An Evidence-Based Approach

Robert E. Pieroni

CLINICAL PEARLS 512

OVERVIEW 513
Terminology 513
Epidemiology 513

DIFFERENTIAL DIAGNOSIS 513

RISK FACTORS 513
Braden Scale 513

STAGING 515
Saucerization of Pressure Damage 515
Reverse (Healing) Staging 516

INCIDENCE/PREVALENCE 516

COMPLICATIONS 516

PREVENTION 516
Injury Prevention 516
Long-term Care Prevention 519
Staffing 519
Education (Physicians) 519
Education (Nurses) 519
Nursing Home Quality Initiative 520
Communication 521

AGENCY FOR HEALTHCARE RESEARCH AND QUALITY PREDICTION AND PREVENTION RECOMMENDATIONS 521
Strength of Evidence 521
Use of Risk Assessment Tools and Risk Factors 521
Skin Care And Early Treatment 521
Mechanical Loading and Support Surfaces 522
Education 522

AGENCY FOR HEALTHCARE RESEARCH AND QUALITY RECOMMENDATIONS FOR TREATMENT 522
Assessment 522
Managing Tissue Loads 523
Ulcer Care 524
Managing Bacterial Colonization and Infection 525
Surgical Repair of Pressure Ulcers 525
Education and Quality Improvement 526

SPECIFIC MANAGEMENT STRATEGIES 526
Pressure Ulcer Scale for Healing Tool 526
Wound Healing 526
Pain Management 526
Mental Status 527
Restraints 527
Support Surfaces 527

Debridement 527
Dressings 528
Medications 528
Nutrition 528
Dehydration 528
Surgery 528

CONCLUSION 528

CLINICAL PEARLS

- The prevention of pressure ulcers is considered a marker for quality of care.
- Patients with pressure ulcers often suffer the psychosocial effects of pain, depression, social isolation, and decreased quality of life.
- Patients should not be allowed to lie on skin that has been reddened by pressure.
- Of the numerous pressure ulcer risk factors, the two major ones that can be influenced by clinicians are nutrition and tissue loading.
- Turning schedules need to be individualized; some patients may need to be turned more frequently than every 2 hours.
- Studies have demonstrated decreased pressure ulcer incidence in health care facilities that have instituted the recommendations of the federal agency formerly known as the Agency for Health Care Policy and Research (AHCPR), and now known as the Agency for Healthcare Research and Quality (AHRQ), including pressure ulcer risk assessment and care protocols.
- Because muscle and subcutaneous tissue are more susceptible to pressure than the epidermis, pressure ulcers are often worse than they appear and are often understaged.
- The AHCPR/AHRQ pressure ulcer guidelines continue to represent the standard for comprehensive pressure ulcer management used by regulating and accrediting bodies.
- The process of healing is by granulation, contraction, and re-ephithelialization and scar tissue formation; open ulcers never return to Stage I.
- Excess weight can mask nutritional deficiencies; even morbidly obese patients can be severely malnourished, placing them at further risk for the development of pressure ulcer.
- A static support surface may be effective in patients who can spontaneously reposition themselves; otherwise, a dynamic surface is preferable.
- Patients should be placed on a dynamic support surface if there are limited positioning options or if the patient bottoms out on a static surface.
- Patients with large Stage III or IV pressure ulcers should be strongly considered for a dynamic support surface.
- Use of dynamic support surfaces in high-risk patients with pressure ulcers has resulted in both improved outcomes and cost savings.
- Hospitalized patients placed on air-fluidized beds have demonstrated significant decreases in pressure ulcer size.
- Electrotherapy may be considered for clean Stages III and IV pressure ulcers when there is no improvement after a month of otherwise optimal treatment.
- Surgical debridement is the most rapid and efficient method to remove necrotic debris; with ongoing infection, sharp debridement is required.
- With eschars, penetration of enzymatic agents is decreased; before enzyme application, softening by autolysis or cross-hatching by sharp incision is needed.
- Open pressure ulcers can lose considerable fluid and protein, contributing to dehydration and malnutrition; increased catabolism, especially with infected pressure ulcers, can further deplete nutrients.
- When a pressure ulcer does not heal, always consider a possible infection, including osteomyelitis.

Pressure ulcers, although affecting all age-groups, are more common in the elderly and can result in considerable pain, suffering, expense, litigation, morbidity, and possibly, death. The purpose of this chapter is to provide the reader with an overview of the widely accepted, evidence-based guidelines, *Pressure Ulcers in Adults: Prediction and Prevention* (Clinical Practice Guideline No. 3)[1] and *Treatment of Pressure Ulcers* (Clinical Practice Guideline No. 15),[2] both prepared by the federal agency formerly known as the Agency for Health Care Policy and Research (AHCPR). (AHCPR has since become the Agency for Healthcare Research and Quality [AHRQ]. While the guidelines may still sometimes be referred to as *AHCPR guidelines*, we use the current agency name, AHRQ, here.)

The following case study underscores several important aspects in the prevention of pressure ulcers in at-risk patients.

CASE ONE

Mrs. R., a 78-year-old, was admitted to our medical center with respiratory failure requiring ventilation. Additionally, she had breast cancer that had metastasized to her spine, resulting in paraplegia. Other problems included type 2 diabetes mellitus and hypertensive arteriosclerotic cardiovascular disease. She was on numerous medications at home, several of which were found to be inappropriate for her age and medical conditions and were discontinued. On admission, nutritional parameters, including serum prealbumin and red blood cell count, were found to be low. Her blood urea nitrogen (BUN) and serum glucose levels were high. Her food and fluid intake were optimized, pain was controlled, and diabetes and hypertension were better regulated. The nursing staff closely followed hospital and national guidelines including skin inspection, turning, repositioning, surface support, and infection control, among other measures. She was also closely followed up by the dietary and physical therapy departments. Several pulmonary infections and urinary tract infections (UTIs) were promptly diagnosed and treated. Physicians frequently complimented the nursing staff on their excellent care of the patient.

Despite her metastasic cancer and other comorbid conditions, the patient survived for several more years. Although she was at extremely high risk for the development of pressure ulcers, as noted on her initial pressure ulcer assessment, the patient died peacefully with completely intact skin.

All members of a multidisciplinary medical team worked closely to ensure Mrs. R.'s comfort and to prevent complications. In addition to her initial suboptimal nutrition, hydration, and diabetic control, Mrs. R. had other risk factors for developing pressure ulcers, including immobility from her paralysis, frequent infections, and the need for continued ventilator support, among other medical problems. Close collaborative efforts on a continuous basis prevented the development of any pressure ulcers.

OVERVIEW

Terminology

Although the terms *pressure ulcer* and *decubitus ulcer* have been used interchangeably, technically the latter (from the Latin *decumbere,* meaning "to lie down") refers to ulcers over bony prominences while the patient is supine (e.g., over the occupit, sacrum, or heels). A pressure ulcer that results from excess pressure while a patient is seated would not be classified as a decubitus ulcer. *Pressure ulcer* is therefore the preferred terminology because it applies to all wounds caused by excessive pressure over bony prominences.

Many sites may be involved in pressure ulcers. Almost 95% form on the lower portion of the body, with approximately 65% in the pelvic area and 30% in the lower extremities. Common sites include sacrum, coccyx, ischium, ilial crest, trochanter, lateral malleolus, lateral foot, and heel.

Epidemiology

It has been estimated that from 1 to 3 million adults in the United States may be affected by pressure ulcers. The elderly, because of possible skin changes with aging, as well as increased likelihood of comorbid states, have a higher incidence of pressure ulcer development, with as many as 70% of pressure ulcers developing in patients older than 70.[3,4]

Estimates of pressure ulcer management costs in the United States have ranged from $1.3 to $6.8 billion dollars annually. Treating a severe pressure ulcer and its sequelae can cost in excess of $250,000. The cost in human suffering is incalculable. Pressure ulcer prevention guidelines can significantly decrease such costs and may considerably increase ulcer-free days at minimal cost.[4–6]

DIFFERENTIAL DIAGNOSIS

In addition to pressure ulcers, the main type of dermal ulcers (e.g., ischemic, venous, and neuropathic), as well as some clinical features and modes of treatment, are shown in Table 37.1.

RISK FACTORS

Scores of risk factors and comorbid states that may enhance susceptibility to pressure ulcers have been described. The extrinsic risk factors (e.g., pressure, friction, and shear) often act in combination. Both intensity and duration of pressure are important in the development of pressure ulcer. Table 37.2 summarizes the conditions associated with pressure ulcers.

Braden Scale

The Braden Scale (see Fig. 37.1) is an assessment tool to determine a patient's risk level for developing skin breakdown.[7] It has been tested in both acute-care and long-term care settings and has demonstrated high interrater reliability.[8,9] The Braden score may range from 6

TABLE 37.1
DIFFERENTIAL DIAGNOSIS OF SKIN ULCERS

Condition	Dx	Rx
Pressure ulcers (707.*x* by site)	Develop in pressure areas	Decrease pressure, optimize conditions
Ischemic ulcers (440.23)	Decreased pulses, start in extremities	Enhance arterial flow, control pain
Venous ulcers (454.0)	Leg edema and ulcers	Control edema, avoid maceration
Neuropathic ulcers (357.9)	Diminished pain or sensation on metatarsal head, diabetes	Offload pressure, treat infection

The numbers provided in parenthesis refer to ICD-9 numbers. Dx, diagnosis; Rx, therapy.
Adapted from Takahashi, Kiemele, et al. Wound care for elderly patients: Advances and clinical applications for practicing physicians. *Mayo Clin Proc*. 2004;79(2):260–267.

BRADEN SCALE FOR PREDICTING PRESSURE SORE RISK

Patient's Name ______________ Evaluator's Name______________ Date of Assessment

SENSORY PERCEPTION Ability to respond meaningfully to pressure-related discomfort	**1. Completely Limited** Unresponsive (does not moan, flinch, or grasp) to painful stimuli, due to diminished level of consciousness or sedation OR limited ability to feel pain over most of body.	**2. Very Limited** Responds only to painful stimuli. Cannot communicate discomfort except by moaning or restlessness OR has a sensory impairment which limits the ability to feel pain or discomfort over ½ of body.	**3. Slightly Limited** Responds to verbal commands, but cannot always communicate discomfort or the need to be turned OR has some sensory impairment which limits ability to feel pain or discomfort in 1 or 2 extremities.	**4. No Impairment** Responds to verbal commands. Has no sensory deficit which would limit ability to feel or voice pain or discomfort.				
MOISTURE Degree to which skin is exposed to moisture	**1. Constantly Moist** Skin is kept moist almost constantly by perspiration, urine, etc. Dampness is detected every time patient is moved or turned.	**2. Very Moist** Skin is often, but not always moist. Linen must be changed at least once a shift.	**3. Occasionally Moist:** Skin is occasionally moist, requiring an extra linen change approximately once a day.	**4. Rarely Moist** Skin is usually dry, linen only requires changing at routine intervals.				
ACTIVITY Degree of physical activity	**1. Bedfast** Confined to bed.	**2. Chairfast** Ability to walk severely limited or non-existent. Cannot bear own weight and/or must be assisted into chair or wheelchair.	**3. Walks Occasionally** Walks occasionally during day, but for very short distances, with or without assistance. Spends majority of each shift in bed or chair.	**4. Walks Frequently** Walks outside room at least twice a day and inside room at least once every two hours during waking hours.				
MOBILITY Ability to change and control body position	**1. Completely Immobile** Does not make even slight changes in body or extremity position without assistance.	**2. Very Limited** Makes occasional slight changes in body or extremity position but unable to make frequent or significant changes independently.	**3. Slightly Limited** Makes frequent though slight changes in body or extremity position independently.	**4. No Limitation** Makes major and frequent changes in position without assistance.				
NUTRITION Usual food intake pattern	**1. Very Poor** Never eats a complete meal. Rarely eats more than ¾ of any food offered. Eats 2 servings or less of protein (meat or dairy products) per day. Takes fluids poorly. Does not take a liquid dietary supplement OR is NPO and/or maintained on clear liquids or IV's for more than 5 days.	**2. Probably Inadequate** Rarely eats a complete meal and generally eats only about ½ of any food offered. Protein intake includes only 3 servings of meat or dairy products per day. Occasionally will take a dietary supplement OR receives less than optimum amount of liquid diet or tube feeding.	**3. Adequate** Eats over half of most meals. Eats a total of 4 servings of protein (meat, dairy products) per day. Occasionally will refuse a meal, but will usually take a supplement when offered OR is on a tube feeding or TPN regimen which probably meets most of nutritional needs.	**4. Excellent** Eats most of every meal. Never refuses a meal. Usually eats a total of 4 or more servings of meat and dairy products. Occasionally eats between meals. Does not require supplementation.				
FRICTION & SHEAR	**1. Problem** Requires moderate to maximum assistance in moving. Complete lifting without sliding against sheets is impossible. Frequently slides down in bed or chair, requiring frequent repositioning with maximum assistance. Spasticity, contractures or agitation leads to almost constant friction.	**2. Potential Problem** Moves feebly or requires minimum assistance. During a move skin probably slides to some extent against sheets, chair, restraints or other devices. Maintains relatively good position in chair or bed most of the time but occasionally slides down.	**3. No Apparent Problem** Moves in bed and in chair independently and has sufficient muscle strength to lift up completely during move. Maintains good position in bed or chair.					
				Total Score				

Figure 37.1 Braden Scale. NPO, no oral intake; TPN, total parenteral nutrition.

TABLE 37.2
INTRINSIC RISK FACTORS AND COMORBID STATES ASSOCIATED WITH PRESSURE ULCER DEVELOPMENT

Immobility	Increased age
Inability to reposition	Medications (e.g., steroids, NSAIDs)
Decreased activity level	Spinal cord/brain injury
Impaired sensation	Diabetes mellitus
Malnutrition	Vascular disorder, CVA
Dehydration	Incontinence of urine and feces
Edema	Cognitive impairment
Decreased albumin and prealbumin level	Decreased blood pressure, shock
Previous pressure ulcers	Anemia
Recent fractures/surgery	Febrile illness
Very obese or thin patient	Renal disease
Low BMI	Vitamin/mineral deficiency
High CSI	CNS-active medications, oversedation
High Apache II scores	Decreased ADLs
Decreased lymphocyte count	Paralysis
Decreased nocturnal spontaneous movements	Cachexia
Overly dry or moist skin	Restraints (physical and chemical)
Psychosocial problems	Contractures
Smoking	Foley catheter

NSAIDs, nonsteroidal anti-inflammatory drugs; CVA, cerebral vascular accident; BMI, body mass index; CSI, comprehensive severity index; CNS, central nervous system; ADL, activity of daily living.

(highest pressure ulcer risk) to 23 (lowest risk). Patients with scores <18 are considered at risk.[10] Factors included in the Braden Scale are sensory perception, moisture, activity, mobility, nutrition, friction, and shear.

STAGING

Saucerization of Pressure Damage

At pressures above the capillary filling pressure of 32 mm Hg, arteriolar perfusion is jeopardized. Pressure at the skin surface has a cone-shaped radiation, resulting in much greater internal distribution. The skin is actually less susceptible to damage than the subcutaneous tissue is. Subcutaneous tissue, in turn, is better protected than muscle, which is most vulnerable to pressure damage. Therefore, on examining the skin we frequently see just the tip of the iceberg as far as tissue damage.[11]

The multidisciplinary National Pressure Ulcer Advisory Panel (NPUAP), formed in 1987, is an independent, nonprofit organization established to evaluate areas of concern in pressure ulcer management. NPUAP's pressure ulcer staging system,[12] the most frequently used, has been adopted by the AHRQ guideline panels. The NPUAP staging system is:

Stage I:

Pressure ulcers are observable pressure-related alterations of intact skin whose indicators, as compared to adjacent or opposite body areas, may include changes in skin temperature (i.e., warmth or coolness), tissue consistency (i.e., firmness or bogginess), and/or sensation (i.e., pain, itching). The pressure ulcer appears as a defined area of persistent redness in lightly pigmented skin, whereas in darker skin tones, the pressure ulcer may have persistent red, blue, or purple hues.

Stage II:

Pressure ulcers are associated with partial-thickness skin loss involving epidermis, dermis, or both. The ulcer is superficial and presents clinically as an abrasion, blister, or shallow crater.

Stage III:

Pressure ulcers are associated with full-thickness skin loss involving damage to, or necrosis of, subcutaneous tissue that may extend down to, but not through, the underlying fascia. The pressure ulcer presents clinically as a deep crater, with or without undermining of the adjacent tissue.

Stage IV:

Pressure ulcers are associated with full-thickness skin loss with extensive destruction, tissue necrosis, or damage to muscle, bone, or supporting structures (e.g., tendon, joint, or capsule). Undermining and sinus tracts may also be associated with Stage IV pressure ulcers. (The above is adapted from National Pressure Ulcer Advisory Panel (NPUAP). *NPUAP position on reverse staging of pressure ulcers, in Advanced Wound Care,* Vol. 8. 1998:32).

Because skin is a not a uniform organ, its appearance or thickness varies according to anatomic site. On average, a pressure ulcer that is approximately 2 mm or deeper and is located on the trunk, pelvic girdle, ankle, or heel is usually classified at least as a Stage III. This depth approximates that of a US nickel or a house key. Initial pressure ulcer staging is important because the ulcer is not restaged as it heals.

Reverse (Healing) Staging

The NPUAP has issued a position statement[12] against using back staging or reverse staging. For example, a healing Stage IV pressure ulcer would not be progressively downstaged to III, II, and so on, as it heals. A healing pressure ulcer is replaced with scar tissue because dermis, subcutaneous fat, and muscle cannot be regenerated. Therefore, restaging as an ulcer heals does not describe the physiologic changes that occur. If a previously healed pressure ulcer reopens, the prior staging diagnosis should be used (i.e., once an ulcer is Stage IV, it will always remain Stage IV).

NPUAP recommends[12] that pressure ulcers also be described by size, the presence of granulation tissue, and the presence of infection and that an appropriate pressure ulcer healing tool (e.g., the Pressure Ulcer Scale for Healing [PUSH] tool [see Fig. 37.2]) also be used.

INCIDENCE/PREVALENCE

Values for pressure ulcer incidence, (i.e., new cases occurring over a specified period) and prevalence (a cross-sectional count of cases at a specific time point) may vary considerably among different patient populations, among treatment facilities, and with differences in methodology used for calculating pressure ulcers. Some high-risk populations, such as quadriplegics, are obviously more prone to develop pressure ulcers. AHRQ and NPUAP panels have compiled statistics for pressure ulcer incidence and prevalence in different care settings, as shown in Table 37.3.

COMPLICATIONS

Clinicians often surrender to a defeatist attitude about pressure ulcers because of the oversimplified conception that ulcers reflect a patient's age and/or disease process. The presence of pressure ulcers may compromise the care for other medical needs. Coexistent malnutrition and dehydration contribute to further development of pressure ulcer and result in a lethal vicious cycle. Complications of pressure ulcers include the following: Protein loss, malnutrition, anemia, dehydration, electrolyte disturbances, pain, suffering, disfigurement, psychological distress, suicide, social isolation and stigmatization, increased lengths of stay, decreased quality of life, squamous cell carcinoma, susceptibility to future pressure ulcers, maggot infestation, multiorgan failure, risk to others (e.g., from infection by methicillin-resistant *Staphylococcus aureus* [MRSA] or vancomycin-resistant enterococci [VRE]), delay in treating other disorders, infections (e.g., bacteremia, cellulitis, fasciitis, endocarditis, osteomyelitis, septic arthritis, sinus tract infections, abscesses, tetanus, meningitis), and death.

Bed-bound patients who develop pressure ulcers are almost twice as likely to die. Twenty years ago it was estimated that >60,000 deaths occur yearly from pressure ulcers and their complications. Once a pressure ulcer develops, the patient may have a twofold to sixfold increase in chance of dying.[13,14]

PREVENTION

Prevention of pressure ulcers is an area of growing concern to all physicians, but especially to geriatricians. Pressure ulcers are largely preventable. Some clinicians feel that pressure ulcers are completely preventable with appropriate care.[15–17] Should a pressure ulcer develop, after early recognition and treatment with a comprehensive regimen, nearly all Stage IV pressure ulcers can be avoided.[18]

Injury Prevention

When evaluating potentially preventable medical injuries in the hospitalized aged, Rothschild et al.[19] reviewed the literature on six preventable injury categories: Pressure ulcers, nosocomial infections, falls, adverse drug reactions, delirium, and surgical complications. The authors found that treatment variables that predispose to the development of pressure ulcer include nurse staffing ratios, repositioning frequency, medication selection, and type of surface support. They recommend quality management programs with multidisciplinary approaches to prevent injuries. Physicians and other health care workers with specialized training in fall prevention can help reduce injuries and ulcers by up to one third. Staff education can decrease pressure

TABLE 37.3
INCIDENCE (I) AND PREVALENCE (P) OF PRESSURE ULCERS

Reference	Acute Care	Long-term Care	Home Care	Critical Care
NPUAP 2001	I: 7%–38%	7%–23.9%	16.5%–17%	8%–40%
NPUAP 2001	P: 10%–18%	23%–28%	0%–29%	—

NATIONAL PRESSURE ULCER ADVISORY PANEL

Pressure Ulcer Scale for Healing (PUSH)

PUSH Tool 3.0

Patient Name ______________________ Patient ID# ______________

Ulcer Location ______________________ Date ______________

Directions:
Observe and measure the pressure ulcer. Categorize the ulcer with respect to surface area, exudate, and type of wound tissue. Record a sub-score for each of these ulcer characteristics. Add the sub-scores to obtain the total score. A comparison of total scores measured over time provides an indication of the improvement or deterioration in pressure ulcer healing.

LENGTH X WIDTH (in cm^2)	0 0	1 < 0.3	2 0.3 – 0.6	3 0.7 – 1.0	4 1.1 – 2.0	5 2.1 – 3.0	**Sub-score**
		6 3.1 – 4.0	7 4.1 – 8.0	8 8.1 – 12.0	9 12.1 – 24.0	10 > 24.0	
EXUDATE AMOUNT	0 None	1 Light	2 Moderate	3 Heavy			**Sub-score**
TISSUE TYPE	0 Closed	1 Epithelial Tissue	2 Granulation Tissue	3 Slough	4 Necrotic Tissue		**Sub-score**
							TOTAL SCORE

Length x Width: Measure the greatest length (head to toe) and the greatest width (side to side) using a centimeter ruler. Multiply these two measurements (length x width) to obtain an estimate of surface area in square centimeters (cm^2). Caveat: Do not guess! Always use a centimeter ruler and always use the same method each time the ulcer is measured.

Exudate Amount: Estimate the amount of exudate (drainage) present after removal of the dressing and before applying any topical agent to the ulcer. Estimate the exudate (drainage) as none, light, moderate, or heavy.

Tissue Type: This refers to the types of tissue that are present in the wound (ulcer) bed. Score as a "4" if there is any necrotic tissue present. Score as a "3" if there is any amount of slough present and necrotic tissue is absent. Score as a "2" if the wound is clean and contains granulation tissue. A superficial wound that is reepithelializing is scored as a "1". When the wound is closed, score as a "0".

4 – **Necrotic Tissue (Eschar):** black, brown, or tan tissue that adheres firmly to the wound bed or ulcer edges and may be either firmer or softer than surrounding skin.

3 – **Slough:** yellow or white tissue that adheres to the ulcer bed in strings or thick clumps, or is mucinous.

2 – **Granulation Tissue:** pink or beefy red tissue with a shiny, moist, granular appearance.

1 – **Epithelial Tissue:** for superficial ulcers, new pink or shiny tissue (skin) that grows in from the edges or as islands on the ulcer surface.

0 – **Closed/Resurfaced:** the wound is completely covered with epithelium (new skin).

www.npuap.org
11F

PUSH Tool Version 3.0: 9/15/98

Figure 37.2 Pressure Ulcer Scale for Healing (PUSH) tool. (*continued*)

NATIONAL PRESSURE ULCER ADVISORY PANEL

Pressure Ulcer Healing Chart

To monitor trends in PUSH Scores over time
(Use a separate page for each pressure ulcer)

Patient Name________________________________ Patient ID#______________

Ulcer Location ________________________________ Date ______________

Directions:
Observe and measure pressure ulcers at regular intervals using the PUSH Tool.
Date and record PUSH Sub-scores and Total Scores on the Pressure Ulcer Healing Record below.

Pressure Ulcer Healing **Record**														
Date														
Length x Width														
Exudate Amount														
Tissue Type														
PUSH Total Score														

Graph the PUSH Total Scores on the Pressure Ulcer Healing Graph below.

PUSH Total Score	Pressure Ulcer Healing **Graph**													
17														
16														
15														
14														
13														
12														
11														
10														
9														
8														
7														
6														
5														
4														
3														
2														
1														
Healed = 0														
Date														

www.npuap.org
11F

PUSH Tool Version 3.0: 9/15/98

Figure 37.2 *(continued)*

TABLE 37.4
FACTORS AFFECTING A HEALTH CARE FACILITY'S RISKS RELATING TO PRESSURE ULCERS

Factor	Issues
Medical Record	■ Evidence of assessment of relevant factors relating to a pressure ulcer ■ Documentation of initial assessment and problem definition by a qualified clinician ■ Documentation of periodic follow-up, the frequency of which is related to the pressure ulcer progress, possible complications, and patient's overall status and treatment goals ■ Apparent basis for selecting various treatments or for not treating identified conditions or situations ■ Clear indication of factors felt to be associated with delayed pressure ulcer healing or with a patient with pressure ulcer who is declining medically
Staff and Practitioner	■ A cooperative approach in preventing and managing pressure ulcers ■ Sufficient equipment, supplies, and staffing to provide appropriate pressure ulcer care ■ Administration and nursing management who fully support the staff's efforts to prevent and manage pressure ulcers appropriately ■ Active and cooperative physician participation in pressure ulcer management ■ Consistent policies and procedures that reflect current standards, with guidelines and options for pressure ulcer care and appropriate follow-up ■ Documentation explaining reasons for possible deviations from policies and procedures ■ All staff having access to correct procedures ■ Evidence of relevant, ongoing staff training in basic aspects of pressure ulcer management ■ Evidence of a review of actual performance of functions and tasks

Adapted from American Medical Directors Association (AMDA). *Pressure ulcer therapy companion: Clinical practice guideline*. Columbia, MD: (available at: www.amda.com); 1999.

ulcers by 50%.[19] They further noted that physical restraints are associated with the development of pressure ulcer.

Long-term Care Prevention

Horn et al.[20] reported results of the National Pressure Ulcer Long-Term Care Study, in which >1,500 residents from 95 US long-term care facilities were evaluated. Findings indicated that numerous patient, treatment, and facility factors were associated with higher incidence of pressure ulcer. These factors included higher initial disease severity, history of a recent pressure ulcer, significant weight loss, eating difficulties, and urinary catheter use. Factors associated with diminished likelihood of developing pressure ulcers included nutritional intervention, use of antidepressants, use of disposable briefs, increased nurse and aide time devoted to patient care, and lower Licensed Practical Nurses (LPNs) turnover rates. This study underscores the decreased quality of life and increased morbidity and mortality associated with pressure ulcers. Long-term care facilities can lower pressure ulcer incidence by implementing comprehensive prevention protocols.[20]

Over the years, hundreds of empiric remedies have been used to treat pressure ulcers, some with untoward results. Parish et al.[21] listed several of these including sugar, egg whites, dried blood, castor and cod liver oils, mutton tallow, and vegetable poultices made from carrots, turnips, and charcoal. Unfortunately, even today some publications have recommended outmoded remedies such as drying and massage of pressure ulcers.

Staffing

Recent national studies have reported that many US health care facilities, such as nursing homes, are often understaffed and unable to provide ample care to their patients. Suboptimal care may result in increased incidence of pressure ulcers and falls, as well as contribute to malnutrition and dehydration. Physicians caring for at-risk patients should be alert to this national dilemma and do their best to optimize patient care.

The American Medical Directors Association (AMDA)[22] has developed a comprehensive list of factors that may affect a health care facility's risks relating to pressure ulcers, as shown in Table 37.4.

Education (Physicians)

Kimura and Pacala[23] found that most family physicians felt that knowledge concerning pressure ulcers might be enhanced by additional exposure to elderly patients, more rigorous geriatric training in residencies, and greater knowledge of AHRQ guidelines. The physicians who had been introduced to the guidelines displayed a better knowledge of pressure ulcer management.[23]

Education (Nurses)

O'Brien[24] reported that appropriate knowledge of pressure ulcer care has not consistently filtered down to health care workers. Using a pressure ulcer knowledge test, O'Brien found that nursing staffs (Registered Nurses,

LPNs, and Certified Nurse Assistants/Aides) perform better when knowledgeable about the causative factors associated with pressure ulcers and the modalities of pressure ulcer treatment and classification systems. The author emphasized the need for continuous updated education of nursing personnel, who share the medical, moral, and legal responsibility to advocate for their patients in pressure ulcer prevention and therapy.[24]

Nursing Home Quality Initiative

The Nursing Home Quality Initiative (NHQI) is an initiative to improve nursing home quality of care using principles of continuous quality improvement. The Secretary of Health and Human Services (HHS) noted that although care of nursing home patients has improved, considerably more remains to be done. The percentage of patients with pain or in physical restraints has decreased but there has been no significant decline in pressure ulcers. Nursing homes are now publicly graded on the proportion of patients who have potentially preventable problems. Additionally, long-term care facilities are being provided with guidance by consultants on quality care, and more attention is being focused on decreasing pressure ulcers and restraint usage.[25]

Healthy People 2010 also includes for the first time, a pressure ulcer objective, underscoring a growing national concern. The objective of Healthy People 2010 is to reduce the proportion of nursing home patients with a current diagnosis of pressure ulcer, from a baseline of 16/1,000 (1997 data) to 8/1,000 patients. This goal of a 50%

Pressure Ulcers: Nursing Home Communication with Physician

Resident:________ **Age:**____ **Sex:**____ **Date:**________

Diagnoses: ________

Current Medications: ________

Allergies: ________

Vital Signs: Temp: ____ **Pulses:**____ **Resp:** ____ **BP:** ____/____

Pressure Ulcer Description					
Location 1:____			**Location 2:**____		
Size: Length____ Width____ Depth____			**Size:** Length____ Width____ Depth____		
Stage #:			**Stage #:**		
	Yes	No		Yes	No
Exudate	☐	☐	Exudate	☐	☐
Serous	☐	☐	Serous	☐	☐
Serosanguineous	☐	☐	Serosanguineous	☐	☐
Purulent	☐	☐	Purulent	☐	☐
Sinus tract	☐	☐	Sinus tract	☐	☐
Tunneling	☐	☐	Tunneling	☐	☐
Undermining	☐	☐	Undermining	☐	☐
Necrotic tissue	☐	☐	Necrotic tissue	☐	☐
Slough	☐	☐	Slough	☐	☐
Eschar	☐	☐	Eschar	☐	☐
Granulation	☐	☐	Granulation	☐	☐
Epithelialization	☐	☐	Epithelialization	☐	☐
Pain (If yes, perform pain assessment)	☐	☐	Pain (If yes, perform pain assessment)	☐	☐
Pain Intensity Score____			Pain Intensity Score____		

RELATED FACTORS	PHYSICIAN'S COMMENTS/TREATMENT ORDER
Mobility Bed mobility ☐ No assist ☐ Some assist ☐ Extensive assist Chair mobility ☐ No assist ☐ Some assist ☐ Extensive assist Support services used ☐ Yes ☐ No Type of support service used:____	☐ OT consult for positioning devices
Bowel/Urinary Incontinence Is pressure ulcer exposed to urine and/or fecal contaminants? ☐ Yes ☐ No	
Nutritional Status Adequate oral intake? ☐ Yes ☐ No Current Height____ Current Weight____ BMI____ (if available via dietary consult) Recent weight loss?____	☐ Dietary consult

Used with permission — *This material was developed by the QIO Program for CMS'NHQI and is intended as general information. Any individual using the material must consider the possibility of human error, changes in medical sciences, and the need to use clinical judgment in each specific case.*

Figure 37.3 Instrument for communication between nursing homes and physicians, developed for the Quality Improvement Organization.

reduction in pressure ulcer prevalence has been achieved in numerous long-term care facilities, including Veterans Affairs hospitals.[26]

Communication

Communication among all health care workers involved in patient care is vital, but all too often inadequate. This is especially true in regard to patients at risk for the development of pressure ulcer. Accurate documentation of skin disorders before admission, or early on admission, to a health care facility not only assists in adequately planning for patients' medical needs but can also prevent accusations of negligence on the part of the treating facility and its medical team.[27,28] An example of a useful instrument for communication between nursing homes and physicians, developed for the Quality Improvement Organization (QIO) by the Centers for Medicare & Medicaid Services (CMS), is shown in Figure 37.3.

AGENCY FOR HEALTHCARE RESEARCH AND QUALITY PREDICTION AND PREVENTION RECOMMENDATIONS

Because of the clinical importance of pressure ulcers, AHRQ, a key agency of the U.S. Department of Health and Human Services, was charged with the preparation of guidelines germane to prevention and treatment of pressure ulcers. A total of six monographs were written on pressure ulcers, three on their prevention and three on treatment. The *Clinical Practice Guidelines* give recommendations with supporting information, figures, tables, and references. The *Quick Reference Guides for Clinicians* are shortened versions of the *Clinical Practice Guidelines*. The consumer versions, available in both English and Spanish, are booklets for the general public. The monographs may be obtained free of charge from the AHRQ Publication Clearinghouse (1-800-358-9295).

The first AHRQ pressure ulcer guideline[1] (henceforth referred to as A92) developed was *Pressure Ulcers in Adults: Prediction and Prevention*. This guideline's purpose is to assist in identifying adults at risk for developing pressure ulcers and to define early preventive interventions. The guideline can also be used to assist in the treatment of Stage I pressure ulcers. Goals that were targeted in the recommendations made by the 13-member expert panel are:

1. to identify at-risk patients needing prevention and the specific factors placing them at increased risk
2. to maintain and improve the tolerance of tissues to pressure
3. to protect against the untoward effects of pressure, friction, and shear
4. to reduce pressure ulcer incidence through education programs.

Strength of Evidence

Most clinical guidelines for pressure ulcer management have been based on published evidence and face validity of various practices, as well as professional judgment. For example, turning and repositioning at-risk patients is a practice with high face validity; however, there are no randomized controlled trials that examine its effectiveness in the absence of other interventions.[29] Therefore, many well-accepted practices have received lower strength of evidence gradings. Several AHRQ recommendations have been upgraded by more recent national and international guidelines, using evidence-based gradings, by organizations such as the NPUAP[8,12] and the Wound, Ostomy and Continence Nurses Society (WOCN).[4]

The technology assessment group of ECRI (formally the Emergency Care Research Institute), an independent nonprofit health service agency, evaluated and summarized the A92 recommendations and AHRQ's clinical practice guideline on pressure ulcer treatment[2] (henceforth referred to as A94) and found the guidelines to be, in essence, valid and current.[30,31] Adaptation of these summary prevention recommendations, prioritized from highest to lowest strengths of evidence for each category, are shown below.

Use of Risk Assessment Tools and Risk Factors

- Promptly assess patients at risk for developing pressure ulcers for additional risk factors by using a validated risk assessment tool, such as the Braden Scale or Norton Scale. Periodically reassess pressure ulcer risk (Evidence Level A).
- Document all risk assessments (Evidence Level C).

Skin Care And Early Treatment

- Avoid massaging over bony prominences (Evidence Level B).
- Perform systematic skin inspections on all patients at risk for pressure ulcers at least daily, with special attention to bony prominences. Document results (Evidence Level C).
- Cleanse the skin routinely and at the time of soiling. Individualize the frequency of skin cleansing. Avoid hot water, and use a mild cleansing agent. During the cleansing process, use care to minimize the force and friction to the skin (Evidence Level C).
- Minimize environmental factors that can dry the skin such as low humidity and cold exposure. With dry skin, moisturizers can be helpful (Evidence Level C).
- Minimize skin exposure to moisture from incontinence, perspiration, or pressure ulcer drainage; with uncontrolled moisture, absorbent, quick-drying underpads or briefs can be used, as can topical agents that act as moisture barriers (Evidence Level C).
- Minimize skin injury from friction and shear by proper positioning, transferring, and turning techniques.

Friction injuries can also be reduced by the use of lubricants (such as corn starch and creams), protective films (such as transparent film dressings and skin sealants), and protective dressings (such as hydrocolloids), as well as protective padding (Evidence Level C).

- When apparently well-nourished patients do not consume adequate protein or calories, caregivers should attempt to discover factors compromising intake and then offer support with eating. Nutritional supplements or support may be needed. If dietary intake remains inadequate and if consistent with overall therapy goals, consider more aggressive nutritional interventions (e.g., enteral or parenteral feedings) (Evidence Level C).
- For nutritionally compromised patients, institute a plan of nutritional support and/or supplementation that meets the patients' needs (Evidence Level C).
- If the potential exists for improving the patient's mobility and activity status, institute rehabilitation efforts that are consistent with treatment goals. Maintaining current activity level, mobility, and range of motion is an appropriate goal for most patients (Evidence Level C).
- Monitor and document interventions and outcomes (Evidence Level C).

Mechanical Loading and Support Surfaces

- Reposition any patient in bed who is felt to be at risk for developing pressure ulcers, at least every 2 hours if consistent with overall patient goals. Use a written schedule for systematically turning and repositioning (Evidence Level B).
- Place any patient assessed to be at risk for developing pressure ulcers, when lying in bed, on a pressure-reducing device, such as foam, static air, or alternating air, gel, or water mattress (Evidence Level B).
- For patients in bed, use positioning devices such as pillows or foam wedges to keep bony prominences (such as knees or ankles) from direct contact. Use a written plan for turning and repositioning (Evidence Level C).
- Completely immobile bedridden patients should have a care plan that includes the use of devices that totally relieve heel pressure, most commonly by raising heels off the bed. Do not use donut-type devices (Evidence Level C).
- When the side-lying position is used in bed, avoid positioning directly upon the trochanter (Evidence Level C).
- Keep the head of the bed at the lowest degree of elevation consistent with medical needs and other restrictions. Limit the time the head of the bed is elevated (Evidence Level C).
- Use a lifting device such as a trapeze or bed linen to move (and not drag) a patient, who cannot assist during the transfer and change of position, in bed (Evidence Level C).
- Any patient at risk for the development of pressure ulcer should avoid uninterrupted sitting in chair or wheelchair. The patient should be repositioned, shifting the points under pressure, at least hourly, or be placed in bed if consistent with overall management goals. Patients who are able should be taught to shift weight every 15 minutes (Evidence Level C).
- For chair-bound patients, use a pressure-reducing device (e.g., foam, gel, air, or a combination). Do not use donut-type devices (Evidence Level C).
- Positioning of chair-bound patients should include consideration of postural alignment, weight distribution, balance, stability, and relief from pressure (Evidence Level C).
- A written plan for use of positioning devices and schedules can be helpful for chair-bound patients (Evidence Level C).

Education

- Educational programs for pressure ulcer prevention should be structured, organized, comprehensive, and directed to all levels of health care providers, patients, family, or other caregivers (Evidence Level A).
- Educational programs for pressure ulcer prevention should include information on the following items: Etiology and risk factors for pressure ulcers, risk assessment tools, assessment of skin, selection and use of support surfaces, personalized skin care programs, demonstration of positioning to decrease tissue breakdown, and data collection and documentation (Evidence Level B).
- The educational program should describe each person's role and be updated regularly to incorporate appropriate techniques and technologies (Evidence Level C).

  (The above was adapted from ECRI summary of A92 Guidelines [2001]).

AGENCY FOR HEALTHCARE RESEARCH AND QUALITY RECOMMENDATIONS FOR TREATMENT

AHRQ's A94 clinical practice guideline on pressure ulcer treatment[2] has also been validated after extensive use and published reviews of its recommendations.[32–34] The A94 treatment panel developed comprehensive clinical algorithms to help clinicians understand decision points and appropriate management principles in treating pressure ulcers. Summary treatment recommendations adapted from A94, and ECRI 1998,[30] and prioritized from highest to lowest strengths of evidence for each category, are shown below.

Assessment

- Assess pressure ulcers initially for location, stage, size, sinus tracts, undermining, tunneling, exudates, necrotic tissue, presence or absence of granulation tissue, and epithelialization (Evidence Level C).

- Reassess pressure ulcers at least weekly. If the condition of the patient or of the pressure ulcer deteriorates, reevaluate the treatment plan promptly (Evidence Level C).
- A clean pressure ulcer should show evidence of some healing within 2 to 4 weeks. If progress cannot be demonstrated, reevaluate the adequacy of the overall treatment plan, as well as adherence, making necessary changes (Evidence Level C).

Assessing the Patient with a Pressure Ulcer

History and Physical Examination

- Perform a complete history and physical because a pressure ulcer should be assessed in the context of the patient's overall physical and psychosocial health (Evidence Level C).

Nutritional Assessment and Management

- Ensure adequate dietary intake to prevent malnutrition if it is compatible with the patient's wishes. Consider use of laboratory markers such as prealbumin (Evidence Level B).
- Perform an abbreviated patient nutritional assessment, at least every 3 months, for patients at risk for malnutrition (e.g., those unable to take food by mouth or who experience an involuntary weight change) (Evidence Level C).
- Encourage dietary intake or supplementation if a patient with a pressure ulcer is malnourished. If dietary intake remains inadequate, impractical, or impossible, nutritional support (usually tube feeding) should be used to put the patient into positive nitrogen balance (approximately 30 to 35 calories/kg/day and 1.25 to 1.50 g of protein/kg/day) according to the goals of care (Evidence Level C).
- Use vitamin and mineral supplements if deficiencies are suspected (Evidence Level C).

Pain Assessment and Management

- Assess all patients for pain related to the pressure ulcer or its treatment (Evidence Level C).
- Manage pain by controlling or managing the pain source (e.g., covering pressure ulcers, adjusting support surfaces, repositioning.) Provide analgesia as needed and as appropriate (Evidence Level C).

Psychosocial Assessment and Management

- All patients being treated for pressure ulcers should have a psychosocial assessment to determine their ability and motivation to understand and adhere to the treatment program. The assessment should include, but not be limited to, the following:
- Mental status, learning ability, depression, social support, polypharmacy or overmedication, alcohol and/or drug abuse, goals, values, and lifestyle, sexuality, ethnicity and culture, and stressors.
- Periodic reassessment is recommended (Evidence Level C).
- Assess resources (e.g., skill and availability of caregivers, finances, and equipment) of patients being treated for pressure ulcers in the home (Evidence Level C).
- Arrange interventions to meet identified psychosocial needs and goals. Plan follow-up in cooperation with the patient and caregiver (Evidence Level C).

Managing Tissue Loads

While in Bed

Positioning Techniques

- Avoid positioning patients on a pressure ulcer (Evidence Level C).
- Use a positioning device to raise a pressure ulcer off the support surface. If the patient is no longer at risk for developing pressure ulcers, these devices may decrease the need for pressure-reducing overlays, mattresses, and beds. Avoid using donut-type devices (Evidence Level C).
- Develop a written repositioning schedule (Evidence Level C).
- Avoid positioning immobile patients directly on trochanters; use devices such as pillows and foam wedges that totally relieve pressure on the heels, most commonly by raising the heels off the bed (Evidence Level C).
- Use positioning devices, such as pillows or foam, to prevent direct contact between bony prominences (such as knees or ankles) (Evidence Level C).
- Maintain the head of the bed at the lowest degree of elevation consistent with medical conditions or other restrictions. Limit the time the head of the bed is elevated (Evidence Level C).

Support Surfaces

- Use a static support surface if a patient can assume a variety of positions without bearing weight on the pressure ulcer and without "bottoming out" (Evidence Level B).
- Use a dynamic support surface if the patient cannot assume a variety of positions without bearing weight on the pressure ulcer, if the patient fully compresses the static support surface, or if the pressure ulcer is not healing (Evidence Level B).
- Assess all patients with existing pressure ulcers to determine the risk of developing additional pressure ulcers. If the patient remains at risk, use a pressure-reducing surface (Evidence Level C).
- If a patient has large Stage III or IV pressure ulcers on multiple turning surfaces, a low–air-loss bed or an air-fluidized bed may be indicated (Evidence Level C).
- When excess moisture on intact skin can result in maceration and skin breakdown, a support surface providing

airflow can be important in drying the skin and preventing additional pressure ulcers (Evidence Level C).

While Sitting

Positioning Techniques

- A patient with a pressure ulcer on a sitting surface should avoid sitting. If pressure on the ulcer can be relieved, limited sitting can be allowed (Evidence Level C).
- Consider postural alignment, weight distribution, balance, stability, and pressure relief when positioning sitting patients (Evidence Level C).
- Reposition the sitting patient so that the points under pressure are shifted at least hourly. If this schedule cannot be kept or is inconsistent with overall treatment goals, return the patient to bed. Patients who are able should be taught to shift weight every 15 minutes (Evidence Level C).

Ulcer Care

Debridement

- Remove devitalized tissue in pressure ulcers when appropriate for the patient's condition and goals (Evidence Level C).
- Select the debridement method most appropriate for the patient's condition and goals. Sharp, mechanical, enzymatic, and/or autolytic debridement may be used when there is no urgent clinical need for drainage or removal of devitalized tissue. If there is urgent need for debridement (e.g., with advancing cellulitis or sepsis), sharp debridement is necessary (Evidence Level C).
- Use clean, dry dressings for 8 to 24 hours after sharp debridement associated with bleeding; then reinstitute moist dressings. Clean dressings can be used in conjunction with mechanical or enzymatic debridement techniques (Evidence Level C).
- Heel pressure ulcers with dry eschar need not be debrided if they do not have fluctuance, edema, erythema, or drainage. Assess these wounds daily to monitor for pressure ulcer complications that would require debridement (i.e., fluctuance, edema, erthyema, and drainage) (Evidence Level C).
- Prevent or manage pain from debridement as needed (Evidence Level C).

Wound Cleansing

- Do not clean pressure ulcers with skin cleansers or antiseptic agents (e.g., povidone iodine, iodophor, sodium hypochlorite solution [Dakin solution], hydrogen peroxide, or acetic acid) (Evidence Level B).
- Use enough irrigation pressure to enhance wound cleansing without traumatizing the pressure ulcer bed. Safe and effective pressure ulcer irrigation pressures range from 4 to 15 psi (Evidence Level B).
- Cleanse pressure ulcers initially and with each dressing change (Evidence Level C).
- Use minimal mechanical force when cleansing the pressure ulcer with gauze, cloth, or sponges (Evidence Level C).
- Use normal saline to cleanse most pressure ulcers (Evidence Level C).
- Consider whirlpool treatment for cleansing pressure ulcers containing thick exudates, slough, or necrotic tissue; discontinue whirlpool when the pressure ulcer is clean (Evidence Level C).

Dressings

- Use a dressing that keeps the pressure ulcer bed continuously moist. Wet-to-dry dressings should be used only for debridement (Evidence Level B).
- Use clinical judgment in selecting a type of moist dressing suitable for the pressure ulcer. Studies of different types of moist wound dressings have shown differences in pressure ulcer healing outcomes (Evidence Level B).
- Consider caregiver time when selecting a dressing (Evidence Level B).
- Select a dressing that keeps the surrounding intact (periulcer) skin dry while keeping the pressure ulcer moist (Evidence Level C).
- Select a dressing that controls exudates but does not desiccate the pressure ulcer bed (Evidence Level C).
- Eliminate pressure ulcer dead space by loosely filling cavities with dressing material. Avoid overpacking the pressure ulcer (Evidence Level C).
- Monitor dressings applied near the anus because they are difficult to keep intact (Evidence Level C).

Adjunctive Therapies

- Consider a treatment course with electrotherapy for Stages III and IV pressure ulcers that have been unresponsive to conventional therapy. Electrical stimulation may also help recalcitrant Stage II ulcers (Evidence Level B).
- The therapeutic efficacy of hyperbaric oxygen, infrared, ultraviolet, low-energy laser irradiation, and ultrasound has not been sufficiently established to allow recommendation of these therapies for pressure ulcer treatment at this time (Evidence Level C).
- The therapeutic efficacy of miscellaneous topical agents (e.g., sugar, vitamins, and hormones), growth factors, and skin equivalents has not been sufficiently established to warrant recommendation at this time (Evidence Level C).

- The therapeutic efficacy of systemic agents other than antibiotics has not been sufficiently established to allow their recommendation for pressure ulcer treatment (Evidence Level C).

Managing Bacterial Colonization and Infection

Pressure Ulcer Colonization and Infection

- Minimize pressure ulcer colonization and increase healing by effective pressure ulcer cleansing and debridement (Evidence Level A).
- Consider initiating a 2-week trial of topical antibiotics for clean pressure ulcers that are not healing or are producing exudates after 2 to 4 weeks of optimal patient care. Antibiotics should be effective against gram-negative, gram-positive, and anaerobic organisms (e.g., silver sulfadiazine and triple antibiotic) (Evidence Level A).
- Start appropriate systemic antibiotic therapy for patients with bacteremia, sepsis, advancing cellulitis, or osteomyelitis (Evidence Level A).
- Do not use topical antiseptics (e.g., povidone iodine, iodophor, sodium hypochlorite [Dakin solution], hydrogen peroxide, acetic acid) to decrease bacterial count in pressure ulcer tissue (Evidence Level B).
- If purulence or foul odor is present, more frequent cleansing and, possibly, debridement are needed (Evidence Level C).
- Do not use swab cultures to diagnose pressure ulcer infection because all pressure ulcers are colonized (Evidence Level C).
- Obtain quantitative bacterial cultures of soft tissue and evaluate the patient for osteomyelitis when the pressure ulcer does not respond to topical antibiotic therapy (Evidence Level C).
- Systemic antibiotics are not required for pressure ulcers with clinical signs of local infection only (Evidence Level C).
- Protect pressure ulcers from exogenous sources of contamination (e.g., feces) (Evidence Level C).

Infection Control

- When treating pressure ulcers follow body substance isolation precautions or an equivalent system appropriate for the health care setting and the patient's condition (Evidence Level C).
- Use clean gloves for each patient. When treating multiple pressure ulcers on the same patient, treat the most contaminated pressure ulcer last (e.g., in the perianal region). Remove gloves and wash hands between patients (Evidence Level C).
- Use sterile instruments to debride pressure ulcers (Evidence Level C).
- Disposal of contaminated dressings in the home should be done consistent with local regulations (Evidence Level C).

Surgical Repair of Pressure Ulcers

Patient Selection

- Determine patient need and suitability for surgical repair when clean Stage III or IV pressure ulcers do not respond to optimal patient care. Possible candidates are medically stable and appropriately nourished, and can tolerate surgical loss of blood and postoperative immobility. Quality of life, patient preferences, goals of therapy, recurrence risk, and expected rehabilitative outcome are additional considerations (Evidence Level C).

Controlling Factors that Impair Healing

- Promote successful surgical closure by controlling or correcting factors that can impair healing, such as smoking, spasticity, levels of bacterial colonization, incontinence, and UTI (Evidence Level C).

Surgical Procedures

- Use the most effective and least traumatic method to repair the pressure ulcer defect. Pressure ulcers can be closed by direct closure, skin grafting, skin flaps, musculocutaneous flaps, and free flaps. To minimize recurrence, the choice of surgical technique should be based on the patient's needs and overall goals (Evidence Level C).
- Prophylactic ischiectomy is not recommended because it frequently causes perineal ulcers and urethral fistulas, which are more threatening than the ischial pressure ulcers (Evidence Level C).

Postoperative Care

- Assess for pressure ulcer recurrence as an ongoing component of care. Caregivers should provide education and encourage adherence to pressure reduction measures, daily skin examination, and intermittent relief techniques (Evidence Level A).
- Minimize pressure to the surgical site by using an air-fluidized bed, a low–air-loss bed, or a Stryker frame for a minimum of 2 weeks. Assess postoperative viability of the surgical site as clinically indicated. The patient should slowly increase periods of time spent sitting or lying on the flap to increase its tolerance to pressure. To determine the degree of tolerance, monitor the flap for pallor or redness, or both, that does not resolve after 10 minutes of pressure relief (Evidence Level C).

Education and Quality Improvement

Education

Prevention and Treatment: A Continuum

- Design, develop, and implement educational programs for patients, caregivers, and health care providers that reflect a continuum of care. The program should begin with a structured, comprehensive, and organized approach to prevention and should end in effective treatment protocols promoting healing and preventing recurrence (Evidence Level C).
- Educational programs should identify individuals who are responsible for pressure ulcer treatment and describe each person's role. Information presented and degree of participation expected should be appropriate for the audience (Evidence Level C).

Assessing Tissue Damage

- Educational programs should emphasize the need for accurate, consistent, and uniform assessment, description, and documentation of extent of tissue damage (Evidence Level C).
- The following information should be included when developing an educational program on pressure ulcer treatment (Evidence Level C):
  - Etiology and pathology
  - Risk factors
  - Uniform terminology for stage of tissue damage based on specific classification
  - Principles of wound healing
  - Principles of nutritional support regarding tissue integrity
  - Individualized program of skin care
  - Principles of cleansing and infection control
  - Principles of postoperative care including positioning and support surfaces
  - Principles of prevention to reduce recurrence
  - Product selection (i.e., categories and uses of support surfaces, dressings, topical antibiotics, etc.)
  - Effects or influence of the physical and mechanical environment on the pressure ulcer and management strategies
  - Mechanisms to accurately document and monitor pertinent data, including treatment interventions and healing progress.

Quality Improvement

- Convene an interdisciplinary committee of knowledgeable and interested persons to address quality improvement in pressure ulcer management (Evidence Level C).
- Identify and monitor the occurrence of pressure ulcers to determine their incidence and prevalence. This information can serve as a baseline to the development, implementation, and evaluation of therapy protocols (Evidence Level C).

SPECIFIC MANAGEMENT STRATEGIES

Pressure Ulcer Scale for Healing Tool

The NPUAP has developed an excellent tool, the PUSH tool, to rapidly and reliably monitor alterations in pressure ulcer status. The tool has been validated in several large studies. Until recently, no instrument was available to efficiently monitor the healing of pressure ulcers. The PUSH tool is simple to use and monitors three parameters that best describe healing (i.e., wound size, amount of exudate and tissue type) at regular intervals. Scoring helps determine the need for careful reassessment of the both pressure ulcer and the patient's condition.[12]

Wound Healing

Sholar and Stadlemann[35] describe wound healing as the result of multiple processes that overlap into three phases (i.e., inflammatory, proliferative, and maturation phases). Wound infection is probably the most common cause of poor pressure ulcer healing. Although all open wounds have some degree of bacterial contamination, the size of the bacterial inoculum, as well as host immune defenses, determine whether infection sets in. Adequate debridement in patients with normal host defense mechanisms is essential to healing, even in the face of a high bacterial burden. Malnutrition limits neovascularization and fibroblast proliferation, as well as humoral and cellular immune response. Provision of adequate protein is essential for the healing of cutaneous wounds.

NSAIDs interfere with the arachidonic cascade necessary for healing. Steroids suppress inflammation and impair healing. If these medicines must be used, pressure ulcer prevention measures should be intensified.[35]

Pain Management

The Joint Commission on Accreditation of Healthcare Organizations (JCAHO) has designated pain as the fifth vital sign. Persistent pain may afflict 45% to 80% of long-term care patients. Similar to conditions such as arthritis, previous fracture sites, and neuropathies, pressure ulcers can also result in considerable pain.[36] Dallam et al.[37] reported that only 2% of patients reporting pain from pressure ulcers were receiving analgesics. The degree of pain was found to correlate with the stage of a pressure ulcer. More recently, Won et al.[38] reported that 25% of nursing home patients with persistent pain received no analgesics. Often there was inadequate compliance with geriatric prescribing recommendations.[38]

Many patients with pressure ulcers are unable to express the extent of pain they are experiencing. Obviously, the pain should be eliminated to the extent possible. Sometimes, simultaneous interventions are necessary; for example, a combination of repositioning, covering the pressure ulcer, and systemic analgesia may be needed for pressure ulcer relief.

Mental Status

Mental status evaluation of patients is important in determining pressure ulcer risk, especially in those who are sedated or have mobility limitations. Patients with impaired mentation may be unable to change positions, perceive discomfort from pain, move spontaneously, be motivated to move, remember to move, or become educated about their condition. Care providers should be alert to these limitations and intensify appropriate corrective and preventative measures. (Adapted from Maklebust J, Sieggreen M. *Pressure ulcers: Guidelines for prevention and management,* 3rd ed. Springhouse, PA: Springhouse Corporation; 2001.)

Restraints

The Omnibus Reconciliation Act of 1987 (OBRA-87) stated that a nursing home patient has the right to be free from physical and chemical restraints if used for staff convenience or disciplinary reasons and if not needed to treat the patient's medical disorder. OBRA-87s explicit goal for this reform is to allow nursing home patients to attain the highest practical physical, mental, and psychological well-being. Decreased use of restraints, both physical and chemical, can reduce the incidence of pressure ulcer and other complications that have been associated with restraint use.[39]

Support Surfaces

Evidence has shown that specially designed surfaces effectively prevent pressure ulcer development in high-risk patients. Revis[40] noted that specialized support surfaces, available for beds and wheelchairs, can maintain tissues at pressures <32 mm Hg. Specialized surfaces include foam devices, air-filled devices, and low–air-loss beds. Regardless of the choice of support surface, turning and repositioning the patient remain the cornerstones for pressure ulcer prevention and treatment.[40]

Ayello and Braden[41] have recommended that in high-risk patients consideration should be given to increased turning frequency and provision of pressure-reducing support surfaces. For those at very high risk, in addition to increased frequency of turning, a pressure-relieving surface may be used, especially in patients with intractable pain and pain on turning, as well as for immobilized or malnourished patients. Again, a specialty bed should not be considered a substitute for an appropriate turning schedule.[41] Select characteristics of classes of support surfaces, as summarized by the A94 treatment panel, are shown in Table 37.5.

Debridement

Debridement is the removal of devitalized tissue and foreign matter from wounds such as pressure ulcers. Several methods have been used for this purpose (Adapted from A94):

1. *Autolytic debridement:* The use of synthetic dressings to cover a pressure ulcer and allow eschar to self-digest by the action of enzymes present in wound fluids.
2. *Enzymatic or chemical debridement:* The topical application of proteolytic enzymes to break down devitalized tissue.
3. *Mechanical debridement:* The removal of foreign material and devitalized or contaminated tissue from a pressure ulcer by physical forces rather than by chemical (enzymatic) or natural (autolytic) forces. Examples include wet-to-dry dressings, pressure ulcer irrigation, whirlpool, and dextranomers. The latter (dextranomers) are highly hydrophilic dextran-polymer beads that are poured into secreting pressure ulcers to absorb wound exudates and act as a debriding agent.

TABLE 37.5
SUPPORT DEVICES

Performance Characteristics	Air-Fluidized	Low–Air-Loss	Alternating Air	Static Flotation (Air or Water)	Foam	Standard Mattress
Increased support area	Yes	Yes	Yes	Yes	Yes	No
Low moisture retention	Yes	Yes	No	No	No	No
Reduced heat accumulation	Yes	Yes	No	No	No	No
Shear reduction	Yes	?	Yes	Yes	No	No
Pressure reduction	Yes	Yes	Yes	Yes	Yes	No
Dynamic area	Yes	Yes	Yes	No	No	No
Cost per day	High	High	Moderate	Low	Low	Low

Reprinted from Bergstrom N, Bennett MA, Carlson CE, et al. *Treatment of pressure ulcers.* Clinical Practice Guideline No. 15. Rockville, MD: U.S. Department of Health and Human Services. Public Health Service, Agency for Health Care Policy and Research, AHCPR Publication No. 95–0652. December, 1994.

4. *Sharp debridement:* The removal of foreign material or devitalized tissue by a sharp instrument such as a scalpel. Laser debridement is also considered a type of sharp debridement.

Dressings

Dressings are materials applied to a pressure ulcer, for both wound protection and absorption of drainage. The A94 panel described the following types of dressings:

- *Alginate dressing.* A nonwoven absorptive dressing made from seaweed.
- *Film dressing.* A clear, adherent, nonabsorptive, polymer-based dressing that is permeable to both oxygen and water vapor but not to water.
- *Foam dressing.* A sponge-like polymer dressing that may or may not be adherent; it may be impregnated or coated with other materials and has absorptive properties.
- *Gauze dressing.* A cotton or synthetic fabric dressing that is absorptive and permeable to water, water vapor, and oxygen; gauze dressings may be impregnated with petrolatum, antiseptics, or other agents:
  - *Wet-to-dry saline gauze.* A dressing technique in which gauze moistened with normal saline is applied wet to the pressure ulcer and removed once the gauze becomes dry and adheres to the wound bed.
  - *Continuously moist saline gauze.* A dressing technique in which gauze moistened with normal saline is applied to the pressure ulcer and remoistened often enough to remain moist. Its goal is to maintain a continuously moist pressure ulcer environment.
- *Hydrocolloid dressing.* An adhesive, moldable wafer made from a carbohydrate-based material, usually with a waterproof backing. This dressing is usually impermeable to oxygen, water, and water vapor and has absorptive properties.
- *Hydrogel dressing.* A water-based, nonadherent, polymer-based dressing having absorptive properties.
- *Pastes/powders/beads.* Agents formulated primarily to fill pressure ulcer cavities and which may have some absorptive properties. (Adapted from A94)

Medications

Drugs that can cause excess sedation, such as long-acting benzodiazepines and muscle relaxants, should generally be avoided in elderly patients. Also, all barbiturates (except phenobarital when used for seizure control), as well as sedating antihistamines, such as diphenhydramine, hydroxyzine, and cyproheptadine, are potentially dangerous because they may contribute to sedation and worsen dementia. The analgesic activity of propoxyphene (Darvon) is little more than that of acetaminophen and it carries potential narcotic adverse effects caused by its many active metabolites. These drugs can cause oversedation, decreased mobility, falls resulting in hip fractures, and increased pressure ulcer development.[42]

Nutrition

There is a strong association between nutrition and skin integrity.[43] Nutrition is an essential host factor for pressure ulcer healing, and the importance of dietary protein in the healing process cannot be overemphasized.[11] Hypoproteinemia and anemia decrease oxygen supply to the skin, and dehydration results in dry, fragile skin.

Early recognition and treatment of involuntary weight loss and protein energy malnutrition are of critical importance in both preventing and treating chronic wounds of all types. A decreased lean muscle mass will not only augment pressure ulcer development but also diminish healing. Open pressure ulcers perpetuate catabolism and exude proteins, further impairing nutrition and retarding healing.[44]

Dehydration

Dehydration is potentially life-threatening and is associated with increased propensity to develop pressure ulcers. It can also negatively impact healing. Among the many conditions associated with dehydration are febrile illnesses, diarrhea, vomiting, poorly controlled diabetes, and fluid restrictions, as well as diuretic and laxative use. Patients with mental impairment, cerebral vascular accidents (CVAs), and arthritis and those who are sedated often require assistance with eating and drinking. Patients with dysphagia should be evaluated by speech therapists.[45]

Surgery

Sorenson et al. of the Copenhagen Wound Healing Center recently discussed the surgical treatment of pressure ulcers.[46] The authors noted that most patients with Stages I and II pressure ulcers would likely benefit from more conservative treatment, whereas patients with Stages III and, especially, IV pressure ulcers might require surgery. The authors described various types of flaps and skin grafting and noted that thorough debridement before reconstruction, as well as control of underlying disease, quality postoperative support, and sufficient pressure relief, were mandatory for successful treatment of pressure ulcers.[46]

CONCLUSION

It is well established that pressure ulcers and their associated morbidity and mortality are, to a great extent, preventable. Even if a pressure ulcer develops, with appropriate care it need not progress. Unfortunately, despite excellent guidelines for both prevention and treatment of pressure ulcers, health workers responsible for caring for at-risk patients are often either unaware of the AHRQ recommendations or fail to consistently adhere to them. The societal costs, both economically and in terms of human suffering, are immeasurable. By using the AHRQ guidelines[1,2] that have been discussed in detail in this chapter, as well as recommendations offered by organizations such as NPUAP,[8,12] WOCN,[4] and AMDA,[13] physicians caring for the elderly should be much better prepared to cope with this potentially devastating disorder.

REFERENCES

1. Bergstrom N, Allman RM, Carlson CE, et al. *Pressure ulcers in adults: Prediction and prevention.* Clinical Practice Guidelines No. 3., Rockville, MD. U.S. Department of Health and Human Services. Agency for Health Care Policy and Research, AHCPR Publication No. 92-0047. May, 1992.
2. Bergstrom N, Bennett MA, Carlson CE, et al. *Treatment of pressure ulcers.* Clinical Practice Guideline No. 15. Rockville, MD: U.S. Department of Health and Human Services. Public Health Service, Agency for Health Care Policy and Research, AHCPR Publication No. 95-0652. December, 1994.
3. O'Neil C. Prevention and treatment of pressure ulcers. *J Pharm Pract.* 2004;17(2):137–148.
4. Wound, Ostomy and Continence Nurses Society (WOCN). *Guidelines for prevention and management of pressure ulcers.* Glenview, IL: 2003.
5. Lyder CH. Pressure ulcer prevention and management.. *JAMA.* 2003;289(2):223–226.
6. Xakellis GC, Frantz RA. The cost-effectiveness of interventions for preventing pressure ulcers. *J Am Board Fam Pract.* 1996;9(2):79–85.
7. Braden B., Bergstrom N. www.bradenscale.com; 1988.
8. National Pressure Ulcer Advisory Panel (NPUAP). Cuddigan, J, Ayello EA, Sussman C. *Pressure ulcers in America: Prevalence, incidence, and implications for the future.* Reston, VA: NPUAP; 2001.
9. www.spanamerica.com/main_med_glossary.html.
10. Maklebust J, Sieggreen M. *Pressure ulcers: Guidelines for prevention and management,* 3rd ed. Springhouse, PA: Springhouse Corporation; 2001.
11. Tomas. www.eMedicine.com; 2001.
12. National Pressure Ulcer Advisory Panel(NPUAP). *NPUAP position on reverse staging of pressure ulcers, in Advanced Wound Care,* Vol. 8. 1998:32.
13. American Medical Directors Association (AMDA). *Pressure ulcers: Clinical practice guidelines,* 1996.
14. Ferguson M, Cook A, Rimmasch H, et al. Pressure ulcer management: The importance of nutrition. *Med Surg Nurs.* 2000;9(4):163–175, quiz 176–177.
15. Kosiak, M, Prevention and rehabilitation of pressure ulcers. *Decubitus.* 1991;4(2):60–62,64,66, passim.
16. Olshansky K. Essay on knowledge, caring, and psychological factors in prevention and treatment of pressure ulcers. *Adv Wound Care.* 1994;7(3):64–68.
17. Levine JM, Totolos E. Pressure ulcers: A strategic plan to prevent and heal them. *Geriatrics.* 1995;50(1):32–37, quiz 38–39.
18. Brem H, Lyder C. Protocol for the successful treatment of pressure ulcers. *Am J Surg.* 2004;188(Suppl 1A):9–17.
19. Rothschild JM, Bates DW, Leape LL. Preventable medical injuries in older patients. *Arch Intern Med.* 2000;160(18):2717–2728.
20. Horn SD, Bender SA, Fergusson ML, et al. The National Pressure Ulcer Long-Term Care Study: Pressure ulcer development in long-term care residents. *J Am Geriatr Soc.* 2004;52(3):359–367.
21. Parish, LC, Witkowski JA, Crissey JT, et al. *The decubitus ulcer: Year book medical publishers,* Chicago, IL: 1983:39.
22. American Medical Directors Association (AMDA). *Pressure ulcer therapy companion: Clinical practice guideline.* Columbia, MD: (available at: www.amda.com); 1999.
23. Kimura S, Pacala JT. Pressure ulcers in adults: Family physicians' knowledge, attitudes, practice preferences, and awareness of AHCPR guidelines. *J Fam Pract.* 1997;44(4):361–368.
24. O'Brien D, Beity J, Fey J. Perceived need for education vs. actual knowledge of pressure ulcer care in a hospital nursing staff. *Dermatol Nurs.* 1999;11(2):125–128.
25. Department of Health & Human Services. www.hhs.gov/news/press/2004pres/20041222.html; 2004.
26. Healthy People 2010. Objective 1–16. In: *Healthy people 2010; January 2000;* Washington DC: U.S. Department of Health and Human Services; 2000.
27. Shepard MA, Parker D, DeClercque N. The under-reporting of pressure sores in patients transferred between hospital and nursing home. *J Am Geriatr Soc.* 1987;35(2):159–160.
28. Bennett RG, O'Sullivan J, De Vito EM, et al. The increasing medical malpractice risk related to pressure ulcers in the United States. *J Am Geriatr Soc.* 2000;48(1):73–81.
29. Agostini JV, Baker DI, Bogardus ST, et al. *Prevention of pressure ulcers in older patients: Chapter 27.* Web address: www.ahcpr.gov/clinic/pfsafety/chap27.htm; 2001.
30. ECRI. www.guideline.gov/summary/sumary.aspx?doc_id=810&nabr=8&string=pressure; 1998.
31. ECRI. www.guideline.gov/summary/sumary.aspx?doc_id=810&nabr=8&string=pressure; 2001.
32. Cervo FA, Cruz AC, Posillico JA. Pressure ulcers. Analysis of guidelines for treatment and management. *Geriatrics.* 2000; 55(3):55–60, quiz 62.
33. Shekelle PG, Ortiz E, Rhodes S, et al. Validity of the Agency for Healthcare Research and Quality clinical practice guidelines: How quickly do guidelines become outdated? *JAMA.* 2001; 286(12):1461–1467.
34. Ortiz, O, Eccles M, Grimshaw J, et al. *Current validity of clinical practice guidelines. Technical Review 6 (Contract No. 290-97-0001 to the Southern California Evidence-based Practice Center at RAND).* AHRQ Publication No. 02–0035, Rockville, MD: Agency for Healthcare Research and Quality; 2002.
35. Sholar AC, Stadlemann W. *Wound Healing, Chronic Wounds.* Available at: www.emedicine.com/plastic/topic477.htm, 2003.
36. Frampton KK. *Vital Sign #5: Pain assessment and management in LTC requires a thorough, team-oriented care plan, in caring for the ages.* 2004:26–35.
37. Dallam L, Smyth C, Jackson BS, et al. Pressure ulcer pain: Assessment and quantification. *J Wound Ostomy Continence Nurs.* 1995;22(5):211–215, discussion 217–218.
38. Won AB, Lapane KL, Vallow S, et al. Persistent nonmalignant pain and analgesic prescribing patterns in elderly nursing home residents. *J Am Geriatr Soc.* 2004;52(6):867–874.
39. Winzelberg GS. The quest for nursing home quality: Learning history's lessons. *Arch Intern Med.* 2003;163(21):2552–2556.
40. Revis DR. *Decubitus ulcers.* (Available at: www.emedicine.com/med/topic2709.htm); 2004.
41. Ayello EA, Braden B. *Advances in skin wound care.* May-June. Vol. 15(3), 2002:125–131.
42. Fick DM, et al. Updating the Beers criteria for potentially inappropriate medication use in older adults: Results of a US consensus panel of experts. *Arch Intern Med.* 2003;163(22):2716–2724.
43. Gibbon RB, *Nutritional aspects of wound management, in Home Health Care Consultant.* 2000:19–22.
44. Demling R. *Nutrition and wound healing,* Wayne, PA: HMP Communication; Vol. 13(4): Supplement D, July/August; 2001: 3D–21D.
45. Hoffman NB. Dehydration in the elderly: Insidious and manageable. *Geriatrics.* 1991;46(6):35–38.
46. Sorensen JL, Jorgensen B, Gottrup F. Surgical treatment of pressure ulcers. *Am J Surg.* 2004;188(Suppl 1A):42–51.

Neoplastic Disease

38

Kenneth G. Schellhase

CLINICAL PEARLS 530
Prevention 530
Screening 530
Survivors 531

BURDEN OF CANCER IN THE ELDERLY 531

CANCER-RELATED CARE AS PART OF PRIMARY CARE 531

CHAPTER GOALS AND STRUCTURE 531

PRIMARY PREVENTION OF CANCER 532
Lung Cancer and Smoking Cessation 532
Skin Cancer and Limiting Sun Exposure 533
Diet, Obesity, and Cancer Risk 533
Environmental Hazards 533
Chemoprevention of Cancer 533

SECONDARY PREVENTION: SCREENING FOR CANCER 534
Criteria for Appropriate Screening 534
Inappropriate Screening 534
Cancer Screening in Geriatric Patients: Special Considerations 534
Selected Cancer Screening Recommendations 537
Breast Cancer Screening 537
Cervical Cancer Screening 537
Colorectal Cancer Screening 537
Prostate Cancer Screening 539
Screening for Other Selected Cancers 539

ROUTINE CARE OF THE CANCER SURVIVOR 539
The Cancer Survivorship Phenomenon 539
Cancer Survivorship Model 540
Surveillance Care Guidelines 541
Breast Cancer Surveillance 541
Prostate Cancer Surveillance 541
Colorectal Cancer Surveillance 543

PREVENTIVE CARE AND HEALTH MAINTENANCE IN CANCER SURVIVORS 545

CLINICAL PEARLS

Prevention

- Few interventions other than smoking cessation are known to be effective for cancer prevention.
- Most cancer prevention studies are performed in younger populations. Caution should be used when generalizing these results to older populations.
- While evidence of an association is strong, a causal link between obesity and cancer risk has not been established nor is there evidence that weight loss will reduce cancer risk.
- Residential radon exposure is an overlooked environmental health risk.
- The US Surgeon General estimates that within 10 years of quitting smoking the risk of lung cancer is reduced to half that of a current smoker.

Screening

- Evidence regarding the benefit of screening interventions should be held to a high standard.
- Screening in the geriatric patient requires balancing life expectancy with the anticipated benefits and risks of screening.
- Randomized trials suggest that it takes at least 5 years before there is a mortality benefit from screening tests.
- For most cancers, we lack clear evidence about when to stop screening.

- There continue to be multiple acceptable options for colorectal cancer screening.
- Despite the high mortality burden of lung and ovarian cancers, routine screening for these diseases is still not recommended.

Survivors

- There are roughly 10 million cancer survivors in the United States today, triple the number from 30 years ago.
- Most cancer survivors are elderly.
- Primary care physicians can, and should, provide routine cancer survivor care for their patients.
- Most cancer surveillance regimens are fairly straightforward.
- Guidelines for common cancers can help primary care physicians provide appropriate routine follow-up testing in cancer survivors.

BURDEN OF CANCER IN THE ELDERLY

Despite advances in prevention, detection, and treatment, cancer is still an enormous health burden in the United States, and this burden is particularly heavy for the elderly. Table 38.1 shows the incidence and mortality rates, as well as ICD-9 codes, for a number of cancers common in the elderly. More than half of all new cancer diagnoses are in patients older than 65. Cancer is the most common cause of death for both men and women aged 60 to 79, and the second leading cause of death in patients aged 80 and older.[1] Additionally, the word "cancer" evokes a special dread (and among some, still a certain stigma) like few other diseases. Consequently, the very discussion of cancer can have important emotional dimensions for our patients, which we should not underestimate.

CANCER-RELATED CARE AS PART OF PRIMARY CARE

Primary care physicians have a critical role to play in providing cancer-related care throughout the lifespan of their geriatric patients. To provide some perspective, Figure 38.1 depicts the cancer care continuum. The continuum starts with the prevention and screening/symptom phases, comprising typical primary care services that are of an indefinite and continuous duration. These services include primary prevention of cancer, cancer screening, and evaluation of presenting symptoms. If cancer is detected by screenings or symptoms, patients move from this continuity model to the acute-care model of the diagnosis phase, where definitive diagnostic maneuvers may be performed by primary or specialty physicians, depending on the particular cancer. Patients then move to the treatment phase. The treatment phase is characterized by episodic care, with a duration usually measured only in months. In this phase, the treatment of cancer by surgery, chemotherapy, or radiation therapy is typically managed by specialists, with the exception of certain skin cancers. After treatment, patients enter the survivorship phase, another period of indefinite duration where the continuity-based follow-up care provided to cancer survivors takes the form of chronic disease care. In addition to showing the importance of primary care physicians in the cancer-related care of the geriatric patient with cancer, Figure 38.1 shows that care uniquely provided by cancer-related specialists occupies a critical, although relatively brief, period in the cancer care continuum.

CHAPTER GOALS AND STRUCTURE

The goal of this chapter is to guide primary care physicians in caring for patients in the three main parts of the cancer

TABLE 38.1
COMMON MALIGNANCIES IN THE GERIATRIC POPULATION (>65 Y)

Cancer Site	Incidence[a]	Mortality[a]	ICD-9 Codes
Prostate	940.9	33.9	185.0
Breast (female)	416.7	30.9	174.0–174.9
Colon and rectum	332.2	25.0	153.0–154.8
Lung/bronchus	319.5	52.5	162.0–162.9
Bladder	115.8	4.8	188.0–188.7
Uterus/corpus	97.0	4.7	182.0–182.8
Non-Hodgkin lymphoma	72.3	7.3	200.0–200.8, 202.0–202.2, 202.8–202.9
Pancreas	64.5	10.7	157.0–157.9
Leukemia	59.4	8.0	204.0–208.9
Stomach	53.2	6.5	151.0–151.9
Ovary	52.9	9.4	183.0–183.9
Oral cavity/pharynx	46.0	3.6	141.0–146.9

[a]Age-adjusted rate per 100,000 population.

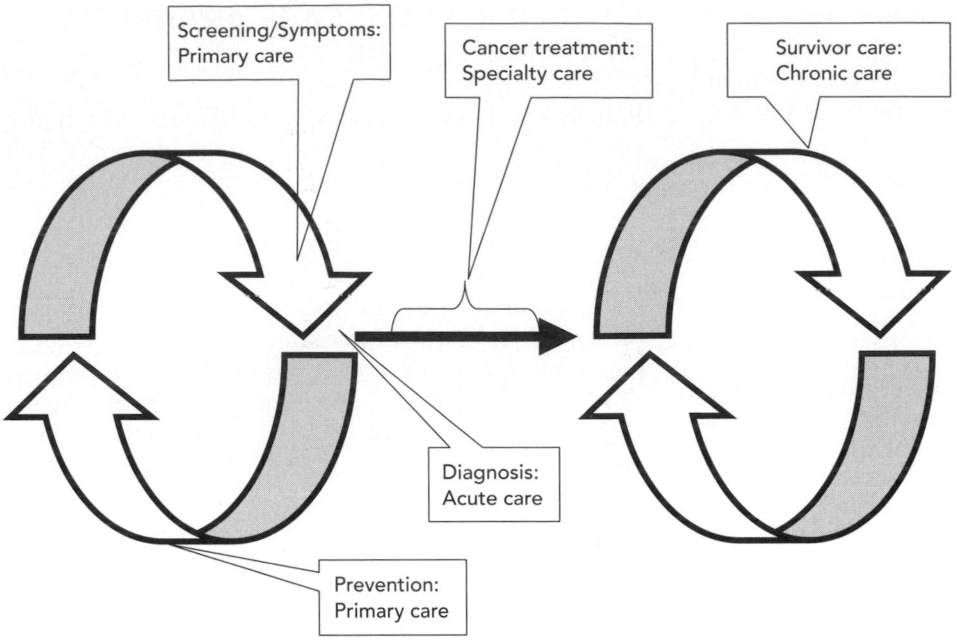

Figure 38.1 Cancer continuum.

care continuum in Figure 38.1: (i) Cancer prevention services, (ii) cancer screening services, and (iii) routine care of the cancer survivor. Therefore, the section "Primary Prevention of Cancer" focuses on effective interventions that may reduce the risk of getting cancer. The section "Secondary Prevention: Screening for Cancer" presents evidence-based recommendations for prevention and screening services for common cancers, with consideration given to the appropriate use of screening in elderly populations with limited life expectancy. The section "Routine Care of the Cancer Survivor" is an acknowledgment of the relatively recent phenomenon of tremendous growth in the number of cancer survivors, most of whom are elderly. This section examines the role of the primary care physician in the care of the cancer survivor in the context of a chronic disease model and presents recommendations for routine follow-up care of survivors of common cancers.[1,2]

Clinical issues surrounding the workup, diagnosis, or treatment of cancer will not be addressed in this chapter. Although many primary care physicians will work up and definitively diagnose cancer, these broad areas are beyond the scope of this text. Additionally, while many generalist physicians may feel comfortable with the initial management of potential cancer recurrence as well as late effects and complications of treatment, these areas are also beyond the scope of this chapter.

PRIMARY PREVENTION OF CANCER

Most studies of the primary prevention of cancer, whether by lifestyle interventions, chemoprevention or other means, focus on nongeriatric populations. The rationale for this is simple: Younger populations are thought to be more likely to benefit because these preventive interventions will take years to have an impact on cancer risk. Carcinogenesis is thought to start slowly, many years before clinically evident cancer is noted. In other words, if an 80-year-old smoker does not have some smoking-related cancer, getting him to stop smoking is not likely to have a large impact on his risk of dying from cancer. Therefore, the evidence of any benefit for the primary prevention of cancer will be limited for the elderly. However, our patients still come to us wanting to know what they can do to decrease their risk of cancer. The following discussion reviews the potential benefit of common cancer prevention interventions.

Lung Cancer and Smoking Cessation

Cigarette smoking is the greatest preventable cause of disease in the United States, most notably leading to increased risk of death from lung and many other cancers and to increased risk of heart disease (Evidence Level A). Lung cancer is by far the leading cause of cancer death in both men (32% of all cancer deaths in 2004) and women (25% of all cancer deaths in 2004), with a dismal 15% overall 5-year survival rate.[1] In addition, there is evidence that exposure to secondhand cigarette smoking also increases cancer risk. Although nicotine is highly addictive, there are effective methods to aid patients with smoking cessation, including nicotine replacement, antidepressant medications, and behavioral interventions.[3] Recently, Medicare adopted a policy to reimburse physicians for smoking cessation counseling for Medicare enrollees who currently smoke and have a smoking-related illness. The sooner patients accomplish and sustain smoking cessation, the sooner they will accrue the health benefits of having stopped smoking. The US

Surgeon General estimates that the risk of lung cancer is reduced to half that of a current smoker within 10 years of quitting.[4] The time lag until health benefits accrue to recipients of secondhand smoke is unknown.

Skin Cancer and Limiting Sun Exposure

Skin cancer is the most common form of neoplasm in the United States, with over 1 million cases annually.[5] In 2004, melanoma was expected to account for 55,000 skin cancers and nearly 8,000 deaths.[1] Mortality from other forms of skin cancer is rare, although given the generally high incidence of skin cancer, the overall burden of suffering from these other forms is substantial. There is limited evidence suggesting that significant sun exposure early in life is associated with increased risk of skin cancer in adulthood and that counseling to limit sun exposure may be effective at reducing ultraviolet light exposure. However, there is no direct evidence linking interventions to limit ultraviolet light exposure (e.g., protective clothing or sunscreen) with decreased skin cancer incidence or death. Patients may nonetheless be motivated to limit sun exposure given the possibility of benefit, lack of harm, and concerns about premature aging of the skin from extensive exposure (Evidence Level C).

Diet, Obesity, and Cancer Risk

The evidence supporting a link between high fruit and vegetable consumption and decreased risk of cancer has been conflicting, with early reports suggesting benefit, but more recent research indicating less-certain effects on risk. Despite uncertain benefits, some professional organizations endorse fruit and vegetable consumption as a way to lower cancer risk[5] (Evidence Level C). However, these diets may be recommended in elderly patients on other clinical grounds (e.g., part of a balanced diet, prevention of constipation, beneficial effects on lipids from fiber), and in moderation, there is little risk of harm for the typical patient.

Emerging literature now links obesity to increased risk of several types of cancer[6] (Evidence Level B). To date, this evidence comes only from observational studies, so thus far obesity has not been shown to be causally related to cancer risk. It has also not been shown that interventions in obese individuals that decrease body weight result in reduced cancer risk. Therefore, we clearly lack the evidence at this time to recommend weight loss to patients as a means to reduce cancer risk. However, there are numerous other clinical grounds on which to recommend maintaining healthy body weight.

Environmental Hazards

There are ubiquitous environmental hazards—other than secondhand smoke—that may contribute to cancer risk, although most environmental health issues have historically been addressed at the level of the public health system. Patients at particular risk for environmental exposures, such as asbestos, can usually be identified through obtaining careful social and occupational histories. However, one environmental health issue that is often overlooked, yet appropriately addressed at the level of the individual patient, is ionizing radiation from residential radon gas exposure. Radon is the second leading cause of lung cancer, after cigarette smoking, and is estimated to cause 5% to 10% of lung cancers in the United States (Evidence Level B). Radon results from the natural radioactive decay of uranium in the soil, and its exposure occurs most commonly in the basement level of private homes through small foundation cracks. High soil radon levels are more common in the upper Midwest of the United States but can occur anywhere. Residential radon exposure has been shown in multiple meta-analyses to be correlated with increased lung cancer risk.[7] The Environmental Protection Agency (www.epa.gov) offers detailed advice to homeowners on how to test for and correct problems with radon gas. Currently, there is no evidence that radon abatement programs will reduce lung cancer risk.

Chemoprevention of Cancer

The possibility of chemoprevention of cancer through the use of vitamin supplements or a number of pharmaceuticals (e.g., aspirin) has received significant attention in recent years. Despite a number of large observational studies of various chemopreventive agents showing an association between the intake of these substances and reduced cancer risk, no consistent evidence has emerged from randomized trials that would support recommending chemoprevention for the primary prevention of cancer in average-risk patients (Evidence Level B). Indeed, the U.S. Preventive Services Task Force (USPSTF) has recently recommended against the use of β-carotene for cancer prevention owing to the evidence of increased lung cancer risk in heavy smokers using this supplement.[3]

There has been some preliminary evidence from observational studies suggesting a role for both cyclo-oxygenase-2 (COX-2) inhibitors and 3-hydroxy-3-methylglutaryl coenzyme A reductase inhibitors (statins) in cancer prevention[8,9] (Evidence Level B). Randomized cancer prevention trials of these agents may take place in the near future, although in the case of COX-2 inhibitors, this may depend on further clarification of cardiovascular risks. Nevertheless, it is critical for physicians to bear in mind the higher standards of evidence demanded by the ethical foundations of screening and prevention (discussed in the section "Secondary Prevention: Screening for Cancer") before prescribing or endorsing such preventive interventions.

While the USPSTF has recommended against using tamoxifen for chemoprevention in women at average risk for breast cancer, there may be a role for this drug as primary prevention in women at high risk for breast cancer, as indicated by family history or genetic testing

(Evidence Level B). However, given the higher risk of thromboembolic events and other harms or adverse effects in geriatric patients, the risks of tamoxifen use for primary prevention are likely to outweigh the expected benefits in this age-group.[10] Consequently, any decision to use tamoxifen as primary breast cancer prevention in geriatric patients should not be pursued without prior consultation with an oncologist and thorough consideration of the particular patient.

SECONDARY PREVENTION: SCREENING FOR CANCER

Criteria for Appropriate Screening

Screening for cancer—the attempt to find preclinical disease in asymptomatic patients—has long been central to providing primary care services to geriatric patients. Because virtually any test could be used as a screening test, general criteria have been developed by clinical epidemiologists to guide the appropriate use of screening tests; these criteria can be applied to potential cancer screening tests as well as for other disease screening. As summarized in Table 38.2, when employing screening tests, we must consider disease factors such as prevalence and burden of illness, patient factors such as the willingness to undergo testing, test factors such as accuracy of results, and social factors such as cost-effectiveness.

All these domains must be considered in determining whether to recommend screening (or preventive interventions) on a population basis. Often, the most difficult criterion for which direct evidence needs to be established is the requirement that treatment of patients with screen-detected disease must lead to better outcomes than treatment of patients with clinically detected disease. Apart from this, there is no justification to expose patients to the risks that are inherent in any screening program. This is critical to remember because the ethical foundation for screening and preventive interventions differs from the ethical foundation of "traditional" medical care composed of diagnosis and treatment, and this difference demands a higher standard of evidence demonstrating the benefit of screening tests.[11] Reasons for this include the following: (a) Most screened patients will not benefit from screening, (b) most patients suffering harm from screening will never benefit from it, and (c) historically, screening has occurred because it has been advocated by physicians and not sought by patients.

TABLE 38.2
CRITERIA FOR APPROPRIATE SCREENING

1. Disease must be sufficiently prevalent
2. Morbidity and mortality must be of sufficient concern to public health
3. Test must be sufficiently sensitive and specific
4. Test must be safe and acceptable to patients
5. Diagnostic workup for a positive screen must be acceptable given the number of false positives (risk of harm must be minimal)
6. Treatment of screen-detected disease must improve outcomes
7. Screening must be relatively cost effective compared to other accepted clinical preventive services

Inappropriate Screening

Many physicians have had at least one patient who has elected to undergo helical (low-dose) computed tomography (CT) scanning for lung cancer screening or possibly even the "whole body" CT scan or magnetic resonance imaging that is typically performed at free-standing for-profit imaging centers in major metropolitan areas. While lung cancer screening through helical CT scan does hold legitimate promise as an appropriate screening test, the evidence of its beneficial effect on lung cancer mortality is still very preliminary, and the magnitude of potential harms ensuing from false-positive workups should not be underestimated. Large National Institute of Health–sponsored clinical trials currently under way may provide the needed evidence. In the absence of this evidence, patients should be encouraged to enroll in clinical screening trials but to otherwise refrain from self-referral for these services. Indeed, the use of full-body CT screening is a clear-cut example of inappropriate screening. There is no current evidence of its benefit to patients and there are no large clinical screening trials under way; yet there is evidence of harm to patients from this screening modality.[12]

Cancer Screening in Geriatric Patients: Special Considerations

Most of the large, well-designed studies of screening efficacy that provide support to current cancer screening recommendations (e.g., breast cancer, colorectal cancer) were performed in populations with middle-aged to "young" elderly patients up to around age 70. Yet these patients continue to seek and receive cancer screening well beyond the age for which we have good supporting data. In general terms, one would expect the benefits of screening to decline with advancing age for at least three reasons:[13]

1. Tumors tend to be less aggressive in older patients, so these patients are more likely to die from other comorbid conditions (e.g., cardiovascular disease) rather than from cancer.
2. Increasing comorbidity and frailness from advancing age may make the diagnostic workup for a positive screen fraught with risk, or the rigors and side effects of definitive treatment may become unacceptable.
3. The potential harms of screening weigh more heavily, in view of points 1 and 2.

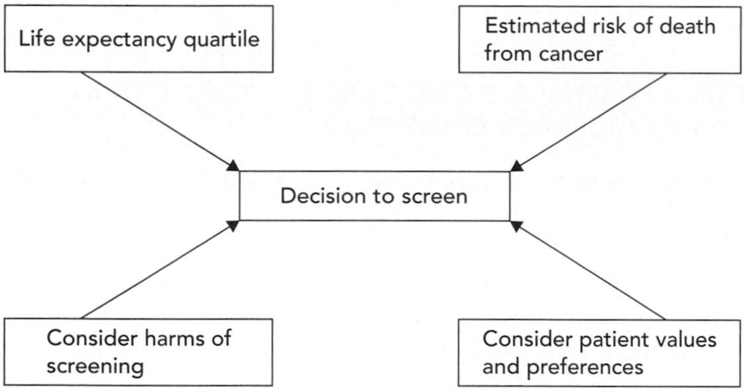

Figure 38.2 Individualized cancer screening in the elderly. (Based on: Walter LC, Covinsky KE. Cancer screening in elderly patients: A framework for individualized decision making. *JAMA.* 2001;285(21):2750–2756.).

However, because overall cancer incidence rises with increasing age, the predictive value of a positive screen is greater—that is, a positive screen is more likely to represent real disease. Further, we see increasing numbers of surprisingly healthy patients in their eighties and beyond, which complicates generic recommendations about the correct age at which cancer screening must be stopped. Given these competing considerations, Walter and Covinsky have proposed a conceptual framework to help individualize decisions about screening in elderly patients.[14] Summarized in Figure 38.2, this framework includes quantitative assessments based on life expectancy and estimates of risk reduction from screening that must be blended with qualitative judgments about potential harms of screening and patient preferences, in order to arrive at a more informed, individualized decision about whether to proceed with screening.

For the reader's convenience, quantitative estimates of life expectancy and likelihood of benefit from screening tests are reproduced from the Walter and Covinsky article, and shown in Tables 38.3 and 38.4 respectively. Life expectancy data were generated from standard US life tables and are expressed in tertiles of high, medium, and low. Risk of dying from a given cancer was determined from the National Cancer Institute's Surveillance, Epidemiology, and End Results (SEER) cancer registry data. The authors

TABLE 38.3

RISK (PERCENTAGE) OF DYING FROM CANCER IN REMAINING LIFETIME FOR MEN AND WOMEN AT SELECTED AGES AND LIFE EXPECTANCY QUARTILES[a]

	Age 50 (y)			Age 70 (y)			Age 75 (y)			Age 80 (y)			Age 85 (y)			Age 90 (y)		
	Life Expectancy of Women (y)																	
	40	**33**	**24.5**	**21.3**	**15.7**	**9.5**	**17**	**11.9**	**6.8**	**13**	**8.6**	**4.6**	**9.6**	**5.9**	**2.9**	**6.8**	**3.9**	**1.8**
Cancer																		
Breast	4.4	3.1	2.0	3.3	2.2	1.2	2.8	1.8	0.9	2.4	1.5	0.7	1.9	1.2	0.6	1.4	0.8	0.4
Colorectal	3.8	2.2	1.0	3.5	2.0	0.9	3.3	1.9	0.9	3.0	1.8	0.8	2.5	1.6	0.8	1.8	1.0	0.5
Cervical	0.34	0.26	0.18	0.22	0.15	0.08	0.19	0.12	0.07	0.15	0.10	0.05	0.12	0.07	0.04	0.08	0.05	0.02
	Life Expectancy of Men (y)																	
	36	**28.5**	**19.6**	**18**	**12.4**	**6.7**	**14.2**	**9.3**	**4.9**	**10.8**	**6.7**	**3.3**	**7.9**	**4.7**	**2.2**	**5.8**	**3.2**	**1.5**
Cancer																		
Colorectal	4.1	2.3	1.0	3.8	2.1	0.9	3.5	1.9	0.8	3.2	1.8	0.8	2.7	1.6	0.8	2.0	1.1	0.5

[a]Life expectancy quartiles correspond to upper, middle, and lower quartiles as presented in the Figure. Data are presented as percentages. Risks for 50-year-old patients are included for comparison. Risks were calculated by multiplying life expectancy by age-specific cancer mortality rates from Surveillance, Epidemiology, and End Results (SEER) *Cancer Statistics Review 1973–1996*. Since cancer screening in the United States among elderly patients remains low, these cancer mortality risks approximate those expected for patients who have not received regular cancer screeing. For example, to estimate the risk of dying of breast cancer for an 80-year-old woman with a life expectancy of 8.6 years, we multiplied the annual breast cancer mortality rate for women aged 80 to 84 years (157/100,000) by 5 = 0.785%. Next we multiplied the annual mortality rate for women older than age 80 years (200.5/100,000) by 3.6 = 0.722% and added these numbers to get the overall risk of 1.5%.

TABLE 38.4

NUMBER NEED TO SCREEN OVER REMAINING LIFETIME TO PREVENT ONE CANCER-SPECIFIC DEATH FOR WOMEN AND MEN AT SELECTED AGES AND LIFE EXPECTANCY QUARTILES[a]

	RRR (95% CI)	Age 50 (y)			Age 70 (y)			Age 75 (y)			Age 80 (y)			Age 85 (y)			Age 90 (y)		
Life Expectancy of Women (y)																			
Screening test		**40**	**33**	**24.5**	**21.3**	**15.7**	**9.5**	**17**	**11.9**	**6.8**	**13**	**8.6**	**4.6**	**9.6**	**5.9**	**2.9**	**6.8**	**3.9**	**1.8**
Mammography	0.26 (0.17–0.34)[a]	95	133	226	142	242	642	176	330	1,361	240	533	—	417	2,131	—	1,066	—	—
Papanicolaou smear	0.60[b]	533	728	1,140	934	1,521	4,070	1,177	2,113	8,342	1,694	3,764	—	2,946	15,056	—	7,528	—	—
Fecal occult blood	0.18 (0.01–0.32)[c]	145	263	577	178	340	1,046	204	408	1,805	262	581	—	455	2,326	—	1,163	—	—
Life Expectancy of Men (y)																			
Screening test		**36**	**28.5**	**19.6**	**18**	**12.4**	**6.7**	**14.2**	**9.3**	**4.9**	**10.8**	**6.7**	**3.3**	**7.9**	**4.7**	**2.2**	**5.8**	**3.2**	**1.5**
Fecal occult blood[d]	0.18 (0.01–0.32)[c]	138	255	630	177	380	1,877	207	525	—	277	945	—	554	—	—	2,008	—	—

Life expectancy quartiles correspond to upper, middle, and lower quartiles as presented in the Figure. The NNS is based on the baseline risk of dying of a screen-detectable cancer (Table 38.1), the relative risk reduction (RRR) of the screening test, and the life expectancy over which the patient is expected to be screened. Patients with life expectancies of less than 5 years are unlikely to derive any survival benefit from cancer screening, which is denoted by ellipses. The numbers for 50-year-old patients are included for comparison. For example, we first estimated the risk of dying of breast cancer for an 80-year-old woman with a life expectancy of 8.6 years who has regular mammography screening during this period. We assumed a 5-year lag before mortality benefit starts. We multiplied the annual breast cancer mortality rate for women aged 80 years to 84 (157/100,000) by 5, which equals 0.785%. Next we multiplied the annual rate for women older than age 85 years (200.5/100,000) by 3.6 and reduced this number by 26% (the RRR of mammography), which equals 0.534%. Adding these numbers together gives an estimated risk of 1.319%. Since the estimated risk of dying of breast cancer without screening is 1.5068% (Table 38.1), the absolute risk of dying of breast cancer without screening is 1.5068% minus 1.319%, which is 0.1878%. The NNS is 1/0.001878 and equals 533.

[a]RRR estimate for breast cancer mortality from a meta-analysis of screening mammography in women aged 50 to 74 years.

[b]RRR estimate represents mid point of reported mortality reductions from population-based studies of screening Papanicolaou smears in women aged 20 through 79 years since no randomized controlled trials have been done.

[c]RRR estimate for colorectal cancer mortality from a randomized study of screening biennial fecal occult blood testing (nonrehydrated) in people aged 45 to 75 years.[10]

[d]Alternative methods for colorectal cancer screening, such as colonoscopy, would have lower numbers to treat since the RRR of these tests are probably higher than that of fecal occult blood testing. Fecal occult blood testing is presented since it is the only test for colorectal cancer screening that has been studied in randomized controlled trials.

RRR, relative risk reduction.

chose cancers for which there was convincing evidence, and a plausible numerical estimate, for the benefits of screening. Therefore, we do not see estimates for cancers of the prostate, lung, ovary, and so on.

To illustrate how to use these data, consider the case of a robust 75-year-old man who has no chronic medical problems and whom you therefore judge to have better-than-average life expectancy for his age (i.e., high tertile). Table 38.3 tells us that his estimated life expectancy is 14.2 years, and he has a 3.5% risk of dying from colorectal cancer during the remainder of his life. These data are the basis for the calculations in Table 38.4 but can also give patients a quantitative basis as they consider their values and preferences regarding cancer screening. From Table 38.4, we can determine that among 75-year-old men with this life expectancy, the number needed to screen (NNS) by fecal occult blood testing (FOBT) is 207 in order to prevent one death from colorectal cancer. Because the NNS is the inverse of the absolute risk reduction (ARR), we can calculate the ARR from FOBT to be $1/207 \approx 0.005$, or a decrease in the risk of colorectal cancer death of approximately 0.5% for this healthy 75-year-old man.

It is noteworthy that the estimates in these tables rely on data from randomized screening trials showing that it takes at least 5 years on average before there is any mortality benefit at all from screening tests. Given this, let us then consider the case of a 75-year-old man who suffers from numerous serious comorbid conditions and was judged to be in the low tertile of life expectancy. From Table 38.4, we see that if this man had worse-than-average life expectancy, one should consider not screening for colorectal cancer, because his predicted remaining lifespan of 4.9 years is less than the amount of time it will take before he is likely to see any benefit of screening.

Selected Cancer Screening Recommendations

With the foregoing ethical considerations in mind, this section presents recommendations for cancer screening from three respected, nonspecialty-based organizations. These recommendations, summarized in Table 38.5, are for average-risk patients and not for those who may belong to higher-risk groups. The recommendations provided also implicitly, if not explicitly, pertain to geriatric patients. Specific recommendations for older patients will be noted where they exist. Table 38.5 also provides information about Medicare coverage for certain cancer screening services, subject to standard deductibles and copayments. For new enrollees beginning January 1, 2005, Medicare will also pay for one introductory "Welcome to Medicare" visit, which is intended to involve a variety of preventive and screening services (see http://www.medicare.gov/health/physicalexam.asp). This is the first time Medicare has covered a health maintenance office visit, and it is an excellent opportunity to provide primary and secondary cancer preventive services.

The USPSTF and the Canadian Task Force on Preventive Health Care (CTFPHC)[15] take similar methodologic approaches, using an explicit and rigorous evidence-based approach when evaluating a given screening test. The evaluation and grading scheme for both the groups allows for an indeterminate category when the quantity or quality of evidence is not convincing enough to definitively recommend for or against screening. The American Cancer Society (ACS) also has a formal guideline development process that employs assessment of the evidence, but where the evidence is uncertain, the ACS approach may rely more on expert opinion than on the USPSTF or CTFPHC. In presenting a variety of viewpoints, the intent is that the reader will be able to choose a screening strategy for individual patients, which is informed by a range of reasonable options.

Breast Cancer Screening

As seen in Table 38.5, there is general consensus on the appropriateness of mammography as the mainstay for breast cancer screening. There is less certainty about the proper interval between screenings, but all three organizations allow that screening as often as annually is appropriate (Evidence Level A). With regard to the use of clinical breast examinations and breast self-examinations, there is less general agreement. Atypically, the CTFPHC does endorse clinical breast examinations despite a firm lack of evidence of any mortality benefit. Breast self-examinations receive a weak endorsement from the ACS. Mammography is reimbursed annually by Medicare.

The USPSTF does not make specific recommendations about the age at which mammography in older women may be stopped, but it does note that women older than 70 with significant comorbidities that alter life expectancy would be unlikely to benefit from screening. Similarly, the ACS does not cite a specific age, but rather recommends individualizing screening recommendations in older women on the basis of a judgment about potential risks and benefits while considering health status. The CTFPHC makes a positive screening recommendation only up to age 69 and does not comment on older women.

Cervical Cancer Screening

Cervical cancer screening is endorsed by the ACS, CTFPHC, and USPSTF (Evidence Level A). There are modalities beyond the original Papanicolaou (Pap) smear by which cervical cancer is screened, including liquid-based tests such as the ThinPrep introduced in the mid-1990s (Table 38.5). The ThinPrep is now the most commonly used method of cervical cancer screening in the United States, and it is the only U.S. Food and Drug Administration–approved method of human papilloma virus testing. The recommended interval between conventional Pap testing varies between 1 year (ACS) and 3 years (USPSTF and CTFPHC), although for women older than 30, the ACS does allow a 2- or 3-year interval testing by conventional Pap or ThinPrep if the patient has had three consecutive normals. Given the relatively limited experience with liquid-based cervical cell–sampling methods, neither the USPSTF nor the CTFPHC found sufficient evidence to make recommendations about their use. Medicare will cover cervical cancer screening on a biennial basis.

All three organizations address the issue of cessation of screening for older women, with the USPSTF and ACS specifying age 65 and 70, respectively, as a stopping point for screening in women who have had recent normal screening. The CTFPHC makes a recommendation to screen only up to age 69 and implicitly, by default, does not endorse screening beyond that age. Cessation of screening after hysterectomy, performed for reasons other than cancer, is supported by both the USPSTF and the ACS (Evidence Level A).

Colorectal Cancer Screening

Over the past 5 years, the options for colorectal cancer screening have become more complicated with the emergence of data supporting the use of colonoscopy for screening.[16] Despite being a time-honored practice, digital rectal examination (DRE) with FOBT has not been shown to be effective in reducing colorectal cancer mortality. Beyond that, physicians have several options for colorectal cancer screening (Table 38.5). Of these, only the three-sample FOBT use is currently supported by multiple randomized trials showing cancer mortality benefit (Evidence Level A). All three organizations endorse the three-sample FOBT, although the ACS notes that its preferred use is

TABLE 38.5
SELECTED CANCER SCREENING RECOMMENDATIONS

Cancer Site	Screening Test	Recommended Screening for Average-Risk Geriatric Patients: USPSTF[3]	CTFPHC[15]	ACS[5]	Medicare Coverage of Screening Test
Breast	Mammography	*Recommend* q12–33 mo	*Recommend* q1–2y up to age 69	*Annually*	Annually
	Clinical breast examination	*Insufficient evidence* to recommend for or against	*Recommend* q1–2y up to age 69	*Annually*	Not reimbursed separately from examination
	Breast self-examination	*Insufficient evidence* to recommend for or against	*Recommend against*	*Optional*	N/A
Cervical	Papanicolaou smear or "ThinPrep" test (liquid-based cytology)	Up to age 65: *Strongly recommend* Pap q3 y After age 65: *Recommend against* Pap if patient had recent normal test ThinPrep: *Insufficient evidence* to recommend for or against	*Recommend* Pap q3y up to age 69 No recommendation regarding ThinPrep	*Annually by Pap or biennially by ThinPrep* But if patients have had three consecutive normals they may test every 2–3 y by Pap or ThinPrep May stop after age 70 if at least three consecutive normal tests	Biennially (with coverage of biennial pelvic examination)
	HPV testing	*Insufficient evidence* to recommend for or against	Not addressed	Optional: add HPV test to Pap or ThinPrep and screen q3 y	
	Screening after total hysterectomy	*Recommend against* in women who had surgery for benign disease	Not addressed	Not necessary unless surgery for cervical cancer	
Colorectal	DRE	Not addressed	Not addressed	Not addressed	Not reimbursed separately from examination
	FOBT	*Strongly recommend* annually	*Recommend* q1–2y	*Annually*, preferred in combination with flex-sig	Annually
	Flexible sigmoidoscopy (flex-sig)	*Strongly recommend*	*Recommend*	*Every 5 y*, preferred in combination with FOBT	Every 4 y
	Double contrast barium enema	*Strongly recommend*	Not addressed	*Every 5 y*	Every 4 y
	Colonoscopy	*Strongly recommend*	*Insufficient evidence* to recommend for or against	*Every 10 y*	Every 10 y, but not within 4 y of flex-sig
Prostate	DRE	*Insufficient evidence* to recommend for or against	*Insufficient evidence* to recommend for or against	"Offer" annually[a]	Not reimbursed separately from examination
	Prostate-specific antigen test	*Insufficient evidence* to recommend for or against	*Recommend against*	"Offer" annual[a]	Annually
	Transrectal ultrasound	Not addressed	*Recommend against*	Not addressed	Not covered for screening
Ovary	Ca-125 test Imaging	*Recommend against* both	*Recommend against* both	Not addressed	—
Lung	Chest radiography Sputum cytology Helical chest CT scan	*Insufficient evidence* to recommend for or against	*Insufficient evidence* to recommend for or against	Not addressed	—
Skin	Physical examination	*Insufficient evidence* to recommend for or against	Not addressed	Not addressed	—

[a]For men with at least 10 years, life expectancy.
USPSTF, United States Preventive Services Task Force; CTFPHC, Canadian Task Force on Preventive Health Care; ACS, American Cancer Society; HPV, human papilloma virus; FOBT, fecal occult blood test; DRE, digital rectal examination; CT, computed tomography.

in conjunction with flexible sigmoidoscopy (flex-sig). All three organizations also endorse flex-sig screening, but the USPSTF and CTFPHC found insufficient evidence to recommend a screening interval for this test (Evidence Level B). In practice in the United States, the frequency of flex-sig screening is typically every 5 years, in line with the ACS recommendation. There is no randomized trial evidence that the combination of flex-sig with FOBT is superior to either modality used alone.

While still only supported by observational evidence rather than randomized trial data, the USPSTF (as well as the ACS) recommends colonoscopy as another screening option, despite the risks of conscious sedation and higher rates of colonic perforation than flex-sig (Evidence Level B). Randomized trials are currently under way to evaluate the effectiveness of both screening colonoscopy and screening flex-sig, which will hopefully provide more definitive guidance on the relative value of these different modalities. If colonoscopy becomes the preferred method of colorectal cancer screening, issues of access to this service will arise because there are currently not enough trained colonoscopists to meet this demand. However, with newer modalities showing potential as screening tests, such as virtual colonoscopy (a radiologic procedure), it may be that the undersupply of colonoscopists will be short-lived.

Although rarely used in comparison with other screening modalities, the double contrast barium enema (DCBE) is also an acceptable alternative for the USPSTF and the ACS, and it may be preferred by some patients (Evidence Level B). The ACS specifies a 5-year screening interval for DCBE, but the USPSTF did not find sufficient evidence to determine an optimal interval.

With the addition, in 2001, of coverage for colonoscopy once every 10 years (in average-risk persons), Medicare now pays for each of the screening tests discussed in the preceding text.

There is little guidance about when to stop screening for colorectal cancer. Only the FOBT effectiveness trials included patients up to age 80, but for other test types, there is no direct evidence of effectiveness after age 70. Given that on average it takes 5 years from the time of colorectal cancer screening to detect a mortality benefit, it is reasonable to offer screening services to those patients with at least a 5-year life expectancy.

Prostate Cancer Screening

The controversy over whether to screen for prostate cancer has been passionate for more than a decade, with little progress toward a consensus on the basic value of screening. The prostate-specific antigen (PSA) test was originally developed in the late 1970s as a way to monitor tumor recurrence among patients who had been treated for prostate cancer. In subsequent years, it came into use secondarily as a screening tool for the general population, based on results from observational studies. Large, high-quality randomized trials of prostate cancer screening are under way in the United States and Europe, and results are expected in the next few years. Despite this prospect, some original proponents of PSA screening have recently declared the era of PSA screening over because of poor test performance characteristics.[17]

The lack of good data on the effectiveness of PSA screening is reflected in the recommendations shown in Table 38.5. Both the USPSTF and CTFPHC either recommend against or find insufficient evidence for PSA testing and DRE. The ACS suggests, somewhat ambiguously, that these interventions only be "offered" to patients, rather than making a clear recommendation for or against their use (Evidence Level C). Transrectal ultrasound for prostate cancer screening is uncommon, and only the CTFPHC addressed this modality with a recommendation against its use. Despite all the uncertainty about its value as a screening tool, Medicare has covered annual PSA screening since 2000.

Screening for Other Selected Cancers

Unlike the cancers discussed previously, screening for cancers of the lung, ovary, and skin is not typically done in a systematic, population-based fashion. However, the disease burden of these cancers is substantial owing to either high incidence or high mortality, and systematic screening for these diseases is an issue that our patients often wish to discuss. The ACS' screening recommendations do not address screening for lung, ovary, or skin cancer. From Table 38.5, it should also be evident that there is little enthusiasm among the USPSTF or the CTFPHC for screening for these cancers. Both these organizations explicitly oppose ovarian cancer screening with currently available testing modalities. With regard to lung cancer screening, the USPSTF and CTFPHC find insufficient evidence on which a recommendation may be based. For the USPSTF, this is a change from a prior unequivocal recommendation against screening and represents the new uncertainty introduced by initial promising results of helical CT chest imaging as a lung cancer–screening tool. As noted previously, however, more definitive data for helical CT screening is years away.

ROUTINE CARE OF THE CANCER SURVIVOR

The Cancer Survivorship Phenomenon

Over the past few decades, improved therapeutics (and in some cases, mass screening) have changed cancer into a disease that is no longer an automatic death sentence for many patients. Correspondingly, there has been an explosion in the number of individuals considered to be cancer "survivors." In 2001, there were an estimated 9.8 million cancer survivors in the United States, more than triple the number from 30 years earlier.[18] Cancer survivorship has important implications for the geriatric population, with >60% of survivors aged 65 or older. In addition, we are seeing increasing numbers of long-term survivors, with nearly one in seven survivors having been diagnosed at least 20 years earlier.

With large and increasing numbers of cancer survivors in primary care practices over long periods of time, it is critical that primary care physicians understand the unique health care needs of this population and their own important role in providing them. Figure 38.1 provides some perspective on this role, highlighting the limited time that the care of cancer survivors is out of the domain of primary care. This section will explore general considerations in understanding the care of the cancer survivor and will discuss how to approach routine screening—also known as "surveillance"—for cancer recurrence in the common, survivable cancers of the breast, prostate, and colon.

Cancer Survivorship Model

Multiple factors with complex interactions may influence a given individual's probability of surviving cancer. Figure 38.3 presents a model that highlights some of these variables and their interactions. These factors can be divided into patient-level and health-system-level factors. Patient factors that influence survival include disease characteristics such as tumor type, stage, and grade and patient characteristics such as comorbid conditions, socioeconomic status, and race. Health-system factors that influence survival include the appropriateness and timeliness of initial cancer treatment as well as other variables that affect quality of care. Lastly, follow-up care after cancer treatment, including routine surveillance for cancer recurrence, plays a role in cancer survival. Primary care physicians can, and should, have an important influence on the appropriate provision of routine follow-up care for cancer survivors.

This role is more easily understood when cancer survivor care is understood simply as another form of chronic disease care, which involves long-term routine follow-up care in a continuity relationship, judicious application of primary, secondary, and tertiary prevention, and the recognition and management of disease progression and complications. These elements of chronic disease care find clear application in cancer survivor care:

1. Long-term routine follow-up and continuity promotes the regular checkups recommended for survivors.
2. Appropriate prevention in survivors pertains to both the proper use of surveillance testing and general preventive and screening interventions in survivors.
3. Recognition and management of disease progression in survivors consist of initial workup, referral, and coordination of care for cancer recurrence—all services commonly provided in primary care.
4. Recognition and management of disease complications in survivors consist of workup of both disease complications and late effects of cancer treatment. Whether primary care physicians manage these complications directly or seek consultation is more variable.

Indeed, when aware of what constitutes appropriate routine cancer surveillance care, primary care physicians can play the central role in ensuring that cancer survivors receive that care. While recognition and management of disease recurrence and complications are important, an adequate discussion of these topics is beyond the scope of this chapter.

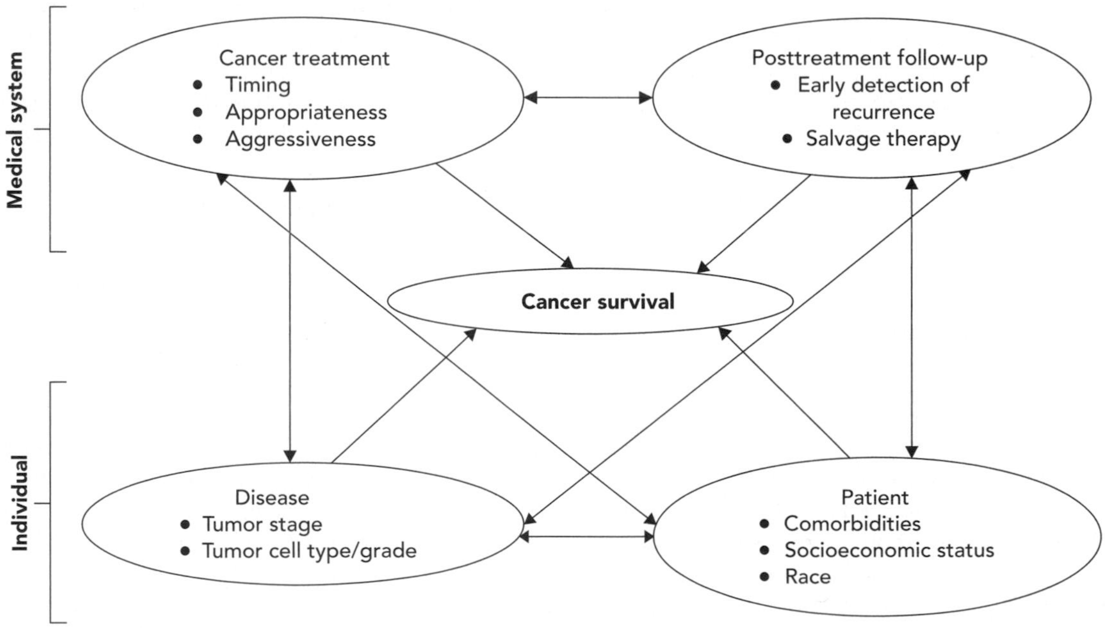

Figure 38.3 Conceptual model of cancer survival.

Surveillance Care Guidelines

Two oncology specialty societies have expended considerable effort in developing guidelines for the care of cancer survivors: The National Comprehensive Cancer Network (NCCN) and the American Society for Clinical Oncology (ASCO). The guidelines of these societies will provide the basis for the recommendations presented in this text. The development of available guidelines has used evidence-based approaches where possible. However, research on care for cancer survivors is relatively sparse, so expert opinion and consensus-based approaches have also been used. In some cases, these organizations' guidelines will diverge, as is the case for general cancer screening. The intent is to provide differing views to give the reader a range of reasonable options from which to choose.

Breast Cancer Surveillance

Breast cancer is the most common cancer in US women, with an estimated 216,000 new cases in 2004. Over the past few decades, breast cancer survival has improved, and now the overall 5-year survival rate is 87%.[1] This in turn leads to a large survivor population, with an estimated 2.2 million breast cancer survivors in 2001. However, despite a relatively good 5-year survival rate, breast cancer survivors continue to be at risk for recurrent disease. The cancer recurrence rate is approximately 1% to 2% per year, and this rate is linear over time—that is, the risk of recurrence does not decrease over time. This highlights the importance of surveillance for recurrence among breast cancer survivors.

The key provisions of surveillance care for breast cancer survivors are highlighted in Table 38.6. Breast cancer surveillance is straightforward, consisting only of periodic office visits (Evidence Level C) and annual mammography (Evidence Level B). Mammography should be performed on the contralateral breast, as well as on any residual tissue on the ipsilateral side. There are minor differences between NCCN and ASCO regarding the exact frequency of office visits, but a twice-yearly schedule for the first 5 years is consistent with both. At those visits, an interval history and directed physical examination should be performed. The interval history should include a cancer-relevant review of systems, eliciting constitutional symptoms, such as unintended weight loss or pronounced fatigue, from patients. Patients should also be asked about common symptoms of metastatic disease, such as bone pain, abdominal pain, new or unusual headache, or lymph node enlargement. Finally, symptoms of local breast cancer recurrence should be sought, such as palpable masses or pain in the breast or chest wall.

Randomized trials in the 1990s found that there is no survival benefit and no quality-of-life benefit of more aggressive surveillance with routine use of CT scans, bone scans, or blood work in asymptomatic survivors.[19,20] Despite this fairly simple surveillance regimen, recent research on survivors suggests that up to a third fail to receive annual mammography and that there is substantial overuse of nonrecommended tests.[21] No randomized trials of the mortality benefit of mammography or office visits have been done; therefore, we do not have any direct evidence of the benefit of these interventions for breast cancer survivors. This is not likely to change, because such trials are not likely to be done for ethical reasons.

Chemoprevention of Breast Cancer Recurrence

Many postmenopausal breast cancer survivors with tumors positive for estrogen or progesterone receptors may be eligible for adjuvant hormonal therapy, such as tamoxifen, or the newer, and possibly even more effective, aromatase inhibitor agents, such as anastrozole or letrozole.[22] These adjuvant regimens should normally be initiated by the patient's surgeon or oncologist, usually last 5 years postcancer diagnosis, and offer a clear mortality advantage. Given the potential benefits, these agents are the standard of care in eligible patients, and primary physicians should ensure that patients have discussed with their cancer treatment team whether such therapy would be appropriate in their case (Evidence Level A).

Prostate Cancer Surveillance

Prostate cancer is the most common cancer in US men, representing 33% of all (nonskin) cancer diagnoses in men and accounting for 230,000 new cases in 2004.[1]

TABLE 38.6
BREAST CANCER SURVEILLANCE GUIDELINES

	2004 National Comprehensive Cancer Network Guidelines	1998 American Society of Clinical Oncology Guidelines
History and physical examination	q4–6 mo × 5 y, then annually	q3–6 mo × 3 y, then q6–12 mo × 2 y, then annually
Imaging	Mammography annually	Mammography annually
Procedures	None recommended	None recommended
Blood work	None recommended	None recommended

Considering all stages, the 5-year survival is 98%, although for patients with distant disease at the time of diagnosis, the 5-year survival drops to 34%. This high survival rate leads to a large prostate cancer survivor population, estimated around 1.7 million in 2001. Over time, the risk of recurrent disease becomes substantial: By 5 years after cancer diagnosis, the risk of recurrence is 7% for patients treated with radical prostatectomy and 24% in patients who received radiation therapy. At 10 years after diagnosis, recurrence rates are 31% for prostatectomy and 44% for radiation therapy.

The approach to surveillance care for prostate cancer survivors varies by the therapeutic approach taken toward the patient. Many patients will choose aggressive management of their disease with a presumptive intention for cure, which involves definitive treatment by prostatectomy or radiation therapy. However, given the indolent nature of many prostate carcinomas, and the likelihood of elderly men dying with prostate cancer rather than dying from it, some patients may elect "expectant management" of their disease. Under this approach, patients forego definitive treatment for presumptive cure and are instead monitored clinically.

Prostate cancer survivors who have had definitive treatment for cure have a relatively straightforward surveillance care strategy (see Table 38.7). Most survivors should have an annual interval history and physical examination (Evidence Level C). However, for those patients with tumor, node, and metastasis (TNM) tumor-staging classification of N1 or M1 indicating distant spread of disease, these visits should be scheduled every 3 to 6 months. Under either schedule, patients should have a review of systems with attention to constitutional symptoms such as anorexia and weight loss, as well as more disease-specific questions about decreased urine flow, difficulty with initiating micturition, hematuria, and bone pain. Physical examination should include a DRE with prostate palpation if the gland is still present. Neither imaging nor any procedures are necessary on a routine basis. In patients without evidence of distant disease, blood testing for PSA tumor antigen levels should be done every 6 months for the first 5 years after diagnosis and annually thereafter (Evidence Level C). In patients with N1 or M1 disease staging, PSA testing should be done every 3 to 6 months in conjunction with office visits. Rising PSA levels in any patient treated for cure are an indication for further workup and consultation with the patient's urologist. Additionally, any patient treated with radical prostatectomy should have undetectable PSA levels within a few months after surgery. Consequently, any detectable level of PSA should be considered suspicious for either primary treatment failure or recurrence and should be managed accordingly.

Patients who have chosen expectant management should also receive cancer surveillance care (Table 38.7). Regardless of life expectancy, surveillance care consists of a periodic evaluation with an interval history and physical examination (Evidence Level C). The elements of this office visit should be similar to those described in the preceding text for definitively managed patients. Patients with life expectancy of <10 years should be evaluated once or twice yearly. No specific tests are required for surveillance care in this group. The purpose of such surveillance is to identify patients with advancing disease who may benefit from palliative interventions. Patients with an estimated life expectancy of 10 years or more, who may be candidates for definitive interventions at a later date, should have an interval history and physical one to two times a year. These patients require additional elements of care

TABLE 38.7

PROSTATE CANCER SURVEILLANCE GUIDELINES

2004 National Comprehensive Cancer Network Recommendations for patients who had definitive therapy

History and physical examination	DRE annually If T1 or N1 disease, DRE q3–6 mo[a]
Imaging	None recommended
Procedures	None recommended
Blood work	PSA q6 mo × 5 y, then yearly If T1 or N1 disease, PSA q3–6 mo[a]

2004 National Comprehensive Cancer Network Recommendations for patients using expectant management:

Life expectancy ≥10 y:	*Life expectancy <10 y*:
■ PSA q6 mo	■ Clinical evaluation q6–12 mo
■ DRE q6 mo	
■ Repeat prostate biopsy in 1 y, then periodically	

Definitive therapy is either surgery or radiation therapy for prostate cancer.
Expectant management is clinical observation and monitoring, without surgery or radiation.
[a]History, physical, and PSA testing every 3–6 months for patients having T1 or N1 disease (or greater), based on TNM-staging designation.
DRE, digital rectal examination; PSA, prostate-specific antigen test.

for surveillance. Blood testing for PSA levels should be performed every 6 months (Evidence Level C). Rising PSA levels should prompt urologic consultation. Lastly, a repeat prostate biopsy is recommended at 1 year postdiagnosis and periodically thereafter (Evidence Level C). No routine imaging is indicated. If progressive disease is discovered in these patients, they may still be eligible to consider definitive therapy again or may be eligible for palliative interventions.

The evidence base to support PSA testing in prostate cancer survivors is very limited. PSA testing came into clinical use in the 1980s as a replacement for other prostate cancer tumor markers that are used to monitor the recurrence or progression of the disease.[23] However, it is not known whether PSA surveillance testing is effective, because no randomized clinical trials that evaluate whether the use of PSA testing in survivors reduces prostate cancer mortality have been published. For ethical reasons, it is unlikely that such studies will be done. Clinical trials evaluating the relative effectiveness of different prostate cancer surveillance regimens have also not been done, so the optimal content, frequency, and duration of prostate cancer surveillance is not known.

Colorectal Cancer Surveillance

Colorectal cancer is the third most common cancer in both men and women in the United States, with an estimated 151,000 new cases in 2004.[1] With more than 55,000 total deaths in 2004, colon cancer is also the third leading cause of cancer death in both men and women, after lung and prostate cancers in men and lung and breast cancers in women. Across all patients regardless of stage, tumor type, or location (i.e., colon, rectum, or anus), the 5-year survival is 62%. While lower than the 5-year survival of breast or prostate cancer, this fairly high survival rate coupled with high incidence has led to an estimated 1 million colorectal cancer survivors as of 2004. Approximately 90% of colorectal cancer recurrences occur in the first 5 years after diagnosis, and consistent follow-up and surveillance in this period is important.

Surveillance regimens for colorectal cancer are somewhat complex. They vary by the professional organization (ASCO vs. NCCN) promoting them. They also differ somewhat according to the anatomic site of the cancer, with separate recommendations for colon, rectal, and anal cancers. The suggested surveillance for each will be considered in order.

Colon Cancer

All colon cancer survivors should have periodic office visits and surveillance colonoscopy. Routine blood work is also recommended in selected patients. The exact frequency of office visits for interval history and physical examination varies between ASCO and NCCN, but a reasonable schedule would be every 1 to 6 months in the first 3 years after cancer diagnosis, every 6 months for the next 2 years, and annually thereafter. At these visits, patients should be asked about constitutional symptoms such as unintended weight loss and increasing fatigue. More specific reviews of systems should include questions regarding hematochezia, change in stool caliber or patterns, and abdominal pain. Directed physical examination should include stool guaiac testing for occult blood, abdominal and liver palpation, and examination of vital signs, skin, and mucus membranes for evidence of anemia (Evidence Level C).

Surveillance colonoscopy is central to colon cancer survivor care (see Table 38.8) (Evidence Level A). Recommendations vary somewhat on the frequency of this surveillance. A more aggressive approach would be colonoscopy 1 year after diagnosis, to be repeated in 1 year if findings were positive or every 3 years if it were negative. A less aggressive approach is to simply perform colonoscopy every 3 to 5 years after diagnosis. There are no data showing that the more frequent colonoscopy schedule leads to decreased colon cancer mortality.

The only routine surveillance blood work recommended by NCCN and ASCO is carcinoembryonic antigen (CEA) testing (Evidence Level B). However, this testing is only recommended in certain patients who have stage II or III disease or TNM tumor stage classification of T2 that designates tumors which invade the muscularis propria (see Table 38.8).[24] Further, among stage II/III or T2 patients, CEA testing should be done only in those who would be both able and willing to undergo further substantial intervention (e.g., surgical resection of isolated hepatic metastases) to treat recurrent disease if discovered through elevated CEA levels. In appropriate patients, CEA testing should be done every 3 months for the first 2 years after diagnosis and then every 3 to 6 months until 5 years from diagnosis. Currently, routine imaging in colon cancer survivors is not recommended, although abdominal CT scan may be considered in patients at extremely high risk of recurrence, such as those having a poorly differentiated tumor.

Previous versions of these guidelines did recommend additional routine surveillance, such as routine imaging with both abdominal CT scan and chest radiography, and routine liver function testing and blood counts. The evidence regarding the elements to include in a colon cancer surveillance strategy is difficult to interpret and, at times, conflicting. On the basis of the meta-analyses of randomized trials, it appears that, in general, intensive surveillance confers survival benefits compared to nonintensive surveillance. Yet, the definition of "intensive" has varied considerably among studies of the efficacy of colon cancer surveillance programs, and currently the beneficial elements of intensive programs are unknown, as there are little or no data that isolate the effect of individual tests.[25] Perhaps due to the growing influence of evidence-based methods, the guidelines have evolved to include what is essentially a moderately intensive approach

TABLE 38.8
COLON AND RECTAL CANCER SURVEILLANCE GUIDELINES

	2004 National Comprehensive Cancer Network Guidelines	2000 American Society of Clinical Oncology Guidelines
History and physical examination	q3 mo for 2 y, then q6 mo for 3 y	q3–6 mo for 3 y, then annually
Imaging	*None recommended*[a]	*None recommended*
Procedures	Colonoscopy in 1 y, then repeat in 1 y if positive, or q3 y if negative[b]	Colonoscopy q3–5 y
Blood work	CEA[c] q3 mo for 2 y, then q6 mo for 3 y for T2 or greater lesions	CEA[c] q2–3 mo for stage II or III for ≥ 2 y

[a]For colon cancer only, may consider abdominal CT scan if "high risk" for recurrence (e.g., poorly differentiated tumor).
[b]For colon cancer only, greater frequency if obstructive lesion or unprepped bowel.
[c]Only done if patient is a candidate for further intervention, e.g., resection of metastases.
CT, computed tomography; CEA, carcinoembryonic antigen testing.

to surveillance, excluding those elements of surveillance for which there is the least amount of supporting data.

Rectal Cancer

Surveillance care for rectal cancer is similar to that of colon cancer (see Table 38.9). All rectal cancer survivors should have regular office visits that follow the same schedule described in the section "Colon Cancer." An appropriate interval history should include questions about constitutional symptoms of weight loss and fatigue, specific symptoms such as hematochezia, pain with defecation, changes in bowel patterns or caliber, and any symptoms suggestive of rectal obstruction (Evidence Level C).

No routine imaging is recommended for rectal cancer surveillance, and, unlike colon cancer, there are no special considerations for high-risk patients. Just as in colon cancer, the cornerstone or rectal cancer surveillance is follow-up colonoscopy. The schedule for surveillance colonoscopy mirrors that of colon cancer (Evidence Level A). The more aggressive approach is an initial examination 1 year after diagnosis, which is to be repeated in 1 year if positive or every 3 years if negative. Unlike colon cancer, there is no provision for even more frequent examinations on the basis of the presence of an obstructive primary lesion. The less aggressive approach would simply be colonoscopy every 3 years. Recommendations for routine blood work are exactly the same as for colon cancer: For CEA, testing is recommended only in patients with stage II/III or T2 disease and among that group, only in those who are able and willing to undergo further definitive interventions should CEA testing discover recurrent disease. In patients who meet these criteria, the schedule for CEA testing is the same as for colon cancer surveillance detailed above (Evidence Level B).

Surveillance for rectal cancer is separated here from colon cancer to allow clarification of some subtle differences in recommendations. However, the research on which these surveillance strategies are based is the same for both cancers, because both colon and rectal cancers have been studied together. Hence, the same uncertainties about the relative efficacy of different colon cancer surveillance strategies also apply to rectal cancer surveillance.

Anal Cancer

Only NCCN breaks out separate guidelines for anal cancers (Table 38.9). Office visits for interval history and physical examination are recommended every 3 to 6 months for 5 years after cancer diagnosis. At these visits, patients

TABLE 38.9
ANAL CANCER SURVEILLANCE GUIDELINES (NATIONAL COMPREHENSIVE CANCER NETWORK)

History and physical examination	DRE, inguinal node palpation q3–6 mo for 5 y
Imaging	If T3–T4, consider abdominal CT scan q6 mo for 5 y
Procedures	Anoscopy q3–6 mo for 5 y
Blood work	None recommended

T3, T4, Tumor characteristics according to Tumor, Node, Metastasis disease-staging designation; DRE, digital rectal examination; CT, computed tomography.

should be asked about constitutional symptoms, such as weight loss and fatigue. Directed review of systems should focus on hematochezia, change in stool caliber, pain with defecation, inguinal lymph node enlargement, and symptoms suggestive of anal obstruction. Physical examination should include DRE for masses and occult blood, and inguinal lymph node palpation (Evidence Level C). Anoscopy should be performed every 3 to 6 months for 5 years after diagnosis, rather than full colonoscopy as is recommended in colorectal cancer (Evidence Level C). No routine blood work is recommended.

PREVENTIVE CARE AND HEALTH MAINTENANCE IN CANCER SURVIVORS

With a few exceptions, the approach to providing routine preventive care and screening among cancer survivors relies on the same principles one would employ in a population of geriatric patients who were not cancer survivors. Therefore, in cancer survivors treated for presumptive cure, recommendations for screening are the same as for the general population, including periodic screening for lipid disorders as well as for other cancers (e.g., colorectal cancer screening in a breast cancer survivor). However, it is also critical to keep in mind that these recommendations are tempered by the same considerations about when it is appropriate to stop screening, as discussed in the section "Secondary Prevention: Screening for Cancer" of this chapter. Additionally, for survivors who are *BRCA* oncogene carriers, more intensive mammography screening of remaining breast tissue (e.g., some would suggest every 6 months) may be considered even without the evidence of its benefit.

Preventive services such as counseling regarding tobacco cessation and seat belt use and influenza and pneumococcal pneumonia vaccination should also be offered to cancer survivors. One exception to general health maintenance principles is that patients who have had chemotherapy that included alkylating agents should be vaccinated against pneumococcal pneumonia even if they are younger than 65.

REFERENCES

1. Jemal A, Tiwari RC, Murray T, et al. Cancer statistics. *CA Cancer J Clin*.2004;54(1):8–29.
2. National Cancer Institute. *SEER CanQues cancer prevalence database surveillance, epidemiology, and end results program*.2004.
3. U.S. Preventive Services Task Force. *Guide to clinical preventive services*.2004.
4. The Office of the Surgeon General. *The health benefits of smoking cessation: A report of the surgeon general*. Rockville, MD: U.S. Department of Health and Human Services;1990.
5. American Cancer Society. *Cancer prevention & early detection, facts & figures*. Atlanta, GA: American Cancer Society;2004.
6. Calle EE, Rodriguez C, Walker-Thurmond K, et al. Overweight, obesity, and mortality from cancer in a prospectively studied cohort of U.S. adults. *N Engl J Med*.2003;348(17):1625–1638.
7. Wakeford R. The cancer epidemiology of radiation. *Oncogene*.2004;23(38):6404–6428.
8. Jakobisiak M, Golab J. Potential antitumor effects of statins (Review). *Int J Oncol*.2003;23(4):1055–1069.
9. Kismet K, Akay MT, Abbasoglu O, et al. Celecoxib: A potent cyclooxygenase-2 inhibitor in cancer prevention. *Cancer Detect Prev*.2004;28(2):127–142.
10. Fisher B, Wickerham DL, Kavanagh M, et al. Tamoxifen for prevention of breast cancer: Report of the National Surgical Adjuvant Breast and Bowel Project P-1 Study. *J Natl Cancer Inst*.1998;90(18):1371–1388.
11. Ewart RM. Primum non nocere and the quality of evidence: Rethinking the ethics of screening. *J Am Board Fam Pract*.2000;13(3): 188–196.
12. Brenner DJ, Elliston CD. Estimated radiation risks potentially associated with full-body CT screening. *Radiology*.2004;232(3): 735–738.
13. Welch HG. *Should I be tested for cancer? maybe not and here's why*. Berkeley, CA: University of California Press;2004:224.
14. Walter LC, Covinsky KE. Cancer screening in elderly patients: A framework for individualized decision making. *JAMA*.2001; 285(21):2750–2756.
15. Canadian Task Force on Preventive Health Care. *CTFPHC systematic reviews and recommendations*.2004.
16. Lieberman DA, Weiss DG, Bond JH, et al. Use of colonoscopy to screen asymptomatic adults for colorectal cancer. *N Engl J Med*.2000;343(3):162–168.
17. Stamey TA, Caldwell M, McNeal JE, et al. The prostate specific antigen era in the United States is over for prostate cancer: What happened in the last 20 years? *J Urol*.2004;172(4 Pt 1): 1297–1301.
18. Rowland J, Mariotto A, Aziz N, et al. Cancer survivorship–United States, 1971–2001. *Morb Mortal Wkly Rep*.2004;53(24):526–529.
19. Rosselli Del Turco M, Palli D, Cariddi A, et al. Intensive diagnostic follow-up after treatment of primary breast cancer. A randomized trial. National research council project on breast cancer follow-up. *JAMA*.1994;271(20):1593–1597.
20. The GIVIO Investigators. Impact of follow-up testing on survival and health-related quality of life in breast cancer patients. A multicenter randomized controlled trial. *JAMA*.1994;271(20): 1587–1592.
21. Schapira MM, McAuliffe TL, Nattinger AB. Underutilization of mammography in older breast cancer survivors. *Med Care*.2000; 38(3):281–289.
22. Howell A, Cuzick J, Baum M, et al. Results of the ATAC (Arimidex, Tamoxifen, Alone or in Combination) trial after completion of 5 years' adjuvant treatment for breast cancer. *Lancet*.2005;365(9453):60–62.
23. Stamey TA, Yang N, Hay AR, et al. Prostate-specific antigen as a serum marker for adenocarcinoma of the prostate. *N Engl J Med*.1987;317(15):909–916.
24. Compton CC, Greene FL. The staging of colorectal cancer: 2004 and beyond. *CA Cancer J Clin*.2004;54(6):295–308.
25. Pfister DG, Benson AB 3rd, Somerfield MR. Clinical practice. Surveillance strategies after curative treatment of colorectal cancer. *N Engl J Med*.2004;350(23):2375–2382.

Hematology

39

Gerald L. Logue

CLINICAL PEARLS 546

ANEMIA 547
Normocytic Anemia 547
Microcytic Anemia 547
Macrocytic Anemia 548

THROMBOCYTOPENIA AND NEUTROPENIA 549

SCREENING FOR BLEEDING PRIOR TO SURGERY/THE PROLONGED PARTIAL THROMBOPLASTIN TIME 550

PLASMA CELL DISORDERS 551
Multiple Myeloma 551
Monoclonal Gammopathy of Unknown Significance 551
Plasmacytoma and Other Plasma Cell Proliferative Diseases 551

MYELOPROLIFERATIVE DISEASES 552
Erythrocytosis 552
Thrombocytosis 552
Leukocytosis 552

VENOUS THROMBOSIS 553

CLINICAL PEARLS

- Anemia should be evaluated for its cause in all patients without assuming that it is a natural consequence of aging.
- The most common cause of anemia (approximately 50%) is secondary to systemic disease, referred to as *anemia of chronic disease.*
- Normocytic anemia requires an evaluation of the patient's entire status, including the presence of thyroid or renal disease.
- Patients with early iron deficiency may have normocytic anemia.
- A low serum ferritin always means iron deficiency.
- Iron deficiency in older patients should be diagnosed definitively because it is often associated with gastrointestinal (GI) malignancy.
- Marked reduction in mean corpuscular volume (MCV) with nearly normal red blood cell counts is usually caused by thalassemia minor.
- Patients with iron deficiency, who are refractory to iron therapy, should be tested for gluten-induced enteropathy.
- Nonmegaloblastic macrocytic anemia is common and should be considered when a high MCV is noted.
- Patients with macrocytic anemia should have a reticulocyte count done to exclude hemolytic anemia.
- Initial evaluation of thrombocytopenia requires careful evaluation of the peripheral blood smear.
- Heparin-induced thrombocytopenia may produce paradoxical arterial and venous thrombosis. Patients on heparin should have platelet counts monitored daily.
- Drug-induced thrombocytopenia is common in older patients.
- Chronic neutropenia is often well tolerated without infections in older individuals.
- The most important information regarding the risk of bleeding with surgery is a history of prior bleeding.
- A prolonged partial thromboplastin should be initially evaluated with a "mixing study."
- Older patients with prolonged partial thromboplastin time (PTT) due to antiphospholipid antibodies are not at increased risk of bleeding with surgery.
- Screening for multiple myeloma can be done with serum and urine electrophoreses. Ninety-nine percent of patients with multiple myeloma will test positive. Negative tests essentially exclude the diagnosis.
- Approximately one quarter of patients with monoclonal gammopathy of unknown significance will progress to

a more aggressive plasma cell proliferative disease in 10 years.

- Cigarette smoking produces erythrocytosis by causing chronic carbon monoxide poisoning.
- Patients with erythrocytosis should be carefully examined for splenomegaly, which is often associated with a myeloproliferative disease.
- Measurement of erythropoietin is important in determining the cause of erythrocytosis.
- Patients with thrombocytosis should be screened for iron deficiency and GI or pulmonary neoplasia.
- Venous thrombosis in older patients does not generally require screening for underlying inherited thrombophilic states unless there is a family history of clotting.

ANEMIA

Anemia occurs with increasing frequency in older patients. There are two competing theories regarding this observation. One is that decreased production of red cells is a natural consequence of the aging process (presbypoiesis). The decreasing amount of marrow dedicated to hematopoiesis as aging progresses lends support to this theory. Children have active hematopoiesis in all bones, including long bones. But with aging the proportion of marrow that produces blood diminishes. Animal models suggest that the number of hematopoietic stem cells lessens with age.

A second theory of anemia in older patients is that the elderly accumulate chronic diseases that are associated with secondary anemia. There are certainly many healthy older individuals who have normal blood counts. From a practical point of view, anemia should be evaluated in all patients because treatable illnesses are often identified; that is, anemia should not be attributed to age alone.[1]

Anemia in older patients is associated with increased morbidity and mortality independent of concurrent diseases. Exogenous therapeutic erythropoietin has improved the life of many patients with concurrent diseases such as renal failure, cancer, and human immunodeficiency virus (HIV), as well as those undergoing cancer therapy. At this point, there are no studies to suggest that erythropoietin is useful to treat anemia in older patients who do not have a specific disease indication, but studies are ongoing.[2]

To evaluate the causes of anemia in older patients, it is useful to categorize it according to the size of the red cells (the mean red cell volume or mean corpuscular volume [MCV]) as determined by automated blood counting.

Normocytic Anemia

Normocytic anemia accounts for most patients who have low red cell counts, including some who are anemic secondary to other systemic diseases. The differential diagnosis of normocytic anemia includes a large number of primary hematologic diseases such as multiple myeloma, aplastic anemia, and myelodysplastic syndrome. Normocytic anemia is also common in many chronic diseases, requiring careful consideration of the entire clinical status. Early iron deficiency can present with normocytic anemia, but continued iron-deficient hematopoiesis will eventually cause the MCV to fall.

Evaluation of normocytic anemia may require a bone marrow examination. Myelodysplastic syndromes usually present with anemia in older individuals. These syndromes include refractory anemia with and without ringed sideroblasts. The latter present a hypercellular bone marrow with increased red cell precursors. Refractory anemia with excess blast cells may resemble acute leukemia and needs to be monitored for further transformation. Myelodysplastic syndromes are associated with prior chemotherapy and toxic chemical exposure. Current therapy is directed at blood cell support but newer therapeutic approaches are being tested.[3]

Microcytic Anemia

The differential diagnosis of anemia with a low MCV is outlined in Table 39.1. Iron deficiency is a common consideration and is almost always due to blood loss in older patients. There are multiple tests available to determine a patient's iron status. Measurement of serum ferritin is useful because there are very few false positives (if patients have a low serum ferritin, they are very likely to be iron deficient) (Evidence Level C).[1] In contrast, there is an incidence of false negatives with a serum ferritin. Some patients with iron deficiency may have normal ferritin.

Serum iron and iron-binding capacity have a higher incidence of false positives than ferritin; that is, patients may have low serum iron and low iron saturation but may not be iron deficient. Serum iron measurements also have a relatively high incidence of false negatives because serum iron may change relatively quickly and transiently after an intake of oral iron. Detection of bone marrow iron stores are generally felt to be a "gold standard" for determining a patient's iron status, but the procedure is more invasive.

Oral iron therapy should be used in older patients if at all possible (Evidence Level A).[4] Parenteral iron preparations are available but carry increased risks of complications in older patients. The gastrointestinal (GI) symptoms of cramping and bowel irregularity seen with oral iron preparations diminish after the first 1 to 2 weeks of therapy. Patients who continue to be iron deficient despite oral iron therapy should be tested for glutin-sensitive enteropathy (celiac disease).

Thalassemic syndromes are disorders of globin chain synthesis. There are two types of globin chains in the most prevalent adult hemoglobin (hemoglobin A): α Chains and β chains. Disordered production of globin chain synthesis is usually inherited but rare instances of acquired disorders have been seen in myelodysplastic

TABLE 39.1
DIFFERENTIAL DIAGNOSIS OF COMMON BLOOD DYSCRASIAS

Microcytic Anemia	Macrocytic Anemia		Plasma Cell Proliferative Diseases	Myeloproliferative Diseases	Differential Diagnosis of Thrombocytosis
Iron deficiency (280.9)	Nonmegaloblastic macrocytic anemia (281.9)	Megaloblastic anemia (281.3)	Monoclonal gammopathy of unknown significance (273.1)	Polycythemia vera (238.4)	GI bleeding (578.9)
β Thalassemia minor (282.49)	Liver disease (573.9)	Cytotoxic chemotherapy (V58.1)	Multiple myeloma (203.00)	Primary thrombocythemia (238.7)	Iron deficiency (280.9)
α Thalassemia minor (282.49)	High reticulocyte count	HIV therapy	Isolated plasmacytoma (238.6)	Myelofibrosis (205.10)	Cancer of many sites (199.0)
Anemia secondary to inflammatory processes	Hypothyroidism (244.9)	B_{12} deficiency (281.1)	Primary amyloidosis with monoclonal immunoglobulin	Chronic myelogenous leukemia (205.1)	Chronic infections
Lead poisoning (984.9)	—	Folate deficiency (281.2)	—	—	Myeloproliferative diseases (238.7)
Sideroblastic anemia (285.0)	—	Myelodysplastic syndromes (238.7)	—	—	—

Differential Diagnosis of Erythrocytosis

Relative erythrocytosis (normal red cell mass but reduced plasma volume) (289.0)	Erythrocytosis with increased erythropoietin. 1. Arterial hypoxemia (799.0) 2. Congenital heart disease (746.9), chronic lung disease (518.89) 3. Chronic carbon monoxide poisoning (tobacco smoking) (986) 4. Erythropoietin producing tumors 5. Inherited hemoglobinopathy with increased oxygen affinity	Erythrocytosis with decreased or absent erythropoietin (polycythemia vera) (238.4)

GI, gastrointestinal; HIV, human immunodeficiency virus.

syndromes. β Thalassemia minor is the reduced ability to produce β chains. These patients have mild, asymptomatic anemia with a low MCV and can be mistakenly diagnosed as being iron deficient. Iron therapy is contraindicated in these patients because they tend to have abnormally enhanced iron absorption and the potential to develop iron overload (hemosiderosis). These patients can be diagnosed by measuring the amount of the two other types of hemoglobin found in healthy adults (i.e., quantitation of Hb A_2 and Hb F) or hemoglobin electrophoresis. Because Hb A_2 and Hb F do not have β chains, they will be present in greater amounts in patients with β thalassemia.

Thalassemia due to the decreased production of α globin chains is more difficult to diagnose. These patients will appear clinically identical to patients with β thalassemia minor, except that their hemoglobin A_2 and F levels will be normal. α Thalassemia should be suspected in patients with long-standing mild anemia with marked reduction in MCV but with normal iron stores.

Other causes of anemia with reduced MCV include anemia secondary to chronic inflammatory diseases. These patients have a disorder of iron reutilization. They have increased iron stores but macrophages do not release iron efficiently for red cell production. Anemia with a low MCV can also be seen in lead poisoning and rarely in myelodysplastic syndromes such as sideroblastic anemia. In the latter, there is an acquired defect in iron metabolism, which leads to pathologic iron depositions in mitochondria of developing erythroid cells, producing "ringed sideroblasts."

Macrocytic Anemia

The differential diagnosis of anemia with a high MCV is outlined in Table 39.1. It is important to distinguish megaloblastic anemia from the various causes of macrocytic anemia without a megaloblastic process. The latter disorders are more common than diseases with megaloblastosis. Megaloblastic anemia is caused by a variety of processes which alter the synthesis of deoxyribonucleic acid (DNA). This inhibition of DNA synthesis in turn causes an impaired nuclear maturation and a morphologic abnormality of the marrow and blood, which is described as megaloblastic anemia.

Megaloblastic anemia was originally described in patients with deficiencies of vitamin B_{12} or folate. Vitamin B_{12} and folate are required for normal synthesis of DNA precursors. B_{12} and folate deficiencies are easily treated and should be excluded in all patients with macrocytic anemia. Serum B_{12} level is an accurate and inexpensive analysis. In adults, folate deficiency is caused by inadequate diet and should be suspected from the diet history. Serum folate levels are accurate but change rapidly with folate intake. Red cell folate levels are also available. These levels are more stable because they reflect folate concentrations when the red cells were produced.

B_{12} is a coenzyme for maintenance of nerve tissue, and severe neurologic disease results from long-standing B_{12} deficiency. The syndrome includes peripheral neuropathy, degeneration of dorsal spinal columns, and cortical disease leading to dementia. Neurologic manifestations of B_{12} deficiency can occur without blood abnormalities, and excessive folate intake will "mask" the hematologic findings but have no effect on the neurologic disease.

Treatment of macrocytic anemia is usually a lifetime issue. Vitamin B_{12} is given parenterally for B_{12} deficiency states at doses of 100 μg subcutaneously daily for a week and then monthly. Folate supplementation should be started only after B_{12} has been started to avoid increased neurologic problems. Patients should be considered for endoscopy every 5 years to rule out gastric carcinoma. While the anemia is reversible, the neurologic deficits of B_{12} deficiency are often not (Evidence Level A).

In modern medicine, megaloblastic anemia is often iatrogenic. Many therapeutic agents interfere with the DNA synthesis and produce macrocytic anemia. Patients receiving HIV therapy and a variety of cytotoxic therapies for cancer or autoimmune diseases may develop macrocytosis.

Nonmegaloblastic macrocytic anemia is quite common and serves to confuse the diagnosis of anemia with a high MCV. Patients with anemia and a high MCV should have a reticulocyte count. Hemolytic anemia with a high reticulocyte count will produce macrocytosis. Younger red cells (reticulocytes) are larger, becoming smaller as they age. Therefore, a higher proportion of younger red cells will lead to a high MCV.

Liver disease also commonly produces a high MCV, usually up to an MCV of approximately 105. This macrocytosis is associated with the finding of target cells in peripheral blood. The cause of this macrocytosis is altered plasma lipids, which lead to increased cell membrane, target cells, and an elevated MCV. Anemia in these patients is often multifactorial because alcohol, dietary deficiency, and GI bleeding may be present in these patients. Patients with macrocytic anemia should also be tested for thyroid disease.

THROMBOCYTOPENIA AND NEUTROPENIA

Thrombocytopenia in older adults may be associated with diseases that have relatively high morbidity or mortality. Therefore, the underlying cause should be sought aggressively. A careful history of drugs should be taken, including both prescribed and over-the-counter medications. Physical examination should include evaluation for enlarged lymph nodes, spleen, and purpura or other signs of bleeding.

Evaluation of thrombocytopenia should include microscopic study of a peripheral blood film. This should be done in a qualified laboratory or by an appropriate physician. Some of the possible findings in the smear are listed in Table 39.2. The first step is to verify that the platelet count is low. There are several situations in which automated cell counters will show falsely low platelet counts (so-called pseudothrombocytopenia). In these situations, abnormal platelet clumping occurs *in vitro*, and platelet clumps will usually be seen in the peripheral blood smear.

Evaluation of red cell morphology is extremely important when working up patients with thrombocytopenia. If fragmented red cells (schistocytes) are found, the differential diagnosis includes life-threatening diseases such as thrombotic thrombocytopenic purpura, hemolytic uremic syndrome, disseminated intravascular coagulation, or other types of microangiopathic hemolytic anemia. Other lab tests, which would be helpful, include serum lactate dehydrogenase, haptoglobin, and bilirubin. These patients usually require hospitalization for rapid diagnosis and for therapeutic interventions. Other types of red cell morphology may include microspherocytes, seen in autoimmune hemolytic anemia, which may accompany immune thrombocytopenia.

The peripheral blood white cell morphology is also helpful when evaluating thrombocytopenia. Patients with hematologic malignancies or pathologic processes involving the marrow may have immature white blood cells in the periphery. These patients require a bone marrow to further define the pathologic process. Patients with allergies or

TABLE 39.2
POSSIBLE PERIPHERAL BLOOD FINDINGS IN THROMBOCYTOPENIA

1. Pseudothrombocytopenia
2. Red cell fragmentation (schistocytes)
3. Microspherocytes
4. Immature white blood cells
5. Atypical mononuclear cells

immune reactions associated with thrombocytopenia may also have atypical mononuclear cells similar to those with infectious mononucleosis.

If the examination of the peripheral blood shows only thrombocytopenia without other cell abnormalities, drug-induced thrombocytopenia should be considered. Drug-induced thrombocytopenia is generally of two types: Mild, asymptomatic, and severe with purpura. Mild drug-induced thrombocytopenia can be caused by agents such as anticonvulsants and some antibiotics. These patients usually have platelet counts in the range of 50 to 150,000. In contrast, severe thrombocytopenia with purpura and bleeding occurs with drugs such as quinine, quinidine, and procainamide. This so-called quinine purpura usually has a rapid onset and a platelet count <20,000. The offending agent should be discontinued immediately because this reaction may become life threatening. Thrombocytopenia should abate within 3 to 5 days of stopping the drug.

Immune thrombocytic purpura (ITP) occurs in adults of all ages, including older patients. ITP will be idiopathic in many cases, but it can be associated with an underlying disease. Lymphoproliferative diseases such as Hodgkin disease, non-Hodgkin lymphoma, or lymphocytic leukemia may be present. These patients may have enlarged lymph nodes or hepatosplenomegaly. Other diseases associated with ITP include rheumatologic conditions such as systemic lupus erythematosus. Initial therapy of these patients usually includes corticosteroids such as prednisone, and additional treatments are often given including intravenous gammaglobulin or therapy for lymphoproliferative diseases.[5]

Heparin-induced thrombocytopenia is a unique entity that may be associated with thrombosis. As mentioned elsewhere, all patients receiving heparin should have platelet counts measured carefully. A reduction in the platelet count requires discontinuation of the heparin. Low–molecular-weight heparin can usually be substituted when heparin-induced thrombocytopenia is noted. Patients with heparin-induced thrombocytopenia should never receive even small doses of heparin again (Evidence Level A). Very small amounts of heparin may be sufficient to trigger this reaction.[6]

Neutropenia is often found in acutely ill patients and may be associated with overwhelming bacterial infection. If neutropenia is seen in association with fever, aggressive use of antibiotics should be undertaken. Chronic neutropenia may be the result of adverse drug reactions or other systemic diseases. Neutropenia can also be an early sign of a myelodysplastic syndrome or other bone marrow malignancy. Bone marrow examination may be necessary to evaluate patients with chronic neutropenia. Finally, neutropenia may be associated with rheumatologic conditions such as rheumatoid arthritis. Chronic neutropenia in these settings is often well tolerated in older patients. If there is no history of infection, no specific therapy may be needed for the chronic neutropenia.

SCREENING FOR BLEEDING PRIOR TO SURGERY/THE PROLONGED PARTIAL THROMBOPLASTIN TIME

Physicians caring for older patients are often asked to screen them for bleeding disorders before surgery. The most useful information in this process is a careful history about prior bleeding (see Table 39.3 for screening questions). In the absence of a bleeding history, screening tests are likely to produce false-positive rather than true-positive results. Preoperative screening should include a complete blood count with platelet count, prothrombin time, and activated partial thromboplastin time (PTT). If these tests are normal in a patient with no history of bleeding, a bleeding disorder is extremely unlikely (Evidence Level C).[7]

A common laboratory abnormality in older patients is a prolonged activated PTT. A prolonged PTT should be followed with a mixing study in which the patient's plasma is mixed with an equal amount of normal plasma and the activated PTT is repeated. If the test corrects immediately after mixing, the patient is confirmed to be deficient in a clotting factor. Some older patients exhibit the so-called lupus anticoagulants. In these patients, immediate mixing study does not correct the PTT because an inhibitor in the patient's plasma interferes with the clotting reaction of the normal plasma *in vitro*. Lupus anticoagulants are usually antiphospholipid antibodies and do not cause clinical bleeding. Most lupus anticoagulants have no clinical sequela except a rare increased tendency to clot. If there is no history of thrombosis, a prolonged PTT owing to a so-called lupus anticoagulant should not deter surgery (Evidence Level B).

Older patients rarely acquire autoimmune antibodies to clotting factors, but if they do, it is usually factor VIII. These patients will have active bleeding and a prolonged PTT that will correct with an immediate mix as described in the preceding text, but the mixed reaction of the patient and normal plasma will be prolonged after incubation of 1 to 2 hours. Patients with acquired factor VIII inhibitors require aggressive immunosuppressive therapy to reduce the antibody. In most cases, a hematology consult should be considered before surgery is considered.

TABLE 39.3

QUESTIONS TO EXPLORE BLEEDING HISTORY

1. Prolonged or excessive bleeding after dental extractions
2. Excessive bleeding after prior surgery
3. Prior blood transfusions
4. Family history of bleeding disorder
5. Excessive bleeding following trauma
6. Excessive bleeding following labor and delivery

PLASMA CELL DISORDERS

Plasma cell proliferative disorders are seen predominantly in older individuals. These diseases are characterized by the production of monoclonal immunoglobulins, which can be detected in serum or urine. Plasma cell proliferative disorders vary from asymptomatic laboratory abnormalities to rapidly progressive illnesses with high mortality. Their differential diagnosis is listed in Table 39.1.[8]

Multiple Myeloma

The most severe of these diseases is multiple myeloma. Multiple myeloma is a plasma cell malignancy that occurs predominantly in older individuals. It produces symptoms involving multiple organ systems as shown in Table 39.4. This disease is an uncommon cause of common complaints. Bone pain in multiple myeloma arises from osteolytic lesions in the spine or proximal long bones. This pain may present with signs of spinal cord compression. New-onset bone pain or changes in a previous stable pattern of pain should lead to the suspicion of multiple myeloma. Bone x-rays and screening of plasma and urine proteins should be ordered. Bone scans are insensitive to these lesions.

Multiple myeloma may also present with other laboratory abnormalities. Anemia is common and often occurs early in the disease. Leukopenia and thrombocytopenia are less common but may also be found. Multiple myeloma is sometimes diagnosed during the workup of normocytic anemia. The bone marrow usually shows increased numbers of atypical plasma cells. If the multiple myeloma responds to treatment, the anemia usually resolves.

Hypercalcemia also occurs in patients with multiple myeloma, apparently secondary to mobilization of calcium from involved bone lesions. The abnormal plasma cells produce factors that increase the osteolytic activity. Patients with unexplained hypercalcemia should be screened for the plasma or urine proteins of multiple myeloma. Other manifestations of multiple myeloma include renal failure, which may also occur before the disease is evident. Immunoglobulin light chains and hypercalciuria are both able to cause direct damage to renal tubular cells.

TABLE 39.4
CLINICAL MANIFESTATIONS OF MULTIPLE MYELOMA—AN UNCOMMON CAUSE OF COMMON PROBLEMS

1. Bone pain
2. Hypercalcemia
3. Anemia
4. Renal failure
5. Bacterial infection

Patients with multiple myeloma are susceptible to bacterial infections. Early in the disease, a small set of patients with multiple myeloma will show marked susceptibility to encapsulated bacteria. These patients may have recurrent infections with streptococcal pneumonia, including infections in atypical sites. Later in the course of multiple myeloma, patients are susceptible to gram-negative infections.

The median survival is 3 to 4 years, but approximately 50% of patients have a good treatment response with up to a sevenfold increase in survival. Prednisone (1 mg per kg) should be started at the time of diagnosis to control the hypercalciuria (Evidence Level B). Most patients will receive melphalan or cyclophosphamide. Patients younger than 70 may be considered for autologous peripheral stem cell support, which has largely replaced bone marrow transplant as a treatment for multiple myeloma. Treatment of multiple myeloma requires a comprehensive approach and is usually conducted under the direction of a hematologist or in a cancer center.[9]

Monoclonal Gammopathy of Unknown Significance

Monoclonal gammopathy of unknown significance occurs almost exclusively in older individuals and is seen with increased frequency in the eighth and ninth decades. This disorder was previously called *benign monoclonal gammopathy* because in many patients there is no disease progression beyond the presence of a monoclonal immunoglobulin "spike" in the serum. Long-term follow-up of several large groups of patients has been described. After 10 years of follow-up, approximately 50% of patients would have died of other causes. Of those who were alive, approximately one half (25% of the initial group) will remain unchanged, without disease progression. The other 25% of the initial group will have progressed to one of the other plasma cell proliferative diseases, usually multiple myeloma. Therefore, patients with monoclonal gammopathy but without manifestations of multiple myeloma should be followed by repeat serum protein studies every 6 to 12 months (Evidence Level A). A progressive increase in the amount of abnormal protein usually predicts disease progression.

Plasmacytoma and Other Plasma Cell Proliferative Diseases

Occasionally, elderly individuals will present with plasma cell proliferation localized to one area. Usually these occur in the bones of the axial skeleton. These patients lack evidence of generalized multiple myeloma at other sites. These tumors are usually quite sensitive to radiation therapy and, if successfully treated, abnormal serum proteins should disappear (Evidence Level B). Some of these patients will apparently be cured with this treatment, whereas others progress to multiple myeloma.[8]

Abnormal monoclonal proteins can also be found in patients with other organ system diseases. Some patients with primary amyloidosis have abnormal monoclonal serum proteins and may benefit from therapy for multiple myeloma. Occasionally, patients with lymphoproliferative disease and rheumatologic conditions will have an associated monoclonal serum protein. This protein does not change the prognosis of the underlying disease.

MYELOPROLIFERATIVE DISEASES

Myeloproliferative diseases are more common in older patients and usually present with a differential diagnosis of elevated blood counts. These diseases are characterized by unregulated proliferation of blood cell precursors. In each situation, the diagnosis of elevated blood counts in older patients includes myeloproliferative diseases as well as other problems for which the abnormal blood counts occur as a secondary process.

Erythrocytosis

Diseases included in the differential diagnosis of erythrocytosis are shown in Table 39.1. A mild increase in red blood counts can occur in patients who have chronic reduction of plasma volume. In these patients, the red cell mass is normal but other factors such as the chronic use of diuretics or lack of adequate fluid intake may lead to mild concentration of red cell counts, usually with hematocrits in the 50% to 55% range. Generally, patients with hematocrits above 55% have an elevation of their red cell mass.

Patients with elevated red cell counts should have a history taken to determine occupation, tobacco use, and family history of high blood counts. Physical examination should include evaluation for hepatosplenomegaly. Routine lab tests including white cell count, platelet count, and plasma erythropoietin are useful. In a number of situations, the patient will have elevated erythropoietin in the presence of increased red cell production; that is, the marrow responds appropriately to an abnormal external stimulus. A common cause of elevated erythropoietin is tobacco smoking and the subsequent chronic carbon monoxide exposure. Patients with heavy smoking exposure from cigarettes, cigars, or pipes often have carboxyhemoglobin levels in the range of 5% or higher. Carboxyhemoglobin cannot carry oxygen, triggering increased erythropoietin production with elevated red cell counts. Increased erythropoietin production occurs in patients with arterial hypoxemia due to chronic lung disease. Ectopic erythropoietin can be produced by some tumors, such as renal cell carcinoma. Also, familial erythrocytosis occurs in patients with some inherited hemoglobinopathies. These hemoglobins bind oxygen tighter than normal hemoglobin and lead to increased erythropoietin production and increased red cell counts.

Erythrocytosis, in the face of low or absent erythropoietin, occurs when the marrow red cell precursors lose their sensitivity to erythropoietin. This autonomous proliferation occurs in polycythemia vera. Polycythemia vera is a myeloproliferative disease in which the unregulated growth of precursor cells produces increased red cells, often with elevated white cell and platelet production. The patients may present with plethora and often have a peculiar intense itching, especially after showering in warm water. They often have splenomegaly on physical examination.[10]

Polycythemia vera is a chronic disease associated with increased risk of thrombosis and bleeding. Early treatment with therapeutic phlebotomy may be successful in some patients, but others develop thrombocytosis requiring cytotoxic therapy. Late complications include transformation to acute leukemia or progression to a form of bone marrow failure characterized by intense bone marrow fibrosis (myelofibrosis).

Thrombocytosis

Elevated platelet counts occur in multiple clinical situations. A list of the associated diseases with thrombocytosis is shown in Table 39.1. GI bleeding and/or chronic iron deficiency often produce thrombocytosis. Treatment of the iron deficiency will resolve the elevated platelet count. Thrombocytosis also occurs in some patients with an underlying solid tumor, sometimes before the cancer becomes otherwise evident. Finally, thrombocytosis is a manifestation of several myeloproliferative disorders.

Patients with unexplained thrombocytosis should have a history taken for weight loss and GI or chest symptoms. A physical examination should include evaluation of enlarged lymph nodes and hepatosplenomegaly. Screening for GI and chest malignancy should be routine. Patients should also be screened for iron deficiency. If no underlying disease is present, the thrombocytosis may be caused by a primary myeloproliferative disease.

Thrombocytosis that is not due to a myeloproliferative disease usually does not have overt clinical consequences, but thrombocytosis associated with myeloproliferative diseases causes arterial and venous occlusive disease. This appears to be related to platelet abnormalities associated with myeloproliferative disease. In older patients, thrombocytosis caused by a myeloproliferative disease such as polycythemia vera or primary thrombocythemia should be treated with agents to reduce the platelet count. Untreated, these patients are more likely to develop strokes, heart attacks, and GI bleeding.

Leukocytosis

Granulocytic leukocytosis often presents a diagnostic problem in older patients. History should include symptoms of acute or chronic infection such as fever, night sweats, or weight loss. Physical examination should include evaluation for lymphadenopathy and hepatosplenomegaly. Leukemoid reactions can also occur with tumors such as lung or GI cancer.

Most patients with granulocytic leukocytosis do not have a leukemic process, but the differential diagnosis includes chronic myelogenous leukemia (CML). Patients with CML usually have anemia and splenomegaly, and confirmation of the diagnosis requires finding a specific unique genetic abnormality, the *BCR-ABL* gene. The treatment of this disease has recently been improved by a new agent that interferes with the product of this oncogene. The tyrosine kinase inhibitor imatinib (Gleevec) produces significant responses in most patients.[11]

Lymphocytic leukemia also occurs in older patients, usually due to chronic lymphocytic leukemia or other variants of lymphoproliferative diseases. These patients may have enlarged lymph nodes or hepatosplenomegaly. Specific diagnosis is usually accomplished by flow cytometry of the abnormal lymphoid cells to define their surface antigens. Treatment of chronic lymphocytic leukemia depends heavily on the presence of anemia, thrombocytopenia, or degree of infiltration of organs by the lymphoid tissue.[12]

VENOUS THROMBOSIS

Venous clotting disorders, such as deep vein thrombosis and pulmonary embolism, are common in the elderly. The factors that predispose to thrombosis are listed in Table 39.5. Immobilization commonly leads to venous thrombosis, so it is now routine to anticoagulate older patients following hip or knee surgery. Long bus, train, or airline rides also predispose to thrombosis. Tobacco smoking and estrogen therapy also increase the risk.

Venous thrombosis is sometimes seen in patients with occult neoplasm. Adenocarcinoma of the lung and pancreas can produce the so-called Trousseau syndrome, in which recurrent thrombosis may precede the manifestation of the tumor by months.

Inherited thrombophilic diseases are also associated with venous clotting. The most common inherited thrombophilic disease is due to factor V Leiden. This abnormal clotting factor, a variation of factor V, is resistant to inhibition by the natural clotting inhibitor, activated protein C (APC). APC resistance is usually detected in clotting disorders of younger patients but the abnormality is common and may remain undetected in older individuals as well. In addition to factor V Leiden, other identified thrombophilic diseases include abnormalities of protein S, protein C, and antithrombin III. Acquired lupus anticoagulants may also manifest with increased clotting. Generally, screening for these thrombophilic states is indicated in older patients only if there is a family history of thrombosis in younger relatives.[13]

Treatment of deep vein thrombosis is intended to prevent extension of the clot and/or prevent pulmonary embolism. Anticoagulation should be given for at least 4 months and the associated predisposing factors be reduced as much as possible.[14,15]

TABLE 39.5
FACTORS PREDISPOSING TO VENOUS THROMBOSIS

1. Prolonged immobilization
2. Estrogen therapy
3. Tobacco smoking
4. Obesity
5. Thrombocytosis
6. Occult malignancy
7. Inherited thrombophilias

REFERENCES

1. Ania BJ, Suman VJ, Fairbanks VF, et al. Incidence of anemia in older people: An epidemiologic study in a well defined population. *J Am Geriatr Soc.* 2003;45:825–831.
2. Pennix BW, Guralnik JM, Onder G, et al. Anemia and decline in physical performance among older persons. *Am J Med.* 2003;115:104–110.
3. Guralnik J, Eisenstaedt R, Ferrucci F, et al. Prevalence of anemia in persons 65 years and older in the US: Evidence for high rate of unexplained anemia. *Blood.* 2004;15:2263–2268.
4. Goodnough L, Skikne B, Brugnora C. Erythropoietin, iron and erythropoiesis. *Blood.* 2000;96:823–833.
5. Cines DB, Blanchette VS. Immune thrombocytopenic purpura. *N Engl J Med.* 2002;346:995.
6. Warkentin T. Heparin induced thrombocytopenia. *Circulation.* 2004;110:454–458.
7. Kojouri K, Vesely S, Terrell D, et al. Splenectomy for adult patients with idiopathic thrombocytopenic purpura: A systematic review to assess long-term platelet count responses, prediction of response, and surgical complications. *Blood.* 2004;104:2623–2634.
8. Dimopoulos M, Moulopoulis L, Maniatas A, et al. Solitary plasmacytoma of bone and asymptomatic multiple myeloma. *Blood.* 2000;96:2037–2044.
9. Hideshima T, Bergsagel P, Kuehl W, et al. Advances in the biology of multiple myeloma: Clinical applications. *Blood.* 2004;104:607–618.
10. Spivak J. Polycythemia vera myths, mechanisms, and management. *Blood.* 2002;100:4272–4290.
11. Kantarjian H, Sawyers C, Hochhaus A, et al. Hematologic and cytogenetic responses to imatinib mesylate in chronic myelogenous leukemia. *N Engl J Med.* 2002;346:645–652.
12. Shanafelt T, Geyer S, Kay N. Prognosis at diagnosis: Integrating molecular biologic insights into clinical practice for patients with CLL. *Blood.* 2004;103:1202–1210.
13. Seligsohn U, Lubetsky A. Genetic susceptibility to venous thrombosis. *N Engl J Med.* 2001;344:1222–1226.
14. Hirsh J, O'Donell M, Weitz J. New anticoagulants. *Blood.* 2005;105:453–463.
15. Ridker P, Goldhaber S, Danielson E, et al. Long-term, low-Intensity warfarin therapy for the prevention of recurrent venous thromboembolism. *N Engl J Med.* 2003;348:1425–1434.

Common Infections in the Elderly

40

William A. Woolery

- **CLINICAL PEARLS 554**
- **AGING IN THE IMMUNE SYSTEM 554**
- **EPIDEMIOLOGY 555**
- **CLINICAL FEATURES OF INFECTIONS IN THE ELDERLY 555**
- **LABORATORY/DIAGNOSIS 556**
- **SPECIFIC INFECTIONS 556**
  - Urinary Tract Infections 556
  - Sepsis 557
  - Varicella Zoster Virus Infection 557
  - Viral Hepatitis 558
  - Severe Acute Respiratory Syndrome 558
  - West Nile Fever 558
  - Human Immunodeficiency Virus 558
  - Influenza 559
- **CUTANEOUS INFECTIONS 559**
  - Pressure Ulcers 559
- **IMMUNIZATIONS 560**
- **COMMUNITY-ACQUIRED RESISTANT PATHOGENS 561**
- **CONCLUSION 561**

CLINICAL PEARLS

- The skin undergoes changes that predispose the host to a variety of infectious insults.
- Innate immunity does not appear to be affected by aging, but several changes occur with acquired immunity.
- Infectious diseases account for approximately one third of all deaths in individuals older than 65.
- Only 60% of older adults develop leukocytosis even with a serious infection.
- Thirty percent of elderly women and 10% of elderly men experience bacteriuria in their lifetimes.
- Asymptomatic bacteriuria in the elderly does not require treatment.
- Prostatitis in elderly patients should be treated for 6 to 12 weeks.
- Management of an elderly patient with sepsis involves the prompt administration of IV fluids and broad-spectrum antibiotics.
- Famciclovir may be the antiviral agent of choice for herpes zoster.
- Human immunodeficiency virus (HIV) infection does occur in the elderly. Up to age 70, homosexuality ranks first as a co-factor to infection. Heterosexual transmission is an increasing risk.
- Rimantadine for influenza treatment has few central nervous system (CNS) side effects and is not dependent on renal excretion.
- Fifty percent of individuals older than 60 do not have sufficient levels of antitoxin antibodies to protect against tetanus or diphtheria.

AGING IN THE IMMUNE SYSTEM

Immune senescence can create an inefficient immune response. Clinically, immune senescence potentiates the colonization of the elderly, particularly the ill, by more virulent microorganisms and sets the stage for more serious infections.[1]

Several anatomic and physiologic changes occur with aging that compromise the ability to ward off infections. The first line of defense, the skin and mucosal lining, undergo important changes that predispose the host to a variety of infectious insults.[2,3] The epidermis thins, resulting in a decreased production of Langerhans cells, interleukin-1, and thymocyte-activity factor. As a result, cellulitis and infected decubitus ulcers become more likely. Mucocutaneous tissue production of secretory Immunoglobin A (IgA), a predominant immunoglobulin of the mucosal immune system, does not appear to be reduced with aging.[1,2]

A normal immune response is comprised of two independent processes. Innate (natural) immunity is comprised of neutrophils, macrophages, and natural killer cells, which do not require prior sensitization to respond to a foreign antigen.[1–3] However, repeated exposure to a specific antigen does not enhance these cells' response. The second type, acquired immunity, requires the activation of the immune system following the exposure to an antigen. The acquired immune response involves cells of lymphoid lineage, T cells (cellular immunity) and B cells (humoral immunity) stimulated to the production of a variety of antigen-specific compounds. Repeated exposure to the antigen enhances the immune response.[3]

Innate immunity does not appear to be greatly affected by aging. However, there are several changes that occur with acquired immunity. There is a decreased production of interleukin-2 (IL-2) and IL-2-induced T cells. The number of circulating and antigen-responsive B cells also decreases. Dysfunctional B lymphocytes produce less effective and fewer antibodies. As a result, the quality, quantity, and memory of antigen-specific molecules is adversely affected. These effects combine to blunt the response to vaccination, and increase the likelihood of infection in the elderly. Humoral antibody unresponsiveness accounts, in part, for the increased incidence and high mortality associated with pneumonia, influenza, infectious endocarditis, and tetanus in the elderly.[4]

EPIDEMIOLOGY

Infectious diseases account for approximately one third of all deaths in individuals older than 65. Ninety percent of all deaths due to pneumonia occur in people older than 65.[5] Influenza and pneumonia are the fourth leading causes of death in the elderly. Bacteremia is the ninth leading cause.

As the population ages and travel becomes easier, a greater variety of pathogens emerge as potential health concerns in the elderly. Hanta and Ebola virus, herpes simplex type 6, methicillin-resistant *Staphylococcus aureus* (MRSA), penicillin-resistant *Staphylococcus pneumoniae* (PRSP), vancomycin-resistant enterococci (VRE), and multiple drug-resistant, gram-negative bacilli (MDRGNB), Cryptosporidium, and severe acute respiratory syndrome (SARS) will trigger a larger portion of morbidity and mortality in the elderly. Compared to young, healthy adults, mortality from any specific infections in the elderly may be 20 to 25 times greater.[6] Table 40.1 lists common infections seen in the elderly.

CLINICAL FEATURES OF INFECTIONS IN THE ELDERLY

Infections in the elderly may present in an atypical, unusual, and nonclassical fashion, yet early diagnosis and treatment greatly lowers the morbidity and mortality in this population.[7] The signs and symptoms of infection that are common in younger patients are frequently less obvious or even absent in older patients. Only 60% of older adults develop leukocytosis with a serious infection, yet the absence of such response does not rule out an infectious process. Nuchal rigidity may be absent in geriatric patients with bacterial meningitis and peritoneal signs may be absent in elderly patients with intra-abdominal infections. In all elderly patients with any infection, there may be a complete disassociation of the clinical signs and symptoms with the severity of the illness.[7,8]

There are several factors associated with the atypical presentation of infection in the elderly. Coexisting diseases may mask or alter the normal immune response to infection in the elderly while increasing the risk of infection. The inability of a patient to cognitively interpret signs and symptoms may be complicated by an inability to communicate. Normally, nonpathogenic or weakly pathogenic organisms may become virulent in the elderly. Lastly, an altered physiologic response can create an atypical presentation.[9,10]

Fever, like many physiologic functions, normally exhibits a circadian rhythm. Early morning values are lowest, 36.1°C (97.0°F), rising to temperatures of 37.4°C (99.3°F) in the late afternoon.[5,11,12] This cyclic variation has two important consequences in the elderly. First, febrile responses associated with a disease state, although superimposed on the normal circadian variation, peak in the late afternoon or early evening. Therefore, the patient cannot be considered to be afebrile until the temperature pattern has been monitored for at least 24 hours. Second, small temperature elevations >37.0°C (98.6°F) are often recorded in healthy individuals. It has been recommended that a temperature elevation of 2°C (1.1°F) from the baseline temperature be used as a true indicator of fever (Evidence Level C). However, in the elderly, a core temperature of 37.8°C (100.0°F) associated with a decline of mental functioning is highly suggestive of an infectious process.[11,12] A blunted or absent febrile response occurs in 20% to 30% of geriatric patients, particularly in individuals 75 years or older. The presence of fever should not be taken lightly, as up to 10%

TABLE 40.1
DIFFERENTIAL DIAGNOSIS OF COMMON INFECTIONS WITH ICD-9 CODES

Systemic Infections	**Organ Specific**
Immune deficiency (279.3)	Pneumonia (486)
Sepsis (995.91)	Pneumonitis (486)
SIRS (995.90)	Urinary infections (599.0)
West Nile fever (066.40)	Prostatitis (601.9)
HIV (V08)	Bacteriuria (791.9)
Influenza (487.1)	Asymptomatic bacteria (791.9)
	Upper respiratory infection (465.9)
	Gastroenteritis (558.9)
Microbe Specific	**Cutaneous**
PRSP (V09.0)	Cellulitis (682.9)
MRSA (V09.0)	Shingles (herpes zoster) (053.9)
VRE (V09.8)	Herpes simplex (054.9)
MDRGNB (V09.90)	Encephalitis (323.9)
VISA (V09.8)	Hepatitis (573.3)
	Pyodermas (686.00)
	Folliculitis (704.8)
	Furuncles (680.9)
	Carbuncles (680.9)
	Hidradenitis suppurativa (705.83)
	Erysipelas (035)
	Pressure ulcers (707.00)

SIRS, systemic inflammatory response syndrome; HIV, human immunodeficiency virus; PRSP, penicillin-resistant *streptococcus pneumoniae*; MRSA, methicillin-resistant *Staphylococcus aureus*; VRE, vancomycin-resistant Enterococci; MDRGNB, multiple drug-resistant gram-negative bacilli; VISA, vancomycin-resistant/intermediate *S. aureus*

of febrile patients older than 60 who present to an emergency department die within 1 month, compared to 1% to 5% of younger individuals. The clinician should also keep in mind that fever may occur as a result of noninfectious processes.

LABORATORY/DIAGNOSIS

Although a thorough history and physical is the cornerstone for the management and treatment of patients, this may be very difficult in the elderly patient. The incidence of confusion and delirium increases in the infected patient and compromises the accuracy of history in many cases.[13]

The white blood cells (WBC) and band percentage have a high predictability of bacteremia (sepsis) in the elderly. Generally, a WBC count of >11,000 with a bandemia of 6% or greater is highly predictive of bacteremia.

A chest radiography (CXR) is useful to confirm the diagnosis of pneumonia, but the predictive value of a sputum Gram stain and culture is debated. Urinalysis is a simple test to obtain, but interpreting the results should be done carefully. Negative urinalysis results are more useful in excluding a urinary tract infection than positive results are in diagnosing an infection. Blood cultures from two separate sites should be obtained on all febrile hospitalized patients. Afebrile elderly individuals presenting with an acute functional decline and leukocytosis with bandemia or pulmonary infiltrate should also have blood cultures obtained.

SPECIFIC INFECTIONS

Pneumonia, a major infectious disease in the elderly, is discussed in detail in Chapter 30.

Urinary Tract Infections

Urinary tract infections (UTIs) are the most common bacterial infection in the elderly. Up to 30% of elderly women and 10% of elderly men experience bacteriuria in their lifetimes. Elderly individuals are predisposed to UTIs because of age-associated anatomic changes in the genitourinary tract and immunologic function.[14] Elderly women have an increased incidence of bladder prolapse, which causes incomplete bladder emptying and urinary stasis. Prostate enlargement in men causes outflow obstruction and urinary stasis. Stagnant urine is a potential microbial culture medium for the colonization and growth of bacteria and subsequent bacteriuria. Adding to stasis is the aging kidney's inability to excrete high urea loads, resulting in less concentrated urine and diminished antibacterial properties.

Uncomplicated UTIs are caused by a fairly predictable group of susceptible microorganisms. Complicated UTIs are usually associated with anatomic or functional abnormalities of the genitourinary tract. The diagnosis of UTI is partially based on a quantitative urine culture yielding >100,000 (10^5) colony-forming units or bacteria per mL of urine.[15]

Asymptomatic UTI is the presence of bacteriuria without dysuria, polyuria, new-onset incontinence, pyuria, new-onset mental status changes, fever, and suprapubic tenderness. Asymptomatic UTIs are frequently transient in nature. Most experts agree that asymptomatic UTIs in the elderly do not require treatment (Evidence Level B). However, those elderly patients with asymptomatic bacteriuria who are scheduled to undergo invasive genitourinary procedures or surgery should receive prophylactic antibiotic therapy. In this case, therapy is initiated to prevent urosepsis rather than for the treatment of the bacteriuria.

Uncomplicated symptomatic UTIs should be treated. The goal of treatment is to alleviate symptoms and not necessarily sterilize the urine. The antibiotics of choice include trimethoprim (TMP)—sulfamethoxazole (SMZ), first generation cephalosporins, nitrofurantoin, or quinolones. Ampicillin or amoxicillin provide good coverage for enterococcal infections. In renally compromised elderly patients, an extended spectrum cephalosporin or quinolone at a reduced dose, for at least 7 days, is the preferred therapy.[16]

Empiric therapy for complicated UTI should include third-generation cephalosporin, aztreonam, quinolones, or aminoglycosides (Evidence Level A). One dose monotherapy is not recommended due to the high rate of recurrence.

Patients with indwelling urinary catheters have polymicrobial urine. After approximately 1 month, these patients become bacteriuric. Antimicrobial therapy is reserved for those patients who develop clinical signs of infection. The antibiotics of choice for these symptomatic patients with indwelling urinary catheters are TMP/SMZ, quinolones, and an augmented penicillin. The treatment should continue for 7 days. Prolonged therapy in those individuals will lead to the emergence of more resistant microorganisms.[15,16]

Prolonged treatment of UTIs in the elderly is generally discouraged. There are a few exceptions. Prostatitis in elderly male patients should be treated for 6 to 12 weeks because antibiotics penetrate noninflamed prostate glands poorly, and the condition is subject to recurrence (Evidence Level B). Long-term therapy in those patients with large unremovable struvite renal stones is also recommended to suppress recurrent infections and prevent the enlargement of the stone(s).

Prevention of recurrent UTIs in the elderly lies primarily with the management of comorbid conditions to the extent that this can be accomplished. Avoidance of indwelling urinary catheters and condom catheters, whenever possible, decreases the frequency of bacteriuria substantially. Unfortunately, there is no compelling evidence to support the use of cranberry juice to prevent infections.

Sepsis

Bacteremia is defined as the presence of bacteria in the blood stream, and sepsis or septicemia is the physiologic syndrome and systemic inflammatory response to an infection or endotoxic product. Sepsis is the fifth leading cause of death in those older than 65.[15] Mortality approximates 50% in individuals older than 65 and nearly 100% in the very old.[17] Mortality is greatest in those elderly individuals with a nongenitourinary source of infection. Primary sources of sepsis in the elderly are the genitourinary tract, lungs, skin, and biliary tract. Gram-negative bacteremia causes two thirds of sepsis in the elderly.

There are no pathognomonic signs and symptoms of sepsis in the elderly.[1] The classic triad of tachycardia, rigors, and hypotension are rare in most elderly individuals. Elderly individuals with new-onset falls, altered mental status, oliguria, and abdominal pain should raise a suspicion for sepsis. Tachypnea, although a nonspecific sign, is frequently present in the elderly patient presenting with bacteremia or sepsis.

The systemic inflammatory response syndrome (SIRS) is the generalized physiologic response to inflammation (burns, trauma) or infection. An individual must have two or more of the following criteria for the diagnosis of SIRS:

- Temperature >38.4°C (101.0°F) or <35.6°C (96.1°F)
- Heart rate >90 beats per minute
- Respiratory rate >20 breaths per minute
- WBCs >12,000 per mm^3 or >10% bands.[1]

Sepsis is diagnosed when an individual meets the SIRS criteria and has documented positive blood cultures.

The management of an elderly patient with sepsis is in the prompt administration of IV fluids and broad-spectrum antibiotics. A third-generation cephalosporin, imipenem/cilastin, ticarcillin/clavulanate with or without an aminoglycoside, aztreonam, or parenteral fluoroquinolone is generally adequate coverage until definitive culture results are available (Evidence Level A). Vancomycin or linezolid (Zyvox) should be added when MRSA is a concern. Fluid deficits should be calculated and administered aggressively but cautiously in the elderly, who often have coexistent cardiovascular problems.

Varicella Zoster Virus Infection

Varicella zoster virus (VZV) is a deoxyribo nucleic acid (DNA) virus that belongs to the herpes virus family. It is six times more common in those older than 80 compared to those younger than 50. VZV causes two distinct clinical syndromes: Primary disseminated infection (chicken pox), and reactivation of the latent virus in the dorsal root ganglion (herpes zoster or "shingles").[1,6,7]

Diagnosis can be facilitated by fluorescin/conjugated monoclonal antibody to VZV assay. The test takes 2 hours but accurately differentiates VZV from herpes simplex virus (HSV).

Herpes zoster (shingles) develops in patients with previous exposure to VZV. Shingles probably reflects a patient's waning acquired immunity status. The severity of the disease and its complications increase with age and comorbid conditions. Age, severity of acute pain, rash severity, sensory impairment, and location (trigeminal nerve involvement) are all predictors of the development of postherpetic neuralgia, which develops in up to 75% of those older than 70. Once postherpetic neuralgia develops, the treatment of pain is generally disappointing.

The treatment of acute VZV infection should be initiated within 72 hours of the onset of rash. Oral acyclovir has been the standard of treatment for several years.[1,11] However, valacyclovir (Valtrex) and famciclovir (Famvir) may prove to be better agents for therapy. The most dramatic treatment results with acyclovir are in those patients with fever and those older than 67 (Evidence Level B). Acyclovir, valacyclovir, and famciclovir all require dose reduction in renal-impaired patients. Famciclovir's active metabolite, pencidovir triphosphate, has an intracellular half-life >9 hours, compared with 0.9 hours for acyclovir triphosphate. Coupled with demonstrated reduction in postherpetic neuralgia and dosing three times a day, famciclovir may be the antiviral agent of choice (Evidence Level B). Corticosteroids do not appear to improve the clinical outcomes.

Patients with disseminated VZV, zoster encephalitis, zoster pneumonitis, ocular involvement, and those who are significantly immunocompromised should receive intravenous acyclovir. The intravenous dosing of acyclovir requires renal dose adjustment due to potential nephrotoxicity.

Research on the VZV vaccine in adults suggests that the induction of an immunity in adults compared to children is more difficult. Although not yet approved for use in adults to prevent the recurrence of varicella zoster, it appears that a two-dose regimen will be required.

Viral Hepatitis

Hepatitis A virus (HAV) is a ribonucleic acid (RNA) virus transmitted by the fecal-oral route. Most elderly individuals older than 80 are seropositive. With advanced age, the clinical manifestations of HAV are more severe with prolonged cholestasis. Although HAV deaths in the United States are uncommon, 70% of deaths are in individuals older than 50. HAV vaccination appears to confer almost 100% seroconversion in elderly individuals.

Hepatitis B virus (HBV) is a DNA virus transmitted by parenteral or sexual means. Transfusion-related HBV infection is now uncommon. Acute HBV infection in the elderly is generally a mild cholestatic-like infection. However, the development of a chronic carrier state occurs more often in those individuals infected later in life and the rate of hepatocellular carcinoma increases in the elderly. Treatment of HBV infections is generally supportive in nature.[9,10] HBV vaccination provides only 50% seroconversion in individuals older than 60.

Hepatitis C virus (HCV) is an RNA virus transmitted parenterally (and possibly sexually) in the elderly individual. HCV accounts for most acute viral hepatitis in older adults. The major risk factor for HCV is the receipt of blood or blood product transfusion before 1990, when routine screening of the nation's blood supply began. The clinical signs of acute HCV infection are generally mild and flulike. Fulminant HCV hepatitis is uncommon. The development of chronic liver disease is very common, and it is associated with an increase in risk for hepatocellular carcinoma.[1,10] Treatment of HCV requires combination therapy with α-interferon and ribavirin, but response rates are generally poor in elderly individuals. Therapy should be reserved for those individuals with type 1 genotype, low RNA viral titer, and minimal hepatic fibrosis on liver biopsy.

The importance of hepatitis E and G have yet to be determined in the elderly.

Severe Acute Respiratory Syndrome

With the availability of world travel to endemic areas, the geriatrician must ask about travel in patients who present with an upper respiratory type infection.[18] Elderly patients with SARS appear to have a prolonged incubation period of 14 to 21 days and may present with nausea and vomiting accompanying respiratory symptoms. The presence of fever of >38°C (100°F) (one of the generally accepted clinical criteria for SARS) may not be evident in the elderly patient. The mortality rate increases with age to >75% in those age 85 and older.[19] The side effects of treatment with ribavirin and high-dose corticosteroids may not be well tolerated.

West Nile Fever

West Nile Fever (WNF) is a zoonotic disease that is transmitted to humans by mosquitoes and has shown increased incidence across the United States over the past several years. Clinical features of WNF include fever, diarrhea, and rash. Forty percent present with confusion, and 50% with headaches.[20] A decline in consciousness preceded all fatal outcomes. Mortality approximates 25%. In those elderly survivors, 70% returned to baseline functioning. Treatment is supportive.

Human Immunodeficiency Virus

Human immunodeficiency virus (HIV) infection does occur in the elderly. Thirty percent of new cases older than 65 are women. Up to the age of 70, homosexuality ranks first, intravenous drug use second, blood transfusion third, and heterosexual transmission fourth, as cofactors to infection.[9–11] Important history includes blood transfusion before 1984, but 20-plus years post-blood screening, very few new-onset transfusion-related cases will occur. Other history should include sexual preferences, condom use, and intravenous drug use. Heterosexual transmission is an increasing risk as many elderly remain sexually active late in life. Infected elderly individuals have a higher mortality rate compared to their younger cohorts. Age is a factor, but the failure to diagnose HIV early in the elderly is the primary reason for an accelerated course and increased mortality rate.

Treatment usually requires triple-drug therapy, two nucleoside reverse transcriptase inhibitors (RTI) and one protease inhibitor. The financial cost and adverse side effects profile may preclude elders from participating in triple-drug regimens[21,22] (Evidence Level A).

Influenza

Influenza viruses are RNA viruses classified as A, B, or C. Influenza C is a nonvirulent form, B is a risk primarily to children, and A attacks persons of all ages. Influenza A is a major cause of morbidity and mortality in the elderly. The presence of one high-risk comorbid medical condition increases the risk of death from influenza to almost 40-fold.[1,9]

The signs and symptoms of influenza A infections in the elderly include rapid onset of headache, myalgias, fever, cough, and sore throat. Most individuals recover in 7 to 10 days, but elderly adults may develop persistent fatigue that may last for several weeks. Individuals older than 70 have a 75% change of developing pneumonia.

There are four antiviral agents approved for the treatment of influenza A. All four agents, amantadine (Symmetrel), rimantadine (Flumadine), zanamivir (Relenza), and oseltamivir (Tamiflu) must be taken within 48 hours of the onset of symptoms to be effective. Since most elderly elect to treat "flu-like" illnesses at home, the window of opportunity frequently has passed by the time they seek care. Rimantadine is more expensive but has fewer central nervous system (CNS) side effects and is less dependent on renal excretion. Amantadine and oseltamivir both require dosage adjustment in elderly patients with impaired renal function. Table 40.2 reviews treatments for influenza infections.

Influenza vaccine is made from egg-grown viruses that are purified and inactivated. The current vaccines contain viral antigens from two type A and one type B virus. Influenza vaccination is indicated for all elderly individuals and those who care for elderly individuals. The vaccination reduces the risk of infection 50% to 60% in elderly individuals. The only contraindication to vaccination is a previous history of Guillain–Barré syndrome or an anaphylactic hypersensitivity to eggs. People who eat eggs or products that contain eggs can be vaccinated safely. Nasal vaccination with FluMist is not yet recommended in the elderly.

CUTANEOUS INFECTIONS

Elderly individuals are at increased risk for skin infections because of their impaired immunity and the coexistence of multiple comorbid conditions. Superficial skin infections (primary pyodermas) occur in all age-groups, but are more common in the community-dwelling elderly patient. Localized *S. aureus* include: Folliculitis, furuncles, carbuncles, and hidradenitis suppurativa. Most of these infections can be treated effectively with conservative measures with antistaphylococcal antibiotics (cloxacillin, first generation cephalosporins, clindamycin, minocycline).[2,3] Erysipelas is a primary pyoderma caused by group A, C, or G streptococci. Erysipelas most commonly involves the cutaneous lymphatic vessels of the face.

Uncommon microbes can cause cellulitis. *Pasteurella multocida* from dog or cat bites is treated with TMP/sulfamoxole (SMX). *Enteromonas* hydrophilia from contaminated freshwater or after the application of leeches; *Vibrio vulnificus* after ingestion of contaminated oysters or other shellfish causes characteristic bullous skin lesions that can mimic gas gangrene and are treated with doxycycline. Elderly individuals with underlying cirrhosis are particularly susceptible.[23]

Erysipeloid is a localized subacute cellulitis caused by the gram-positive bacilli, *Erysipelothrix rhusiopathiae. Erysipelothrix* is acquired from the handling of contaminated animals or fish, usually following some trauma to the skin. Treatment is with penicillin.

Nodular lymphangitis is characterized by the superficial nodules of the subcutaneous lymphatics and is caused by *Sporothrix schenckii* or *Mycobacterium marinum. Sporothrix* is a fungus that is found in the soil and occurs primarily in gardeners. Treatment is with itraconazole. The *M. marinum* occurs both in fresh and salt water. Most cases occur in those individuals who have contact with fresh or saltwater aquariums, swimming pools, or fish. Treatment is usually with doxycycline or TMP/SMX.

Pressure Ulcers

Pressure ulcers develop in elderly patients from direct pressure and resulting skin and subcutaneous ischemia.[1] Greater than two thirds of pressure ulcers occur in people older than 70. Malnutrition and fecal/urinary incontinence, and limited mobility are risk factors for the development of pressure ulcers. Pressure ulcers are staged to reflect the layers of tissues involved: Stage 1—skin intact with observable pressure-related ulcerations; stage 2—partial thickness loss of intact skin involving the epidermis or dermis; stage 3—full skin thickness loss with subcutaneous necrosis; stage 4—full skin thickness loss with extensive damage to underlying muscle, tendon, or bone.

Pressure ulcers generally yield polymicrobial culture results. The most commonly found bacteria are *S. aureus*, gram-negative rods, *Bacteroides fragilis, Proteus mirabilis*, and

TABLE 40.2
INFLUENZA TREATMENT

Adults >65 y of Age	Normal Renal Function
Documented influenza A	Amantadine 100 mg daily for 3–5 d Rimantadine 100 mg daily for 3–5 d Zanamivir two inhalations (10 mg) twice daily for 3–5 d Oseltamivir 75 mg twice daily for 3–5 d
Prophylaxis	Unvaccinated patient exposed to influenza A Amantadine/rimantadine 100 mg daily for 1 wk postexposure Zanamivir and oseltamivir are not approved in patients for whom vaccination is contraindicated. Amantadine 100 mg daily for 10–12 wks during the influenza season
Renal impairment	Amantadine
Creatinine clearance	
20–30 mL/min	200 mg twice wkly
10–20 mL/min	100 mg thrice wkly
<10 mL/min	100 mg every 7 d

anaerobes. Left untreated or inadequately treated, they can result in secondary cellulitis, necrotizing fasciitis, contiguous osteomyelitis, bacteremia, sepsis, endocarditis, and rarely tetanus.[24]

The key to the management and treatment of pressure ulcers is prevention. Relief of pressure and shearing forces is essential for healing. If this is not accomplished, healing will not occur. Reduction in the bacterial count of the wound also promotes healing. Topical antibiotic therapy may lower bacterial counts but penetrate deep ulcers poorly. The multitude of "cleaning solutions" used (hydrogen peroxide, povidone/iodine, boric acid, Dakin solution) all have antiseptic properties but most cause damage to surrounding healthy tissues. If these agents are used, they should be highly diluted. Some long-term care facilities use a mixture of 50% normal saline, 25% hydrogen peroxide, and 25% Dakin solution.

Hydrogel or hydrocolloid dressings reduce the need for frequent dressing changes. Mechanical or chemical debridement of the wound is necessary before the reapplication of an occlusive dressing.

A relatively new treatment modality, negative-pressure wound therapy (NPWT) was developed in 1990.[25] The effect of this negative pressure results in quicker closure and resolution of the pressure ulcer. NPWT is contraindicated in those wounds caused by malignancy, untreated contiguous osteomyelitis, unexplored fistulas, or overexposed blood vessels or organs. Inadequately prepared wound beds with eschar formation, freshly debrided wounds without adequate hemostasis, and desiccated wounds are not candidates for NPWT.

When secondary cellulitis, osteomyelitis, or sepsis is a concern, treatment with systemic antibiotics is recommended. Clindamycin or metronidazole plus quinolone, aztreonam, or ticarcillin/clavulanic acid provides good coverage for the variety of bacteria found in pressure ulcers. (For more on pressure ulcers, see Chapter 37.)

IMMUNIZATIONS

Most elderly individuals have been immunized for a variety of diseases at some point in their lifespan. However, they still require some immunizations even though adverse effects can occur at any age.[1,9] A hypersensitivity reaction, local or systemic, can occur due to the inherent immunogenic substances contained in the vaccine and the toxoids. This is of particular concern in those immunoglobulins of equine (botulism antitoxin, many antivenoms) or egg (influenza) origin. Known hypersensitivity to a vaccine or toxoid component is a contraindication to its use; however, if important, a prevaccination skin prick test can determine a hypersensitivity response.

Influenza and pneumonia prophylaxis have been discussed in Chapter 30. Fifty percent of individuals older than 60 do not have sufficient levels of antitoxin antibodies to protect against tetanus or diphtheria. Elderly patients who have been primarily immunized need booster doses of tetanus and diphtheria toxoid (TD) at 10-year intervals throughout their lives (Evidence Level A). Those without primary immunization need two IM doses of TD given 1 month apart, followed by a booster dose at 10-year intervals. A TD booster dose is recommended for those patients with a contaminated or severe puncture wound, in whom more than 5 years have lapsed since the last dose. Hepatitis A vaccination in the elderly is generally reserved for those individuals traveling to endemic countries, sexually active homosexual men, IV drug users, food handlers, and those with chronic liver disease. Hepatitis B vaccination is recommended for sexually active homosexual men, sexual contacts of hepatitis B carriers, and health care personnel.

Lyme disease vaccination is not recommended in those individuals older than 70. It is recommended only in those individuals who engage in activities that result in frequent or prolonged exposure to tick-infested areas. Use of the varicella vaccine has not been approved in elderly individuals.[1]

COMMUNITY-ACQUIRED RESISTANT PATHOGENS

As the baby-boomer generation ages, old bugs such as *Chlamydia pneumoniae, Mycobacterium tuberculosis, Streptococcus pneumoniae,* and new bugs such as *Cryptosporidium* and *Legionella* are emerging as important pathogens. The most common resistant bacteria in the elderly include: PRSP, MRSA, VRE, MDRGNB, and vancomycin-resistant/intermediate *Staphylococcus aureus* (VISA).[26,27] Although these bacteria are most likely to be isolated from acute care or long-term care facilities, increasingly the elderly experience short stays in facilities for acute care and rehabilitation. Predictably these bacteria will become more common in the outpatient arena.

By definition, MRSA is resistant to methicillin (nafcillin, oxacillin) but these bacteria are usually resistant to all cephalosporins and quinolones as well. Therefore, vancomycin is the drug of choice for MRSA eradication. The recent emergence of VISA requires treatment with Synercid (quinupristin and dalfopristin), a streptogramin, or the new oxazolidine (linezolid, Zyvox) (Evidence Level B). Synercid is available only in an intravenous preparation and requires no dosage adjustment for geriatric patients. Linezolid (Zyvox) is available in both oral and intravenous forms. This antibiotic is active against MRSA, PRSP, and VRE. The U.S. Food and Drug Administration (FDA) recently granted proprietary review to an investigational agent, Dalbavancin, a second-generation lipoglycopeptide agent in the same class as vancomycin. Dalbavancin is administered once a week for the treatment of complicated skin and soft tissue infections caused by MRSA.

PRSP is more prevalent in those individuals younger than 5 and older than 65. In some communities, 28% of pneumococci isolates are now resistant to penicillin and >40% are resistant to TMX/SMX and erythromycin. Pneumonococcal resistance to quinolones is uncommon, but ciprofloxacin has the least activity against PRSP, while levofloxacin, gatifloxacin, and moxifloxacin have the highest activity (lowest minimum inhibitory concentrations [MICs]).

VRE infections in the elderly are becoming more common. Most isolates of VRE are *Enterococcus faecium*, usually type VAN A or VAN B. Over the past 25 years, most enterococcal isolates have become resistant to β-lactams with increasing resistance to aminoglycoside antibiotics. Treatment of VRE is dependent on the strain (VAN A, VAN B) and the specific resistance pattern to other antibiotics. The treatment combinations have met with limited success. Synercid may be the drug of choice for multiresistant VRE. However, Synercid is only bacteriostatic for VRE and, therefore, resistant strains have already appeared.

MDRGNB are most frequently encountered in elderly individuals with UTIs. Urine isolates of MDRGNB are more common in older individuals with poor functional status, multiple comorbidities, recent antimicrobial exposure or indwelling urinary catheters. Because of the common resistance to β-lactam antibiotics, many clinicians have opted to begin treatment of symptomatic UTIs with quinolone antibiotics.

CONCLUSION

As the current "baby-boomer" generation ages, those individuals 65 years and older will approach 70 million by the year 2035. We must find more advanced approaches of intervention that will reduce the morbidity and mortality associated with infectious processes in the elderly. This will be accomplished through a combination of new antibiotics classes, faster and more sensitive diagnostic techniques, and the development of immune modulators or vaccines.

Primary care providers, geriatric fellows, and geriatricians must be trained to quickly recognize infectious disease. The early and appropriate treatment of pneumonia, severe symptomatic UTIs, necrotizing tissue infections, bacterial meningitis, systemic VZV and sepsis/septic shock can greatly decrease the morbidity and mortality associated with these conditions.

REFERENCES

1. Yoshikawa TT, Norman DC, eds. *Infectious disease in the aging: A clinical handbook*. Totowa, NJ: Humana Press; 2001.
2. High KP. Immunity and infection in older adults. Infectious disease society of America. *Annual meeting*. Boston, MA; 2004.
3. Cantrell M, Norman DC. Infections. In: Duthie EH, Katz PR. *Practice of geriatrics*, 3rd ed. Philadelphia, PA: WB Saunders; 1998:410–420.
4. Crossley KB, Peterson PK. Infections in the elderly. *Clin Infect Dis*. 1996;221:209–215.
5. Crossley KB, Peterson PK. Infections in the elderly—new developments. *Curr Clin Top Infect Dis*. 1998;18:75–100.
6. Mouton CP, Bazaldua OV, Pierce B, et al. Common infections in older adults. *Am Fam Physician*. 2001;63:257–268.
7. Stollerman GH. Infectious diseases. In: Cassel CK, et al. ed. *Geriatric medicine*, 3rd ed. New York, NY: Springer-Verlag; 1997: 599–626.
8. Beers MH, Berkow R, eds. *The merck manual of geriatrics*, 3rd ed. Whitehouse Station, NJ: Merek Research Laboratories; 2000.
9. Wilson LA. Infections of the elderly. In: Gallo JJ, ed. *Reichel's care of the elderly: Clinical aspects of aging*, 5th ed. Philadelphia, PA: Lippincott Williams & Wilkins; 1999:296–307.
10. Corpuz, MO. Infections in the elderly. In: Dharmarajan TS, Norman RA, ed. *Clinical geriatrics*. New York, NY: The Parthenon Publishing Group; 2003:475–486.
11. Katz ED, Carpenter CR. Fever and immune function in the elderly. In: Meldon SW, Ma OJ, Woolard RH, eds. *Geriatric emergency medicine*, 1st ed. New York, NY: The McGraw-Hill Companies; 2004:55–64.
12. Simon HB. Hyperthermia, fever, and fever of undetermined origin. In: Dale DC, Federman DO, ed. *ACP medicine*, Vol 2. New York, NY: WebMD; 2004:1431–1442.

13. Cantrell M, Norman DC. Management of common clinical infectious problems. In: Evans JG, Williams TF, ed. *Oxford textbook of geriatric medicine*. Oxford: Oxford University Press; 1992:60–69.
14. Malani PN. Diagnosis and management of urinary tract infections in older women. *Clin Geriatr*. 2005;13(4):47–53.
15. Rajagopalan S, Moron D. Infectious disease emergencies. In: Yoshikawa TT, Norman DC, ed. *Acute emergencies and critical care of the geriatric patient*. New York, NY: Marcel Dekker; 2000:337–355.
16. Orenstein R, Wong ES. Urinary tract infections in adults. *Am Fam Physician*. 1999;59(5):1225–1234,1237.
17. Gavazzi G, Mallaret MR, Couturier P, et al. Bloodstream infection: Differences between young-old, old, and old-old patients. *J Am Geriatr Soc*. 2002;50:1667–1673.
18. Kong TK, Dai DLK, Leung MF, et al. Severe Acute Respiratory Syndrome (SARS) in elders. *J Am Geriatr Soc*. 2003;51:1182.
19. Tee AKH, On HML, Hui KP, et al. Atypical SARS in geriatric patient. *Emerg Infect Dis*. 2004;10(2)
20. Berner YN, Lang R, Chowers MY. Outcome of west nile fever in older adults. *J Am Geriatr Soc*. 2002;50:1844–1846.
21. Wellons MF, Sanders L, Edwards LJ, et al. HIV infection: Treatment outcomes in older and younger adults. *J Am Geriatr*. 2002;50:603–607.
22. Wachtel TJ, Stein MD, Robin DL. HIV Infection in older people. In: Gallo JJ, ed. *Reichels care of the elderly: Clinical aspects of aging*, 5th ed. Philadelphia, PA: Lippincott Williams & Wilkins; 1999: 309–314.
23. Elgart ML. Skin infections and infestations in geriatric patients. *Clin Geriatr Med*. 2002;18(1):89–101.
24. Weinberg JM, Scheinfeld NS. Cutaneous infections in the elderly: Diagnosis and management. *Dermatol Ther*. 2003;16: 195–205.
25. Gupta S. Guidelines for managing pressure ulcers with negative pressure wound therapy. Supplement. *Caring for the Aged*. 2005; 6(1):1–16.
26. Yoshikawa TT. Antimicrobial resistance and aging: Beginning at the end of the antibiotic era? *J Am Geriatr Soc*. 2002;50:S206–S209.
27. Strausbaugh LJ. Emerging health-care associated infections in the geriatric population. *Emerg Infect Dis*. 2001;7(2):268–271.

Common Gastrointestinal Disorders in the Elderly

41

Kristen M. Robson *Anthony Lembo*

CLINICAL PEARLS 563

PEPTIC ULCER DISEASE 564
Nonsteroidal Anti-inflammatory Drugs 564
Helicobacter pylori 564
Non–Helicobacter pylori, Non–Nonsteroidal Anti-inflammatory Drug Ulcers 564
Clinical Features 565
Complications 565
Diagnosis 565
Treatment 565
Summary 565

DISORDERS OF THE GALLBLADDER AND BILIARY TRACT 565
Age-Related Changes in the Biliary Tract 565
Gallbladder Disease 566

ESOPHAGEAL DYSPHAGIA 568
Age-Related Physiologic Changes of the Esophagus 568
Dysphagia 568
Motility Disorders 570
Mechanical Causes 571

CONSTIPATION 571
Definition of Constipation 572
Pathophysiology 572
Diagnosis 573
Management 573

FECAL INCONTINENCE 574
Etiology 574
Evaluation 574
Diagnosis 574
Treatment 575

GASTROESOPHAGEAL REFLUX DISEASE 575
Pathophysiology 575
Diagnosis 576
Evaluation 576
Treatment 576

CLINICAL PEARLS

- The elderly may not present with typical symptoms of peptic ulcer disease, such as abdominal pain and dyspepsia.
- The mainstay of therapy for cholangitis are broad-spectrum antibiotics, relief of biliary obstruction and biliary drainage.
- Choledocholithiasis in elderly patients can be adequately treated by endoscopy with clearance of the bile duct and does not necessarily need to be followed by cholecystectomy.
- In elderly patients with nonacute dysphagia, it is often helpful to obtain a barium esophagram as the first imaging study.

- Patients should be directly asked about fecal incontinence, as many patients are reluctant to bring it up with their caregivers.
- The hallmark symptoms of gastroesophageal reflux disease (GERD) are heartburn and regurgitation.
- An upper endoscopy should be considered in patients with suspected GERD who have had symptoms longer than 5 years to exclude erosive esophagitis, esophageal stricture, or Barrett's esophagus.
- Among the elderly who complain of constipation, the most common symptom is that of excessive straining and hard stools.
- Increasing dietary fiber to 20 to 25 g per day is often effective in treating mild to moderate constipation.
- Patients are often reluctant to discuss this problem with their physician due to social embarrassment.
- Anorectal biofeedback therapy, which involves retraining the pelvic floor and the abdominal wall musculature, has been shown to improve symptoms in two thirds of patients with fecal incontinence.

The physiologic function of the gastrointestinal (GI) tract is generally maintained with aging. Nevertheless, GI symptoms and diseases are particularly common in the elderly. New GI symptoms in elderly patients should be investigated to determine if pathology exists. The evaluation of symptoms in an elderly patient should be performed in a timely fashion. Elderly patients may not be able to compensate or withstand the effects of a GI illness as compared to their younger counterparts.

PEPTIC ULCER DISEASE

Peptic ulcer disease (PUD) can affect patients of all ages. Although the approach to the management of PUD is similar in both younger and older patients, there may be an increased risk of morbidity and mortality in elderly patients.[1] In addition, data from the National Health Interview Survey suggest that increasing age is a risk factor for PUD.[2] There are three major mechanisms that contribute to the development of PUD: Nonsteroidal anti-inflammatory drugs (NSAIDs), *Helicobacter pylori* infection, and acid.

Nonsteroidal Anti-inflammatory Drugs

The elderly take NSAIDs more frequently than any other age-group. Nearly 40% of elderly persons receive at least one prescription for NSAIDs each year, and 1% to 8% of these patients are hospitalized because of a GI complication secondary to NSAIDs within the first year of use.[3]

NSAIDs inhibit the synthesis of prostaglandins by the gastric mucosa. Prostaglandins E_2 and I_2, the principal prostaglandins of the stomach, perform several functions that protect the gastric mucosa. These prostaglandins inhibit gastric acid secretion, increase mucosal blood flow, and promote the secretion of bicarbonate and mucus.[1] The cyclooxygenase-2 (COX-2) inhibitors have been shown to have less GI toxicity than the traditional NSAIDs due to their affinity for COX-2 over COX-1.[1] In a double-blind outcome trial of over 8,000 patients with arthritis, COX-2–specific inhibitors (coxibs) decreased complications of an upper GI event (bleeding, perforation, obstruction, or symptomatic ulcer).[4]

The efficacy of proton pump inhibitors (PPIs) has been assessed in patients who present with ulcers associated with NSAID use. One study compared the use of placebo versus lansoprazole in patients taking low-dose aspirin who had a history of ulcer disease. If present, *H. pylori* was first eradicated. Ulcer recurred in 15% of the placebo group versus 2% of the lansoprazole group at a median duration of 1 year[5] (Evidence Level B).

Helicobacter pylori

The prevalence of *H. pylori* infection increases with advancing age, reaching levels of 40% to 60% in asymptomatic elderly individuals and over 70% in elderly patients with GI illness. The eradication of *H. pylori* may prevent the progression of intestinal metaplasia and gastric atrophy.[6] There are several tests available to diagnose *H. pylori*. Nonendoscopic tests include the immunoglobulin G antibody test, the ^{13}C-urea breath test, and the stool antigen test. Endoscopic tests include biopsy for rapid urease testing and histologic examination. Treatment of *H. pylori* is discussed in the subsequent text.

Non–Helicobacter pylori, Non–Nonsteroidal Anti-inflammatory Drug Ulcers

A prospective study of nearly 2,400 patients with duodenal ulcers revealed that 27% were *H. pylori* negative and denied NSAID use. What is the etiology of such ulcers? Other common causes of ulcers, such as Crohn's disease or hypersecretory states, should be considered as well as unreported NSAID use.

CASE ONE

Mr. C. is an 81-year-old who presents to his primary care physician complaining of black stools and weakness. One month before presentation, he began taking ibuprofen as a sleeping aid. He was also taking an enteric-coated aspirin daily. He denies nausea, abdominal pain, hematemesis, chest pain, or shortness of breath. His hematocrit on admission to the hospital is 30%, and his baseline is 43%. He is placed on intravenous PPI. Upper endoscopy is performed, and this reveals a duodenal ulcer. The serology for *H. pylori* is negative. The patient does well, and oral intake is resumed. He is discharged from the hospital on PPI and with the recommendation to avoid nonsteroidal anti-inflammatory medications.

Clinical Features

The presentation of PUD usually is epigastric abdominal pain, typically postprandial. The pain is often relieved with food or over-the-counter antacids. The elderly, however, are prone to atypical dyspeptic symptoms. In one report, 65% of patients older than 80 years who presented with upper GI bleeding secondary to PUD had no pain upon presentation.[7] In another study of elderly patients with PUD, 35% of patients reported no abdominal pain, as compared with 8% of younger patients with either gastric or duodenal ulcers diagnosed by endoscopy.[8] The lack of the typical presenting symptoms of PUD in the elderly may lead to a delay in diagnosis and contribute to a higher mortality rate of complicated ulcer disease.

Complications

For both gastric and duodenal ulcers, the most common complication is bleeding, followed by perforation. Both of these complications may occur more frequently in the elderly. GI hemorrhage and perforation from PUD carry an overall 30% mortality rate for patients older than 65 years. Complicated PUD may result in higher mortality rates in the elderly compared to their younger counterparts.[9] Factors that may contribute to the increase in the complication rates of PUD in the elderly include atypical presentations of PUD that may lead to a delay in diagnosis, as well as the presence of comorbid conditions.[9]

Diagnosis

The primary method for diagnosing both gastric and duodenal ulcers is upper endoscopy. Endoscopy has been shown to be safe in elderly patients, with complication rates similar to those in younger patients.[10] Although duodenal ulcers are typically not followed-up with upper endoscopy, all gastric ulcers require repeat endoscopy after several weeks of therapy to assure healing and that the ulcer was not malignant. PUD can also be diagnosed by upper GI series using a double contrast technique.[1]

All patients with PUD, whether young or old, should be tested for *H. pylori* infection. A variety of methods can be used, including both invasive and noninvasive testing (see Table 41.1).

Treatment

The treatment of PUD is first directed to the removal of potential causes such as the *H. pylori* infection and the discontinuation of NSAIDs. Paramount to the treatment of PUD is acid suppression to heal the ulcer as well as to provide maintenance therapy. PPIs are more effective in healing ulcers than are histamine-2 receptor antagonists. One study that examined the healing rates of duodenal ulcers treated with omeprazole 40 mg daily reported 93% healing at 2 weeks, and nearly 100% healing at 4 weeks[11] (Evidence Level A).

TABLE 41.1
***HELICOBACTER PYLORI*: METHODS OF TESTING**

Noninvasive Testing	Invasive Testing (Endoscopic Biopsy)
Serum IgG *Helicobacter pylori* antibody	Rapid urease test
^{13}C-urea breath test	Histologic examination
Stool antigen test	

IgG, immunoglobulin G.

For patients who develop peptic ulcers secondary to NSAIDs, the NSAIDs should be discontinued. If this is not a reasonable option, there is evidence that the coadministration of a PPI can reduce the risk of ulcer recurrence[5] (Evidence Level A).

When a *H. pylori* infection is identified in the setting of PUD, the bacteria should be eradicated. A minimum of a 1-week PPI-based triple therapy regimen, including clarithromycin, amoxicillin, and/or nitroimidazoles, is highly effective and well tolerated in elderly patients. The main factors attributed to treatment failure in the elderly are noncompliance and antibiotic resistance.[6]

Summary

PUD can present in elderly patients in an atypical manner. This may lead to a delay in diagnosis. The elderly remain at risk for PUD not only because of the widespread use of NSAIDs but also because of the increased prevalence of *H. Pylori* as compared to younger patients.

DISORDERS OF THE GALLBLADDER AND BILIARY TRACT

Age-Related Changes in the Biliary Tract

The overall prevalence of gallstone disease in the elderly, by ultrasound, is 26.7%. Advanced age is also associated with a higher rate of calcified pigment stones.[12] The lithogenicity of bile is thought to change as a result of age-related changes in biliary metabolism. Increased cholesterol saturation of bile and reduced gallbladder emptying are contributing factors[13] (see Table 41.2).

Some studies demonstrate that the diameter of the common bile duct increases with advancing age. In a prospective study of over 1,000 patients between the age of 60 and 96, a small but statistically significant increase in the caliber of the common bile duct was demonstrated with increasing age. In another study by Bachar et al. of 51 patients undergoing abdominal ultrasonography, an

TABLE 41.2
AGE-RELATED CHANGES IN THE BILIARY TRACT

1. Increased prevalence of gallstones
2. Increased common bile duct diameter
3. Increased lithogenicity of bile
4. Increased incidence of pigment stones

Adapted from Ross SO, Forsmark CE. Pancreatic and biliary disorders in the elderly. *Gastroenterol Clin North Am.* 2001;30(2):531–545.

age-dependent change in the diameter of the common bile duct was demonstrated. This study suggested that the upper normal limit of duct size in the elderly be set at 8.5 mm.[14,15]

CASE TWO

A 78-year-old woman presented to the emergency room with fever, right upper quadrant pain and abnormal liver function tests. Her pain began after eating a fatty meal. She denied weight loss or early satiety. Ultrasonography revealed a dilated common bile duct. The patient was given intravenous antibiotics and admitted to the hospital. Endoscopic retrograde cholangiography was performed (see Fig. 41.1). This showed a dilated common bile duct and choledocholithiasis. Sphincterotomy was performed, followed by basket retrieval of the stone. The patient did well and finished a course of antibiotics. She was discharged on a low fat diet with plans for outpatient follow-up.

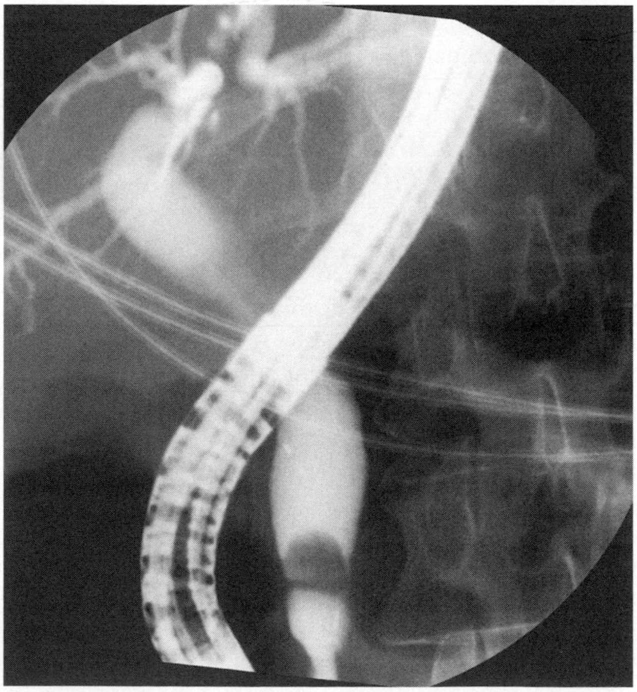

Figure 41.1 Common bile duct stone.

Gallbladder Disease

Cholelithiasis and Acute Cholecystitis

The prevalence of gallstones increases with age. In a large population-based study, the prevalence in the 50- to 65-year-old age-group was 13.7%, as compared to 1.7% in the 18- to 25-year-old age-group.[16] As in younger patients, therapy for asymptomatic gallstones found in elderly patients is not indicated (Evidence Level B). Elderly patients with cholelithiasis are more likely than younger patients to present with an acute complication of gallstones, such as acute cholecystitis, gallstone pancreatitis, or common bile duct stones.[17]

Clinical Manifestations

Acute cholecystitis commonly presents as constant right upper quadrant abdominal pain that may radiate to the back or right shoulder. Nausea, emesis, and anorexia may be associated symptoms, and fatty food ingestion may have preceded the onset of pain. Symptoms such as fever and prolonged pain (i.e., hours) should alert the clinician to the likelihood of acute cholecystitis as opposed to a limited attack of biliary colic.

Patients with acute cholecystitis tend to have fever, tachycardia, and an overall ill appearance, as well as peritoneal signs on physical examination. A "Murphy's sign" may also be present. The patient is asked to inspire deeply while the gallbladder fossa is palpated. As the gallbladder descends, the patient typically experiences increased discomfort. The sensitivity of the Murphy's sign, however, may be decreased in the elderly.[18]

Complications

There is a high rate of complications of untreated cholecystitis. The most common complication of acute cholecystitis is gangrenous cholecystitis (up to 20% of cases), which occurs more frequently in older patients. Sepsis is typically present in patients with gallbladder gangrene, and subsequent gallbladder perforation occurs in 2% of cases.[19] The additional complications of acute cholecystitis are listed in Table 41.3.

Diagnostic Testing

In the patient with symptoms of cholecystitis, laboratory work often shows a leukocytosis with an increased percentage of bands. Abnormalities in liver function tests, including hyperbilirubinemia and elevated alkaline phosphatase, should raise the suspicion for complicating factors such as cholangitis or choledocholithiasis.

The initial imaging study is usually ultrasonography, which can often confirm the diagnosis. The presence of gallbladder stones, gallbladder wall thickening or edema, and a "sonographic Murphy's sign" all support the diagnosis of cholecystitis. A systematic review of 30 studies of ultrasonography for the evaluation of gallstones and acute cholecystitis demonstrated that the sensitivity

TABLE 41.3
COMPLICATIONS OF ACUTE CHOLECYSTITIS

1. Gangrenous cholecystitis
2. Gallbladder perforation
   a. Localized perforation: pericholecystic abscess
   b. Free perforation: generalized peritonitis (associated with high mortality)
3. Cholecystenteric fistula: More often secondary to pressure necrosis from gallstones
4. Gallstone ileus: Results from passage of a stone through a fistula, leading to mechanical small bowel obstruction
5. Emphysematous cholecystitis
   a. Secondary infection of the gallbladder with a gas-forming organism such as *Clostridium* sp
   b. May lead to gallbladder perforation

Adapted from Zakko SF, Afdhal NH. Clinical features of acute cholecysitis. In: Rose Bd, ed. UpToDate. Waltham, MA: UpToDate; 2006.

and specificity of ultrasound for the detection of gallstones were in the range of 84% and 99%, respectively. The sensitivity and specificity for acute cholecystitis were 88% and 80%, respectively.[20]

Cholescintigraphy (also referred to as hepatic iminodiacetic acid [HIDA] scan) can be helpful if the ultrasound is inconclusive. A technetium-labeled HIDA is administered intravenously and is then selectively taken up by hepatocytes and excreted into the bile. This agent will enter the gallbladder if the cystic duct is patent and will be visualized within 30 to 60 minutes. The test is positive if the gallbladder is not visualized secondary to the cystic duct obstruction from gallbladder edema or an obstructing gallstone. The sensitivity and specificity of this nuclear medicine test are approximately 97% and 90%, respectively.[20,21]

An abdominal computed tomography (CT) scan can demonstrate findings associated with acute cholecystitis such as gallbladder wall edema and pericholecystic stranding. A CT scan can be helpful when complications of acute cholecystitis are suspected or when alternative diagnoses are being considered.[22]

Treatment

Laparoscopic cholecystectomy is the treatment of choice for symptomatic cholecystitis. In a retrospective study of patients undergoing laparoscopic cholecystectomy, elderly patients were significantly more likely than younger patients to present with acute cholecystitis, gallstone pancreatitis, and common bile duct stones. The open conversion rate in elderly patients with complicated gallstone disease was significantly higher compared to younger patients. Elderly patients with uncomplicated gallstone disease, however, appeared to be excellent candidates for laparoscopic cholecystectomy. The study concluded that early conversion or open cholecystectomy may be indicated in the elderly with acute complications of cholelithiasis.[17]

Because of increased complications from acute cholecystitis in elderly patients, percutaneous cholecystomy may be considered as an alternative therapy in the acute setting. In an uncontrolled trial, percutaneous cholecystomy was performed in a group of elderly patients who were at high risk for surgery due to a variety of comorbid conditions. Percutaneous cholecystomy was successful in 95% of patients, with low morbidity and overall zero mortality.[23]

Gallbladder Carcinoma

As in gallstone disease, gallbladder carcinoma, although uncommon overall, occurs more frequently in the elderly. In a study of 4,500 autopsies in Japan, the incidence of gallbladder carcinoma was 2.1%. From 50% to 88% of patients with gallbladder carcinoma have gallstones.[24,25]

Choledocholithiasis and Cholangitis

Acute cholangitis is a potentially life-threatening infection of the biliary tree. Choledocholithiasis is the most common cause of infection, which is characterized by fever, jaundice, and abdominal pain.[26,27] Confusion and hypotension can occur in patients with suppurative cholangitis. Hypotension may be the only manifestation in elderly patients.[28]

Diagnostic Testing and Treatment

Ultrasound is generally recommended as the first imaging study in patients suspected of having cholangitis. Endoscopic retrograde cholangiopancreatography (ERCP) is utilized both to establish the diagnosis and to provide therapeutic intervention with sphincterotomy, stone removal, and/or stent insertion. Magnetic resonance cholangiopancreatography is emerging as an excellent tool in the evaluation of choledocholithiasis, particularly in patients whose symptoms of cholangitis are not severe and when the risks of ERCP are high.[28,29] Magnetic resonance cholangiopancreatography can also be considered in patients with suspected choledocholithiasis in the absence of cholangitis.

As in younger patients, the first line of therapy for cholangitis includes intravenous broad spectrum antibiotics to cover gram-negative organisms, for the relief of biliary obstruction and providing biliary drainage. Supportive measures such as the administration of intravenous fluids and close monitoring are also important. Biliary drainage can be accomplished mainly by ERCP. Percutaneous drainage or surgical decompression are occasionally used. In an uncontrolled study of the management of acute cholangitis in patients older than 80, the morbidity and mortality rates of methods for drainage were compared. Endoscopic drainage was associated with the lowest rates of morbidity and mortality (17% and 6%), followed by percutaneous drainage (36% and 9%), and surgical drainage, which was associated with rates of 88% and 25% (Evidence Level C). It should be noted, however, that morbidity and mortality rates for all interventions were significantly higher in older patients than in younger patients.[27]

For patients with a gallbladder, cholecystectomy usually follows endoscopic treatment for choledocholithiasis. For elderly patients, especially those at high risk for surgery, endoscopic sphincterotomy alone may be the treatment of choice. In a study of the long-term outcome of endoscopic treatment for choledocholithiasis, this approach was found to be relatively favorable. No significant risk factors for cholecystitis as a late complication were identified.[30]

ESOPHAGEAL DYSPHAGIA

Age-Related Physiologic Changes of the Esophagus

Although the esophagus generally ages well under normal conditions, changes can be documented. Age-related changes in the oropharynx and esophagus are listed in Table 41.4. *Presbyesophagus* is a term that formerly described age-related changes in the esophageal body. It is now felt, however, that these changes in motility are most likely secondary to medical conditions found in the elderly. These medical conditions include neurologic disorders, diabetes mellitus, and the effects of medications.[31]

TABLE 41.4
AGE-RELATED PHYSIOLOGIC CHANGES OF THE OROPHARYNX AND ESOPHAGUS

1. Decreased upper esophageal sphincter pressure
2. Delays in upper esophageal sphincter relaxation after deglutition
3. Decreased amplitude of esophageal body contractions
4. Nonperistaltic contractions
5. Diminished visceral perception
6. Hiatal hernia

From Greenwald DA. Aging, the gastrointestinal tract, and the risk of acid-related disease. *Am J Med.* 2004;117(5A):8S-13S.

Dysphagia

Dysphagia is the sensation of impaired passage of either solids or liquids from the mouth to the stomach. Dysphagia is a common symptom that can affect patients of all ages, but it may be more common in older patients. In one study, the prevalence of dysphagia appeared to increase with age, and at least 10% of people older than age 50 complained of some dysphagia.[32,33] Dysphagia is an alarm symptom and requires prompt evaluation to determine the etiology and to provide therapy. Dysphagia in elderly patients should not be attributed to normal aging without further prompt evaluation.[34,35]

Dysphagia can be classified into two types: Oropharyngeal and esophageal (transfer and transport dysphagia). Oropharyngeal dysphagia arises from diseases of the upper esophagus and pharynx or from upper esophageal sphincter dysfunction. Esophageal dysphagia arises within the body of the esophagus or the lower esophageal sphincter, and it is most commonly due to a mechanical cause or motility disturbance.[34] The focus of this section will be on esophageal or transport dysphagia.

CASE THREE

Mr. B. is a 79-year-old with a long history of heartburn. He occasionally takes over-the-counter antacids. He presented with gradually progressive dysphagia to solid food only and no weight loss. An upper endoscopy revealed a short esophageal stricture proximal to a hiatal hernia and mucosal changes consistent with erosive esophagitis. The stricture was dilated endoscopically with a balloon. He was placed on a PPI. His dysphagia and heartburn resolved.

Careful history is important in the evaluation of elderly patients with dysphagia. Dysphagia should be distinguished from odynophagia, which refers to pain with swallowing in contrast to difficulty swallowing. A variety of mechanical and neuromuscular disorders are associated with esophageal dysphagia. There are three main factors that can help determine the source of dysphagia:

1. The type of food that produces symptoms (i.e., solids, liquids, or both)
2. The temporal progression of symptoms (intermittent vs. progressive)
3. Associated symptoms or findings, such as heartburn.

Dysphagia to both solids and liquids at the onset of the symptoms is suggestive of but not diagnostic of a motility disorder. Dysphagia for solids that progresses to include liquids is more likely to reflect a mechanical obstruction.[36] Symptoms such as heartburn may suggest the presence of a complication of gastroesophageal reflux disease (GERD), such as a benign or a malignant stricture. There are numerous conditions that present with esophageal dysphagia (see Table 41.5). The more common causes will be reviewed here.

TABLE 41.5
DIFFERENTIAL DIAGNOSIS OF GASTROINTESTINAL COMPLAINTS

Causes of Constipation (564.00)	Causes of Fecal Incontinence (787.91)	Conditions Associated with Esophageal Dysphagia
Slow transit constipation (564.01) Defecatory disorders (536.9) Normal transit constipation (564.00)	Infectious (009.2) Inflammatory bowel disease (569.9) Radiation enteritis (558.1) Short-gut syndrome (579.3) Carcinoid syndrome (259.2) Celiac disease (579.0)	Achalasia (530.0) Hypermotility or spastic motility disorders (536.8/564.9) Diabetes mellitus (250.00) Systemic sclerosis (710.0)
Mechanical obstruction Colon cancer (239.0) Rectocele (male 564.49) (female 618.04) Sigmoidocele Stricture (569.2) Extrinsic compression	*Neurologic conditions* Multiple sclerosis (340) Strokes (434.91) Diabetes (250.00) Central nervous system disorders (e.g., dementia, strokes, tumors, myelomeningoceles, spinal cord lesions)	*Mechanical causes (luminal)* Peptic stricture (537.9) Malignancy (i.e., adenocarcinoma) Radiation-induced injury Medication-induced esophagitis/stricture
Metabolic and endocrine Diabetes mellitus (250.00) Hypothyroidism (244.9) Hyperthyroidism (242.90) Hypokalemia (276.8) Pregnancy (V22.2) Pheochromocytoma (194.0) Panhypopituitarism (253.2) Porphyria (277.1) Heavy metal poisoning (e.g., lead, mercury, arsenic intoxication)	*Overflow incontinence* Fecal impaction (560.39) Neoplasm (239.9)	*GERD (530.81)*
Medications Calcium channel blockers (e.g., verapamil) μ-Opioid agonists (loperamide, morphine, fentanyl) Anticholinergics (e.g., antispasmodics, antipsychotics, tricyclic antidepressants, antiparkinsonian drugs) Anticonvulsants (e.g., phenobarbital, carbamazepine, phenytoin) Antacids (e.g., aluminum- or calcium-containing antacids) 5-HT_3 antagonists (e.g., alosetron) Iron supplements Nonsteroidal anti-inflammatory agents (e.g., ibuprofen) Diuretics (e.g., furosemide) Chemotherapeutics (e.g., vinca derivatives)	*Pelvic floor denervation* Obstetrical injury of the pudendal nerve (959.14) Chronic straining leading to descending-perineum syndrome Rectal prolapse (569.1)	*Extrinsic compression* Enlarged aorta (dysphagia aortica) (447.8) Enlarged left atrium (429.3) Aberrant subclavian artery (747.60) Mediastinal mass (786.6)
Neuropathies and myopathies Systemic sclerosis (710.0) Amyloidosis (277.3) Dermatomyositis (710.3) Multiple sclerosis (340) Parkinson disease (332.0) Spinal cord injury (952.9) Autonomic neuropathy (337.9) Chagas disease (086.2) Intestinal pseudo-obstruction (564.89) Cerebrovascular accidents (434.91) Shy-Drager syndrome (333.0)	*Anal sphincter injury (959.19)* Obstetrical injury (665.9) Anorectal surgery (959.19) Accidental injury (959.9)	

GERD, gastroesophageal reflux disease.

Motility Disorders

Achalasia

Achalasia is an idiopathic esophageal motility disorder characterized by the incomplete relaxation of the lower esophageal sphincter. It is accompanied by lack of peristalsis of the esophageal body. Patients commonly present with dysphagia to both solids and liquids, but they may also complain of chest pain, regurgitation, and weight loss. The onset of achalasia is typically between the ages of 20 and 40 years, but a second peak occurs in the elderly. Achalasia results from a loss of the myenteric neurons controlling esophageal smooth muscle function.[37–39] Clinical findings include a functional obstruction of the esophagus that is evident on barium esophagram. The classic appearance is that of a "bird beak" of the lower esophageal sphincter secondary to the incomplete relaxation of the lower esophageal sphincter coupled with the progressive dilation of the esophageal body (see Fig. 41.2). Manometric studies reveal normal to high baseline lower esophageal sphincter pressure with incomplete relaxation following wet swallows. The esophageal body typically displays the absence of peristalsis with low amplitude, simultaneous contractions. It is important that endoscopy be performed in these patients, mainly to rule out malignancy of the gastroesophageal junction or the distal esophagus (i.e., pseudoachalasia).[37] Other causes of pseudoachalasia include amyloidosis, sarcoidosis, and Chagas disease. In patients with a clinical triad of age >50 years, dysphagia of <1 year duration, and weight loss >7 kg, pseudoachalasia or secondary achalasia should be suspected.[31] If the clinical suspicion of secondary achalasia is high despite a negative upper endoscopy, a CT scan of the chest or endoscopic ultrasound should be performed.

There are several treatments for patients with achalasia. Medical therapy includes trials of agents such as nitrates and calcium channel blockers, but these agents have no certain benefit.[40] Pneumatic dilation, surgical (including laparoscopic) myotomy, and an injection of botulinum toxin are the main therapeutic options. Pneumatic dilation should be considered only in elderly patients who are good surgical candidates if a perforation occurs. Myotomy of the lower esophageal sphincter has been of benefit in selected elderly patients. In the patient with multiple medical problems, botulinum toxin injection into the lower esophageal sphincter can provide temporary symptomatic relief. The endoscopic treatment may need to be repeated when symptoms recur[41] (Evidence Level C).

Spastic Disorders of the Esophagus

Spastic or hypermotility disorders of the esophagus include diffuse esophageal spasm, "nutcracker esophagus," and hypertensive lower esophageal sphincter, and they can present with dysphagia to solids and liquids. Diffuse esophageal spasm usually presents with intermittent symptoms. Barium esophagram can demonstrate a distinctive radiologic pattern, often referred to as "corkscrew" esophagus (see Fig. 41.3). Both calcium channel blockers and low-dose tricyclic antidepressant medications were shown to improve symptoms in small studies of patients with hypermotility disorders.[42,43]

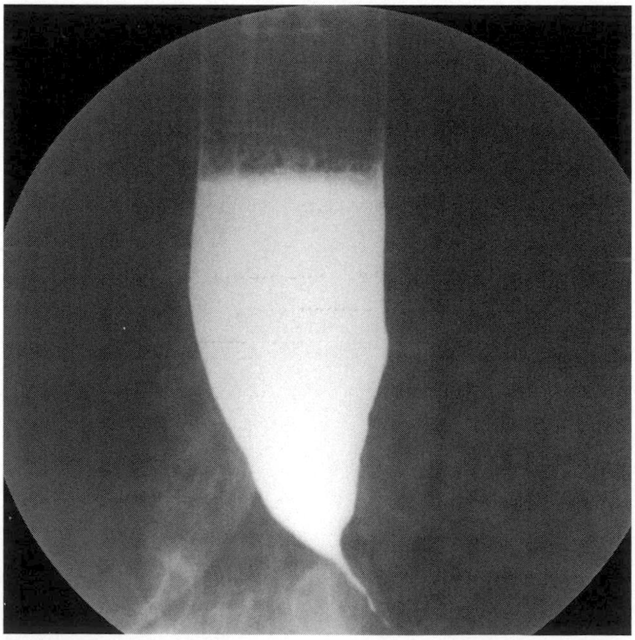

Figure 41.2 Achalasia.

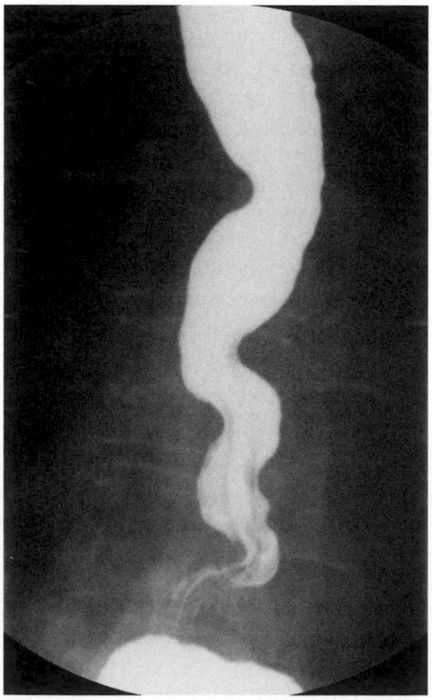

Figure 41.3 Esophageal spasm.

Mechanical Causes

Medication-Induced Esophageal Injury

Several factors account for the increased risk of pill-induced injury of the esophagus in the elderly. Elderly patients take more medications than younger people, they spend more time in a recumbent position, and they are more likely to have motility or anatomic disorders of the esophagus. A number of medications may result in acute esophageal injury (see Table 41.6). In younger patients, antibiotics are most commonly associated with pill esophagitis; however, in older patients, potassium chloride, alendronate, quinidine, and nonsteroidal anti-inflammatory agents are often the culprits.[31,44] Patients typically present with odynophagia and substernal chest pain. Endoscopy may reveal findings such as erythema, an ulcer or a stricture. Lesions are most frequently found at the midesophagus at the level of the aortic arch or at the lower esophageal sphincter. Most cases of pill esophagitis resolve with the discontinuation of the offending agent. The use of short-term acid suppressing therapy may also be helpful.

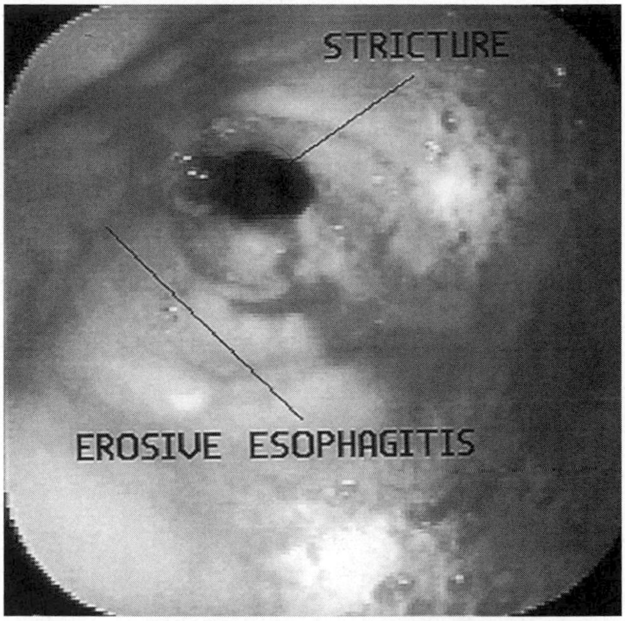

Figure 41.4 Erosive esophagitis with stricture.

Peptic Stricture

A peptic stricture typically presents in a patient with a history of heartburn and slowly progressive dysphagia for solid food.[46] Weight loss is unusual. Endoscopy can provide both diagnosis and exclude malignancy, as well as provide therapy with esophageal dilation (see Fig. 41.4). PPI therapy should be used in those patients who may develop recurrent strictures from long-standing acid reflux.[47] Because of age-related alterations in pain perception, older individuals with severe GERD, and complications such as Barrett's esophagus, erosive esophagitis, or stricture may be asymptomatic or have mild symptoms.[48]

Esophageal Cancer

Esophageal cancer may present with rapidly progressive dysphagia, first for solids and then for liquids, and also with associated weight loss. Squamous cell carcinoma of the esophagus is associated with a history of tobacco and alcohol use. The primary risk factor for adenocarcinoma of the esophagus is Barrett's esophagus, which is secondary to long-standing GERD. The incidence of adenocarcinoma of the esophagus has been increasing in recent years.

In elderly patients who are good operative candidates, surgical resection can be performed. Older patients who are at high risk for surgery may be unresectable. Palliative therapy includes radiation, chemotherapy, or a combination of both. Symptomatic treatment may include the endoscopic placement of a stent. The prognosis of esophageal cancer is poor, with a 5-year survival rate of <5%. Patients with known Barrett's esophagus who undergo endoscopic surveillance have a better prognosis when esophageal cancer is detected.[41]

TABLE 41.6
COMMON CAUSES OF MEDICATION-INDUCED ESOPHAGEAL INJURY IN THE ELDERLY

Tetracyclines
Doxycyclines
Potassium chloride
Quinidine
Alendronate
Nonsteroidal anti-inflammatory medications
Ferrous compounds

Dysphagia Aortica

Degenerative changes of the aorta, such as atherosclerotic disease, may result in the compression of the esophagus. This disorder, which is unique to the elderly, is referred to as "dysphagia aortica." The upper esophagus can be compressed by a thoracic aneurysm, and the atherosclerotic aorta usually affects the more distal portion of the esophagus. This disorder is more common in women because of the presence of kyphosis, particularly in postmenopausal years[41] (see Fig. 41.5).

CONSTIPATION

Constipation affects a substantial portion of the Western population and is particularly prevalent in the elderly. The prevalence of constipation in the general population ranges between 2% and 28% in Western countries. Only

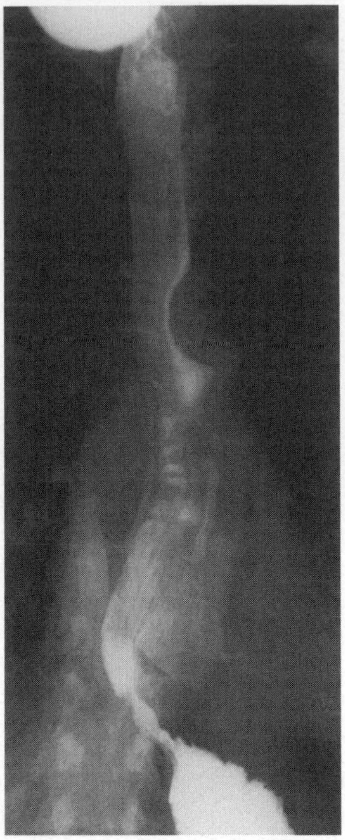

Figure 41.5 Dysphagia aortica.

one third of people with constipation seek medical care for their symptoms;[49] nevertheless, constipation still results in over 2.5 million physician visits, 92,000 hospitalizations,[50] and laxative sales of several hundred million dollars per year in the United States. Eighty-five percent of physician visits for constipation lead to a prescription for laxatives or cathartics. The cost of testing alone in patients with constipation has been estimated to be 6.9 billion dollars annually.[51] An analysis of physician visits for constipation in the United States between 1958 and 1986 found that 31% of patients who required medical attention were seen by general and family practitioners, followed by internists (20%), pediatricians (15%), surgeons (9%), and obstetricians–gynecologists (9%).

The prevalence of self-reported constipation among the elderly ranges between 15% and 30% with most, but not all, studies showing an increase in prevalence with age. Constipation is particularly problematic in nursing home residents, where it is reported in nearly one half of residents and where 50% to 74% use laxatives on a daily basis.[52] Nearly 13% of elderly people entering a nursing home developed a new onset of constipation over 3 months of follow-up. Likewise, hospitalized elderly patients appear to be at a very high risk of developing constipation. A study of a geriatrics ward in the United Kingdom showed up to 42% of the patients have fecal impaction.[53]

TABLE 41.7
ROME II CRITERIA FOR CHRONIC CONSTIPATION

At least 12 wk, which need not be consecutive, in the preceding 12 mo of two or more of the following:

1. Straining >25% of bowel movements
2. Lumpy or hard stools >25% of bowel movements
3. Sensation of incomplete evacuation >25% of bowel movements
4. Sensation of anorectal obstruction/blockage >25% of bowel movements
5. Manual maneuvers to facilitate >25% of bowel movements (e.g., digital evacuation, support of the pelvic floor; and/or
6. Less than three defecations/wk

Loose stools are not present, and there are insufficient criteria for IBS[55]

IBS, irritable bowel syndrome.

Definition of Constipation

Most patients define constipation by a variety of symptoms, including the need for excessive straining, hard stools, unsuccessful defecation, infrequent stools (<3 per week), abdominal discomfort, sense of incomplete bowel evacuation, and excessive time spent on the toilet. Among elderly patients who complain of constipation, the most common complaint is that of excessive straining and hard stools. In a community sample of 209 people aged 65 to 93 years, the main symptom used to define constipation was the need to strain to defecate, while only 3% of men and 2% of women reported that their average bowel frequency was <3 per week.[54] A consensus definition of constipation (Rome II Criteria) (see Table 41.7) has been established, which incorporates the multiple symptoms of constipation.[55]

Pathophysiology

Constipation can result from a systemic or neurologic disorder, mechanical obstruction, or a side effect of medications, and it is frequently multifactorial (Table 41.5). It is particularly important to consider these causes of constipation in elderly patients presenting with new or recent change in symptoms or warning signs such as weight loss or blood in stools. Even in the elderly, constipation is most often due to a disorder in the function of the colon or rectum ("functional constipation") that is not explained by any of these factors.

The role of fiber and exercise in constipation remains controversial. Cross-sectional studies have not linked low fiber intake with constipation. However, increased fiber consumption appears to decrease colonic transit time and increases stool frequency and stool weight. The Nurses Health Study assessed the self-reported bowel habits of 62,036 women between the age of 36 and 61 years. The study found that women who were in the highest quintile of fiber intake and who exercised daily were 68% less likely to report constipation than women who were in the lowest quintile of fiber intake and exercised less than once a week.[56] Immobility, as in a patient who is bed bound, is frequently associated with constipation.

Dehydration has also been associated with slowed colonic transit time and should therefore be considered in the elderly, especially those without free access to water.

Diagnosis

A thorough history and physical examination can exclude most secondary causes of constipation. A careful rectal examination is often the most revealing part of the clinical evaluation and should be performed in every patient presenting with constipation. This includes examining the perianal area for scars, fistula, fissures, and the presence of external hemorrhoids. Next, the perineum should be observed with the patient at rest and while bearing down to evaluate the extent of perineal descent, normally between 1 to 3.5 cm. Reduced descent (<1 cm) may indicate the inability to relax the pelvic floor muscles during defecation; excessive perineal descent (below the plane of the ischial tuberosities or >3.5 cm) may indicate excessive laxity of the perineum, which usually results from childbirth or excessive straining over many years. In more severe cases, excessive perineal descent may result in injury to the sacral nerves from stretch, and denervation, which can lead to reduced rectal sensation and incontinence. Finally, a digital rectal examination should be performed to evaluate for the presence of fecal impaction, anal stricture, and rectal masses. A patulous anal sphincter may suggest trauma or a neurologic disorder impairing sphincter function. Difficulty or inability to insert the finger into the anal canal suggests elevated anal sphincter pressure at rest or anal stricture. Tenderness of the posterior aspect of the rectum may suggest pelvic floor spasm.[57]

Laboratory tests to be considered in elderly patients with constipation include thyroid function tests, calcium, glucose, electrolytes, complete blood count, and urinalysis. A complete examination of the colon is required to exclude structural diseases (e.g., colon cancer, inflammatory bowel disease, and colonic stricture) when there are "alarm symptoms" such as a new onset or worsening of constipation, the presence of blood in stools, weight loss, fevers, nausea, and vomiting. In addition, routine screening colonoscopy or both sigmoidoscopy and barium enema should be considered as part of the recommendations to prevent colorectal cancer.

Management

Therapy consists first of conservative management with increasing fluid intake in dehydrated patients and exercise in sedentary patients able to increase their mobility. Increasing dietary fiber intake to approximately 20 to 25 g per day should be the first treatment choice for most patients (Evidence Level C). Although several studies have confirmed the benefit of fiber in relieving mild to moderate constipation, compliance with fiber supplementation is low due to side effects such as flatulence, distension, bloating, and poor taste. Patients should be instructed to gradually increase their total dietary fiber intake over several weeks. Initially, foods rich in dietary fiber should be increased; if the results from this therapy are disappointing, commercially packaged fiber supplements should be added. Supplemental fiber, especially with psyllium, should be taken with plenty of water because it can form into a thick gel that has been reported to cause intestinal obstruction. Finally, patients should be encouraged to utilize the morning postprandial gastrocolic response and to elevate their feet by 6 to 8 inches when sitting on the toilet to increase the anorectal angle, thereby allowing stool to pass more easily through the distal rectum.

If a trial with an adequate amount of fiber is unsuccessful, then laxatives can be considered. The most commonly used types of laxatives are stool softeners, and osmotic and stimulant laxatives.

Osmotic laxatives are poorly or nonabsorbed substances, which result in the secretion of water in the intestines to maintain isotonicity with plasma. Most osmotic laxatives take several days to work. Saline laxatives contain either magnesium or phosphorus. Patients with renal insufficiency or cardiac dysfunction can experience electrolyte and volume overload from the absorption of sodium, magnesium, or phosphorus.

Another osmotic laxative, lactulose, has been shown to not only increase the frequency of bowel movements but also reduce the number of episodes of fecal impaction and the need for enemas in a study of elderly patients living in a nursing home.[58] A study comparing sorbitol (mean dose of 21 g per day) to lactulose (mean dose of 21 g per day) in ambulatory elderly men with constipation found no difference between the effect of the two compounds with regard to the frequency or the normality of bowel actions or patient preference.[59] Polyethylene glycol (PEG) is an iso-osmotic laxative that is metabolically inert and is able to increase intraluminal and bind water molecules. PEG is not metabolized by colonic bacteria and should therefore be less likely to cause bloating and excessive gas. PEG appears to be effective in relieving constipation and reducing the incidence of fecal impaction in the elderly.[60,61]

Stimulant laxatives increase intestinal motility and intestinal secretion. They begin working within hours and are often associated with abdominal cramps and watery diarrhea. Stimulant laxatives include diphenylmethanes (e.g., phenolphthalein, bisacodyl, and sodium picosulfate) and anthraquinones (e.g., cascara, aloe, and senna). Despite a history of concerns, stimulant laxatives do not appear to have long-term negative effects on the colon.[62] Nevertheless, the elderly are prone to developing dehydration and malabsorption from stimulant laxatives, and caution is therefore warranted.

Tegaserod is a 5-HT_4 receptor partial agonist that increases GI motility and secretion, and reduces visceral hypersensitivity. A study involving 1,264 patients with chronic constipation randomized them to receive either tegaserod 2 or 6 mg, or placebo twice daily for 12 weeks. In this study, a responder was defined as a patient with an increase of one or more complete spontaneous bowel movements per week compared to the baseline during the first 4 weeks of the study. The responder rates for this study were 35.6% for tegaserod 2 mg b.i.d., 40.2% for 6 mg b.i.d., and 26.7% for placebo. The number needed to treat was 7.3 for the 6 mg b.i.d. dose compared with 11.1 for the tegaserod 2 mg b.i.d. Tegaserod 6 mg b.i.d. reduced straining, abdominal bloating/distension, and abdominal pain/discomfort during the 12-week treatment period compared with placebo.[63] Tegaserod does appear to improve symptoms in patients older than 65. However, it should not be used in patients with renal insufficiency, liver disease, or abdominal adhesions, nor in the presence of symptomatic gall bladder disease. No drug/drug interactions have yet been reported with tegaserod[64] (Evidence Level B).

Suppositories and enemas can be an effective and safe treatment of constipation in the elderly. Rare perforations of the rectum or mucosal injury have been reported. The anterior rectum is most vulnerable to trauma from the tip of an enema catheter, and therefore, whenever possible, the enema tip should be directed posteriorly in the rectum. The most commonly used enemas are phosphate enemas, tap water, glycerin, mineral oil, and soap suds enemas. Phosphate enemas have been associated with hyperphosphatemia and hypocalcemia in patients unable to expel the enema. Because water is absorbed in the colon, patients who retain the enema are at risk of developing electrolyte abnormalities (Evidence Level C).

FECAL INCONTINENCE

Fecal incontinence, which is the involuntary release of stool, is a common problem, especially in the elderly. Up to 1% of elderly people report regular episodes of fecal incontinence. Up to 10% of nursing home residents and 30% of hospitalized patients also experience frequent episodes of fecal incontinence. The prevalence of incontinence in epidemiologic studies varies significantly[65] and estimates are likely to underrepresent the true prevalence of fecal incontinence, as patients are often reluctant to discuss this problem with their physician due to embarrassment.[66,99] Factors most significantly associated with fecal incontinence are urinary incontinence, enteral tube feedings, loss of daily living activities, diarrhea, and the need for restraints. Fecal incontinence is the second leading cause of nursing home placement.

Etiology

Because continence has multiple overlapping mechanisms, the cause of fecal incontinence is often multifactorial. The major mechanisms involved in maintaining continence include anal sphincter function, rectal sensation, compliance, the anorectal angle, the consistency of stool, and mental state.

Causes of particular concern in the elderly include fecal incontinence due to injury to the pudendal nerve from years of repetitive straining. Childbirth trauma to the anal sphincter can predispose patients to fecal incontinence in later life. Diabetes can result in reduced internal anal sphincter resting pressure, and these patients frequently have altered motility from autonomic neuropathy, leading to either diarrhea or constipation. Patients who have had radiation to the pelvic area are at risk for radiation proctitis that can impair the compliance of the rectum, leading to increased urgency and even incontinence. Fecal impaction is a common cause of fecal incontinence in the elderly by inhibiting the internal anal sphincter and permitting the leakage of liquid stool around the impaction. Risk factors for fecal impaction in the elderly include alterations in mental function, immobility, rectal hyposensitivity, multiple medications, and inadequate intake of fluids and dietary fiber.

Evaluation

The history should initially focus on determining the onset, duration, frequency, severity of symptoms, and precipitating events, and obtaining the history of prior vaginal delivery, anorectal surgery, pelvic irradiation, diabetes, neurologic disease, and whether the incontinence occurs with diarrhea. The physical examination should include the inspection of the perianal area for fistulae, prolapsing hemorrhoids, or rectal prolapse. Perianal sensation should be tested by evoking the anocutaneous reflex (anal wink sign), which is done by gently stroking the area adjacent to the anus and observing for the contraction of the external anal sphincter. The absence of this reflex suggests nerve damage and interruption of the spinal reflex. A digital examination can assess for rectal mass or fecal impaction, and can provide a crude assessment of the anal sphincter resting tone. Patients should be instructed to bear down and to then squeeze against the finger, which permits the appreciation of the movement and angle of the puborectalis muscle, pelvic floor descent, and squeeze pressure. However, the accuracy of these components of the physical examination are highly dependent upon experience and correlate poorly with the objective measures of anorectal function.

Diagnosis

Most patients should undergo an inspection of their distal colon and the anus with flexible sigmoidoscopy or colonoscopy, depending on when their last examination was performed. An anoscopy should be performed if the anal canal is not well-visualized during endoscopy. Other tests available measure the specific components of anorectal function. Anorectal manometry measures the resting and squeeze pressure of the anal sphincter, the rectoanal inhibitory reflex, threshold of conscious rectal sensation, and rectal compliance.[67] Pudendal nerve terminal latency is usually performed during anorectal manometry and measures whether there has been damage to the nerve. Endorectal ultrasound evaluates for anatomic defects in the anal sphincter and is most useful for establishing the diagnosis in patients in whom the medical history or manometric findings suggest occult sphincter injury.

Treatment

The approaches most commonly used for the treatment of fecal incontinence are: Medical therapy, biofeedback, and surgery. Medical therapy aims at reducing stool frequency and improving stool consistency with fiber and antidiarrheal drugs. Fiber therapy or bulking agent is particularly helpful in patients who have low-volume, loose stools. It can, however, exacerbate incontinence in patients with decreased rectal compliance (such as those with radiation proctitis or a rectal stricture). Stool frequency can be reduced with antidiarrheal drugs such as loperamide.[68]

Patients who have stool impaction should be disimpacted and treated with a bowel regimen (i.e., rectal suppositories, and laxatives) to prevent recurrent impaction. Patients who have incontinence related to mental dysfunction or physical disability may benefit from assistance with a regular defecation program similar to that for patients with fecal impaction.

Biofeedback therapy involves retraining the pelvic floor and the abdominal wall musculature, similar to the technique used to treat patients with urinary incontinence. The general mechanisms by which biofeedback may improve fecal incontinence are: Improved contraction of the striated muscles of the pelvic floor, enhancement of the ability to perceive rectal distension, and improved coordination of the sensory and strength components that are required for continence. The overall average probability of improvement for patients treated with biofeedback is approximately 67%.[69] A large prospective controlled study found no significant benefit of nine 40- to 60-minute sessions over 6 months with a specialist nurse offering advice on diet, fluids, techniques to improve evacuation, bowel training, and titration of antidiarrheal medications.[70] The overall improvement with biofeedback was 54% compared with 53% with standard care. Therefore, conservative measures may be as effective as biofeedback for fecal incontinence. Nevertheless, the 2004 guideline issued by the American College of Gastroenterology recommends biofeedback in patients with weak sphincters and/or impaired rectal sensation[67] (Evidence Level C).

Surgical treatment for fecal incontinence is reserved for patients with severe symptoms who have failed medical and biofeedback therapy. Some of the therapies that have been described include direct sphincter repair, plication of the posterior part of the sphincter, anal encirclement, implantation of an artificial sphincter, and muscle transfer procedures with or without electrical stimulation. Colostomy may be the only option in patients with intractable symptoms who are not candidates for any other therapy, or in whom other treatments have failed.

Electrical stimulation of the sacral nerve roots can restore continence in patients with structurally intact muscles. An electrode inserted into the S3 sacral foramen provides low-grade stimulation through a chronic stimulator implanted under the anterior abdominal wall. The mechanism of action is not entirely clear, but physiology studies in patients with sacral nerve stimulation have shown improvement in the resting and squeeze pressures of the anal sphincter as well as improved rectal sensation. Recent studies suggest that the device improves incontinence, with only minor adverse effects.[71] Therefore, sacral nerve stimulation may be considered in patients who fail conventional treatment and before sphincter replacement or stoma creation[72] (Evidence Level C).

GASTROESOPHAGEAL REFLUX DISEASE

GERD is a chronic condition that is the result of increased gastric contents refluxing into the esophagus. The hallmark symptoms of GERD, heartburn and regurgitation, are experienced weekly by 14% of the adult US population.[73] GERD can impair the sufferers' quality of life and it is associated with a number of complications including asthma, hoarseness, Barrett's metaplasia, and adenocarcinoma of the esophagus.[74,75] The total annual US health care costs associated with GERD are estimated to be in excess of $9.8 billion.[76]

The prevalence of GERD symptoms in the elderly is similar to that of the younger people.[73] In contrast, complications of GERD, such as esophagitis, Barrett's or esophageal stricture, are significantly higher in the elderly. A study by Collen et al. found that patients with GERD older than 60 years were more likely to have esophageal mucosal disease (i.e., erosive esophagitis, Barrett's esophagus) than those younger than 60 years (81% vs. 47%, respectively).[77]

The higher prevalence of GERD-related complications in the elderly is likely due to an increase in esophageal acid exposure. Huang et al. found elderly patients with typical reflux symptoms had a greater amount of acid reflux in the esophagus as measured by 24-hour pH study, and more severe esophagitis on endoscopy than did younger patients with similar symptoms.[78] The elderly appear to have reduced esophageal pain sensitivity, which results in delayed presentation and the higher GERD-related complications.[79]

Pathophysiology

GERD is most often due to a defect in the antireflux barrier, which includes the lower esophageal sphincter. The most common cause of reflux is due to the transient relaxation of the lower esophageal sphincter that is not accompanied by a swallow. An increase in the frequency of these relaxations results in acid refluxing into the distal esophagus and GERD. It is not, however, known whether this changes with age.

The antireflux barrier can also be defective due to a weakened lower esophageal sphincter as a result of calcium channel blockers, anticholinergic agents, nitrates, theophylline, benzodiazepines, and antidepressants.[78] The final mechanism to cause a defective antireflux barrier is a hiatal hernia, which reduces the lower esophageal sphincter pressure and impairs distal esophageal clearance. Hiatal hernias are more common in the elderly, reaching 60% in patients older than 60.[80]

Other causes of GERD include abnormal esophageal peristalsis, reduced salivary production, delayed gastric emptying due to comorbid medical conditions such as diabetes mellitus or Parkinson disease, and the use of multiple medications. For example, the elderly appear to have impaired esophageal clearance of acid. Compared to younger people, the elderly have a significant decrease in the amplitudes of contraction in the esophagus. They also have more frequent simultaneous and irregular contractions.[81] Likewise, the elderly also have a decrease in the production of salivary bicarbonate, which helps to neutralize acid in the esophagus.[82]

Diagnosis

The most common presentation of GERD is the presence of heartburn and regurgitation. Other common symptoms associated with GERD include nausea and belching. Heartburn is typically described as a burning sensation that begins in the epigastric area and rises into the substernal region. It can radiate to the neck or throat region. Bending forward, lying flat, or eating a large fatty meal frequently exacerbates the symptoms. The diagnosis of GERD is made on the basis of the presence of these symptoms.

Extraesophageal symptoms from GERD are also common in the elderly.[45] These include globus sensation, atypical chest pain, laryngitis, chronic cough, asthma, pulmonary aspiration, and hoarseness.[83] Frequently, extraesophageal symptoms are the only symptoms of GERD. In these patients, the diagnosis of GERD can be more difficult to establish.

Patients who present with warning symptoms such as difficulty swallowing or dysphagia, weight loss, or anemia suggest the presence of complications from GERD, such as esophageal stricture or cancer. These patients should be thoroughly evaluated rather than empirically treated.

Evaluation

Several diagnostic tests are available for evaluating a patient with GERD. Barium swallow and upper endoscopy are useful to evaluate the anatomy of the esophagus. An upper endoscopy is the preferred test to evaluate for mucosal injury. Ambulatory 24- or 48-hour esophageal pH monitoring is useful when the diagnosis of GERD is questioned or when quantification of acid reflux is required. Esophageal manometry, which measures the lower esophageal sphincter pressure and contractions in the esophagus, is reserved for only those patients undergoing antireflux surgery or with dysphagia not explained by upper endoscopy. Esophageal impedance allows for the detection of both acid and nonacid reflux. The PPI test can be used to help confirm the diagnosis of GERD, especially in patients with atypical chest pain. The test consists of a short course (i.e., 1 to 7 days) of high-dose PPI therapy (e.g., omeprazole 60 mg per day).[84]

Diagnostic tests are generally not required to make the diagnosis of GERD. In contrast to younger people, an upper endoscopy should be considered in most patients with suspected GERD, independent of the severity or duration of symptoms. An aggressive approach to the elderly is warranted due to the high prevalence of complications from GERD, and the poor correlation between symptom severity and complications.

Treatment

The goal of treatment for GERD is to reduce symptoms, heal esophagitis, and manage complications.[85] The range of treatments currently available for the treatment of GERD is listed in Table 41.8. Lifestyle modifications should be recommended as the initial strategy, but they are rarely sufficient. These include elevating the head of the bed 6 to 8 inches, avoiding eating at least 3 hours prior to lying down, discontinuing smoking, avoiding foods known to relax the lower esophageal sphincter (such as peppermint, onion, alcohol, coffee, and caffeine). Weight loss and loose fitting clothes may also be helpful. Medications known to weaken the lower esophageal sphincter should be avoided when possible. Obesity is a risk factor for GERD; however, studies have not conclusively shown improvement in GERD symptoms with weight loss. Nevertheless, weight loss should be recommended in patients who are overweight.

Medications are frequently required to control symptoms and avoid complications associated with GERD. Antacids may be helpful on an as-needed basis in patients with mild intermittent symptoms. Frequent use of antacids may cause hypercalcemia, hypermagnesia, and diarrhea.

Histamine-2 receptor antagonists (H_2-blockers) are sold over the counter and, like antacids, are helpful for patients with mild intermittent symptoms. The most common H_2-blockers sold over the counter are cimetidine, ranitidine, famotidine, and nizatidine. They can be taken up to four times per day but are best used as needed. The dose of H_2-blockers should be reduced in patients with renal insufficiency. Side effects, especially in the elderly, are common. Delirium, dizziness, and confusion have been reported with H_2-blockers.[86,87] Likewise, gynecomastia,

TABLE 41.8
THERAPIES FOR GASTROESOPHAGEAL REFLUX DISEASE (GERD)

Lifestyle modifications
Elevate head of the bed 6–8 inches or a Styrofoam wedge under the mattress
Avoid eating 3 h prior to lying down
Avoid smoking
Reduce caffeine, alcohol, peppermint, fatty foods
Avoid medications known to inhibit the lower esophageal sphincter (e.g., calcium channel blockers, nitrates, theophylline, β-blockers, bisphosphonates)
Avoid tight fitting garments
Medications
Antacids—e.g., aluminum/magnesium hydroxide
H_2-receptor antagonists—e.g., cimetidine, ranitidine, famotidine, and nizatidine
Proton pump inhibitors—e.g., omeprazole, esomeprazole, pantoprazole, lansoprazole, rabeprazole
Surgery
Laparoscopic Nissen fundoplication
Endoscopic therapies
NDO plicator
Stretta
Enteryx
EndoCinch

impotency, anemia, and cardiac arrhythmias have been reported. Cimetidine interacts with the metabolism of warfarin, benzodiazepines, and phenytoin, and therefore dose adjustments are necessary.

Patients who do not respond to these therapies or those with complications from GERD should be treated and maintained with a PPI (Evidence Level B). Current PPIs include omeprazole, esomeprazole, lansoprazole, pantoprazole, and rabeprazole. PPIs are more effective than antacids or H_2-blockers in suppressing acid[88] and are generally well tolerated. No adjustment in dose in elderly patients is needed. PPIs are generally dosed once per day, although patients with atypical or ear, nose, and throat symptoms frequently require twice daily doses. Prolonged acid suppression with PPIs may induce bacterial overgrowth and may decrease vitamin B_{12} absorption.[89]

Most patients can be managed successfully with medical therapies. However, symptoms or complications of GERD occasionally require surgical or endoscopic therapies. The most common antireflux surgery performed is a laparoscopic Nissen fundoplication. Age alone is not an exclusion.[90] Careful patient selection is mandatory and should include preoperative esophageal manometry, prolonged ambulatory esophageal pH recording, and potentially a gastric emptying study. Nissen fundoplication has been associated with morbidity in up to 5% of patients, including gas, bloating, and dysphagia.[91] Furthermore, reoperation due to complications and/or recurrent reflux is necessary in 13% of patients.[92] The long-term durability of surgery is not established. One study reported 63% of Nissen fundoplication patients use antisecretory medications at a mean follow-up of 10.6 years.[93]

An ongoing study with 5-year follow-up comparing open Nissen fundoplication to omeprazole 20 mg per day has found surgery to be superior to omeprazole for the treatment of erosive esophagitis.[94] However, if the dose of omeprazole was increased during periods of relapse, the two therapeutic strategies were not statistically different (Evidence Level B).

Several endoscopic therapies for the treatment of GERD have recently been approved. The Stretta (Curon Medical Inc., Sunnyvale, CA) utilizes radio frequency energy to create submucosal thermal lesions in the smooth muscles of the lower esophageal sphincter.[95] As the thermal lesions heal, scar tissue forms and the resulting tissue contraction is thought to increase resistance to acid reflux. The EndoCinch (Bard Endoscopic Technologies, Billerica, MA) utilizes a transoral flexible endoscopic suturing device to plicate the gastroesophageal junction.[96] This device places a submucosal suture to form a "neoesophagus" to accentuate the valvular mechanism at the gastroesophageal junction. The Enteryx utilizes an injection of a biopolymer (Enteric Medical Technology, Palo Alto, CA) under fluoroscopy into the lower esophageal sphincter.[97] The NDO plicator utilizes an endoscopic full-thickness plication device near the gastroesophageal junction.[98]

Most of the studies performed to date with endoscopic therapies have included patients with relatively mild GERD who do not have a significant hiatal hernia and who respond to medical therapies. It is not known how effective these therapies would be on refractory patients; the long-term efficacy of these relatively new therapies is also not known. Therefore, while endoscopic therapies offer a less invasive method of enhancing the antireflux barrier, caution is warranted until further studies are completed.

REFERENCES

1. Linder JD, Wilcox CM. Acid peptic diseases in the elderly. *Gastroenterol Clin North Am*. 2001;30(2):363–376.
2. Everhart JE, Byrd-Holt D, Sonnenberg A. Incidence and risk factors for self-reported peptic ulcer disease in the United States. *Am J Epidemiol*. 1998;147(6):529–536.
3. Griffin MR. Epidemiology of nonsteroidal anti-inflammatory drug-associated gastrointestinal injury. *Am J Med*. 1998;104(3A): 23S–29S.
4. Laine L, Bombardier C, Hawkey CJ, et al. Stratifying the risk of NSAID-related upper gastrointestinal clinical events: Results of a double-blind outcomes study in patients with rheumatoid arthritis. *Gastroenterologia*. 2002;123:1006–1012.
5. Lai KC, Lam SK, Wong BC, et al. Lansoprazole for prevention of recurrence of ulcer complications from long-term low-dose aspirin use. *N Engl J Med*. 2002;346(26):2033–2038.
6. Pilotto A, Malfertheiner P. Review article: An approach to Helicobacter pylori infection in the elderly. *Aliment Pharmacol Ther*. 2002;16:683–691.

7. Wilcox CM, Clark WS. Features associated with painless peptic ulcer bleeding. *Am J Gastroenterol.* 1997;92(8):1289–1292.
8. Clinch D, Banerjee AK, Ostick G. Absence of abdominal pain in elderly patients with peptic ulcer. *Age Ageing.* 1984;13:120–123.
9. Glinsky NH. Peptic ulcer disease in the elderly. *Gastroenterol Clin North Am.* 1990;19:255–271.
10. Eshchar J, Pavlotzki MM, Cohen L, et al. Gastrointestinal endoscopy in octogenarians. *J Clin Gastroenterol.* 1986;8:520–524.
11. Maton PN. Omeprazole. *N Engl J Med.* 1991;324(14):965–975.
12. Lirussi F, Nassuato G, Passera D, et al. Gallstone disease in an elderly population: The Silea Study. *Eur J Gastroenterol Hepatol.* 1999;11(5):485–491.
13. Jansen PL. Liver disease in the elderly. *Best Pract Res Clin Gastroenterol.* 2002;16(1):149–158.
14. Perret RS, Sloop GD, Bourne JA. Common bile duct measurements in an elderly population. *J Ultrasound Med.* 2000;19(11):727–730.
15. Bachar GN, Cohen M, Belensky A, et al. Effect of aging on the adult extrahepatic bile duct. *J Ultrasound Med.* 2003;22:879–882.
16. Kratzer W, Kachele V, Mason RA, et al. Gallstone prevalence in Germany. *Dig Dis Sci.* 1998;43(6):1285–1291.
17. Magnuson TH, Ratner LE, Zenilman ME, et al. Laparoscopic cholecystectomy: Applicability in the geriatric population. *Am Surg.* 1997;63(1):91–96.
18. Adedeji OA, McAdam WA. Murphy's sign, acute cholecysitis and elderly people. *J R Coll Surg Edinb.* 1996;41:88–89.
19. Reiss R, Nudelman I, Gutman C, et al. Changing trends in surgery for acute cholecystitis. *World J Surg.* 1990;14:567–571.
20. Shea JA, Berlin JA, Escarce JJ, et al. Revised estimates of diagnostic test sensitivity and specificity in suspected biliary tract disease. *Arch Intern Med.* 1994;154:2573–2581.
21. Zakko SF, Afdhal NH. Clinical features and diagnosis of acute cholecystitis. In: Rose BD, ed. UpToDate. Waltham, MA: UpToDate; 2006.
22. Fidler J, Paulson EK, Layfield L. CT evaluation of acute cholecystitis: Findings and usefulness in diagnosis. *Am J Roentgenol.* 1996;166:1085–1088.
23. Borzellino G, deManzoni G, Ricci F, et al. Emergency cholecystostomy and subsequent cholecystectomy for acute gallstone cholecystitis in the elderly. *Br J Surg.* 1999;86:1521–1525.
24. Ross SO, Forsmark CE. Pancreatic and biliary disorders in the elderly. *Gastroenterol Clin North Am.* 2001;30(2):531–545.
25. Kimura W, Shimada H, Kuroda A, et al. Carcinoma of the gallbladder and extrahepatic bile duct in autopsy cases of the aged, with special reference to its relationship to gallstones. *Am J Gastroenterol.* 1989;84:386–390.
26. Gigot JF, Leese T, Dereme T, et al. Acute cholangitis: Multivariate analysis of risk factors. *Ann Surg.* 1999;209:435–438.
27. Sugiyama M, Atomi Y. Treatment of acute cholangitis due to choledocholithiasis in elderly and younger patients. *Arch Surg.* 1997;132(10):1129–1133.
28. Afdhal NH. Acute cholangitis. In: Rose BD, ed. UpToDate. Waltham, MA: UpToDate; 2006.
29. Chan Y, Chan AC, Lam WW, et al. Choledocholithiasis: Comparison of MR cholangiography and endoscopic retrograde cholangiography. *Radiology.* 1996;200(1):85–89.
30. Saito M, Tsuyuguchi T, Yamaguchi T, et al. Long-term outcome of endoscopic papillotomy for choledocholithiasis with cholecystolithiasis. *Gastrointest Endosc.* 2000;51(5):540–545.
31. Sallout H, Mayoral W, Benjamin SB. The aging esophagus. *Clin Geriatr Med.* 1999;15(3):439–456.
32. Robson KM, Glick ME. Dysphagia and advancing age: Are manometric abnormalities more common in older patients? *Dig Dis Sci.* 2003;48(9):1709–1712.
33. Lindgren S, Janzon L. Prevalence of swallowing complaints and clinical findings among 50–79 year old men and women in an urban population. *Dysphagia.* 1991;6(4):187–192.
34. Fass R. Approach to the patient with dysphagia. In: Rose BD, ed. UpToDate. Waltham, MA: UpToDate; 2006.
35. Shamburek RD, Farrar JT. Disorders of the digestive system in the elderly. *N Engl J Med.* 1990;322(7):438–443.
36. Castell DO, Donner MW. Evaluation of dysphagia: A careful history is crucial. *Dysphagia.* 1987;2(2):65–71.
37. Shaker R, Staff D. Esophageal disorders in the elderly. *Gastroenterol Clin North Am.* 2001;30(2):335–361.
38. Sonnenberg A, Massey BT, McCarty DJ, et al. Epidemiology of hospitalization for achalasia in the United States. *Dig Dis Sci.* 1993;38:233–244.
39. Goldblum JR, Rice TW, Richter JE. Histopathologic features in esophagomyotomy specimens from patients with achalasia. *Gastroenterology.* 1996;111:648–654.
40. Gelfond M, Rozen P, Gilat T. Isosorbide dinitrate and nifedipine treatment of achalasia: A clinical, manometric and radionuclide evaluation. *Gastroenterology.* 1982;83(5):963–969.
41. Farrell JJ, Friedman LS. Esophageal diseases in the elderly. *Clin Perspect Gastroenterol.* 2001;4(6):363–368.
42. Cattau EL Jr, Castell DO, Johnson DA, et al. Diltiazem therapy for symptoms associated with nutcracker esophagus. *Am J Gastroenterol.* 1991;86(3):272–276.
43. Clouse RE, Lustman PJ, Eckert TC, et al. Low-dose trazadone for symptomatic patients with esophageal contraction abnormalities. A double-blind, placebo-controlled trial. *Gastroenterology.* 1987;92(4):1027–1036.
44. Bott S, Prakash C, McCallum RW. Medication-induced esophageal injury: Survey of the literature. *Am J Gastroenterol.* 1987;82(8): 758–763.
45. Raiha I, Manner R, Hietanen E, et al. Radiographic pulmonary changes of gastro-esophageal reflux disease in elderly patients. *Age Ageing.* 1992;21(4):250–255.
46. Greenwald DA. Aging, the gastrointestinal tract, and risk of acid-related disease. *Am J Med.* 2004;117(5A):8S–13S.
47. Metz DC. Managing gastroesophageal reflux disease for the lifetime of the patient: Evaluating long-term options. *Am J Med.* 2004;117(5A):49S–55S.
48. Collen MJ, Abdulian JD, Chen YK. GERD in the elderly: More severe disease that requires aggressive therapy. *Am J Gastroenterol.* 1995;90(7):1053–1057.
49. Pare P, Ferrazzi S, Thompson WG, et al. An epidemiological survey of constipation in canada: Definitions, rates, demographics, and predictors of health care seeking. *Am J Gastroenterol.* 2001; 96:3130–3137.
50. Sonnenberg A, Koch TR. Physician visits in the United States for constipation: 1958 to 1986. *Dig Dis Sci.* 1989;34:606–611.
51. Locke GR 3rd, Pemberton JH, Phillips SF. American Gastroenterological Association. AGA technical review on constipation. *Gastroenterology.* 2000;119:1766–1778.
52. Talley NJ, Fleming KC, Evans JM, et al. Constipation in an elderly community: A study of prevalence and potential risk factors. *Am J Gastroenterol.* 1996;91:19–25.
53. Read NW, Celik AF, Katsinelos P. Constipation and incontinence in the elderly. *J Clin Gastroenterol.* 1995;20:61–70.
54. Campbell AJ, Busby WJ, Horwath CC. Factors associated with constipation in a community based sample of people aged 70 years and over. *J Epidemiol Community Health.* 1993;47:23–26.
55. Thompson WG, Longstreth GF, Drossman DA, et al. Functional bowel disorders and functional abdominal pain. *Gut.* 1999;45(suppl 2):II43–II47.
56. Dukas L, Willett WC, Giovannucci EL. Association between physical activity, fiber intake, and other lifestyle variables and constipation in a study of women. *Am J Gastroenterol.* 2003;98: 1790–1796.
57. Lembo A, Camilleri M. Chronic constipation. *N Engl J Med.* 2003;349:1360–1368.
58. Sanders JF. Lactulose syrup assessed in a double-blind study of elderly constipated patients. *J Am Geriatr Soc.* 1978;26:236–239.
59. Lederle FA, Busch DL, Mattox KM, et al. Cost-effective treatment of constipation in the elderly: A randomized double-blind comparison of sorbitol and lactulose. *Am J Med.* 1990;89:597–601.
60. Loening-Baucke V, Krishna R, Pashankar DS. Polyethylene glycol 3350 without electrolytes for the treatment of functional constipation in infants and toddlers. *J Pediatr Gastroenterol Nutr.* 2004;39:536–539.
61. Corazziari E, Badiali D, Bazzocchi G, et al. Long term efficacy, safety, and tolerability of low daily doses of isosmotic polyethylene glycol electrolyte balanced solution (PMF-100) in the treatment of functional chronic constipation. *Gut.* 2000;46:522–526.
62. Muller-Lissner SA, Kamm MA, Scarpignato C, et al. Myths and misconceptions about chronic constipation. *Am J Gastroenterol.* 2005;100:232–242.

63. Kamm MA, Muller-Lissner S, Talley NJ, et al. Tegaserod for the treatment of chronic constipation: A randomized, double-blind, placebo-controlled multinational study. *Am J Gastroenterol.* 2005;100:362–372.
64. Muller-Lissner S, Holtmann G, Rueegg P, et al. Tegaserod is effective in the initial and retreatment of irritable bowel syndrome with constipation. *Aliment Pharmacol Ther.* 2005;21:11–20.
65. Macmillan AK, Merrie AE, Marshall RJ, et al. The prevalence of fecal incontinence in community-dwelling adults: A systematic review of the literature. *Dis Colon Rectum.* 2004;47:1341–1349.
66. Johanson JF, Lafferty J. Epidemiology of fecal incontinence: The silent affliction. *Am J Gastroenterol.* 1996;91:33–36.
67. Rao SS. American College of Gastroenterology Practice Parameters Committee. Diagnosis and management of fecal incontinence. *Am J Gastroenterol.* 2004;99:1585–1604.
68. Tuteja AK, Rao SS. Review article: Recent trends in diagnosis and treatment of faecal incontinence. *Aliment Pharmacol Ther.* 2004;19:829–840.
69. Palsson OS, Heymen S, Whitehead WE. Biofeedback treatment for functional anorectal disorders: A comprehensive efficacy review. *Appl Psychophysiol Biofeedback.* 2004;29:153–174.
70. Norton C, Chelvanayagam S, Wilson-Barnett J, et al. Randomized controlled trial of biofeedback for fecal incontinence. *Gastroenterology.* 2003;125:1320–1329.
71. Matzel KE, Stadelmaier U, Hohenberger W. Innovations in fecal incontinence: Sacral nerve stimulation. *Dis Colon Rectum.* 2004;47:1720–1728.
72. Jarrett ME. Neuromodulation for constipation and fecal incontinence. *Urol Clin North Am.* 2005;32:79–87.
73. Locke GR 3rd, Talley NJ, Fett SL, et al. Prevalence and clinical spectrum of gastroesophageal reflux: A population-based study in Olmsted County, Minnesota. *Gastroenterology.* 1997; 112:1448–1456.
74. Farup C, Kleinman L, Sloan S, et al. The impact of nocturnal symptoms associated with gastroesophageal reflux disease on health-related quality of life. *Arch Intern Med.* 2001;161:45–52.
75. Kulig M, Leodolter A, Vieth M, et al. Quality of life in relation to symptoms in patients with gastro-oesophageal reflux disease–an analysis based on the ProGERD initiative. *Aliment Pharmacol Ther.* 2003;18:767–776.
76. Sandler RS, Everhart JE, Donowitz M, et al. The burden of selected digestive diseases in the United States. *Gastroenterology.* 2002;122:1500–1511.
77. Collen MJ, Abdulian JD, Chen YK. Gastroesophageal reflux disease in the elderly: More severe disease that requires aggressive therapy. *Am J Gastroenterol.* 1995;90:1053–1057.
78. Huang X, Zhu HM, Deng CZ, et al. Gastroesophageal reflux: The features in elderly patients. *World J Gastroenterol.* 1999;5:421–423.
79. Fass R, Pulliam G, Johnson C, et al. Symptom severity and oesophageal chemosensitivity to acid in older and young patients with gastro-oesophageal reflux. *Age Ageing.* 2000;29:125–130.
80. Stilson WL, Sanders I, Gardiner GA, et al. Hiatal hernia and gastroesophageal reflux. A clinicoradiological analysis of more than 1,000 cases. *Radiology.* 1969;93:1323–1327.
81. Ferriolli E, Oliveira RB, Matsuda NM, et al. Aging, esophageal motility, and gastroesophageal reflux. *J Am Geriatr Soc.* 1998;46: 1534–1537.
82. Sonnenberg A, Lepsien G, Muller-Lissner SA, et al. When is esophagitis healed? esophageal endoscopy, histology and function before and after cimetidine treatment. *Dig Dis Sci.* 1982;27:297–302.
83. Raiha IJ, Impivaara O, Seppala M, et al. Prevalence and characteristics of symptomatic gastroesophageal reflux disease in the elderly. *J Am Geriatr Soc.* 1992;40:1209–1211.
84. Fass R. Empirical trials in treatment of gastroesophageal reflux disease. *Dig Dis.* 2000;18:20–26.
85. DeVault KR, Castell DO. The Practice Parameters Committee of the American College of Gastroenterology. Updated guidelines for the diagnosis and treatment of gastroesophageal reflux disease. *Am J Gastroenterol.* 1999;94:1434–1442.
86. Nickell PV. Histamine-2 receptor blockers and delirium. *Ann Intern Med.* 1991;115:658.
87. Cantu TG, Korek JS. Central nervous system reactions to histamine-2 receptor blockers. *Ann Intern Med.* 1991;114: 1027–1034.
88. Vigneri S, Termini R, Leandro G, et al. A comparison of five maintenance therapies for reflux esophagitis. *N Engl J Med.* 1995; 333:1106–1110.
89. Howden CW. Vitamin B12 levels during prolonged treatment with proton pump inhibitors. *J Clin Gastroenterol.* 2000;30:29–33.
90. Trus TL, Laycock WS, Wo JM, et al. Laparoscopic antireflux surgery in the elderly. *Am J Gastroenterol.* 1998;93:351–353.
91. Hookman P, Barkin JS. Surgical complications of laparoscopic fundoplication for gastroesophageal reflux disease: Call for reevaluation of surgical criteria. *Am J Gastroenterol.* 2000;95: 3305–3308.
92. Lafullarde T, Watson DI, Jamieson GG, et al. Laparoscopic Nissen fundoplication: Five-year results and beyond. *Arch Surg.* 2001;136:180–184.
93. Spechler SJ, Lee E, Ahnen D, et al. Long-term outcome of medical and surgical therapies for gastroesophageal reflux disease: Follow-up of a randomized controlled trial. *JAMA.* 2001;285:2331–2338.
94. Lundell L, Miettinen P, Myrvold HE, et al. Continued (5-year) followup of a randomized clinical study comparing antireflux surgery and omeprazole in gastroesophageal reflux disease. *J Am Coll Surg.* 2001;192:172–179; discussion 179–181.
95. Triadafilopoulos G, DiBaise JK, Nostrant TT, et al. The Stretta procedure for the treatment of GERD: 6 and 12 month follow-up of the U.S. open label trial. *Gastrointest Endosc.* 2002;55:149–156.
96. Swain P, Park PO. Endoscopic suturing. *Best Pract Res Clin Gastroenterol.* 2004;18:37–47.
97. Johnson DA. Enteryx implant for gastroesophageal reflux disease. *Curr Treat Options Gastroenterol.* 2005;8:51–57.
98. Pleskow D, Rothstein R, Lo S, et al. Endoscopic full-thickness plication for the treatment of GERD: A multicenter trial. *Gastrointest Endosc.* 2004;59:163–171.
99. Madoff RD, Parker SC, Varma MG, et al. Faecal incontinence in adults. *Lancet.* 2004;364:621–632.

Index

A

Abandonment, 96, 100
Abdominal aortic aneurysm, 173–174
  follow-up, 174
  imaging, 173–174
  management of, 174
  physical examination, 173
Abusive caregivers, 30
Acceptance and adaptation, 61
Acceptance coping, 31
ACE inhibitors, 42, 74, 354, 358–359, 397, 445, 449–450
  and hypertension, 313
ACE-I therapy, 340–341
Acetaminophen (Tylenol), 45, 47, 55–56, 93, 166, 217, 279, 282, 284
  and Alzheimer disease, 247
Acetylcholine, 5
Acetylcholinesterase, 5
Achalasia, 570
Achlorhydria, 8
Acid–base balance, disorders of, 430–431
Acid-fast bacilli (AFB), 410
Acoustic admittance, 140
Acoustic impedance, 140
Acoustic neuromas, 142
Acquired immunodeficiency virus (AIDS), 198
Acral lentiginous maligna, 507
ACSs, *See* Acute coronary syndromes (ACSs),
Actinic keratoses (solar keratoses), 503–504
Activated protein C (APC), 553
Activities of daily living (ADLs), 112, 114
  and stroke, 365
Acupuncture, 52
Acute coronary syndromes (ACSs), 342–343
  high-risk characteristics of, 335
Acute glomerulonephritis (AGN), 420
Acute grief, 60
Acute ischemic stroke:
  assessing and managing risk of complications following, 370
  complications, 371
  general care following, 370
  general medical care of the patient with, 369–370
Acute pain, 50, 51
Acute renal insufficiency/failure, 420–421
  causes of, 420–421
  intrarenal etiologies of, 420
  postrenal acute renal failure (obstruction), 421
  prerenal, 420
Adalimumab, 465
A-delta fibers, 49
Adhesive capsulitis of the shoulder, 280, 283–284
  follow-up, 284
  imaging, 283
  management of, 284
  physical examination, 283
  workup/keys to diagnosis, 283–284
Adjuvant medications, 56–57
ADLs, *See* Activities of daily living (ADLs),
α-Adrenergic blockers, and hypertension, 313, 314
Adult Protective Services, 96–98, 104–106
Advanced sleep-phase syndrome (ASPS), 263
Adverse drug events, 18
Adynamic bone disease (ABD), 299, 305, 308
Ageism, 10
Agency for Healthcare Research and Quality (AHRQ), 512
  prediction and prevention recommendations, 521–522
    education, 522
    mechanical loading and support surfaces, 522
    Risk Assessment Tools and, 521
    skin care and early treatment, 521–522
    strength of evidence, 521
  recommendations for treatment for pressure ulcers, 522–526
    assessment, 522–523
    education and quality improvement, 525–526
    managing bacterial colonization and infection, 524–525
    managing tissue loads, 523
    surgical repair of pressure ulcers, 525
    ulcer care, 524
Age-related macular degeneration (ARMD), 121, 123–125
  choroidal neovascular membrane (CNVM), 123–124
    laser therapy for, 124–125
    reducing risk for, 124
  defined, 123
  dry form of, 121, 123
  intravitreal injections of inhibitors to vascular endothelial growth factor (VEGF), 125
  photodynamic therapy, 124
  retinal pigment epithelium (RPE), 123
  wet form of, 121, 123, 132
Aging:
  age-related physiologic changes, 9
  behavior observation, 15–16
    arm and hand movements, 16
    eye contact, 15
    facial expression, 15
    mouth and smile, 15–16
    sitting and standing postures, 16
  body composition, 4
  changes:
    in the cardiovascular system, 6–7
    in the gastrointestinal system, 7–8
    in height, 4
    in the nervous system, 5
    in the respiratory system, 7
    in the special senses, 6
  clinically relevant differences between young and old people, 4–9
  clinician's perspective, changes in, 10–12
  defined, 4
  function, importance of, 11–12
  geriatric assessment, performing, 12–15
  hematopoietic tissues, 8–9
  how the body ages, 4
  increase in biologic and psychological uniqueness on, 4
  musculoskeletal changes, 5
  normal, 4
  and pain, 48
  physiology, 9
  presentation of illness, 10
  reviewing our perceptions of, 2
  skin and connective tissue, 4–5
Agnosia, 112
α-agonists, 178, 183
AHRQ, *See* Agency for Healthcare Research and Quality (AHRQ),
Albumin, 200

Alcohol abuse/alcoholism, 82, 83–84, 111, 112
and aging, 83
alcohol metabolism, age-related changes that affect, 83
and dementia, 250
early onset drinkers, 83
and heart failure, 361
and insomnia, 258–259
late-onset drinkers, 83
and sleep disorders, 259
Alcohol withdrawal, and benzodiazepines, 87
Alendronate, 298
Alfuzosin (Uroxatral), 190
Allergic conjunctivitis, 131
Allergic contact dermatitis, 491, 496–498
Allopurinol, 43
and weight loss, 118
Alprazolam (Xanax), 44
Alteration of sleep, and pain, 49
Altered pattern of illness, 10
Altered response to illness, 10
Alternative therapies, 52
Aluminum-induced osteomalacia, 301
Alzheimer disease, 19, 30–32, 236, 238–249
and caregivers, 31–32
common diagnoses, 242
defined, 242–243
genetics of, 244
incidence and prevalence, 243
laboratory, 244
management of, 245, 246–247
alternative treatments, 246
lifestyle, 245
medications, 245–246
pathophysiology of, 242–243
Ronald Reagan Alzheimer's Breakthrough Act of 2004, 31
time course of, 243–244
and weight loss, 111, 112, 119
workup/keys to diagnosis, 244
Alzheimer's Association, 31–32, 38
Amantadine (Symmetrel), 559
Ambulatory care, 19
American Academy of Orthopedic Surgeons, 155
American Association for Geriatric Psychiatry, 29
American College of Cardiology (ACC), 74
American Geriatrics Society, 29, 155
American Heart Association (AHA), 74
American Medical Association (AMA), 29
American Psychiatric Association, 29
Practice Guidelines, 270
American Society of Addiction Medicine Patient Placement Criteria, 86
American Society of Anesthesiologist (ASA), 76
American Tinnitus Association (ATA), 144
American Urological Association Symptom Index (AUASI), 176
Ametropia, 122
Aminoglycosides, 144
Amiodarone, 43, 349, 445, 458, 460
Amitriptyline (Elavil), 44, 57, 282
Amorolfine, 502
Amoxapine, 57
Amoxicillin, 47, 77
Ampicillin, 77
Amputation, and peripheral arterial disease (PAD), 323, 331–332
indications for, 331
postoperative care, 332
preoperative evaluation/ risk reduction, 332
preoperative risks, 332
results of, 331–332
β-amyloid plaques, and dementia, 236, 243, 247
Amyloidosis, 469–470
Anaerobes, 560
Anal cancer, 545
Analgesic medications, dosing, 48
Androgen deficiency, 200–201
Androgen deprivation, and prostate cancer, 193
Androgen level, 4
Anemia, 9, 339, 422, 547–549
defined, 547
macrocytic, 546, 548–549
megaloblastic, 549
microcytic, 547–548
nonmegaloblastic macrocytic, 546
normocytic, 546, 547
Anesthesia, 81
Anesthetic gels, 54–55
Anger, 61
caregivers, 36
Angina, *See also* Stable angina, defined, 338
Angiography, 328
Angioplasty/stenting, 321, 328, 332–333
indications for, 332
patient monitoring/ secondary prevention, 333
perioperative risks, 333
postoperative care, 333
preoperative evaluation/ risk reduction, 333
results of, 332–333
Angiotensin II, 358
Angiotensin receptor blocking agents, *See* ACE inhibitors,
Angiotensin-receptor blockers (ARBs), 42, 358, 450
and hypertension, 312–313
Anhedonia, 61
Ankle-brachial index (ABI)/Doppler pressures, 450
Annulus fibrosis, 163
Anorectal biofeedback therapy, 564
Anorexia, 111, 113
Anorexia tardive, 111
Anterior ischemic optic neuropathy (AAION), 130–131
Antianginal agents, 341
Antiarrhythmics, in treatment of heart failure, 360–361
Antibiotics, 173
Anticholinergic drugs, 20, 183
and delirium, 226, 229
Anticholinergic medications, 177
Anticipatory grief:
assessing/assisting, 64–65
defined, 60
Anticonvulsants, 56, 57
and dementia, 250
Antidepressants, 46, 56, 93, 119, 132, 177, 214–216
and insomnia, 258
Antihistamines, 177, 527
and weight loss, 118
Antihypertensive agents, 43
Antihyperuricemic agents, 472
Anti-inflammatory agents, 93
Antioxidants, and Alzheimer disease, 247
Antiplatelet agents, and stroke, 373–374
Antiplatelet therapy, 329
Antipsychotics, 177
Antispasmodics, 57
Anti-SS-A/Ro antibodies, 466
Anti-SS-B/La antibodies, 466
Antithrombotic treatment with warfarin or aspirin, 375
Anulus fibrosus, 167
Anxiety, 266
comorbidity in schizophrenia, 266, 267
differential diagnosis of, 272–273
disease course, 274
generalized anxiety disorder (GAD), 272
diagnostic criteria for, 272
genetics, 272
late-age, 272
treatment, 273–274
management of, 273–274
pathophysiology of, 272
phobias, 266, 272
and weight loss, 112
workup, 273
Aortic aneurysms, 163
Aortic regurgitation, 345
Aortic stenosis (AS), 336, 339, 344–345
diagnostic testing, 344
etiology of, 344
management of, 344–345
pathophysiology, 344
signs/symptoms of, 344
Aortic valve disease, 337
Aortic valve replacement surgery, 345
Apnea–hypopnea index (AHI), 411
Appetite, and pain, 49
ARBs, *See* Angiotensin-receptor blockers (ARBs),
Area Agency on Aging, 38
Aripiprazole (Abilify), 271

ARMD, *See* Age-related macular degeneration (ARMD),
Armpit hair growth rate, 5
Arms crossed on chest, 16
Arrhythmias, 147, 347–353
  atrial fibrillation, 347–350
  bradyarrhythmias, 352–353
  common medications used to treat, 349
  ventricular arrhythmias, 350–352
Arterial blood gas (ABG) analysis, 397
Arterial dissection or trauma, 325
Arterial oxygen tension, 400
Arteriography, 328
Arteriovenous fistulae, 339
Articular cartilage, 277
AS, *See* Aortic stenosis (AS),
Aspiration pneumonia, and oral diseases, 488–489
Aspirin, 53–54, 55, 338, 342
  and Alzheimer disease, 247
  combining clopidogrel and, 373–374
Assertive Community Treatment (ACT) teams, 271
Assistive listening devices, 142–143
Asthma, 395–396
  cough-variant, 395, 397
  diagnosis of, 400
  epidemiology of, 400
  stepwise approach for managing, in adults, 401
  treatment of, 400–402
Astigmatism (distorted vision), 122
Asymptomatic bacteriuria, 18, 175, 183, 185–186, 554
Atenolol, 349
  and tremor, 387, 388
Atherosclerosis, cardiovascular disease, and stroke, and oral conditions, 488
Atherosclerotic occlusive disease, incidence and prevalence of, 321
Atherothrombotic microembolism (blue-toe syndrome), 325
Atorvastatin, 317, 338
Atrial fibrillation (AF), 79, 336, 347–350, 375
  etiology of, 347–348
  incidence and prevalence, 347
  management of, 348
  medications, 348–350
  pathophysiology of, 347
  percutaneous/surgical interventions, 350
  physical examination for, 348
  workup/keys to the diagnosis, 348
At-risk drinkers, 83
  contents of brief interventions for, 85–86
  feedback on, 86
Atrophic gastritis, and weight loss, 111
Atrophic vaginitis, 434–435
Attentive perioperative care, 73
Atypical antidepressants, 218
Atypical depression, 208
Auditory brainstem response (ABR), 141
Auditory evoked potentials, 141
Aural rehabilitation, 143
Autoimmune thyroiditis, 457
Azithromycin, 77
Azotemia, 415–416, 418–419
Aztreonam, 560

B
Back pain, 50
Baclofen (Lioresal), 56
Bacteremia, 557
Bacterial endocarditis, prophylactic antibiotic regimens for patients at risk for, 77
Bacterial infections, 499–503
Bacterial vaginosis, 436–437
Bacteroides fragilis, 559
β-agonists, 402–403
Balance, 148
  gait and balance assessment tools, 156–158
Barbiturates, 92
Bartholin gland carcinoma, 437
Basal cell carcinoma, 504–506
Basal systolic murmur, 335
Belladonna alkaloids (Donnatal), 45
Benazepril, 358
Benign positional vertigo (BPV), 148
Benign prostatic hyperplasia (BPH), 175–176, 187–191
  management of, 188–191
  medications for, 189–190
  surgery, 190–191
  watchful waiting, 189
  workup, 188
Benzodiazepines, 20, 43, 78, 92, 260, 266–275, 527
  and alcohol withdrawal, 87
  chronic use of, 84
  complications of, 274
  and delirium, 229
  and insomnia, 260–261
  and tremor, 390
Bereavement, 58–72
  anticipatory grief, assessing/assisting, 64–65
  bereavement register, establishing, 64
  communicating with older bereaved patients, 69
  complicated grief, 61–62
    cognitive-behavior therapy for, 70
    defined, 58, 60
    diagnosis of, 63
    diagnostic criteria for, 62
    symptoms of, 58, 62
    treating, 70–71
  defined, 60
  depression, diagnosis of, 63
  family-focused grief therapy, 70
  as health risk, 58–59
  high-risk patients, identifying, 64
  monitoring for poor bereavement outcome, 70
  normal grief, 60–61
    defined, 60
    diagnosis of, 63
    symptoms of, 62
  pharmacotherapy, 69–70
  terminology, 60
  traumatic grief treatment, 70
  and weight loss, 111–112
Bereavement care, 62–71
  attending the funeral, 67–68
  dying patients:
    common concerns of, 65
    counseling, 66
    providing support to the family of, 66–67
  functional assessment, 68
  gradually shifting to palliative care, 58, 62–63
  grieving process, assisting in, 68–70
  letter of condolence, 67–68
  normal physical changes in final stages of life, 67
Bereavement register, 58
Bethanechol, 177
Bevacizumab (Avastin), 125
BHP, *See* Benign prostatic hyperplasia (BPH),
Bicalutamide, 194
Biceps tendon rupture, 277, 280, 286–287
  follow-up, 287
  imaging, 286
  management of, 286–287
  physical examination, 286–287
  workup/keys to diagnosis, 286–287
Bile acid-binding resins, and lipid disorders, 317–318
Biliary tract disorders, 565–568
  age-related changes in the biliary tract, 565–566
Bilirubin excretion, 8
Binswanger disease, 247
Bioavailable testosterone, 204
Biofeedback therapy, and fecal incontinence, 575
Bipolar depression, 210
Bipolar disorder, 209–210
Bisoprolol, 358
Bisphosphonates, 298–299, 307
Bladder:
  capacity, 176
  distended, 73
  functions of, 177
Bladder cancer, 179
Bladder record (voiding diary), 181
Bladder training (habit training), 181
Blepharochalasis, 131
Blepharoptosis, 131
α-blockers, 177, 182, 189–190
  and hypertension, 313
β-blockers, 73, 75, 78, 93, 341, 342, 354, 386, 402, 449
  and hypertension, 313
  and insomnia, 258
  in treatment of heart failure, 359
Blood glucose, self-monitoring of, 451

Blood pressure, 7, 46
Blood urea nitrogen (BUN), 42, 175, 181, 229
Blood vessel changes, 7
Blood vessels, 7, 163
Blood volume, 8
BMD, *See* Bone mineral density (BMD),
BMI, *See* Body mass index (BMI),
Bodily energy requirements, 109–110
Body cell mass, 109
Body composition, and aging, 4
Bone disease, recognition of, in high-risk populations, 308
Bone growth, 5
Bone infection, and lower back pain, 172–173
Bone loss, 5
Body Mass Index (BMI), 109
Bone mineral density (BMD):
  defining osteoporosis by, 295
  testing, 295–296
Bonney (or Marshall) test, 181
Botulin toxin, and tremor, 390
Bowel resections, 73
Bowen disease, 505
Bowlby theory of attachment, 60
Braden Scale, 513–515
Bradyarrhythmias, 352–353
Bradycardia, 335
Brain dysfunction, 80
Brain natriuretic peptide (BNP), 357
Brain weight, decline in, 5
Branch retinal vein occlusions (BRVOs), 126–127
Brandt-Daroff exercise, 153
Breast cancer recurrence, chemoprevention of, 541
Breast cancer surveillance, 541
Breast disease, 441–443
  breast cancer, 433–434
  breast infections, 442
  breast mass evaluation at the end of life, 443
  inflammatory carcinoma, 443
  lumps, 441–442
  nipple discharge, 442
  Paget disease of the breast, 442
Breathing techniques, 52
Breslow tumor thickness, 507
Bright light therapy, 259–260
British Geriatrics Society, 155
Bronchial hyperreactivity (BHR), 397
Bronchiectasis, 398
Bronchodilators, and insomnia, 258
Bronchogenic carcinoma, 398
Bullous impetigo, 499
Bullous lesions, 498–499
Bullous pemphigoid, 436
Bumetanide, 358
BUN, *See* Blood urea nitrogen (BUN),
Buprenorphine, 87
Bupropion, 218–219
Burning mouth syndrome (stomatopyrosis), 487
Buspirone, 266
Butabarbital, 93
Butorphanol, 93

C

Cachexia, 109, 113, 119
Cadmium, 300
Caffeine, and insomnia, 258–259
CAGE questionnaire, 85, 214
Calcimimetics, 305
  and primary hyperparathyroidism (PHPT), 305
Calciphylaxis, 306
Calcitonin, 298
Calcitriol therapy, 307
Calcium acetate, 307
Calcium, and osteoporosis, 297
Calcium channel blockers, 79
  and hypertension, 313, 314
  in treatment of heart failure, 360
Calluses and corns of the foot, 291
Calmette-Guérin (BCG) vaccine, 409
Cancer, 50, 97
  breast cancer recurrence, chemoprevention of, 541
  breast cancer surveillance, 541
  burden of, in the elderly, 531
  cancer survivorship model, 540–541
  cancer survivorship phenomenon, 539–540
  chemoprevention of, 533–534
  colorectal cancer surveillance, 543–545
  common malignancies in the geriatric population, 531
  and complicated grief, 61
  diet, obesity, and cancer risk, 533
  environmental hazards, 533
  primary prevention of, 532–534
  prostate cancer surveillance, 541–543
  screening for, 530–531, 534–539, *See also* Cancer screening
  secondary prevention of, 534–535
  surveillance care guidelines, 541
Cancer screening, 433–434, 534–539
  breast cancer screening, 537
  cervical cancer screening, 537
  colorectal cancer screening, 537–539
  criteria for, 534
  in geriatric patients, 534–537
  inappropriate, 534
  of lung/ovary/skin, 539
  prostate cancer screening, 539
  screening recommendations, 537
Candida vaginitis, 436
Candidiasis, 500
  oral, 485–486
Capsaicin, 54
Capsaisin, 132
Captopril, 358
  and weight loss, 118
Carbamazepine (Tegretol), 56, 57
  and weight loss, 118
Carbamide peroxide (Debrox), 139
Carbon monoxide diffusion capacity, 7
Carcinoma, 163
Carcinomas of the vulva, 437
Cardiac catheterization, 346
Cardiac contractility, 7
Cardiac disease, 335–353, 402
  arrhythmias, 347–353
  cardiovascular system, normal age-related changes in, 336–337
  coronary heart disease (CHD), 336, 337–338
  valvular heart disease, 344–347
Cardiac dysrhythmias, 336
Cardiac rhythm disturbances, postoperative, 79
Cardioembolic stroke, reducing the risk of thrombosis for, 375–376
Cardiomyopathies, 347
Cardiovascular disease (CVD):
  and diabetes mellitus (type 2), 449
  and oral conditions, 488
  and weight loss, 111
Cardiovascular medications, and delirium, 21
Cardiovascular problems, postoperative management, 79
Cardiovascular system, 10
  and aging, 6–7
  blood pressure, 7
  normal age-related changes in, 336–337
  preoperative assessment and management, 74–76
  and stresses, 7
Care, 18–27
  ambulatory, 19
  chronic disease, common complications of, 20
  constipation, 25
  end of life, 26
  functional decline and rehabilitation, 25–26
  hospital programs, 19
  infections, 22–25
  in the long-term care facility, 19–20
  medication management, 20–22
  organization of, 19–20
  palliative, 26
  patient-centered care model, 19
  pressure ulcers, 25
  transitions in, 20
Caregivers, 28
  abusive, 30
  anger, 36
  Caregiver Self-assessment Questionnaire, 35–36, 38
  classification of, 30
  guidelines/recommendations for working with, 29
  office-based caregiving support, 28–39
  physician:
    caregiver assessment, 36–37
    caregiver education, 38
    caregiver guide to office visits, 37
  physicians' concern about, 29
  reduction of the burden of, 31–32

Caregiving:
effects of, 30–31
research, 31
styles of, 30
Carisoprodol (Soma), 44, 56
Carotidynia, 482–483
Cartilage, 277
Carvedilol, 349, 358
Cataracts, 121–123
cortical, 122–123
extraction, 73, 123
nuclear, 122
posterior subcapsular, 123
Catecholamines, and aging, 462
Catheterized patients, 175
infections in, 186–187
Caudate nucleus, 5
Cefazolin, 77
Celecoxib (Celebrex), 53, 54
Celiac disease, and weight loss, 111
Cellulitis, 497
Central nervous system (CNS), 49
disorders, 112
stimulants, and insomnia, 258
Central retinal vein occlusions (CRVOs), 126–127
role of retinal photocoagulation in, 127
Centrally acting agents, and hypertension, 313, 314
Cerebellar intention tremor, 383
Cerebellar tremor, treatment for, 393
Cerebral hemorrhage, presence of, 367–369
Cerebrovascular disease, 363–376
Cerivastatin, 317
Cervical cancer, 439–440
Cervical dizziness, 149
Cervical spondylosis, 280, 281–282
follow-up, 282
imaging, 282
management of, 282
physical examination, 281
workup/keys to diagnosis, 281–282
Cervical sprain, 279–281
follow-up, 281
imaging, 279
management of, 279–281
Cervical vertebrae, arthritis of, 482
C-fibers, 49
CHD, *See* Coronary heart disease (CHD),
Chest pain, differential diagnosis of, in patients with, 338
Chest radiograph (CXR), 397
Chest wall, age-related changes in, 399
Chest X-ray, and heart failure, 357
Chin stroking, 16
Chiropractic healing, 52
Chlamydia, 198, 436
Chlamydia pneumoniae, 407, 462, 561
Chlordiazepoxide (Librium), 44
Chlordiazepoxide–amitriptyline (Limbitrol), 44
Chlorophyllin, 175
Chlorpheniramine (Chlor-Trimeton), 45
Chlorpropamide (Diabinese), 45, 452–453
Chlorzoxazone (Paraflex), 44
Cholecystectomy, 73
Choledocholithiasis/cholangitis, 563–564, 567–568
diagnostic testing and treatment, 567–568
Cholelithiasis/acute cholecystitis, 566–567
clinical manifestations, 566
complications, 566–567
diagnostic testing, 566–567
treatment of, 567
Cholesteatoma, 139
Cholesterol, 46
Cholestyramine, 300, 341
Choline acetyltransferase, 5
Choline magnesium trisalicylate (Trilisate), 53, 54
Cholinesterase inhibitors, 42
and Alzheimer disease, 245–246
and dementia, 237, 247
Choroidal neovascular membrane (CNVM), 123–125
laser therapy for, 124–125
reducing risk for, 124
Chronic ambulatory peritoneal dialysis (CAPD), 423
Chronic arterial insufficiency, 508
Chronic bronchitis, 397
defined, 402
Chronic CHF, 397
Chronic disease, 113
common complications of, 20
management of, 18, 73
Chronic heart disease, 19
Chronic kidney disease, 421–423
causes of, 421–422
hypertension, control of, 422
nutritional modifications, 422–423
Chronic lymphocytic thyroiditis, 457
Chronic memory impairment, *See* Memory impairment, chronic,
Chronic myelogenous leukemia (CML), 553
Chronic neutropenia, 546
Chronic obstructive pulmonary disease (COPD), 19, 396
diagnosis of, 403
epidemiology, 403
and oral diseases, 488–489
prevalence of, 402
treatment of, 403–404
Chronic pain management, goal of, 48
Chronic pancreatitis, and weight loss, 111
Chronic phase of normal grief, defined, 60
Chronic venous insufficiency, 324
Chronologic age *vs.* biologic age, 1
Chylomicrons, 315
Ciclopirox (Penlac), 502
Cigarette smoking, and erythrocytosis, 547
Cilostazol, and peripheral arterial disease (PAD), 330
Cimetidine, 43
Cinacalcet, 307
Ciprofloxacin, 43
Circadian rhythm sleep disorders, 263
Circadian rhythmicity, 255
Citalopram, 216
Clarithromycin, 77
Clark anatomic level of invasion, 507
Clidinium–chlordiazepoxide (Librax), 44, 45
Clindamycin, 77, 560
Clinical Institute Withdrawal Assessment (CIWA), 87–88
Clinical interview (taking the history), 1
Clinically significant macular edema (CSME), 126
Clofibrate, and lipid disorders, 318
Clofibrozil, 341
Clomipramine, 57
Clonazepam (Klonopin), 56
and rapid eye movement sleep behavior disorder, 264
Clonidine, 87, 441
Clopidogrel, 342, 373
Clostridium difficile diarrhea, 24–25
Clozapine (Clozaril), 271
CNS, *See* Central nervous system (CNS),
Cochlea, 135
Cochlear echoes, 141
Cochlear implants, 142
Cockcroft-Gault method, 77
Codeine, 55
Codfish vertebrae, 302
Cognitive ability, 5
Cognitive behavioral therapies, 52
Cognitive heart failure, hypertension, age, diabetes, and stroke ($CHADS_2$), 375
Colitis, and complicated grief, 61
Collagen, 5, 277
Collagen vascular disease, 172
Colon cancer, 543–544
Colonic disorders, and weight loss, 111
Colonization and infection, pressure ulcers, 524–525
Colorectal cancer:
anal cancer, 545
colon cancer, 543–544
rectal cancer, 544
surveillance, 543–545
Comfort, Alex, 197
Communication techniques, 68–69
Comorbid depression, 93
Complementary therapies, 52
Complicated grief, 61–62
cognitive-behavior therapy for, 70
defined, 58, 60
diagnosis of, 63
diagnostic criteria for, 62
symptoms of, 58, 62
treating, 70–71

Complications, 73
  bleeding, 79
  cardiac, in noncardiac surgery, 74–75
  of chronic disease, 20
  pulmonary, 76–77
Compression, 141
Compression fractures, 162, 163, 170–171
  follow-up, 171
  imaging, 171
  management of, 171
  physical examination, 171
Compression technique, 141
Computed tomography (CT) scan, 162, 172–173, 181, 229, 236, 244, 282, 419
  and hemorrhage, 366–368
Conditioning, and degeneration of muscles/bones, 5
Conduction abnormalities, 335
Conductive hearing loss, 136, 142
Congestive heart failure (CHF), 396
Conjunctivitis, 131
Connective tissue, and aging, 4–5
Constipation, 25, 48, 371, 564, 571–574
  defined, 572
  diagnosis of, 572–573
  management of, 573–574
  pathophysiology, 572
  Rome II criteria for, 572
  self-reported, prevalence of, 572
  and weight loss, 111–112, 119
Contact dermatitis (eczematoid/irritant dermatitis), 435
Context, and interpretation of behavior, 15
Continuous dizziness, 151
Continuous positive airway pressure (CPAP), 262, 411
Contradictions, and interpretation of behavior, 15
COPD, *See* Chronic obstructive pulmonary disease (COPD),
Coping styles, caregivers, 30
Corneal changes, 6
Corns and calluses, 280, 291, 509
Coronary arteries, 6
Coronary artery bypass surgery (CABG), 342
Coronary artery disease (CAD), peripheral arterial disease (PAD) compared to, 323
Coronary heart disease (CHD), 336–338, 339
  ACE-I therapy, 340–341
  acute coronary syndromes (ACSs), 342–343
  alternative treatments, 342
  differential diagnosis of, 337–338
  lifestyle recommendations, 340
  management of, 340
  medications, 340–341
  mnemonic for, 335
  percutaneous/surgical interventions, 342
  primary prevention of, clinical trials for, 314
  signs/symptoms of 337
  stable angina, 338–339
  unstable angina, risk of death or nonfatal myocardial infarction in patients with, 343
Corporate sponsorship of new diseases, 197
Cortical β-adrenergic receptors, 5
Cortical cataracts, 122–123
Corticosteroid (Prednisone), 53
Corticosteroids, 78, 132
  eye medications, 466
  and insomnia, 258
  and rheumatoid arthritis, 465
  and scleroderma, 468
Cortisol, and delirium, 226
Cough:
  common causes of, 395
  as symptom, 397
Council for Nutrition's Clinical Strategies in Long-Term Care, 113
COX-2 inhibitors, 45, 54
Credé maneuver, 182
CREST syndrome, 468
Creutzfeldt-Jakob disease (CJD), and dementia, 250
Crossed arms, 16
Crotamiton 10% cream, 437
Cryosurgery, 506
Cryptosporidium, 555, 561
Cutaneous infections, 559–560
Cutaneous-evoked tinnitus, 143
CVD, *See* Cardiovascular disease (CVD),
Cyclobenzaprine (Flexeril), 44
Cyclooxygenase-2 (COX-2) NSAIDs, 45
Cyclophosphamide, 551
Cyproheptadine (Periactin), 45, 118, 119
Cystitis, 179
Cystourethrocele, 438
Cytochrome P-451 enzymes, 217
Cytokines, 462–463
  proinflammatory, 464

D

Dakin solution, 560
Darifenacin (Enablex), 182
Debridement, pressure ulcers, 524
Deconditioning, and dizziness, 150
Decongestants, and insomnia, 258
Decubitus ulcer, *See* Pressure ulcers,
Deep breathing exercises, 79
Deep pressure ulcers, 25
Deep somatic pain, 49
Deep vein thrombosis, 326, 553
Degenerative disc disease, 166–167
  follow-up, 167
  imaging, 167
  management of, 167
  physical examination, 167
Delirium, 18, 46, 225–235
  adverse consequences, 225–226
  antipsychotic mediation, 225
  behavior assessment and intervention, 21
  clinical features of, 227–229
  confusion assessment method (CAM) features of, 228
  defined, 225, 227
  Delirium Prevention Trial, 232
  differential diagnosis of, 228–230
  epidemiology of, 226
  evaluation of the patient with, 229
  incidence and prevalence, 226
  interventions, 225
  and intraoperative blood loss, 80
  and medications, 225
  medications associated with, 22
  nonpharmacologic approaches to management, 233–234
  pathophysiology of, 226–227
  pharmacologic approaches to management, 234
  postoperative, 80
  predisposing risk factors, 225
  prevention of, 231–232
  risk factors, 20, 229–231
    pneumonic, 230
    postoperative delirium, 231
    predisposing and precipitating, 230–231
  signs/symptoms of 227–228
  treatment of, 225, 232–234
Delta (slow-wave) sleep, 255
Dementia, 112, 229, 266, 267
  Alzheimer disease, 238–249
  and β-amyloid plaques, 236, 243
  behavioral problems in, 250–251
  caregiver burden screen, 251
  caregivers, 251
  causes of, 249
  changes in sleep with, 264
  and cholinesterase inhibitors, 237
  and Creutzfeldt-Jakob disease (CJD), 250
  defined, 237
  and depression, 241–242
  differential diagnosis of, 237, 241–242
  and hyperthyroidism, 250
  non-Alzheimer disease dementia, 246–249
    dementia associated with Parkinson disease, 247–248
    frontotemporal dementia, 237, 242
    Lewy body dementia, 237, 242, 247
    mixed dementia, 249
    vascular dementia, 237, 242, 246–247
    white matter dementia, 248–249
  and oral diseases, 489
  prevalence of, 236, 237
  screening for, 238
  and serotonin reuptake inhibitors (SSRIs), 249, 250
  signs/symptoms of 239–241

syphilis, 249
and toluene inhalation, 249
treating behavioral problems, 250
and urinary incontinence, 175, 176, 178–180, 182
and urinary tract infections (UTIs), 183–184, 186–187
white matter, 242
Demodex folliculorum, 509
Denial, 61
Dental decay (caries), 474, 477–479
management of, 479
prevention of, 478
Dental hygiene, 7
Deoxyribonucleic acid (DNA), 549
Depression, 10
acute phase management, 215
monitoring in, 219
antidepressants, 46, 56, 93, 119, 132, 177, 214–216
assessment for, 210
atypical, 208
atypical antidepressants, 218–219
bipolar disorder, 209–210
causes of, 221–223
bereavement, 222
chronic illness, 221–222
declining health and function, 221
gender differences, 222
informal caregiving, 222
retirement, 221
comorbid, 93
continuation phase management, 219–220
cultural considerations, 211
defined, 208–210
and diabetes, 445
diagnosing, 63, 210–214
differential diagnosis of, 61, 213–214
dual agents, 215, 217, 218
duration of treatment, 215
dysthymia, 209
and elder abuse, 98
evaluation and treatment of, 207–223
Geriatric Depression Scale (GDS), 212
heterocyclic antidepressants, 217–218
major, 208–209
management of symptoms, 219
with mania, 208
minor, 208
and pain, 49
poststroke, assessing and managing, 372
referral to a mental health counselor or therapist, 220
screening tools, 211–212
seasonal affective disorder (SAD), 208, 209, 215
serotonin reuptake inhibitors (SSRIs), 215–217, 218
dosing, 217
and drug-drug interactions and half-lives, 216–217
side effects, 217
as side effect of medication, 207
signs/symptoms of 210–211
and sleep disturbance, 219
social support and environment, 214
substance-induced, 213–214
and suicide, 214
symptoms of, 62
treatment of, 70–71, 214–220
maintenance phase of, 220
and urinary incontinence, 178
and weight loss, 111–112, 119
Dermabrasion, 504
Dermatitis medicamentosa, 509
Dermatologic conditions, 491–509
acrochordons, 495
allergic contact dermatitis, 491, 496
bacterial/parasitic/fungal infections, 499–503
benign lesions, 494–495
bullous lesions, 498–499
cellulitis, 497
cherry hemangiomas, 495
corns and calluses, 509
dermatitis, 496–498
dermatitis medicamentosa, 509
differential diagnosis of, 493
fungal infections, 492
herpes zoster (shingles), 491, 499–500, 558
intrinsic versus extrinsic changes of aging, 491–492
itraconazole, 491
keratoacanthoma, 496
lichen simplex, 497–498
melanoma, 491
milia, 494
miscellaneous skin conditions, 509
neurodermatitis, 497–498
photoaging, 492–494
premalignant and malignant lesions, 503–508
rosacea, 509
scabies, 492
sebaceous hyperplasia, 494–495
seborrheic dermatitis, 496
of the scalp (dandruff), 491
seborrheic keratoses, 491, 495
secondary skin changes, 491
senile purpura (ecchymosis), 495
solar lentigines, 494
squamous and basal cell carcinoma, 491
stasis dermatitis, 497
terbinafine, 491
ulceration, 492
vascular disease, skin manifestations of, 508–509
venous lakes (benign venous angiomas), 495–496
xerosis, 492, 496
Dermatosis papulosa nigra, 495
Desipramine, 57
Detrusor hyperactivity, 175, 179–182
Detrusor muscle, 177
Detrusor underactivity, 179
Diabetes, 51, 340, 445–461, 471
and depression, 445
and hearing difficulty, 138
and oral conditions, 488
and urinary incontinence, 455
and weight loss, 111
Diabetes mellitus, 172, 402, 445
and peripheral arterial disease (PAD), 329
type 2, 446–456
alternative or integrative medicine, 454–455
aspirin therapy, 454
and cardiovascular disease (CVD), 449
comorbidity concerns, 455
course/timeline, 447
description/definition of problem, 446
diabetes education, 451
dyslipidemia, 456
foot care/neuropathy, 450–451
genetics, 447
hypertension, 455–456
and influenza and pneumococcal immunization, 451
insulin therapy, 453–454
lifestyle recommendations, 451–452
management of, 448–449
medications, 452–454
oral medications, 452–453
pathophysiology, 446–447
and peripheral arterial disease (PAD), 449–450
and retinopathy, 450
risk factors for, 447–448
signs/symptoms of 447
systems impacted by, 447
workup/keys to diagnosis, 448
Diabetes (type 1 and 2), 471
Diabetic macular edema, 126
Diabetic neuropathy, 326
Diabetic retinopathy, 125–126
Diagnosis, 11–12
final prescribing criteria considering, 44
Diagnostic and Statistical Manual of Mental Disorders, Fourth Edition (DSM-IV), 199, 203, 210–211, 213
features of delirium, 227
and GAD, 272
and schizophrenia, 269
Dialysis, 80, 423
Diarrhea, and weight loss, 111
Diastolic heart failure, 47
Diazepam (Valium), 44
and dizziness, 153
Diclofenac potassium, 53
Diclofenac sodium, 53, 504
Dicyclomine (Bentyl), 45, 182
Diet, and cancer risk, 533
Dietary fiber, 564
and constipation, 573
Diethylstilbestrol, 193

Diflunisal, 53
Digestive enzymes, 338–339
Digitalis, 61
Digoxin, 43, 349, 358
  in treatment of heart failure, 359
Digoxin (Lanoxin), 44
  and weight loss, 118
Dihydrotestosterone (DHT), 188
Dilantin, 43
Dilated cardiomyopathy, 339
Diltiazem, 341, 349
Diphenhydramine, 527
Diphenhydramine (Benadryl), 45
  and insomnia, 261
Diphtheria, 554
Dipyridamole (Persantine), 44, 45
Disease, understanding the difference between illness and, 11
Disk compression, 4
Disopyramide (Norpace, Norpace CR), 44
Disruptive problem behaviors, 31
Diuretics:
  and hypertension, 313
  and insomnia, 258
  in treatment of heart failure, 357–358
Diverticuli, 8
Dix-Hallpike maneuver, 148, 152
Dizziness, 147–148
  benign positional vertigo (BPV), 148
    treatment of, 152–153
  Brandt-Daroff exercise, 153
  cervical, 149
  conditions leading to, 149
  continuous, 151
  defined, 148
  differential diagnosis of, 148–150
  in the elderly, 148–153
  episodic, 151
  hyperventilation syndrome, 150
  impact on function, 152
  incidence and prevalence, 151
  management of, 152–153
  medications for, 153
  multiple sensory impairments, 150
  normal gait and balance, 148
  pathophysiology, 150–151
  physical deconditioning, 150
  postural, 149
  prognosis for, 152
  psychologic factors, 150
  signs/symptoms of 151
  and stroke, 150
  subtypes of, 151
  vestibular rehabilitation, 152
  workup/keys to the diagnosis, 152
Dofetilide, 349
Domestic violence, 100
Donepezil, and Alzheimer disease, 246
Dopamine, 458
  and delirium, 226
Dosing, 47
Dosing errors, and prescribing errors, 22
Douglas, Kirk, 31
Doxepin (Sinequan), 44, 56, 57
Dronabinol, and weight loss, 118, 119
Drug toxicity, 46
Drug-induced osteomalacia, 299–300
Drug-induced thrombocytopenia, 546, 550
Drug-resistant *Streptococcus pneumoniae* (DRSP), 407–408
Dual agents, 215, 217, 218
Duloxetine (Cymbalta), 56, 57
Dupuytren contracture/disease, 277, 280, 287–288
  follow-up, 288
  imaging, 288
  management of, 288
  physical examination, 288
Dutasteride (Avodart), 190
DXA scan, bone density measurement by, 306
Dying patients:
  bereavement care:
    counseling, 66
    providing support to the family of, 66–67
Dynamic Gait Index (DGI), 157
Dysequilibrium, 149, 151
Dysgeusia, and weight loss, 111
Dyslipidemia, 341
  and peripheral arterial disease (PAD), 329
Dysmotility syndromes, and weight loss, 111
Dyspareunia, 203
Dysphagia, and weight loss, 111
Dysplastic nevi, 507
Dyspnea, 395, 403
  common causes of, 396
  defined, 396
Dysthymia, 208, 209
Dystonic tremor, treatment for, 393

E

Eagle syndrome, 483
Early-onset drinkers, 83
Ebola virus, 555
Echocardiography, 345, 346
ED, *See* Erectile dysfunction (ED),
Edentulousness, 111–112
Eggs, anaphylactic hypersensitivity to, and influenza vaccination, 559
Elder abuse/elder mistreatment, 95–107
  Academic Geriatric Experts Recommendation, 102
  caregiver issues, 99
  case studies, 98, 100
  clinical assessment, 102–105
    capacity *vs.* competence, 105
    history, 102
    laboratory, 105
    mental capacity, assessing, 104–105
    physical examination, 102–104
    setting, 102
  cultural issues, 99
  defined, 95
  and dependency, 99
  documentation, 106
  domestic violence, 100
  family situations, 99
  financial exploitation, 96, 101
  as a geriatric syndrome, 97–98
  incidence/prevalence, 96–97
  interventions, 105
  management of, 105–106
    principles, 105
    recommendation, 106
    reporting, 106
  mortality rates, 97
  National Clinical Guidelines Recommendation Statement, 101–102
  neglect, 96, 100–101
    abandonment, 96, 100
    self-neglect, 101
  physical abuse, 96, 99–100
  practical clinician tool, 102
  psychological abuse, 96, 100
  public health issues, 96
  red flags, 99
  risk factors for, 98–99
  screening for, 101–102
  sexual abuse, 100
  social isolation, 98
  and stress, 99
  terminology, 96–99
  types of, 99–100
  vulnerability, 98
  when to suspect, 98
Elderly people:
  general principles to improve care of, 2–4
  generalist physicians caring for, responsibilities of, 74
Electrocardiogram, 356–357, 397
Electroencephalography (EEG), 411
Electromyography (EMG), 411
Electronystagmography (ENG), 144
Electrooculography (EOG), 411
Elevated intraocular pressure (IOP), 121, 129
Elimite, 437
Emmetropia (neutral refraction), 122
Emotional distancing, 32
Emphysema, 397
Enalapril, 358
End of life care, 26
Endocarditis, 76
EndoCinch (Bard Endoscopic Technologies), 577
Endocrine disease, prevalence of, 445–446
Endocrine disorders, 446
Endolymphatic hydrops (Ménière disease), 145
Endolymphatic potential, 136
Endometrial cancer, 439
Endometrial hyperplasia, 441
Endorphins, and delirium, 226
End-stage organ dysfunction, 50
End-stage renal disease (ESRD), 305–308, 421, 423

Enemas, 574
Enterocele, 438
Enterococcus, 175, 183, 184, 187
Enteromonas hydrophilia, 559
Enteryx (Enteric Medical Technology), 577
Environmental conditions, and clinician-patient communication, 3
Episodic dizziness, 151
Erectile dysfunction (ED), 196, 197, 201–202
  assessment, 202
  treatment of, 202
Erythrocytosis, 547, 552
Erythromycin, 43
Erythroplasia of Queyrat, 505
Erythropoietin, 547
Escapist–wishful thinking coping strategies, 32
Escherichia coli, and urinary tract infections (UTIs), 183
Escitalopram, 216
Esmolol, 349
Esophageal dysphagia, 568–571
  achalasia, 570
  age-related physiologic changes of the esophagus, 568
  dysphagia, 568–570
  dysphagia aortica, 571
  esophageal cancer, 571
  mechanical causes, 570–571
  medication-induced esophageal injury, 570–571
    causes of, 571
  motility disorders, 570
  peptic stricture, 571
  spastic disorders of the esophagus, 570
Esophageal motility, 7
Esophagus, 7–8
  age-related physiologic changes of, 568
Essential (ET) tremor, 382–383
Essential hypertension, 310
Estazolam, and insomnia, 261
Estrogen, 178, 194
  and sexual function, 201
Estrogen level, 4
Eszopiclone, 69–70
  and insomnia, 261
Etanercept, 465
Ethacrynic acid, 358
Ethambutol, 410
Etidronate, 301
Etodolac, 53
Eurax, 437
Evaluation of pain, 50–51
Eversion/inversion of the lid margins, 131
Exercise, 52
  for herniated nucleus pulposus (disc), 167–169
  Kegel pubococcygeus muscle, for detrusor hyperactivity, 181–182
  for low back sprain/strain, 166
  and recovery, 92
  for spinal stenosis, 170
Exercise-induced leg pain:
  differential diagnosis of the patient with, 323–324
    chronic venous insufficiency, 324
    nerve root compression, 323
    osteoarthritis, 323
    popliteal artery adventitial cystic disease, 324
    popliteal artery entrapment syndrome, 324
    venous claudication, 324
Extended-release morphine (Kadian), 55
Eye contact, 15
Ezetimibe, 341
  and lipid disorders, 317–318

F

FABER maneuver, 164
Facet joints, 163
Facial expression, 15
Facial grimacing, 51
Factor V Leiden, 553
"Fading Memory" (Coe), 28
Failure to thrive, 109
Fallopian tube cancer, 440
Falls, 147, 154–160
  activity and environmental causes of, 155
  assistive devices, 159–160
  conditions leading to, 149
  etiology and risk factors, 154–155
  fall evaluation, 156
  fall-prevention education, 159
  gait and balance assessment tools, 156–158
  hip protectors, 160
  impact on function, 154
  impaired vision, improving, 160
  incidence and prevalence, 154
  interventions, 158–159
    exercise, 158–159
    home modifications, 159
  management of, 158–160
  medications for, 155, 159–160
  multifactorial approach to preventing, 158
  multifactorial fall-intervention trials, 158
  and pain, 49
  pathophysiology, 154
  safer footwear, wearing, 160
  vitamin D supplementation, 160
  workup/keys to the diagnosis, 155–156
Famciclovir, 554
Family Caregiver Alliance of the National Center for Caregiving, 30
Family-focused grief therapy, 70
Fascia, 163
Fatigue, and pain, 49
Fecal incontinence, 574–575
  and biofeedback therapy, 575
  diagnosis of, 574
  etiology of, 574
  evaluation, 574
  surgical treatment for, 575
  treatment of, 574–575
Fecal occult blood testing, 114
Feet, joint changes/flattening of the arches, 4
Fenofibrate, and lipid disorders, 318
Fenoprofen, 53
Fentanyl patch, 55
Fever, and infection, 172
Fibric acid, and lipid disorders, 317–318
Financial exploitation, 96, 101
Finasteride (Proscar), 190
Finger gestures, 16
Flavoxate (Urispas), 182
Floating, symptoms of, 151
Fluid and nutrition management, postoperative, 80
FluMist, 559
Fluoride, 301
Fluoroquinolones, 47
Fluoxetine (Prozac), 47, 216, 441
  and insomnia, 258
Flurazepam (Dalmane), 43, 44
  and insomnia, 261
Flurbiprofen, 53
Fluvastatin, 317
Fluvoxamine, 441
Folate, and reduction of homocysteine levels, 342
Folate deficiency, 549
Folate supplementation, 57
Foot care/neuropathy, and diabetes mellitus (type 2), 450–451
Fosinopril, 358
Frailty and Injuries: Cooperative Studies of Intervention Techniques (FICSIT) trials, 159
Free radical scavengers, and Alzheimer disease, 247
Frontotemporal dementia, 237, 242, 248
Frozen shoulder, *See* Adhesive capsulitis of the shoulder,
Fullerton Advanced Balance Scale (FAB), 158
Function, importance of, 11–12
Functional capacity, activities helping to stratify patients according to, 75
Functional decline, 18, 25–26
Functional impairment, prevention of, 18
Functional Pain Scale rating, 51
Fungal infections, 499–503
Furosemide, 358

G

GABA (γ-aminobutyric acid), 226
Gabapentin (Neurontin), 56–57, 435, 441
  and tremor, 389–390

GAD, *See* Generalized anxiety disorder (GAD),
Gadolinium, 142
Gait, 148
Gait and balance assessment tools, 156–158
  Dynamic Gait Index (DGI), 157
  Fullerton Advanced Balance Scale (FAB), 158
  Modified Clinical Test of Sensory Interaction and Balance (mCTSIB), 157–158
  Performance-Oriented Mobility Assessment (POMA), 157
  test selection, 156
  "Timed Up and Go test" (TUG), 155–157
  "walkie-talkie" test, 158
Gallbladder disease, 10, 566–568
  choledocholithiasis and cholangitis, 566–567
  cholelithiasis and acute cholecystitis, 566–567
  gallbladder carcinoma, 567
Garlic, and blood pressure/cholesterol levels, 342
Gastric cytoprotection, and stroke, 374
Gastric motility, 8
Gastroesophageal reflux, 111
Gastroesophageal reflux disease (GERD), 397, 564, 570–571, 575–577
  diagnosis of, 576
  evaluation, 576
  and histamine-2 receptor antagonists (H_2-blockers), 576
  medical therapies, 577
  and obesity, 576
  pathophysiology, 575–576
  prevalence of GERD symptoms in the elderly, 575
  therapies for, 576
  treatment of, 576–577
Gastrointestinal disorders, 563–578
  anorectal biofeedback therapy, 564
  cholangitis, 563
  choledocholithiasis, 563
  constipation, 564, 571–574
  and dietary fiber, 564
  differential diagnosis of, 569
  disorders of the gallbladder and biliary tract, 565–568
  esophageal dysphagia, 568–571
  fecal incontinence, 574–575
  gastroesophageal reflux disease (GERD), 397, 564, 570–571, 575–577
  nonacute dysphagia, 563
  peptic ulcer disease (PUD), 563, 564–565
Gastrointestinal system:
  and aging, 7–8
  esophagus and stomach, 7–8
  liver and pancreas, 8
  small and large intestine, 8
Gaze-evoked tinnitus, 143
Gemfibrozil, 341
  and lipid disorders, 316–317
Gene typing, 236
General paralysis of the insane, use of term, 268–269
Generalized anxiety disorder (GAD), 272, 274
  diagnostic criteria for, 272
Gentamicin, 77
GERD, *See* Gastroesophageal reflux disease (GERD),
Geriatric assessment, performing, 12–16
  appearance, 12–13
  dress (diagnostic clues from clothing), 13–14
  language, 14–15
Geriatric clinicians:
  healing atmosphere, creating, 3
  psychology of, 2–3
  showing reverence for patients, 3
Geriatric Depression Scale, 108, 114
Geriatric wasting, *See* Wasting,
Gestures, 16
GI effects, 57
Ginkgo biloba:
  and Alzheimer disease, 247
  and treatment of tinnitus, 144
Glaucoma, 6, 121, 129–310
  alternative surgeries for, 130
  normal tension (NTG), 130
  primary open-angle (POAG), 129
  side effects of eye drops for, 129
Gleason grade, 176, 192–193
Glenohumeral arthritis, 282
Glipizide, 452
Glomerular filtration rate (GFR), 450
Glomerulonephritis, 465
Glucocorticoids, 458
  and aging, 462
α-Glucosidase inhibitors, 453
Glutamate, and delirium, 226
Glutamic acid decarboxylase, 5
Glyburide, 452
Glycemic control, 448
Gonorrhea, 198
Gout, 471–472
Gram-negative rods, 559
Graves disease, 459, 461
Graves speculum, 432–433
Graying of hair, 5
Grief reactions, 60–61, 68
  misdiagnosis of, 60
Grieving process, assisting in, 68–70
Griseofulvin, 502
Growth hormone, as orexigenic agent, 118–119
Guillain-Barré syndrome, 451
  and influenza vaccination, 559
Guilt, 61
Gynecology, 432–444
  breast disease, 441–443
  cancer screening, 433–434
  examination in the elderly patient, 432–433
  hormone replacement therapy, 440–441
  mammograms, 433–434
  Pap (Papanicolaou) smears, 433, 436
  upper genital tract, disorders of, 438–440
  vulva/vagina disorders, 434–438

H

Haloperidol, 229
HALT, 92
Handheld tympanometry/audiometry test, 139–140
Hanta virus, 555
Hashimoto thyroiditis, 457, 471
HDL cholesterol, 315, 456
Headache, 50, 57
Healed perforation, tympanic membrane, 139
Health care proxy, 18
Health care services, 73
Health Insurance Portability And Accountability Act (HIPAA), 106
Hearing aids, 142
Hearing Handicap Inventory for the Elderly (HHIE), 138
Hearing loss, 6, 134–146
  assistive listening devices, 142–143
  aural rehabilitation, 143
  aural/hearing rehabilitation programs, 134
  case studies, 136
  cochlear implants, 142
  conditions causing, 136
  conductive, 142
  differential diagnosis of, 136
  dizziness and balance, 144–145
    diagnostic testing, 144–145
    history, 144
    management of, 145
  functional hearing deficits, 134
  hearing aids, 134, 142
  hearing and aging, 135–136
  high-resolution computed tomography, 134
  interpreting audiogram results for, 141
  magnetic resonance imaging (MRI), 134
  management of, 142–143
  Ménière disease, 145
  physical examination for, 139–142
    handheld tympanometry/audiometry test, 139–140
    nuclear magnetic resonance imaging (MRI), 142
    pure-tone audiogram, 140–141
    special tests for populations with testing challenges, 141
    speech recognition, 141
    ticking watch, 139
    tuning fork tests, 139
    tympanometry, 140
    whispered voice, 139

presbycusis, 136–143
rehabilitation, 142
screening for, 138–139
self-help groups for, 143
sensorineural, 142
tinnitus, 143–144
Heart failure, 79, 340, 354–361
comorbidity, 361
defined, 354
etiology of, 355
hospice, 361
medications, 354, 358
nonpharmaceutical therapies, 361
pathophysiology of, 355
signs/symptoms of 356–357
brain natriuretic peptide (BNP), 357
chest X-ray, 356
echocardiogram, 356–357
electrocardiogram, 356
renal insufficiency, 357, 420
symptoms of, 354
systolic and diastolic dysfunction, 355–356
treatment of, 357–361
angiotensin receptor blocking agents, 359
angiotensin-converting enzyme inhibitors, 358–359
antiarrhythmics, 360–361
β-blockers, 359
calcium channel blockers, 360
digoxin, 359
diuretics, 357–358
hydralazine and oral nitrates, 360
spironolactone, 359–360
Heart muscle, 6
Heart Outcomes Prevention Evaluation (HOPE) trial, 340–341
Heart valves, 6
Height, changes in, 4
Helical CT scan, 534
Helicobacter pylori infection, 462, 564–565
Hematology, 546–552
anemia, 546, 547–549
anemia of chronic disease, 546
blood dyscrasias, differential diagnosis of, 548
myeloproliferative diseases, 552–553
neutropenia, 549–550
partial thromboplastin time (PTT), 550
plasma cell disorders, 551–552
screening for bleeding prior to surgery, 550
thrombocytopenia, 549–550
venous thrombosis, 553
Hematopoiesis, 8
Hematopoietic tissues, 8–9
Hematuria, 183, 414, 416–418
Hemiretinal vein occlusion (HRVO), 126–127
Hemophilus influenzae, 406–407
Hemoptysis, 398
causes of, 398
Heparin, 342
Heparin-induced thrombocytopenia, 546, 550
Heparinoids, 373
Hepatic metabolism, 41–42
Hepatic toxicity, 335
Hepatitis:
B, 198
isoniazid-induced, 396
Hepatitis A virus (HAV), 558
Hepatitis B virus (HBV), 558
Hepatitis C virus (HCV), 558
Herniated nucleus pulposus (disc), 167–169
follow-up, 169
imaging, 168–169
management of, 168–169
physical examination, 168
Herpes, 198
Herpes simplex type, 6, 555, 556, 558
Herpes zoster ophthalmicus (shingles), 131–134
Herpes zoster (shingles), 499–500, 558
differential diagnosis of, 500
treatment of, 500
Heterocyclic antidepressants, 217–218
Heterocyclics, 215
Hidden patients, use of term, 31
High blood pressure, 46
and complicated grief, 61
as grief reaction, 60
hypertension, 74
High-Frequency Pure-Tone Average (PTA) Scale, 138
Hip fracture, 10
Hip protectors, 160
Histamine blockers, 119
Histamine-2 receptor antagonists (H_2-blockers), and gastroesophageal reflux disease (GERD), 576
HIV, *See* Human immunodeficiency virus (HIV) infection,
HIV testing, 114
HIV/AIDS, *See* Human immunodeficiency virus/acquired immunodeficiency syndrome (HIV/AIDS),
Hodgkin disease, 550
Hollenhorst plaques, 128
Homeopathic healing, 52
Homeostenosis, 396
Hopelessness, 61
Hormonal changes, 4
Hormone replacement therapy (HT), 304–305, 440–441
and primary hyperparathyroidism (PHPT), 304–305
risks and benefits, 440–441
vasomotor symptoms, alternative treatments for, 441
Hormone treatment, and prostate cancer, 193
Hospice, 361
Hospice, and heart-failure patients, 361
Hospital Elder Life Program (HELP), 232
HT, *See* Hormone replacement therapy (HT),
Human immunodeficiency virus (HIV) infection, 50, 172, 558–559
Human immunodeficiency virus/acquired immunodeficiency syndrome (HIV/AIDS), 196, 198, 554
Huperzine A:
and Alzheimer disease, 247
and dementia, 247
Hutchinson sign, 132
Hydralazine, 358
in treatment of heart failure, 360
Hydrochlorothiazide, 358
Hydrocodone, 55
Hydromorphone, 55
3-Hydroxy-3-methylglutaryl coenzyme A reductase inhibitors (statins), 317, 341
Hydroxyzine (Vistaril, Atarax), 22, 45, 436, 497, 528
Hyoscyamine (Levsin, Levsinex), 45
Hypercalcemia, 307, 424, 551
Hypercalciuria, 551
Hypergammaglobulinemia, 339
Hyperglycemia, 78, 424, 448
and stroke outcomes, 369
Hyperkalemia, 415, 428–429
Hyperlipidemia, 340
management of, 316–318
drug therapy, 316–317
specific lipid-lowering agents, 317–318
Hypernatremia, 426–427
Hyperopia (farsightedness), 122
Hyperparathyroidism, 293, 422–423
Hyperphosphatemia, 422–423
Hypertension, 309–314, 340, 421, 446, 455–456
antihypertensive medications, 313
complications, 311
defined, 310
differential diagnosis of, 311
essential, 310
isolated systolic, 310–311
treatment of, 314
management of, 312–314
combinations, 314
drug treatment, 312–314
lifestyle modification, 312
and peripheral arterial disease (PAD), 329
preoperative assessment and management, 74
risk factors for developing, 310
secondary, physical findings in, 311
workup/keys to the diagnosis, 311
Hyperthyroidism, 78, 459–461
and dementia, 250

Hyperthyroidism (*continued*)
description/definition of problem, 459
imaging, 460
impact on function, 459
laboratory/diagnostic procedures, 460
management of, 460–461
medications, 460–461
pathophysiology, 459
physical examination, 460
risk factors of, 460
signs/symptoms of 459
subclinical, 460
surgical interventions, 461
systems impacted by, 459
and weight loss, 111
workup/keys to diagnosis, 460
Hypertrophic cardiomyopathy, 339
Hyperventilation syndrome, 150
Hyperviscosity syndromes, 339
Hypoactive sexual desire disorder, 200–202
Hypocalcemia, 422–423
Hypoglycemia, 45
and stroke outcomes, 369
Hypokalemia, 415, 421, 424, 428
causes of, 429
manifestations of, 429
Hyponatremia, 424–426
with contracted extracellular fluid volume (primary salt depletion), 424–425
in the elderly, 426
with expanded extracellular fluid volume (dilutional hyponatremia), 425–426
with normal extracellular fluid volume (syndrome of inappropriate antidiuretic hormone), 426
Hypotension, 81, 335
Hypothyroidism, 457–459
alternative or integrative medicine, 459
and dementia, 250
description/definition of problem, 457
etiology and course/timeline, 457–458
general measures, medications, and patient monitoring, 458
and hearing difficulty, 138
imaging and diagnostic procedures, 458
impact on function, 457
laboratory, 458
lifestyle recommendations, 459
management of, 458–459
pathophysiology and genetics, 457
physical examination, 458
prevalence/gender, 457
risk factors of, 458
signs/symptoms of 457
systems impacted by, 457
and weight loss, 111
workup/keys to diagnosis, 458
Hypoxemia, 81, 339

I

Ibuprofen, 53–54, 55
Ibutilide, 349
ICD-9 coding, 213
ICSD Diagnostic and Coding Manual, 256–257
Ifosfamide, 300
Illness, understanding the difference between disease and, 11
Imipramine (Tofranil), 56, 57, 182
Immune and inflammatory disease, 462–472
aging of the immune system, 464
autoimmune diseases, 462
classification of, 462
cytokines, 462–463
Interleukin (IL)-1s, 463
nonrheumatoid diseases with immune etiology, 468–472
amyloidosis, 469–470
diabetes (type 1 and 2), 471
gout, 471–472
Hashimoto thyroiditis, 457, 471
multiple sclerosis, 470–471
polymyalgia rheumatica and giant cell arteritis, 468–469
soft-tissue rheumatism, 471
vasculitis, 468–469
pro- and anti-inflammatory cytokines, examples of, 463
rheumatoid arthritis, 462, 464–468
tumor necrosis factor (TNF-α), 463
Immune thrombocytic purpura (ITP), 551
Impatience, in clinician-patient communication, 4
Impending death, signs of, 26
Impingement syndrome, 280, 284–285
follow-up, 285
imaging, 285
management of, 285
physical examination, 284–285
workup/keys to diagnosis, 284–285
Incontinence, *See* Urinary incontinence,
Independent living, 1, 12
Individualized medical care, 1
Indomethacin (Indocin), 44
Infection, 22–25, 554–561
in catheterized patients, 186–187
clinical features of, 555–556
Clostridium difficile diarrhea, 24–25
community-acquired resistant pathogens, 561
cutaneous, 559–560
differential diagnosis of, 556
epidemiology, 555
human immunodeficiency virus (HIV), 558–559
immune system, aging in, 554–555
immunizations, 560–561
influenza, 558–559
laboratory/diagnosis, 556
and lower back pain, 172–173
follow-up, 173
imaging, 173
management of, 173
physical examination, 172–173
pneumonia, 24
sepsis, 557
severe acute respiratory syndrome, 558
urinary tract, 20, 22–24, 556–557
viral hepatitis, 558
viral infections, 557–558
West Nile Fever (WNF), 558
Inferior vena cava, 163
Inflammatory bowel disease, and weight loss, 111
Inflammatory carcinoma, 443
Infliximab, 465
Influenza, 406–408, 558–559
and diabetes mellitus (type 2), 451
treatment of, 560
virus classifications, 559
Informal caregivers, 30
Inner conflict, signs of, 16
Insomnia, 257–258, 396, 410
differential diagnosis of, 258
drug and alcohol dependency, 258–259
management of, 259
and medical problems, 258
nonpharmacologic treatment, 259–260
bright light therapy, 259–260
multicomponent behavioral therapy, 259
progressive muscle relaxation, 259
sleep hygiene education, 259
sleep restriction therapy, 259
stimulus control, 259
pharmacologic treatment, 260–261
poor sleep hygiene, 259
and psychiatric disorders, 258
and recovery, 92
restless legs syndrome (RLS), 259
treatment for, 254
treatment of, 254
Institutionalization, and weight loss, 112
Instrumental activities of daily living (IADLs), 112, 114
Instrumental coping response, 31
Insulins, 78, 452
characteristics of, 455
Interdisciplinary comprehensive assessment, 18
Interleukin (IL)-1s, 463
Intermediate-density lipoprotein, LDL, 315
International Classification of Sleep Disorders (ICSD), 256–258
Interstitial lung disease (ILD), 397
Intestine, 8
Intraocular lens implantation, 73

Intravenous glycoprotein IIb/IIIa inhibitors, 342
Intravitreal triamcinolone acetonide AQ5 (Kenalog) injection, and diabetic macular edema, 126
Invasive epidermoid carcinoma, 437
Iron deficiency, 546
Ischemia, systemic diseases potentially exacerbating, 339
Ischemic arterial ulcers, 508
Ischemic heart disease, as grief reaction, 60
Ischemic occlusion of a cerebral artery, 365
Isoflavones, 441
Isolated systolic hypertension, 310–311
  treatment of, 314
Isolation, and weight loss, 111–112
Isoniazid-induced hepatitis, 396
Isosorbide dinitrate, 358
Itai–Itai disease, 300
Ivermectin (Stromectol), 437

J

Joint replacements, 73, 79
Joints, pain in, 49

K

Kegel exercises, 181–182
Keratoacanthoma, 503
Keratotic scabies, 502–503
Ketoconazole, 194, 502
Ketoprofen (Orudis), 53
Kidney diseases, differential diagnosis of, 416
Kidney failure, postoperative management, 79–80
Kidney, 4
  preoperative assessment and management, 77–78
Korsakoff syndrome, 249
Kubler-Ross stages of grief, 60
Kwell, 437

L

L. pneumophila, 406
L4 nerve root, 164
L5 nerve root, 164
Lachs, Dr. Mark, 97
Lactulose, 56, 573
Langerhans cells, reduction of, 4
Lanoxin, 43
Laparoscopic cholecystectomy, and symptomatic cholecystitis, 567
Large artery atherosclerosis, 365
Large intestine, 8
Large perforation, tympanic membrane, 139
Laser in situ keratomileusis (LASIK), 122
Latent tuberculosis infection (LTBI):
  defined, 408
  diagnosis and treatment of, 409–410
Late-onset drinkers, 83
  risk factors for, 84
LDL cholesterol, 315, 456
Leg pain:
  differential diagnosis of the patient at rest with, 324–326
    arterial dissection or trauma, 325
    atherothrombotic microembolism (blue-toe syndrome), 325
    deep venous thrombosis, 326
    diabetic neuropathy, 326
    peripheral bypass graft occlusion, 325
    peripheral emboli, 325
    thromboangiitis obliterans (Berger disease), 325
    thrombosed popliteal artery aneurysm, 326
Legionella sp., 407, 561
Lentigo maligna melanoma, 507
Letter of condolence, 58, 67–68
Leukemia, 339
Leukocytosis, 552–553, 554
Levine, Carol, 38
Levodopa, and weight loss, 118
Levothyroxine, 461
Lewy body dementia, 237, 242
Lichen sclerosus, 435
Lichen simplex, 497–498
Lid ectropion/entropion, 131
Lidocaine (Lidoderm), 45, 57, 132
Ligamentous sprains, 278
Ligaments, 163
Lindane lotion (Kwell), 437
Linguistic analysis, 1
Lipid disorders, 309, 314–318
  age-related cholesterol metabolism, 315
  hyperlipidemia, management of, 316–318
  lipid lowering:
    agents for, 316–317
    benefits of, in the elderly, 315
  primary prevention, 315–316
  screening for, 315
  secondary prevention, 316
Lipoproteins, 315
Lisinopril, 338, 358
Lithium, 460
Liver, 4, 8
Liver disease, 549
LMWH, 373
Long-term care, 30
Long-term care facility, 19–20
Long-term interdisciplinary management, 18
Lorazepam (Ativan), 43, 44
  and alcohol withdrawal, 87
Loss and bereavement, *See* Bereavement care; Grief,
Loss, defined, 60
Loud talkers, 139
Lovastatin, 317
Low back sprain/strain, 163, 165–166
  follow-up, 166
  imaging, 166
  management of, 166
  physical examination, 166
Low-density lipoprotein cholesterol (LDL-C), 338
Lower back pain, 162–174
  abdominal aortic aneurysm, 173–174
  compression fracture, 170–171
  degenerative disc disease, 166–167
  differential diagnosis of, 165–174
  herniated nucleus pulposus (disc), 167–169
  history, 163–164
  incidence/frequency of, 162–163
  infection, 172–173
  low back sprain/strain, 165–166
  lumbar segment, anatomy of pain in, 163
  metastatic disease, 171–172
  nerve root examination, 162
  normal aging of the back, 163
  physical examination, 164–166
  specific causes of, 165–174
  spinal stenosis, 169–170
Low-vision rehabilitation, 132
Lumbar spine, 163, 166
Lumps, in the breast, 441–442
Lung, age-related changes in, 398–399
Lung cancer, and smoking cessation, 532–533
Lung capacity, 7
Lung elasticity, 7
Lupus, 465–466
Luteinizing hormone (LHJ), 204
Lyme disease vaccination, 561
Lymphocytic leukemia, 550, 553
Lymphoproliferative diseases, 550

M

Macrocytic anemia, 546, 548–549
Macronutrients, and weight loss, 119
Macular degeneration, *See* Age-related macular degeneration (ARMD),
Magnesium laxatives, 56
Magnetic resonance imaging (MRI), 134, 142, 162, 172–173, 229, 236, 245, 267, 282, 419
  and hemorrhage, 366–368
Major depression, 208–209
Malabsorption, and weight loss, 111
Malignancy, 10
Malignant melanoma, 437
Malnutrition, 10
Mammograms/mammography, 433–434, 541
Manic depressive illness, 208, 209–210, *See* Bipolar disorder
Manual dexterity, 12
Matrix metalloproteinases, 338–339
Maximum oxygen consumption (VO_2max), 7
McGill Pain Inventory, 51
Mean bronchiolar diameter, 398
Mean corpuscular volume (MCV), 546
Meclizine, and dizziness, 153
MedAmerica, 95
Medicaid program, 30

Medicare program, 19, 30, 114
Medication dosing, 47
Medication error, 22
Medication management, 20–22
adverse drug events at home, 20–21
adverse drug events in the hospital, 21–22
adverse drug events in the nursing home, 22
Megaloblastic macrocytic anemia, 549
Megestrol acetate, and weight loss, 118–119
Meglitinides, 452–453
Melanocytes, 4
Melanomas, 495
clinical features of, 507
excisional biopsy, 507–508
nodular type, 507
risk factors for, 507
staging, 507
types of, 507
visceral metastasis, 508
Melatonin, and insomnia, 261
Melphalan, 551
Memantine, and Alzheimer disease, 246
Membrane fluidity changes, 5
Memory impairment, chronic, 236–252
normal memory aging, 237–239
Ménière disease, 145, 149
laboratory and imaging, 145
management of, 145
Meperidine (Demerol), 45
Meprobamate (Miltown, Equanil), 44
Metabolic acidosis, causes of, 430
Metabolic alkalosis, 430–431
Metabolic bone disease, 293–308
osteomalacia, 293, 299–302
osteoporosis, 293–299
primary hyperparathyroidism, 293, 303–305
renal osteodystrophy, 293, 305–308
Metabolism:
preoperative assessment and management, 77–78
and weight loss, 113
Metastatic disease, and back pain, 162, 171–172
follow-up, 172
imaging, 172
management of, 172
physical examination, 172
Metaxalone (Skelaxin), 44
Metformin, 453
Methadone, 55, 56
Methicillin-resistant *Staphylococcus aureus* (MRSA), 555, 561
Methimazole, 460
Methocarbamol (Robaxin), 44
Methotrexate, and rheumatoid arthritis, 465
Methyldopa (Aldomet), 44, 441
Methyldopa–hydrochlorothiazide (Aldoril), 44
Methyphenidate, as orexigenic agent, 118
Metoclopramide, 119
Metolazone, 357, 358
Metrolol/Metrolol XL, 338, 349, 358
Metronidazole, 560
Michigan Alcoholism Screening Test (MAST), 85
Microcytic anemia, 547–548
Milkman syndrome, 302
Mini Nutritional Assessment (MNA), 114, 117
Mini-Mental Status Examination (MMSE), 61, 108, 114, 236, 238, 239–241
Minimum Data Set (MDS), 19
Minor depression, 208, 209
Miquimod, 504
Mirtazapine, 118–119, 215, 217, 218
and dementia, 250
Mitral regurgitation, 345–346
diagnostic testing, 346
etiology of, 345–346
management of, 346
pathophysiology, 346
signs/symptoms of 346
Mitral stenosis, 346–347
diagnostic testing, 346
etiology of, 346
management of, 346–347
signs/symptoms of 346
Mitral valve disease, 337
Mitral valve repair, 335–336
Mixed dementia, 249
Modification of Diet in Renal Disease study group, 78
Modified Clinical Test of Sensory Interaction and Balance (mCTSIB), 157–158
Mohs micrographic surgery, 506–507
Monoamine oxidase inhibitors (MAOIs), 55
Monoclonal gammopathy of unknown significance, 546–547, 551
Mononuclear cells, 9
Monovision with laser in situ keratomileusis (LASIK), 122
Morphine, 55–56
Motility disorders, esophagus, 570
Mourning, defined, 60
Mouth, 15–16
MRI, *See* Magnetic resonance imaging (MRI),
Multi-infarct dementia, 19
Multinodular goiter (MNG), 459
Multiple drug-resistant, gram-negative bacilli (MDRGNB), 555, 561
Multiple myeloma, 551
Multiple sclerosis, 470–471
and hearing difficulty, 138, 142
and weight loss, 111
Multiple sleep latency test (MSLT), 256
Murray, Thomas, 38
Muscle mass, 77
Muscle relaxants, 45–46, 56, 527
Muscle strains, 278
Muscle weight, decrease in, 5
Muscles, 163
Musculoskeletal changes, 5
Musculoskeletal problems, 276–292
adhesive capsulitis of the shoulder, 283–284
articular cartilage injuries, 278
biceps tendon rupture, 277, 286–287
cervical spondylosis, 281–282
cervical sprain, 279–281
changes in musculoskeletal tissue with aging, 277
corns and calluses of the foot, 291
Dupuytren contracture/disease, 277, 287–288
history, 278–279
impingement syndrome, 284–285
of the shoulder, 277
injury, general areas of, 277–278
ligamentous sprains, 278
mechanism of injury, 277
muscle strains, 278
olecranon bursitis, 277, 287
osteoarthritis, 19, 48, 163, 277, 323
of the hip, 280, 288–289
of the knee, 280, 289–290
of the shoulder, 280, 282–283
plantar fasciitis, 277, 290–291
prevalence of, 277
rotator cuff rupture/tear, 285–286
Spurling maneuver, 277
tendon injuries, 278
Musculoskeletal system disorders, 462
Mycobacterium tuberculosis, 561
Mycobacterium tuberculosis bacillus, 407
Mycoplasma pneumoniae, 406
Myeloproliferative diseases, 552–553
erythrocytosis, 552
leukocytosis, 552–553
thrombocytosis, 552
Myocardial infarction (MI), 336
Myocardial ischemia, atypical symptoms of, 335
Myopia (nearsightedness), 122
Myxedema, 10

N

Nabumetone (Relafen), 53
Nadolol, and tremor, 389
Naproxen (Naproxyn/Aleve), 53, 54
Narcolepsy, 256, 264
Narcotic analgesics, 93
and constipation, 48
Narcotics, 20
and delirium, 229
National Association of Adult Protective Services Administrators (NAAPSA), consensus statement, 105
National Center for the Prevention of Elder Abuse, 97
National Center on Elder Abuse, 96
National Elder Abuse Incidence Study, 96-97, 98

National Health and Nutrition Examination Survey (NHANES), 138
National Institutes of Health Stroke Scale, 366, 367
National Kidney Foundation, 78
National Pressure Ulcer Advisory Panel (NPUAP), 515–516
Nausea, and weight loss, 111
NDO plicator, 577
Neer and Hawkins impingement signs, 284
Negative self-image, 61
Negative-pressure wound therapy (NPWT), 560
Neglect, 96, 100–101
  abandonment, 96, 100
  self-neglect, 101
Neoplastic disease, 530–545
  cancer:
    breast cancer recurrence, chemoprevention of, 541
    breast cancer surveillance, 541
    burden of, in the elderly, 531
    cancer survivorship model, 540–541
    cancer survivorship phenomenon, 539–540
    chemoprevention of, 533–534
    colorectal cancer surveillance, 543–545
    diet, obesity, and cancer risk, 533
    environmental hazards, 533
    primary prevention of, 532–534
    prostate cancer surveillance, 541–543
    screening for, 530–531, 534–539, *See also* Cancer screening
    secondary prevention of, 534–535
    surveillance care guidelines, 541
  cancer-related care as part of primary care, 531
  lung cancer, and smoking cessation, 532–533
  prevention of, 530
  skin cancer, and limiting sun exposure, 533
  survivors, 531
Neovascularization, 126
Nephropathy, and diabetes mellitus (type 2), 450
Nerve roots, 162–164
  compression of, 323
  evaluations of the sensory and motor functions of, 281
Nervous system, and aging, 5
Neurodermatitis, 497–498
Neuroimagining, 229
Neurologic abnormalities, and degeneration of muscles/bones, 5
Neuromuscular pain, diagnosis of, 50
Neuropathic pain, 48–50
Neuropathic tremor, 384
Neuroplasticity, 49
Neurotransmitter changes, 5
Neutropenia, 549–550
Neutrophils, 9
Niacin, and lipid disorders, 317–318
Nicotinic acid, and lipid disorders, 317
Nifedipine therapy, 345
Night splints, and plantar fasciitis, 291
Nipple discharge, 442
Nissen fundoplication, 577
Nitrates, 341, 342
N-methyl-D-aspartate (NMDA) receptors, 53
Nociceptive pain, 48–50
Nonacute dysphagia, 563
Non-Alzheimer disease dementia, 247–249
  frontotemporal dementia, 237, 242, 248
  Lewy body dementia, 247
  mixed dementia, 249
  white matter dementia, 242–243, 248–249
Nonarteritic anterior ischemic optic neuropathy (NAION), 130
Nonbenzodiazepine CNS depressants, 260
Noncardiac surgery:
  cardiac complications of, 74–75
  clinical predictors of increased perioperative cardiac risk for, 75
  delaying for additional testing and management, 75
  risks of cardiac complications associated with, 76
Noncardioembolic stroke, reducing the risk of thrombosis for, 374–375
Non-Hodgkin lymphoma, 550
Nonmegaloblastic macrocytic anemia, 546, 549
Nonopioid pain medications, 53–54
Nonpresyncopal lightheadedness, 151
Nonproliferative diabetic retinopathy (NPDR), 125–126
Nonrapid eye movement (NREM) sleep, 255
Nonrheumatoid diseases with immune etiology, 468–472
  amyloidosis, 469–470
  diabetes (type 1 and 2), 471
  gout, 471–472
  Hashimoto thyroiditis, 471
  multiple sclerosis, 470–471
  polymyalgia rheumatica and giant cell arteritis, 468–469
  soft-tissue rheumatism, 471
  vasculitis, 468–469
Nonsteroidal anti-inflammatory drugs (NSAIDs), 42–43, 46, 48, 53–54, 54, 93, 166, 279, 282, 283, 284, 285, 286, 287, 288, 289, 357, 376, 421
  and peptic ulcer disease, 564
  and soft-tissue rheumatism, 471
Nonverbal cues, techniques to improve, 3
Norepinephrine and dopamine reuptake inhibitors (NDRIs), 56
Normal grief, 60–61
  defined, 58, 60
  diagnosis of, 63
  differential diagnosis of, 61
  symptoms of, 62
Normal tension glaucoma (NTG), 130
Normocytic anemia, 546, 547
Nortriptyline, 57
Norwegian scabies, 502–503
Nose twitching, 16
NSAIDs, *See* Nonsteroidal anti-inflammatory drugs (NSAIDs),
Nuclear cataracts, 122
Nuclear thyroid scanning with radioactive iodine (RAI), 460
Nurse practitioner, 20
Nursing homes, 19–20
Nutrition, 78
  and dementia, 251
  and degeneration of muscles/bones, 5
  and pressure ulcers, 528
Nutritional frailty, 110
Nutritional osteomalacia, 299

O

Obesity
  and cancer risk, 533
  and gastroesophageal reflux disease (GERD), 576
  and heart failure, 361
  and obstructive sleep apnea, 262
  and pressure ulcers, 512
Observing behaviors, 15
Obstructive nephropathy, 80
Obstructive sleep apnea, 254, 262–263
  clinical symptoms of, 262
  laboratory evaluation, 262
  treatment of, 262
Occlusive disease of the renal arteries, 421
Occupational therapy, 52
1-Octanol, and tremor, 390
Office-based caregiver support, 28–39
Olanzapine (Zyprexa), 271
Olecranon bursitis, 277, 280, 287
Onychomycosis, 500–502
Open hands, 16
Operative therapy, 73
Ophthalmic zoster, 500
Opioid addiction, 87
Opioid analgesics, 55–56
Opioid pain medications, 55–56
Optic nerve head edema, 130
Oral acyclovir, 132
Oral cancer, 474, 483–485
Oral candidiasis, 485–486
  signs/symptoms of, 486
Oral conditions, 474–489
  and aspiration pneumonia/chronic obstructive pulmonary disease, 488–489

Oral conditions (*continued*)
and atherosclerosis, cardiovascular disease, and stroke, 488
burning mouth syndrome (stomatopyrosis), 487
and dementia, 489
dental decay (caries), 474, 477–479
and diabetes, 488
diet and nutrition, 481
intraoral physical examination, 475–477
medical management of, 479–480
oral cancer, 474, 483–485
oral candidiasis, 485–486
oral cavity, evaluation of, 475–477
oral health, 474–475
oral medicine, 483
oral mucositis, 485
orofacial conditions, 474
orofacial pain, 482–483
periodontal disease, 474, 479–481
perioperative considerations, 487–488
root surface caries, 478
root surface dental decay, 474
and systemic disease, 487
traumatic lesions, 486–487
xerostomia, 474, 481–482
Oral estrogens (Premarin), 178
Oral iron therapy, 547
Oral mucositis, 485
Oral problems, and weight loss, 111
Orchiectomy, 193
Organ of Corti, 135–136
and age-related hearing loss, 136
Organization of care, 19–20
Orgasmic disorders, 203
Original Folstein Mini-Mental State Exam, 238
Oropharynx, age-related physiologic changes of, 568
Orthopnea, 397
Orthostatic tremor, 384
treatment for, 384, 390–391, 393
Orthotic devices, 52
OSA syndrome, 262
Oseltamivir (Tamiflu), 559
Osmotic laxatives, and constipation, 573
Osteitis fibrosa, 305
Osteitis fibrosa cystica, 303
Osteoarthritis, 19, 48, 163, 323
of the hip, 280, 288–289
follow-up, 289
imaging, 288
management of, 288–289
physical examination, 288
workup/keys to the diagnosis, 288–289
of the knee, 280, 289–290
follow-up, 290
imaging, 289
management of, 289–290
physical examination, 289
workup/keys to the diagnosis, 289–290
of the shoulder, 280, 282–283
follow-up, 283
imaging, 283
management of, 283
physical examination, 282–283
workup/keys to diagnosis, 282–283
Osteomalacia, 293, 299–302
aluminum-induced, 301
defined, 299
drug-induced, 299–300
management of, 302
nutritional, 299
rarity of, 305
and vitamin D, 300–302
workup/keys to diagnosis, 301–302
Osteopenia, 170
Osteophytes, 170
Osteoporosis, 47, 97, 170, 293–299, 402
bone mineral density (BMD):
defining osteoporosis by, 295
testing, 295–296
defined, 293
diagnosis of, 294
and involuntary weight loss, 113
laboratory testing for secondary causes of, 296
management of, 296–299
medications, 42
nutritional counseling, 297
pharmacologic therapy, 297–298
bisphosphonates, 298–299, 307
calcitonin, 298
hormone therapy (HT), 297
recombinant human PTH (hPTH), 297, 300, 301
selective estrogen receptormodulators (SERMs), 297
teriparatide, 299
physical examination, diagnostic signs in, 296
risk factors for osteoporotic fractures, 295
type I or II, 293
who should be tested, 296
workup/keys to diagnosis, 295–296
Otitis media, 140
Otoacoustic emissions (OAEs), 141
Ovarian cancer, 440
Oxybutynin (Ditropan/Ditropan XL), 44, 182
Oxycodone, 55
Oxytrol patch, 182

P

PAD, *See* Peripheral arterial disease (PAD),
Paget disease, 437
Pain, 73
acute, 50, 51
back, 50
barriers leading to underreporting of, 50
case studies, 49
classification of, 49–50
controlling, 48–58
coping strategies, 51
defined, 48
effects of, 49
and elder abuse, 98
emotional and psychosocial impact of, 51
evaluation of, 50–51
in the cognitively impaired, 51
as "fifth vital sign," 48
headache, 50
mechanism of, 49
neuropathic, 48–50
nociceptive, 48–50
patient's report of, 48
persistent, 50, 55–56
physical effects of, 49
and recovery, 93
secondary to a concomitant disease, 51
severity of, 50–51
social supports, 51
undermanaged, 51
vascular, 50
Pain management, 47, 48–49, 51
clarification of perceptions of, 52
goals of, 51–57
and impending death, 26
nonpharmacologic pain therapies, 52–53
pharmacologic management, 53–57
self-report, 51
strategies, 52
surgical intervention, 57
Pain questionnaires, 51
Pain scales, 48
Palatal tremor, 384
Palliative care, 18, 26
gradually shifting to, 58, 62–63
Pallor, 51
Palm movements, 16
Pancreas, 8, 163
Panretinal photocoagulation (PRP), 126
Pap (Papanicolaou) smears, 433, 436
Paradoxical sleep, 255
Paranoid disorders, and weight loss, 111–112
Paraphrenia, 267
Parasitic infection, 499–503
and weight loss, 111
Parathyroid surgery, 304
Parathyroidectomy, 307
Parenteral anticoagulants, and stroke, 373
Parkinson disease, 10
dementia associated with, 247–248
Parkinson disease (PD), treatment algorithms for, 391
Paroxetine (Paxil), 56
and insomnia, 258
Pasteurella multocida, 559

Patient Bill of Rights, 205
Patient Health Questionnaire-2 (PHQ-2), 210–211
Patient Health Questionnaire-9 (PHQ-9):
Patient-centered care model, 19
Patients:
  hearing impaired, 3
  showing reverence for, 3
  sitting, importance of, 3–4
  visual information, improving for, 3
Paxil-CR, 441
PC-SPES, 194
pDXA, 296
Peabody, Francis Ward, 3
Pederson speculum, 432
Pediculosis, 502
Pediculosis capitis, 503
Pediculosis pubic, 503
Pegaptanib sodium (Macugen), 125–126
Pellagra, 249
Penicillin-resistant *Staphylococcus pneumoniae* (PRSP), 555, 561
Pentazocine (Talwin), 44, 45
Pentoxifylline, and peripheral arterial disease (PAD), 329
Peptic ulcer disease (PUD), 563, 564–565
  clinical features, 565
  complications of, 565
  diagnosis of, 565
  Helicobacter pylori infection, 564
    methods of testing, 565
  non-*Helicobacter pylori* infection/non-nonsteroidal anti-inflammatory drug users, 564–565
  and nonsteroidal anti-inflammatory drugs (NSAIDs), 564
  treatment of, 565
  and weight loss, 111
Perceptive knowledge, sharing, 3
Percutaneous balloon mitral valvuloplasty (commissurotomy), 347
Percutaneous coronary intervention (PCI), 342
Performance-Oriented Mobility Assessment (POMA), 157
Periaortic lymph nodes, 163
Periodic limb movement disorder (PLMD), 256, 262–263
Periodontal disease, 474, 479–481
  management of, 480
  signs/symptoms of, 479–480
  and weight loss, 112
Periodontitis, 488
Peripheral arterial disease (PAD), 320–333
  amputation, 323, 331–332
  angioplasty/stenting, 321, 332–333
  defined, 321
  and diabetes mellitus (type 2), 449–450
  etiology of and risk factors for, 323
  evaluation of the patient with, 323–324
  exercise-induced leg pain, differential diagnosis of the patient with, 323–324
  history, 326
  impact on functional status, 323
  impact on survival, 323
  incidence and prevalence of, 323
  laboratory examinations, 327
  leg pain, differential diagnosis of the patient at rest with, 324–326
  management of, 328–330
    antiplatelet therapy, 329
    cilostazol, 330
    diabetes mellitus, 329
    dyslipidemia, 329
    foot ulcer prevention, 329
    hypertension, 329
    lifestyle recommendations, 328
    medications, 328, 329–330
    pentoxifylline, 329
    tobacco abuse, 328–329, 547
  pathophysiology of, 322–323
  percutaneous intervention, 321
  perioperative β-blockade, 321
  physical examination for, 327
  radiologic studies, 327–328
  revascularization, 321, 330–331
  symptoms of, 321
  topics associated with, 322
Peripheral bypass graft occlusion, 325
Peripheral emboli, 325
Peripheral vascular disease, 51
Peristalsis, 7
Permethrin 5% cream, 437
Perphenazine–amitriptyline (Triavil), 44
Persistent pain, 50
Persistent to chronic pain, 50
Pfeiffer Short Portable Mental Status Questionnaire, 236, 239, 240
Pharmacodynamic changes, 42
Pharmacologic management:
  adjuvant medications, 56–57
  nonopioid pain medications, 53–54
  opioid pain medications, 55–56
  topical agents, 54–55
Phenoxybenzamine (Dibenzyline), 182
Phenylbutazone (Butazolidin), 44
Phenytoin (Dilantin), 43, 56, 57, 458
Phobias, 266, 272
Phospholipids, 315
PHPT, *See* Primary hyperparathyroidism (PHPT),
Physical abuse, 96, 99–100
Physical therapies, 52
Physician assistant, 20
Physician, attitudes regarding aging and death, 2
Physician's role, in caregiving, 32–36
Phytoestrogens, 441
Pinching the bridge of the nose, 16
Pineal β-adrenergic receptors, 5
Pipelle endometrial biopsy device, 439
Pitch discrimination, 7
Plantar fasciitis, 277, 280, 290–291
  follow-up, 291
  imaging, 290
  management of, 290–291
  physical examination, 290
  workup/keys to the diagnosis, 290–291
Plasma cell disorders, 551–552
  monoclonal gammopathy of unknown significance, 551
  multiple myeloma, 551
  plasmacytoma and other plasma cell proliferative diseases, 551–552
Plasmacytoma and other plasma cell proliferative diseases, 551–552
Platelet numbers, 9
Pleuritic chest pain, 397–398
PLMD, *See* Periodic limb movement disorder (PLMD),
PLMS index, 263
Pneumococcal immunization, and diabetes mellitus (type 2), 451
Pneumonia, 18, 20, 24, 396, 405–408, 560
  causative organisms in the elderly, 406–407
  community-acquired, empiric management of, 407
  diagnostic evaluation, 405–406
  pathophysiology and clinical presentation, 405
  pneumococcal polysaccharide vaccine, 408
  prevalence of, 405
  prophylaxis, 408
  treatment of, 407–408
Polyarthritis, 465
Polycythemia vera, 552
Polyethylene glycol (MiraLax), 56
Polymyalgia rheumatica, 10
  and giant cell arteritis, 468–469
Polypharmacy, 18, 20, 455
Polyuria, 424
Popliteal artery adventitial cystic disease, 324
Popliteal artery entrapment syndrome, 324
Positron emission tomography (PET), 143
Posterior subcapsular cataracts, 123
Postherpetic neuralgia, 500
Postmenopausal bleeding, 438–439
Postoperative cognitive decline, 73, 80–81
Poststroke depression, assessing and managing, 372
Postural dizziness, 149
Postural hypotension, 45
Posture, 4
Potassium balance:
  commentary, 427–428
  disorders of, 427–430

Potassium balance (*continued*)
hyperkalemia, 428–429
hypokalemia, 428
Poverty, and weight loss, 111, 112
pQCT, 296
Practical problem solving, 31
Pravastatin, 317
Prednisone, 194, 551
Premature ejaculation, 203
Preoccupation with death, 61
Preoperative assessment and management, 73, 74–79
cardiovascular system, 74–76
kidney and metabolism, 77–78
neuropsychiatric concerns, 78–79
respiratory system, 76–77
Preproliferative diabetic retinopathy (PDR), 126
Presbycusis, 6, 136–143
management of, 142–143
assistive listening devices, 142–143
aural rehabilitation, 143
cochlear implants, 142
hearing aids, 142
medical, 142
rehabilitation, 142
physical examination, 139–142
screening, 138–139
Presbyesophagus, 7
Presbyopia, 6, 122
Prescribed substances, 83–84
Presentation of disease, 10
Pressure touch thresholds, 6
Pressure ulcers, 25, 511–528, 559–560
Agency for Healthcare Research and Quality (AHRQ):
prediction and prevention recommendations, 521–522
recommendations for treatment, 522–526
Braden Scale, 513–515
complications, 516
differential diagnosis of, 513
epidemiology, 513
guidelines, 512
healing process, 512
health care facility's risks relating to, 519
incidence/prevalence, 516
management of, 526–528
adjunctive therapies, 524
colonization and infection, 524–525
debridement, 524, 527
dehydration, 528
dressings, 524, 527
education, 525–526
history and physical examination, 523
infection control, 525
medications, 527
mental status evaluation, 526
nutrition, 528
nutritional assessment and management, 523
pain assessment and management, 523
pain management, 526
positioning techniques, 523–524
pressure ulcer scale for healing tool (PUSH tool), 516–517, 526
psychosocial assessment and management, 523
quality improvement, 526
restraints, 526–527
support surfaces, 512, 523, 527
surgery, 525, 528
tissue load management, 523–524
wound cleansing, 524
wound healing, 526
Nursing Home Communication with Physician (form), 520
and obesity, 512
and pain, 49
Pressure Ulcer Healing Chart, 518
prevention of, 511–529
communication, 520–521
injury prevention, 516
long-term care prevention, 516–519
nurse education, 519–520
Nursing Home Quality Initiative (NHQI), 520
physician education, 519
staffing, 519
risk factors for, 512, 513–515
staging:
reverse (healing) staging, 515–516
saucerization of pressure damage, 515
terminology, 513
Presyncopal lightheadedness, 151
Prevention of Events with Angiotensin Converting Enzyme Inhibition (PEACE) trial, 341
Primary care physician, 19
Primary hyperparathyroidism (PHPT), 293, 303–305
calcimimetics, 305
defined, 303
hormone replacement therapy (HT), 304–305
and inherited syndromes, 303
and kidney abnormalities, 303
laboratory assessment of patients with, 304
management of, 304–305
parathyroid surgery, 304
sestamibi-single photon emission computed tomography (SPECT) imaging, 304
skeletal involvement in, 303
treatment of, 304
workup/keys to the diagnosis, 303–304
Primary open-angle glaucoma (POAG), 129
Primary writing tremor, treatment for, 393
Primidone, and tremor, 387–390
Principles of Assessment and Management of Elder Abuse Tool, 105
Prions, 249
Proactive case management, 68
Pro-Banthine, 182
Probenecid, 472
Problem drinkers, 83
Problem drugs, 43–46
Progestational agents, and weight loss, 119
Prognosis, 11
Prolonged partial thromboplastin, 546
Promethazine–dexchlorpheniramine (Polaramine), 45
Pronto, 437
Propanolol, 349
Propantheline (Pro-Banthine), 45
Prophylactic regimens, 79
Propoxyphene (Darvon), 44, 527
Propranolol, and tremor, 387–388, 390
Propylthiouracil (PTU), 460
PROspective Study of Pravastatin in the EldeRly at Risk (PROSPER), 341
Prostate, 4
Prostate cancer, 176, 191–194
defined, 191–192
management of, 193–194
risk of, and age, 191
workup, 191
Prostate cancer surveillance, 541–543
Prostate glands, 188
Prostate-specific antigen (PSA), 176
Prostatitis, 554
Protease inhibitor, 559
Proteinuria, 415, 417
Proton pump inhibitors, 119
Protriptyline, 57
Pseudodendritic keratopathy, 132
Pseudothrombocytopenia, 549–550
Psoriasis, 435
Psoriatic arthritis, 468
Psychiatric disorders, prevalence of among younger *vs.* older adults, 268
Psychoactive agents, 43
Psychoactive medications, and delirium, 229
Psychoeducative group program, 32
Psychogenic tremor, 384
Psychological abuse, 96, 100
Psychology of the examiner, 2–3
Psychotropic medications, 46
and weight loss, 112
PTA, 141
Pubic hair growth rate, 5
Pubic lice (phthirus pubis), 437
Public health issues, 96
PUD, *See* Peptic ulcer disease (PUD),
Pulmonary and thromboembolic problems, postoperative management, 79
Pulmonary disease, 395–412
asthma, 395–396
cough-variant, 395, 397

diagnosis, 400
epidemiology of, 400
stepwise approach for managing, in adults, 401
treatment, 400–402
chronic obstructive pulmonary disease (COPD), 396, 402–405
cough, common causes of, 396
dyspnea, 395
common causes of, 396
hemoptysis, 398
homeostenosis, 396
isoniazid-induced hepatitis, 396
methacholine challenge testing, 396
pleuritic chest pain, 397–398
pneumonia, 396, 405–408
prevention of, 396
respiratory system, normal age-related changes in, 399–400
sleep-disordered breathing, 410–411
tuberculosis (TB), 407–410
two-step purified protein derivative skin test, 396
Pulmonary embolism, 396
Pulmonary embolus (PE), 365
Pulmonary function, age-related changes in, 399–400
Pulmonary function testing (PFT), 397, 403
Pulmonary valve disease, 337
Pulsatile tinnitus, 143
Pure-tone audiogram, 140–141
PUSH (pressure ulcer scale for healing tool), 516–517, 526
Pyrazinamide (PZA), 409–410
Pyrethrin (Nix), 437
Pyuria, 183, 416
and casts, 418

Q

Quadriplegia, and weight loss, 111
Quantitative ultrasound (QUS), 296
Quazepam, and insomnia, 261
Quetiapine (Seroquel), 271
Quinapril, 358
Quinine purpura, 550
Quinolone, 560

R

Radiation therapy, and prostate cancer, 193
Radioactive iodine (RAI), 460
Radon, 533
Raloxifene, 297–298
Ramipril, 358
Ramsay-Hunt Syndrome, 499
Ranibizumab (Lucentis), 125–126
Rapid eye movement (REM) sleep, 255
behavior disorder (RBD), 263–264
Rate-control over rhythm-control strategy, 336
Rational drug therapy, 40–47
adverse drug reactions, 42–43
case studies, 42, 46–47
clinical strategies, 46–47
pharmacokinetics, 41–42
polypharmacy, 42
specific problem drugs in the elderly, 43–46
Reagan, Ronald, 30–31
Recombinant human PTH (hPTH), 297, 300, 301, 307
Rectal cancer, 544
Red eye, 131
5α-reductase inhibitors, 189–190
Rehabilitation, 25–26
emphasizing the benefits of, 2
hearing loss, 142
Relaxation techniques, 52
Renal cholesterol embolization, 421
Renal failure, and weight loss, 111
Renal function, 414–431
acid–base balance, disorders of, 430–431
acute renal insufficiency or failure, 420–421
azotemia, 415–416, 418–419
chronic kidney disease, 421–423
dialysis, 423
disorders of sodium and water balance, 423–427
end-stage renal disease, 421, 423
hematuria, 183, 414, 416–418
hyperkalemia, 415
hypernatremia, 426–427
hypokalemia, 415
hyponatremia, 424–426
imaging techniques, 419
kidney diseases, differential diagnosis of, 416
laboratory tests, 419
multiple myeloma/light chain cast nephropathy, 415
nonsteroidal anti-inflammatory drugs (NSAIDs), 415
with normal aging, 415
occlusive disease of the renal arteries, 421
potassium balance:
commentary, 427–428
disorders of, 427–430
hyperkalemia, 428–429
hypokalemia, 428
pyuria, 414
renal biopsy, 420
renal cholesterol embolization, 421
renal disease, clinical presentations of, 415–419
renal vascular disease, 421
serum urea nitrogen (SUN), 414–415, 420, 424–426
syndrome of inappropriate antidiuretic hormone secretion (SIADH), 217, 415, 424
transplantation, 423
urinary abnormalities, 417–418
Renal insufficiency, 357
Renal osteodystrophy, 293, 305–308
defined, 305
end-stage renal disease (ESRD), 305–308
management of, 306–308
and vitamin D, 307
workup/keys to the diagnosis, 305–306
Renal physiology, changes in, 42
Renal toxicity, 335
Renal vascular disease, 421
Reserpine (Serpasil), 45
Resident assessment protocols (RAPs), 19
Respiratory complications, 73
Respiratory depressants, 254
Respiratory disturbance index (RDI), 411
Respiratory muscles, age-related changes in, 399
Respiratory reserve, loss of, 400
Respiratory system:
and aging, 7
preoperative assessment and management, 76–77
Restless legs syndrome (RLS), 259, 262–263
Retinal arterial occlusive disease, 128–129
Retinal changes, 6
Retinal photocoagulation therapy, 127
Retinal venous occlusive disease, 126–127
Retinopathy, and diabetes mellitus (type 2), 450
Retrocochlear hearing loss, 136
Revascularization, 321, 330–331
indications for, 330
patient monitoring/ secondary prevention, 331
perioperative risks, 330
postoperative care, 331
preoperative evaluation/ risk reduction, 330–331
procedures, 73
results of, 330
Reverse transcriptase inhibitors (RTI), 559
Reversible disease in chronically ill people, search for, 11
Rheumatoid arthritis, 47, 48–49, 462, 464–468
cytokines, proinflammatory, 464
diagnosis of, 464
psoriatic arthritis, 468
revised diagnostic criteria for classification of, 464
scleroderma, 467–468
Sjögren syndrome, 465–467
systemic lupus erythematosus (SLE or lupus), 465–466
treatment of, 464–465
Rheumatoid disease, 172
Rhinophyma, 509
Ribonucleic acid (RNA) synthesis, 8
Rickets, 299
Rid, 437

Rifampin, 409–410
Rimantadine (Flumadine), 554, 559
Rinne tuning fork test, 139
Risedronate, 298
Risk indices, 73
Risperidone (Risperdal), 271
RLS, *See* Restless legs syndrome (RLS),
Rofecoxib (Vioxx), 54
Rosacea, 509
Rosuvastatin, 317
Rotator cuff rupture/tear, 280, 285–286
  follow-up, 286
  imaging, 286
  management of, 286
  physical examination, 285–286
  workup/keys to diagnosis, 285–286
Rubral tremor, 384
  treatment for, 393

S

S1 nerve root, 164
Saccharated ferric oxide, 300
Sacral nerve roots, electrical stimulation of, and fecal incontinence, 575
SAD, *See* Seasonal affective disorder (SAD),
Sadness, 60
Saliva, 481
Salsalate (Disalcid), 53, 54
Sarcopenia, 25, 109, 113
Sarcoptes scabiei (itch mite), 437
SARS, *See* Severe acute respiratory syndrome (SARS),
Scabies, 437, 502–503
Scalp hair growth rate, 5
Schirmer test, 466
Schizophrenia, 266–271
  defined, 267
  diagnostic criteria, 270
  differential diagnosis of, 268–269
  disease course, 271
  genetics, 268
  late-age, pathophysiology in, 267–268
  management of, 270–271
  mortality rates, 271
  paraphrenia, 267
  Schizophrenia Patient Outcomes Research Team (PORT) guidelines, 270
  workup, 269–270
Schwabach Test, 139
Schwabach tuning fork test, 139
Scleroderma, 467–468
Scopolamine, and dizziness, 153
Seasonal affective disorder (SAD), 208, 209, 215
Sedating antihistamine, 260
Selective benzodiazepine-receptor antagonists (SBRAs), 69–70
Selective serotonin reuptake inhibitors (SSRIs), 45, 52, 55, 57, 70, 93, 200, 215–217, 242, 249, 273
  and weight loss, 112, 119
Self-neglect, 101
Senna concentrate (Senokot), 56
Sensorineural hearing loss, 136, 142
Separation distress, 61
Sepsis, 557
Serotonin, and delirium, 226
Serotonin, binding sites for, 5
Serotonin reuptake inhibitors, 218
Serotonin–norepinephrine reuptake inhibitors (SNRIs), 56
Serotonin-2 antagonist reuptake inhibitors (SARIs), 56
Serous otitis media, 139
Sertraline (Zoloft), 56, 216, 441
  and insomnia, 258
Serum albumin, 53, 78
Serum intact PTH (iPTH), 305–306
Serum urea nitrogen (SUN), 414–415, 420, 424–426
Sestamibi-single photon emission computed tomography (SPECT) imaging, 304
Sevelamer, 307
Severe acute respiratory syndrome (SARS), 555, 558
Severe aortic regurgitation, 335
Severe aortic stenosis, 75–76
  symptoms of, 335
Sex hormone–binding globulin (SHBG), 200
Sexual abuse, 100
Sexual disorders, classification of:
  erectile dysfunction (ED), 196, 201–202
  hypoactive sexual desire disorder, 200–202
  orgasmic disorders, 203
  sexual arousal disorder in women, 202–203
  sexual aversion disorder, 199–200
  sexual pain disorders, 203
Sexual dysfunction, drugs associated with, 201
Sexual health, defined, 197
Sexual hyperexpression, 205
Sexuality and older adults, 196–206
  history taking and evaluation, 203–204
  human immunodeficiency virus/acquired immunodeficiency syndrome (HIV/AIDS), 196, 198
  myths of aging and sexuality, 197–198
  prevalence of sexual activity with aging, 198–199
  sex and environmental issues, 205
  sexual disorders, classification of, 199–203
  sexually transmitted diseases (STDs), 196, 198
Shingles, *See* Herpes zoster (shingles),
Shock, 60–61
Short Michigan Alcoholism Screening Test—Geriatric Version (SMAST—G), 85
Shouting, to hearing-impaired patients, 3
Sickle cell disease, 339
Sidewise palms, 16
Simvastatin, 317
Single photon emission computed tomography (SPECT), 244
Sinus tachycardia, suppression of, 335
Sitting postures, 16
Sjögren syndrome, 466–467
  manifestations of, 467
Skin, and aging, 4–5
Skin cancer, and limiting sun exposure, 533
Skin ulcers, *See* Pressure ulcers,
Skull, 5
Sleep disorders, 254–266
  advanced sleep-phase syndrome (ASPS), 263
  changes in sleep with normal aging, 255
  circadian rhythm sleep disorders, 263
  circadian rhythmicity, 255
  classification and ICD-9 codes, 257
  classification of, 256–257
  delta (slow-wave) sleep, 255
  diagnostic approach/assessment of, 255–256
  drugs that interfere with sleep, 256
  etiology of sleep problems, 254
  evaluation of older patients with sleeping difficulties, 257
  insomnia, 257–258
    treatment for, 254
  International Classification of Sleep Disorders (ICSD), 256–258
  narcolepsy, 256, 264
  nonrapid eye movement (NREM) sleep, 255
  paradoxical sleep, 255
  periodic limb movement disorder (PLMD), 262–263
  polysomnography, referral for, 254
  rapid eye movement (REM) sleep, 255
  rapid eye movement (REM) sleep behavior disorder, 263–264
    treatment of, 264
  respiratory depressants, 254
  restless legs syndrome (RLS), 262–263
  sleep architecture, 255
  sleep diary, 256
  sleep hygiene, 254
  sleep in the nursing home, 264–266
  sleep stages, 255
  sleep-disordered breathing, 261–262
    obstructive sleep apnea, 254, 262
Sleep fragmentation, 411
Sleep hygiene, 259
Sleep-disordered breathing, 410–411
  diagnosis, 411
  obstructive sleep apnea, 410–411
  sleep patterns, changes in, 411
  treatment of, 411

Small intestine, 8
Smell, sense of, 6
Smiles, interpreting, 15–16
Smoking cessation, 84–85
nicotine withdrawal, 89
Social withdrawal, and pain, 49
Sodium, 423–427
Soft-tissue rheumatism, 471
Solifenacin (VESIcare), 182
Somatic pain, 49
Spastic disorders of the esophagus, 570
Special senses, changes in, 6
vision, 6
Specific task and dystonic tremors tremor, 384
Speech discrimination, 7
testing, 141
Speech recognition tests, 141
Speech recognition threshold (SRT), 141
Spinal stenosis, 163, 169–170
defined, 169–170
follow-up, 170
imaging, 170
management of, 170
physical examination, 170
Spine, forward bending of, 4
Spiritual healing, 52
Spironolactone, 354, 358
in treatment of heart failure, 359–360
Spiritual support, and recovery, 92
Spondees, 141
Sprains, defined, 279
Spurling maneuver, 277
Squamous cell carcinoma, 504–506
SSRIs, *See* Selective serotonin reuptake inhibitors (SSRIs),
Stable angina, 338–339
defined, 338
diagnostic procedures, 339
etiology of, 339
laboratory, 339
pathophysiology of, 338–339
physical examination for, 339
risk factors for, 339
workup/keys to the diagnosis, 339–340
Standing postures, 16
Stapes, 135
Staphylococcus aureus, 406–407, 499, 516, 559, 561
Stasis dermatitis, 497
Statins, 317
Steepling the fingers, 16
Stenting, *See* Angioplasty/stenting,
Stereotypes, about aging and elderly people, 2
Steroids, 78
Stevens-Johnson syndrome, 498–499
Stomach, 7–8
Straight leg raise, 164, 168, 170
Stratum corneum, 4
Streptococcus pneumoniae, 406–407, 561
Stroke, 19, 51, 363–377
acute ischemic stroke:
assessing and managing risk of complications following, 370
complications, 371
general care following, 370
general medical care of the patient with, 369–370
aspiration pneumonia risk, assessing and managing, 370
cardioembolic, reducing the risk of thrombosis for, 375–376
cerebral hemorrhage, presence of, 367–369
classification of, 364–365
comorbid coronary heart disease (CHD), assessing, 372
complications associated with, 365
conditions causing stroke-like symptoms, 364
deep vein thrombosis risk, 365
assessing and managing, 371
description/definition of problem, 364
diagnostic studies as confirmation of, 367
differential diagnosis of, 364
focal brain dysfunction, evidence of, 367
hemorrhagic, 365, 366–368
impact on function, 365
incidence and prevalence, 365
lifestyle recommendations, 373
management of, 368–376
determining appropriate location and intensity of, 368
medications, 373–374
antiplatelet agents, 373–374
gastric cytoprotection, 374
parenteral anticoagulants, 373
thrombolytic agents, 373
warfarin, 374
National Institutes of Health Stroke Scale, 366, 367
noncardioembolic, reducing the risk of thrombosis for, 374–375
and oral conditions, 488
pathophysiology, 364–365
patient education, 376
patient monitoring/secondary prevention, 374–376
poststroke depression, assessing and managing, 372
pressure ulcer risk, assessing and managing, 372
prevention of, 363
prognosis for, 368
pulmonary embolus (PE), 365
recurrent, assessing and reducing risk, 374
rehabilitation needs, multidisciplinary assessment of function and determination of, 372
risk factors for, 365
signs/symptoms of 364, 366
stroke syndrome, development of, 367
stroke unit, 369
surgical interventions, 374
systems impacted by, 365
thrombolysis, criteria for, 368
thrombolytic the, 363
tissue oxygenation, 370
urinary tract infection (UTI), 365
assessing and managing, 371
and weight loss, 111
workup/keys to the diagnosis, 366–368
Subacute bacterial endocarditis, and weight loss, 111
Subclinical hyperthyroidism, 460
Substance dependence:
diagnosis of substance abuse *vs.*, 85–86
Diagnostic and Statistical Manual of Mental Disorders, 4/e (DSM-IV) criteria for, 86
Substance use disorders, 82–94
alcohol abuse, 82, 83–84
and aging, 83
alcohol metabolism, age-related changes that affect, 83
early onset drinkers, 83
late-onset drinkers, 83
alcohol withdrawal, signs/symptoms of, 87
biomedical conditions and complications, 89
early intervention, 90
emotional/behavioral conditions and complications, 89–90
epidemiology, 83
intensive outpatient treatment/partial hospitalization, 90
management of, 85–89
acute intoxication or withdrawal potential, 87
diagnosis of substance abuse *vs.* substance dependence, 85–86
screening and assessment, 85
medically managed intensive inpatient treatment, 90
opioid addiction, 87
outpatient treatment, 90
prescribed substances, 83–84
readiness to change (resistance to treatment), 90
and recovery, 92
recovery:
anxiety disorders, 93
common medical problems in, 92–93
depression, 93
over-the-counter and prescription medication use, 93
pain, 93
sleep disorders, 92
red flags, 85
relapse risk, 90
residential/inpatient treatment, 90

Substance use disorders (*continued*)
risk factors for, 82
tobacco use, 84–85
and peripheral arterial disease (PAD), 328–329
treatment of, 90–92
abstinence, 82, 91
compulsive behavior, 92
emotional symptoms, 92
exercise, 92
family and relationship issues, 92
goals of, 91
legal issues, 92
leisure activities, 92
meeting attendance, 91–92
physical health, 92
primary care of the patient in recovery, 91
spiritual support, 92
sponsor contact, 92
Substance-induced depression, 213–214
Subsyndromal depression, 208
Subthreshold depression, 209
Sulfonylurea, 452–453
Suicide:
and complicated grief, 61
and depression, 214
as grief reaction, 60
Sulindac (Clinoril), 53, 54
SUN, *See* Serum urea nitrogen (SUN),
Superficial spreading melanoma, 507
Suppositories, 574
Surgical excision, skin cancers, 506
Surgical intervention, 57
for pain, 57
Surgical patient management, 73–81
operative risk, decline in, 74
postoperative management of, 79–81
cardiovascular problems, 79
delirium and postoperative cognitive decline, 80–81
fluid and nutrition management, 80
kidney failure, 79–80
pulmonary and thromboembolic problems, 79
Swallowing, 7
Sweating, 51
Symptom evaluation, 19
Symptom management, 1
Symptomatic aortic stenosis, 335
Syncope, 147–148
conditions leading to, 149
course/timeline, 154
differential diagnosis of, 153
in the elderly, 153–154
etiology of, 147
incidence and prevalence, 153–154
pathophysiology, 153
workup/keys to the diagnosis, 154
Syndrome of inappropriate antidiuretic hormone secretion (SIADH), 217, 415, 424
Syphilis, 198
Syphilis dementia, 250
Systemic lupus erythematosus (SLE or lupus), 465–466
Systolic hypertension, 46–47

T

Tachyarrhythmias, 339
Tachycardia, 51
Tai Chi trials, 159
Tamsulosin (Flomax), 176, 182, 190
Taste sensitivity, 6
TB, *See* Tuberculosis (TB),
TB skin testing, 114
Tear production, reductions in, 131
Tegaserod, 573–574
Temazepam (Restoril), 44
Temporal variation, 61
Tendinosis, 278
Tendon injuries, 278
Terazosin (Hytrin), 182
Terbinafine, 502
Teriparatide, 299
Testosterone, 204
deficiency, 200–201
as orexigenic agent, 118–119
Tetanus, 554
Thalassemic syndromes, 547–548
Theophylline, 61
and insomnia, 258
Thiazide-induced hypokalemia, 43
Thiazolidinediones, 453
36-Hour Day, The (Mace/Rabins), 38
Thromboangiitis obliterans (Berger disease), 325
Thrombocytopenia, 546, 549–550
Thrombocytosis, 339, 547, 552
Thrombolytic agents, and stroke, 373
Thrombolytic therapy, 363
Thrombosed popliteal artery aneurysm, 326
Thyroid disease:
hyperthyroidism, 459–461
hypothyroidism, 457–459
Thyroid disorders, 460–461
Thyroid storm, 459
Thyroidectomy, 461
Thyroid-stimulating hormone (TSH) level, 114
Thyroxine, 458
Ticarcillin/clavulanic acid, 560
Ticking watch test, 139
Timed Up and Go test" (TUG)D 155–157
Tinea cruris, 500–501
Tinea pedis, 500–501
Tinidazole, 436
Tinnitus, 136, 143–144
cutaneous-evoked, 143
defined, 143
gaze-evoked, 143
laboratory and imaging, 143–144
management of, 144
physical examination for, 143
pulsatile, 143
tinnitus retraining therapy (TRT), 144
Tissue plasminogen activator (tPA), 369
Tizanidine (Zanaflex), 56, 57
Tobacco abuse, and peripheral arterial disease (PAD), 328–329, 547
Tobacco use, 84–85
and peripheral arterial disease (PAD), 328–329
Tolterodine (Detrol), 182
Topical agents, 54–55
Topical salicylates, 54
Topiramate (Topamax), and tremor, 389–390
Torsemide, 358
Touch, sense of, 6
Toxic epidermal necrolysis (TEN), 499
Tramadol (Ultram), 53, 55
Trandolapril, 358
Transcutaneous electrical nerve stimulation (TENS), 52
Transient ischemic attack (TIA), *See also* Stroke,
defined, 364
Transitional care, 20
Transplantation, kidneys, 423
Transrectal ultrasound (TRUS), and prostate cancer, 191–192
Transurethral resection of the prostate (TURP), 182
and benign prostatic hyperplasia (BPH), 190–191
Traumatic grief treatment, 70
Trazodone, 219, 237
and dementia, 250
Tremor, 112, 378–394
action and postural, 381, 383–384
bilateral brain stimulation, 393
cerebellar, 393
cerebellar intention, 383
defined, 379
differential diagnosis of, 379–381
dystonic, treatment for, 393
essential (ET), 379, 382–383
general measures for, 386–387
history, 384–385
laboratory tests, 385
lifestyle and therapy, 387
management of, 386–393
medications, 386–388
atenolol, 387, 388
β-blockers, 386, 387
benzodiazepines, 390
botulin toxin A, 390
gabapentin (Neurontin), 389–390
nadolol, 389
1-Octanol, 390
primidone, 387–390
topiramate (Topamax), 389–390
neuropathic, 384
orthostatic, 384
palatal, 384
Parkinson disease (PD), 378
Parkinsonian rest, 381
patient resources, 393
physical examination for, 385
primary writing, treatment for, 393
psychogenic, 384

rubral, 384
treatment for, 393
special studies, 385–386
specific task and dystonic tremors, 384
surgery, 393
syndromes, 378, 381–383
physical examination features of, 385
toxic/metabolic, 378, 381–382
treatment of, 390–392
Wilson disease, 384
workup and diagnosis of patients with, 384–386
Tretinoin, 504
Triazolam (Halcion), 44
Trichomonas, 198, 436
Tricuspid valve disease, 337
Tricyclic antidepressants (TCAs), 20, 55–56, 92, 132, 435
Tricyclics, and weight loss, 119
Trifluridine (Viroptic), 132
Triglycerides/triglyceride levels, 46, 315
Trimethoprim–sulfamethoxazole, 47
Trolamine polypeptide oleate (Cerumenex), 139
Trospium (Sanctura), 182
Trousseau syndrome, 553
Trypsin secretion, 8
Tube feeding, 116–118
Tuberculin positivity, criteria, 409
Tuberculosis (TB), 10, 398, 407–410
active, clinical presentation, diagnosis, and treatment of, 410
latent tuberculosis infection (LTBI), diagnosis and treatment of, 409–410
tuberculin positivity, criteria for, 409
tuberculin skin testing, 408–409
and weight loss, 111
TURP, *See* Transurethral resection of the prostate (TURP),
Two-step purified protein derivative skin test, 396
Tympanic membrane (TM), 135
Tympanograms, 139–141
Tympanometry, 140

U

Ulcerative colitis, and complicated grief, 61
Ultrasound, and choledocholithiasis/cholangitis, 567
Undermanaged pain, 51
Underreporting of illness, 10
Unfractionated heparin (UFH), 373
Unstable angina, risk of death or nonfatal myocardial infarction in patients with, 343
Upper genital tract disorders, 438–440
cervical cancer, 439–440
endometrial cancer, 439
fallopian tube cancer, 440
ovarian cancer, 440
physiologic changes, 438
postmenopausal bleeding, 438–439
prolapse, 438
Uricosuric drugs, 472
Urinary abnormalities, 417–418
hematuria, 416–418
nephrotic syndrome:
causes of, due to glomerular disease, 418
defined, 417
proteinuria, 415, 417
pyuria and casts, 418
Urinary catheters, 175
Urinary disorders, 175–195
benign prostatic hyperplasia (BPH), 175–176, 187–191
prostate cancer, 176, 191–194
urinary incontinence, 175, 176–183
urinary tract infections, 175, 183–187
Urinary incontinence, 175, 176–183, 371
adult diapers, 185
causes of, 178
detrusor hyperactivity, 179–182
detrusor underactivity, 179
established, 179–180
management of, 181–183
normal aging, 176–177
and pain, 49
pathophysiology, 177–178
reversible causes of, 178–179
workup, 180–181
Urinary tract infections (UTIs), 20, 22–24, 175, 183–187, 556–557
asymptomatic bacteriuria, 183, 185–186
choice of treatment, 191
disease background, 183
infections in catheterized patients, 186–187
initial antibiotic choices in elderly patients with, 184
management of, 184–185
secondary causes of, 183
workup, 183–184
U.S. Preventive Services Task Force (USPSTF), 155, 210
UTIs, *See* Urinary tract infections (UTIs),
Uveitis, 132

V

Vaginal bleeding, 438–439
Vaginismus, 203
Valdecoxib (Bextra), 53, 54
Valerian, and insomnia, 261
Valsalva maneuver, 182
Valvular heart disease, 75–76, 336, 344–347
aortic regurgitation, 345
aortic stenosis (AS), 344–345
mitral regurgitation, 345–346
mitral stenosis, 346–347
Vancomycin, 77
Vancomycin-resistant enterococci (VRE), 516, 555, 561
Varicella zoster virus (VZV), 557–558
Vascular abnormalities, and degeneration of muscles/bones, 5
Vascular dementia, 237, 242
Vascular diseases, 172
hypertension as marker for, 74
skin manifestations of, 508–509
Vascular endothelial growth factor (VEGF), 125
Vascular pain, 50
Vasculitis, 468–469
classification of, 469
Vasodilators, and hypertension, 313, 314
VEGF, 126
Venlafaxine, 215, 217, 218
and insomnia, 258
Venlafaxine (Effexor), 56, 57, 441
Venous claudication, 324
Venous insufficiency ulcers, 508
Venous thrombosis, 547, 553, *See also* Deep vein thrombosis
Ventilation-perfusion (V/Q) mismatch, 7
Ventricular arrhythmias, 350–352
defined, 350
diagnostic procedures, 351
etiology and risk factors, 351
incidence and prevalence, 351
laboratory, 351
management of, 351
medications, 351–352
pathophysiology of, 351
percutaneous/surgical interventions, 352
physical examination for, 351
signs/symptoms of 351
workup/keys to the diagnosis, 351
Ventry and Weinstein Scale, 138
Verapamil, 341, 349
Verrucous carcinoma, 438
Vertebrae, 163
growth of, 4
Vertebral periosteum, 163
Vertigo, 142, 151
and hearing loss, 142
and Ménière disease, 145, 149
Very low-density lipoprotein (VLDL), 315
Vestibular Disorders Association (VEDA), 145
Vestibular dysfunction, 148–149
Vestibular rehabilitation therapy, 147
Vestibular schwannomas, 144–145
Vestibular–ocular pathway, 144
Vestibulo–ocular reflex, 144
Vibrio vulnificus, 559
Video nystagmography, 144
Viral hepatitis, 558
Viral infections, 557–558
Viruses, 406–407
Vision, 6
Visual impairment, 112, 121–133
and aging, 121

Visual impairment (*continued*)
anterior ischemic optic neuropathy (AAION), 130–131
cataracts, 121–123
diabetic retinopathy, 125–126
in the elderly, conditions causing, 122
elevated intraocular pressure (IOP), 121, 129
eyelid problems, 131
glaucoma, 121, 129–310
herpes zoster ophthalmicus (shingles), 131–134
low-vision rehabilitation, 132
macular degeneration, 121
red eye, 131
refractive error, 121–123
retinal arterial occlusive disease, 128–129
retinal venous occlusive disease, 126–127
tear production, reductions in, 131
and weight loss, 111
Vitamin B_6, and reduction of homocysteine levels, 342
Vitamin B_{12}, 549
and dementia, 245
and reduction of homocysteine levels, 342
Vitamin C, and Alzheimer disease, 247
Vitamin D:
and osteomalacia, 300–302
and osteoporosis, 297
and renal osteodystrophy, 307
Vitamin E, and Alzheimer disease, 247
Voiding record, 181
Vomiting, and weight loss, 111
Vulvar lichen planus, 435–436
Vulva/vagina disorders, 434–438
atrophic vaginitis, 434–435
bacterial vaginosis, 436–437
Bartholin gland carcinoma, 437
bullous pemphigoid, 436
cancer, 437–438
Candida vaginitis, 436
carcinomas of the vulva, 437
contact dermatitis (eczematoid/irritant dermatitis), 435
invasive epidermoid carcinoma, 437
lichen sclerosus, 435
malignant melanoma, 437
Paget disease, 437
psoriasis, 435
pubic lice (phthirus pubis), 437
scabies, 437
Trichomonas infection, 436
verrucous carcinoma, 438
vulvar lichen planus, 435–436
vulvodynia, 435
Vulvodynia, 435

W

"Walkie-talkie" test, 158
Warfarin, 43, 371, 374
and stroke, 374
Wasting, 109, 113
Watchful waiting, defined, 193
Water balance, 423–427
Weber test, 139
Weber tuning fork test, 139
Weight loss, 108–120
anorexia tardive, 111
antidepressants, trial of, 108
assessment, 113–114
biochemical changes, 113
causes of, 110–112
and depression, 108
energy demand, 108
gastrointestinal causes of, 111–112
hormonal changes, 113
inflammatory/infectious/chronic diseases as causes of, 112
involuntary, 108
oral problems associated with, 111
and osteoporosis, 113
malabsorption, 111
management of, 115–119
environmental factors, 118
medications, 118–119
nutritional interventions, 115–116
physical activity, 118
tube feeding, 116–118
medications as cause of, 112
and mental status, 108
and metabolism, 113
mortality risk, 108
neurologic causes of, 112
nutritional frailty, 110
nutritional intervention, 108
physiology of, 112–113
psychiatric causes of, 112
resting energy expenditure (REE), 108
terminology, 109–110
testing for, 114
weight change, 110
weight maintenance, 108
weight reduction (voluntary weight loss), 115
West Nile Fever (WNF), 558
Whispered voice test, 139
White cells, 9
White matter dementia, 242–243, 248–249
Wilson disease, 384
Wishfulness coping, 32
Wishfulness–intrapsychic coping, 32
Wrist actigraphy, 256

X

Xerophthalmia, 466
Xerosis, 496
Xerostomia, 466, 474, 481–482
X-ray radiation therapy, 506

Z

Zaleplon, 69–70
and insomnia, 261
Zanamivir (Relenza), 559
Zinc sulfate, and venous insufficiency ulcers, 508
Ziprasidone (Geodan), 271
Zolpidem (Ambien), 44, 92
and insomnia, 261